The Amygdala

A functional analysis

Second edition

Edited by

John P. Aggleton

School of Psychology, Cardiff University, UK

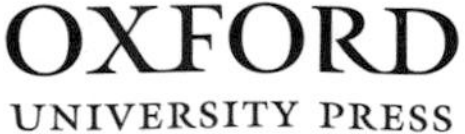

OXFORD
UNIVERSITY PRESS

Oxford University Press, Great Clarendon Street, Oxford OX2 6DP

Oxford University Press is a department of the University of Oxford.
It furthers the University's objective of excellence in research, scholarship, and education by publishing worldwide in

Oxford New York

Auckland Bangkok Buenos Aires Cape Town Chennai
Dar es Salaam Delhi Hong Kong Istanbul Karachi Kolkata
Kuala Lumpur Madrid Melbourne Mexico City Mumbai Nairobi
São Paulo Shanghai Taipei Tokyo Toronto

Oxford is a registered trade mark of Oxford University Press in the UK and in certain other countries

Published in the United States by Oxford University Press Inc., New York

First edition published by A Wiley-Liss (As The Amygdala: Neurological Aspects of Emotion, Memory, and Mental Dysfunction), 1992
Second edition published by Oxford University Press, 2000

Reprinted 2001, 2003

A catalogue record for this book is available from the British Library

Library of Congress Cataloging in Publication Data

(Data available)

1 3 5 7 9 10 8 6 4 2

ISBN 0 19 850501 9 (Hbk)

Printed in Great Britain on acid-free paper by Biddles Ltd, *www.biddles.co.uk*

Preface

To understand how our emotions work, it is necessary to understand a brain structure called the amygdala. This is because the amygdala (the name literally means almond) is involved in the ways that our likes and dislikes are formed, how our emotions affect our actions and our memories, and how we interact socially with others. Not surprisingly, malfunctions of the amygdala are thought to contribute to a number of disorders that affect personality, these include Alzheimer's disease, autism, and schizophrenia. This book provides the first comprehensive analysis of this fascinating brain structure for nearly a decade, a decade in which the brain sciences have advanced at an unprecedented rate. As a consequence, this book will be of value both to the expert and to the newcomer interested in brain mechanisms of emotion and memory.

In spite of its undoubted importance, the amygdala had remained relatively under-researched. This situation has finally changed. The advent of new techniques for examining brain function, combined with a number of conceptual breakthroughs, has led to new insights into the contributions of the human amygdala to emotion and memory. At the same time, complementary research using animals is allowing researchers to uncover the mechanisms underlying these processes.

The present book provides a comprehensive insight into different levels of research on the amygdala. To do this, the knowledge of leading world experts on different aspects of amygdala function has been brought together in a single book. One consequence of the increase in amygdala research means that chapters are devoted to topics that barely existed when the last book on the amygdala was published (e.g. functional imaging, studies of facial processing after amygdala damage, cytotoxic lesions of the primate amygdala, long-term potentiation and depression). Another consequence of the growth of amygdala research is that it is not feasible to bring together all amygdala-related issues in a single volume. For this reason, there is a deliberate emphasis on the functions of the amygdala.

Twenty five years ago I began my first research on the amygdala, and the initial excitement and fascination that I felt then has never waned. As the primary goals of this book are to inform and to promote future amygdala research, I can only hope that this book will help others to appreciate this enigmatic structure.

Finally, I would like to thank the following for all their help and support in compiling this volume: Jane Aggleton, Nicky Thomas, Lorraine Awcock and all the contributing authors.

(dedicated to P.C.A. 1920–1998)

Contents

List of contributors

Ralph Adolphs Department of Neurology, Division of Cognitive Neuroscience, University of Iowa College of Medicine, 200 Hawkins Drive, Iowa City, IA 52242-1053, USA

John P. Aggleton School of Psychology, Cardiff University, PO Box 901, Park Place, Cardiff CF10 3YG, UK

Jocelyne Bachevalier Department of Neurobiology and Anatomy, University of Texas Health Science Center, Houston, TX 77030, USA

Robert A. Barton Evolutionary Anthropology Research Group, Department of Anthropology, University of Durham, 43 Old Elvet, Durham DH1 3HN, UK

Mark G. Baxter Department of Psychology, Harvard University, Cambridge, MA 02138, USA

Larry Cahill Center for the Neurobiology of Learning and Memory, University of California, Qureshey Research Laboratory, Irvine, CA 92697-3800, USA

Rudolf N. Cardinal Department of Experimental Psychology, University of Cambridge, Downing Street, Cambridge CB2 3EB, UK

Paul F. Chapman Cardiff School of Biosciences, Cardiff University, PO Box 911, Museum Avenue, Cardiff CF10 3US, UK

Sumantra Chattarji National Centre for Biological Sciences, Tata Institute of Fundamental Research, Bangalore, India

Tiffany W. Chow UCLA School of Medicine, 710 Westwood Plaza, Los Angeles, CA 90095-1769, USA

Jeffrey L. Cummings UCLA School of Medicine, 710 Westwood Plaza, Los Angeles, CA 90095-1769, USA

Michael Davis Emory University School of Medicine, Department of Psychiatry, 1639 Pierce Drive, Atlanta, GA 30322, USA

Raymond J. Dolan Wellcome Department of Cognitive Neurology, Queen Square, London WC1N 3BG, UK

Yadin Dudai Department of Neurobiology, The Weizmann Institute of Science, Rehovot 76100, Israel

Alexander Easton Department of Experimental Psychology, University of Oxford, South Parks Road, Oxford OX1 3UD, UK

Barry J. Everitt Department of Experimental Psychology, University of Cambridge, Downing Street, Cambridge CB2 3EB, UK

Barbara Ferry Center for the Neurobiology of Learning and Memory and Department of Neurobiology and Behavior, University of California, Qureshey Research Laboratory, Irvine, CA 92697-3800, USA

Sandra E. File Psychopharmacology Research Unit, Neuroscience Research Centre, GKT School of Biomedical Sciences, King's College London, UK

David Gaffan Department of Experimental Psychology, University of Oxford, South Parks Road, Oxford OX1 3UD, UK

Michela Gallagher Department of Psychology, Johns Hopkins University, 3400 North Charles Street, Baltimore, MD 21218, USA

Jeremy Hall Department of Experimental Psychology, University of Cambridge, Downing Street, Cambridge CB2 3EB, UK

Raphael Lamprecht Department of Neurobiology, The Weizmann Institute of Science, Rehovot 76100, Israel

Joseph LeDoux W.M. Keck Laboratory of Neurobiology, Center for Neural Science, New York University

He Li Department of Psychiatry, Uniformed Services University of the Health Sciences, Bethesda, Maryland, USA

James L. McGaugh Center for the Neurobiology of Learning and Memory and Department of Neurobiology and Behavior, University of California, Irvine, CA 92697-3800, USA

Elisabeth A. Murray Laboratory of Neuropsychology, National Institute of Mental Health, 49 Convent Drive, Bethesda, MD 20892, USA

John A. Parkinson Department of Anatomy, University of Cambridge, Downing Street, Cambridge CB2 3DY, UK

Asla Pitkänen Epilepsy Research Laboratory, A. I. Virtanen Institute for Molecular Sciences, University of Kuopio, PO Box 1627, FIN-70 211 Kuopio, Finland

R.M. Post Biological Psychiatry Branch, National Institute of Mental Health, Bldg 10/3N212, 9000 Rockville Pike, Bethesda, MD 20892, USA

Trevor W. Robbins Department of Experimental Psychology, University of Cambridge, Downing Street, Cambridge CB2 3EB, UK

Edmund T. Rolls University of Oxford, Department of Experimental Psychology, South Parks Road, Oxford OX1 3UD, UK

Benno Roozendaal Center for the Neurobiology of Learning and Memory and Department of Neurobiology and Behavior, University of California, Irvine, CA 92697-3800, USA

Richard C. Saunders Laboratory of Neuropsychology, National Institute of Mental Health, 49 Convent Drive, Bethesda, MD 20892, USA

Martina Sitcoske-O'Shea Biological Psychiatry Branch, National Institute of Mental Health, Bldg 10/3N212, 9000 Rockville Pike, Bethesda, MD 20892, USA

Daniel Tranel Department of Neurology, Division of Cognitive Neuroscience, University of Iowa College of Medicine, 200 Hawkins Drive, Iowa City, IA 52242-1053, USA

Almira Vazdarjanova Center for the Neurobiology of Learning and Memory and Department of Neurobiology and Behavior, University of California, Irvine, CA 92697-3800, USA

Susan R.B. Weiss Biological Psychiatry Branch, National Institute of Mental Health, Bldg 10/3N212, 9000 Rockville Pike, Bethesda, MD 20892, USA

1 The amygdala—what's happened in the last decade?

John P. Aggleton[1] and Richard C. Saunders[2]

[1]*School of Psychology, Cardiff University, Cardiff CF10 3YG, UK and*
[2]*Laboratory of Neuropsychology, National Institute of Mental Health, Building 49, Bethesda, MD 20892, USA*

Summary

Research on the amygdala has more than doubled in the last decade. During that time, new techniques and new questions have had a considerable impact on our understanding of this structure. A dominant theme has been the convergence of findings from studies of rodents and studies of primates, including humans. This has been aided by advances in brain imaging and the discovery of specific cognitive deficits that accompany amygdala damage in humans. These advances are now making it possible to appreciate the likely contribution of the amygdala to various psychopathologies, including schizophrenia, that affect emotional and social behaviour. This review also considers in detail the contributions of the amygdala to olfactory processes as they highlight the diversity of functions associated with this structure.

1.1 Introduction

In the eight years since the last book devoted to the amygdala was published (Aggleton, 1992a), there has been a doubling in the number of scientific papers concerning this brain region (Figure 1.1). The need for a new book stems directly from the volume of new research and new ideas that have appeared in recent years. By considering some of the major issues and discoveries that have emerged over the last decade, the structure and logic behind this book will become clearer. At the same time, we will take the opportunity to consider some of the issues that emerge from the experimental data described in this book, but which do not have specific sections devoted to them.

1.2 Does the amygdala exist?

It may seem absurd to start with this question, giving that an entire book on the amygdala must surely mean *de facto* that the amygdala exists. There is no doubt that a set of brain

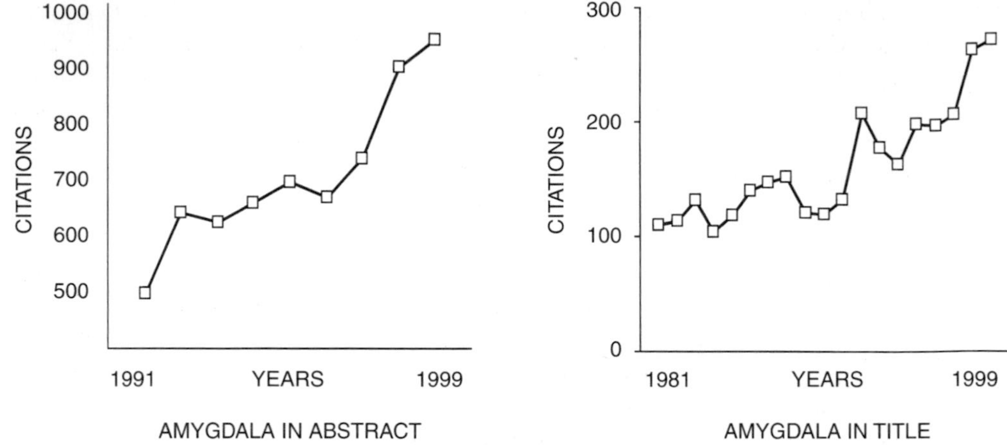

Figure 1.1 Graphs showing the increase in the number of scientific papers in which the terms amygdala/amygdalar/amygdaloid are used in the Abstract (1991–1999) or the Title (1981–1999). Data are taken from BIDS (Bath Information Data Services, Bath University).

nuclei that together are called the amygdala exists in the mammalian brain, the term 'amygdala' originally being used by Burdach (1819). Later descriptions, especially those by Johnston (1923), were central in defining the extent of the nuclear group referred to as the amygdala or amygdala complex. While the extent of the amygdala has been questioned in later studies, most notably by the concept of an 'extended amygdala' as proposed by Alheid and Heimer (1988), the notion that it is a structural unit has largely gone unchallenged.

The traditional view, that it is meaningful to regard the amygdala nuclei as forming a single entity, was challenged by Swanson and Petrovich (1998) in a recent, provocative review. Central to their argument are the facts that cell groups within the amygdala are derived from different regions, that these groups can be distinguished by their connectivity and by the distributions of neurotransmitters within each grouping, and that as a consequence they can be distinguished functionally (Figure 1.2). The four nuclear (and functional) groups in the rat brain which Swanson and Petrovich (1998) describe comprise; (i) the central nucleus (autonomic); (ii) the medial nucleus (accessory olfactory system); (iii) the cortical and basomedial nuclei (main olfactory system); and (iv) the lateral and basolateral nuclei (frontotemporal cortical system).

It is undeniable that there is some logic in this proposal, and further support may be found in a consideration of the electrophysiological properties, including LTP, of different parts of the amygdala (Chapman and Chattarji, Chapter 3). Indeed, a review of the topics covered in this book reveals that there is much more focus on what Swanson and Petrovich (1998) refer to as the 'autonomic' and 'frontotemporal' systems than on the 'olfactory' systems, again suggestive of fundamental, underlying divisions. Indeed, for this very reason, we have included an extended section in this review specifically devoted to the amygdala and olfactory processing to compensate for this imbalance. At the same time, evidence in this book also highlights the value of regarding the amygdala as a structural entity. Perhaps key to this issue are the extrinsic and intrinsic amygdala connections. Each amygdala nucleus has a unique set of extrinsic connections, and this applies not only to nuclei in the different functional groupings proposed by Swanson and Petrovich (1998) but also to nuclei within the same grouping. Indeed, this can now be extended to the connections of subregions *within* individual amygdala nuclei (Pitkänen, Chapter 2), as different portions of the same nuclei have different patterns of extrinsic connections. In addition, it has been known for a long time that there are dense intra-amygdala connections (Aggleton, 1985; Pitkänen, Chapter 2) and these serve to integrate the activities of the different nuclei (Figure 1.3). Importantly, these connections cut across the divisions proposed by Swanson and Petrovich (1998) to such an extent that in order to understand one division it will be necessary to understand another (e.g. central and basolateral nuclei, LeDoux, Chapter 7; Gallagher, Chapter 8). This important point is reiterated throughout this volume, even if it is possible to dissociate, and even doubly dissociate, some functions within the amygdala (Everitt *et al.*, Chapter 10).

Other evidence that different divisions within the amygdala combine to form an overall entity comes from an analysis of the volume of different components of the amygdala, and their relationships to the volume of 16 major brain structures across 43 primate species (Barton and Aggleton, Chapter 14). When the amygdala is divided into a central/medial and a basolateral/cortical division, it is found that the only significant correlations for these amygdala subregions are with each other, and not with the other regions. This again speaks to the integrity of the structure. There is also the pragmatic reason that techniques used to investigate 'amygdala' function often lack sufficient anatomical resolution or specificity to distinguish between subregions within the structure. This is especially pertinent to research on the human amygdala. Rather than discount all such information, it is better to include it, but with the caveat that it may cut across functional entities within the amygdala.

A related point is that different regions within the amygdala may contribute to different aspects of the same overall function. This is most evident in the study of fear conditioning where interactions between the basolateral amygdala and central nucleus are so critical for different attributes of the learning process (Davis, Chapter 6; Le Doux, Chapter 7). Such findings underline the value of treating the amygdala as an integrated structural unit, while recognizing the value of challenging and reappraising long-held beliefs concerning the nature of this complex of multiple nuclei.

1.3 Connectional analyses of the amygdala

Our understanding of the major connections of the primate amygdala has changed relatively little in the last few years (Amaral *et al.*, 1992), and recent advances have consisted largely of refinements of existing knowledge rather than the discovery of new connections (e.g. Carmichael and Price, 1995; Stefanacci *et al.*, 1996; McDonald, 1998). For this reason, there is no chapter devoted to this topic. Instead, a series of diagrams (Figures 1.3–1.6) that present summary information are provided for reference purposes. The first of these figures (Figure 1.3) shows the major intrinsic connections of the amygdala in the macaque monkey. Two features are of special note. The first is the striking tendency for information to pass

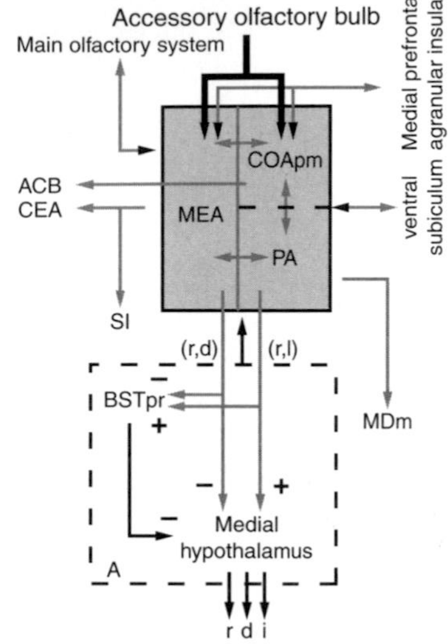

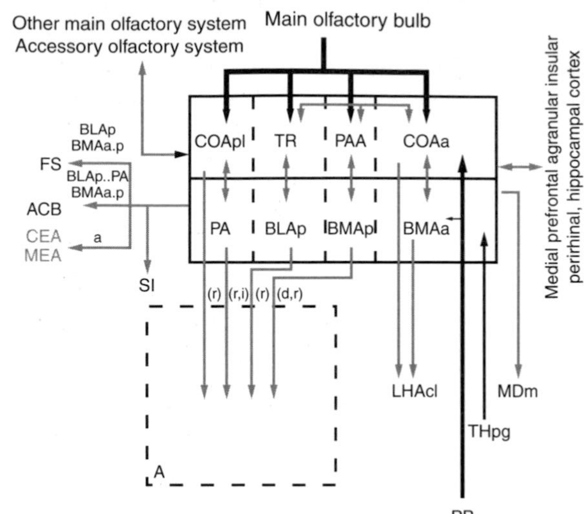

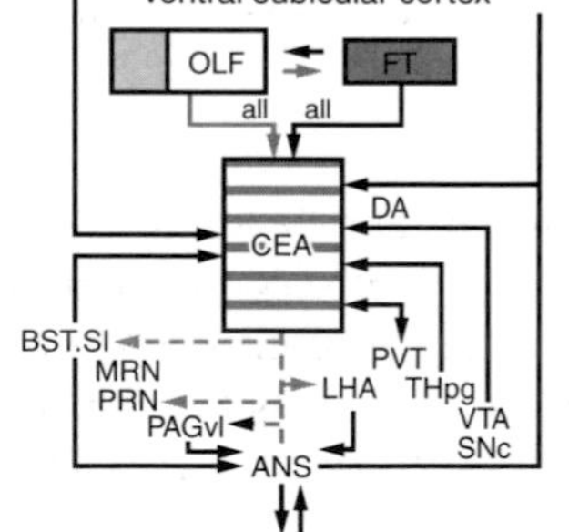

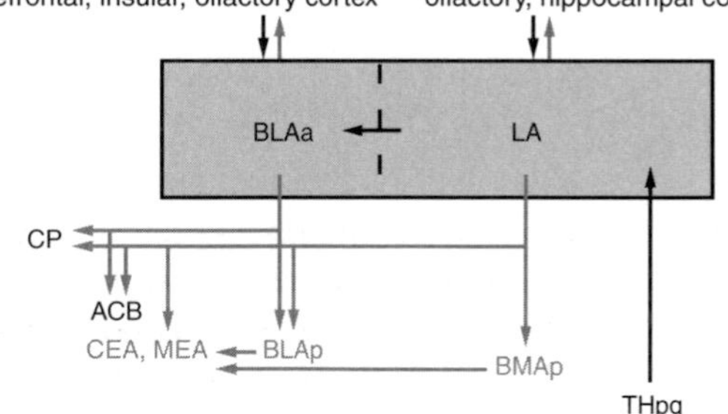

Figure 1.2 The major anatomical connections of the four functional systems associated with the amygdala as described by Swanson and Petrovich (1998). The sets of anatomical connections reveal the importance of the links between; (i) the olfactory systems, amygdala, and hypothalamus; (ii) autonomic system, central nucleus, and brainstem; and (iii) frontal and temporal cortices with basolateral nuclei and striatum. Abbreviations: ACB, nucleus accumbens; ANS, brainstem autonomic centres; BLAa, p, basolateral nucleus—anterior, posterior parts; BMAa,p, basomedial nucleus—anterior, posterior parts; BST, bed nucleus stria terminalis; CEA, central nucleus amygdala; COA a, pl,pm, cortical nucleus amygdala—anterior, posterior lateral, posterior medial parts; CP, caudoputamen; d, medial hypothalamic defensive system; DA, dopamine; FS, fundus of striatum; FT, frontotemporal component of amygdala; i, medial hypothalamic ingestive behavioural system; LA, lateral nucleus amygdala; LHA, lateral hypothalamic area; MEA, medial nucleus amygdala; MDm, mediodorsal nucleus thalamus; MRN,

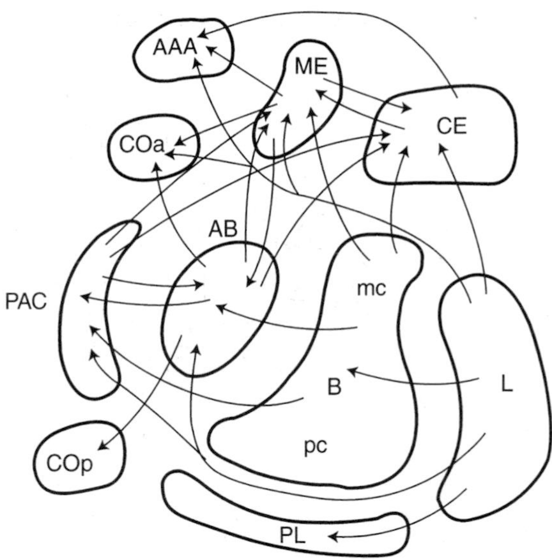

Figure 1.3 Schematic diagram showing the main intra-amygdala connections in the macaque monkey. Abbreviations: AAA, anterior amygdala area; AB, accessory basal nucleus; CE, central nucleus; COa,p cortical nucleus, anterior and posterior parts; B mc, pc, basal nucleus, magnocellular and parvicellular parts; L, lateral nucleus; PAC, periamygdaloid cortex; PL, paralamellar part of basal nucleus.

in a lateral to medial direction, the second is for information to pass in a ventral to dorsal direction. The lateral to medial flow, which includes particularly dense projections from the lateral nucleus to the basal and accessory basal nuclei (Aggleton, 1985; Pitkänen and Amaral, 1991), ensures that inputs from sensory association cortices gain access across the structure (Amaral *et al.*, 1992). Recent studies are now revealing the pattern of intranuclear connections in the primate brain (Bonda, 2000).

The major cortical connections of the primate amygdala are shown in Figures 1.4 and 1.5, the subcortical connections in Figures 1.6 and 1.7. These show how the amygdala can interact with information from every sensory modality. While these figures highlight the extent of the connections of the amygdala nuclei, they do not depict their relative densities. The basal

---

mesencephalic reticular nucleus; OLF, olfactory components of amygdala; PA, posterior nucleus amygdala; PAA, piriform–amygdala area; PAG, periaqueductal grey; PB, parabrachial nucleus; PRN, pontine reticular nucleus; PVT, paraventricular nucleus thalamus; r, medial hypothalamic reproductive behaviour system; SI, substantia innominata; SNc, substantia nigra, pars compacta; THpg, thalamus perigeniculate region; TR postpiriform transition area; VTA, ventral tegmentalarea. Reprinted from Trends in Neuroscience, 21, 329, 1998, with permission from Elsevier Science. See also Plate section for colour reproduction.

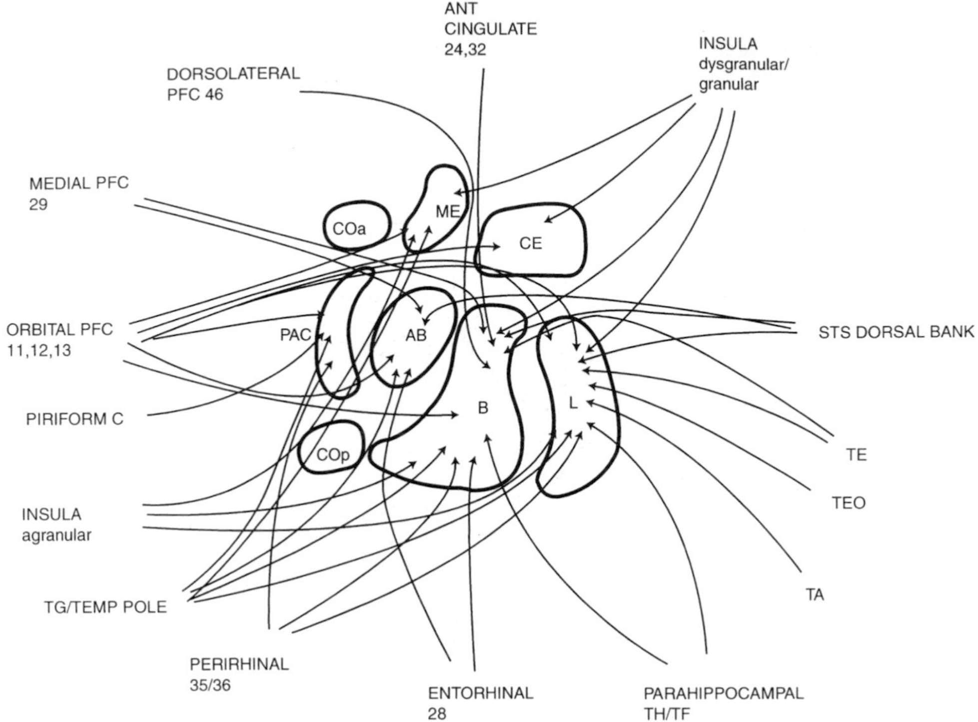

Figure 1.4 Schematic diagram showing the array of cortical inputs to the amygdala of the macaque monkey (hippocampal inputs are shown in Figure 1.6). Abbreviations of amygdala nuclei are as in Figure 1.3.

nucleus is, for example, the principal source of many of the amygdala–cortical projections, even though there may be minor contributions from other nuclei (Amaral and Price, 1984). It is perhaps no understatement to say that the single, most important advance concerning the primate amygdala over the last 25 years has been the discovery of so many amygdala–cortical connections.

An innovative way of depicting the relationship of the amygdala with the cerebral cortex can be seen in a connectional analysis (Figure 1.8) in which the relative positions of different cortical regions are determined by the extent of shared connections and their weighting (density). By using an approach based on non-metric multidimensional scaling, Young and his co-workers (Young *et al.*, 1994) were able to depict the relationship of the primate amygdala to the cerebral cortex. Its central position, in striking contrast to, for example, the hippocampus, is a reflection of the fact that the amygdala receives highly processed sensory information and is in a position to integrate information both across and within modalities. Through its subcortical connections, the amygdala can also affect autonomic, hormonal, and motor function. The richness of its connections is mirrored by the richness of the neurotransmitters and neuromodulators that are present in the amygdala. Although this level of

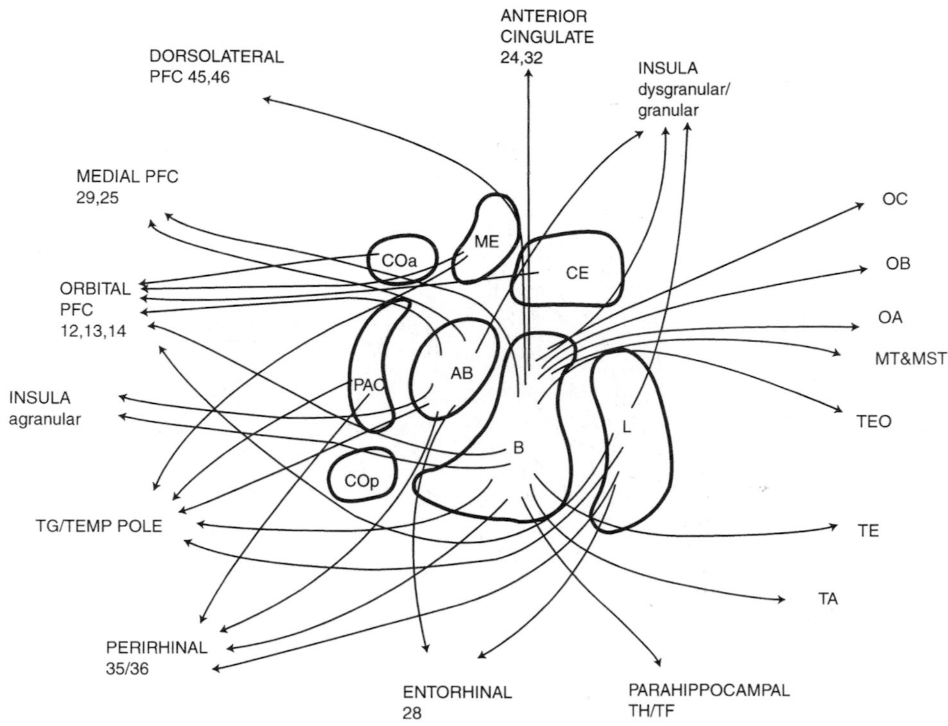

Figure 1.5 Schematic diagram showing the array of cortical projections from the amygdala of the macaque monkey (hippocampal projections are shown in Figure 1.7). Abbreviations of amygdala nuclei are as in Figure 1.3.

complexity will make progress difficult in our attempts to understand the amygdala, it is a feature that needs to be incorporated when appreciating its probable functions.

While a chapter devoted to the connections of the primate amygdala has not been included, a comprehensive review of the connections of the rat amygdala is provided (Pitkanen, Chapter 2). Extraordinary advances have occurred in our understanding of the nuclear connections of the rat amygdala, so that a new level of analysis is possible. As a consequence, the extra-amygdala connections of cytoarchitectonically defined subregions *within* individual nuclei can be catalogued in a comprehensive manner (Pitkänen, Chapter 2). This also extends to the description of intrinsic connections within individual nuclei. A future challenge will be to re-analyse the connections of the primate amygdala to this level of resolution.

1.4 The amygdala and olfactory processing

As already noted, this chapter has an extended section devoted to the amygdala and olfaction, and one of its goals is to highlight the diversity of functions associated with amygdala

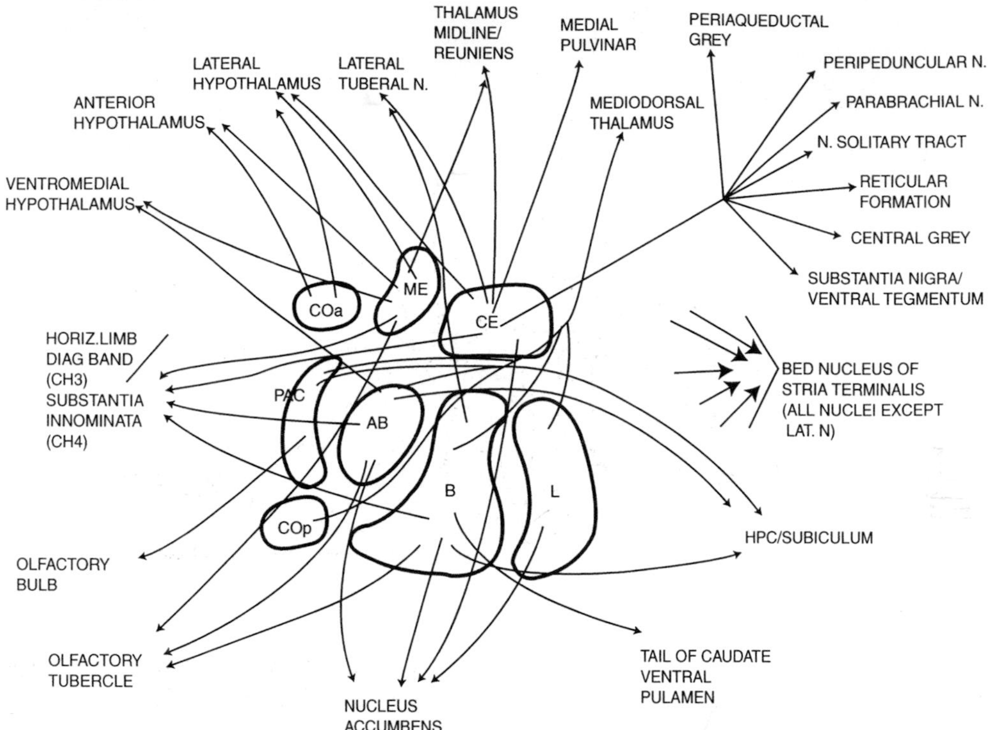

Figure 1.6 Schematic diagram showing the array of subcortical inputs from the amygdala of the macaque monkey. Abbreviations of amygdala nuclei are as in Figure 1.3.

activity. It has long been recognized that the only sensory modality to gain direct access to the amygdala is smell, as all other modalities reach the amygdala in a stepwise manner via sensory association cortices (Figure 1.4). The amygdala receives direct inputs from the main olfactory bulbs, and these connections appear similar across species such as the rat and the macaque monkey. In both species, the olfactory bulb projects principally to the anterior cortical nucleus and the periamygdaloid cortex (Turner *et al.*, 1978; Carmichael *et al.*, 1994; McDonald, 1998). In the rat, there also appear to be lighter, additional projections to parts of the medial nucleus and the anterior amygdaloid area (McDonald, 1998). In addition, the primary olfactory cortex (piriform cortex) projects directly to the amygdala in both rodents and monkeys (Carmichael *et al.*, 1994; McDonald, 1998), and the arrangement of these inputs is shown in Figures 1.2 and 1.4.

Most mammalian species, including rats, mice, and New World monkeys, also possess a vomeronasal organ (Keverne, 1999). This chemoreceptor organ is sited at the base of the nasal cavity and its sensory neurons innervate the accessory olfactory bulb. The accessory olfactory bulb projects to a number of sites including the amygdala and medial hypothalamus. The inputs to the amygdala terminate in the medial nucleus and the posterior cortical nucleus, and these same nuclei project to the medial hypothalamus. There is considerable

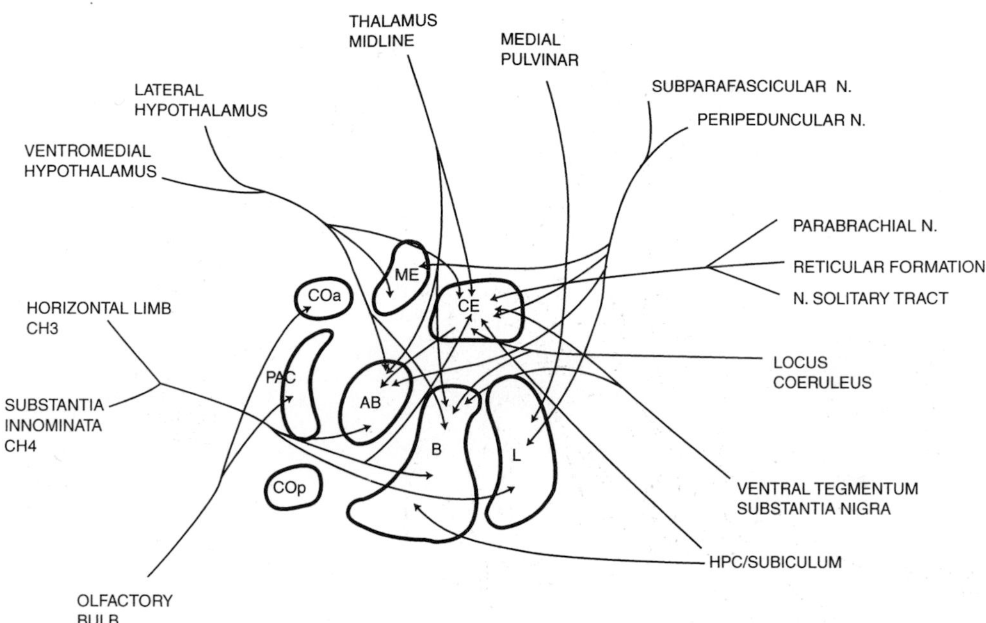

Figure 1.7 Schematic diagram showing the array of subcortical projections to the amygdala of the macaque monkey. Abbreviations of amygdala nuclei are as in Figure 1.3.

evidence demonstrating the importance of the vomeronasal organ in pheromone detection, although this does not preclude the olfactory receptors from also having a functional role in detecting certain pheromones. Through these routes, the amygdala has been shown to have a key role in aspects of social signalling and reproductive behaviour, and this has been demonstrated most clearly in rodent species. Many of these effects are via the amygdala's efferents to the medial hypothalamus (Numan, 1994). It should be noted that while the vomeronasal organ is present in foetal humans, it has proved difficult to show that it has a functional role in adult humans and apes (MontiBloch *et al.*, 1998; Keverne, 1999).

A striking feature of some of the structures linked to the accessory olfactory system is that they exhibit sexual dimorphism. Thus within the rat amygdala, the medial nucleus and the closely related bed nucleus of the stria terminalis (BNST) both show gender differences in volume (Hines *et al.*, 1992). In fact, the volumes of the posterodorsal region of the medial nucleus and the encapsulated region of BNST are almost twice as large in male than female rats (Hines *et al.*, 1992). These nuclei are also neurochemically sexually dimorphic (e.g. for levels of substance P, cholecystokinin, and vasopressin). In addition, the medial nucleus shows differences in its neuronal architecture, with male rats possessing more shaft synapses in the medial molecular layer and more dendritic spines in the ventral molecular layer (Nishizuka and Arai, 1981, 1983). The posteromedial portion of the cortical amygdala nucleus also receives a direct input from the accessory olfactory bulb, and again this portion of the nucleus is larger and contains more neurons in male than female rats (VinaderCaerols *et al.*, 1998).

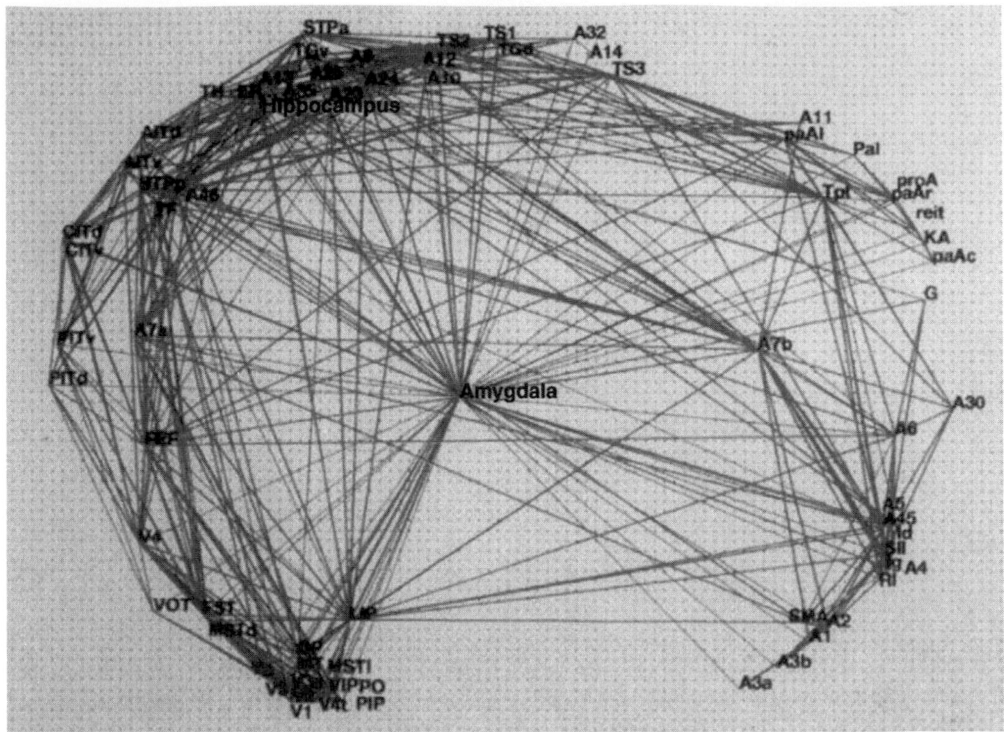

Figure 1.8 Topological organization of entire macaque cerebral cortex. A total of 758 connections between 72 areas is represented, of which 136 (18%) are one-way. Reciprocal connections are shown in red, one-way connections from left to right are in grey, and one-way connections from right to left are in blue (from Young *et al.*, 1994). See also Plate section for colour reproduction.

By virtue of their reception of both olfactory and vomeronasal system inputs, the medial amygdala nuclei are well positioned to regulate the effects of chemosensory signals on social behaviour in rodents. Furthermore, many of the medial and cortical amygdala neurons are androgen and oestrogen sensitive, and are connected not only to each other but also to other sexually dimorphic nuclei in the medial preoptic area (Newman, 1999). The interactions between these various components are highly organized, as shown by anatomical studies of the Syrian hamster (Coolen and Wood, 1998). In this species, the anterior division of the medial nucleus has widespread connections with olfactory/chemosensory regions, while the posterior division of the medial nucleus is heavily interconnected with steroid-responsive brain regions (Coolen and Wood, 1998). These two divisions also have different connections with the preoptic area and the BNST. At the same time, these two divisions of the medial nucleus are interconnected with each other (Coolen and Wood, 1998; Pitkänen, Chapter 2), thus helping the integration of chemosensory and hormonal signals to control social and sexual behaviour. Indeed, in the hamster, this integration within the medial amygdala appears to be essential for mating behaviour (Wood and Coolen, 1997). Furthermore, crossed lesion studies in rats have helped to show the importance of the interaction between the medial amygdala and medial preoptic area for mating behaviour in the male rat (Kondo and Arai, 1995). Not surprisingly, some authors have grouped the corticomedial amygdala nuclei with the BNST to create an 'extended medial amygdala' that is involved in the control of sexually dimorphic behaviour, often via its links with the medial hypothalamus (Newman, 1999). These functions include the regulation of behaviour by olfactory information, including its effects upon sexual, aggressive and maternal behaviour.

Initial attempts to uncover the importance of the medial amygdala for chemosensory signals that control social and sexual behaviour relied largely on the lesion technique. Some of the first evidence came from studies of male hamsters showing that lesions of the medial nucleus, but not of the basolateral nuclei, eliminated mating behaviour and severely reduced the male's investigation of the female hamster's anogenital region (Lehman *et al.*, 1980). Conversely, the decrease in mating that follows castration in male hamsters can be partially reversed by the infusion of testosterone into the medial nucleus (Coolen and Wood, 1999). Lesions in the same nucleus also affect the female hamster as they eliminate the normal preference to explore male odours and to scent-mark in response to odour cues, even though they do not appear to affect the ability to distinguish between the odours of individual male animals (Petrulis and Johnstone, 1999). The medial nucleus is also critically involved in rat mating behaviour, and this again relates to the involvement of chemosensory signals. Thus, although lesions of the posterior medial nucleus do not affect reflexive penile erections, they do reduce copulatory behaviour and eliminate erections evoked by the odours of oestrous females (Kondo *et al.*, 1998). In contrast, the effects of medial amygdala lesions on female rats appear more subtle as they appear to spare many aspects of female sexual behaviour (Masco and Carrer, 1980).

The problem with the lesion approach is that it can only identify regions that are critical for a given behaviour, and may therefore fail to identify other areas that contribute. To avoid this problem, researchers increasingly have used the expression of immediate early genes (IEGs) such as c-*fos* to help identify pathways that enable olfactory cues to influence social and sexual behaviour in rodents. Anogenital investigation of female rats by males leads to increased IEG activation in the posterodorsal division of the medial amygdala and BNST (Coolen *et al.*, 1997). Similarly, exposure to pheromonal cues from oestrous rats leads to increased Fos immunoreactivity in both male and female rats throughout the olfactory circuits, including the medial amygdala, BNST, and medial preoptic area (Bressler and Baum, 1996; Pfaus and Heeb, 1997). It should be noted, however, that the IEG responses of male rats to oestrous female rats appear to comprise a combination of effects, so that volatile cues from absent oestrous females are processed via the main olfactory system while chemosensory cues from oestrous bedding activate the accessory olfactory system (Kelliher *et al.*, 1999). Intriguingly, even a previously neutral odour that has been paired repeatedly with the presentation of sexually receptive females leads to increased Fos induction in the posterodorsal medial amygdala (Pfaus and Heeb, 1997). Finally, it is not surprising that the same areas that are activated by olfactory stimuli are also activated by copulatory stimuli in both male and female rodents, across a range of species (Pfaus and Heeb, 1997). For example, Fos induction is increased markedly in the lateral part of the posterodorsal medial amygdala of the rat following ejaculation (Pfaus and Heeb, 1997).

In some rodents, the smell of an unfamiliar male conspecific can interrupt pregnancy (the Bruce effect). The initial learning of the male mate (so that an unfamiliar animal can be recognized) involves the establishment of an olfactory memory in the accessory olfactory bulb. In some species, the amygdala also appears to be involved as lesions of the amygdala can disrupt this olfactory memory for a particular mate (Demas *et al.*, 1997). The amygdala is also involved in rodent parental behaviour, aspects of which are also triggered by olfactory and chemosensory signals. For example, studies of rat maternal behaviour implicate the medial nucleus of the amygdala (Numan, 1994), while c-*fos* studies underline the importance of olfactory signals for activating the medial amygdala during interactions with pups (Fleming and Walsh, 1994). This parental involvement is not restricted to rats as lesions of the medial nucleus reduce contact with pups by male prairie voles (Kirkpatrick *et al.*, 1994a), while exposure to a pup (which provides visual, tactile, auditory, and olfactory cues) induces c-*fos* activation in the medial nucleus in both male and female prairie voles (Kirkpatrick *et al.*, 1994b). Indeed, evidence from a range of rodent species indicates that those medial amygdala nuclei in which olfactory and vomeronasal system transmission is modulated by populations of oestrogen- and androgen-sensitive neurons form part of a larger integrated system that controls both male and female sexual and parental behaviour, as well as some forms of aggression (Newman, 1999). Many these actions are via its connections with the medial preoptic area.

The parental studies so far described have focused on rodents, where offspring typically are born at a very immature stage of development and require much care. A very different set of problems occur in mammals that give birth to precocial young, where the offspring may be mobile shortly after birth. One problem posed by gregarious species that are synchronous breeders (e.g. many ungulates) is that the mother must be able to recognize its offspring to prevent their becoming lost. Studies of parturition in sheep have revealed the complex interplay of signals, including chemosensory signals, that are vital for this crucial aspect of maternal behaviour (Kendrick *et al.*, 1997). The medial amygdala is one of a series of structures (olfactory bulb, BNST, and medial preoptic area) that coordinate the olfactory recognition of offspring. The stimulus involves airborne odours rather than pheromones, and learning initially is triggered by the release of hormones (e.g. oxytocin) as a result of vaginocervical stimulation at birth. This hormone facilitates the olfactory memory formation in the olfactory bulb. Oxytocin acts on several other sites, including the amygdala, where it helps to reduce aversive responses to both neonates and their odours (Kendrick *et al.*, 1997).

As in rodents, there is the possibility that the human amygdala contributes to gender-specific aspects of smell, and in particular the action of pheromones. The principal evidence for human pheromones comes from studies on the effects of olfactory stimuli upon the menstrual cycle (Stern and McClintock, 1998). There is, however, some controversy as to whether the adult human vomeronasal organ is functional and the extent to which it may contribute to chemosensory communication (MontiBloch *et al.*, 1998; Keverne, 1999). It is quite likely, therefore, that human pheromonal responses are mediated via the olfactory bulb and its outputs (which include the medial amygdala). Care should be taken, however, not to overemphasize this possible role, as human reproductive behaviour, unlike that of rodents, is not tied in an obligatory manner to olfactory cues (Keverne, 1999).

In contrast to its clear involvement in social/sexual behaviour signalled by chemosensory inputs, the amygdala appears less important for other forms of olfactory-related behaviour (i.e. non-pheromonal). For example, Slotnick (1985) found that combined electrolytic lesions of the posterior lateral olfactory tract and anterior amygdala in rats had no effect on the retention or learning of new olfactory discrimination tasks. Likewise, Eichenbaum *et al.* (1986) reported that bilateral amygdala lesions did not affect the learning of multiple odour discriminations (see also Slotnick and Schoonover, 1992). At first sight, the failure of amygdala lesions to show impaired performance appears surprising given the connections of the olfactory system, and reports that approximately 40% of rat amygdala neurons respond to olfactory stimuli (Cain and Bindra, 1972). The reason for the lack of clear deficits would appear to stem, in part, from the existence of parallel olfactory inputs to other regions (e.g. piriform cortex, orbitofrontal cortex, entorhinal cortex, and thalamic nucleus medialis dorsalis) that can compensate for the loss of amygdala olfactory routes. At the same time, the olfactory tests used so far presumably lack sufficient specificity to detect those particular aspects of olfactory function that are dependent on the amygdala.

In order to avoid these problems, researchers have turned to studies of amygdala activation during olfactory tasks. In a recent study, a total of 229 neurons in the lateral and basolateral nuclei were recorded in rats during olfactory discrimination learning (Schoenbaum *et al.*, 1999; see Gallagher, Chapter 8). Of these neurons, 60 were found to show selective responses depending on whether a particular olfactory cue was paired with a pleasant or an unpleasant outcome. This selectivity often appeared early in learning and many units could be reversed, indicating that the amygdala neurons encoded the motivational significance of the cues (Gallagher, Chapter 8). This evidence for the involvement of the basolateral amygdala as learning progresses also accords with c-*fos* imaging data. In a study comparing different stages of olfactory discrimination learning by rats (Hess *et al.*, 1997), it was found that initial exploration (no specific odours) led to raised medial (medial, anterior, and posterior cortical nuclei) and, to a lesser extent, raised basolateral activation. In contrast, central nucleus levels stayed low. When cued olfactory discrimination training began, there was a switch producing high basolateral but relatively low medial activation. Finally, in overtrained rats, the differences between these amygdala divisions were reduced (Hess *et al.*, 1997). This study shows that the balance of amygdala activation shifts in a dynamic manner that is dependent on the task demands and upon the stages of learning. As a typical learning experiment would involve multiple stages, it is readily apparent that lesion studies are unlikely to identify specific contributions relating to specific stages of learning.

The contribution of the primate amygdala, and in particular the human amygdala, to olfactory processing remains poorly understood. While group studies have shown that extensive, unilateral temporal lobectomies can disrupt olfactory identification (Rausch and Serafetinides, 1975) and the recall of odours (Rausch *et al.*, 1977), these studies provide little direct evidence for the specific involvement of the amygdala. Reports on the effects of surgery to remove just the amygdala or parts of the amygdala typically have described no disruption to the sense of smell (Scoville *et al.*, 1953; Chitonondh, 1966; Narabayashi, 1977), although these studies lack proper test details. In a more systematic study, odour identification was examined in three groups of unilateral temporal lobe resection cases where the site of surgery had been divided into (i) primarily neocortical, (ii) amygdalohippocampectomy, and (iii) anterior temporal lobe with encroachment on the amygdala or hippocampus (Jones-Gotman *et al.*, 1997). All three groups were impaired, but no clear correlations could be drawn between the presence of an impairment and amygdala damage. The finding that unoperated epileptic cases were also impaired led the authors to emphasize the potential importance of the piriform cortex (Jones-Gotman *et al.*, 1997).

More direct evidence for the contribution of the human amygdala has come from electrophysiological studies that have confirmed the responsiveness of amygdala neurons to odours (Andy and Jurko, 1975) and shown that amygdala activity can lead to olfactory auras (Andy *et al.*, 1975). In a series of patients about to undergo right temporal lobe surgery, amygdala responses to familiar odours were examined prior to surgery (Hughes *et al.*, 1972). Similar patterns of amygdala activity were noticed for similar smells, while judgements of odour intensity appeared to relate to the amplitude of frequency components. Differences were found both for the pleasant–unpleasant dimension and for the high–low intensity dimension (Hughes *et al.*, 1972).

There are also a small number of single-case clinical studies that implicate the amygdala region in aspects of olfactory processing. Andy *et al.* (1975) described a woman who had received an extensive, bilateral amygdalotomy that had involved the entorhinal cortex in one hemisphere. While her detection of odours was largely unchanged, her identification of odours was impaired (Andy *et al.*, 1975). Similarly, the famous case H.M., in whom the amygdala, entorhinal cortex, and hippocampus were removed bilaterally (Corkin *et al.*, 1997), also shows olfactory deficits as he is severely impaired at odour identification, discrimination, and matching, although he can detect weak odours and appreciate odour intensity (Eichenbaum *et al.*, 1983). In both cases, the pathology was not limited to the amygdala, and it may be that the combination of amygdala and entorhinal pathology is critical for identification. More specifically, a single case described by Jones-Gotman and Zatorre (1993) implicated the right amygdala in recognition memory for odours. Finally, two patients with relatively circumscribed, bilateral amygdala pathology as a result of Urbach–Wiethe disease performed quite poorly in a task where specific odours had to be associated with specific drawings (Markowitsch *et al.*, 1994), but it is unclear whether this deficit was specific for odour associations.

The conclusion to be drawn from these and related clinical studies (Eslinger *et al.*, 1982) is that the involvement of the human amygdala in olfaction is often not made apparent by lesion studies. As in rodents, this presumably reflects the presence of multiple olfactory projection routes, i.e. parallel routes to orbitofrontal, thalamic, and other temporal regions. The solution is to look at functional imaging studies and to devise more selective tests. As a first step, Zald and Pardo (1997) reported that exposure to a highly aversive odorant produces a strong increase in cerebral blood flow as measure by positron emission tomography (PET) in both amygdalae, as well as the left orbitofrontal cortex. The left amygdala and left orbitofrontal activations were highly intercorrelated, while less aversive odours failed to activate the amygdala (Zald and Pardo, 1997). Of particular interest was the finding that activity within the left amygdala was associated significantly with subjective ratings of aversiveness, suggesting that amygdala activity is related to the perceived hedonic value of the stimulus. Further tests were conducted with pleasant smells (fruits, spices, and florals), but these only produced a non-significant increase in blood flow in the right anterior amygdala/periamygdaloid area (Zald and Pardo, 1997). It would appear that the amygdala is activated when olfaction engages strong emotional reactions, although it remains to be determined if these effects are confined to aversive odours (for tastes, see Rolls, Chapter 13). Finally, aversive odours can affect amygdala activation via associative processes. In a functional magnetic resonance imaging (fMRI) study, it was found that the presentation of a neutral face that previously had been paired with an aversive odour led to a decrease in amygdala activity in a group of 12 normal subjects (Schneider *et al.*, 1999), providing parallels with data from rats (Gallagher, Chapter 8). Interestingly, the opposite pattern (i.e. increased amygdala activation) was found in a group of 12 subjects suffering from social phobia (Schneider *et al.*, 1999).

The discovery that aversive smells and their associations can activate the amygdala may help to explain other ways in which smells can influence memory. In a real world study (Aggleton, unpublished findings), we examined the long-term retention of specific smells by people who previously had visited a museum (Jorvik Viking Museum, York, UK) where these same smells were used to help recreate the experience of visiting a Viking city. While people who had visited the museum many years before nearly always recalled that there had been smells, only those that were rated independently as being the most aversive (e.g. the smell of a Viking latrine!) were remembered consistently. We also found that these same smells acted as effective contextual cues to help subjects to recall details of the museum, even though they had not visited it for many years (Aggleton and Waskett, 1999). This raises the intriguing possibility that the amygdala not only enhances learning when a subject is emotionally aroused by visual events (see Cahill, Chapter 12), but that arousing smells may also be effective contextual cues through a similar process.

1.5 Plastic mechanisms within the amygdala

The involvement of the amygdala in associative learning (Davis, Chapter 6; Gallagher, Chapter 8; Everitt *et al.*, Chapter 10) strongly suggests that plastic changes occur within the amygdala. One candidate mechanism is long-term potentiation (LTP), the opposite of which is long-term depression (LTD). LTP was first demonstrated in the amygdala by Racine *et al.* in 1983, but the first *in vivo* demonstration was not until 1990 (Clugnet and LeDoux, 1990). Such studies have provoked considerable interest in LTP and LTD within the amygdala (Chapman and Chattarji, Chapter 3). Of particular interest has been the finding of a link between fear conditioning and LTP within the amygdala (Davis, Chapter 6). At the same time, evidence for differences between amygdala LTP and hippocampal LTP (Chapman and Chattarji, Chapter 3) has helped to highlight the multiple forms of LTP that exist.

While plastic changes within the amygdala inevitably must contribute to its role in learning, it is less immediately obvious that such changes will also contribute to other activities generated by the amygdala. A striking example is 'kindling' (Weiss *et al.*, Chapter 4), which provides an experimental model of temporal lobe epilepsy. The key stage is the transformation of a previously subconvulsive seizure into one which is able to induce convulsive behaviour. Much is now known about the candidate processes that underlie kindling, and their similarities to and differences from LTP (Weiss *et al.*, Chapter 4). Intriguingly, these plastic mechanisms within the amygdala might not only contribute to learning and epilepsy, but might also be involved in clinical conditions such as post-traumatic stress disorder and major psychosis (Weiss *et al.*, Chapter 4). The plastic mechanisms also appear to be involved in the formation of drug-associated cues that can have such a powerful influence on the behaviour of drug addicts (Everitt *et al.*, Chapter 10).

1.6 Neurotoxic lesions of the amygdala

In 1988, Dunn and Everitt served notice that some of the effects classically attributed to amygdala damage might in fact be a consequence of damage to fibres of passage passing through or immediately adjacent to the structure. As a consequence of their study, the impact of amygdala damage on conditioned taste aversion learning by rats was questioned (Dunn and Everitt, 1988; Lamprecht and Dudai, Chapter 9). While this initial study was in rats, it is perhaps in studies with macaque monkeys that the impact of using neurotoxins to minimize the effects of fibre damage when making amygdala lesions is having the most dramatic consequences (Baxter and Murray, Chapter 16; Easton and Gaffan, Chapter 17).

It had long been known that the traditional means of removing the amygdala by aspiration resulted in additional damage to portions of perirhinal cortex, entorhinal cortex, piriform cortex, and temporal stem, and the possible impact of this additional damage could be examined by selective removal of just this region (Murray, 1992). What had always remained uncertain was whether there were additional effects of amygdalectomy as a result of white matter damage (principally to fibres of passage). The most direct way to examine this was to make cytotoxic lesions of the entire amygdala, but until MRI guidance could be used for non-human primates this class of experiment was simply not practical (Saunders *et al.*, 1990). With the introduction of this technique, it is becoming increasingly clear that the effects of selective amygdala neuron lesions are far more restricted than the effects of amygdala lesions made by conventional methods (Baxter and Murray, Chapter 16; Easton and Gaffan, Chapter 17). This process of re-examining amygdala lesion effects is not yet complete, but it has already forced a complete reconsideration of the contributions of this region to object recognition, stimulus–stimulus associations and reward–object associations. At the same time, it is clear that neurotoxic amygdala neuron lesions do alter affective responses, typically causing a decrease in reactivity (Meunier *et al.*, 1999). This research has numerous implications. These include a new light on the apparent discrepancies between the effects of amygdala damage in humans and in non-human primates (Aggleton and Young, 1999), and a reconsideration of the effects of disconnecting temporal cortical sites (Easton and Gaffan, Chapter 17).

1.7 The effects of amygdala pathology in humans

A review of the effects of amygdala pathology in humans published 8 years (Aggleton, 1992b) failed to find any consistent effects upon memory, learning, or perception. Indeed, the most striking finding was the *lack* of effect on cognitive abilities, with changes in emotionality being the only consistent theme. A possible exception was evidence of a differential impairment on tests of recognition memory for faces and words (Warrington, 1984). While normal performance was observed for word recognition, modest deficits were found for face recognition (Aggleton, 1992b). This was taken as evidence that amygdala damage might impair some aspects of visuospatial memory, but nothing more specific could be determined from the literature at that time.

This situation changed dramatically a few years later with the publication of two key papers (Adolphs *et al.*, 1994; Young *et al.*, 1995). Both papers described cases with bilateral amygdala damage, but with very different aetiologies. The cases did, however, share a remarkable, common feature: a deficit in identifying certain facial expressions of emotion (Adolphs *et al.*, 1994; Young *et al.*, 1995). In case S.M. described by Adolphs *et al.* (1994), this impairment was found to be highly selective as the identification of fear was impaired while other expressions were intact (Adolphs and Tranel, Chapter 18). Indeed this subject seemed to lack the concept of fear. In case D.R. (Young *et al.*, 1995), consistent deficits were also found when identifying fearful expressions, although she showed some difficulty with faces of disgust and anger as well (Calder *et al.*, 1996). Case D.R. also had a selective difficulty in identifying sounds associated with fearful states (Scott *et al.*, 1997). This specific link with fear is consistent with studies of rodents that had already highlighted the importance of the amygdala for fear conditioning (Davis, Chapter 6; LeDoux, Chapter 7), while the involvement in face perception provided one of the first functional routes by which to test the contributions of the human amygdala to different aspects of information processing. This latter approach has been adapted both for studies analysing the effects of pathological damage (Adolphs and Tranel, Chapter 18), and for studies using brain imaging techniques in normal (Dolan, Chapter 19) and abnormal subjects (Baron-Cohen *et al.*, 1999; Phillips *et al.*, 1999). This role in face perception also provides a link between the changes in affective and social behaviour, observed in both humans (Aggleton, 1992b; Aggleton and Young, 1999) and monkeys (Bachevalier, Chapter 15), and amygdala damage.

Another key breakthrough can be traced directly back to research on rats that had investigated how certain drugs such as adrenaline (epinephrine), opioids, and GABAergic antagonists could modulate memory when injected systemically (McGaugh *et al.*, 1992). Through careful research, it became evident that these effects were associated with the way in which arousing situations (e.g. aversive conditioning) promote effective memories, and that the amygdala has a key role in these processes (McGaugh *et al.*, 1992, Chapter 11). This raises the question of whether the amygdala is involved in the modulation of memory that can occur in humans experiencing emotionally arousing events. The findings from both clinical and imaging studies strongly indicate that this is so (Cahill, Chapter 12), and this has opened up another new avenue by which to explore the functions of the human amygdala. While this process might be beneficial in aiding the recall of potentially important, highly arousing events, it may also be detrimental when such events cannot be forgotten. Not surprisingly, it has been proposed that amygdala activation might contribute to post-traumatic stress syndrome (Weiss *et al.*, Chapter 4), but such a link is largely hypothetical at present. There is, however, more direct evidence that implicates amygdala dysfunction in a range of other disorders that are characterized by abnormal affect.

It has long been appreciated that the amygdala has a key role in primate social behaviour (Bachevalier, Chapter 15) and it has been assumed that it also has an important role in human social interactions. Support for this includes the recent studies of facial processing (Adolphs *et al.*, 1998, 2000; Adolphs and Tranel, Chapter 18; Dolan, Chapter 19). This evidence leads to the prediction that dysfunctions of the amygdala might result in abnormal social behaviour and social intelligence. This proposal has been examined most thoroughly with regard to autism and Asperger's syndrome, where evidence is growing that interactions between the amygdala and the frontal lobes may have a key, contributory role (Baron-Cohen *et al.*, 1999; Bachevalier, Chapter 15).

The advent of imaging techniques has offered new ways of investigating the contribution of the amygdala to other disorders that alter affect. Mood induction experiments in normal subjects have, for example, shown changes in amygdala activation. The most consistent finding is that induction of a sad mood is associated with increased metabolic activity in the left amygdala (Grodd *et al.*, 1995; Schneider *et al.*, 1995). These findings can be linked to the report of a positive correlation between depression severity and left amygdala blood flow (Drevets *et al.*, 1992) in unipolar depressed patients. Interestingly, the same study found evidence for increased amygdala blood flow in depressed patients who were in remittance, suggesting that this may be a trait marker. A different PET study also found amygdala activity to be positively correlated with extent of depression, but this time the correlation was found for the right amygdala (Abercrombie *et al.*, 1998). Evidence that core amygdala nuclei show bilateral reductions of volume in depressed patients (Sheline *et al.*, 1998) underlines the need to resolve these PET differences and determine the extent of the amygdala's contribution to affective disorders. At the same time, there is growing evidence that the amygdala is also involved in anxiety states, some of the most important evidence coming from studies of the sites of actions of anti-anxiety drugs (File, Chapter 5).

The growing understanding of the involvement of the human amygdala in affective and cognitive processes is helping researchers to identify the ways in which amygdala pathology might contribute to various dementing disorders. It has been known for a long time that amygdala pathology occurs in the early stages of Alzheimer's disease (Chow and Cummings, Chapter 20), and it is now evident that amygdala pathology is found in other dementing disorders such as vascular dementia, dementia with Lewy bodies, Parkinson's disease with dementia, and frontotemporal dementia (Chow and Cummings, Chapter 20). The difficulty is that all of these conditions are associated with pathology in multiple sites (Braak *et al.*, 1994, 1997; Chow and Cummings, Chapter 20), and so complex interactions will occur with the functional breakdown of multiple systems. For this reason, the contributions of the amygdala are so much harder to discern, yet at the same time they are likely to be all the more devastating.

Finally, there have been frequent proposals that amygdala dysfunction contributes to psychotic states, most notably schizophrenia (Stevens, 1973; Reynolds, 1992). From what we know of the likely functions of the amygdala, it is not unreasonable to suspect that abnormalities of some or the whole of this complex might contribute to schizophrenia. Perhaps the most obvious link concerns the changes in affect and social behaviour observed in monkeys with amygdala damage (Aggleton and Young, 1999; Meunier *et al.*, 1999;

Bachevalier, Chapter 15), and the negative symptoms of schizophrenia. A pertinent example comes from studies on the effects of early amygdala damage in macaque monkeys on emotional and social interaction (Malkova *et al.*, 1997; Bachevalier, Chapter 15). In these monkeys, the amygdala was removed during the first week of life (Malkova *et al.*, 1997). While they appeared not to have the classic amygdala syndrome (loss of fear and emotionality), they were clearly abnormal in their social interaction as demonstrated by their inappropriate social interactions, increased withdrawal, less contact, and abnormal contacts. Humans with amygdala damage also show mild decreases in emotional reactivity and evidence of disruption to social behaviour (Aggleton and Young, 1999; Adolphs and Tranel, Chapter 18). Other parallels are seen in the performance of recognition memory tests for words and faces, as both patients with schizophrenia and patients with bilateral amygdala damage show disproportionate problems with face recognition memory (Aggleton and Shaw, 1996). The discovery that amygdala pathology impairs the identification of emotional faces (Adolphs *et al.*, 1999; Adolphs and Tranel, Chapter 18) provides another apparent similarity with schizophrenia (Cramer *et al.*, 1992), as does the involvement of the amygdala in olfaction and evidence of olfactory identification deficits in schizophrenia (Hurwitz *et al.*, 1988). While these examples suggest that amygdala dysfunction contributes to features of schizophrenia, this form of evidence is at best indirect and has to be interpreted alongside evidence of dysfunctions in other structures.

A more direct approach has been to look for evidence of morphometric changes in the amygdala of schizophrenic subjects using MRI or post-mortem studies. The most consistent abnormality revealed by MRI is lateral ventricular enlargement (Chua and McKenna, 1995), while shrinkage of the adjacent grey matter of the medial temporal lobes is one of the most often reported grey matter changes (Bogerts *et al.*, 1993; McCarley *et al.*, 1999). It is generally considered that the hippocampal formation is the region of primary change, but even this is not a consistent feature (Chua and McKenna, 1995; Lawrie and Abukmeil, 1998; Nelson *et al.*, 1998). Where separate measurements of amygdala volume have been reported, the results have been inconsistent, with only some studies reporting decreased amygdala volume (Weinberger, 1995). An interesting variant has been to look at non-psychotic relatives of schizophrenics, and MRI evidence has again been found of medial temporal lobe shrinkage that probably involves the amygdala (Keshaven *et al.*, 1997; Seidman *et al.*, 1999). Such findings suggest that structural abnormalities in this region are associated with vulnerability to schizophrenia. Unfortunately, all of the above studies are limited by the fact that the volume of the amygdala is extremely difficult to determine as some of its borders lack visible landmarks (but see Convit *et al.*, 1999), and for this reason parts of the hippocampal formation are often included within amygdala measurements. Finally, because these investigations have examined the whole of the amygdala, it is possible that critical damage within a functional subregion (Swanson and Petrovich, 1998) may have been overlooked.

Like MRI studies, evidence from post-mortem examinations of the amygdala in schizophrenic brains is suggestive but not conclusive. Abnormalities include a marked decrease of receptors for thyrotrophin-releasing hormone (Lexow *et al.*, 1994), and decreases in cholecystokinin and asymmetric dopamine levels (Reynolds, 1992). At the same time, normal levels have been reported for neurotensin, methionine-enkephalin, vasoactive intestinal polypeptide, and 5-HT_3 (Zech *et al.*, 1986; Reynolds, 1992; Abidargham *et al.*, 1993). In all of these histochemical studies, there is the need to demonstrate whether these changes have a causal role, or whether they merely reflect a consequence of the disorder.

Other evidence comes from rare examples of schizophrenic-like psychosis associated with amygdala pathology (Emsley and Paster, 1985; Sumi *et al.*, 1992; Fudge *et al.*, 1998). The two cases described by Emsley and Paster (1985), who both showed prominent paranoid symptoms, are of interest as they both suffered from Urbach–Wiethe disease and, as a consequence, had bilateral calcifications in the amygdala. These psychotic symptoms are not, however, a typical feature of the disease (Adolphs and Tranel, Chapter 18). Furthermore, in none of these cases was the pathology restricted to the amygdala. Other data suggesting a link between abnormal amygdala function and psychosis are from temporal lobe epilepsy patients in whom emotional changes and psychotic symptoms are sometimes associated with the seizures (Slater and Beard, 1963; Gold *et al.*, 1994). Indeed, Heath (1954), in his in-depth recording studies, reported abnormal amygdala and hippocampal activity in schizophrenic patients. These findings raise the intriguing possibility that abnormal medial temporal firing in schizophrenics may produce kindling-like effects in the amygdala (Weiss *et al.*, Chapter 4).

The advent of functional imaging has provided a new means of investigating the possible contribution of the amygdala to psychotic states. Under states of emotional stimulation, amygdala activation is reduced remarkedly in the brains of schizophrenic patients (Schneider *et al.*, 1995, 1998). A recent fMRI study that examined responses to different facial expressions of emotion (Phillips *et al.*, 1999) also found evidence of abnormal amygdala activity, but only to certain expressions and only in specific subgroups (non-paranoid) of schizophrenic subjects. These imaging findings might indicate that amygdala function is itself abnormal, or they could result from the amygdala's interactions with regions that are dysfunctional and this abnormality is reflected in a normal amygdala. This caveat is important as the amygdala has extensive interactions with other areas implicated in the pathogenesis of schizophrenia, including the hippocampal formation, the prefrontal cortex, and the ventral striatum. While these connections serve to increase the likelihood of amygdala involvement, they also increase the possibility that reduced amygdala activation could be a result of a primary dysfunction elsewhere.

One of the first, and still one of the most influential proposals is that schizophrenics suffer an underlying abnormality in the dopaminergic system (Snyder, 1974; Grace, 1993; Willner, 1997). This idea was founded primarily on the discovery that the most effective antipsychotic drug therapies are antidopaminergics, and that their potency correlates with their ability to block dopamine receptors. More recently, clinical pathological data have been published that are consistent with abnormalities of the dopamine system (Breier *et al.*, 1997; Willner, 1997; Joyce and Gurevich, 1999). For these reasons, it is of note that the amygdala receives a dopaminergic input from the ventral tegmentum and the dorsal pars compacta of the substantia nigra. Within the amygdala, dopaminergic fibres are most numerous in the central, basal, and lateral nuclei (Sadikot and Parent, 1990). Furthermore, there is evidence that schizophrenics show increased levels of dopamine in the left amygdala (Reynolds, 1992). While it is possible that abnormalities in this connection contribute to the disorder, e.g. paranoid delusions (Fibiger, 1991), other amygdala connections have also been linked with dopaminergic theories of schizophrenia. These connections include the direct projections to the ventral striatum, which preferentially terminate in nucleus accumbens, and the amygdala's projections back to substantia nigra (Russchen *et al.*, 1985; Haber and Fudge, 1997). This network of direct and indirect connections between the amygdala and ventral striatum provides a means by which the amygdala can modulate dopamine-related behaviours (Haber and Fudge, 1997).

A persistent problem for the dopamine theory is the fact that shizophrenia is associated with abnormalities in multiple sites. Notable among them is the prefrontal cortex, and studies of cognitive changes and functional imaging have continued to confirm its likely importance (Weinberger *et al.*, 1986, 1988; Frith, 1992; Weinberger and Berman, 1996). The challenge, therefore, is to bring together seemingly disparate pathologies in a manner consistent with the disorder. Abnormalities of the prefrontal cortex can, in fact, be readily linked to limbic dysfunction in the temporal lobes as these areas have extensive reciprocal connections. This still leaves the problem of how dopamine therapy might alleviate symptoms generated by dysfunctions in these regions, and a theory is needed that is able to bring the various strands of evidence together. Recent developmental studies are now providing such a theoretical framework.

There is growing evidence that increased vulnerability to schizophrenia is acquired early in life. It has therefore been suggested that early damage to the medial temporal lobe, particularly in the rostral hippocampal regions including the entorhinal cortex, results in abnormal prefrontal cortical function and abnormal dopamine regulation within the striatum. Consistent with this are numerous accounts that the pathology in schizophrenia does not seem to be progressive and that it occurs early during development of the medial temporal cortex, resulting in alterations in the cellular organization of the entorhinal cortex and the hippocampus (Jakob and Beckman, 1986; Arnold *et al.*, 1991). The maldevelopment of the medial temporal lobe then results in abnormal prefrontal cortical function and dopamine regulation (Weinberger, 1995). While there is little direct clinical evidence for this theory, there is a growing body of supportive experimental work with animals. It has, for example, been demonstrated in rodents that after neonatal lesions of the ventral hippocampus, dopamine-related behaviour is abnormal after the animal reaches puberty (Lipska *et al.*, 1992). Changes in dopamine levels and receptors are also reported to be abnormal after these early limbic lesions. It has also been demonstrated that cognitive behaviours related to prefrontal functions are abnormal in these same animals (Moghadem *et al.*, 1999). Furthermore, in non-human primates, it has now been demonstrated that neonatal lesions of the medial temporal lobe, including the amygdala and hippocampal formation, result in abnormal dopamine function in the ventral striatum (Saunders *et al.*, 1998). These animals, when tested as adults and compared with animals receiving similar lesions as adults, showed hyperdopaminergic activity in the caudate nucleus when the prefrontal cortex was stimulated. This abnormal increase in the striatum after frontal cortical stimulation was reduced in the presence of antidopaminergics (e.g. haloperidol, and clozapine) (Kolachana, unpublished). In schizophrenic patients, a neuronal marker for normal cortical development, *N*-acetylaspartate (NAA), has been shown to be abnormal (Bertolino *et al.*, 1996). A similar decrease in NAA in the prefrontal cortex has also been shown in these same monkeys with early medial temporal limbic lesions (Bertolino *et al.*, 1997). Furthermore, these same animals show abnormal emotional and social behaviour (Malkova *et al.*, 1997; Bachevalier, Chapter 15). Other relevant evidence comes from findings that limbic, including amygdala, inputs to nucleus accumbens 'gate' both frontal–striatal and hippocampal–striatal inputs (Grace, 1993; Mulder *et al.*, 1998; Rosenkranz and Grace, 1999). It is therefore argued that in schizophrenia, limbic–frontal dysfunctions give rise to abnormalities in the dopamine-rich striatum that may be direct (via limbic inputs) or indirect (via prefrontal dysfunctions). In this way, the seemingly disparate malfunctions associated with schizophrenia can be incorporated into a single theoretical framework (Weinberger, 1995).

In conclusion, it can be seen that the problem with identifying the involvement of the amygdala in schizophrenia is not the lack of evidence but rather sifting out the potentially misleading evidence. At the same time, there is the added problem of understanding amygdala dysfunction against a background of presumed dysfunctions in other systems. The goal of most experimental research in the late 20th century was to isolate and explore *individual* brain structures or systems. The challenge for future studies of psychopathology will be to understand the interactions that occur when *multiple* systems malfunction, be it in dementias or in psychosis.

References

Abercrombie, H.C., Schaefer, S.M., Larson, C.L., Oakes, T.R., Lindgren, K.A., Holden, J.E., Perlman, S.B., Turski, P.A., Krahm, D.D., Benca, R.M., and Davidson, R.J. (1998) Metabolic rate in the right amygdala predicts negative affect in depressed patients. *NeuroReport*, 9, 3301–3307.

Abidargham, A., Laruelle, M., Lipska, B., Jaskiw, G.E., Wong, D.T., Robertson, D.W., Weinberger, D.R., and Kleinman, J.E. (1993) Serotonin 5-HT_3 receptors in schizophrenia—a postmortem study of the amygdala. *Brain Research*, 616, 53–57.

Adolphs, R., Tranel, D., Damasio, H., and Damasio, A.R. (1994) Impaired recognition of emotion in facial expressions following bilateral damage to the human amygdala. *Nature*, 372, 669–672.

Adolphs, R., Tranel, D., and Damasio, A.R. (1998) The human amygdala and social judgment. *Nature*, 393, 470–474.

Adolphs, R., Tranel, D., Hamann, S., Young, A.W., Calder, A.J., Phelps, E., Anderson, A., Lee, G.P., and Damasio, A.R. (2000) Recognition of facial emotion in nine individuals with bilateral amygdala damage. *Neuropsychologia*, in press.

Aggleton, J.P. (1985) A description of intra-amygdaloid connections in old world monkeys. *Experimental Brain Research*, 57, 390–399.

Aggleton, J.P. (1992a) *The Amygdala: Neurobiological Aspects of Emotion, Memory, and Mental Dysfunction*. Wiley-Liss; New York.

Aggleton, J.P. (1992b) The functional effects of amygdala lesions in humans: a comparison with findings from monkeys. In *The Amygdala: Neurobiological Aspects of Emotion, Memory, and Mental Dysfunction* (ed. J.P. Aggleton), pp. 485–503. Wiley-Liss, New York.

Aggleton, J.P. and Shaw, C. (1996) Amnesia and recognition memory: a re-analysis of psychometric data. *Neuropsychologia*, 34, 51–62.

Aggleton, J.P. and Waskett, L. (1999) The ability of odours to serve as state-dependent cues for real-world experiences: can Viking smells aid the recall of Viking experiences. *British Journal of Psychology*, 90, 1–7.

Aggleton, J.P. and Young, A.W. (1999) The enigma of the amygdala: concerning its contribution to human emotion. In *Cognitive Neuroscience of Emotion* (eds R.D. Lane and L. Nadel), pp. 106–128. Oxford University Press, New York.

Alheid, G.F. and Heimer, L. (1988) New perspectives in basal forebrain organisation of special relevance for neuropsychiatric disorders: the striatopallidal, amygdaloid, and corticopetal components of substantia innominata. *Neuroscience*, 1, 1–39.

Amaral, D.G. and Price, J.L. (1984) Amygdalo-cortical projections in the monkey (*Macaca fascicularis*). *Journal of Comparative Neurology*, 230, 465–496.

Amaral, D.G., Price, J.L., Pitkänen, A., and Carmichael, S.T. (1992) Anatomical organization of the primate amygdaloid complex. In *The Amygdala: Neurobiological Aspects of Emotion, Memory, and Mental Dysfunction* (ed. J.P. Aggleton), pp. 1–66. Wiley-Liss, New York.

Andy, O.J. and Jurko, M.F. (1975) The human amygdala: excitability state and aggression. In *Neurosurgical Treatment in Psychiatry, Pain, and Epilepsy* (eds W.H. Sweet, S. Obrador and J.G. Martin-Rodriguez), pp. 417–427. University Park Press, Baltimore.

Andy, O.J., Jurko, M.F., and Hughes, J.R. (1975) The amygdala in relation to olfaction. *Confinia Neurologica*, 37, 215–222.

Arnold, S.E., Hyman, B.T., Van Hoesen, G.W., and Damasio, A.R. (1991) Some cytoarchitectural abnormalities of the entorhinal cortex in schizophrenia. *Archives of General Psychiatry*, 48, 625–632.

Baron-Cohen, S., Ring, H.A., Wheelwright, S., Bullmore, E.T., Brammer, M.J., Simmons, A., and Williams, S.C.R. (1999) Social intelligence in the normal and autistic brain: an fMRI study. *European Journal of Neuroscience*, 11, 1891–1898.

Bertolino, A. Nawroz, S., Mattay, V.S., Duyn, J.H., Moonen, C.T.W., Barnett, A.S., Frank, J.A., Tedeschi, G., and Weinberger, D.R. (1996) A specific pattern of neurochemical pathology in schizophrenia as assessed by multislice proton magnetic resonance spectroscopic imaging. *American Journal of Psychiatry*, 153, 1554–1563.

Bertolino, A., Saunders, R.C., Mattay, A., Bachevalier, J., Frank, J., and Weinberger,D.R. (1997) Altered development of prefrontal neurons in rhesus monkeys with neonatal mesial temporo-limbic lesions: a proton magnetic resonance spectroscopic imaging study. *Cerebral Cortex*, 7, 740–748.

Bogerts, B., Lieberman, J.A., Ashtari, M., Bilder, R.M., Degreef, G., Lerner, G., Johns, C., and Masiar, S. (1993) Hipocampus–amygdala volumes and psychopathology in chronic schizophrenia. *Biological Psychiatry*, 33, 236–246.

Bonda, E. (2000) Organization of connections of the basal and accessory basal nuclei in the monkey amygdala. *European Journal of Euroscience*, **12**, 1971–1992.

Braak, H., Braak,E. Yilmazer, D., de Vos, R.A.I., Jansen, E.N.H., Bohl, J., and Jellinger, K. (1994) Amygdala pathology in Parkinson's disease. *Acta Neuropathologica*, 88, 493–500.

Braak, H., Griffing, K., and Braak,E. (1997) Neuroanatomy of Alzheimer's disease. *Alzheimer's Research*, 3, 235–247.

Brier, A., Saunders, R.C., Su, T.-P., Carson, R.E. Kolachana, B.S., de Bartolomeis, A., Weisenfeld, N., Malhotra, A.K., Eckelman, W.C., and Pickar, D. (1997) Schizophrenia is associated with elevated amphetamine-induced synaptic dopamine concentrations. *Proceedings of the National Academy of Sciences of the United States of America*, 94, 2569–2574.

Bressler, S.C. and Baum, M.J. (1996) Sex comparison of neuronal fos immunoreactivity in the rat vomeronasal projection circuit after chemosensory stimulation. *Neuroscience*, 71, 1063–1072.

Burdach, K.F. (1819–1822) *Vom Baume und Leben des Gehirns*. Leipzig.

Cain, D.P. and Bindra, D. (1972) Responses of amygdala single units to odours in the rat. *Experimental Neurology*, 35, 98–110.

Calder, A.J., Young, A.W., Rowland, D., Perrett, D.I., Hodges, J.R., and Etcoff, N.L. (1996) Facial emotion recognition after bilateral amygdala damage: differentially severe impairment of fear. *Cognitive Neuropsychology*, 13, 699–745.

Carmichael, S.T. and Price, J.L. (1995) Limbic connections of the orbital and medial prefrontal cortex in Macaque monkeys. *Journal of Comparative Neurology*, 363, 615–61.

Carmichael, S.T., Clugnet, M.-C., and Price, J.L. (1994) Central olfactory connections in the Macaque monkey. *Journal of Comparative Neurology*, 346, 403–434.

Chitonondh, H. (1966) Stereotaxic amygdalotomy in the treatment of olfactory seizures and psychiatric disorders with olfactory hallucinations. *Confinia Neurologica*, 27, 181–196.

Chua, S.E. and McKenna, P.J. (1995) Schizophrenia—a brain disease? *British Journal of Psychiatry*, 166, 563–582.

Clugnet, M.C. and LeDoux, J.E. (1990) Synaptic plasticity in fear conditioning circuits—induction of LTP in the lateral amygdala by stimulation of the medial geniculate body. *Journal of Neuroscience*, 10, 2818–2824.

Convit, A., McHugh, P., Wolf, O.T., deLeon, M.J., Bobinski, M., DeSanti, S., Roche, A., and Tsui, W. (1999) MRI volume of the amygdala: a reliable method allowing separation from the hippocampal formation. *Psychiatry Research—Neuroimaging*, 90, 113–123.

Coolen, L.M. and Wood, R.I. (1998) Bidirectional connections of the medial amygdaloid nucleus in the Syrian hamster brain: simultaneous anterograde and retrograde tract tracing. *Journal of Comparative Neurology*, 399, 189–209.

Coolen, L.M. and Wood, R.I. (1999) Testosterone stimulation of the medial preoptic area and medial amygdala in the control of male hamster sexual behavior: redundancy without amplification. *Behavioural Brain Research*, 98, 143–153.

Coolen, L.M., Peters, H.J.P.W., and Veening, J.G. (1997) Distribution of Fos immunoreactivity following mating versus anogenital investigation in the male rat brain. *Neuroscience*, 77, 1151–1161.

Corkin, S., Amaral, D.G., Gonzalez, R.G., Johnson, K.A., and Hyman, B.T. (1997) H.M.'s medial temporal lobe lesion: findings from magnetic resonance imaging. *Journal of Neuroscience*, 17, 3964–3979.

Cramer, P., Bowen, J. and O'Neill, M. (1992) Schizophrenics and social judgement. Why do schizophrenics get it wrong? *British Journal of Psychiatry*, 160, 481–487.

Demas, G.E., Williams, J.M., and Nelson, R.J. (1997) Amygdala but not hippocampal lesions impair olfactory memory for mate in praire voles (*Microtus ochrogaster*). *American Journal of Physiology—Regulatory Integrative and Comparative Physiology*, 42, 1683–1689.

Drevets, W.C., Videen, T.O., Price, J.L., Preskorn, S.H., Carmichael, S.T., and Raichle, M.E. (1992) A functional anatomical study of unipolar depression. *Journal of Neuroscience*, 12, 3628–3641.

Dunn, L.T. and Everitt, B.J. (1988) Double dissociations of the effects of amygdala and insular cortex lesions on conditioned taste aversion, passive avoidance and neophobia in the rat using the excitoxin ibotenic acid. *Behavioral Neuroscience*, 102, 3–23.

Eichenbaum, H., Fagan, A., and Cohen, N.J. (1986) Normal olfactory discrimination learning set and facilitation of reversal learning after medial-temporal damage in rats: implications for an account of preserved learning abilities in amnesia. *Journal of Neuroscience*, 6, 1876–1884.

Emsley, R.A. and Paster, L. (1985) Lipoid proteinosis presenting with neuropsychiatric manifestations. *Journal of Neurology, Neurosurgery, and Psychiatry*, 48, 1290–1292.

Eslinger, P.J., Damasio, A.R., and Van Hoesen, G.W. (1982) Olfactory dysfunction in man: anatomical and behavioral aspects. *Brain and Cognition*, 1, 259–285.

Fibiger, H.C. (1991) The dopamine hypothesis of schizophrenia and mood disorders: contradictions and speculations. In *The Mesolimbic Dopamine System: From Motivation to Action* (eds P. Willner and J. Scheel-Kruger), pp. 615–637 John Wiley & Sons, Chichester, UK.

Fleming, A.S. and Walsh, C. (1994) Neuropsycholgy of maternal behavior in the rat—c-fos expression during mother–litter interactions. *Psychoneuroendocrinology*, 19, 429–443.

Frith, C. (1992) *The Cognitive Neuropsychology of Schizophrenia*. Lea, Hove, UK.

Fudge, J.L., Powers, J.M., Haber, S.N., and Caine, E.D. (1998) Considering the role of the amygdala in psychotic illness: a clinicopathological correlation. *Journal of Neuropsychiatry and Clinical Neurosciences*, 10, 383–394.

Gold, J.M., Hermann, B.P., Randolph, C., Wyler, A.R., Goldberg, T.E., and Weinberger, D.R. (1994) Schizophrenia and temporal lobe epilepsy. *Archives of General Psychiatry*, 51, 265–272.

Grace, A.A. (1993) Cortical regulation of subcortical dopamine systems and its possible relevance to schizophrenia. *Journal of Neural Transmission—General*, 9, 111–134.

Grodd, W.W., Schneider, F., Klose, U., and Nagele, T. (1995) Functional magnetic-resonance imaging of psychological functions with experimentally induced emotion. *Radiologe*, 35, 283–289.

Haber, S.N. and Fudge, J.L. (1997) The interface between dopamine neurons and the amygdala: implications for schizophrenia. *Schizophrenia Bulletin*, 23, 471–482.

Heath, R.G. (1954) *Studies in Schizophrenia*. Harvard University Press, Cambridge, Massachusetts.

Hess, U.S., Gall, C.M., Granger, R., and Lynch, G. (1997) Differential patterns of c-*fos* mRNA expression in amygdala during successive stages of odor discrimination learning. *Learning and Memory*, 4, 262–283.

Hines, M., Allen, L.S., and Gorski, R.A. (1992) Sex differences in subregions of the medial nucleus of the amygdala and the bed nucleus of the stria terminalis of the rat. *Brain Research*, 579, 321–326.

Hughes, J.R., Hendrix, D.E., Andy, O.J., Wang, C., Peeler, D., and Wetzel, N. (1972) Correlations between electrophysiology and subjective reponses to odorants as recorded from the olfactory bulb, tract and amygdala of waking man. In *Neurophysiology Studied in Man* (ed. G.G. Somjen), pp. 260–279, Amsterdam Excerpta Medica.

Hurwitz, T., Kopala, L., Clark, C., and Jones, B. (1988) Olfactory deficits in schizophrenia. *Biological Psychiatry*, 23, 123–128.

Jakob, H. and Beckman, H. (1986) Prenatal development disturbances in the limbic allocortex in schizophrenics. *Neural Transmission*, 65, 303–326.

Johnston, J.B. (1923) Further contributions to the study of the evolution of the forebrain. *Journal of Comparative Neurology*, 35, 337–481.

Jones-Gotman, M. and Zatorre, R.J. (1993) Odor recognition memory in humans: role of right temporal and orbitofrontal regions. *Brain and Cognition*, 22, 189–192.

Jones-Gotman, M., Zatorre, R.J., Cendes, F., Olivier, A., Andermann, F., McMacking, D., Staunton, H., Siegel, A.M., and Wieser, H.-G. (1997) Contribution of medial versus lateral temporal-lobe structures to human odour identification. *Brain*, 120, 1845–1856.

Joyce, J.N. and Gurevich, E.V. (1999) D-3 receptors and the actions of neuroleptics in the ventral striatopallidal system of schizophrenics. *Annals of the New York Academy of Sciences*, 877, 595–613.

Kelliher, K.R., Liu, Y.C., Baum, M.J., and Sachs, B.D. (1999) Neuronal Fos activation in olfactory bulb and forebrain of male rats having erections in the presence of inaccessible estrous females. *Neuroscience*, 92, 1025–1033.

Keverne, E.B. (1999) The vomeronasal organ. *Science*, 286, 716–720.

Kendrick, K.M., Da Costa, A.P.C., Broad, K.D., Ohkura, S., Guevara, R., Levy, F., and Keverne, E.B. (1997) Neural control of maternal behaviour and olfactory recognition of offspring. *Brain Research Bulletin*, 44, 383–395.

Keshaven, M.S., Montrose, D.M., Pierri, J.N., Dick, E.L., Rosenberg, D., Talagala, L., and Sweeney, J.A. (1997) Magnetic resonance imaging and spectroscopy in offspring at risk for schizophrenia: preliminary studies. *Progress in Neuro-Psychopharmacology and Biological Psychiatry*, 21, 1285–1295.

Kirkpatrick, B., Carter, C.S., Newman, S.W., and Insel, T.R. (1994a) Axon sparing lesions of the medial nucleus of the amygdala decrease affiliative behaviors in the prairie vole (*Microtus ochrogaster*): behavioral and anatomical specificity. *Behavioral Neuroscience*, 108, 501–513.

Kirkpatrick, B., Kim, J.W., and Insel, T.R. (1994b) Limbic system fos expression associated with paternal behavior. *Brain Research*, 658, 112–118.

Kondo, Y. and Arai, Y. (1995) Functional association between the medial amygdala and the medial preoptic area in regulation of mating-behaviour in the male rat. *Physiology and Behavior*, 57, 69–73.

Kondo, Y., Sachs, B.D., and Sakuma, Y. (1998) Importance of the medial amygdala in rat penile erection evoked by remote stimuli from estrous females. *Behavioural Brain Research*, 91, 215–222.

Lawrie, S.M. and Abukmeil, S.S. (1998) Brain abnormality in schizophrenia—a systematic and quantitative review of volumetric magnetic resonance imaging studies. *British Journal of Psychiatry*, 172, 110–120.

Lehman, M.N., Winans, S.S., and Powers, J.B. (1980) Medial nucleus of the amygdala mediates chemosensory control of male hamster sexual behaviour. *Science*, 210, 557–560.

Lexow, N., Joyce, J.N., Kim, S.J., Phillips, J., Casanova, M.F., Bird, E.D., Kleinman, J.E., and Winokur, A. (1994) Alterations in the TRH receptors in temporal-lobe of schizophrenics—a quantitative autoradiographic study. *Synapse*, 18, 315–327.

Lipska, B.K., Jaskiw, G.E., Chrapusta, S., Karoum, F., and Weinberger, D. (1992) Ibotenic acid lesion of the ventral hippocampus differentially affects dopamine and its metabolites in the nucleus accumbens and prefrontal cortex in the rat. *Brain Research*, 585, 1–6.

Malkova, L.. Mishkin, M., Suomi, S., and Bachevalier, J. (1997) Socioemotional behavior in adult rhesus monkeys after early versus late lesions of the medial temporal lobe. *Annals of the New York Academy of Sciences*, 807, 538–540.

Markowitch, H.J., Calabrese, P., Wurker, M., Durwen, H.F., Kessler, J., Babinsky, R. Brechtelsbauer, D., Heuser, L., and Gehlen, W. (1994) The amygdala's contribution to memory—a study on two patients with Urbach–Wiethe disease. *NeuroReport*, 5, 1349–1352.

Masco, D.H. and Carrer, H.F. (1980) Sexual receptivity in female rats after lesion or stimulation of different amygdaloid nuclei. *Physiology and Behavior*, 24, 1073–1080.

McCarley, R.W., Wible, C.G., Frumin, M., Hirayasu, Y., Levitt, J.J., Fischer, I.A., and Shenton, M.E. (1999) MRI anatomy of schizophrenia. *Biological Psychiatry*, 45, 1099–1119.

McDonald, A. J. (1998) Cortical pathways to the mammalian amygdala. *Progress in Neurobiology*, 55, 257–332.

McGaugh, J.L., Introini-Collison, I.B., Cahill, L., Kim, M., and Liang, K.C. (1992) Involvement of the amygdala in neuromodulatory influences on memory storage. In *The Amygdala: Neurobiological Aspects of Emotion, Memory, and Mental Dysfunction* (ed. J.P. Aggleton), pp. 431–451. Wiley-Liss, New York.

Meunier, M., Bachevalier, J., Murray, E.A., Malkova, L., and Mishkin, M. (1999) Effects of aspiration versus neurotoxic lesions of the amygdala on emotional responses in monkeys. *European Journal of Neuroscience*, 11, 4403–4418.

Moghadem, B., Aultman, J., Weinberger, D.R., and Lipska, B.K. (1999) Neonatal damage of the ventral hippocampus impairs acquisition of a working memory task. *Society for Neuroscience Abstracts*, 29, 1891.

MontiBloch, L., Jennings White, C., and Berliner, D.L. (1998) The human vomeronasal system—a review. *Annals of the New York Academy of Sciences*, 855, 373–389.

Mulder, A.B., Hodenpijl, M.G., and Lopes da Silva, F.H. (1998) Electrophysiology of the hippocampal and amygdaloid projections to the nucleus accumbens of the rat: convergence, segregation, and interaction of inputs. *Journal of Neuroscience*, 18, 5059–5102.

Murray, E.A. (1992) Medial temporal lobe structures contributing to recognition memory: the amgydaloid complex versus the rhinal cortex. In *The Amygdala: Neurobiological Aspects of Emotion, Memory, and Mental Dysfunction* (ed. J.P. Aggleton), pp. 453–470. Wiley-Liss, New York.

Narabayashi, H. (1977) Stereotaxic amygdalectomy for epileptic hyperactivity—long range results in children. In *Topics in Child Neurology* (eds M.E. Blaw, I. Rapin, and M. Kinsbourne), pp. 319–331. Spectrum Publications, New York.

Nelson, M.D., Saykin, A.J., Flashman, L.A., and Riordan, H.J. (1998) Hippocampal volume reduction in schizophrenia as assessed by magnetic resonance imaging—a meta-analytic study. *Archives of General Psychiatry*, 55, 433–440.

Newman, S.W. (1999) The medial extended amygdala in male reproductive behavior—a node in the mammalian social behavior network. *Annals of the New York Academy of Sciences*, 877, 242–257.

Nishizuka, M. and Arai, Y. (1981) Sexual dimorphism in synaptic organisation in the amygdala and its dependence on neonatal hormone environment. *Brain Research*, 212, 31–38.

Nishizuka, M. and Arai, Y. (1983) Regional difference in sexually dimorphic synaptic organization of the medial amygdala. *Experimental Brain Research*, 49, 462–465.

Numan, M. (1994) A neural circuitry analysis of maternal behavior in the rat. *Acta Paediatrica*, 83, 19–28.

Petrulis, A. and Johnston, R.E. (1999) Lesions centred on the medial amygdala impair scent marking and sex-odor recognition but spare discrimination of individual odours in female golden hamsters. *Behavioral Neuroscience*, 113, 345–357.

Pfaus, J.G. and Heeb, M.M. (1997) Implications of immediate early gene induction in the brain following sexual stimulation of female and male rodents. *Brain Research Bulletin*, 44, 397–407.

Phillips, M.L., Williams, L., Senior, C., Bullmore, E.T., Brammer, M.J., Andrew, C., Williams, S.C.R., and David, A.S. (1999) A differential neural response to threatening and non-threatening negative facial expressions in paranoid and non-paranoid schizophrenics. *Psychiatry Research—Neuroimaging*, 92, 11–31.

Pitkänen, A. and Amaral, D.G. (1991) Demonstration of projections from the lateral nucleus to the basal nucleus of the amygdala: a PHA-L study in the monkey. *Experimental Brain Research*, 83, 465–470.

Racine, R.J., Milgram, N.W., and Hafner, S. (1983) Long term potentiation phenomena in the rat limbic forebrain. *Brain Research*, 260, 217–231.

Rausch, R. and Serafetinindes, E.A. (1975) Specific alterations of olfactory function in humans with temporal lobe lesions. *Nature*, 255, 557–558.

Rausch, R., Serafetinindes, E.A., and Crandall (1977) Olfactory memory in patients with anterior temporal lobectomy. *Cortex*, 13, 445–452.

Reynolds, G.P. (1992) The amygdala and the neurochemistry of schizophrenia. In *The Amygdala: Neurobiological Aspects of Emotion, Memory, and Mental Dysfunction* (ed. J.P. Aggleton), pp. 561–574. Wiley-Liss, New York.

Rosenkranz, J.A. and Grace, A.A. (1999) Modulation of basolateral amygdala neuronal firing and afferent drive by dopamine receptor activation *in vivo*. *Journal of Neuroscience*, 15, 11027–11039.

Russchen, F.T., Bakst, I., Amaral, D.G., and Price, D.L. (1985) The amygdalostriatal projections in the monkey. An anterograde tracing study. *Brain Research*, 29, 241–257.

Sadikot, A.F. and Parent, A. (1990) The monaminergic innervation of the amygdala in the squirrel monkey brain: An immunohistochemical study. *Experimental Brain Research*, 81, 443–446.

Saunders, R.C., Aigner, T.G., and Frank, J. A. (1990) Magnetic resonance imaging of the rhesus monkey brain—use for stereotaxic surgery. *Experimental Brain Research*, 81, 443–446.

Saunders, R.C., Kolachana, B.S., Bachevalier, J., and Weinberger, D.R. (1998) Neonatal lesions of the medial temporal lobe disrupt prefrontal cortex regulation of striatal dopamine. *Nature*, 393, 169–171.

Scott, S., Young, A.W., Calder, A.J., Hellawell, D.J., Aggleton, J.P., and Johnson, M. (1997) Auditory recognition of emotion after amygdalotomy: impairment of fear and anger. *Nature*, 385, 254–257.

Scoville, W.B., Dunsmore, R.H., Liberson, W.T., Henry, C.E., and Pepe, E. (1953) Observations on medial temporal lobotomy and uncotomy in the treatment of psychotic states. *Association Research into Nervous and Mental Disorders*, 31, 347–369.

Schneider, F., Gur, R.E., Mozley, L.H., Smith, R.J., Mozley, P.D., Censits, D.M., Alavi, A., and Gur, R.C. (1995) Mood effects on limbic blood flow correlate with emotional self-rating. *Psychiatry Research—Neuroimaging*, 61, 265–283.

Schneider, F., Weiss, U., Kessler, C., Salloum, J.B., Posse, S., Grodd, W., and Muller-Gartner, H.W. (1998) Differential amygdala activation in schizophrenia during sadness. *Schizophrenia Research*, 34, 133–142.

Schneider, F., Weiss, U., Kessler, C., Muller-Gartner, H.W., Posse, S., Salloum, J.B., Grodd, W., Himmelman, F., Gaebel, W., and Birbaumer, N. (1999) Subcortical correlates of differential classical conditioning of aversive emotional reactions in social phobia. *Biological Psychiatry*, 45, 863–871.

Schoenbaum, G., Chiba, A.A., and Gallagher, M. (1999) Neuronal encoding in orbitofrontal cortex and basolateral amygdala during olfactory discrimination learning. *Journal of Neuroscience*, 19, 1876–1884.

Seidman, L.J., Faraone, S.V., Goldstein, J.M., Goodman, J.M., Kremen, W.S., Toomey,R., Tourville, J., Kennedy, D., Makris, N., Caviness, V.S., and Tsuang, M.T. (1999). Thalamic and amygdala–hippocampal volume reductions in first-degree relatives of patients with schizophrenia: an MRI based morphometric analysis. *Biological Psychiatry*, 46, 941–954.

Sheline, Y.I., Gado, M.H., and Price, J.L. (1998) Amygdala core nuclei volumes are dcreased in recurrent major depression. *NeuroReport*, 9, 2023–2028.

Slater, E. and Beard, A.W. (1963) The schizophrenia-like psychoses of epilepsy. *British Journal of Psychiatry*, 109, 95–150.

Slotnick, B.M. (1985) Olfactory discrimination in rats with anterior amygdala lesions. *Behavioral Neuroscience*, 99, 956–963.

Slotnick, B.M. and Schoonover, F.W. (1992) Olfactory pathways and the sense of smell. *Neuroscience and Biobehavioral Reviews*, 16, 453–472.

Snyder, S.H. (1974) *Madness and the Brain*. McGraw-Hill, New York.

Stefanacci, L., Suzuki, W.A., and Amaral, D.G. (1996) Organization of connections between the amygaloid complex and the perirhinal and parahippocampal cortices in Macaque monkeys. *Journal of Comparative Neurology*, 375, 552–582.

Stern, K. and McClintock, M.K. (1998) Regulation of ovulation by human pheromones. *Nature*, 392, 177–179.

Stevens, J.R. (1973) An anatomy of schizophrenia? *Archives of General Psychiatry*, 29, 2177–2189.

Sumi, S.M., Bird, T.D., Nochlin, D., and Raskind, M.A. (1992) Familial presenile dementia with psychosis associated with cortical neurofibrillary tangles and degeneration of the amygdala. *Neurology*, 42, 120–127.

Swanson, L. W. and Petrovich, G. D. (1998) What is the amygdala? *Trends in Neurosciences*, 21, 323–331.

Turner, B.H., Gupta, K.C., and Mishkin, M. (1978) The locus and cytoarchitecture of the projection areas of the olfactory bulb in *Macaca mulatta. Journal of Comparative Neurology*, 177, 381–396.

VinaderCaerols, C., Collado, P., Segovia, S., and Guillamon, A. (1998) Sex differences in the posteromedial cortical nucleus of the amygdala in the rat. *NeuroReport*, 9, 2653–2656.

Warrington, E.K. (1984) *The Recognition Memory Test*. NFER-Nelson, Windsor, UK.

Weinberger, D.R. (1995) From neuropathology to neurodevelopment. *Lancet*, 346, 552–557.

Weinberger, D.R. and Berman, K.F. (1996) Prefrontal function in schizophrenia: confounds and controversies. *Philosophical Transactions of the Royal Society of London, Series B*, 351, 1495–1503.

Weinberger, D.R., Berman, K.F., and Zec, R.F. (1986) Physiological dysfunction of dorsolateral prefrontal cortex in schizophrenia. I. Regional blood flow evidence. *Archives of General Psychiatry*, 43, 114–124.

Weinberger, D.R., Berman, K.F., and Illowsky, B. (1988) Physiological dysfunction of dorsolateral prefrontal cortex in schizophrenia. III. A new cohort and evidence for a monaminergic mechanism. *Archives of General Psychiatry*, 45, 609–615.

Willner, P. (1997) The dopamine hypothesis of schizophrenia: current status, future prospects. *International Clinical Psychopharmacology*, 12, 297–308.

Wood, R.I and Coolen, L.M. (1997) Integration of chemosensory and hormonal cues is essential for sexual behaviour in the male Syrian hamster: role of the medial amygdaloid nucleus. *Neuroscience*, 78, 1027–1035.

Young, A.W, Aggleton, J.P., Hellawell, D.J., Johnson, M., Broks, P., and Hanley, J.R. (1995) Face processing impairments after amygdalotomy. *Brain*, 118, 15–24.

Young, M.P., Scannell, J.W., Scannell, Burns, G.A.P.C., and Blakemore, C. (1994) Analysis of connectivity: neural systems in the cerebral cortex. *Reviews in the Neurosciences*, 5, 227–249.

Zald, D.V. and Pardo, J.V. (1997) Emotion, olfaction, and the human amygdala: amygdala activation during aversive olfactory stimulation. *Proceedings of the National Academy of Sciences of the United States of America*, 94, 4119–4124.

Zech, M., Roberts, G.W., Bogerts, B., Crow, T.J., and Polak, J.M. (1986) Neuropeptides in the amygdala of controls, schizophrenics and patients suffering from Huntington's chorea: an immunohistochemistry study. *Acta Neuropathologica*, 71, 259–266.

2 Connectivity of the rat amygdaloid complex

Asla Pitkänen

Epilepsy Research Laboratory, A. I. Virtanen Institute for Molecular Sciences, University of Kuopio, PO Box 1627, FIN-70 211 Kuopio, Finland

Summary

The rat amygdala is a nuclear complex composed of 13 nuclei and cortical regions and their subdivisions. Recent anterograde and retrograde studies demonstrate that each nucleus, and even each nuclear subdivision is uniquely interconnected with other amygdaloid nuclei or brain areas. A view emerging from anatomical studies proposes that functional studies of the amygdala, including lesion and imaging studies, would benefit from analyses at the nuclear and subdivisional levels. This review summarizes the principles of amygdala neuronal wiring, and based on that attempts to predict the functional consequences when some of the amygdala nuclei or subdivisions are damaged.

2.1 Introduction

The amygdala is a multinuclear complex located at the medial edge of the temporal lobe. There has been a renaissance of interest in the amygdala over the past 5–10 years due largely to new imaging data on humans demonstrating the role of the amygdala in determining the emotional significance of sensory signals (Adolphs *et al.*, 1994; Bonda *et al.*, 1996; Scott *et al.*, 1997; Zald and Pardo, 1997) and in modulating the memory of emotionally arousing events (see Cahill and McGaugh, 1998; Hamann *et al.*, 1999; Cahill, Chapter 12). j39These functions are essential for successful coping in the everyday social environment (Adolphs *et al.*, 1998; Morris *et al.*, 1998). Progress in understanding the functions of the human amygdala, however, was preceded by fundamental work performed in many laboratories investigating the neuronal pathways involved in the emotional and motivational behaviour of the rat (Davis, 1992; LeDoux, 1992; McGaugh *et al.*, 1992; Gallagher and Holland, 1994). For these studies, knowledge of the connectivity of the rat amygdaloid complex has been a key element in testing the behavioural and electrophysiological hypotheses that were generated regarding the possible contribution of the amygdala to various components of emotional behaviour. Recent studies, in which various amygdaloid nuclei were selectively lesioned (e.g. Killcross *et al.*, 1997) or in which electrophysiological responses were recorded in different amygdaloid nuclei during a behavioural task (e.g. Rogan and LeDoux, 1996; Killcross *et al.*, 1997), have generated a further need for a more detailed understanding of amygdaloid connectivity at nuclear, divisional, and cellular levels. Such information is critical for continued progress in amygdala research.

The various amygdaloid nuclei and cortical areas differ cytoarchitectonically, chemoarchitectonically, and connectionally. Consistent with anatomical data, various nuclei or nuclear groups also differ functionally. For example, major outputs to functional systems generating experiential, motor, mnemonic, autonomic, or endocrine responses originate largely in different nuclei (Russchen, 1986). In fact, it has been proposed that the amygdala is neither anatomically nor functionally a single unit but should be divided, with its parts included in various other functional systems (Swanson and Petrovich, 1998). Others suggest expanding the amygdala both dorsally and medially based on various anatomical criteria to encompass the concept of the 'extended amygdala' (Alheid *et al.*, 1995). Thus, the following questions are raised. What kinds of information does each amygdaloid nucleus receive? How independently can each nucleus evaluate that information? What kinds of responses do various amygdaloid nuclei independently generate via direct amygdalofugal output connections? Is it necessary for several nuclei within the amygdala to work together for the generation of a behaviour with multiple nuances?

The cytoarchitectonics and chemoarchitectonics of the rat amygdala have been reviewed extensively by de Olmos *et al.* (1985) and Alheid *et al.* (1995) and, therefore, these features of the amygdaloid nuclei are not included in this review. Connectivity of the rat amygdala has been reviewed extensively by de Olmos *et al.* (1985) and Price *et al.* (1987). New data regarding the organization of intra-amygdaloid connections in the rat were reviewed by Pitkänen *et al.* (1997). The latest developments in our understanding of the organization of corticoamygdaloid projections in the rat were evaluated elegantly by McDonald (1998). These reviews form a highly valuable database regarding different aspects of the rat amygdala, particularly because some of the reviews extensively compare rat data with those from cat and monkey (Price *et al.*, 1987; McDonald, 1998; see also Amaral *et al.*, 1992; Pare and Smith, 1998).

This review summarizes the connectivity data obtained from the rat amygdaloid complex over the past 25 years, and derives the principles underlying the organization of these amygdaloid circuitries. Some of these principles were proposed previously by Russchen (1986). We give particular emphasis to more recent studies using sensitive anterograde tracing techniques such as *Phaseolus vulgaris* leucoagglutinin (PHA-L), biotinylated dextran amine (BDA), or biocytin. These methods provide information about the distribution and density of projections within the various amygdaloid nuclei that is more detailed than the tracer data obtained using horseradish peroxidase (HRP) or radioactive amino acids. First, a summary of the inputs, outputs, and intra-amygdaloid connections of each amygdaloid nucleus is presented. Then we describe the major principles determining the organization of intra-amygdaloid, afferent, and efferent connections that can be derived from the connectional data available for the rat amygdala. Finally, there is a discussion of what the anatomy might predict about the functional consequences of damage or 'knockout' of various amygdaloid nuclei due to disease processes affecting the central nervous system.

2.2 Intra-amygdaloid, afferent, and efferent connections of different amygdaloid nuclei

2.2.1 Nomenclature

In this review, the amygdaloid complex is partitioned into various nuclei and cortical areas based on the nomenclature described by Price *et al.* (1987) with modifications (Pitkänen *et al.*, 1997; Jolkkonen and Pitkänen, 1998b). One of the major advantages of using this nomenclature is that the naming of presumed homologous portions of the amygdala is similar in different species, including the rat, cat (Price *et al.*, 1987), monkey (Amaral *et al.*, 1992), and human (Sorvari *et al.*, 1995). This similarity is potentially helpful for interspecies comparisons. Briefly, the deep nuclei include the lateral nucleus, basal nucleus, and accessory basal nucleus. The superficial nuclei include the anterior cortical nucleus, bed nucleus of the accessory olfactory tract, medial nucleus, nucleus of the lateral olfactory tract, periamygdaloid cortex, and posterior cortical nucleus. The remaining nuclei include the anterior amygdaloid area, central nucleus, amygdalohippocampal area, and the intercalated nuclei. The location of the different amygdaloid regions is shown in Figure 2.1. A comparison of the nomenclature used here with that used in the two major atlases of the rat brain (Paxinos and Watson, 1986; Swanson, 1992) is presented in Table 2.1. Templates in Figures 2.2–2.21 were modified from the atlas of Paxinos and Watson (1986) except for the lateral view of the cerebral cortex, which was adopted from a recent review by McDonald (1998).

2.2.2 Interpretation of connectional data: methodological aspects

Data included in this review come from studies in which the amygdaloid connections were labelled by injecting anterograde or retrograde tracers into various amygdaloid nuclei or extra-amygdaloid areas. Interpretation of the existence and density of pathways based on retrospective analysis of literature is, however, subject to various errors. Therefore, it is critical to understand the methodological bias of the tracing methods used, the description of pathways, and, consequently, the data presented in this review. This is particularly important when interpreting the connectivity data presented in Figures 2.2–2.21.

It is generally acknowledged that the distribution and density of labelling depend on: (i) the size of the tracer injection; (ii) the spread of the tracer to adjacent regions; (iii) the uptake of the tracer by passing fibres (HRP and radioactive amino acids); (iv) the diameter of fibres to be labelled; and (v) the biochemical procedure used to detect the tracer. Finally, (vi) in different studies, the definition of the borders of various brain areas may differ which also complicates the interpretation of data (see discussion, for example, in MacDonald, 1998). Tracing the connections of small amygdaloid nuclei and their subdivisions provides a further challenge because it is now apparent that there is a very fine-tuned topography in the organization of afferent, efferent, and intra-amygdaloid connections in each of the amygdaloid nuclei, and even within a nuclear division. For example, a large injection of retrograde tracer (HRP, Ottersen, 1982; fluoro-gold, Jolkkonen and Pitkänen, unpublished findings) into the central nucleus labels few cells in the lateral entorhinal cortex (subfields DLE and DIE according to

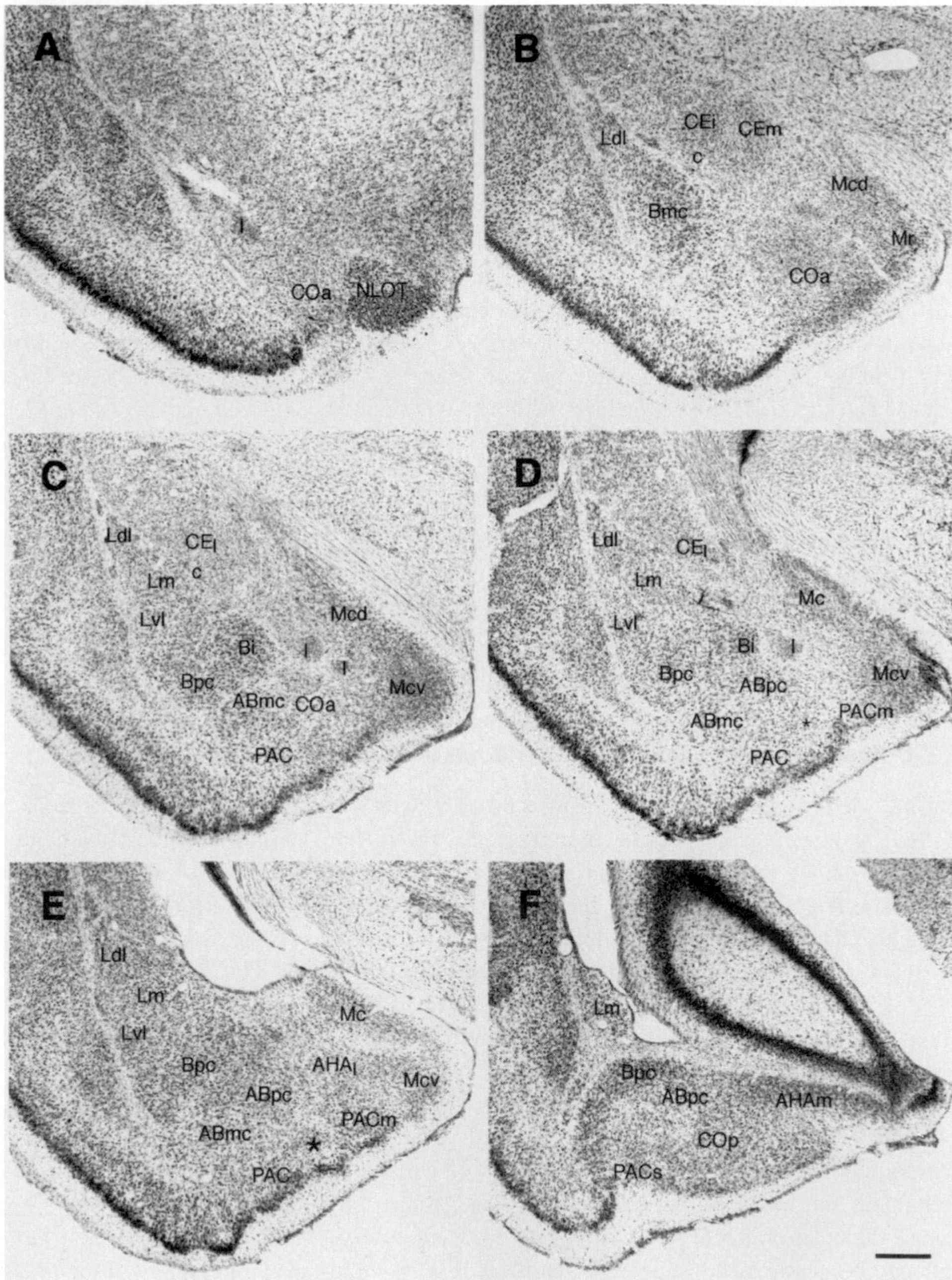

Figure 2.1 Brightfield photomicrographs from thionin-stained coronal sections of the rat amygdaloid complex showing the location of various amygdaloid nuclei and nuclear divisions. Six rostrocaudal levels are presented (A is the most rostral and F the most caudal). For abbreviations, see Table 2.1. Scale bar equals 0.5 mm.

Table 2.1 Amygdaloid nuclei and nuclear divisions: comparison with the nomenclatures that are used in the rat brain atlases of Paxinos and Watson (1986) and Swanson (1992)

	Paxinos and Watson (1986)	*Swanson (1992)*
Deep Nuclei		
lateral nucleus (L)	lateral ncl. (La)	lateral ncl. (LA) (no subdivisions)
dorsolateral division (Ldl)	dorsolateral lateral ncl. (LaDL)	
ventolateral division (Lvl)	ventrolateral lateral ncl. (LaVL)	
medial division (Lm)	ventromedial lateral ncl. (LaVM)	
basal nucleus (B)	basolateral ncl. (BL)	basolateral ncl. (BLA)
magnocellular division (Bmc)	anterior basolateral ncl. (BLA)	basolateral ncl., anterior part (BLAa)
intermediate division (Bi)	included in BLA	included in BLAa
parvicellular division (Bpc)	posterior basolateral ncl. (BLP)	basolateral ncl., posterior part (BLAp)
accessory basal nucleus (AB)	basomedial ncl. (BM)	basomedial ncl. (BMA)
magnocellular division (ABmc)	included in BMP	included in BMAp
parvicellular division (ABpc)	posterior basomedial ncl. (BMP)	basomedial ncl., posterior part (BMAp)
Superficial Nuclei		
nucleus of the lateral olfactory tract (NLOT)	nucleus of the lateral olfactory tract (LOT)	nucleus of the lateral olfactory tract (NLOT)
bed nucleus of the accessory olfactory tract (BAOT)	bed nucleus of accessory olfactory tract (BAOT)	bed nucleus acessory olfactory tract (BA)
anterior cortical nucleus (COa)	layers 1–2 = anterior cortical ncl. (ACo)	layers 1–2 = cortical ncl., anterior part (COAa)
	layer 3 = anterior basomedial ncl. (BMA)	layer 3 = basomedial ncl., anterior part (BMAa)
medial nucleus (M)	medial nucleus (Me)	medial nucleus (MEA)
rostral division (Mr)	anteroventral medial ncl. (MeAV)	medial ncl., anteroventral part (MEAav)
central division		
dorsal part (Mcd)	anterodorsal medial ncl. (MeAD)	medial ncl., anterodorsal part (MEAad)
ventral part (Mcv)	posteroventral medial ncl. (MePV)	medial ncl., posteroventral part (MEApv)
caudal division (Mc)	posterodorsal medial ncl. (MePD)	medial ncl., posterodorsal part (MEApd)

Table 2.1 continued

	Paxinos and Watson (1986)	*Swanson (1992)*
periamygdaloid cortex	cortical ncl. (Co)	cortical ncl. amygdala (COA)
periamygdaloid cortex (PAC)	posterolateral cortical ncl. (PLCo)	cortical ncl., posterior part, lateral zone (COApl)
periamygdaloid cortex, medial division (PACm)	included in PMCo	included in COApl
periamygdaloid cortex, sulcal division (PACs)	included in PLCo	included in COApl
posterior cortical nucleus (COp)	posteromedial cortical nucleus (PMCo)	cortical ncl.,posterior part, medial zone (COApm)
Other Amygdaloid Areas		
anterior amygdaloid area (AAA)	included in dorsal anterior amygdaloid area (AAD)	included in anterior amygdaloid area (AAA)
central nucleus (CE)	central nucleus (Ce)	central ncl. (CEA)
capsular division (CEc)	included in central ncl., lateral division, capsular (CeLC)	included in central ncl., capsular part (CEAc)
lateral division (CE_l)	central ncl., lateral division (CeL)	central ncl., lateral part (CEA_l)
intermediate division (CEi)	central ncl., lateral division, central (CeLCn)	included into CEA_l
medial division (CEm)	central ncl., medial division (CeM)	central ncl., medial part (CEAm)
amygdalo–hippocampal area (AHA)	amygdalohippocampal area (AHi)	
medial division (AHAm)	amygdalohippocampal area, posteromedial (AHiPM)	{ posterior nucleus amygdala (PA)
lateral division (AHA1)	amygdalohippocampal area, anterolateral (AHiAL)	{ included in COApl
intercalated nuclei (I)	intercalated nuclei (I)	intercalated nuclei (IA)

For the location of the various amygdaloid areas, see Figure 2.1.
Abbreviations: ncl. = nucleus.

the nomenclature of Insausti *et al.*, 1997). This contrasts with a recent anterograde PHA-L study by MacDonald and Mascagni (1997) which demonstrated a relatively heavy projection from this same area to the capsular division of the central nucleus. Apparently the capsular division was not involved in the injection site of the retrograde studies and, therefore, the pathway from the entorhinal cortex to the capsular division was undetected. Furthermore, evaluation of the density of projections based on the literature available is also subject to misinterpretation. For example, Ottersen plotted 10–20 retrogradely labelled HRP-positive cells per section in the perirhinal cortex following a large HRP injection into the lateral nucleus of the amygdala (case RB19, Figure 3B, Ottersen, 1982). Recently, Shi and Cassell (1999) injected fluoro-gold into the lateral nucleus and found a substantially larger number of labelled neurons per section in the perirhinal cortex. Consistent with their retrograde tracer data, injection of the anterograde tracer BDA into the corresponding level of the perirhinal cortex produced very heavy labelling in the lateral nucleus of the amygdala (Figures 18 and 4, respectively, in Shi and Cassell, 1999). Therefore, judgement of the density of a projection based only on retrograde tracer studies is difficult. On the other hand, it is often difficult to decide whether a few anterogradely labelled varicose PHA-L-positive fibres (e.g. <5 fibres per section) really represent a functionally significant projection. Finally, camera lucida drawings used to illustrate the pattern of a projection show all axons and terminals labelled throughout the thickness of a section (which might also vary), whereas photomicrographs show largely only the terminals on the surface of a section. This might result in an underestimation of the density of labelling in photomicrographs compared with camera lucida drawings.

With these caveats in mind, data from the literature used to draw the connectivity maps for each of the amygdaloid nuclei were collected separately (Figures 2.2–2.21). The bed nucleus of the accessory olfactory tract, anterior amygdaloid area, and intercalated nuclei are excluded from the description because their connectivity has not been analysed systematically in most of the studies. To shorten the description, references demonstrating a particular projection are included in Figures 2.2–2.21 and explained in Table 2.3. Only the references describing data that cannot be derived from the figures are included in the text. Also, comments on the density and topography of the projections are included in the text. Details of intra-amygdaloid connectivity and corresponding references are shown in Table 2.2. Figure 2.22 summarizes the interamygdaloid connections.

2.2.3 Lateral nucleus

Divisions and location

The lateral nucleus is located at the dorsal aspect of the amygdala, medial to the external capsule and lateral to both the central nucleus (rostrally) and the lateral ventricle (caudally) (Figure 2.1). Ventrally, the lateral nucleus borders the basal nucleus. It has three divisions: dorsolateral, ventrolateral, and medial. Stereological cell counts indicate that the lateral nucleus contains approximately 60 000 neurons (the total number of neurons in the adult rat amygdala is ~600 000), of which 24 000 are in the dorsolateral division, 14 000 in the ventrolateral division, and 22 000 in the medial division (Tuunanen and Pitkänen, 2000; Nissinen and Pitkänen, unpublished findings).

Intranuclear connections

The rostral, middle and caudal portions of the various divisions (dorsolateral, ventrolateral, and medial) of the lateral nucleus do not project to other portions in a given division. Consequently, the information entering one portion of the division does not spread along the rostrocaudal extent of the same division monosynaptically. The dorsolateral division projects to two other divisions of the lateral nucleus. The ventrolateral and medial divisions do not send any substantial projections to each other or to the dorsolateral division. Therefore, at the interdivisional level, the information flow in the lateral nucleus is largely unidirectional (Pitkänen *et al.*, 1997).

Intra-amygdaloid connections

The lateral nucleus receives moderate to heavy inputs from the basal, accessory basal, and medial nuclei as well as from the periamygdaloid cortex (Figure 2.2). Lighter projections originate in other nuclei (Table 2.2). Most of the intra-amygdaloid projections terminate in the medial and ventrolateral divisions (Table 2.2).

The lateral nucleus projects to the basal, accessory basal, central, medial, and posterior cortical nuclei as well as to the periamygdaloid cortex and the amygdalohippocampal area (Figure 2.3). These data suggest that most but not all of the intra-amygdaloid connections of the lateral nucleus are reciprocal (Figures 2.2 and 2.3, Table 2.2). Most of the intra-amygdaloid projections originate in the medial division (Table 2.2).

Interamygdaloid connections

The lateral nucleus does not receive projections from the contralateral amygdala. Also, it does not project to the contralateral amygdala (Figure 2.22).

Extra-amygdaloid inputs

Inputs from other brain areas to the lateral nucleus are summarized in Figure 2.2.

Temporal, insular and parietal cortex. The lateral nucleus receives heavy inputs from a larger number of sensory-related lateral cortical areas than any other amygdaloid nucleus. These projections originate in regions that process either gustatory, visceral, somatosensory, auditory, or visual information. Cortical inputs to the lateral nucleus are organized topographically. For example, heavy projections from the somatosensory (PV, PaRH), gustatory (DIg), or visceral (DIv) cortices terminate most heavily in the rostral portion of the lateral nucleus (dorsolateral and medial divisions), whereas auditory (Te2D, Te3) and visual (Te2) projections are directed to more caudal aspects of the same divisions (McDonald, 1998) (see Figure 2.23). Projections from the perirhinal cortex appear dense throughout the nucleus (McDonald, 1998; Shi and Cassell, 1999).

Frontal cortex. The lateral nucleus also receives projections from the prefrontal cortex, even though most of them are substantially lighter than the projections to the basal nucleus (see below). The infralimbic cortex provides a substantial input to the medial division of the lateral nucleus. Projections from the prelimbic cortex, as well as from the dorsal and ventral agranular insula, are lighter. A few anterograde tracer studies suggest that the lateral orbital cortex and the medial precentral cortex also send a very light input to the lateral nucleus.

Table 2.2 Intra-amygdaloid connections of the rat amygdaloid complex.

ORIGIN OF INPUT	AMYGDALOID AREA RECEIVING AN INPUT																															
	L	Ldl	Lvl	Lm	B	Bmc	Bi	Bpc	AB	ABmc	ABpc	NLOT	BAOT	COa	M	Mr	Mcd	Mcv	Mc	PAC	PACm	PACs	COp	AAA	CE	CEc	CEl	CEi	CEm	AHA	AHAm	AHAl	I
L	●●				●●				●●			●	○	●	●●					●●	●●	●●	●●	●	●●					●●			●
Ldl		●●	●●	●●		●	●	●●		●●	●●	●	○	○		○	●	●	○	●●	●	●	●	○		●●	●	○	●		●	●	○
Lvl		○	●●	○		○	●●	●●		●	●●	○	○	○		○	●	●	○	●	○	●	●	○		●	○	○	○		●●	●●	○
Lm		○	○	●●		●	●●	●		●●	●●	●	○	●		○	●●	●	○	●●	●●	●●	●●	●		●●	●	○	●		●	●	●
B	●●				●●				●			●●	○	●●	●					●	●	●	●	●●	●●					●●			●
Bmc		●	●●	●		●●	●●	●●		●	○	●●	○	●		●	●	○	○	●	●	●	●	●		●	●	○	●		●	●	●●
Bi		●	●	●		●	●●	●		●	●	●●	○	●		○	●	●	○	●	○	●	●	●		●	●	○	●		●	●	●
Bpc		●	●●	●		●●	●●	●●		●	●	●●	○	●●		●	●	●	○	●	●	●	●	●●		●●	●	○	●●		●●	●●	●
AB	●●				●				●●			●	●	●	●●					●●	●	●	●●	●	●●					●●			●
ABmc		●	●	●●		●	●	●		●●	●	●	●	●		●	●	●	●	●●	●	●	●	●		●●	●	○	●●		●	●	●
ABpc		●	●	●●		●	●	●		●	●●	●	●	●		●	●●	●●	●	●	●	●	●●	●		●●	●	○	●●		●●	●	●
NLOT					●●				●●					●	●					●			●		●●								
BAOT																														●●	●●		
COa	●	●	●	●	●●	●	●	●●	●	●	●	●	●	●●	●	●	●	●	●	●	●	●	●	●●	●●	●	●		●●	●	●	●	●
M	●●				●				●●			○	●●	●●	●●					●		●●	●●	●●	●●					●●			●●
Mr																																	
Mcd		○	●●	●●		○	○	●		●●	●●	○	●●	●●		●●	●●	●●	●●	●		●●	●●	●●		●●	○	○	●●		●●	●●	●●
Mcv		○	●●	●●		○	○	○		●●	●●	○	●●	●●		●●	●●	●●	●●	●		●	●●	●●		●	○	○	●		●●	●	●●
Mc		○	○	○		○	○	○		●	●	○	●	●		●●	●●	●●	●●	○		●	●●	●		●●	○	○	●		●●	●	●
PAC	●●	○	●●	●●	●							●		●	●					●●			●		●								
PACm	○	○	○	○																	●●												
PACs	○	○	○	○																		●●											
COp	○	○	○	○	○	○	○	○	●	●	○	○	●●	●	●●	●●	●●	●●	●	●	●	●●	●●	○	○	○	○	○	○	●	○	●	●
AAA									●					●											●					●	●		
CE	○				●				○			○	○	●	○					○	○	○	○	●	●●					●			○
CEc		○	○	○		○	○	●		○	○	○	○	●		○	○	○	○	○	○	○	○	●		●●	●	●	●●		○	○	○
CEl		○	○	○		○	○	●		○	○	○	○	●		○	○	○	○	○	○	○	○	●		●●	●●	●	●●		○	○	○
CEi		○	○	○		○	○	○		○	○	○	○	○		○	○	○	○	○	○	○	○	●		●	●	●●	●		○	○	○
CEm		○	○	○		○	○	●		○	○	○	○	●		○	○	○	○	○	○	○	○	●		●	●	○	●●		●	○	○
AHA	●				●				●			●	●	●	●●					●	●	●	●	●	●●					●●			●
AHAm		○	○	○		○	○	●		○	●	○	●	○		●	●●	○	○	○	○	○	●			●	○	○	○		●●	○	●
AHAl		●	●	○		○	●	●		●	●	●	●	●		●●	●●	●	●	●	●	●	●	●		●	●	○	●●		●●	●●	●●
I																																	

Symbols: ●● moderate to heavy; ● light; ○ projection investigated but not found; empty space, not known. Please note that projections originating in the NLOT, BAOT, Mr, periamygdaloid cortex, AAA or I have not been investigated by using a PHA-L method. Therefore, in these cases the symbol represents the existence of projection, not its density. Projections from one nucleus to another are labeled with grey shading. Projections between divisions are unshaded.
References describing the connections (Table 2.3): 6, 7, 8, 41, 50, 63, 64, 84, 87, 88, 106, 108, 123, 137, 140, 159, 168.

Table 2.3 Reference database for Figures 2.2–2.22 and 2.25, and Table 2.2

1. Price *et al.* 1973; **2**. Scalia and Winans 1975; **3**. de Olmos *et al.* 1978; **4**. de Olmos *et al.* 1985; **5**. Krettek and Price 1978*b*; **6**. Luskin and Price 1983*a*; **7**. Ottersen 1982; **8**. Pitkänen *et al.* 1997; **9**. Luskin and Price 1983*b*; **10**. Rönkkö and Pitkänen, unpublished; **11**. Swizer *et al.* 1985; **12**. Casselland Roberts 1991; **13**. Veening 1978*b*; **14**. Post and Mai 1978; **15**. McDonald 1998; **16**. Turner and Zimmer 1984; **17**. Yasui *et al.* 1991; **18**. Savander *et al.* 1996*a*; **19**. Sun *et al.* 1994; **20**. LeDoux *et al.* 1991; **21**. Romanski and LeDoux 1993; **22**. Mascagni *et al.* 1993; **23**. Shi and Cassell 1997; **24**. McDonald and Mascagni 1996; **25**. Shi and Cassell 1999; **26**. Wyss 1981; **27**. Swanson and Kohler 1986; **28**. Canteras and Swanson 1992; **29**. Cullinan *et al.* 1993; **30**. Van Groen and Wyss 1990*b*; **31**. Philips and LeDoux 1992; **32**. Hurley *et al.* 1991; **33**. Sesack *et al.* 1989; **34**. Brog *et al.* 1993; **35**. McDonald *et al.* 1996; **36**. Carlsen 1989; **37**. Krettek and Price 1977*a*; **38**. Fallon *et al.* 1978; **39**. Cassell and Grey 1989; **40**. McIntyre *et al.* 1996; **41**. Christensen and Frederickson 1998; **42**. Shi and Casell 1998*a*; **43**. Pikkarainen *et al.* 1999; **44**. Sarter and Markowitsch 1984; **45**. Sripanidkulchai *et al.* 1984; **46**. Cassell and Wright 1986; **47**. McDonald and Jackson 1987; **48**. Beart *et al.* 1990; **49**. Kita and Kitai 1990; **50**. Savander *et al.* 1996*b*; **51**. McDonald 1991*a*; **52**. Shinonaga *et al.* 1994; **53**. Conde *et al.* 1995; **54**. Brindley-Reed *et al.* 1995; **55**. Millhouse and Uemura-Sumi 1985; **56**. Savander *et al.* 1997*a*; **57**. Personal observation; **58**. Wallace *et al.* 1989; **59**. Kita and Oomura 1982; **60**. Levine *et al.* 1991; **61**. Cliffer *et al.* 1991; **62**. Burstein and Potrebic 1993; **63**. Canteras *et al.* 1992*a*; **64**. Canteras *et al.* 1995; **65**. Petrovich *et al.* 1996; **66**. Krettek and Price 1974; **67**. Nitecka *et al.* 1979; **68**. Ottersen and Ben-Ari 1979; **69**. LeDoux *et al.* 1985; **70**. McDonald 1987*a*; **71**. Groenewegen 1988; **72**. Cornwall and Phillipson 1988; **73**. Carlsen and Heimer 1988; **74**. Van Vulpen and Verwer 1989; **75**. Su and Bentevoglio 1990; **76**. LeDoux *et al.* 1990; **77**. Turner and Herkenham 1991; **78**. Ray and Price 1992; **79**. Ray *et al.* 1992; **80**. Moga *et al.* 1995; **81**. Namura *et al.* 1997; **82**. Linke *et al.* 1999; **83**. Kelley and Stinus 1984; **84**. Kemppainen and Pitkänen 1998; **85**. Wagner *et al.* 1995; **86**. Swanson 1976; **87**. Otterson 1980; **88**. Pitkänen *et al.* 1995; **89**. Sarter and Markowitsch 1983; **90**. Saper *et al.* 1978; **91**. Krieger *et al.* 1979; **92**. Krettek and Price 1978*a*; **93**. Ono *et al.* 1985; **94**. Newman *et al.* 1996; **95**. McDonald 1987*b*; **96**. Price *et al.* 1991; **97**. Canteras *et al.* 1992*b*; **98**. Canteras *et al.* 1994; **99**. Risold *et al.* 1994; **100**. Gray *et al.* 1989; **101**. Thompson *et al.* 1996; **102**. Prewitt and Herman 1998; **103**. Sun *et al.* 1991; **104**. Datta *et al.* 1998; **105**. Post and Mai 1980; **106**. Jolkkonen and Pitkänen 1998*a*; **107**. Cheung *et al.* 1998; **108**. Savander *et al.* 1995; **109**. Weller and Smith 1982; **110**. Russchen and Price 1984; **111**. Schmued *et al.* 1989; **112**. McDonald 1991*b*; **113**. Berendse *et al.* 1992; **114**. Wright and Groenewegen 1995; **115**. Kirouac and Ganguly 1995; **116**. Wright and Groenewegen 1996; **117**. Shammah-Lagnado *et al.* 1996; **118**. Wright *et al.* 1996; **119**. Deacon *et al.* 1983; **120**. Takagishi and Chiba 1991; **121**. Kelley *et al.* 1982; **122**. Bacon *et al.* 1996; **123**. Krettek and Price 1977*b*; **124**. Beckstead 1978; **125**. Caffe *et al.* 1987; **126**. Van Groen and Wyss 1990*a*; **127**. Phillipson and Griffits 1985; **128**. Calderazzo *et al.* 1996; **129**. McDonald and Mascagni 1997; **130**. Carlsen *et al.* 1985; **131**. Rao *et al.* 1987; **132**. Luiten *et al.* 1985; **133**. Woolf and Butcher 1982; **134**. Luiten *et al.* 1987; **135**. Grove 1988*a*; **136**. Grove 1988*b*; **137**. Nitecka *et al.* 1981*a*; **138**. Ottersen 1981; **139**. Gray 1990; **140**. Savander *et al.* 1997*b*; **141**. Danielson *et al.* 1989; **142**. Zardetto-Smith and Gray 1990; **143**. Li *et al.* 1990; **144**. Rizvi *et al.* 1991; **145**. Rosen *et al.* 1991; **146**. Vertes 1991; **147**. Wallace *et al.* 1992; **148**. Semba and Fibiger 1992; **149**. Bernard *et al.* 1993; **150**. Petrov *et al.* 1994; **151**. Petrovich and Swanson 1997; **152**. Bianchi *et al.* 1998; **153**. Peyron *et al.* 1998; **154**. Beckstead *et al.* 1979; **155**. Saper and Loewy 1980; **156**. Oades and Halliday 1987; **157**. Hallanger and Wainer 1988; **158**. Bernard *et al.* 1989*a*; **159**. Stefanacci *et al.* 1992; **160**. Krukoff *et al.* 1993; **161**. Roder and Ciriello 1993; **162.** Vertes *et al.* 1995; **163**. Shi and Cassell 1998*b*; **164**. Van Bockstaele *et al.* 1996; **165**. Pickel *et al.* 1995; **166**. Vankova *et al.* 1992; **167**. Bernard *et al.* 1989*b*; **168**. Veening 1978*a*; **169**. Takayama and Miura 1991; **170**. Alonso *et al.* 1986; **171**. Haber *et al.* 1985; **172**. Mihailoff *et al.* 1989; **173**. Riche *et al.* 1990; **174**. Nitecka *et al.* 1980; **175**. Simerly and Swanson 1986; **176**. Nitecka 1981; **177**. Behan and Haberly 1999; **178**. Jolkkonen and Pitkänen 1998*b*.

Table 2.4 Abbreviations for Figures 2.2–2.25

Abbreviation	Structure
CORTEX	
AId	Dorsal agranular insular cortex
AIp	Posterior agranular insular cortex
DIg	Gustatory dysgranular insular cortex
DIv	Visceral dysgrandular insular cortex
EC	Entorhinal cortex
GI	Granular insular cortex
Oc1	Primary occipital cortex
Oc2	Secondary occipital cortex
PaRh	Parietal rhinal cortex
PC	Piriform cortex
PRC	Perirhinal cortex
PRCd	Perirhinal cortex, dosal portion
PrCl	Lateral precentral cortex
PrCm	Medial precentral cortex
PRCv	Perirhinal cortex, ventral portion
PV	Parietal ventral area
SI	Primary somatosensory area
SII	Secondary somatosensory area
Te1	Temporal cortex, area 1
Te2	Temporal cortex, area 2
Te2D	Temporal cortex, area 2, dorsal portion
Te3	Temporal cortex, area 3
Te3R	Temporal cortex, area 3, rostral portion
FRONTAL CORTEX	
AC	Dorsal anterior cingulate cortex
AId	Dorsal agranular insular cortex
AIv	Ventral agranular insular cortex
AOB	Accessory olfactory bulb
AON	Anterior olfactory nucleus
DP	Dorsal peduncular cortex
IL	Infralimbic cortex
LO	Lateral orbital cortex
MO	Medial orbital cortex
OB	Olfactory bulb
PL	Prelimbic cortex
PrCm	Medial precentral cortex
TT	Tenia tecta
HIPPOCAMPUS AND SUBICULAR COMPLEX	
CA1	CA1 field of the hippocampus
CA2	CA2 field of the hippocampus
CA3	CA3 field of the hippocampus
DG	Dentate gyrus
EC	Entorhinal cortex
ParaS	Parasubiculum
S	Subiculum
STRIATUM AND BASAL FORBRAIN	
Acc	Nucleus accumbens
BNST	Bed nucleus of stria terminalis
Cd–Pu	Caudate–Putamen
Cl	Claustrum
EP	Endopeduncular nucleus
GP	Globus pallidus
ICa	Islands of Calleja
LS	Lateral septum
MS	Medial septum
NDB	Nucleus of the horizontal limb of the diagonal band
SI	Substantia innominata
OT	Olfactory tubercle
MIDBRAIN	
bPN	Basilar pontine nucleus
CnF	Cuneiform nucleus
CS	Nucleus centralis superior
DR	Dorsal raphe nucleus
LDTg	Laterodorsal tegmental nucleus
LiC	Nucleus linearis caudalis
LL	Lateral lemniscus
PAG	Periaqueductal grey
PPTg	Pedunculopontine tegmental nucleus
R	Raphe nucleus
VTA	Ventral tegmental area
PONS	
A8	A8 dopamine cells
LC	Locus coeruleus
PB	Parabrachial nucleus
RPC	Nucleus reticularis pontis caudalis
sC	Nucleus subcoeruleus
V	Mesencephalic nucleus of trigeminal nerve
MEDULLA	
A1	A1 noradrenaline cells
Amb	Nucleus ambiguus
C1	C1 adrenaline cells
dmX	Dorsal motonnucleus of vagus
GS	Nucleus gigantocellularis
NTS	Nucleus of the solitary tract
pGS	Nucleus paragigantocellularis
Rt	Reticular formation
VII	Facial nucleus

Table 2.4 continued

THALAMUS		HYPOTHALAMUS	
CM	Central medial nucleus	Arc	Nucleus arcuatus
Hab	Habenula	AH	Anterior hypothalamic area/nucleus
IAM	Interanteromedial nucleus	DM	Dorsomedial nucleus
IMD	Intermediodorsal nucleus	LH	Lateral hypothalamus
LP	Lateral posterior nucleus	PaV	Paraventricular nucleus
LT	Lateral terminal nucleus of the accessory optic tract	PeV	Periventricular nucleus
		PH	Posterior hypothalamic area/nucleus
MD	Mediodorsal nucleus	preM	Premamillary nucleus
MG	Medial geniculate nucleus	pFo	Perifornical area
MGm	Medial geniculate nucleus, medial part	PO	Preoptic area/nucleus
PaC	Paracentral nucleus	RCh	Retrochiasmatic area
PaV	Paraventricular nucleus	SCh	Suprachiasmatic nucleus
Pf	Parafascicular nucleus	sM	Supramamillary nucleus
PIN	Posterior intralaminar nucleus	SO	Supraoptic nucleus
PLi	Posterior limitans nucleus	TC	Tuber cinereum
PM	Posteromedian nucleus	tM	Tuberomamillary nucleus
PoM	Posterior thalamic complex, medial group	Tu	Tuberal nucleus
PP	Peripeduncular nucleus	VM	Ventromedial nucleus
PT	Paratenial nucleus		
RE	Reuniens nucleus		
Rh	Nucleus rhomboidus		
SG	Sugrageniculate nucleus		
SN	Substantia nigra		
SPf	Subparafascicular nucleus		
sTh	Nucleus subthalamicus		
VM	Ventromedial nucleus		
VP	Ventral posterior nucleus		
ZI	Zona inserta		

Hippocampal formation. The hippocampal formation is composed of the dentate gyrus, the hippocampus proper (CA3, CA2, and CA1 subfields), the subicular complex (the subiculum, presubiculum, and parasubiculum), and the entorhinal cortex (Amaral and Witter, 1989). Moderate to heavy inputs from the hippocampal formation to the lateral nucleus originate in

Figure 2.2 Cortical, subcortical, and intra-amygdaloid inputs to the lateral nucleus. In Figures 2.2, 2.4, 2.6, 2.8, 2.10, 2.12, 2.14, 2.16, 2.18, and 2.20, the region providing an input to the amygdaloid nucleus is indicated with grey shading. Shading of the abbreviation indicates that the projections originating in that area are moderate to heavy in density (according to the authors cited). The number after the abbreviation refers to the reference(s) demonstrating the existence of that particular projection. The reference database is represented in Table 2.3. Abbreviations are listed in Tables 2.1 and 2.4. Only the known moderate to heavy intra-amygdaloid inputs are indicated with arrows (for lighter projections, see Table 2.2).

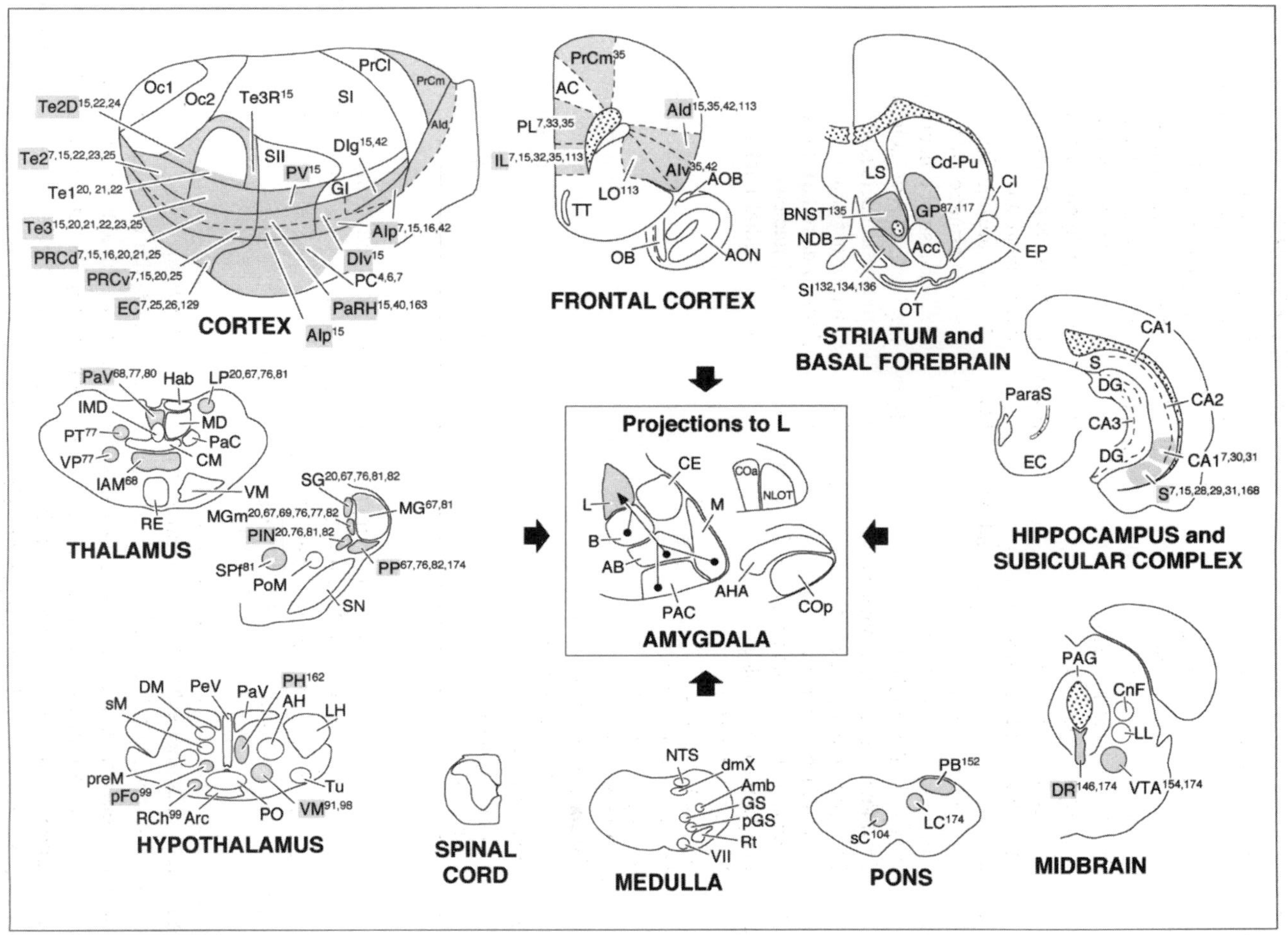
CORTEX
Oc1
Oc2
Te3R[15]
SI
PrCl
PrCm
Ald
Te2D[15,22,24]
Te2[7,15,22,23,25]
Te1[20,21,22]
Te3[15,20,21,22,23,25]
PRCd[7,15,16,20,21,25]
PRCv[7,15,20,25]
EC[7,25,26,129]
SII
PV[15]
Dlg[15,42]
GI
Alp[7,15,16,42]
Dlv[15]
PC[4,6,7]
PaRH[15,40,163]
Alp[15]
FRONTAL CORTEX
PrCm[35]
AC
PL[7,33,35]
IL[7,15,32,35,113]
Ald[15,35,42,113]
Alv[35,42]
AOB
LO[113]
TT
OB
AON
STRIATUM and BASAL FOREBRAIN
LS
Cd-Pu
Cl
BNST[135]
GP[87,117]
NDB
Acc
EP
SI[132,134,136]
OT
HIPPOCAMPUS and SUBICULAR COMPLEX
CA1
S
DG
ParaS
CA2
CA3
EC
DG
CA1[7,30,31]
S[7,15,28,29,31,168]
THALAMUS
PaV[68,77,80]
Hab
LP[20,67,76,81]
IMD
MD
PT[77]
PaC
VP[77]
CM
IAM[68]
VM
RE
SG[20,67,76,81,82]
MG[67,81]
MGm[20,67,69,76,77,82]
PIN[20,76,81,82]
PP[67,76,82,174]
SPf[81]
PoM
SN
Projections to L
CE
COa
NLOT
L
M
B
AB
AHA
PAC
COp
AMYGDALA
HYPOTHALAMUS
DM
PeV
PaV
PH[162]
sM
AH
LH
preM
pFo[99]
RCh[99]
Arc
PO
VM[91,98]
Tu
SPINAL CORD
MEDULLA
NTS
dmX
Amb
GS
pGS
Rt
VII
PONS
PB[152]
sC[104]
LC[174]
MIDBRAIN
PAG
CnF
LL
DR[146,174]
VTA[154,174]

the entorhinal cortex and subiculum. The entorhinal inputs innervate the caudal portion of the medial division most densely (McDonald and Mascagni, 1997). The proximal portion (closest to the CA1 subfield) of the ventral subiculum also provides a heavy input to the medial division of the lateral nucleus (Cullinan *et al.*, 1993). The projection from the CA1 subfield of the hippocampus is light.

Olfactory system. There is some evidence that the lateral nucleus receives a light input from the olfactory cortex, which originates in the ventromedial aspect of the piriform cortex.

Thalamus. The midline and posterior thalamic nuclei provide substantial, topographically organized inputs to the lateral nucleus. The moderate projection from the paraventricular nucleus terminates in the medial and ventrolateral divisions. The paratenial nucleus projects to the medial division. Other midline nuclei that project to the lateral nucleus include the interanteromedial and rhomboid nuclei, but in these latter cases the injection of retrograde tracer into the lateral nucleus might have also involved the basal nucleus (see Figure 13d in Ottersen and Ben-Ari, 1979). More posteriorly, the posterior intralaminar nucleus provides a heavy input to all divisions of the lateral nucleus. The projection from the medial division of the medial geniculate nucleus terminates most heavily in the dorsolateral and ventrolateral divisions of the lateral nucleus. The ventral posterior nucleus projects to the dorsolateral division. In addition, the lateral nucleus receives inputs from the lateral posterior, suprageniculate, and subparafascicular nuclei, as well as from the dorsal aspects of the medial geniculate nucleus.

Hypothalamus. The ventrolateral division of the lateral nucleus receives a substantial input from the ventromedial hypothalamic nucleus. Also, the perifornical area and posterior hypothalamic nucleus provide significant inputs to the lateral nucleus. The projection from the retrochiasmatic area is lighter.

Basal forebrain, striatum, and bed nucleus of the stria terminalis. Both anterograde and retrograde tracer studies indicate that the caudal ventral globus pallidus projects lightly to the lateral nucleus. Another projection originates in the substantia innominata and appears to terminate most heavily in the ventrolateral division. Grove (1988a) reported a light projection from the bed nucleus of the stria terminalis to the lateral nucleus.

Midbrain, pons, and medulla. The lateral nucleus receives a few projections from the tegmentum and more caudal brain areas. These projections originate in the peripeduncular nucleus and ventral tegmental area. The rostral portion of the dorsal raphe provides a heavy input to the lateral nucleus. More caudally, the parabrachial nucleus projects to the medial aspect of the lateral nucleus. Also, the locus coeruleus and nucleus subcoeruleus project to the lateral nucleus.

Figure 2.3 Cortical, subcortical, and intra-amygdaloid outputs of the lateral nucleus. In Figures 2.3, 2.5, 2.7, 2.9, 2.11, 2.13, 2.15, 2.17, 2.19, and 2.21, the region receiving an input from the amygdaloid nucleus is indicated with grey shading. Shading of the abbreviation indicates that the projections terminating in that area are moderate to heavy in density (according to the authors cited). The number after the abbreviation refers to the reference(s) demonstrating the existence of that particular projection. The reference database is represented in Table 2.3. Abbreviations are listed in Tables 2.1 and 2.4. Only the known moderate to heavy intra-amygdaloid outputs are indicated with arrows (for lighter projections, see Table 2.2).

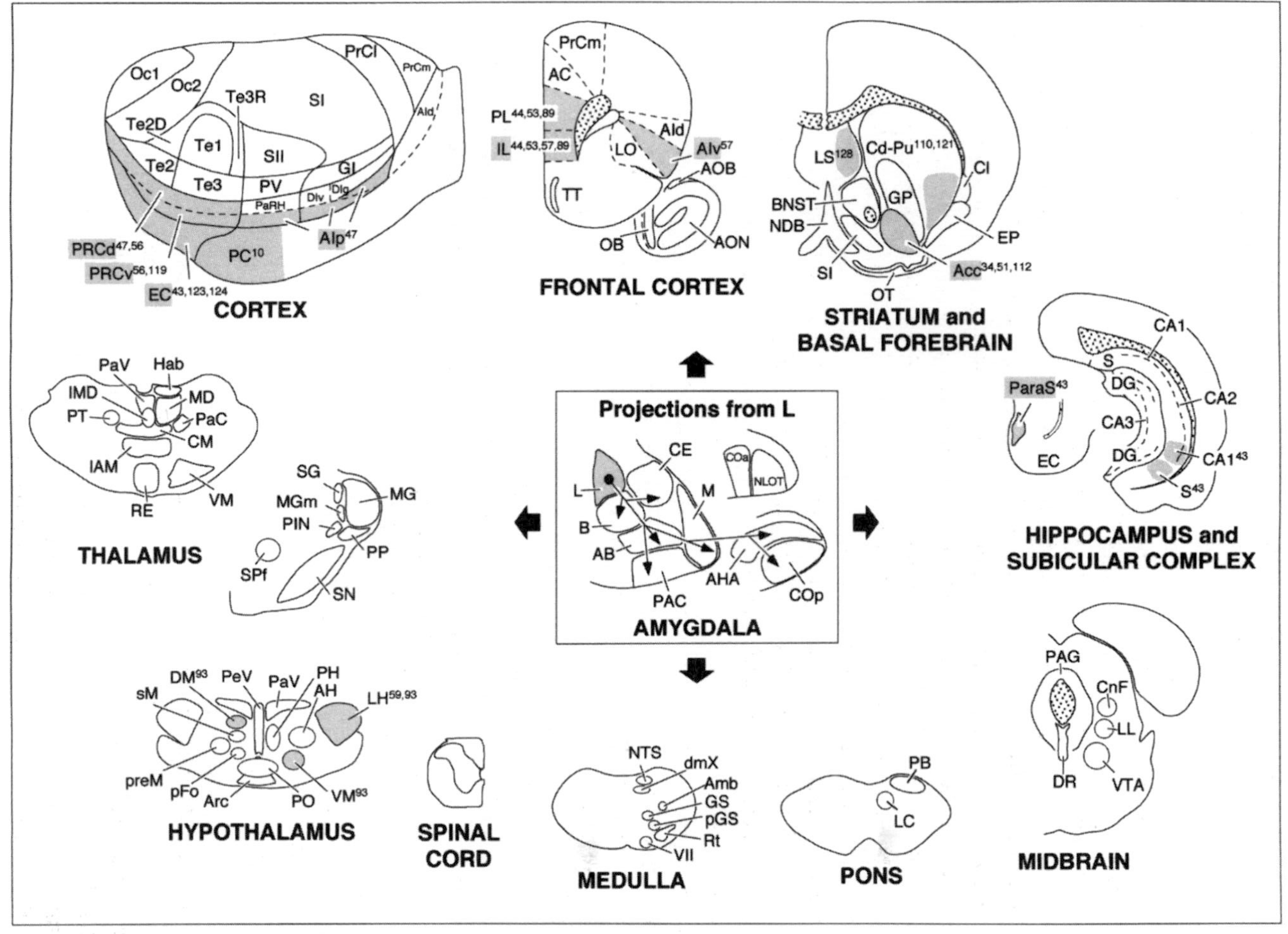

CORTEX
Oc1
Oc2
Te3R
SI
PrCl
PrCm
Ald
Te2D
Te1
SII
Te2
Te3
PV
GI
PaRH
Dlv
Dlg
PRCd[47,56]
PRCv[56,119]
EC[43,123,124]
PC[10]
Alp[47]
FRONTAL CORTEX
PrCm
AC
PL[44,53,89]
IL[44,53,57,89]
Ald
LO
Alv[57]
AOB
TT
OB
AON
STRIATUM and BASAL FOREBRAIN
LS[128]
Cd-Pu[110,121]
Cl
BNST
GP
NDB
EP
SI
OT
Acc[34,51,112]
HIPPOCAMPUS and SUBICULAR COMPLEX
CA1
S
DG
ParaS[43]
CA2
CA3
EC
DG
CA1[43]
S[43]
THALAMUS
PaV
Hab
IMD
MD
PT
PaC
CM
IAM
RE
VM
SG
MGm
MG
PIN
PP
SPf
SN
Projections from L
AMYGDALA
CE
COa
NLOT
L
M
B
AB
AHA
PAC
COp
HYPOTHALAMUS
DM[93]
PeV
PaV
PH
AH
sM
LH[59,93]
preM
pFo
Arc
PO
VM[93]
SPINAL CORD
MEDULLA
NTS
dmX
Amb
GS
pGS
Rt
VII
PONS
PB
LC
MIDBRAIN
PAG
CnF
LL
DR
VTA

Extra-amygdaloid outputs

Cortical and subcortical outputs of the lateral nucleus are summarized in Figure 2.3.

Temporal, insular, and parietal cortex. The spectrum of projections from the lateral nucleus to the cerebral cortex is not as widespread as the number of projections from the cortex to the lateral nucleus (compare Figures 2.2 and 2.3). Based on anterograde tracer studies, the lateral nucleus provides topographically organized heavy inputs to the ventral and dorsal perirhinal cortices. A retrograde tracer study by McDonald and Jackson (1987) shows that the posterior agranular insula also receives input from the lateral nucleus, which is consistent with our observations based on PHA-L injections into the lateral nucleus (unpublished findings).

Frontal cortex. Injections of retrograde tracers into the infralimbic or prelimbic cortex result in neuronal labelling in the lateral nucleus. An anterograde PHA-L tracer study indicated that the rostral portion of the medial division of the lateral nucleus provides a moderate input to the infralimbic cortex as well as to the ventral agranular insula (unpublished findings).

Hippocampal formation. The lateral nucleus also provides direct inputs to the hippocampal formation. The medial division projects heavily to the entorhinal cortex (VIE and DIE subfields; the entorhinal cortex is partitioned according to Insausti *et al.*, 1997). There are light projections to the ventral CA1 and subiculum. The projection to the parasubiculum is heavy, particularly from the caudal portion of the medial division.

Olfactory system. The projection from the lateral nucleus to the olfactory system is meagre and includes only a light projection from the rostral part of the medial division to the caudomedial piriform cortex (Rönkkö and Pitkänen, unpublished findings).

Hypothalamus. Projections from the lateral nucleus to the hypothalamus are light. Retrograde tracer studies suggest that the ventrolateral part of the lateral nucleus projects to the lateral hypothalamic area. The lateral nucleus provides only light projections to the ventromedial and dorsomedial hypothalamic nuclei.

Basal forebrain, striatum, and bed nucleus of the stria terminalis. Retrograde tracer studies indicate that the lateral nucleus provides a substantial input to the nucleus accumbens, particularly to the lateral part of the shell region. Most of the retrogradely labelled neurons were located in the rostral aspect of the medial division of the lateral nucleus (McDonald, 1991b). The lateral nucleus has been reported to project sparsely to the caudoventral aspect of the caudoputamen, and also to the lateral septum.

To summarize, the lateral nucleus receives substantial inputs from the other amygdaloid nuclei, sensory-related lateral cortical areas, prefrontal cortex, hippocampal formation, some midline and posterior thalamic nuclei, and the hypothalamus. The lateral nucleus provides substantial projections to the other amygdaloid nuclei, medial temporal lobe memory system (hippocampal formation and perirhinal cortex), and prefrontal cortex.

2.2.4 Basal nucleus

Divisions and location

The basal nucleus has three divisions: magnocellular, intermediate, and parvicellular. The most rostral part of the basal nucleus, the magnocellular division, is located rostral to the lateral nucleus, medial to the external capsule, and lateral to the central nucleus (Figure 2.1). More caudally, when the intermediate and parvicellular divisions appear, the basal nucleus is located ventral to the lateral nucleus and dorsal to the accessory basal nucleus. Caudally, it is lateral to the lateral ventricle. Stereological cell counts indicate that the entire basal nucleus contains approximately 47 000 neurons, of which 8000 are in the magnocellular division, 7000 are in the intermediate division, and 32 000 are in the medial division (Tuunanen and Pitkänen, 2000).

Intranuclear connections

Unlike the lateral nucleus, each division of the basal nucleus has dense intradivisional projections throughout its rostrocaudal extent. Exceptions include the medial and lateral portions of the parvicellular division, which are not heavily interconnected. Most of the interdivisional connections originate in the parvicellular division. Importantly, the lateral and medial parts of the parvicellular division, which are separated connectionally from each other, project to the intermediate division of the basal nucleus where the inputs converge. Unlike the lateral nucleus, where there are no major reciprocal connections between the nuclear divisions, the magnocellular division of the basal nucleus sends a projection back to the lateral part of the parvicellular division (Table 2.2).

Intra-amygdaloid connections

Based on anterograde tracer studies, the heaviest intra-amygdaloid input to the basal nucleus originates in the lateral and anterior cortical nuclei (Figure 2.4). Lighter projections originate from most of the other amygdaloid nuclei (Table 2.2). Most of the afferent intra-amygdaloid projections terminate in the parvicellular division (Table 2.2).

The basal nucleus projects to the lateral, anterior cortical, and central nuclei as well as to the nucleus of the olfactory tract and the amygdalohippocampal area (Figure 2.5, Table 2.2). Most of the intra-amygdaloid projections originate in the parvicellular division (Table 2.2).

Interamygdaloid connections

The basal nucleus receives a projection from the contralateral basal nucleus. The basal nucleus provides substantial projections to the contralateral amygdala, which terminate in the basal nucleus, central nucleus, nucleus of the lateral olfactory tract, and also in the anterior amygdaloid area (Figure 2.22).

Extra-amygdaloid inputs

Cortical and subcortical inputs to the basal nucleus are summarized in Figure 2.4.

Temporal, insular, and parietal cortex. Cortical inputs to the basal nucleus originate largely in the same regions as projections to the lateral nucleus. Generally, however, their density is lighter. Based on anterograde tracer studies, the basal nucleus receives moderate to heavy inputs from the gustatory (DIg and AIp), visceral (DIv), and somatosensory (PaRH) areas. Projections from the somatosensory areas (SII, PV, PaRH, caudal AIp) innervate the lateral aspect more heavily than the medial aspect of the parvicellular or magnocellular divisions of the basal nucleus (McDonald, 1998). Projections from the auditory and visual cortices are substantially lighter and directed to the magnocellular division. The rostral part of the ventral bank of the perirhinal cortex provides a substantial input to the basal nucleus.

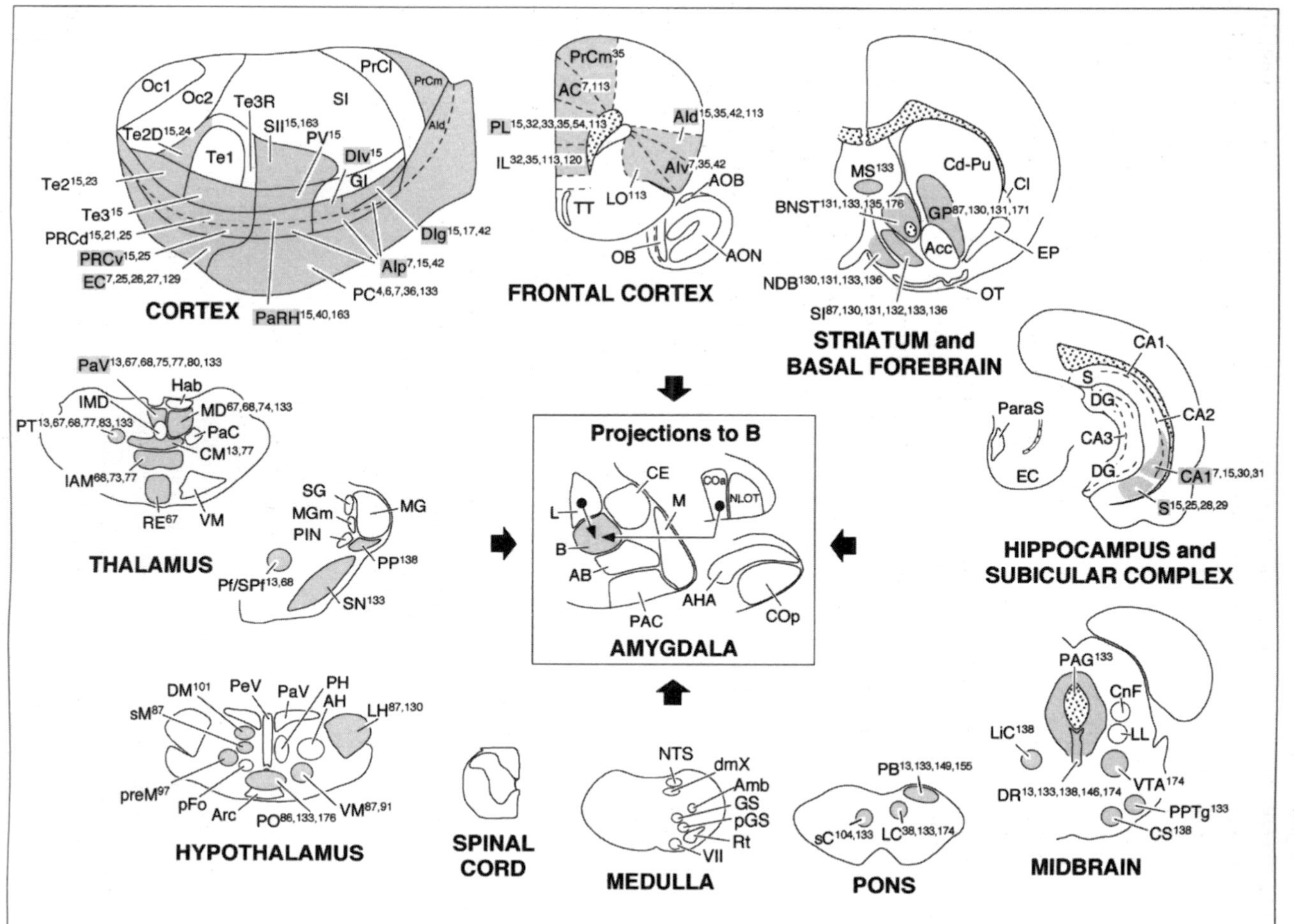

Figure 2.4 Cortical, subcortical, and intra-amygdaloid inputs of the basal nucleus. See legend to Figure 2.2.

Projections from the perirhinal cortex terminate in both the magnocellular and parvicellular divisions (Shi and Cassell, 1999).

Frontal cortex. The medial aspect of the prefrontal cortex provides substantial inputs to the basal nucleus. In most studies, projection from the prelimbic cortex appears heavier than that from the infralimbic cortex. The projection from the prelimbic area innervates the medial aspect of the magnocellular division of the basal nucleus most heavily (McDonald, 1998). Projections from the more dorsally located medial precentral cortex (PrCm) and dorsal anterior cingulate cortex (AC) are lighter. In the lateral prefrontal cortex, the dorsal agranular insula (AId) has a moderate input to the lateral aspects of the magnocellular division and to the lateral portion of the parvicellular division of the basal nucleus. The projection from the ventral agranular insula (AIv) is lighter.

Hippocampal formation. The basal nucleus is the major target for inputs from the hippocampal formation to the amygdaloid complex. Moderate to heavy projections from the entorhinal cortex terminate in the parvicellular division either medially or laterally depending on the location of the injection site in the entorhinal cortex (McDonald and Mascagni, 1996). A PHA-L study by Canteras and Swanson (1992) shows that the projection from the distal (medial) temporal subiculum to the basal nucleus is light and involves only the most caudal portion of the parvicellular division. Cullinan *et al.* (1993) and McDonald (1998), however, found a moderate projection from the proximal (lateral) temporal subiculum to the medial aspect of the basal nucleus, which apparently corresponds to the intermediate division of the basal nucleus or the medial portion of the rostral parvicellular division of the basal nucleus (Figure 3B in Cullinan *et al.*, 1993; Figure 33B in McDonald, 1998). The CA1 subfield of the hippocampus proper that is adjacent to the ventral temporal subiculum also sends a moderate projection to the same region as the proximal part of the subiculum (Figure 34 in McDonald, 1998).

Olfactory system. Retrograde tracer studies suggest that the basal nucleus receives a light olfactory input from the medial aspect of the piriform cortex.

Thalamus. The basal nucleus receives substantial, topographically organized inputs from the midline thalamus. The paraventricular nucleus provides a moderate input to the parvicellular division. The paratenial, centromedial, and interanteromedial nuclei project to the magnocellular division. The reuniens, subparafascicular, parafascicular, and mediodorsal thalamic nuclei also project to the basal nucleus. Some retrograde studies suggest that the medial division of the medial geniculate nucleus might also project to the basal nucleus. This has, however, not been confirmed in more recent anterograde and retrograde tracer studies (LeDoux *et al.*, 1990; Turner and Herkenham, 1991).

Hypothalamus. In general, the hypothalamic inputs to the basal nucleus are light. They originate in the lateral preoptic area, ventromedial nucleus, dorsomedial nucleus, lateral hypothalamic area, premamillary, and supramamillary nuclei.

Basal forebrain, striatum, and bed nucleus of the stria terminalis. Projections from the striatum to the basal nucleus are substantially lighter than the reciprocal projections from the basal nucleus to the striatum. They originate in the ventral globus pallidus. The basal nucleus also receives inputs from the substantia innominata and horizontal limb of the nucleus of the diagonal band. The medial septum and the bed nucleus of the stria terminalis project lightly to the basal nucleus.

Midbrain, pons, and medulla. The basal nucleus receives light projections from the midbrain and pons. These originate in the peripeduncular nucleus, periaqueductal grey, ventral tegmental area, pedunculopontine tegmental nucleus, nucleus centralis superior, and nucleus linearis caudalis. Other projections come from the substantia nigra, dorsal raphe, and locus coeruleus, which provide dopaminergic, serotonergic, and noradrenergic innervation, respectively. The projection from the parabrachial nucleus terminates most heavily in the caudal portion of the parvicellular division. In addition, evidence based on an anterograde tracer study suggests that the cuneiform nucleus provides a light input to the basal nucleus (Hallanger and Wainer, 1988).

Extra-amygdaloid outputs

Projections from the basal nucleus to other brain areas are summarized in Figure 2.5.

Temporal, insular, and parietal cortex. Projections from the basal nucleus to the sensory-related lateral cortical areas are not as widespread as the inputs. Anterograde tracing with HRP demonstrated a substantial projection from the magnocellular division to the posterior agranular insula. Anterograde and retrograde studies suggest that the basal nucleus also projects lightly to the perirhinal cortex.

Frontal cortex. Projections from the basal nucleus to the frontal cortex are more widespread than from any other amygdaloid nucleus. Injections of retrograde tracers into the medial prefrontal cortex label a large number of neurons in the medial aspects of the magnocellular and parvicellular divisions of the basal nucleus, whereas tracer injections into the lateral prefrontal cortex label neurons located more rostrally and laterally. Based on the anterograde tracer data available, the heaviest projection originates in the parvicellular division of the basal nucleus and terminates in the infralimbic cortex. The basal nucleus also projects to the prelimbic cortex and anterior cingulate, as well as to the medial and lateral divisions of the precentral cortex. Injections of retrograde tracers into the somatosensory cortex label only a very few neurons in the basal nucleus (Ray and Price, 1992). The basal nucleus also projects to the ventral and lateral aspects of the frontal cortex, including the medial and lateral orbital cortices, and the agranular insula.

Hippocampal formation. The basal nucleus provides the most widespread amygdaloid projections to the hippocampal formation. Studies using PHA-L as an anterograde tracer show that the medial aspect of the parvicellular division projects moderately or heavily to the entorhinal cortex (subfields AE and VIE). The basal nucleus also provides moderate to heavy inputs to the CA3 and CA1 subfields of the temporal end of the hippocampus, the temporal subiculum, as well as to the parasubiculum. Like the projections to the entorhinal cortex, the heaviest projections originate in the medial portion of the parvicellular division (Pikkarainen *et al.*, 1999). The CA2 subfield also receives a light input from the basal nucleus.

Olfactory system. The projection from the basal nucleus to the olfactory system involves a substantial projection to the olfactory tubercle and light inputs to the caudomedial aspects of the piriform cortex and endopeduncular nucleus. A retrograde tracer injection into the tenia tecta labels very few neurons in the basal nucleus (Cassel and Wright, 1986).

Thalamus. Both the magnocellular and parvicellular divisions of the basal nucleus provide substantial topographically organized inputs to the mediodorsal thalamic nucleus.

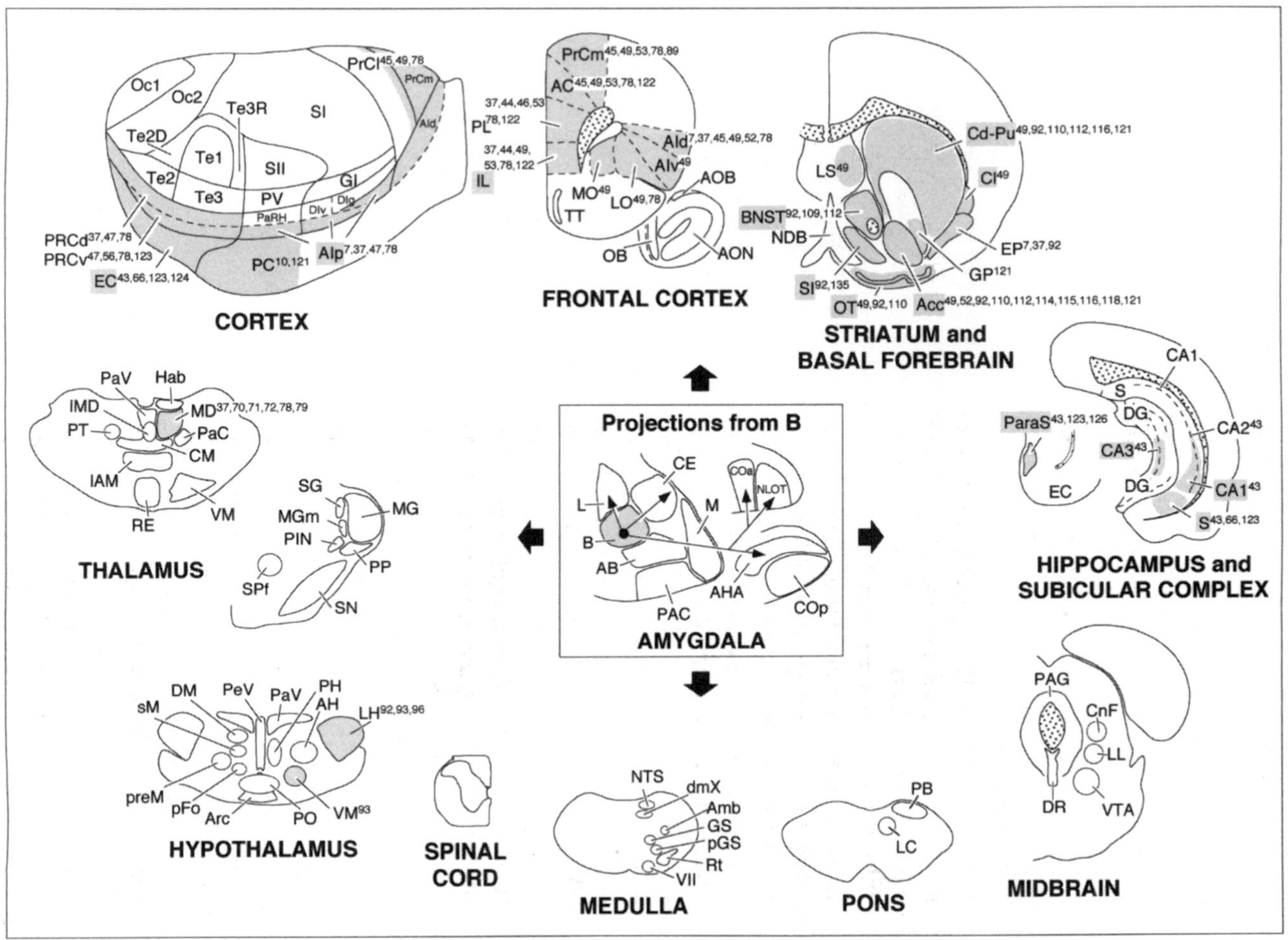

Figure 2.5 Cortical, subcortical, and intra-amygdaloid outputs of the basal nucleus. See legend to Figure 2.3.

Hypothalamus. A few projections from the basal nucleus to the hypothalamus terminate in the lateral hypothalamic area and ventromedial nucleus.

Basal forebrain, striatum, and bed nucleus of the stria terminalis. The basal nucleus is the major source of amygdaloid inputs to the nucleus accumbens and caudate–putamen. Projections originating in the parvicellular division terminate in the rostromedial accumbens, particularly in the shell and in the patches of the medial core region. The projection from the rostral magnocellular division terminates more laterally in the patches of the core compartment. The more caudal magnocellular division appears to project to the patches of the more medially located core region (Wright *et al.*, 1996). Also, the projections to the caudate–putamen are heavy and topographically organized: the magnocellular division projects caudolaterally and the parvicellular division projects rostromedially. A lighter input that terminates in the caudal globus pallidus was also described. The substantia innominata, claustrum, and bed nucleus of the stria terminalis also receive a heavy input from the basal nucleus.

To summarize, the most substantial inputs to the basal nucleus originate in the sensory-related lateral cortical areas, medial and lateral prefrontal cortex, and the hippocampal formation. The basal nucleus provides substantial projections to the medial prefrontal cortex, hippocampal formation, bed nucleus of stria terminalis, substantia innominata, nucleus accumbens, and caudate–putamen.

2.2.5 Accessory basal nucleus

Divisions and location

The accessory basal nucleus has two divisions: magnocellular and parvicellular. The accessory basal nucleus begins caudal to the 'oval-shaped' layer 3 of the anterior cortical nucleus that is called the 'anterior basomedial nucleus' in many descriptions (Table 2.1). The accessory basal nucleus borders the basal nucleus dorsally and the periamygdaloid cortex ventrally. At caudal levels, it is located dorsal to the lateral division of the amygdalohippocampal area (Figure 2.1). Stereological cell counts indicate that the accessory basal nucleus contains approximately 30 000 neurons (Tuunanen and Pitkänen, 2000).

Intranuclear connections

In the accessory basal nucleus, the magnocellular and parvicellular divisions have substantial intradivisional projections. In contrast, the projections between the divisions are meagre, which suggests that one division remains independent of the information entering the other division (Table 2.2).

Intra-amygdaloid connections

The heaviest intra-amygdaloid inputs to the accessory basal nucleus originate in the lateral nucleus and the medial nucleus. In addition, the accessory basal nucleus receives lighter inputs from the anterior cortical nucleus, posterior cortical nucleus, basal nucleus, and the amygdalohippocampal area. Both of the divisions receive heavy intra-amygdaloid inputs (Table 2.2).

The accessory basal nucleus provides substantial intra-amygdaloid inputs to the lateral nucleus, medial nucleus, periamygdaloid cortex, central nucleus, posterior cortical nucleus, and the amygdalohippocampal area. The parvicellular division appears to provide slightly more moderate to heavy intra-amygdaloid projections than does the magnocellular division (Table 2.2).

Interamygdaloid connections

The accessory basal nucleus receives an input from the contralateral accessory basal nucleus. In addition, it projects to the contralateral medial nucleus (Figure 2.22).

Extra-amygdaloid inputs

Cortical and subcortical inputs to the accessory basal nucleus are summarized in Figure 2.6.

Temporal, insular, and parietal cortex. The accessory basal nucleus receives fewer inputs from the sensory-related lateral cortical areas than the lateral or basal nuclei. Moderate to heavy inputs originate in the rostral part of the posterior agranular insula (AIp), the parietal rhinal area (PaRH), and the dorsal bank of the rostral perirhinal cortex. Lighter inputs originate in the gustatory and visceral dysgranular insula (DI), and the ventral bank of the perirhinal cortex.

Frontal cortex. Several PHA-L studies demonstrate a heavy projection from the infralimbic cortex to the accessory basal nucleus. The projection terminates most heavily in the magnocellular division. There are light projections from the prelimbic cortex and ventral agranular insula (AIv) to the accessory basal nucleus (McDonald, 1998).

Hippocampal formation. The accessory basal nucleus receives substantial inputs from the hippocampal formation. These pathways include a moderate projection from the entorhinal cortex to the parvicellular division. Both the proximal and distal aspects of the temporal subiculum provide substantial projections to the magnocellular and parvicellular divisions. There is a light projection from the temporal CA1 subfield of the hippocampus to the accessory basal nucleus.

Olfactory system. Recently, McDonald (1998) described a robust olfactory projection to the accessory basal nucleus in cases where the PHA-L injection involved both the piriform cortex and the endopiriform nucleus. According to a recent anterograde study of Behan and Haberly (1999), the contribution of the endopiriform nucleus to this projection appears meagre. Other studies using retrograde (HRP) or anterograde (radiolabelled amino acids) tracers also indicated that the piriform cortex projects to the accessory basal nucleus.

Thalamus. Injection of retrograde tracers into the accesory basal nucleus produces labelling both in the midline (paraventricular and paratenial nuclei; Ottersen and Ben-Ari, 1979) and posterior thalamic nuclei (LeDoux *et al.*, 1990). Anterograde tracer studies by Turner and Herkenham (1991) and Moga *et al.* (1995) confirmed that the paraventricular nucleus projects to the accessory basal nucleus. A PHA-L study by Turner and Herkenham (1991) suggested that the medial division of the medial geniculate also projects to the accessory basal nucleus. The anterograde labelling appeared rather rostrally, however, and might have also terminated in layer 3 of the anterior cortical nucleus. Furthermore, after injecting retrograde tracers into the accessory basal nucleus, LeDoux *et al.* (1991) did not find any labelled neurons in the medial division of the medial geniculate. They did, however, observe retrogradely labelled neurons in the medial group of the posterior thalamic complex that might have been included in the injection site in the anterograde tracer studies. Also, the subparafascicular nucleus was reported to project to the accessory basal nucleus.

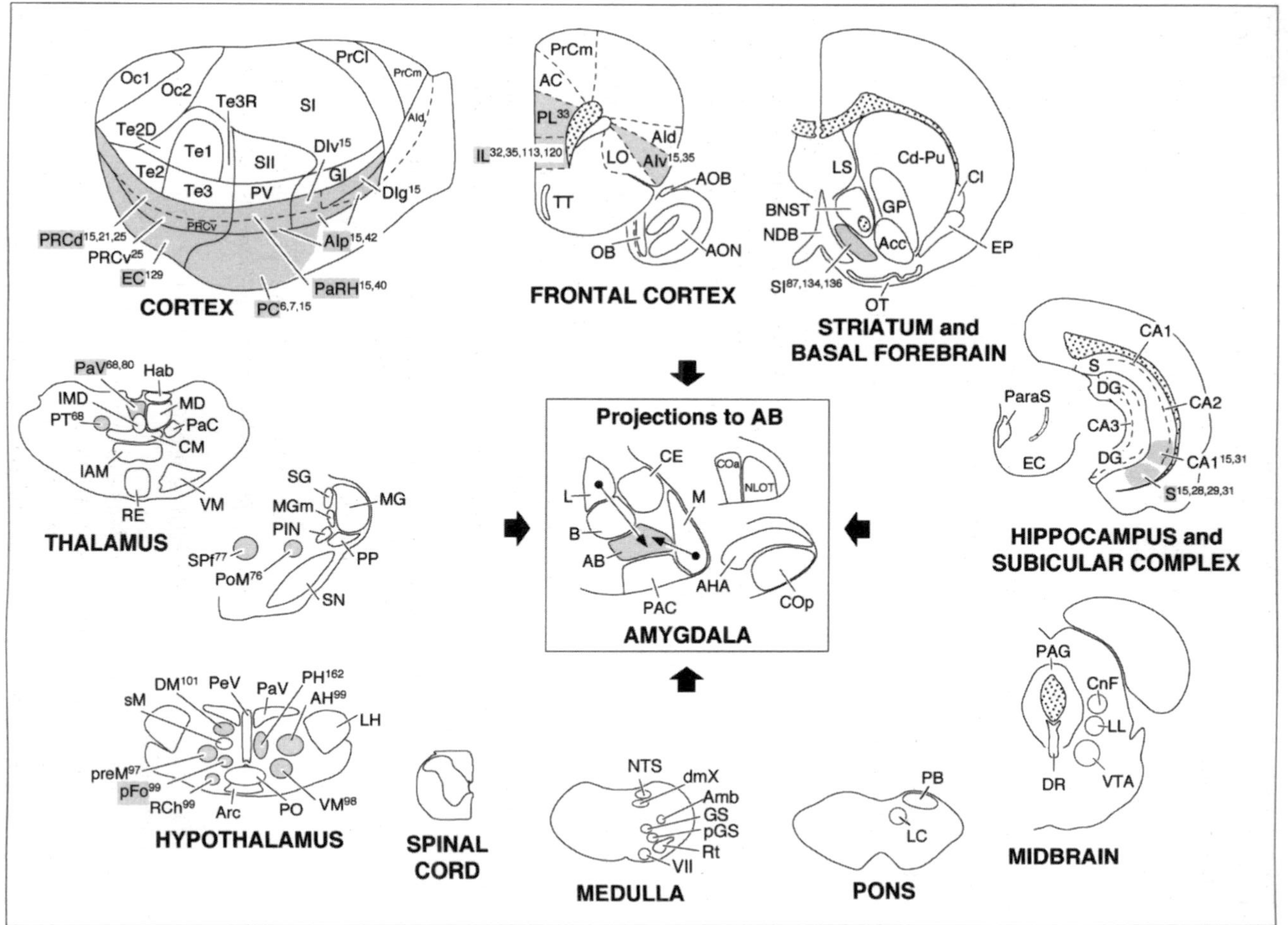

Figure 2.6 Cortical, subcortical, and intra-amygdaloid inputs of the accessory basal nucleus. See legend to Figure 2.2.

Hypothalamus. Most of the projections from the hypothalamus to the accessory basal nucleus are light. These include inputs from the ventromedial nucleus, dorsomedial nucleus, premamillary nucleus, and posterior hypothalamic nucleus. Projections from the perifornical area and also from the retrochiasmatic area are heavier than the projection from the anterior hypothalamic nucleus.

Basal forebrain, striatum, and bed nucleus of the stria terminalis. The substantia innominata projects to the accessory basal nucleus. Other projections from the basal forebrain are meagre.

Midbrain, pons, and medulla. Projections from the midbrain and pons to the accessory basal nucleus are meagre. Saper and Loewy (1980) reported labelling in the 'anterior basomedial nucleus' after injecting radioactive amino acids into the parabrachial nucleus. In their illustrations, however, the labelled area appears to correspond to layer 3 of the anterior cortical nucleus. Similar results were reported by Bernard *et al.* (1993).

Extra-amygdaloid outputs

Cortical and subcortical projections from the accessory basal nucleus are summarized in Figure 2.7.

Temporal, insular, and parietal cortex. The accessory basal nucleus provides a substantial input throughout the rostrocaudal extent of the perirhinal cortex. Other projections to the sensory-related lateral cortical areas are light. These include pathways to the visceral dysgranular insula (DI), somatosensory parietal ventral (PV), and parietal rhinal (PaRH) cortices, the auditory (Te3) and visual (Te2) regions, and also the posterior agranular insula (AIp).

Frontal cortex. The infralimbic cortex receives a moderate input from the accessory basal nucleus, whereas the projections to other regions (PL, AId, and AIv) of the prefrontal cortex are light. One retrograde study suggested that the rostral anterior cingulate cortex (AC) and medial precentral cortex (PrCm) might also receive a light input from the accessory basal nucleus (Conde *et al.*, 1995). These observations, however, have not been confirmed by anterograde tracer studies.

Hippocampal formation. The parvicellular division of the accessory basal nucleus provides moderate inputs to various levels of the hippocampal formation. These include projections to the entorhinal cortex (VIE subfield), temporal aspects of the CA1 subfield and subiculum, and to the parasubiculum.

Olfactory system. Light projections directed to the olfactory system terminate in the anterior olfactory nucleus, olfactory tubercle, and in the caudomedial aspect of the piriform cortex.

Thalamus. The accessory basal nucleus projects lightly to the paraventricular and mediodorsal nuclei of the thalamus.

Hypothalamus. The accessory basal nucleus provides a substantial input to the ventromedial nucleus of the hypothalamus. Lighter projections are directed to several other hypothalamic areas including the medial preoptic area, retrochiasmatic area, anterior hypothalamic area, lateral hypothalamic area, tuberal nucleus, paraventricular nucleus, and dorsomedial nucleus. Labelled terminals were also observed in the premamillary, supramamillary, medial mamillary nuclei, and posterior hypothalamic nucleus.

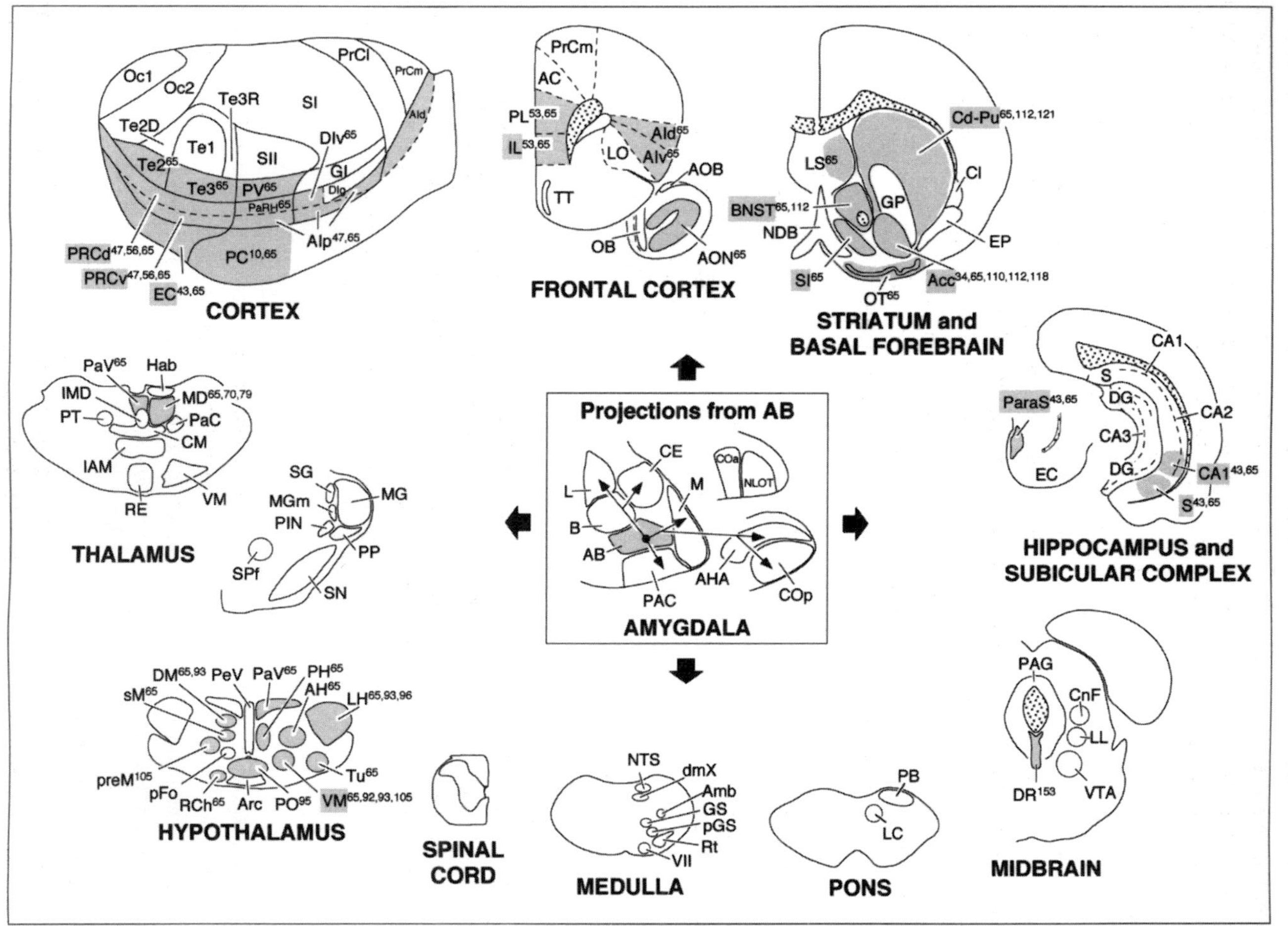

Figure 2.7 Cortical, subcortical, and intra-amygdaloid outputs of the accessory basal nucleus. See legend to Figure 2.3.

Basal forebrain, striatum, and bed nucleus of the stria terminalis. Projections from the accessory basal nucleus to the basal forebrain and striatum are rather extensive, but generally lighter than those originating in the basal nucleus. Moderate to heavy projections terminate in the substantia innominata as well as in the caudate–putamen and shell and core (matrix) compartments of the nucleus accumbens. Also, the bed nucleus of the stria terminalis receives a substantial input from the accessory basal nucleus. The projection to the lateral septum is light.

Midbrain, pons, and medulla. Peyron *et al.* (1998) found very few retrogradely labelled cells in the accessory basal nucleus after injecting choleratoxin B into the dorsal raphe.

To summarize, the heaviest inputs to the accessory basal nucleus originate in the lateral sensory-related cortical areas, hippocampal formation, medial prefrontal cortex, and in some thalamic and hypothalamic nuclei. The accessory basal nucleus provides moderate to heavy inputs to several other amygdaloid nuclei, the sensory-related lateral cortical areas, medial prefrontal cortex, hippocampal formation, hypothalamus, bed nucleus of stria terminalis, substantia innominata, nucleus accumbens, and caudate–putamen.

2.2.6 Central nucleus

Divisions and location

The central nucleus has four divisions: capsular, lateral, intermediate, and medial. It is located at the dorsomedial aspect of the rostral half of the amygdala. It is medial to the lateral and basal nuclei and lateral to the stria terminalis. Caudally, the central nucleus ends when the lateral ventricle appears (Figure 2.1).

Intranuclear connections

Within the central nucleus, each division (except the intermediate division) gives rise to topographically organized intradivisional and interdivisional projections (Table 2.2). Most of these intranuclear connections originate in the lateral and capsular divisions. The lateral division innervates both the capsular and medial divisions. The capsular division projects to the medial division, which sends a light projection back to the capsular division. The lateral division does not receive inputs from other divisions of the central nucleus.

Intra-amygdaloid connections

The central nucleus receives moderate to heavy inputs from the lateral, basal, accessory basal, medial, and anterior cortical nuclei (Figure 2.8). These projections terminate in the capsular and medial divisions (Table 2.2). The few intra-amygdaloid projections originating in the central nucleus are light (Figure 2.9, Table 2.2).

Interamygdaloid connections

The central nucleus receives an input from the contralateral anterior cortical nucleus, the nucleus of the lateral olfactory tract, and the basal nucleus. The central nucleus does not project to the contralateral amygdala (Figure 2.22).

Extra-amygdaloid inputs

Cortical and subcortical inputs directed to the central nucleus are summarized in Figure 2.8.

Temporal, insular, and parietal cortex. Large retrograde injections into the central nucleus often provide relatively little cortical labelling (Ottersen, 1982; personal observations). This might be due to the lack of tracer uptake in the capsular division, which in recent PHA-L studies has been shown to receive inputs from a large number of sensory-related cortical areas (see McDonald, 1998). These areas include the gustatory (DIg) and visceral (DIv) dysgranular cortices which project to the lateral and medial divisions of the central nucleus. In particular, there is a robust projection from the visceral dysgranular insula (DIv) to the lateral division. A light projection from the somatosensory-related area SII, as well as heavier projections from the parietal ventral (PV) and parietal rhinal (PaRH) cortices, terminate in the capsular division. Similarly, McDonald and co-workers (Mascagni *et al.*, 1993; McDonald, 1998) found that the auditory (Te2D and Te3) and visual regions (Te2) provide substantial projections to the capsular division. They also report that the dorsal bank of the perirhinal cortex projects moderately to the capsular division of the central nucleus, whereas the projection from the ventral bank is lighter. A light projection from the posterior agranular insula (AIp) terminates in all divisions of the central nucleus.

Frontal cortex. The central nucleus receives inputs from the medial and lateral prefrontal cortex, most of which appear light in density. Medially, the heaviest projection to the central nucleus originates in the infralimbic area and terminates in the capsular, intermediate, and medial divisions. Light projections from the prelimbic and medial precentral cortex (PrCm) terminate in the capsular division. Laterally, the dorsal agranular insula (AId) provides a substantial input to the lateral division and also lighter projections to other divisions. The ventral agranular insula (AIv) projects lightly to the capsular division.

Hippocampal formation. The entorhinal cortex and the temporal end of the subiculum provide the most substantial projections from the hippocampal formation to the central nucleus. Within the entorhinal cortex, the VIE subfield sends a dense input to the capsular division. In addition, a region located between the periamygdaloid cortex and the entorhinal cortex (called the amygdalo-piriform transition area or partially included in the AE subfield of the entorhinal cortex; see Insausti *et al.*, 1997) provides a robust projection to the lateral division of the central nucleus (Jolkkonen and Pitkänen, 1998b). The proximal temporal subiculum sends a heavy projection to the medial division of the central nucleus (Cullinan *et al.*, 1993). The distal temporal subiculum projects moderately to the capsular division (McDonald, 1998). Finally, Ottersen (1982) reported some labelled neurons in the CA1 subfield of the hippocampus after injecting a retrograde tracer into the central nucleus. More recent anterograde tracer studies, however, have not verified this projection.

Olfactory system. The central nucleus receives light projections from various parts of the olfactory cortex. Retrograde tracer studies suggest that the medial aspect of the piriform cortex projects to the central nucleus. Consistent with these observations, McDonald recently injected PHA-L into the medial piriform cortex/endopiriform nucleus and observed light labelling in the capsular and lateral divisions of the central nucleus (McDonald, 1998). According to a recent anterograde study of Behan and Haberly (1999), the endopiriform nucleus does not contribute to this projection. Retrograde tracer studies suggest that

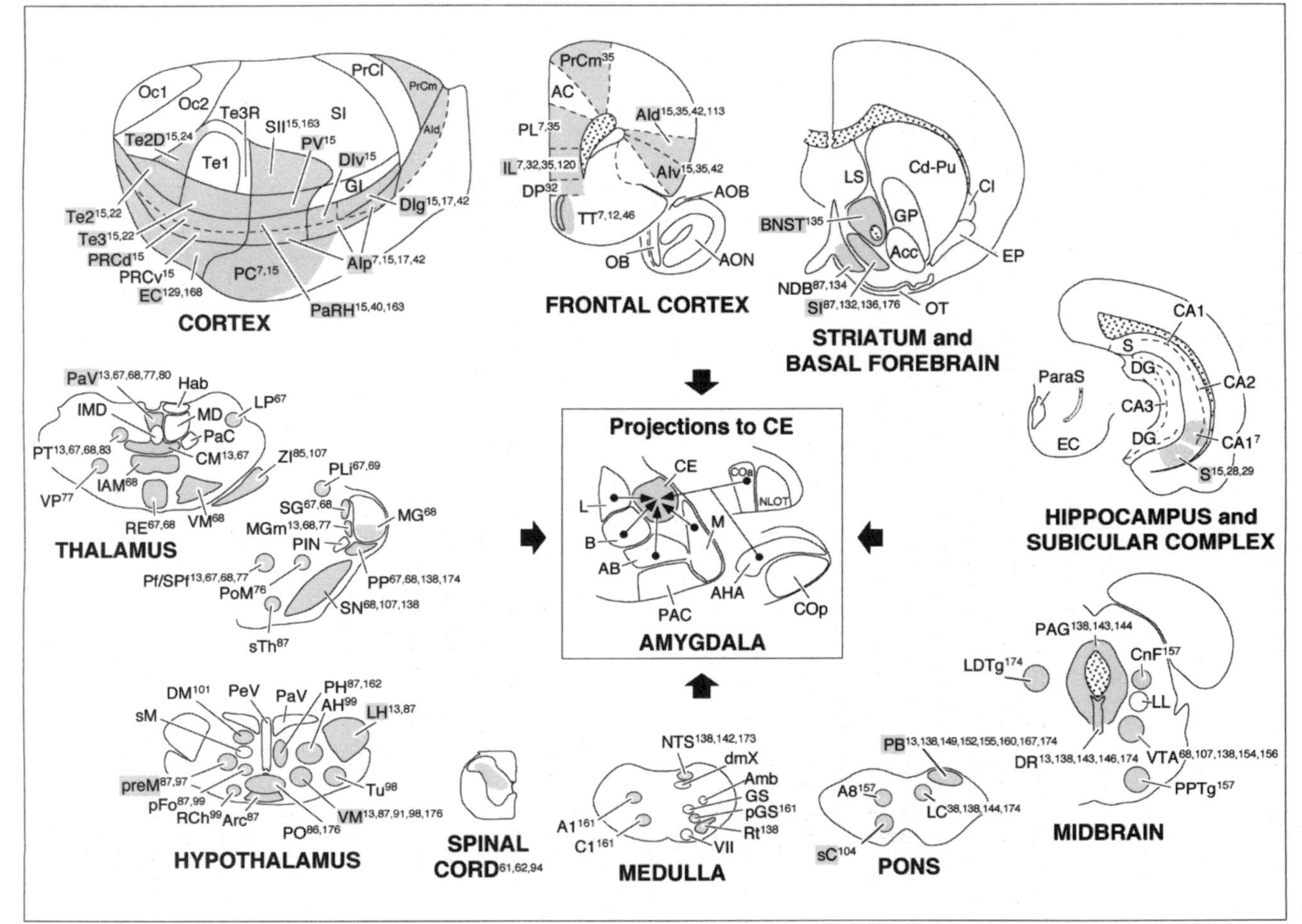

Figure 2.8 Cortical, subcortical, and intra-amygdaloid inputs of the central nucleus. See legend to Figure 2.2.

the central nucleus also receives light projections from the dorsal peduncular cortex and tenia tecta.

Thalamus. Thalamic inputs to the central nucleus originate in the midline region as well as posteriorly, and they terminate largely in the capsular, lateral, or intermediate divisions. In the midline, projections originate in the paraventricular, paratenial, centromedial, inter-anteromedial, and reuniens nuclei. The projection from the paraventricular nucleus appears to terminate in the lateral aspects of the central nucleus (Moga *et al.*, 1995). Rizvi *et al.* (1991) found retrogradely labelled cells in the mediodorsal nucleus after injecting wheat germ agglutinin–HRP (WGA–HRP) into the central nucleus. The injection was relatively large, however, and might have spread to the basal nucleus. More posteriorly, the ventral posterior nucleus, parafascicular and subparafascicular nuclei project to the central nucleus. Also, the lateral posterior, posterior limitans, suprageniculate, ventral aspect of the medial geniculate, and the medial division of the medial geniculate have been reported to project to the central nucleus. However, a retrograde tracer study by Ledoux *et al.* (1990) suggests that the central nucleus does not receive inputs from the suprageniculate and medial division of the medial geniculate (or posterior intralaminar) nuclei. Rather, uptake of anterograde tracer substance by neurons in the medial group of the posterior thalamic complex might have given rise to the projection thought to originate in these thalamic auditory regions. The zona inserta projects to the central nucleus.

Hypothalamus. The hypothalamus provides substantial projections to the central nucleus, many of which terminate in the capsular and medial divisions. Both the ventromedial and ventral premamillary nuclei project heavily to the capsular and medial divisions of the central nucleus. Based on retrograde tracer studies, the lateral hypothalamic area also projects densely to the central nucleus. Lighter projections originate in the lateral preoptic region, arcuate nucleus, retrochiasmatic area (terminates in the capsular division), perifornical area (capsular division), anterior hypothalamic nucleus (capsular division), tuberal nucleus (capsular and medial divisions), dorsomedial nucleus (capsular and medial divisions), and posterior hypothalamic nucleus.

Basal forebrain, striatum, and bed nucleus of the stria terminalis. A retrograde tracer study by Ottersen (1980) shows that the horizontal limb of the nucleus of the diagonal band projects to the central nucleus. Also, the substantia innominata provides an input to the central nucleus that terminates in the medial division. The bed nucleus of the stria terminalis has a substantial projection to the medial division (Grove, 1988a).

Midbrain, pons, medulla, and spinal cord. The central nucleus is the major target for the inputs from the midbrain, pons, and medulla to the amygdaloid complex. After injecting retrograde tracers into the central nucleus, labelled cells are found in substantia nigra (pars compacta), subthalamic nucleus, peripeduncular nucleus, ventral tegmental area, dorsal raphe, locus coeruleus, retrorubral area (A8 cell group), periaqueductal grey, and laterodorsal tegmental nucleus. Anterograde tracer studies also show that the pedunculopontine tegmental nucleus and nucleus cuneiformis provide an input to the central nucleus. More caudally, the parabrachial nucleus provides a heavy topographically organized input to the central nucleus that terminates in the medial, lateral, or capsular division, depending on the location of tracer injection in the parabrachial nucleus (Bernard *et al.*, 1993). The nucleus subcoeruleus recently was reported to provide a substantial input to the medial division. The central nucleus also receives inputs from the nucleus of the solitary tract (including A2 noradrenergic neurons; Zardetto-Smith and Gray, 1990), the mesencephalic and bulbar reticular formation, and from nucleus paragigantocellularis lateralis. Projections from the A1 noradrenergic and C1 adrenergic cell groups in the ventrolateral medulla terminate primarily in the medial division of the central nucleus (Roder and Ciriello, 1993). Finally, there are reports demonstrating that the cervical and lumbar spinal cord project to the central nucleus.

Extra-amygdaloid outputs

The cortical and subcortical outputs of the central nucleus are summarized in Figure 2.9. The central nucleus does not project to the sensory-related lateral cortical areas, frontal cortex, hippocampal formation, or to the olfactory system.

Thalamus. Injection of an anterograde tracer (PHA-L) into the central nucleus labels several nuclei in the midline thalamus. These include the intermediodorsal nucleus, posteromedian nucleus, and centromedian nucleus. Labelled terminals are also found in the mediodorsal nucleus and lateral habenula.

Hypothalamus. The central nucleus provides substantial inputs to a large number of hypothalamic nuclei. Most of the projections originate in the medial division. Moderate to heavy projections are directed to the medial and lateral preoptic area, retrochiasmatic area, lateral hypothalamus, perifornical region, and paraventricular nucleus. Other projections from the central nucleus terminate in the supraoptic nucleus, suprachiasmatic nucleus, arcuate nucleus, anterior hypothalamic area, tuber cinereum, ventromedial nucleus, dorsomedial nucleus, and periventricular nucleus.

Basal forebrain, striatum, and bed nucleus of the stria terminalis. Based on retrograde studies, the substantia innominata receives an input from the central nucleus, which appears to be heavier from the medial than from the lateral division. Phillipson and Griffiths (1985) found a projection from the central nucleus to the nucleus accumbens. The projection was not confirmed, however, in a study by McDonald (1991b). A retrograde tracer study suggested that the lateral septum also receives an input from the central nucleus. The central nucleus projects heavily to the bed nucleus of the stria terminalis. The heaviest projections originate in the lateral and medial divisions and the lighter projections originate in the intermediate and capsular divisions (Sun *et al.*, 1991).

Midbrain, pons, and medulla. The central nucleus provides most of the amygdaloid projections to the midbrain, pons, and medulla. It projects to all divisions of the substantia nigra (lateralis, compacta, and reticularis). In particular, the lateral division projects to the pars lateralis (Vankova *et al.*, 1992). The medial division of the central nucleus projects to the lateral terminal nucleus of the accessory optic tract, central grey, cuneiform nucleus, pedunculopontine tegmental nucleus, and basilar pontine nucleus. Other projections from the central nucleus terminate in the ventral tegmental area, laterodorsal tegmental nucleus, and dorsal raphe. More caudally, the parabrachial nucleus and nucleus of the trigeminal nerve receive heavy inputs from the medial and lateral divisions of the central nucleus. The medial division projects heavily to the nucleus reticularis pontis caudalis. The locus coeruleus, nucleus subcoeruleus, and nucleus retrorubralis (A8) are also innervated by the central nucleus.

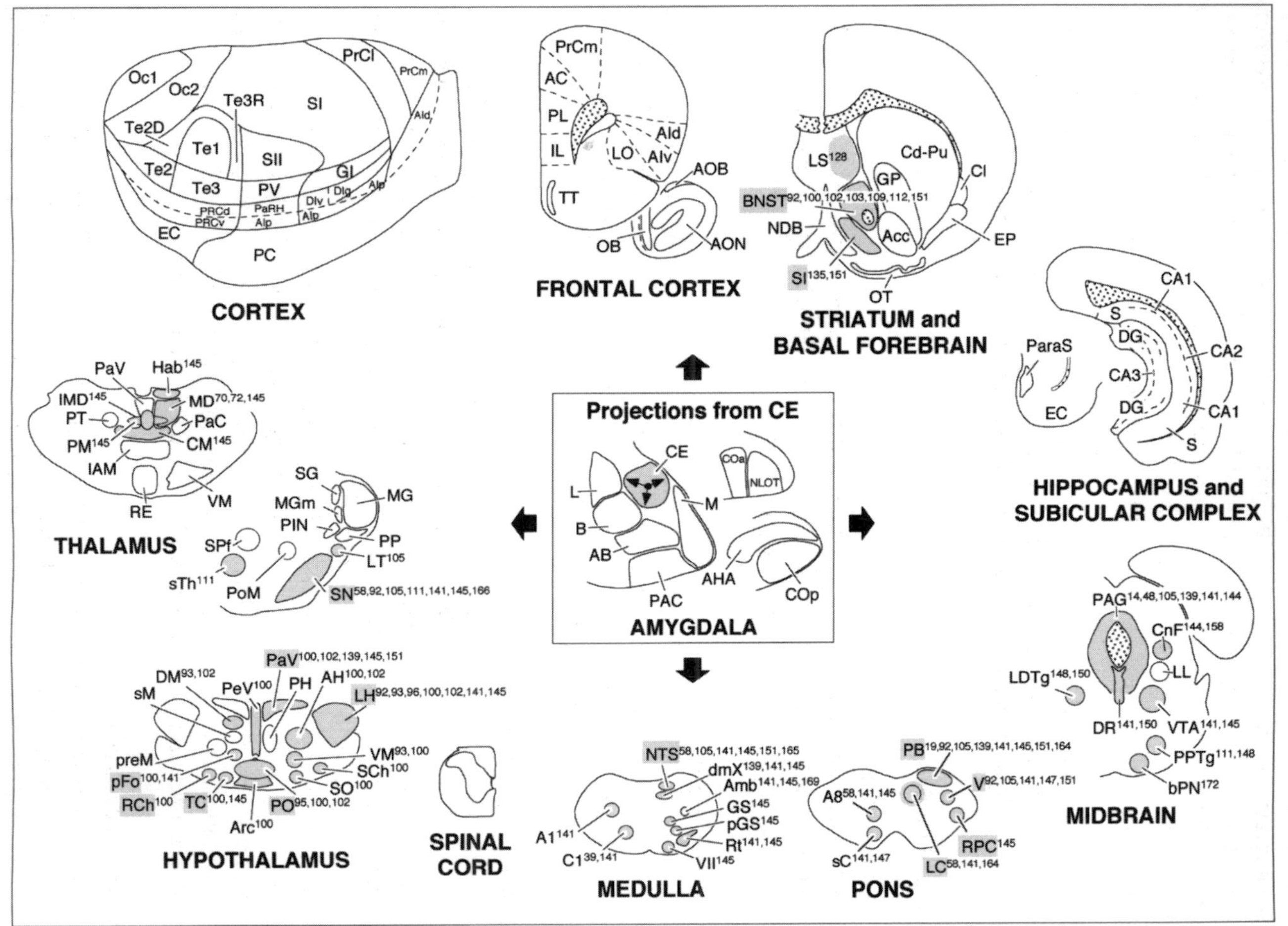

Figure 2.9 Cortical, subcortical, and intra-amygdaloid outputs of the central nucleus. See legend to Figure 2.3.

Finally, in the medulla, the nucleus of the solitary tract receives a heavy input from the medial and lateral divisions of the central nucleus. Other terminals originating in the central nucleus innervate the dorsal motor nucleus of the vagus, nucleus ambiguus (see also the subretrofacial nucleus; Takayama and Miura, 1991), gigantocellular, and paragigantocellular nuclei, parvicellular reticular nucleus, nucleus of the facial nerve, and the A1 noradrenergic and C1 adrenergic cell groups in the ventrolateral medulla.

To summarize, the central nucleus receives moderate to heavy inputs from the lateral sensory-related cortical areas, hippocampal formation, medial and lateral prefrontal cortex, bed nucleus of stria terminalis, substantia innominata, some thalamic nuclei, hypothalamus, and pontine nuclei. The central nucleus provides substantial inputs to the bed nucleus of stria terminalis, many hypothalamic nuclei, and several nuclei in the midbrain, pons, and medulla.

2.2.7 Medial nucleus

Divisions and location

The medial nucleus has three divisions: rostral, central (dorsal and ventral parts), and caudal. The medial nucleus begins at the level of the nucleus of the lateral olfactory tract and extends caudally to where the lateral ventricle begins (Figure 2.1).

Intranuclear connections

Based on a PHA-L study by Canteras *et al.* (1995), the dorsal part of the central division, the ventral part of the central division, and the caudal division all send substantial projections to each other and to the rostral division (Table 2.2). The intranuclear projections of the rostral division are not known.

Intra-amygdaloid connections

The medial nucleus receives moderate to heavy intra-amygdaloid projections from the lateral, accessory basal, and posterior cortical nuclei as well as from the amygdalohippocampal area (Figure 2.10, Table 2.2). Lighter projections originate in the basal nucleus, anterior cortical nucleus, and periamygdaloid cortex. Many of the intra-amygdaloid inputs terminate in the central division (Table 2.2).

The medial nucleus provides substantial intra-amygdaloid inputs to the lateral, accessory basal, central, anterior cortical, and posterior cortical nuclei (Figure 2.11, Table 2.2). Also, the bed nucleus of the accessory olfactory tract and amygdalohippocampal area are innervated. Therefore, many of the intra-amygdaloid connections of the medial nucleus are reciprocal. Most connections originate in the central division (Table 2.2).

Interamygdaloid connections

The medial nucleus receives the largest number of projections from the contralateral amygdala of all the amygdaloid nuclei (Figure 2.22). These include projections from the contralateral accessory basal nucleus, periamygdaloid cortex, nucleus of the lateral olfactory tract, and posterior cortical nucleus. The medial nucleus sends only a very few fibres to the contralateral medial nucleus (Canteras *et al.*, 1995).

Extra-amygdaloid inputs

Cortical and subcortical inputs to the medial nucleus are summarized in Figure 2.10.

Temporal, insular, and parietal cortex. Projections from the sensory-related lateral cortical areas to the medial nucleus are sparse. The posterior agranular insula (AIp) projects to the medial nucleus. This projection has been described as light (Shi and Cassel, 1998a) or strong (McDonald, 1998) in density. The dorsal bank of the perirhinal cortex provides a light input to the medial nucleus.

Frontal cortex. The medial nucleus receives a substantial input from the infralimbic cortex that terminates in the dorsal and ventral parts of the central division. One study also indicates a very light projection from the prelimbic area to the dorsal part of the central division. Laterally, the ventral agranular insula (AIv) provides a light to moderate input to the dorsal part of the central division.

Hippocampal formation. The entorhinal cortex projects lightly to the dorsal part of the central division. Inputs from the proximal and distal parts of the temporal subiculum, however, appear moderate to heavy in density and terminate in the dorsal and ventral parts of the central division. Recently, Christensen and Frederickson (1998) injected sodium selenide into the medial nucleus and found retrogradely labelled cells in the temporal CA1 subfield. This projection, however, has not been observed in anterograde tracer studies.

Olfactory system. The medial nucleus receives inputs from various levels of the olfactory system that include the olfactory bulb, accessory olfactory bulb, and anterior olfactory nucleus. The endopiriform nucleus was shown recently to give rise to a moderate projection to the medial nucleus (Behan and Haberly, 1999). After a sodium selenide injection into the medial nucleus, Christensen and Frederickson (1998) observed a substantial number of retrogradely labelled neurons in layer 2 of the entire mediolateral extent of the piriform cortex.

Thalamus. The medial nucleus receives inputs from the midline and posterior thalamus. Projections in the thalamic midline originate in the paraventricular, centromedian, and reuniens nuclei. The medial nucleus also receives inputs from the paratenial nucleus and ventral posterior thalamic nucleus, as well as from the parafascicular and subparafascicular nuclei. Some retrograde tracer data suggest that the suprageniculate nucleus, the medial division of the medial geniculate nucleus, and the ventral part of the medial geniculate nucleus also project to the medial nucleus. A retrograde tracer study by LeDoux *et al.* (1990), however, suggests that the medial group of the posterior thalamic complex, rather than the more laterally located medial division of the medial geniculate nucleus, projects to the medial nucleus.

Hypothalamus. A large number of hypothalamic nuclei project to the medial nucleus. Moderate to heavy projections originate in the ventromedial and premamillary nuclei. Other hypothalamic regions that project to the medial nucleus include the medial and lateral preoptic area, anterior hypothalamic area, supraoptic nucleus, arcuate nucleus, retrochiasmatic area, tuber cinereum, perifornical area, tuberal nucleus, lateral hypothalamus, dorsomedial nucleus, posterior hypothalamic nucleus, and supramamillary nucleus. In addition, Ottersen (1980) found retrogradely labelled cells around the paraventricular nucleus, but very few within the nucleus.

Basal forebrain, striatum, and bed nucleus of the stria terminalis. Projections from the basal forebrain to the medial nucleus originate in the nucleus of the diagonal band as well

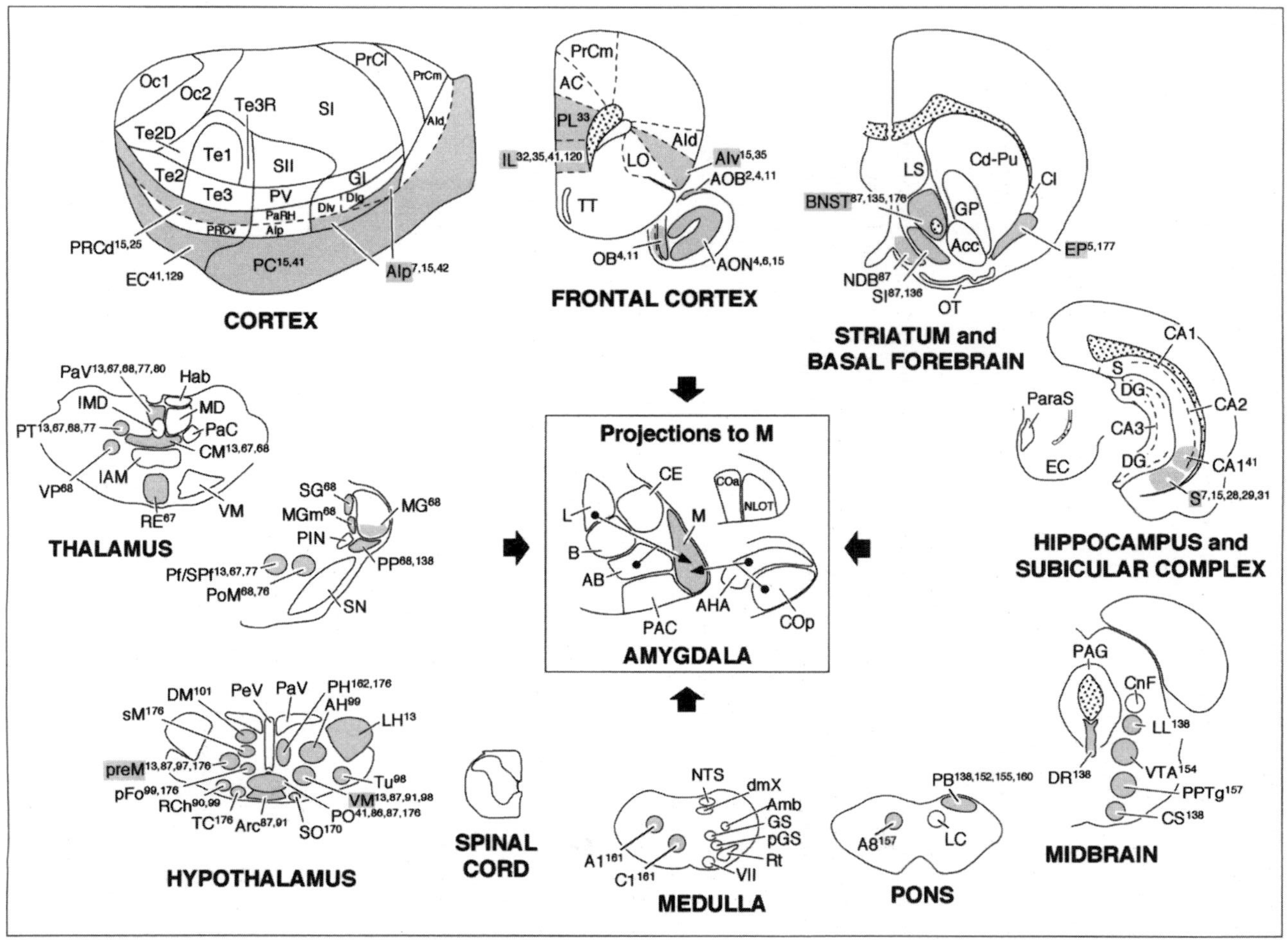

Figure 2.10 Cortical, subcortical, and intra-amygdaloid inputs of the medial nucleus. See legend to Figure 2.2.

as in the substantia innominata, which provide a light input to the medial nucleus. The bed nucleus of the stria terminalis provides a moderate input to the medial nucleus.

Midbrain, pons, and medulla. The medial nucleus receives light projections from the midbrain, pons, and medulla. These include inputs from the peripeduncular nucleus, dorsal nucleus of the lateral lemniscus, retrorubral area (A8), ventral tegmental area, pedunculopontine tegmental nucleus, nucleus centralis superior, dorsal raphe, and parabrachial nucleus. Also, the A1 noradrenergic and C1 adrenergic cell groups in the ventrolateral medulla project lightly to the medial nucleus. Finally, Levine *et al.* (1991) reported a light input from the retina to the medial nucleus.

Extra-amygdaloid outputs

Cortical and subcortical projections of the medial nucleus are summarized in Figure 2.11.

Temporal, insular and parietal cortex. Projections from the medial nucleus to the sensory-related lateral cortical areas are meagre. Both retrograde and anterograde tracer studies show that the medial nucleus provides a light input to the anterior portion of the posterior agranular insula (AIp). After a large retrograde tracer injection into the perirhinal cotrex, some labelled cells have been observed in the medial nucleus (McDonald and Jackson, 1987), but this projection was not reported in a recent PHA-L study (Canteras *et al.*, 1995).

Frontal cortex. The medial nucleus projects lightly to the prefrontal cortex. The innervated areas include the prelimbic and infralimbic cortices medially, as well as the dorsal and ventral agranular insula laterally.

Hippocampal formation. The medial nucleus sends a moderate projection to the entorhinal cortex, particularly to its lateral aspects. These pathways originate in the dorsal and ventral part of the central division and also in the caudal division. There are light projections from the medial nucleus to the temporal end of the CA1 subfield and subiculum, as well as to the parasubiculum.

Olfactory system. Projections from the medial nucleus to the olfactory system are light to moderate in density. A recent anterograde tracer study shows that the central division of the medial nucleus provides moderate inputs to the accessory olfactory bulb, endopiriform nucleus, and piriform cortex. Light inputs are directed to the anterior olfactory nucleus, olfactory tubercle, and tenia tecta (Canteras *et al.*, 1995).

Thalamus. The most prominent projections from the medial nucleus to the thalamus originate in the central division, particularly its dorsal part. Moderate to dense projections terminate in the reuniens, paraventricular, and mediodorsal nuclei. Lighter projections are found in the habenula, paratenial nucleus, subparafascicular nucleus, and zona inserta.

Hypothalamus. All rostrocaudal levels of the hypothalamus receive moderate to heavy projections from the medial nucleus. These are directed to the medial preoptic area and preoptic nucleus, supraoptic nucleus, tuber cinereum, periventricular nucleus, paraventricular nucleus, ventromedial nucleus, tuberal nucleus, lateral hypothalamic area, posterior nucleus, and ventral premamillary nucleus. There are lighter projections to the dorsal hypothalamic area, perifornical area, retrochiasmatic area, arcuate nucleus, anterior hypothalamic area, dorsomedial nucleus, supramamillary, and medial mamillary nuclei.

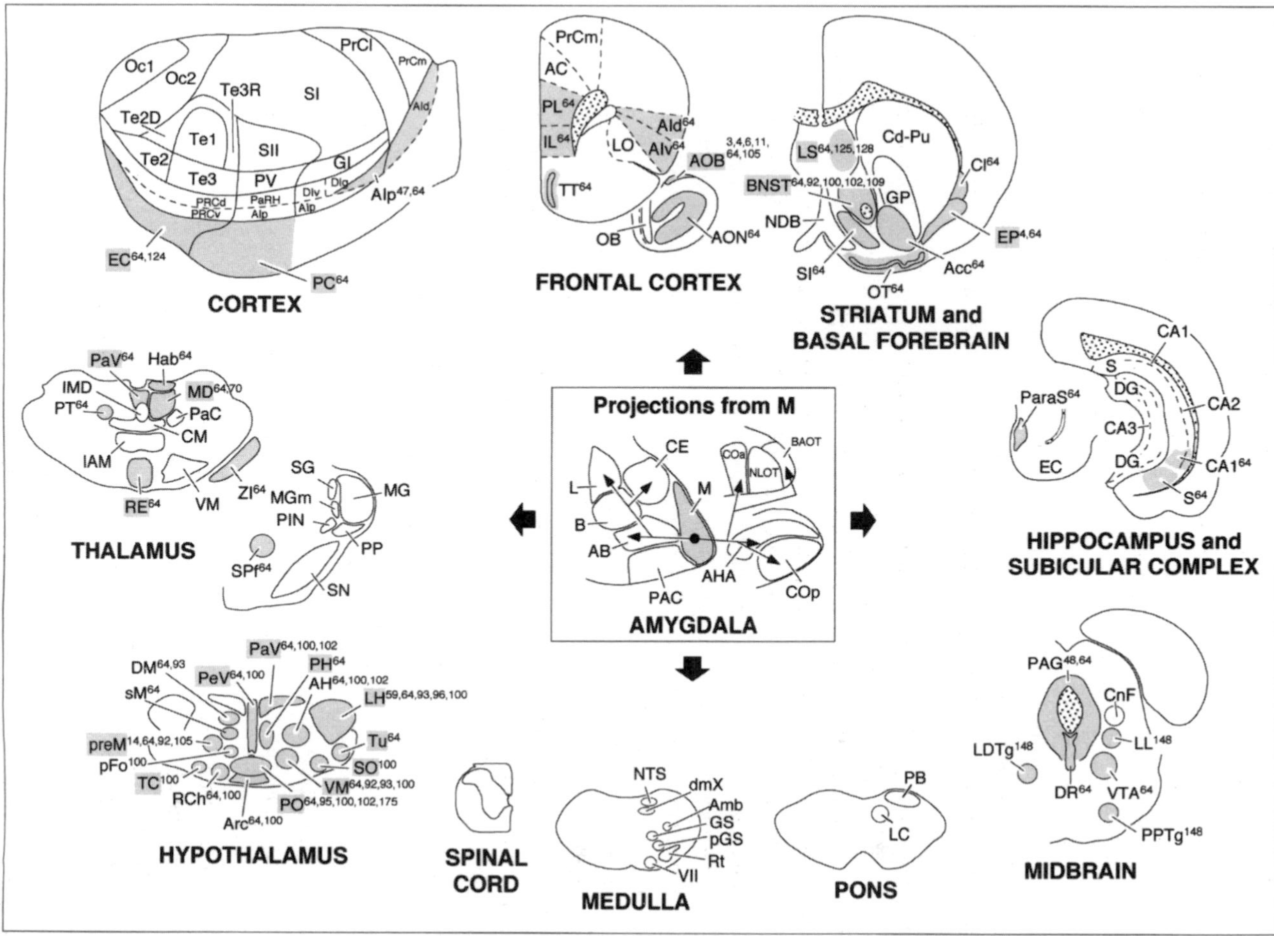

Figure 2.11 Cortical, subcortical, and intra-amygdaloid outputs of the medial nucleus. See legend to Figure 2.3.

Basal forebrain, striatum, and bed nucleus of the stria terminalis. Projections to the substantia innominata, nucleus accumbens, and claustrum are light. The lateral septum, however, receives a substantial input. The medial nucleus also provides a heavy input to the bed nucleus of the stria terminalis.

Midbrain, pons, and medulla. Light projections from the medial nucleus to the midbrain terminate in the central grey, the nucleus of the lateral lemniscus, the ventral tegmental area, various divisions of the raphe nucleus, the pedunculopontine tegmental nucleus, and the laterodorsal tegmental nucleus.

To summarize, the major inputs to the medial nucleus originate in the prefrontal cortex, bed nucleus of stria terminalis, and hypothalamus. The medial nucleus provides moderate to heavy projections to several other amygdaloid nuclei, the olfactory system, bed nucleus of the stria terminalis, thalamus, and hypothalamus.

2.2.8 Anterior cortical nucleus

Location

The anterior cortical nucleus is a three-layered structure. Often the 'oval-shaped' layer 3 is called the 'anterior part of the basomedial nucleus' (see Table 2.1). The anterior cortical nucleus is located ventral to the beginning of the magnocellular division of the basal nucleus. Laterally, it is bordered rostrally by the piriform cortex, and caudally by the periamygdaloid cortex. Rostromedially, it borders with the nucleus of the olfactory tract, and caudomedially with the medial nucleus (Figure 2.1).

Intranuclear connections

A PHA-L injection into layer 3 of the anterior cortical nucleus produces heavy intranuclear projections that do not extend rostrally but are directed more caudally. Therefore, anterior layer 3 projects caudally to the oval-shaped layer 3, but not vice versa.

Intra-amygdaloid connections

The anterior cortical nucleus receives heavy inputs from the basal nucleus and medial nucleus (Figure 2.12, Table 2.2). The anterior cortical nucleus projects heavily to the medial division of the central nucleus and the anterior amygdaloid area (Figure 2.13). It also provides a moderate projection to the lateral portion of the parvicellular division of the basal nucleus (Table 2.2).

Interamygdaloid connections

The anterior cortical nucleus does not receive inputs from the contralateral amygdala. It does, however, project to the contralateral central nucleus (Figure 2.22).

Extra-amygdaloid inputs

Cortical and subcortical inputs to the anterior cortical nucleus are summarized in Figure 2.12.

Temporal, insular, and parietal cortex. The anterior cortical nucleus receives moderate projections from some of the sensory-related lateral cortical areas. These include inputs from

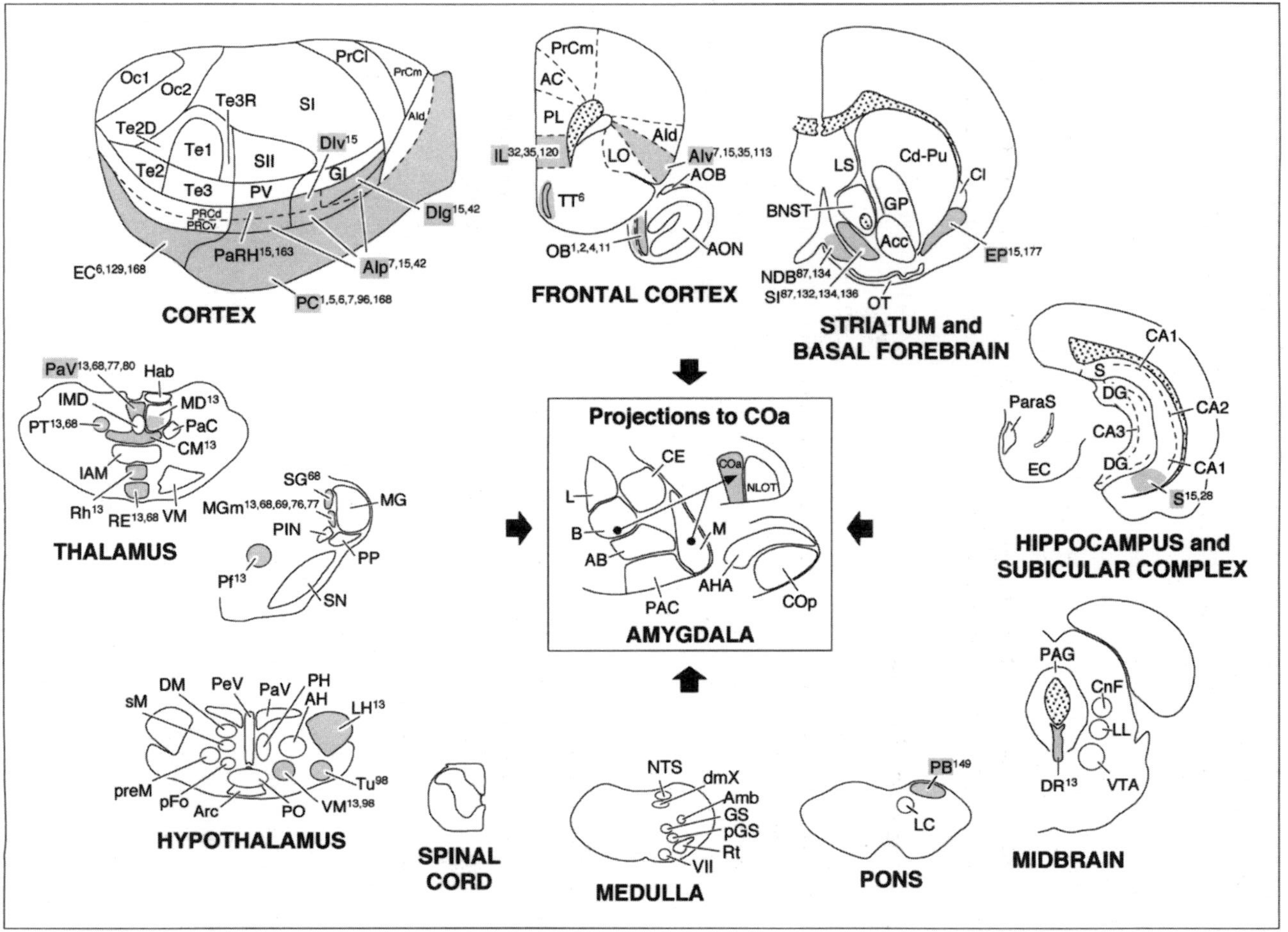

Figure 2.12 Cortical, subcortical, and intra-amygdaloid inputs of the anterior cortical nucleus. See legend to Figure 2.2.

the gustatory dysgranular insula (DIg), visceral dysgranular insula (DIv), as well as the underlying posterior agranular insula (AIp). A projection from the somatosensory-related parietal rhinal area (PaRH) is lighter.

Frontal cortex. Both the medial and lateral prefrontal cortex provide moderate to heavy inputs to the anterior cortical nucleus. Projections originate in the infralimbic cortex and ventral agranular insula (AIv).

Hippocampal formation. Within the hippocampal formation, a moderate projection to the anterior cortical nucleus originates in the proximal portion of the temporal subiculum. The projection from the distal subiculum is light. Also, the lateral entorhinal cortex projects lightly to the anterior cortical nucleus.

Olfactory system. The anterior cortical nucleus receives inputs from several olfactory-related areas, including the olfactory bulb and tenia tecta. Recently, McDonald (1998) showed robust labelling in all layers of the anterior cortical nucleus when a PHA-L injection was placed into the piriform cortex involving the endopiriform nucleus. According to a recent anterograde study of Behan and Haberly (1999), the contribution of the endopiriform nucleus to this projection appears substantial.

Thalamus. The anterior cortical nucleus receives inputs from the midline and posterior thalamus. Inputs from the midline thalamus originate in the paraventricular, centromedian, rhomboid, and reuniens nuclei. Also, the paratenial, mediodorsal, and parafascicular nuclei project to the anterior cortical nucleus. Posteriorly, the suprageniculate and medial division of the medial geniculate nuclei are reported to provide an input to the anterior cortical nucleus.

Hypothalamus. Hypothalamic inputs to the anterior cortical nucleus are meagre. Retrograde and anterograde tracer studies suggest that the anterior cortical nucleus receives light inputs from the lateral hypothalamic area, ventromedial nucleus, and tuberal nucleus.

Basal forebrain, striatum, and bed nucleus of the stria terminalis. Projections from the basal forebrain to the anterior cortical nucleus originate in the substantia innominata and nucleus of the diagonal band.

Midbrain, pons, and medulla. Some evidence from retrograde tracer studies suggests that the medial nucleus receives an input from the dorsal raphe. Anterograde tracer studies show that both layers 2 and 3 receive a moderate projection from the parabrachial nucleus.

Extra-amygdaloid outputs

Cortical and subcortical outputs of the anterior cortical nucleus are summarized in Figure 2.13.

Temporal, insular, and parietal cortex. In general, projections from the anterior cortical nucleus to other cortical areas are lighter and not as widespread as projections from these cortical areas to the anterior cortical nucleus. Light to moderate inputs are directed to the posterior agranular insula (AIp) and there are light inputs to the perirhinal cortex.

Frontal cortex. Light inputs to the prefrontal cortex are found in the infralimbic cortex, and in the dorsal (AId) and ventral (AIv) agranular insula. Light inputs are also directed to the medial and lateral orbital cortices.

Hippocampal formation. The entorhinal cortex, as well as the temporal subiculum and CA1 subfield, receive light projections from the anterior cortical nucleus.

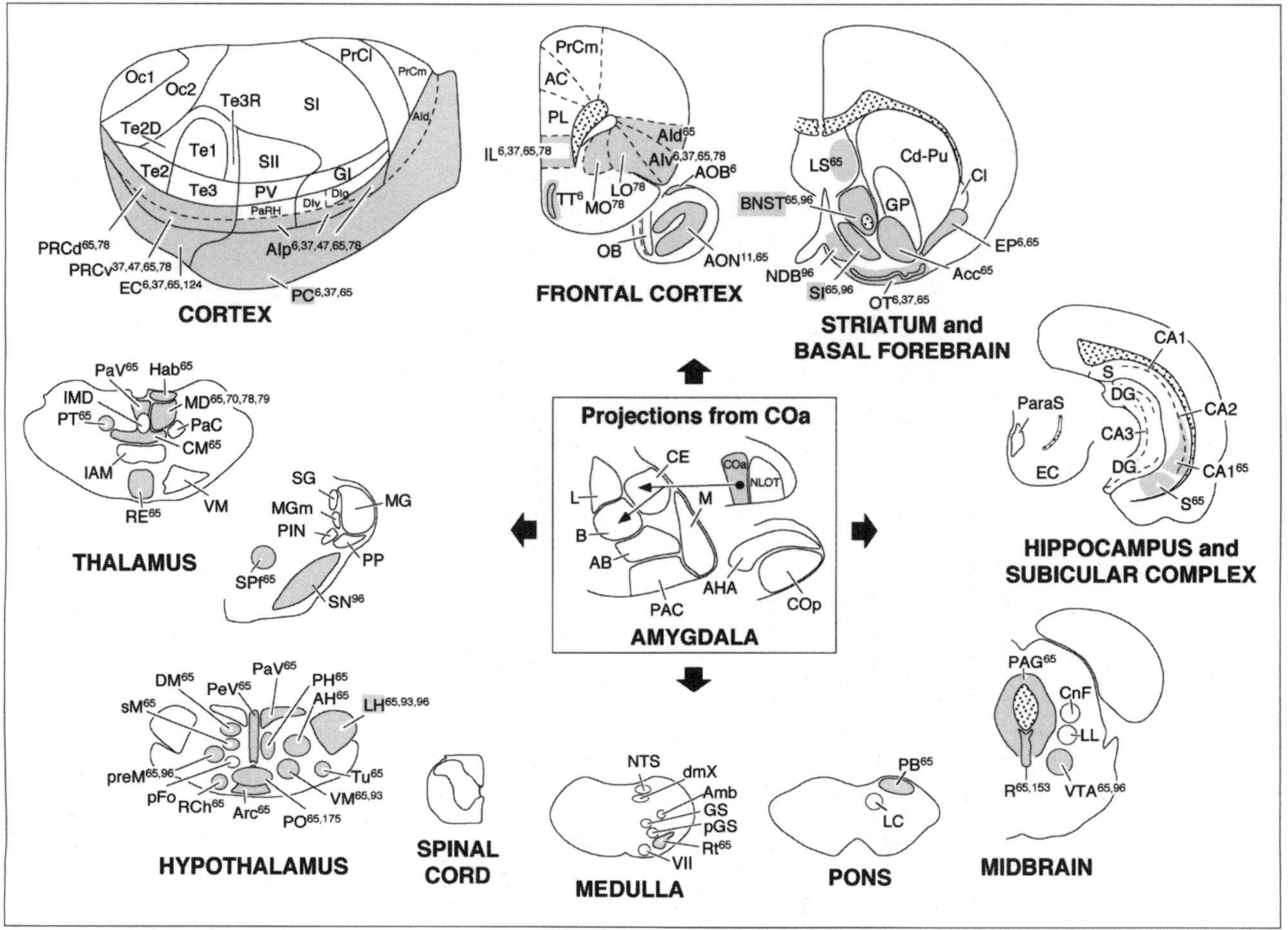

Figure 2.13 Cortical, subcortical, and intra-amygdaloid outputs of the anterior cortical nucleus. See legend to Figure 2.3.

Olfactory system. The anterior cortical nucleus provides projections to various olfactory-related areas. These include a moderate input to the piriform cortex and light inputs to the accessory olfactory bulb, anterior olfactory nucleus, olfactory tubercle, endopiriform nucleus, and tenia tecta.

Thalamus. The anterior cortical nucleus projects to the midline thalamus. Projections terminate in the paraventricular, paratenial, centromedial, and reuniens nuclei. In addition, the anterior cortical nucleus projects to the mediodorsal nucleus and subparafascicular nuclei as well as to the lateral habenula.

Hypothalamus. Layers 2 and 3 (termed 'anterior basomedial nucleus' by Petrovich *et al.*, 1996) of the anterior cortical nucleus project to the hypothalamus. Both layers provide a substantial input to the lateral hypothalamic area. In addition, lighter projections terminate in the lateral and medial preoptic nucleus, arcuate nucleus, retrochiasmatic area, anterior hypothalamic nucleus, ventromedial nucleus, dorsomedial nucleus, periventricular nucleus, paraventricular nucleus, tuberal nucleus, posterior hypothalamic area, supramamillary nucleus, and premamillary nucleus.

Basal forebrain, striatum, and bed nucleus of the stria terminalis. There are substantial projections from the anterior cortical nucleus to the substantia innominata. Lighter projections terminate in the horizontal limb of the nucleus of the diagonal band, lateral septum, and nucleus accumbens. The anterior cortical nucleus also sends a heavy projection to the bed nucleus of the stria terminalis.

Midbrain, pons, and medulla. There are only a few light projections from the anterior cortical nucleus to the midbrain and pons. They terminate in the substantia nigra, periaqueductal grey, ventral tegmental area, central linear nucleus of the raphe, and parabrachial nucleus.

To summarize, the major inputs to the anterior cortical nucleus originate in the gustatory and visceral dysgranular and agranular cortices, prefrontal cortex, paraventricular thalamic nucleus, parabrachial pontine nucleus, and the subiculum. The anterior cortical nucleus provides substantial inputs to the olfactory system, bed nucleus of stria terminalis, and hypothalamus.

2.2.9 Periamygdaloid cortex

Divisions and location

The periamygdaloid cortex can be divided into three divisions: PAC, PACm, and PACs. It is located caudal to the anterior cortical nucleus between the piriform cortex and the medial nucleus. The PAC is the most rostral of the divisions. Caudomedially, the PAC is bordered by the PACm. The PACs is the most caudal subdivision and extends almost to the end of the amygdala. Dorsally, the periamygdaloid cortex borders the accessory basal nucleus (Figure 2.1). The term 'periamygdaloid cortex' is used here to represent all divisions because many details of the connectivity of individual divisions are unknown.

Intranuclear connections

There are no known studies that have focused on the connectivity between the various divisions of the periramygdaloid cortex.

Intra-amygdaloid connections

The heaviest intra-amygdaloid inputs to the periamygdaloid cortex originate in the lateral nucleus, accessory basal nucleus, and in the posterior cortical nucleus (Figure 2.14, Table 2.2). The periamygdaloid cortex projects heavily to the lateral nucleus (Figure 2.15). The density and details of intra-amygdaloid connectivity of the different divisions of the periamygdaloid cortex have not yet been explored in great detail using newer anterograde tracing techniques (Table 2.2).

Interamygdaloid connections

The periamygdaloid cortex receives an input from the contralateral periamygdaloid cortex. In addition to the projection to the contralateral periamygdaloid cortex, it also projects to the contralateral medial nucleus and posterior cortical nucleus (Figure 2.22).

Extra-amygdaloid inputs

Cortical and subcortical inputs of the periamygdaloid cortex are summarized in Figure 2.14.

Temporal, insular, and parietal cortex. The periamygdaloid cortex receives substantial inputs from the sensory-related lateral cortical areas. Light inputs originate in the gustatory dysgranular insula (DIg), visceral dysgranular insula (DIv), somatosensory-related parietal ventral area (PV), and parietal rhinal cortex (PaRH). The ventrally located posterior agranular insula (AIp) and the more caudal perirhinal cortex provide moderate to heavy inputs to the periamygdaloid cortex.

Frontal cortex. In the medial prefrontal cortex, the infralimbic area projects heavily to layer 3 of the periamygdaloid cortex, whereas projections from the prelimbic cortex are meagre. A recent retrograde tracer study by Christensen and Frederickson (1998) shows that the anterior cingulate cortex might also project to the periamygdaloid cortex. Laterally, the ventral agranular insula (AIv) provides a substantial input to the periamygdaloid cortex. Also, the lateral orbital area projects to the periamygdaloid cortex.

Hippocampal formation. Projections from the hippocampal formation to the periamygdaloid cortex are light. They originate in the entorhinal cortex and in the temporal end of the CA1 subfield and subiculum.

Olfactory system. Olfactory inputs to the periamygdaloid cortex originate in the olfactory bulb, endopeduncular nucleus, and piriform cortex. The projections from the piriform cortex and the endopiriform nucleus to the periamygdaloid cortex appear dense (Figure 6, McDonald, 1998; Behan and Haberly, 1999).

Hypothalamus. The few light projections from the hypothalamus to the periamygdaloid cortex originate in the lateral hypothalamic area, preoptic area, and the ventromedial nucleus.

Basal forebrain, striatum, and bed nucleus of the stria terminalis. The nucleus of the diagonal band projects to the periamygdaloid cortex.

Midbrain, pons, and medulla. A retrograde tracer study by Veening (1978b) suggests that the periamygdaloid cortex receives a light input from the dorsal raphe.

Extra-amygdaloid outputs

Cortical and subcortical outputs of the periamygdaloid cortex are summarized in Figure 2.15.

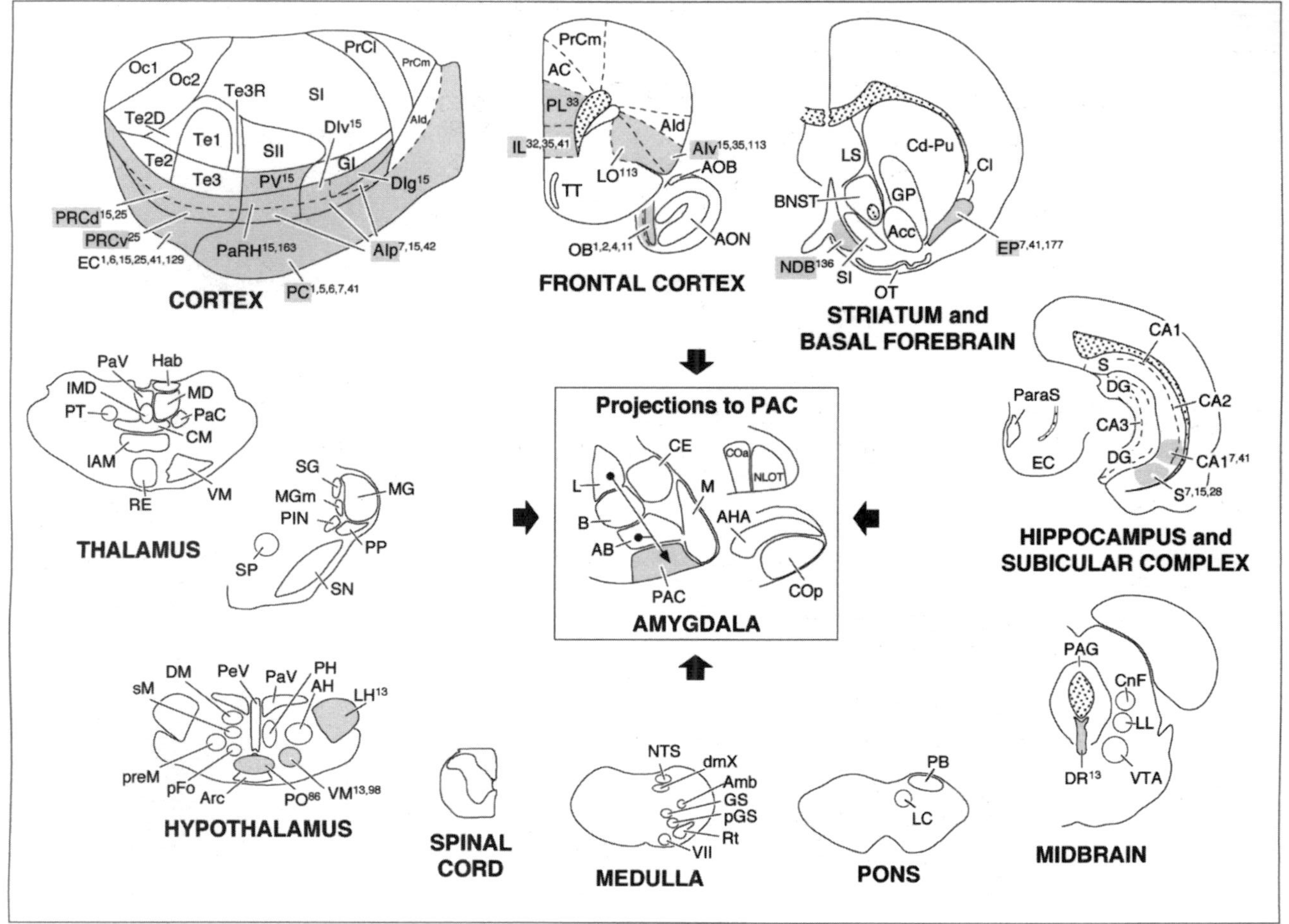

Figure 2.14 Cortical, subcortical, and intra-amygdaloid inputs of the periamygdaloid cortex. See legend to Figure 2.2.

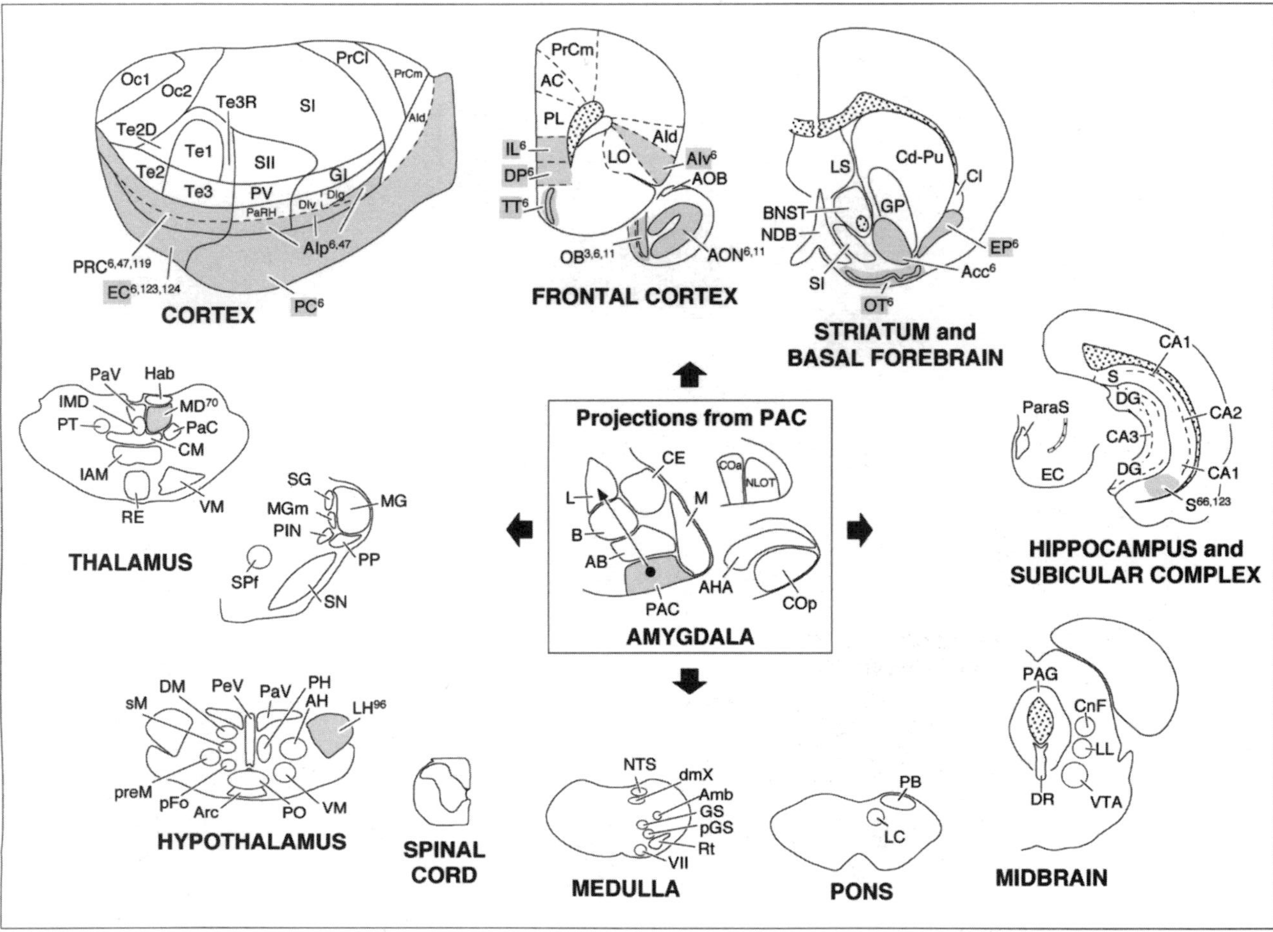

Figure 2.15 Cortical, subcortical, and intra-amygdaloid outputs of the periamygdaloid cortex. See legend to Figure 2.3.

Temporal, insular, and parietal cortex. Injection of radioactive amino acids into the periamygdaloid cortex produces labelling in the sensory-related lateral cortical areas. A light density of silver grains is found in the posterior agranular insula (AIp) and in the perirhinal cortex. Injection of retrograde tracers to the posterior insula as well as the perirhinal cortex have confirmed these observations. The projections originate largely in layer 3.

Frontal cortex. The periamygdaloid cortex provides heavy inputs to the prefrontal cortex. Target regions include the infralimbic cortex medially and the ventral agranular insula (AIv) laterally.

Hippocampal formation. Projections to the hippocampus terminate most heavily in the entorhinal cortex (VIE and DIE subfields). The periamygdaloid cortex also projects to the subiculum.

Olfactory system. The periamygdaloid cortex projects heavily to several olfactory areas. These include the olfactory tubercle, endopiriform nucleus, dorsal peduncular cortex, tenia tecta, and piriform cortex. Also, the olfactory bulb and anterior olfactory nucleus receive a lighter projection from the periamygdaloid cortex.

Thalamus. A retrograde tracer study by McDonald (1987a) shows that the periamygdaloid cortex projects to the mediodorsal thalamic nucleus.

Hypothalamus. A retrograde tracer study indicated that the periamygdaloid cortex projects to the lateral hypothalamus (Price *et al.*, 1991).

Basal forebrain, striatum, and bed nucleus of the stria terminalis. After injecting radioactive amino acids into the periamygdaloid cortex, Luskin and Price (1983a) reported a light density of labelling in the nucleus accumbens.

To summarize, the major inputs to the periamygdaloid cortex originate in the lateral sensory-related cortical areas and prefrontal cortex. The major outputs of the periamygdaloid cortex terminate in the olfactory system and prefrontal cortex.

2.2.10 Posterior cortical nucleus

Location and divisions

The posterior cortical nucleus has three layers, from which layer 2 often appears to fuse with layer 3. The posterior cortical nucleus forms the most caudal part of the amygdaloid complex (Figure 2.1). It borders the amygdalohippocampal area dorsally and the periamygdaloid cortex (sulcal division) laterally.

Intra-amygdaloid connections

The lateral nucleus, accessory basal nucleus, and the medial nucleus provide a heavy intra-amygdaloid input to the posterior cortical nucleus (Figure 2.16, Table 2.2).

The posterior cortical nucleus is the origin of a moderate to heavy projection to the bed nucleus of the accessory olfactory tract, medial nucleus, and the periamygdaloid cortex (Figure 2.17, Table 2.2).

Interamygdaloid connections

The posterior cortical nucleus receives inputs from the contralateral posterior cortical nucleus and the periamygdaloid cortex. Contralaterally, the posterior cortical nucleus projects to the posterior cortical nucleus, the medial nucleus, and the amygdalohippocampal area (Figure 2.22).

Extra-amygdaloid inputs

Cortical and subcortical inputs to the posterior cortical nucleus are summarized in Figure 2.16.

Temporal, insular, parietal, and frontal cortex. Projections from the sensory-related lateral cortices and the prefrontal cortex to the posterior cortical nucleus are meagre. Retrograde and anterograde tracer studies indicate that the rostral posterior agranular insula (AIp) projects lightly to the posterior cortical nucleus. Also, the projection from the infralimbic cortex is composed of only a few fibres.

Hippocampal formation. The entorhinal cortex (VIE subfield) projects heavily to layer 3 of the posterior cortical nucleus. Light projections originate in the temporal CA1 subfield and subiculum.

Olfactory system. The posterior cortical nucleus receives moderate to heavy inputs from several olfactory-related areas. These include projections from the accessory olfactory bulb, endopiriform nucleus, and piriform cortex. A projection from the piriform cortex appears dense, particularly to the deep portion of layer 1 (McDonald, 1998). The anterior olfactory nucleus provides a light input to the posterior cortical nucleus.

Hypothalamus. Projections from the hypothalamus to the posterior cortical nucleus are light. They originate in the preoptic region, retrochiasmatic area, perifornical region, ventromedial nucleus, lateral hypothalamic area, tuber cinereum, posterior hypothalamic nucleus, premamillary nucleus, and supramamillary nucleus.

Basal forebrain, striatum, and bed nucleus of the stria terminalis. The substantia innominata projects to the posterior cortical nucleus. Also, the bed nucleus of the stria terminalis projects to the posterior cortical nucleus. A retrograde study suggests that the claustrum also projects lightly to the posterior cortical nucleus.

Midbrain, pons, and medulla. The nucleus subcoeruleus recently was reported to provide an input to the posterior cortical nucleus.

Extra-amygdaloid outputs

Cortical and subcortical outputs of the posterior cortical nucleus are summarized in Figure 2.17.

Temporal, insular, and parietal cortex. Projections from the posterior cortical nucleus to the lateral cortical areas are meagre. There is evidence that the most lateral aspect of layer 3 provides a light projection to the rostral and caudal posterior agranular insula (AIp), and to the ventral bank of the perirhinal cortex.

Frontal cortex. The posterior cortical nucleus provides moderate inputs to the prefrontal cortex. These projections terminate in the infralimbic cortex medially and in the dorsal (AId) and ventral (AIv) agranular insula laterally.

Hippocampal formation. The posterior cortical nucleus projects moderately to the lateral aspects of the entorhinal cortex and to the CA1 subfield of the temporal end of the hippocampus. Projections to the temporal subiculum or the parasubiculum appear lighter.

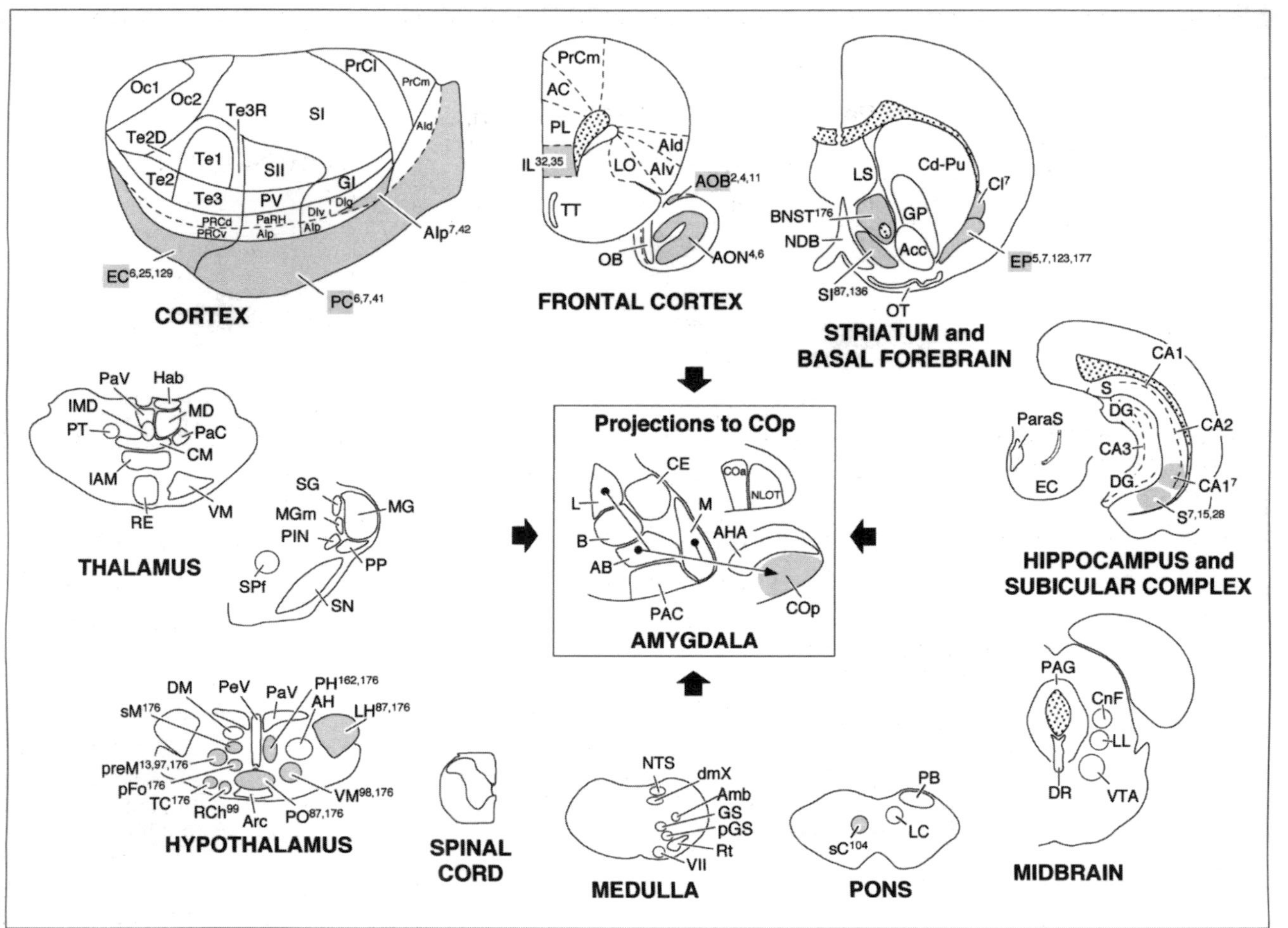

Figure 2.16 Cortical, subcortical, and intra-amygdaloid inputs of the posterior cortical nucleus. See legend to Figure 2.2.

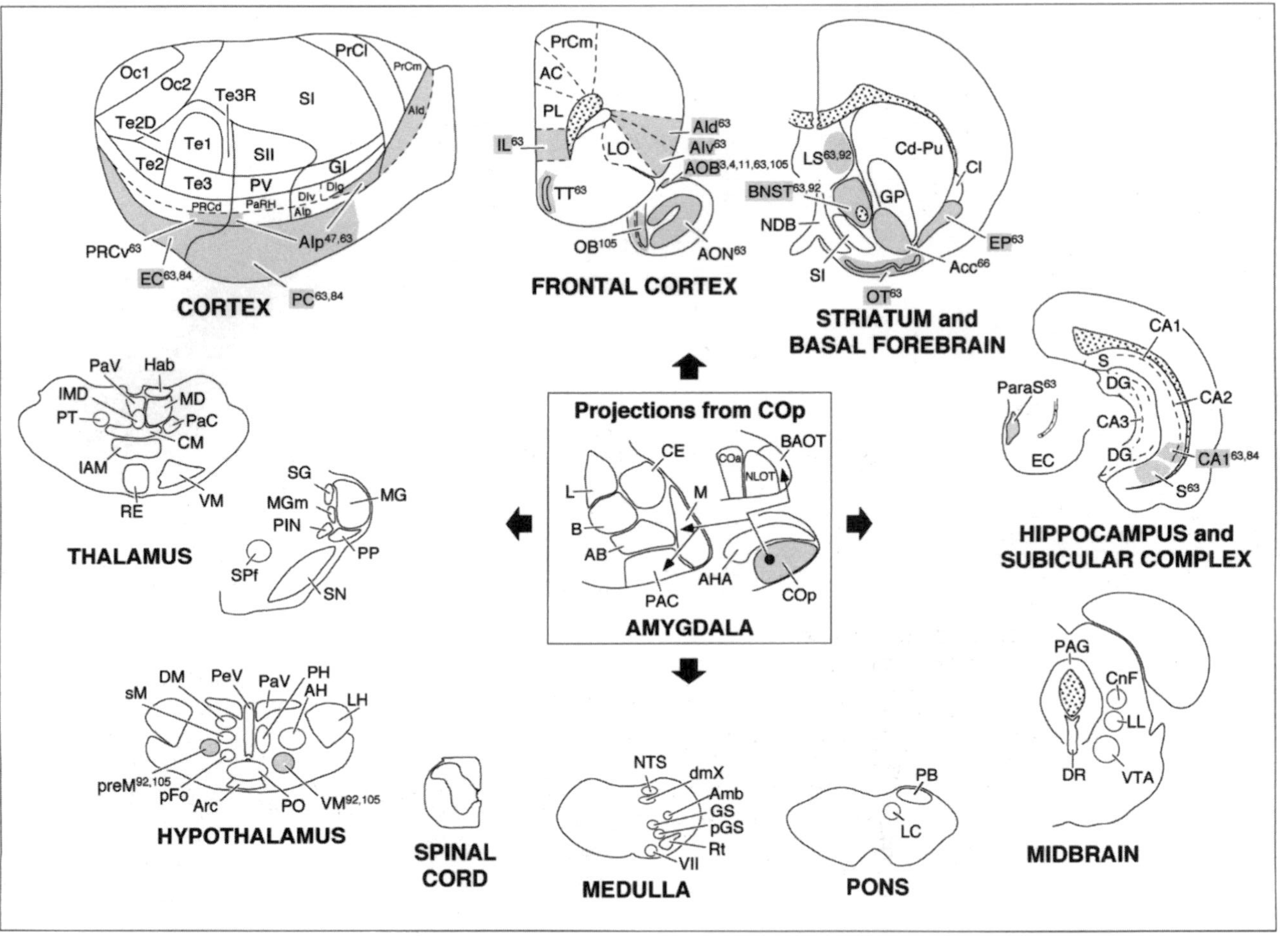

Figure 2.17 Cortical, subcortical, and intra-amygdaloid outputs of the posterior cortical nucleus. See legend to Figure 2.3.

Olfactory system. There are substantial projections to the brain areas processing olfactory information. These include moderate to heavy outputs to the accessory olfactory bulb, olfactory tubercle, endopiriform nucleus, and piriform cortex (Canteras *et al.*, 1992a). Lighter projections terminate in the olfactory bulb, anterior olfactory nucleus, and tenia tecta.

Hypothalamus. There is some evidence that the posterior cortical nucleus projects to the ventromedial and premamillary nuclei of the hypothalamus.

Basal forebrain, striatum, and substantia innominata. The posterior cortical nucleus provides a substantial input to the bed nucleus of the stria terminalis. Lighter projections terminate in the nucleus accumbens, fundus striatum, and lateral septum.

To summarize, the major inputs to the posterior cortical nucleus originate in the olfactory system. The major outputs of the posterior cortical nucleus terminate in the medial temporal lobe memory system, olfactory system, prefrontal cortex, and bed nucleus of stria terminalis.

2.2.11 Amygdalohippocampal area

Location and divisions

The amygdalohippocapal area has two divisions: lateral and medial. The lateral division begins more rostrally by emerging into the space between the medial nucleus dorsally, periamygdaloid cortex ventrally, and the accessory basal nucleus laterally (Figure 2.1). It extends to the caudal end of the amygdala where it lies dorsal to the posterior cortical nucleus.

Intranuclear connections

The lateral division of the amygdalohippocampal area projects heavily to the medial division but not vice versa (Table 2.2).

Intra-amygdaloid connections

The amygdalohippocampal area receives heavy inputs from the lateral nucleus, basal nucleus, accessory basal nucleus, medial nucleus, and bed nucleus of accessory olfactory tract (Figure 2.18, Table 2.2). It provides a substantial input to the medial and central nuclei (Figure 2.19, Table 2.2).

Interamygdaloid connections

The amygdalohippocampal area receives an input from the contralateral posterior cortical nucleus. The amygdalohippocampal area does not provide any substantial contralateral projections (Figure 2.22).

Extra-amygdaloid inputs

Cortical and subcortical inputs to the amygdalohippocampal area are summarized in Figure 2.18.

Temporal, insular, parietal, and frontal cortex. The amygdalohippocampal area does not receive any substantial inputs from the lateral sensory-related cortical areas. Also, projections from the prefrontal cortex are meagre and include only a light input from the infralimbic cortex.

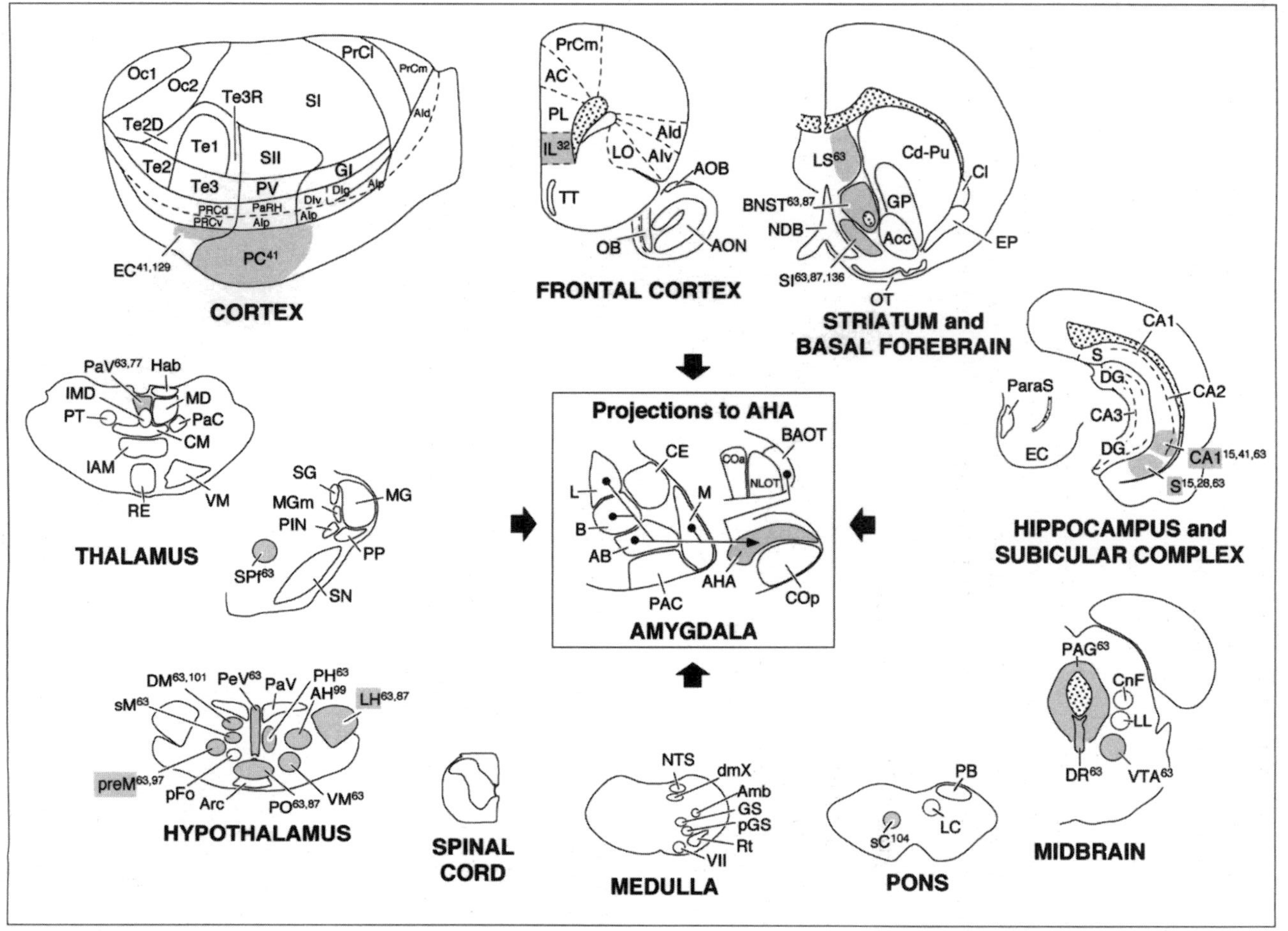

Figure 2.18 Cortical, subcortical, and intra-amygdaloid inputs of the amygdalohippocampal area. See legend to Figure 2.2.

Hippocampal formation. The hippocampal formation, however, provides extensive inputs to the amygdalohippocampal area. A PHA-L study by McDonald and Mascagni (1996) suggests that there is a light projection from the entorhinal cortex to the lateral division of the amygdalohippocampal area. After injecting fluoro-gold into the medial division of the amygdalohippocampal area, Canteras *et al.* (1992a) found substantial labelling in the temporal end of the CA1 subfield and subiculum. Anterograde PHA-L studies have confirmed substantial inputs from the proximal and distal temporal subiculum to the amygdalohippocampal area.

Olfactory system. The retrograde tracer study by Christensen and Fredrickson (1998) suggests that the amygdalohippocampal area receives an olfactory input from the piriform cortex.

Thalamus. Both anterograde and retrograde tracer studies indicate that the paraventricular nucleus of the thalamus projects to the amygdalohippocampal area. In addition, the amygdalohippocampal area receives an input from the subparafascicular nucleus.

Hypothalamus. The medial division of the amygdalohippocampal area receives a heavy input from the ventral premamillary nucleus of the hypothalamus. Retrograde tracer studies also suggest that the projection from the lateral hypothalamic area is substantial. Lighter projections to the amygdalohippocampal area originate in the medial preoptic nucleus, anterior hypothalamic nucleus, ventromedial nucleus, dorsomedial nucleus, periventricular nucleus, posterior hypothalamic nucleus, and supramamillary nucleus.

Basal forebrain, striatum, and bed nucleus of the stria terminalis. Based on the number of retrogradely labelled neurons observed after injecting tracer into the medial division of the amygdalohippocampal area, the substantia innominata, and lateral septum, as well as the bed nucleus of the stria terminalis, it appears that these regions all provide a light to moderate input to the amygdalohippocampal area.

Midbrain, pons, and medulla. The medial division of the amygdalohippocampal area receives light inputs from the periaqueductal grey, ventral tegmental area, and dorsal raphe. Also, the nucleus subcoeruleus projects to the amygdalohippocampal area.

Extra-amygdaloid outputs

Cortical and subcortical outputs of the amygdalohippocampal area are summarized in Figure 2.19.

Temporal, insular, and parietal cortex. Projections from the amygdalohippocampal area to the lateral cortical areas are meagre. Retrograde tracer studies suggest that the projections originate in the lateral aspect of the amygdalohippocampal area and terminate in the anterior portion of the posterior agranular insula (AIp) and perirhinal cortex.

Frontal cortex. The amygdalohippocampal area provides light inputs to the prelimbic and infralimbic regions of the medial prefrontal cortex.

Hippocampal formation. Projections to the hippocampal formation are light and terminate in the entorhinal cortex, as well as in the temporal end of the CA1 subfield and subiculum.

Olfactory system. The amygdalohippocampal area provides light inputs to the olfactory system that terminate in the olfactory tubercle and endopiriform nucleus.

Thalamus. Light inputs from the amygdalohippocampal area to the thalamus terminate in the paraventricular, paratenial, and mediodorsal nuclei.

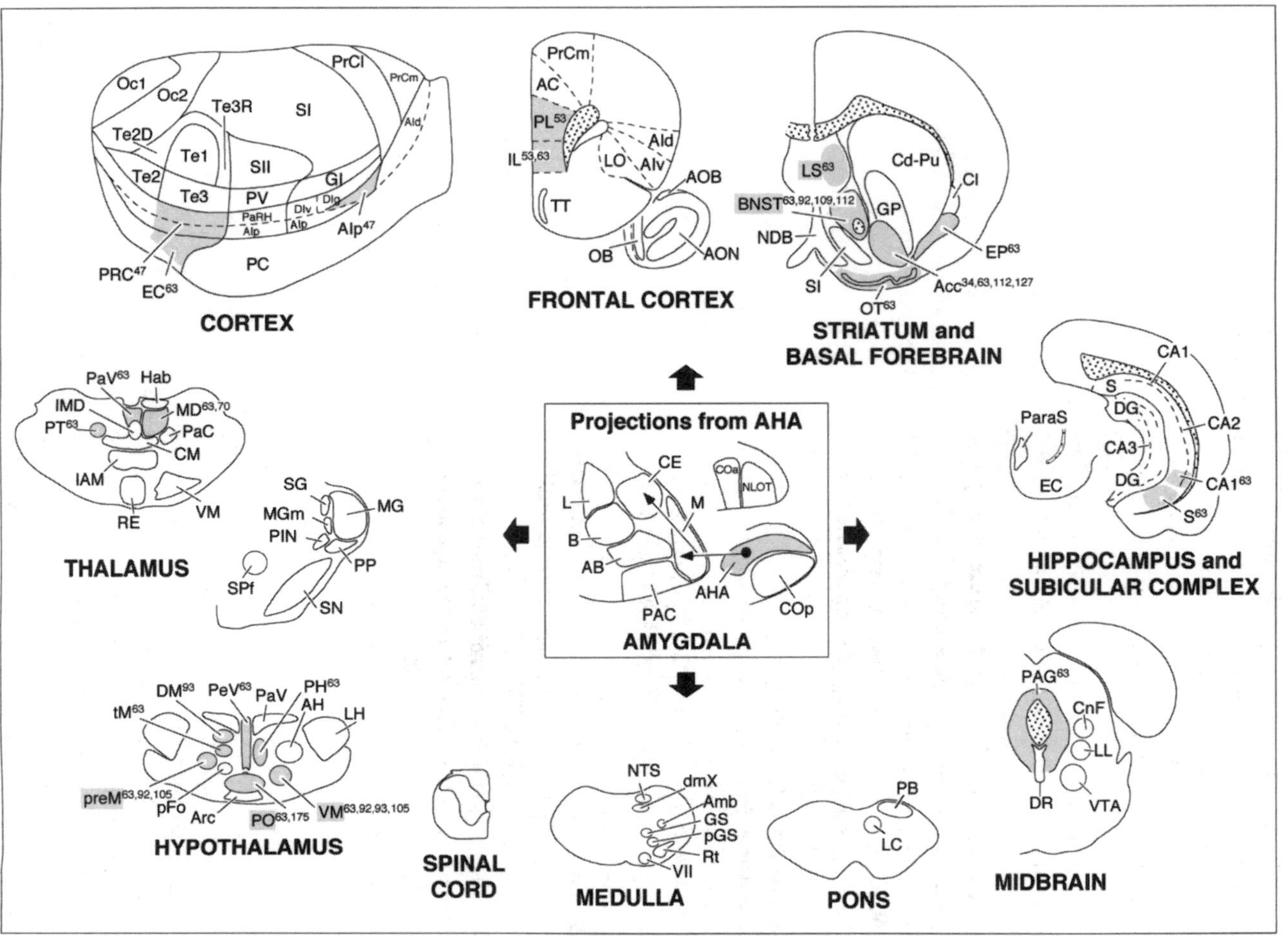

Figure 2.19 Cortical, subcortical, and intra-amygdaloid outputs of the amygdalohippocampal area. See legend to Figure 2.3.

Hypothalamus. The amygdalohippocampal area, particularly the medial division, provides substantial inputs to several hypothalamic nuclei, including the medial preoptic area, ventromedial nucleus, and the premamillary nucleus. Lighter projections terminate in the dorsomedial nucleus, periventricular nucleus, medial mamillary nucleus, tuberomamillary nucleus, and posterior hypothalamic area.

Basal forebrain, striatum, and bed nucleus of the stria terminalis. The amygdalohippocampal area provides a substantial input to the lateral septum. Also, the amygdalohippocampal area projects to the nucleus accumbens. The bed nucleus of the stria terminalis receives a heavy projection.

Midbrain, pons, and medulla. The medial division of the amygdalohippocampal area provides a light input to the rostral periaqueductal grey area.

To summarize, the major inputs to the amygdalohippocampal area originate in the hippocampal formation and hypothalamus. The major outputs of the amygdalohippocampal area terminate in the bed nucleus of stria terminalis and hypothalamus.

2.2.12 Nucleus of the lateral olfactory tract

Location and divisions

The nucleus of the lateral olfactory tract is a three-layered structure that is located in the rostral amygdala, and it is bordered by the anterior cortical nucleus laterally and caudally, and the medial nucleus medially (Figure 2.1).

Intra-amygdaloid connections

The nucleus of the lateral olfactory tract receives a heavy intra-amygdaloid input from the basal nucleus (Figure 2.20, Table 2.2). Data on the efferent intra-amygdaloid connectivity are based on studies with retrograde tracers. These data show that the nucleus of the lateral olfactory tract projects to the basal nucleus, accessory basal nucleus, anterior cortical nucleus, medial nucleus, periamygdaloid cortex, posterior cortical nucleus, and the central nucleus (Table 2.2).

Interamygdaloid connections

The nucleus of the lateral olfactory tract receives an input from the contralateral nucleus of the lateral olfactory tract and basal nucleus. It projects to the contralateral central and medial nuclei, in addition to sending projections to itself (Figure 2.22).

Extra-amygdaloid inputs

Cortical and subcortical inputs to the nucleus of the lateral olfactory tract are summarized in Figure 2.20.

Temporal, insular, and parietal cortex. The posterior agranular insula (AIp) is the only region in the sensory-related lateral cortex that provides an input to the nucleus of the lateral olfactory tract. The projection is moderate in density and terminates primarily in layer 2.

Frontal cortex. In the medial prefrontal cortex, the infralimbic cortex projects lightly to the nucleus of the lateral olfactory tract.

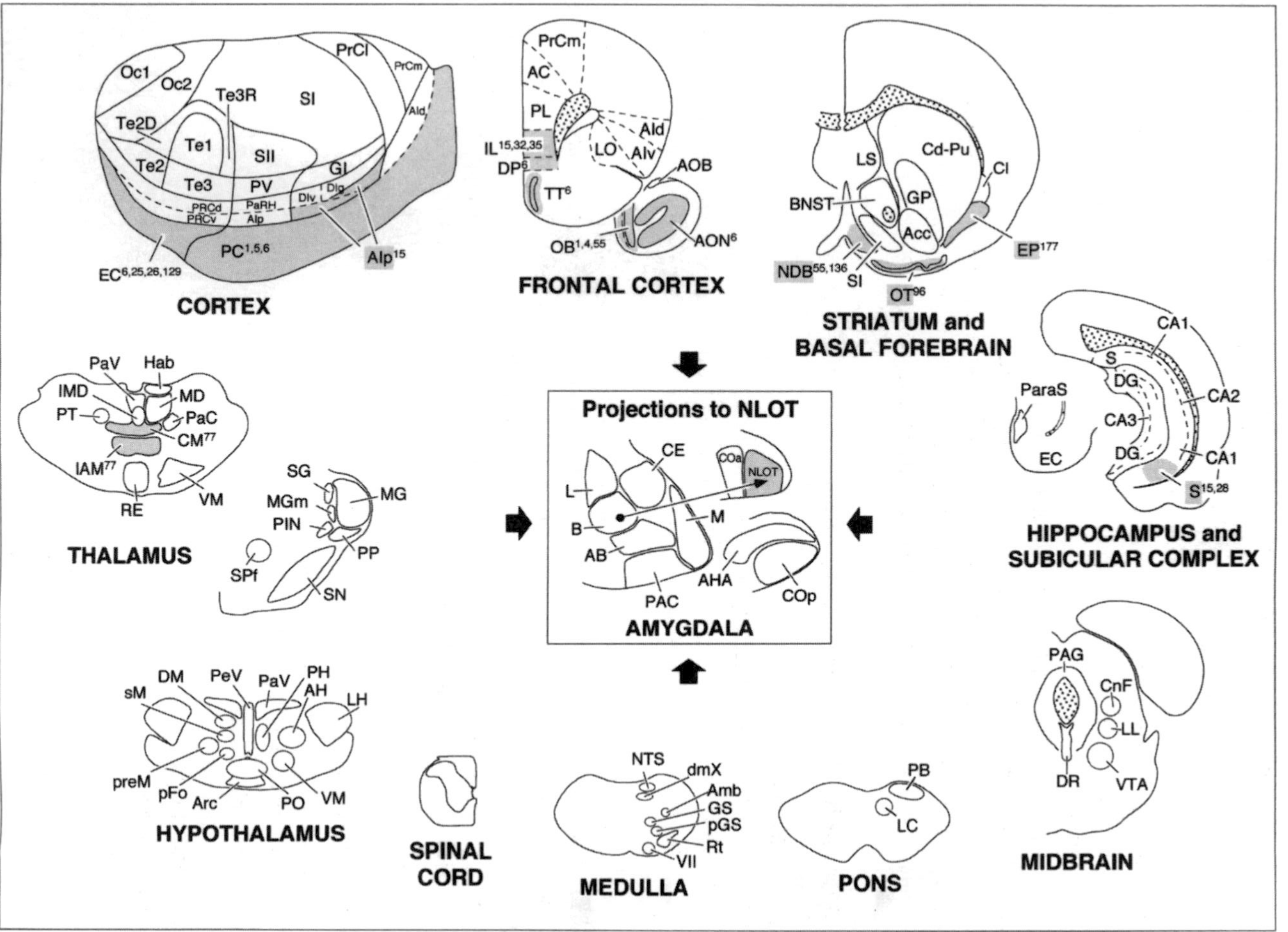

Figure 2.20 Cortical, subcortical, and intra-amygdaloid inputs of the nucleus of the lateral olfactory tract. See legend to Figure 2.2.

Hippocampal formation. The projections from the entorhinal cortex are light, whereas both the proximal and distal aspects of the temporal end of the subiculum provide a moderate input.

Olfactory system. Projections from the olfactory system originate in the olfactory bulb, anterior olfactory nucleus, olfactory tubercle, endopiriform nucleus, dorsal peduncular cortex, tenia tecta, and piriform cortex.

Thalamus. The centromedial and interanteromedial thalamic nuclei are reported to project to the nucleus of the lateral olfactory tract

Basal forebrain, striatum, and bed nucleus of the stria terminalis. The horizontal limb of the nucleus of the diagonal band provides a heavy input to the nucleus of the lateral olfactory tract.

Extra-amygdaloid outputs

Cortical and subcortical outputs of the nucleus of the lateral olfactory tract are summarized in Figure 2.21.

Temporal, insular, and parietal cortex. Layer 3 of the nucleus of the olfactory tract projects to the sensory-related lateral cortical areas including the posterior agranular insula (AIp) and rostral perirhinal cortex.

Frontal cortex. Information about the projections to the prefrontal cortex is based on an injection of radioactive amino acid into the nucleus of the lateral olfactory tract that also lightly involved the anterior cortical nucleus. This injection resulted in labelling in the ventral agranular insula (AIv).

Hippocampal formation. There are some data showing that the nucleus of the lateral olfactory tract projects to the entorhinal cortex (Luskin and Price, 1983a), but this has not been confirmed with specific anterograde tracers.

Olfactory system. Based on radioactive tracer studies, the nucleus of the lateral olfactory tract projects to several levels of the olfactory system including the olfactory bulb, anterior olfactory nucleus, Islands of Calleja within the olfactory tubercle, endopeduncular nucleus, tenia tecta, and piriform cortex.

Thalamus. Injection of a retrograde tracer into the mediodorsal thalamic nucleus results in labelling of scattered cells in the nucleus of the lateral olfactory tract.

Hypothalamus. Injection of anterograde tracer into the nucleus of the lateral olfactory tract results in labelling of the lateral hypothalamic area (Luskin and Price, 1983a). The spread of tracer substance to the neighbouring anterior cortical nucleus, however, might have contributed to this projection.

Basal forebrain, striatum, and bed nucleus of the stria terminalis. A retrograde study by McDonald (1991b) shows that the lateral aspects of the nucleus accumbens and caudate–putamen receive an input from the nucleus of the lateral olfactory tract.

To summarize, the major inputs to the nucleus of the lateral olfactory tract originate in the posterior agranular insula, olfactory tubercle, and subiculum. The major outputs of the nucleus of the lateral olfactory tract terminate in the olfactory system.

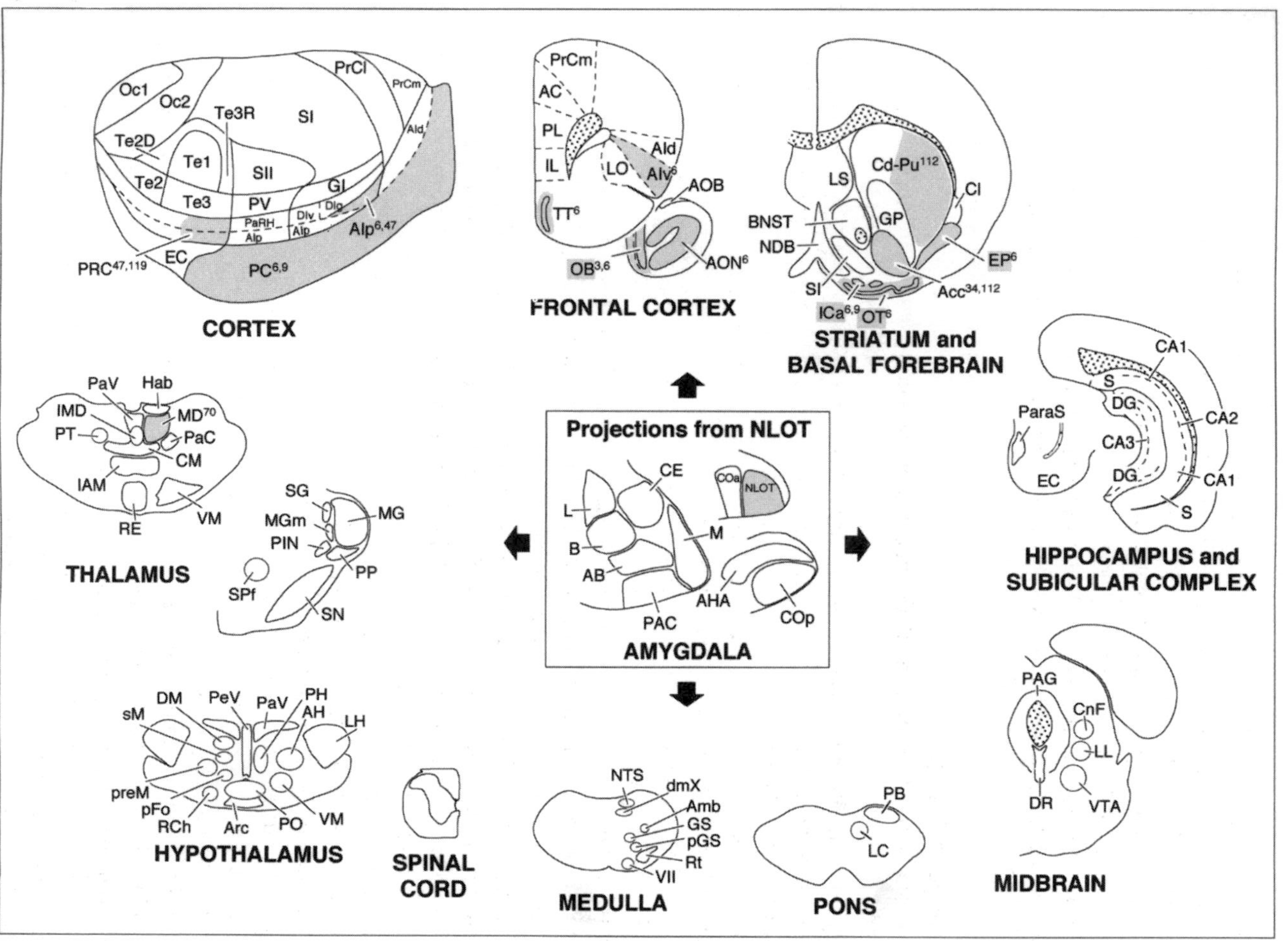

Figure 2.21 Cortical, subcortical, and intra-amygdaloid outputs of the nucleus of the lateral olfactory tract. See legend to Figure 2.3.

2.3 Organization of intra-amygdaloid connections

As has become evident from the previous description of the intra-amygdaloid, afferent, and efferent connections of the various amygdaloid nuclei, the amygdaloid complex is at the interface of information exchange between various functional systems of the brain. The use of sensitive anterograde tracers has provided a tool to obtain an insight into the organization of these connections at the nuclear and divisional level. Data available show that the inputs enter the amygdala via select nuclei or nuclear subdivisions. For example, the projections from many sensory-related cortical areas terminate in the lateral nucleus, and the inputs from the brainstem autonomic centres in the central nucleus. From the input nucleus or division, the information may be distributed to other divisions of the same nucleus by intranuclear connections or to other locations within the amygdala by intra-amygdaloid projections. Finally, the amygdaloid outputs convey the information to other functional systems in the brain such as the temporal lobe memory system, autonomic centres in the brainstem, or the motor system (for a schematic presentation, see Figure 2.27). We will begin the description of the principles of the organization of the amygdaloid pathways by summarizing the organization of intra-amygdaloid connections.

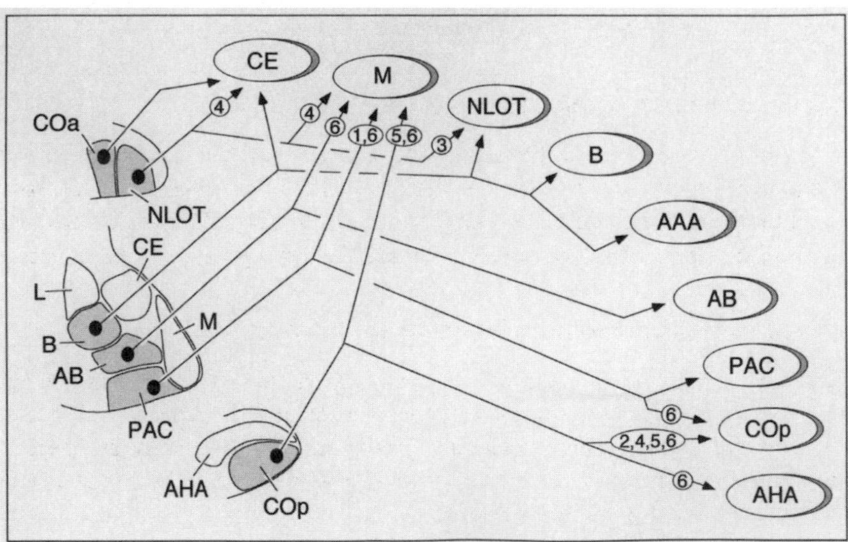

Figure 2.22 Contralateral projections of the amygdala. Data were taken from Savander *et al.* (1997c) and from other references, which are indicated with numbers: [1]Canteras *et al.* (1992a); [2]Krettek and Price (1978b); [3]Luskin and Price (1983a); [4]Nitecka *et al.* (1981b); [5]Ottersen (1982); [6]Christensen and Frederickson (1998). Abbreviations are listed in Table 2.1.

2.3.1 Three levels of intra-amygdaloid connectivity

After entering the amygdala, information can travel to other locations within the amygdala via intra-amygdala connections (Figures 2.2–2.21, Table 2.2). These local pathways have three different levels: intradivisional connections transfer information within a subdivision. For example, the rostral portion of the magnocellular division of the basal nucleus is heavily connected with other portions in that division. Interdivisional connections are links between regions of a particular nucleus. For example, the lateral division of the central nucleus projects to the capsular and medial divisions of the central nucleus. Internuclear pathways connect various amygdaloid nuclei with each other.

2.3.2 Parallel distribution of information within the amygdala

Typically, each amygdaloid nucleus or even a nuclear division gives rise to more than one projection that terminates in different locations of the amygdala. For example, the lateral nucleus, which provides the most substantial intra-amygdala connections, innervates the basal nucleus, the accessory basal nucleus, the medial nucleus, the amygdalohippocampal area, the central nucleus, the posterior cortical nucleus, and the periamygdaloid cortex. Via these different intra-amygdala connections, information entering one nucleus of the amygdala might have representations in various locations within the amygdala and, consequently, become associated with inputs entering these areas from other functional systems of the brain. It is noteworthy that projections originating in different amygdaloid nuclei or nuclear divisions terminate largely in a non-overlapping fashion, which suggests that the intra-amygdaloid connections are organized typically in a point-to-point manner.

2.3.3 Reciprocal intra-amygdala connections

Many of the intra-amygdala connections are reciprocal. For example, most of the amygdaloid nuclei that receive input from the lateral nucleus (e.g. the basal nucleus, the accessory basal nucleus, and the periamygdaloid cortex) project back to the lateral nucleus. These pathways might provide routes by which target neurons regulate the responsiveness of their input regions.

2.3.4 Convergence of intra-amygdala connections in select regions

There are a few nuclei, such as the central nucleus and the amygdalohippocampal area, that receive convergent inputs from several amygdala nuclei but the inputs back to the other amygdala areas are meagre. These nuclei are presumed to act primarily as output stations from the amygdala to other brain regions, to evoke appropriate behavioural responses to stimuli entering via the amygdala.

2.4 Convergence of afferent inputs in the amygdala

The amygdaloid complex receives information from a wide variety of cortical and subcortical areas. How is the information flow to and within the amygdala organized? Recent anterograde tracing data suggest that convergence of information from various functional systems occurs within the amygdaloid complex at three different levels: (i) within the nuclear division; (ii) within the nucleus; or (iii) within the amygdala.

2.4.1 Intradivisional convergence

Tracing of amygdalopetal pathways anterogradely using PHA-L, biocytin, or BDA demonstrates that the inputs from various sources might terminate in the same nuclear division. For example, the dorsolateral division of the lateral nucleus receives information monosynaptically from the gustatory, visceral, somatosensory, auditory, and visual cortical areas (Shi and Cassell, 1997, 1998a,b, 1999; McDonald, 1998). These projections are organized topographically (Figure 2.23A). Projections from the auditory and visual cortices terminate in more caudal portions of the dorsolateral division than do the gustatory, visceral, or somatosensory inputs. Rostrocaudal topography is also apparent in the distribution of projections terminating in the medial division of the lateral nucleus. Some inputs, however, appear to innervate the entire rostrocaudal extent of the division, such as the pathway from the rostral portion of the dorsal perirhinal cortex to the medial division of the lateral nucleus (Shi and Cassell, 1999). In the magnocellular and parvicellular divisions of the basal nucleus, many inputs respect the mediolateral topography (Figue 2.23B). These data suggest that (i) the information entering the amygdala from various sources converges on the same target neuron or the same group of target neurons at the site of the termination of projections, or (ii) some inputs terminating in the different parts of the same nuclear division remain segregated initially. In these cases, the intradivisional connections might provide a pathway for intradivisional convergence.

2.4.2 Intranuclear convergence

Inputs from various functional systems terminate in some division(s) preferentially over others within an amygdaloid nucleus and, therefore, different nuclear divisions are exposed to a different set of incoming information (Figure 2.24). For example, the central nucleus receives inputs from the sensory-related lateral cortical areas that terminate largely in the capsular and lateral divisions. Projections from the medial temporal lobe memory system (subiculum and entorhinal cortex) project preferentially to the capsular and medial divisions. Heavy inputs from the brainstem autonomic nuclei terminate in the lateral or medial divisions. The hypothalamic endocrine centres project to the capsular and medial divisions. Projections from the other amygdaloid nuclei terminate in the capsular and medial divisions (Figure 2.24C). The interdivisional projections provide a route by which the various kinds of information entering the different portions of the nucleus can become associated.

One amygdaloid nucleus can be the site of convergence for information from different levels of the same functional system (Figures 2.24 and 2.25). For example, the lateral nucleus receives afferents from the auditory thalamus (dorsolateral division of the lateral nucleus), auditory-related cortical areas (dorsolateral and medial divisions), as well as from the polymodal perirhinal cortex (medial division) (Figure 2.24A). The basal nucleus, however, receives information from various levels of the hippocampal formation, including the CA1 subfield,

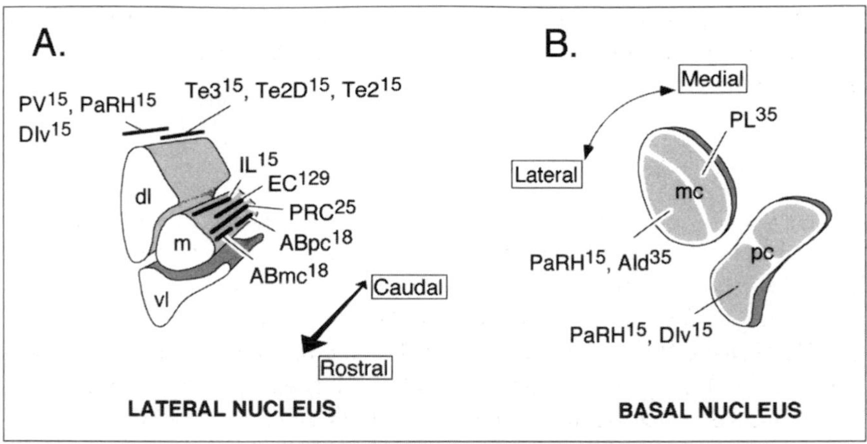

Figure 2.23 Convergence of afferent inputs within the amygdala: intradivisional level. Note that the same division might receive inputs from various sources. The projection fields of different inputs might overlap or terminate in different portions of the same division. In the latter case, the intradivisional projections might provide a route for the association of various kinds of information. (**A**) Auditory (Te3 and Te2D) and visual (Te2) areas innervate more caudal aspects of the dorsolateral division of the lateral nucleus than the visceral (DIv)- and somatosensory (PV, PaRH)-related areas. In the medial division, the projections from the infralimbic cortex (IL) and perirhinal cortex (PRC) terminate throughout most of the rostrocaudal extent of the division. The projections from the entorhinal cortex (EC) innervate the more caudal aspects of the medial division. Intra-amygdaloid inputs from the magnocellular (ABmc) and parvicellular (ABpc) divisions of the accessory basal nucleus terminate in the rostral and caudal parts, respectively. (**B**) Many projections terminating in the basal nucleus respect the mediolateral topography. For example, inputs from the parietal rhinal cortex (PaRH) and dorsal agranular insula (AId) innervate the lateral aspects of the magnocellular division, and inputs from the prelimbic cortex (PL) and visual area Te2 innervate the medial aspect. In the parvicellular division, projections from the parietal rhinal area and visceral dysgranular insula (DIv) terminate in its lateral aspects, and projections from the paratenial thalamic nucleus terminate in the medial aspects. The number after the abbreviation refers to the reference (Table 2.3) demonstrating the topography of that particular projection.

subiculum (magnocellular division), and the entorhinal cortex (parvicellular division) (Figure 2.24B). The functional significance of the convergence of information from the various levels of the same functional system remains to be explored.

2.4.3 Intra-amygdaloid convergence

Even though recent detailed analyses of amygdaloid connectivity indicate that a certain nucleus or even a division receives information from different functional systems, it is apparent that

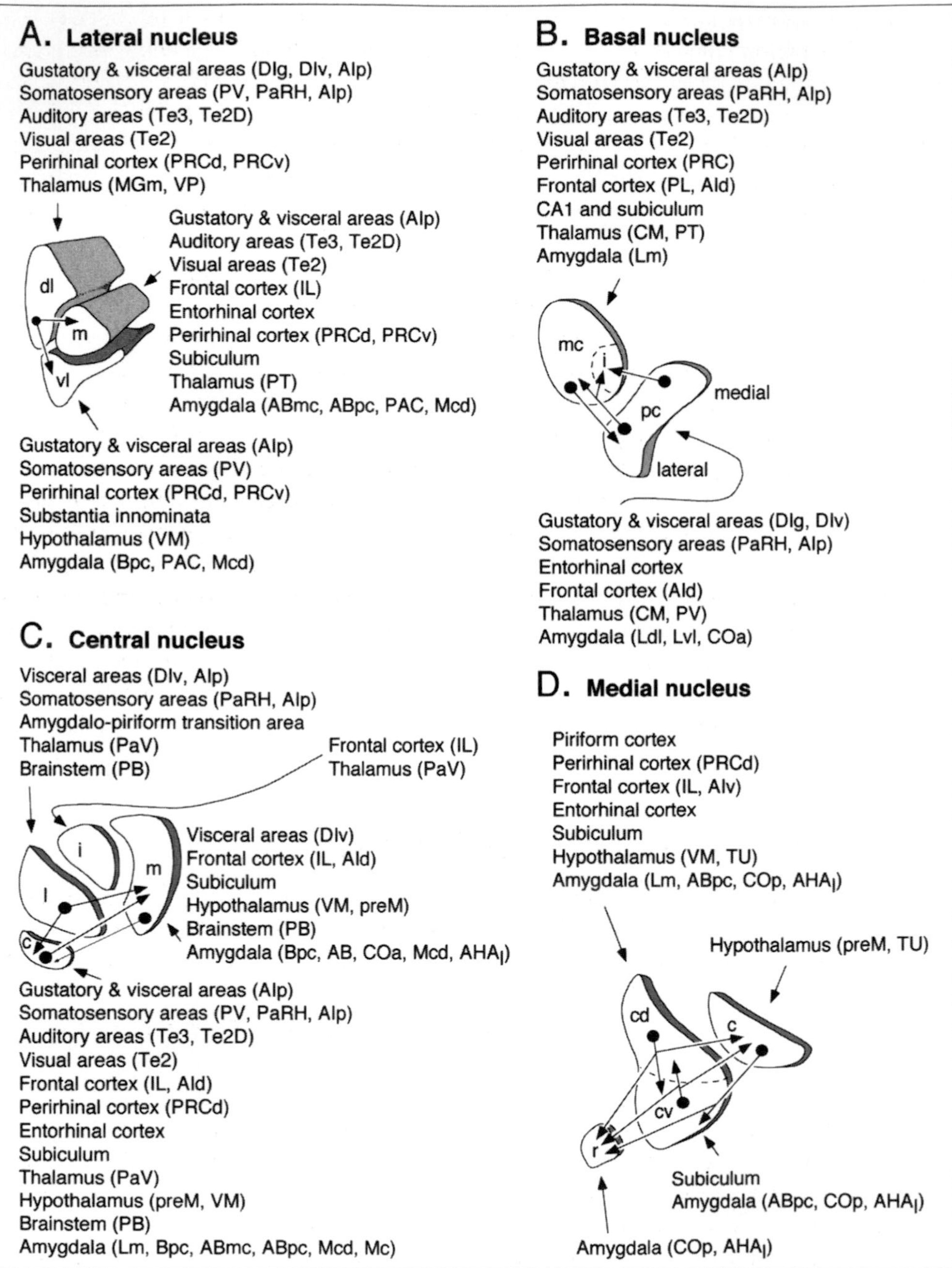

Figure 2.24 Convergence of afferent inputs within the amygdala: intranuclear and intra-amygdaloid level. Examples are presented from the (**A**) lateral nucleus (dl, dorsolateral division; vl, ventrolateral division; m, medial division), (**B**) basal nucleus (mc, magnocellular division; i, intermediate division; pc, parvicellular division), (**C**) central nucleus (c, capsular

there are major differences in the afferent connectivity between the amygdaloid nuclei. The sensory-related information from cortical areas terminates largely in the lateral, basal, accessory basal, central, and anterior cortical nuclei, as well as in the periamygdaloid cortex. The hippocampal formation innervates the lateral, basal, accessory basal, and central nuclei most extensively (Figure 2.25). The largest number of thalamic inputs terminate in the lateral, basal, central, anterior cortical, and medial nuclei. The hypothalamus innervates the central and medial nuclei most extensively, as well as the posterior cortical nucleus and the amygdalo-hippocampal area. Inputs from the bed nucleus of the stria terminalis terminate in the central and medial nuclei. Many of the projections from the midbrain, pons, medulla, and spinal cord, however, terminate almost exclusively in the central nucleus. Therefore, it is likely that the internuclear projections provide a route by which the inputs originating in various major functional systems and terminating in various amygdaloid locations become associated.

The lateral, basal, accessory basal, and medial nuclei appear to provide the largest number of moderate to heavy intra-amygdaloid projections, which suggests that the information directed to these amygdaloid nuclei from the sensory-related lateral cortical areas, frontal cortex, basal forebrain, bed nucleus of the stria terminalis, and hypothalamus becomes distributed efficiently via parallel pathways to different locations within the amygdala. On the other hand, the central nucleus does not provide any major intra-amygdaloid projections, which suggests that the autonomic modulation of intra-amygdaloid information processing is concentrated largely in the central nucleus. Furthermore, this suggests that the association of brainstem information occurs at the late phase of the temporal sequence of the events, during which the information has been travelling within the amygdaloid circuitries and has become modulated by information from various functional systems before leaving the amygdala from the central nucleus.

2.5 Parallel innervation of amygdaloid nuclei

In addition to convergence, parallel distribution of information from the same source to various amygdaloid areas is another typical feature in the organization of amygdaloid inputs. This is typical of cortical afferents, whereas the brainstem or hypothalamic inputs heavily innervate a smaller number of amygdaloid nuclei.

The intranuclear and intra-amygdaloid levels can be separated. An example of parallel distribution of afferent terminals into various divisions of the same nucleus (intranuclear

---

division; l, lateral division; i, intermediate division; m, medial division), and (**D**) medial nucleus (r, rostral division; cd, dorsal part of central division; cv, ventral part of central division; c, caudal division). Note that inputs from various brain areas might terminate in different divisions within the same nucleus. Interdivisional pathways (indicated with arrows) provide a route by which information entering one division might become associated with information in another division of the nucleus. Otherwise, projections might also terminate in the different amygdaloid nuclei (e.g. projections from the posterior agranular insula to the lateral, basal, and central nucleus) and become associated via internuclear projections. For abbreviations, see Tables 2.1 and 2.4.

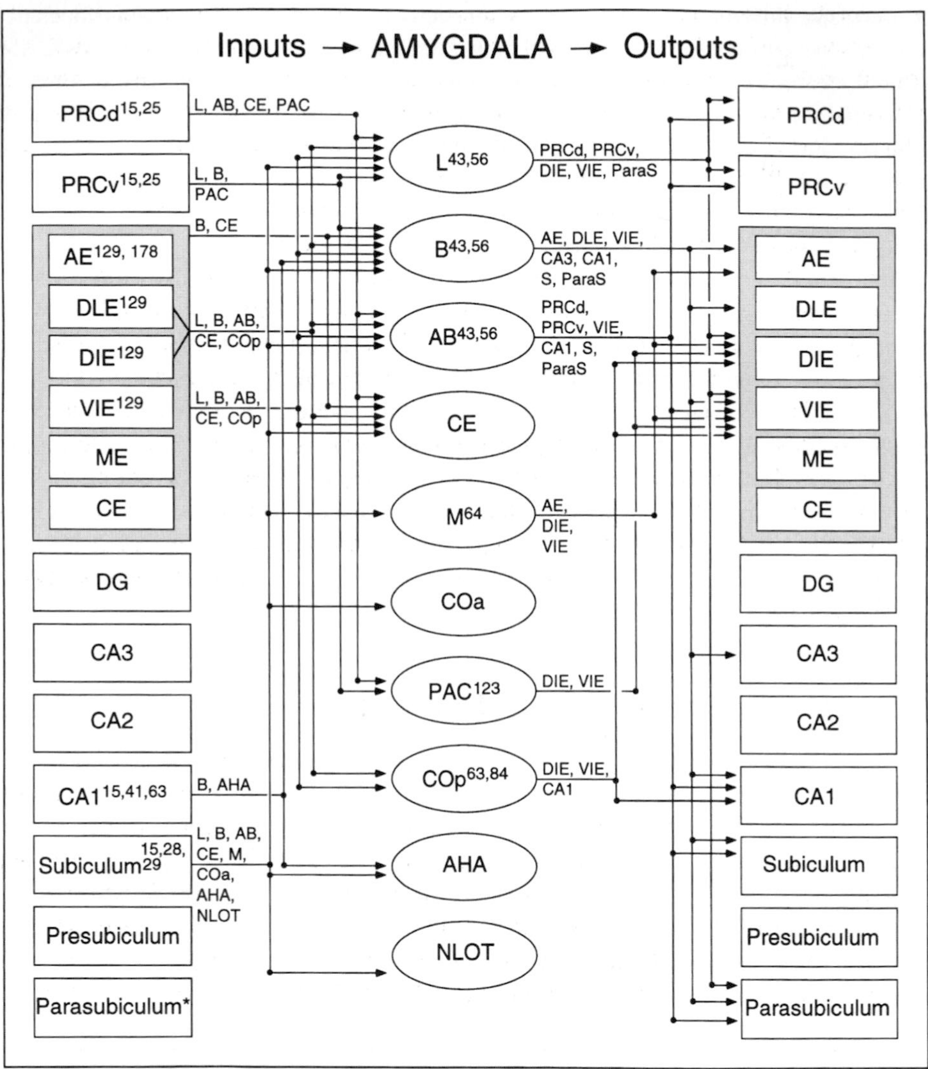

Figure 2.25 Parallel inputs and outputs of the amygdaloid complex with the medial temporal lobe memory system. The schematic figure shows the distribution of projections from the hippocampal formation and the perirhinal cortex (on the left) to the different nuclei of the amygdaloid complex (middle). Projections of the amygdaloid nuclei back to the medial temporal lobe memory system are shown on the right. Only the projections that are moderate to heavy in density are included in the drawing. Note (i) that different regions of the medial temporal lobe memory system project to the amygdaloid complex in parallel. (ii) One region might provide parallel inputs to several amygdaloid nuclei. (iii) Projections from different areas might (a) converge in the same amygdaloid nucleus or (b) remain segregated by terminating in the different amygdaloid nuclei. (iv) The amygdaloid nuclei receiving converging

level) is the projection from the dorsal bank of the perirhinal cortex to all divisions of the lateral nucleus (Shi and Cassell, 1999). At the intra-amygdaloid level, for example, the entorhinal cortex (or even one entorhinal cortex subfield) can innervate the lateral, basal, accessory basal, central, and anterior cortical nuclei, as well as the nucleus of the lateral olfactory tract (Figure 2.25). It is not known whether the parallel inputs represent axon collaterals of the same neuron or whether they come from different neuronal populations. This information, however, is of importance when trying to predict the functional consequences of damage to various amygdaloid nuclei, as will be discussed later.

At the system level, a third class of parallel innervation of the amygdala is observed, i.e. various components of the same functional system (neuronal chain) project to the amygdala. These projections might terminate in the same or different amygdaloid nuclei. For example, inputs from the different levels of the auditory system terminate in the lateral nucleus. The medial part of the medial geniculate nucleus and the posterior intralaminar nucleus project to the dorsolateral division, the auditory-related cortical areas Te2D and Te3 also project to the dorsolateral division, and the dorsal bank of the polymodal perirhinal cortex innervates all divisions of the lateral nucleus. Projections from the medial temporal lobe memory system represent an example where different components of the functional system innervate the amygdala via parallel pathways that terminate either in the same or different amygdaloid nuclei (Figure 2.25).

2.6 Organization of amygdaloid outputs

A first look at the connectivity maps (Figures 2.2–2.21) suggests that there are fewer outputs than inputs in the rat amygdaloid complex. This might relate partially to the amount of data available on amygdaloid efferents obtained by newer anterograde tracing techniques, such as PHA-L or biocytin. Currently, results of comprehensive studies using these techniques are available regarding the outputs of the anterior cortical nucleus (layer 3, which is called the 'anterior part of the basomedial nucleus' by Petrovich *et al.*, 1996), accessory basal nucleus (Petrovich *et al.*, 1996), medial nucleus (Canteras *et al.*, 1995), lateral division of the central nucleus (Petrovich and Swanson, 1997), and from the medial division of the

---

inputs from most of the components of the memory system include the basal, lateral, accessory basal, and central nuclei. (v) Different amygdaloid nuclei provide parallel outputs to different areas of the medial temporal lobe memory system. (vi) One amygdaloid nucleus might innervate different areas of the medial temporal lobe memory system. (vii) The amygdaloid outputs might (a) converge in the same area of the medial temporal lobe memory system or (b) remain segregated. (viii) The areas in the medial temporal lobe memory system in which most of the amygdaloid inputs converge are the rostrolateral aspects of the entorhinal cortex, CA1, subiculum, and parasubiculum. The parasubiculum (asterisk), which is one of the main input regions for the amygdaloid projections, does not provide any substantial projections back to the amygdala (T. Van Groen, personal communication). Superscript numbers are citations to the reference database in Table 2.3. For abbreviations, see Tables 2.1 and 2.4.

amygdalohippocampal area and posterior cortical nucleus (Canteras and Swanson, 1992). As a matter of fact, these nuclei appear to have the most widespread projections to the other brain areas. Therefore, the picture of the connectivity of the amygdaloid outputs might need to be revised after more detailed information becomes available. Based on the data gathered to date, certain principles are apparent in the organization of information outflow from the amygdala that might predict some important aspects of the functional organization of the amygdaloid complex.

2.6.1 Amygdaloid outputs are organized in a point-to-point manner

Projections originating (i) in different divisions of the same nucleus or (ii) in various amygdaloid nuclei appear to terminate in a non-overlapping manner even if they target the same brain area. For example, projections from the different divisions of the medial nucleus to the ventromedial nucleus of the hypothalamus largely innervate different regions of the nucleus (Canteras *et al.*, 1995). Thus, projections from the rostral division of the medial nucleus (anteroventral part of the medial nucleus according to Canteras *et al.*, 1995) terminate most heavily in the central and dorsomedial aspects of the ventromedial nucleus. Projections from the dorsal part of the central division (anterodorsal medial nucleus) terminate in the capsule of the ventromedial nucleus; projections from the ventral part of the central division (posteroventral medial nucleus) terminate both in the capsule and in the dorsomedial and central parts of the ventromedial nucleus; and, finally, projections from the caudal division (posterodorsal medial nucleus) terminate in the capsule surrounding the central and ventrolateral parts of the ventromedial nucleus.

Also, various amygdaloid nuclei might project to the same target area but they appear to terminate in non-overlapping parts in the target area. For example, the medial division of the lateral nucleus projects heavily to the VIE subfield of the entorhinal cortex, as does the parvicellular division of the accessory basal nucleus, but the projections terminate in different layers (layers 3 and 5, respectively) (Pikkarainen *et al.*, 1998). Both the central and medial nuclei project heavily to the paraventricular nucleus of the hypothalamus, but inputs from the central nucleus terminate more caudally than those from the medial nucleus (Gray *et al.*, 1989). These observations suggest that, like the intra-amygdaloid projections, the outputs from the amygdala to other brain areas are also organized in a point-to-point manner.

2.6.2 Amygdaloid nuclei provide parallel outputs to multiple functional systems

Anterograde tracer studies indicate that one nuclear division might project to several functional systems (Figure 2.26). For example, the parvicellular division of the accessory basal nucleus projects within the amygdala (to the lateral, medial, posterior cortical, and central nuclei as well as to the amygdalohippocampal area; Table 2.2) and to the ventromedial nucleus of the hypothalamus, sensory-related cortical areas, such as area 35 of the perirhinal cortex or the VIE subfield of the entorhinal cortex, and to the infralimbic cortex in the medial prefrontal area (Petrovich *et al.*, 1996; Savander *et al.*, 1997a). Whether the same neuron provides axon collaterals to all different target areas or whether they originate from different populations of neurons is not known. There is, however, evidence that the same amygdaloid neuron projects to different brain areas. McDonald (1991a) demonstrated that injection of retrograde tracers to both the prefrontal cortex and the striatum results in double-labelled neurons in the magnocellular and the parvicellular divisions of the basal nucleus.

When the various amygdaloid nuclei are compared with each other, it appears that they differ, first, in the number of functional systems they influence and, secondly, in the type of functional systems to which they project (Figure 2.26). For example, outputs from the lateral nucleus terminate largely in the cortical areas. The accessory basal nucleus provides substantial inputs to the frontal and temporal cortical areas, nucleus accumbens, caudate-putamen, hippocampal formation, and hypothalamus. In the other extreme, the central nucleus innervates primarily only the midbrain/pons/medulla and the hypothalamus. Considering the fact that each of the amygdaloid nuclei receives a large set of incoming information either monosynaptically or via intra-amygdaloid pathways, the pattern of outputs originating in each nucleus (or nuclear division) might actually contribute more to the functional identity of each amygdaloid nucleus (or nuclear division) than the spectrum of inputs it receives. This generates an interesting scenario when considering the functional consequences of nucleus-specific damage in various neurological and psychiatric diseases, as discussed below.

2.6.3 Parallel outputs from various amygdaloid nuclei to the same functional system

It is also of interest that different components of the functional system might receive parallel inputs from various amygdaloid regions. One system investigated in detail is the hippocampal formation (Figure 2.25). The entorhinal cortex receives moderate to heavy inputs from the lateral nucleus, basal nucleus, accessory basal nucleus, medial nucleus, periamygdaloid cortex, and posterior cortical nucleus. The CA1 subfield of the hippocampus is innervated by the basal nucleus, accessory basal nucleus, and posterior cortical nucleus. The subiculum receives substantial inputs from the basal nucleus and accessory basal nucleus, and the parasubiculum receives substantial inputs from the lateral, basal, and accessory basal nuclei. Even though the projections appear to terminate in different layers of the target area, there appears to be a convergence of information from various amygdaloid nuclei in the entorhinal cortex, CA1 subfield, and subiculum. These parallel outputs provide an anatomical basis for the idea that the colouring of emotional memories depends on the activity of individual inputs carrying different kinds of information regarding the internal or external states of the subject at the time of encoding.

Taken together (Figure 2.27), the information coming from a certain brain area may enter the amygdala via one or more amygdaloid nuclei or nuclear divisions. Thereafter, it may become processed within the input region or it may be delivered into one or more amygdaloid regions via intra-amygdaloid circuitries, and, consequently, be modulated in parallel in several amygdaloid locations. Because the projections from many amygdaloid nuclei converge in selective amygdaloid output regions, the behavioural response within one output

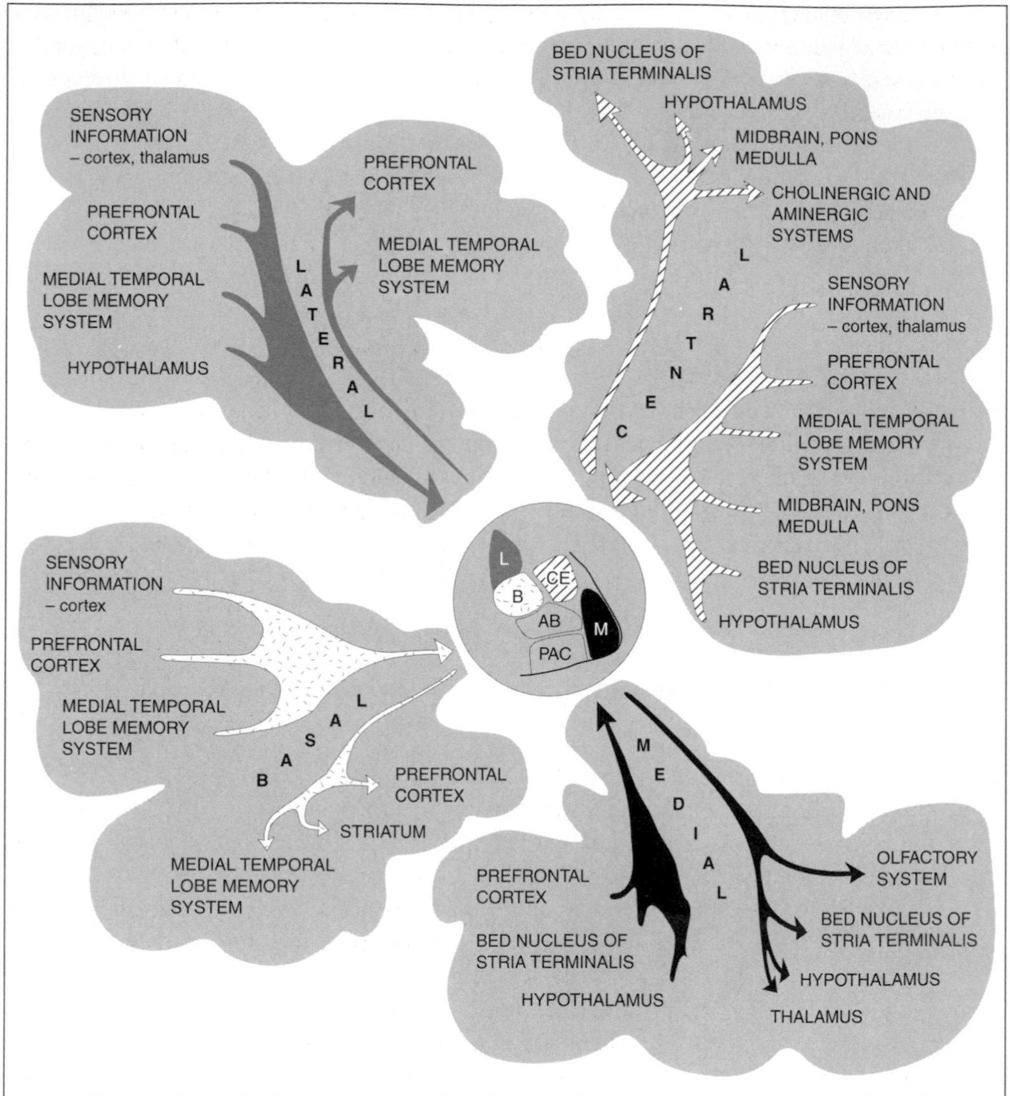

Figure 2.26 Each amygdaloid nucleus is connected to a unique set of other brain areas. In particular, the various amygdaloid nuclei differ in the number and type of functional systems which they influence. For example, outputs from the lateral nucleus terminate largely in the cortical areas. The basal nucleus provides substantial inputs to the frontal cortex, medial temporal lobe memory system, nucleus accumbens, and caudate–putamen. The medial nucleus innervates the prefrontal cortex, bed nucleus of stria terminalis, and hypothalamus. The central nucleus projects to the midbrain/pons/medulla, bed nucleus of stria terminalis, hypothalamus, and ascending cholinergic and aminergic systems. Considering the fact that each of the amygdaloid nuclei receives a large set of incoming information either

station might be the sum of the modulated signal representations. It appears that the same stimulus might activate several output stations which presumably provide the anatomical basis for the expression of different kinds of nuances in the spectrum of responses to emotionally significant stimuli.

2.7 Knock-out of amygdaloid nuclei in brain diseases: what does the anatomy predict about the functional consequences?

The nuclear specificity of amygdaloid damage in brain diseases has received some attention. For example, after status epilepticus or in patients with drug-refractory temporal lobe epilepsy, the medial division of the lateral nucleus and the parvicellular division of the basal nucleus are the most damaged regions, whereas the central nucleus remains rather intact (for a review, see Pitkänen *et al.*, 1998). Similarly, in experimental animal models of status epilepticus induced by electrical stimulation or kainic acid, the amygdaloid damage is nucleus specific. The most easily damaged regions are the medial division of the lateral nucleus, layer 3 of the anterior cortical nucleus, the deep portion of the ventral part of the central divisions of the medial nucleus, the parvicellular division of the basal nucleus, and the accessory basal nucleus. The dorsolateral division of the lateral nucleus, magnocellular division of the basal nucleus, central nucleus, and caudal division of the medial nucleus, however, remain relatively well preserved (Tuunanen *et al.*, 1996). Therefore, many of the cortical input regions, such as the dorsolateral division of the lateral nucleus or the capsular and lateral divisions of the central nucleus, remain preserved in an otherwise heavily damaged epileptic amygdala. Also, many outputs are intact, such as the projections from the magnocellular division of the basal nucleus to the nucleus accumbens and caudate–putamen or the projections from the central nucleus to the hypothalamus and brainstem.

Lesioning of the lateral and basal nuclei in rats impairs conditioning for auditory and contextual cues when the duration of the freezing response is used as a measure (see LeDoux, 1992). A recent study by Vazdarjanova and McGaugh (1998) demonstrates, however, that rats with bilateral excitotoxic lesions to the amygdala (involving the lateral, basal, and accessory basal nuclei, and sparing the central nucleus) retain memory for contextual fear conditioning even though their freezing response is reduced. These observations suggest that epileptic rats with substantial damage in the lateral and basal nuclei would have an impaired freezing response to sensory and contextual cues. Preliminary data on animals with status epilepticus indicate that rats perform poorly in a contextual fear-conditioning task, but perform relatively well in conditioning to a tone when freezing is used as a measure (Nissinen *et al.*, 1998). One idea to be explored further as an explanation of these data is that the nuclei that

---

monosynaptically or via intra-amygdaloid pathways, the pattern of outputs originating in each nucleus might actually contribute more to the functional identity to each amygdaloid nucleus than the spectrum of inputs it receives. For abbreviations, see Table 2.1.

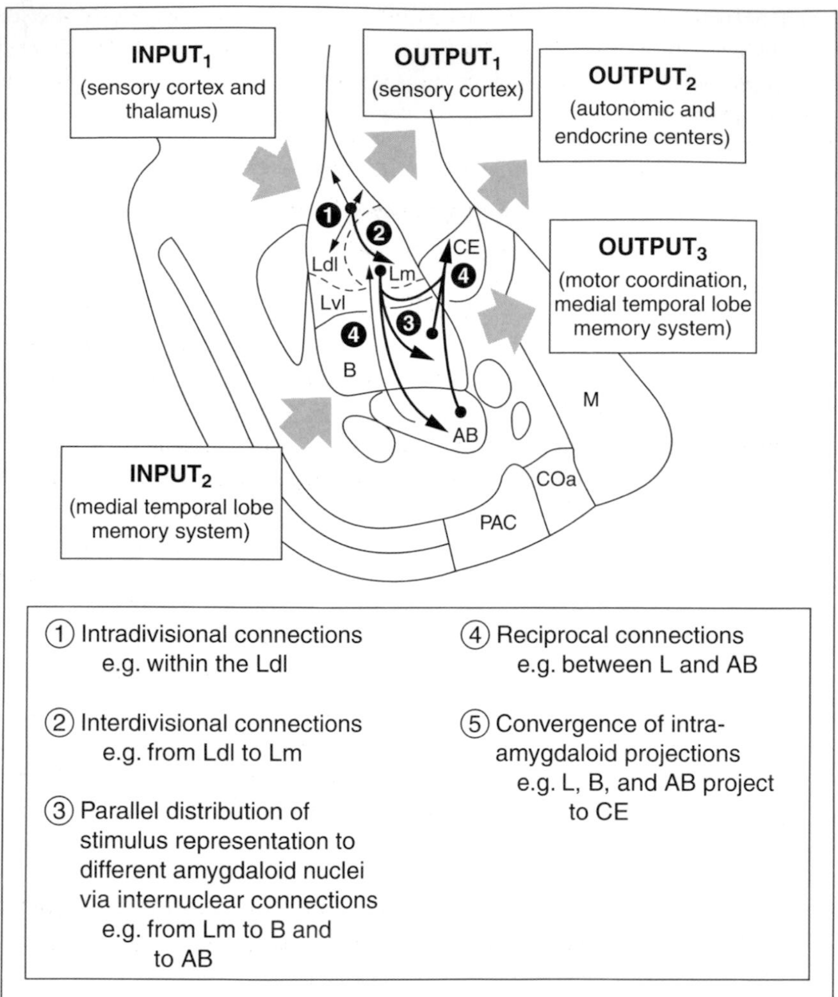

Figure 2.27 Summary of information processing within the intra-amygdaloid circuitries. There are three levels of intra-amygdaloid connectivity: intradivisional, interdivisional, and internuclear. When signals (input1 and input2) enter the amygdaloid complex, they become subject to the intradivisional (e.g. within the dorsolateral division of the lateral nucleus) and interdivisional (e.g. between the dorsolateral division and the medial division of the lateral nucleus) processing that probably determines whether the signal will be distributed to the other amygdaloid nuclei via internuclear connections (e.g. from the lateral nucleus to the basal nucleus). If the intra-amygdaloid projection neurons in a given nucleus elicit action potentials, the signal will have several representations (e.g. information initially represented in the medial division of the lateral nucleus becomes distributed to the parvicellular division of the basal nucleus, accessory basal nucleus, and medial nucleus) and will be modulated in parallel in several amygdaloid locations (e.g. in the parvicellular division of the basal

provide major amygdaloid inputs to the medial temporal lobe memory system are damaged in epileptic rats, whereas the largely intact central nucleus can still evoke freezing as a response to information that it receives directly from the sensory-related cortices and then conveys further to the periaqueductal grey.

In humans, the amygdala recently has been shown to have a critical role in tasks such as the recognition of emotion in visual (Adolphs *et al.*, 1994), auditory (Scott *et al.*, 1997), or olfactory (Zald and Pardo, 1997) stimuli or enhancement of memory for emotionally arousing stimuli (Cahill and McGaugh, 1998). Subjects with amygdaloid damage are impaired in many of these tasks (Cahill, Chapter 12; Adolphs and Tranel, Chapter 18). It has been difficult, however, to pinpoint the specific amygdaloid nucleus critical for these functions using currently available imaging techniques. There is some evidence that in rats as well as in primates, the degree of behavioural impairment depends on the location of the amygdala lesion. For example, lesion studies by Rosvold *et al.* (1954) in monkeys suggest that a post-operative change in social behaviour, particularly increased aggressiveness, depends on whether the lateral and basal nuclei are extensively damaged. On the other hand, a study by Aggleton and Passingham (1981) shows that subtotal amygdaloid lesions involving either the lateral, basal, or more dorsal aspects of the amygdala (anterior cortical, medial, central, or amygdalohippocampal area; Figure 2 in Aggleton and Passingham, 1981) result in only minor behavioural changes in aggression and other aspects of emotional, motivational, and cognitive behaviour. Therefore, when trying to understand the function of the amygdaloid complex, it is difficult to ignore the specific contribution of various amygdaloid nuclei in different aspects of amygdala-mediated behaviour. It remains to be studied, however, to what extent the parallel inputs from sensory-related cortices to various amygdaloid nuclei compensate for partial amygdaloid damage. It is also critical to determine whether the parallel inputs originate in the same or different neurons. If they represent axon collaterals of the same neuron, a small cortical lesion might produce more severe impairment than partial lesioning of the amygdala.

As discussed earlier, the organization of amygdaloid outputs suggests that amygdala-evoked cortical modulation occurs primarily via the lateral nucleus, basal nucleus, accessory basal nucleus, and the periamygdaloid cortex; endocrine modulation via the accessory basal nucleus, central nucleus, and medial nucleus; striatal modulation via the basal and accessory basal

---

nucleus, the signal might become associated with the information from the medial temporal lobe memory system; in the medial nucleus, it might become integrated with information about the internal milieu by connections from the hypothalamus). Reciprocal projections provide a pathway by which the target region might modulate the activity in the input region. Because the projections from many amygdaloid nuclei converge in selective amygdaloid output regions (e.g. in the central nucleus), the behavioural response within one output station might be the sum of the modulated signal representations. Note that the same stimulus might activate several output stations (output1, output2, and output3) which presumably provides the anatomical basis for the expression of different kinds of nuances in the spectrum of responses to emotionally significant stimuli (experiental, mnemonic, motor, endocrine, and autonomic). For abbreviations, see Table 2.1.

nuclei; and autonomic modulation via the central nucleus. Consequently, lesions in the output nuclei might actually produce a more dramatic abnormality in the nuances of emotional behaviour than damage to the input region (except the central nucleus). Considering that the overall behavioural response to an emotionally significant stimulus might be composed of several components, including the emotional experience as well as motor, mnemonic, autonomic, and endocrine responses, the set of amygdaloid nuclei damaged by the disease process might, in fact, be a critical factor in explaining the change in emotional behaviour occurring during the course of the disease.

The anatomical studies performed during the last two decades of the 20th century emphasize the importance of analysing of the amygdaloid connectivity at the nuclear and divisional levels. A more detailed understanding of the amygdaloid pathways at network and single cell levels, analysis of target neurons and receptors for different projections, three-dimensional reconstruction of single neurons, and data on the topographic organization of input and output connections and their quantification will provide a starting point for the generation of a database that can be used to model amygdaloid circuitries and their functions in normal and lesioned brains, and, eventually, to understand the behavioural consequences of nucleus-specific amygdaloid damage in human brain diseases in the new millenium.

Acknowledgements

This study was supported by the Academy of Finland, the Vaajasalo Foundation, and the Sigrid Juselius Foundation. The author thanks Esa Jolkkonen, BMed, Dr Katarzyna Lukasiuk, and Dr Riitta Miettinen for their thoughtful and constructive comments on the manuscript. The secretarial help of Mrs Liisa Marjava is gratefully acknowledged.

References

Adolphs, R., Tranel, D., Damasio, H., and Damasio, A. (1994) Impaired recognition of emotion in facial expressions following bilateral damage to the human amygdala. *Nature*, 372, 669–672.

Adolphs, R., Tranel, D., and Damasio, A.R. (1998) The human amygdala in social judgement. *Nature*, 393, 470–474.

Aggleton, J.P. and Passingham, R.E. (1981) Syndrome produced by lesions of the amygdala in monkeys (*Macaca mulatta*). *Journal of Comparative and Physiological Psychology*, 99, 961–977.

Alheid, G.F., de Olmos, J., and Beltramino, C.A. (1995) Amygdala and extended amygdala. In *The Rat Nervous System* (ed. G. Paxinos), pp. 495–578. Academic Press, California.

Alonso, G., Szafarczyk, A., and Assenmacher, I. (1986) Radioautographic evidence that axons from the area of supraoptic nuclei in the rat project to extrahypothalamic brain regions. *Neuroscience Letters*, 66, 251–256.

Amaral, D.G. and Witter, M.P. (1989) The three-dimensional organization of the hippocampal formation: a review of anatomical data. *Neuroscience*, 31, 571–591.

Amaral, D.G., Price, J.L., Pitkänen, A., and Carmichael, S.T. (1992) Anatomical organization of the primate amygdaloid complex. In *The Amygdala: Neurobiological Aspects of Emotion, Memory, and Mental Dysfunction* (ed. J.P. Aggleton), pp. 1–66. Wiley-Liss , New York.

Bacon, S.J., Headlam, A.J.N., Gabbott, P.L.A., and Smith, A.D. (1996) Amygdala input to medial prefrontal cortex (mPFC) in the rat: a light and electron microscope study. *Brain Research*, 720, 211–219.

Beart, P.M., Summers, R.J., Stephenson, J.A., Cook, C.J., and Christie, M.J. (1990) Excitatory amino acid projections to the periaqueductal gray in the rat: a retrograde transport study utilizing D[^{3}H]aspartate and [^{3}H]GABA. *Neuroscience*, 34, 163–176.

Beckstead, R.M. (1978) Afferent connections of the entorhinal area in the rat as demonstrated by retrograde cell-labeling with horseradish peroxidase. *Brain Research*, 152, 249–264.

Beckstead, R.M., Domesick, V.B., and Nauta, W.J.H. (1979) Efferent connections of the substantia nigra and ventral tegmental area in the rat. *Brain Research*, 175, 191–217.

Behan, M. and Haberly, L.B. (1999) Intrinsic and efferent connections of the endopiriform nucleus in rat. *Journal of Comparative Neurology*, 408, 532–548.

Berendse, H.W., Galis-de-Graaf, Y., and Groenewegen, H.J. (1992) Topographical organization and relationship with ventral striatal compartments of prefrontal corticostriatal projections in the rat. *Journal of Comparative Neurology*, 316, 314–347.

Bernard, J.F., Peschanski, M., and Besson, J.M. (1989a) Afferents and efferents of the rat cuneiformis nucleus: an anatomical study with reference to pain transmission. *Brain Research*, 490, 181–185.

Bernard, J.F., Peschanski, M., and Besson, J.M. (1989b) A possible spino (trigemino)-ponto-amygdaloid pathway for pain. *Neuroscience Letters*, 100, 83–88.

Bernard, J.-F., Alden, M., and Besson, J.-M. (1993) The organization of the efferent projections from the pontine parabrachial area to the amygdaloid complex: a *Phaseolus vulgaris* leucoagglutinin (PHA-L) study in the rat. *Journal of Comparative Neurology*, 329, 201–229.

Bianchi, R., Corsetti, G., Rodella, L., Tredici, G., and Gioia, M. (1998) Supraspinal connections and termination patterns of the parabrachial complex determined by the biocytin anterograde tract-tracing in the rat. *Journal of Anatomy*, 193, 417–430.

Bonda, E., Petrides, M., Ostry, D., and Evans, A. (1996) Specific involvement of human parietal systems and the amygdala in the perception of biological motion. *Journal of Neuroscience*, 16, 3737–3744.

Brindley-Reed, M., Mascani, F., and McDonald, A.J. (1995) Synaptology of prefrontal cortical projections to the basolateral amygdala: an electron microscopic study in the rat. *Neuroscience Letters*, 202, 45–48.

Brog, J.S., Salyapongse, A., Deutch, A.Y., and Zahm, D.S. (1993) The patterns of afferent innervation of the core and shell in the 'accumbens' part of the rat ventral striatum: immunohistochemical detection of retrogradely transported fluoro-gold. *Journal of Comparative Neurology*, 338, 255–278.

Burstein, R. and Potrebic, S. (1993) Retrograde labeling of neurons in the spinal cord that project directly to the amygdala or the orbital cortex in the rat. *Journal of Comparative Neurology*, 335, 469–485.

Caffe, A.R., van Leeuwen, F.W., and Luiten, P.G. (1987) Vasopressin cells in the medial amygdala of the rat project to the lateral septum and ventral hippocampus. *Journal of Comparative Neurology*, 261, 237–252.

Cahill, L. and McGaugh, J.L. (1998) Mechanisms of emotional arousal and lasting declarative memory. *Trends in Neurosciences*, 21, 294–299.

Calderazzo, L., Cavalheiro, E.A., Macchi, G., Molinari, M., and Bentivoglio, M. (1996) Branched connections to the septum and to the entorhinal cortex from the hippocampus, amygdala and diencephalon in the rat. *Brain Research Bulletin*, 40, 245–251.

Canteras, N.S. and Swanson, L.W. (1992) Projections of the ventral subiculum to the amygdala, septum and hypothalamus: a PHAL anterograde track-tracing study in the rat. *Journal of Comparative Neurology*, 324, 180–194.

Canteras, N.S., Simerly, R.B., and Swanson, L.W. (1992a) Connections of the posterior nucleus of the amygdala. *Journal of Comparative Neurology*, 324, 143–179.

Canteras, N.S., Simerly, R.B., and Swanson, L.W. (1992b) Projections of the ventral premammillary nucleus. *Journal of Comparative Neurology*, 324, 195–212.

Canteras, N.S., Simerly, R.B., and Swanson, L.W. (1994) Organization of projections from the ventromedial nucleus of the hypothalamus: a *Phaseolus vulgaris*–leucoagglutinin study in the rat. *Journal of Comparative Neurology*, 348, 41–79.

Canteras, N.S., Simerly, R.B., and Swanson, L.W. (1995) Organization of projections from the medial nucleus of the amygdala: a PHAL study in the rat. *Journal of Comparative Neurology,* 360, 213–245.

Carlsen, J. (1989) New perspectives on the functional anatomical organization of the basolateral amygdala. *Acta Neurologica Scandinavica*, 79, 1–27.

Carlsen, J. and Heimer, L. (1988) The basolateral amygdaloid complex as a cortical-like structure. *Brain Research*, 441, 377–380.

Carlsen, J., Záborszky, L., and Heimer, L. (1985) Cholinergic projections from the basal forebrain to the basolateral amygdaloid complex: a combined retrograde fluorescent and immunohistochemical study. *Journal of Comparative Neurology*, 234, 155–167.

Cassell, M.D. and Gray, T.S. (1989) The amygdala directly innervates adrenergic (C1) neurons in the ventrolateral medulla in the rat. *Neuroscience Letters*, 97, 163–168.

Cassell, M.D. and Roberts, L. (1991) Ultrastructural evidence for an olfactory-autonomic pathway through the rat central amygdaloid nucleus. *Neuroscience Letters*, 133, 100–104.

Cassell, M.D. and Wright, D.J. (1986) Topography of projections from the medial prefrontal cortex to the amygdala in the rat. *Brain Research Bulletin*, 17, 321–333.

Cheung, S., Ballew, J.R., Moore, K.E., and Lookingland, K.J. (1998) Contribution of dopamine neurons in the medial zona incerta to the innervation of the central nucleus of the amygdala, horizontal diagonal band of Broca and hypothalamic paraventricular nucleus. *Brain Research*, 808, 174–181.

Christensen, M.- K. and Frederickson, C.J. (1998) Zinc-containing afferent projections to the rat corticomedial amygdaloid complex: a retrograde tracing study. *Journal of Comparative Neurology*, 400, 375–390.

Cliffer, K.D., Burnstein, R., and Giesler, G.J., Jr (1991) Distributions of spinothalamic and spinotelencephalic fibers revealed by anterograde transport of PHA-L in rats. *Journal of Neuroscience*, 3, 852–868.

Condé, F., Maire-Lepoivre, E., Audinat, E., and Crépel, F. (1995) Afferent connections of the medial frontal cortex of the rat. II Cortical and subcortical afferents. *Journal of Comparative Neurology*, 352, 567–593.

Cornwall, J. and Phillipson, O.T. (1988) Afferent projections to the dorsal thalamus of the rat as shown by retrograde lectin transport—I. The mediodorsal nucleus. *Neuroscience*, 24, 1035–1049.

Cullinan, W.E., Herman, J.P., and Watson, J.S. (1993) Ventral subicular interaction with the hypothalamic paraventricular nucleus: evidence for a relay in the bed nucleus of the stria terminalis. *Journal of Comparative Neurology*, 332, 1–20.

Danielson, E.H., Magnuson, D.J., and Gray, T.S. (1989) The central amygdaloid nucleus innervation of the dorsal vagal complex in rat: a *Phaseolus vulgaris*, leucoagglutinin lectin anterograde tracing study. *Brain Research Bulletin*, 22, 705–715.

Datta, S., Siwek, F., Patterson, E.H., and Cipolloni, P.B. (1998) Localization of pontine PGO wave generation sites and their anatomical projections in the rat. *Synapse*, 30,409–423.

Davis, M. (1992) The role of the amygdala in conditioned fear. In *The Amygdala: Neurobiological Aspects of Emotion, Memory, and Mental Dysfunction* (ed. J.P. Aggleton), pp. 255–306. Wiley-Liss, New York.

Deacon, T.W., Eichenbaum, H., Rosenberg, P., and Eckmann, K.W. (1983) Afferent connections of the perirhinal cortex in the rat. *Journal of Comparative Neurology*, 220, 168–190.

de Olmos, J., Hardy, H., and Heimer, L. (1978) The afferent connections of the main and the accessory olfactory bulb formations in the rat: an experimental HRP-study. *Journal of Comparative Neurology*, 181, 213–244.

de Olmos, J., Alheid, G.F., and Beltramino, C.A. (1985) Amygdala. In *The Rat Nervous System* (ed. G. Paxinos), pp. 317–223. Academic Press, Australia.

Fallon, J.H., Koziell, D.A., and Moore, R.Y. (1978) Catecholamine innervation of the basal forebrain. I. Amygdala, suprarhinal cortex and entorhinal cortex. *Journal of Comparative Neurology*, 180, 509–532.

Gallagher, M. and Holland, P.C. (1994) The amygdala complex: multiple roles in associative learning and attention. *Proceedings of National Academy of Sciences of the United States of America*, 91, 11771–11776.

Gray, T.S. (1990) The organization and possible function of amygdaloid corticotropin-releasing factor pathways. In *Corticotropin-releasing Factor: Basic and Clinical Studies of a Neuropeptide* (eds E.B. De Souza and C.B. Nemeroff), pp. 53–68. CRC Press, Inc., Boca Raton, Florida.

Gray, T.S., Carney, M.E., and Magnuson, D.J. (1989) Direct projections from the central amygdaloid nucleus to the hypothalamic paraventricular nucleus: possible role in stress-induced adrenocorticotropin release. *Neuroendocrinology*, 50, 433–466.

Groenewegen, H.J. (1988) Organization of the afferent connections of the mediodorsal thalamic nucleus in the rat, related to the mediodorsal-prefrontal topography. *Neuroscience*, 24, 379–431.

Grove, E.A. (1988a) Neural associations of the substantia innominata in the rat: afferent connections. *Journal of Comparative Neurology*, 277, 315–346.

Grove, E.A. (1988b) Efferent connections of the substantia innominata in the rat. *Journal of Comparative Neurology*, 277, 347–364.

Haber, S.N., Groenewegen, H.J., Grove, E.A., and Nauta, W.J.H. (1985) Efferent connections of the ventral pallidum: evidence of a dual striato pallidofugal pathway. *Journal of Comparative Neurology*, 235, 322–335.

Hallanger, A.E. and Wainer, B.H. (1988) Ascending projections from the pedunculopontine tegmental nucleus and the adjacent mesopontine tegmentum in the rat. *Journal of Comparative Neurology*, 274, 483–515.

Hamann, S.B., Ely, T.D., Grafton, S.T., and Kilts, C.D. (1999) Amygdala activity related to enhanced memory for pleasant and aversive stimuli. *Nature Neuroscience*, 3, 289–293.

Hurley, K.M., Herbert, H., Moga, M.M., and Saper, C.B. (1991) Efferent projections of the infralimbic cortex of the rat. *Journal of Comparative Neurology*, 308, 249–276.

Insausti, R., Herrero, M.T., and Witter, M.P. (1997) Entorhinal cortex of the rat: cytoarchitectonic subdivisions and the origin and distribution of cortical efferents. *Hippocampus*, 7, 146–183.

Jolkkonen, E. and Pitkänen, A. (1998a) Intrinsic connections of the rat amygdaloid complex: projections originating in the central nucleus. *Journal of Comparative Neurology*, 395, 53–72.

Jolkkonen, E. and Pitkänen, A. (1998b) Projections from the amygdalapiriform transition area to the central nucleus of the amygdala: a PHA-L study in the rat. *Society for Neuroscience Abstracts*, 24, 675.

Kelley, A.E. and Stinus, L. (1984) The distribution of the projection from the parataenial nucleus of the thalamus to the nucleus accumbens in the rat: an autoradiographic study. *Experimental Brain Research*, 54, 499–512.

Kelley, A.E., Domensick, V.B., and Nauta, W.J.H. (1982) The amygdalostriatal projection in the rat—an anatomical study by anterograde and retrograde tracing methods. *Neuroscience*, 7, 615–630.

Kemppainen, S. and Pitkänen, A. (1998) Projections from the posterior cortical nucleus of the amygdala to other temporal lobe areas in rat. *Society for Neuroscience Abstracts*, 24, 676.

Killcross, S., Robbins, T.W., and Everitt, B.J. (1997) Different types of fear-conditioned behaviour mediated by separate nuclei within amygdala. *Nature*, 388, 377–380.

Kirouac, G.J. and Ganguly, P.K. (1995) Topographical organization in the nucleus accumbens of afferents from the basolateral amygdala and efferents to the lateral hypothalamus. *Neuroscience*, 67, 625–630.

Kita, H. and Kitai, S.T. (1990) Amygdaloid projections to the frontal cortex and the striatum in the rat. *Journal of Comparative Neurology*, 298, 40–49.

Kita, H. and Oomura, Y. (1982) An HRP study of the afferent connections of the rat lateral hypothalamic region. *Brain Research Bulletin*, 8, 63–71.

Krettek, J.E. and Price, J.L. (1974) Projections from the amygdala to the perirhinal and entrorhinal cortices and the subiculum. *Brain Research*, 71, 150–154.

Krettek, J.E. and Price, J.L. (1977a) Projections from the amygdaloid complex to the cerebral cortex and thalamus in the rat and cat. *Journal of Comparative Neurology*, 172, 687–722.

Krettek, J.E. and Price, J.L. (1977b) Projections from the amygdaloid complex and adjacent olfactory structures to the entorhinal cortex and to the subiculum in the rat and cat. *Journal of Comparative Neurology*, 172, 723–752.

Krettek, J.E. and Price, J.L. (1978a) Amygdaloid projections to subcortical structures in the basal forebrain and brainstem in the rat and cat. *Journal of Comparative Neurology*, 178, 225–254.

Krettek, J.E. and Price, J.L. (1978b) A description of the amygdaloid complex in the rat and cat with observations on intra-amygdaloid axonal connections. *Journal of Comparative Neurology*, 178, 255–280.

Krieger, M.S., Conrad, L.C.A., and Pfaff, D.W. (1979) An autoradiographic study of the efferent connections of the ventromedial nucleus of the hypothalamus. *Journal of Comparative Neurology*, 183, 785–816.

Krukoff, T.L., Harris, K.H., and Jhamandas, J.H. (1993) Efferent projections from the parabrachial nucleus demonstrated with anterograde tracer *Phaseolus vulgaris* leucoagglutinin. *Brain Research Bulletin*, 30, 163–172.

LeDoux, J.E. (1992) Emotion and the amygdala. In *The Amygdala: Neurobiological Aspects of Emotion, Memory, and Mental Dysfunction* (ed. J.P. Aggleton), pp. 339–352. Wiley-Liss, New York.

LeDoux, J.E., Ruggiero, D.A., and Reis, D.J. (1985) Projections to the subcortical forebrain from anatomically defined regions of the medial geniculate body in the rat. *Journal of Comparative Neurology*, 242, 182–213.

LeDoux, J.E., Farb, C., and Ruggiero, D.A. (1990) Topographic organization of neurons in the acoustic thalamus that project to the amygdala. *Journal of Neuroscience*, 4, 1043–1054.

LeDoux J.E., Farb, C.R., and Romanski, L.M. (1991) Overlapping projections to the amygdala and striatum from auditory processing areas of the thalamus and cortex. *Neuroscience Letters*, 134, 139–144.

Levine, J.D., Weiss, M.L., Rosenwasser, A.M., and Miselis, R.R. (1991) Retinohypothalamic tract in the female albino rat: a study using horseradish peroxidase conjugated to cholera toxin. *Journal of Comparative Neurology*, 306, 344–360.

Li, Y.-Q., Jia, H.-G., Rao, Z.-R., and Shi, J.-W. (1990) Serotonin-, substance P- or leucine-enkephalin-containing neurons in the midbrain periaqueductal gray and nucleus raphe dorsalis send projection fibers to the central amygdaloid nucleus in the rat. *Neuroscience Letters*, 120, 124–127.

Linke, R., de Lima, A.D., Schwegler, H., and Pape, H.-C. (1999) Direct synaptic connections of axons from superior colliculus with identified thalamo-amygdaloid projection neurons in the rat: possible substrates of a subcortical visual pathway to the amygdala. *Journal of Comparative Neurology*, 403, 158–170.

Luiten, P.G.M., Spencer, D.G., Jr, Traber, J., and Gaykema, R.P.A. (1985) The pattern of cortical projections from the intermediate parts of the magnocellular nucleus basalis in the rat demonstrated by tracing with *Phaseolus vulgaris*-leucoagglutinin. *Neuroscience Letters*, 57, 137–142.

Luiten, P.G.M., Gaykema, J., Traber, J., and Spencer, D.G., Jr (1987) Cortical projection patterns of magnocellular basal nucleus subdivision as revealed by anterogradely transported *Phaseolus vulgaris* leucoagglutinin. *Brain Research*, 413, 229–250.

Luskin, M.B. and Price, J.L. (1983a) The topographic organization of associational fibres of the olfactory system in the rat, including centrifugal fibres to the olfactory bulb. *Journal of Comparative Neurology*, 216, 264–291.

Luskin, M.B. and Price, J.L. (1983b) The laminar distribution of intracortical fibers originating in the olfactory cortex of the rat. *Journal of Comparative Neurology*, 216, 292–302.

Mascagni, F., McDonald, A.J., and Coleman, J.R. (1993) Corticoamygdaloid and corticocortical projections of the rat temporal cortex: a *Phaseolus vulgaris* leucoagglutinin study. *Neuroscience*, 57, 697–715.

McDonald, A.J. (1987a) Organization of amygdaloid projections to the mediodorsal thalamus and prefrontal cortex: a fluorescence retrograde transport study in the rat. *Journal of Comparative Neurology*, 262, 46–58.

McDonald, A.J. (1987b) Somatostatinergic projections from the amygdala to the bed nucleus of the stria terminalis and medial preoptic–hypothalamic region. *Neuroscience Letters*, 75, 271–277.

McDonald, A.J. (1991a) Organization of amygdaloid projections to the prefrontal cortex and associated striatum in the rat. *Neuroscience*, 44, 1–14.

McDonald, A.J. (1991b) Topographical organization of amygdaloid projections to the caudatoputamen, nucleus accumbens and related striatal-like areas of the rat brain. *Neuroscience*, 44, 15–33.

McDonald, A.J. (1998) Cortical pathways to the mammalian amygdala. *Progress in Neurobiology*, 55, 257–332.

McDonald, A.J. and Jackson, T.R. (1987) Amygdaloid connections with posterior insular and temporal cortical areas in the rat. *Journal of Comparative Neurology*, 262, 59–77.

McDonald, A.J. and Mascagni, F. (1996) Cortico-cortical and cortico-amygdaloid projections of the rat occipital cortex: a *Phaseolus vulgaris* leucoagglutinin study. *Neuroscience*, 71, 37–54.

McDonald, A.J., Mascagni, F., and Guo, L. (1996) Projections of the medial and lateral prefrontal cortices to the amygdala: a *Phaseolus vulgaris* leucoagglutinin study in the rat. *Neuroscience*, 71, 55–75.

McDonald, A.J. and Mascangni, F. (1997) Projections of the lateral entorhinal cortex to the amygdala: a *Phaseolus vulgaris* leucoagglutinin study in the rat. *Neuroscience*, 445–460.

McGaugh, J.L., Introini-Collison, I.B., Cahill, L., Kim, M., and Liand, K.C. (1992) Involvement of the amygdala in neuromodulatory influences on memory storage In *The Amygdala: Neurobiological Aspects of Emotion, Memory, and Mental Dysfunction* (ed. J.P. Aggleton), pp. 431–452. Wiley-Liss, New York.

McIntyre, D.C., Kelly, M.E., and Staines, W.A. (1996) Efferent projections of the anterior perirhinal cortex in the rat. *Journal of Comparative Neurology*, 396, 302–318.

Mihailoff, G.A., Kosinski, R.J., Azizi, S.A., and Border, B.G. (1989) Survey of noncortical afferent projections to the basilar pontine nuclei: a retrograde tracing study in the rat. *Journal of Comparative Neurology*, 282, 617–643.

Millhouse, O.E. and Uemura-Sumi, M. (1985) The structure of the nucleus of the lateral olfactory tract. *Journal of Comparative Neurology*, 233, 517–552.

Moga, M.M., Weis, R.P., and Moore, R.Y. (1995) Efferent projections of the paraventricular thalamic nucleus in the rat. *Journal of Comparative Neurology*, 359, 221–238.

Morris, J.S., Öhman, A., and Dolan, R.J. (1998) Conscious and unconscious emotional learning in the human amygdala. *Nature*, 393, 467–470.

Namura, S., Takada, M., Kikuchi, H., and Mizuno, N. (1997) Collateral projections of single neurons in the posterior thalamic region to both the temporal cortex and the amygdala: a fluorescent retrograde double-labeling study in the rat. *Journal of Comparative Neurology*, 384, 59–70.

Newman, H.M., Stevens, R.T., and Apkarian, A.V. (1996) Direct spinal projections to limbic and striatal areas: anterograde transport studies from the upper cervical spinal cord and the cervical enlargement in squirrel monkey and rat. *Journal of Comparative Neurology*, 365, 640–658.

Nissinen, J., Halonen, T., and Pitkänen, A. (1998) Emotional behavior at the time of first spontaneous seizures in a model of chronic TLE induced by amygdala stimulation in rats. *Epilepsia*, 39 (Suppl.), 32.

Nitecka, L. (1981) Connections of the hypothalamus and preoptic area with nuclei of the amygdaloid body in the rat: HRP retrograde transport study. *Acta Neurobiologiae Experimentalis*, 41, 53–67.

Nitecka, L., Amerski, L., Panek-Mikuza, J., and Narkiewicz, O. (1979) Thalamoamygdaloid connections studied by the method of retrograde transport. *Acta Neurobiologiae Experimentalis*, 39, 585–601.

Nitecka, L., Amerski, L., Panek-Mikula, J., and Narkiewicz, O. (1980) Tegmental afferents of the amygdaloid body in the rat. *Acta Neurobiologiae Experimentalis*, 40, 609–624.

Nitecka, L., Amerski, L., and Narkiewicz, O. (1981a) The organization of intraamygdaloid connections; an HRP study. *Journal für Hirnforschung*. 22, 3–7.

Nitecka, L., Amerski, L. and Narkiewicz, O. (1981b) Interamygdaloid connections in the rat studied by the horseradish peroxidase method. *Neuroscience Letters*, 26, 1–4.

Oades, R.D. and Halliday, G.M. (1987) Ventral tegmental (A 10) system: neurobiology. 1. Anatomy and connectivity. *Brain Research Reviews*, 434, 117–165.

Ono, T., Luiten, P.G.M., Nishijo, H., Fukuda, M., and Nishino, H. (1985) Topographic organization of projections from the amygdala to the hypothalamus of the rat. *Neuroscience Research*, 2, 221–239.

Ottersen, O.P. (1980) Afferent connections to the amygdaloid complex of the rat and cat: II. Afferents from the hypothalamus and the basal telencephalon. *Journal of Comparative Neurology*, 194, 267–289.

Ottersen, O.P. (1981) Afferent connections to the amygdaloid complex of the rat with some observations in the cat. III. Afferents from the lower brain stem. *Journal of Comparative Neurology*, 202, 335–356.

Ottersen, O.P. (1982) Connections of the amygdala of the rat. Corticoamygdaloid and intraamygdaloid connections as studied with axonal transport of horseradish peroxidase. *Journal of Comparative Neurology*, 205, 30–48.

Ottersen, O.P. and Ben-Ari, Y. (1979) Afferent connections to the amygdaloid complex of the rat and cat. *Journal of Comparative Neurology*, 187, 401–424.

Paré, D. and Smith, Y. (1998) Intrinsic circuitry of the amygdaloid complex: common principles of organization in rats and cats. *Trends in Neurosciences*, 21, 240–241.

Paxinos, G. and Watson, C. (1986) *The Rat Brain in Stereotaxic Coordinates*. Academic Press, New York.

Petrov, T., Krukoff, T.L., and Jhamandas, J.H. (1994) Chemically defined collateral projections from the pons to the central nucleus of the amygdala and hypothalamic paraventricular nucleus in the rat. *Cell and Tissue Research*. 277, 289–295.

Petrovich, G.D. and Swanson, L.W. (1997) Projections from the lateral part of the central amygdalar nucleus to the postulated fear conditioning circuit. *Brain Research*, 763, 247–254.

Petrovich, G.D., Risold, P.Y., and Swanson, L.W. (1996) Organization of projections from the medial nucleus of the amygdala: a PHAL study in the rat. *Journal of Comparative Neurology*, 374, 387–420.

Peyron, C., Petit, J.-M., Rampon, C., Jouvet, M., and Luppi, P.-H. (1998) Forebrain afferents to the rat dorsal raphe nucleus demonstrated by retrograde and anterograde tracing methods. *Neuroscience*, 82, 443–468.

Phillips, R.G. and LeDoux, J.E. (1992) Overlapping and divergent projections of CA1 and ventral subiculum to the amygdala. *Society for Neuroscience Abstracts*, 18, 518.

Phillipson, O.T. and Griffiths, A.C. (1985) The topographic order of inputs to nucleus accumbens in the rat. *Neuroscience*, 16, 275–296.

Pickel, V.M., Van Bockstaele, J.C., Chan, J., and Cestari, D.M. (1995) Amygdala efferents from inhibitory-type synapses with a subpopulation of catecholaminergic neurons in the rat nucleus tractus solitarius. *Journal of Comparative Neurology*, 362, 510–523.

Pitkänen, A., Stefanacci, L., Farb, C.R., Go, C.G., LeDoux, J.E., and Amaral, D.G. (1995) Intrinsic connections of the rat amygdaloid complex: projections originating in the lateral nucleus. *Journal of Comparative Neuorology*, 356, 288–310.

Pitkänen, A., Savander, V., and LeDoux, J.E. (1997) Organization of intra-amygdaloid circuitries in the rat: an emerging framework for understanding functions of the amygdala. *Trends in Neurosciences*, 20, 517–523.

Pitkänen, A., Tuunanen, J., Kälviäinen, R., Partanen, K., and Salmenperä, T. (1998) Amygdala damage in experimental and human epilepsy. *Epilepsy Research*, 328, 233–253.

Pikkarainen, M., Rönkkö, S., Savander, V., Insausti, R., and Pitkänen, A. (1999) Projections from the lateral, basal and accessory basal nuclei of the amygdala to the hippocampal formation in rat. *Journal of Comparative Neurology*, 403, 229–260.

Post, S. and Mai, J.K. (1978) Evidence for amygdaloid projections to the contralateral hypothalamus and the ipsilateral midbrain in the rat. *Cell and Tissue Research*, 191, 183–186.

Post, S. and Mai, J.K. (1980) Contribution to the amygdaloid projection field in the rat. A quantitative autoradiographic study. *Journal of Hirnforschung*, 21, 199–225.

Prewitt, C.M.F. and Herman, J.P. (1998) Anatomical interactions between the central amygdaloid nucleus and the hypothalamic paraventricular nucleus of the rat: a dual tract-tracing analysis. *Journal of Chemical Neuroanatomy*, 15, 173–185.

Price, J.L. (1973) An autoradiographic study of complementary laminar patterns of termination of afferent fibres to the olfactory cortex. *Journal of Comparative Neurology*, 15, 87–108.

Price, J.L., Russchen, F.T., and Amaral, D.G. (1987) The limbic region. II: The amygdaloid complex. In *Handbook of Chemical Neuroanatomy, Vol. 5, Integrated Systems of the CNS, Part I* (eds A. Björklund, T. Hökfelt, and L.W. Swanson), pp. 279–388. Elsevier, Amsterdam.

Price, J.L., Slotnik, B.M. and Revial, M. (1991) Olfactory projections to the hypothalamus. *Journal of Comparative Neurology,* 306, 447–461.

Rao, Z.R., Shiosaka, S., and Tohyama, M. (1987) Origin of cholinergic fibers in the basolateral nucleus of the amygdaloid complex by using sensitive double-labeling technique of retrograde biotinized tracer and immunocytochemistry. *Journal of Hirnforschung*, 5, 553–560.

Ray, J.P. and Price, J.L. (1992) The organization of the thalamocortical connections of the mediodorsal thalamic nucleus in the rat, related to the ventral forebrain–prefrontal cortex topography. *Journal of Comparative Neurology*, 323, 167–197.

Ray, J.P., Russchen, F.T., Fuller, T.A., and Price, J.L. (1992) Sources of presumptive glutamatergic/ aspartatergic afferents to the mediodorsal nucleus of the thalamus in the rat. *Journal of Comparative Neurology,* 320, 435–456.

Riche, D., De Pommery, J., and Menetrey, D. (1990) Neuropeptides and catecholamines in efferent projections of the nuclei of the solitary tract in the rat. *Journal of Comparative Neurology*, 293, 399–424.

Risold, P.Y., Canteras, N.S., and Swanson, L.W. (1994) Organization of projections from the anterior hypothalamic nucleus: a *Phaseolus vulgaris*-leucoagglutinin study in the rat. *Journal of Comparative Neurology*, 348, 1–40.

Rizvi, T.A., Ennis, M., Behbehani, M.M., and Shipley, M.T. (1991) Connections between the central nucleus of the amygdala and the midbrain periaquenductal gray: topography and reciprocity. *Journal of Comparative Neurology*, 303, 121–131.

Roder, S. and Ciriello, J. (1993) Innervation of the amygdaloid complex by catecholaminergic cell groups of the ventrolateral medulla. *Journal of Comparative Neurology*, 332, 105–122.

Rogan, M.T. and LeDoux, J.E. (1996) Emotion: systems, cells, synaptic plasticity. *Cell*, 85, 469–475.

Romanski, L.M. and LeDoux, J.E. (1993) Information cascade from primary auditory cortex to the amygdala: corticocortical and corticoamygdaloid projections of temporal cortex in the rat. *Cerebral Cortex*, 3, 515–532.

Rosen, J.B., Hitchcock, J.M., Sanases, C.B., Miserendino, M.J.D., and Davis, M. (1991) A direct projection from the central nucleus of the amygdala to the acoustic startle pathway: anterograde and retrograde tracing studies. *Behavioral Neuroscience*, 105, 817–825.

Rosvold, H.E., Mirsky, A.F., and Pribram, K.H. (1954) Influence of amygdalectomy on social behavior in monkeys. *Journal of Comparative and Physiological Psychology*, 47, 173–178.

Russchen, F.T. (1986) Cortical and subcortical afferents of the amygdaloid complex. In *Excitatory Amino Acids and Epilepsy* (eds Y. Ben-Ari and R. Schwarcz), pp. 35–52. Plenum Press, New York.

Russchen, F.T. and Price, J.L. (1984) Amygdalostriatal projections in the rat. Topographical organization and fiber morphology shown using the lectin PHA-L as an anterograde tracer. *Neuroscience Letters*, 47, 15–22.

Saper, C.B. and Loewy, A.D. (1980) Efferent connections of the parabrachial nucleus in the rat. *Brain Research*, 197, 291–317.

Saper, C.B., Swanson, L.W., and Cowan, W.M. (1978) The efferent connections of the anterior hypothalamic area of the rat, cat and monkey. *Journal of Comparative Neurology*, 182, 575–600.

Sarter, M. and Markowitsch, H.J. (1983) Convergence of basolateral amygdaloid and mediodorsal thalamic projections in different areas of the frontal cortex in the rat. *Brain Research Bulletin*, 10, 607–622.

Sarter, M. and Markowitsch, H.J. (1984) Collateral innervation of the medial and lateral prefrontal cortex by amygdaloid, thalamic and brain-stem neurons. *Journal of Comparative Neurology*, 224, 445–460.

Savander, V., Go, G.-C., Ledoux, J.E., and Pitkänen, A. (1995) Intrinsic connections of the rat amygdaloid complex: projections originating in the basal nucleus. *Journal of Comparative Neurology*, 361, 345–368.

Savander, V., Go, G.-C., Ledoux, J.E., and Pitkänen, A. (1996a) Intrinsic connections of the rat amygdaloid complex: projections originating in the accessory basal nucleus. *Journal of Comparative Neuorology*, 374, 291–313.

Savander, V., LeDoux, J.E., and Pitkänen, A. (1996b) Topographic projections from the periamygdaloid cortex to select subregions of the lateral nucleus of the amygdala in the rat. *Neuroscience Letters*, 211, 167–170.

Savander, V., Miettinen, M., Rönkkö, S. and Pitkänen, A. (1997a) Projections from the lateral, basal and accessory basal nuclei of the amygdala to the perirhinal and postrhinal cortices: *a Phaseolus vulgaris* leucoagglutinin study in rat. *Society for Neuroscience Abstracts*, 23, 2101.

Savander, V., Miettinen, R., Ledoux, J.E., and Pitkänen, A. (1997b) Lateral nucleus of the rat amygdala is reciprocally connected with basal and accessory basal nuclei: a light and electron microscopic study. *Neuroscience*, 77, 767–781.

Savander, V., LeDoux, J.E., and Pitkänen, A. (1997c) Interamygdaloid projections of the basal and accessory basal nuclei of the rat amygdaloid complex. *Neuroscience*, 76, 725–735.

Scalia, F. and Winans, S.S. (1975) The differential projections of the olfactory bulb and accessory olfactory bulb in mammals. *Journal of Comparative Neurology*, 161, 31–55.

Schmued, L., Phermsangngam, P., Lee, H., Thio, S., Chen, E., Truong, P., Colton, E., and Fallon, J. (1989) Collateralization and GAD immunoreactivity of descending pallidal efferents. *Brain Research*, 487, 131–142.

Scott, S.K., Young, A.W., Calder, A.J., Hellawell, D.J., Aggleton, J.P., and Johnson, M. (1997) Impaired auditory recognition of fear and anger following bilateral amygdala lesions. *Nature*, 385, 254–257.

Semba, K. and Fibiger, H.C. (1992) Afferent connections of the laterodorsal and the pedunculopontine tegmental nuclei in the rat: a retro- and antero-grade transport and immunohistochemical study. *Journal of Comparative Neurology*, 323, 387–410.

Sesack, S.R., Deutch, A.Y., Roth, R.H., and Bunney, B.S. (1989) Topographical organization of the efferent projections of the medial prefrontal cortex in the rat: an anterograde tract-tracing study with *Phaseolus vulgaris* leucoagglutinin. *Journal of Comparative Neurology*, 290, 213–242.

Shammah-Lagnado, S.J., Aldeid, G.F., and Heimer, L. (1996) Efferent connections of the caudal part of the globus pallidus in the rat. *Journal of Comparative Neurology*, 376, 489–507.

Shi, C.-J. and Cassell, M.D. (1997) Cortical, thalamic and amygdaloid projections of rat temporal cortex. *Journal of Comparative Neurology*, 382, 153–175.

Shi, C.-J. and Cassell, M.D. (1998a) Cortical, thalamic and amygdaloid connections of the anterior and posterior insular cortices. *Journal of Comparative Neurology*, 399, 440–468.

Shi, C.-J. and Cassell, M.D. (1998b) Cascade projections from somatosensory cortex to the rat basolateral amygdala via the parietal insular cortex. *Journal of Comparative Neurology*, 399, 469–41.

Shi, C.-J. and Cassell, M.D. (1999) Perirhinal cortex projections to the amygdaloid complex and hippocampal formation in the rat. *Journal of Comparative Neurology*, 406, 299–328.

Shinonaga, Y., Takada, M., and Mizuno, N. (1994) Topographic organization of collateral projections from the basolateral amygdaloid nucleus to both the prefrontal cortex and nucleus accumbens in the rat. *Neuroscience*, 58, 389–37.

Simerly, R.B. and Swanson, L.W. (1986) The organization of neural inputs to the medial preoptic nucleus of the rat. *Journal of Comparative Neurology*, 246, 312–42.

Sorvari, H., Soininen, H., Paljärvi, L., Karkola, K., and Pitkänen, A. (1995) Distribution of parvalbumin-immunoreactive cells and fibers in the human amygdaloid complex. *Journal of Comparative Neurology*, 360, 185–212.

Sripanidkulchai, K., Sripanidkulchai, B., and Wyss, J.M. (1984) The cortical projection of the basolateral amygdaloid nucleus in the rat: anterograde fluorescent dye study. *Journal of Comparative Neurology*, 229, 419–441.

Stefanacci, L., Farb, C., Pitkänen, A., Go, G., LeDoux, J.E., and Amaral, D.G. (1992) Projections from the lateral nucleus to the basal nucleus of the amygdala: a light and electron microscopic PHA-L study in the rat. *Journal of Comparative Neurology*, 323, 586–601.

Su, H.-S. and Bentivoglio, M. (1990) Thalamic midline cell populations projecting to the nucleus accumbens, amygdala and hippocampus in the rat. *Journal of Comparative Neurology*, 297, 582–53.

Sun, N., Roberts, L., and Cassell, M.D. (1991) Rat central amygdaloid nucleus projections to the bed nucleus of the stria terminalis. *Brain Research Bulletin*, 27, 651–666.

Sun, N., Yi, H. and Cassell, M.D. (1994) Evidence for a GABAergic interface between cortical afferents and brainstem projection neurons in the rat central extended amygdala. *Journal of Comparative Neurology*, 340, 43–64.

Swanson, L.W. (1976) An autoradiographic study of the efferent connections of the preoptic region in the rat. *Journal of Comparative Neurology*, 167, 227–256.

Swanson, L.W. (1992) *Brain Maps: Structure of the Rat Brain*. Elsevier, Amsterdam.

Swanson, L.W. and Kohler, C. (1986) Anatomical evidence for direct projections from the entorhinal area to the entire cortical mantle in the rat. *Journal of Neuroscience*, 6, 3010–3023.

Swanson, L.W. and Petrovich, G.D. (1998) What is the amygdala? *Trends in Neurosciences*, 21, 323–330.

Switzer, R.C., de Olmos, J., and Heimer, L. (1985) Olfactory system. In *The Rat Nervous System* (ed. G. Paxinos), pp. 1–35. Academic Press, Sydney.

Takagishi, M. and Chiba, T. (1991) Efferent projections of the infralimbic (area 25) region of the medial prefrontal cortex in the rat: an anterograde tracer PHA-L study. *Brain Research*, 566, 26–39.

Takayama, K. and Miura, M. (1991) Glutamate-immunoreactive neurons of the central amygdaloid nucleus projecting to the subretrofacial of SHR and WKY rats: a double-labeling study. *Neuroscience Letters*, 134, 62–66.

Thompson, R.H., Canteras, N.S., and Swanson, L.W. (1996) Organization of projections from the dorsomedial nucleus of the hypothalamus: a PHA-L study in the rat. *Journal of Comparative Neurology*, 376, 143–173.

Turner, B.H. and Herkenham, M. (1991) Thalamoamygdaloid projections in the rat: a test of the amygdala's role in sensory processing. *Journal of Comparative Neurology*, 313, 295–325.

Turner, B.H. and Zimmer, J. (1984) The architecture and some of the interconnections of the rat's amygdala and lateral periallocortex. *Journal of Comparative Neurology*, 227, 540–557.

Tuunanen, J., Halonen, T., and Pitkänen, A. (1996) Status epilepticus causes selective regional damage and loss of GABAergic neurons in the rat amygdaloid complex. *European Journal of Neuroscience*, 8, 2711–2275.

Van Bockstaele, E.J., Chan, J., and Pickel, V.M. (1996) Input from central nucleus of the amygdala efferents to pericoerulear dendrites, some of which contain tyrosine hydroxylase immunoreactivity. *Journal of Neuroscience Research*, 45, 289–302.

Van Groen, T. and Wyss, J.M. (1990a) The connections of presubiculum and parasubiculum in the rat. *Brain Research*, 518, 227–243.

Van Groen, T. and Wyss, M.J. (1990b) Extrinsic projections from area CA1 of the rat hippocampus: olfactory, cortical, subcortical and bilateral hippocampal formation projections. *Journal of Comparative Neurology*, 302, 515–528.

Van Vulpen, E.H.S., and Verwer, R.W.H. (1989) Organization of projections from the mediodorsal nucleus of the thalamus to the basolateral complex of the amygdala in the rat. *Brain Research*, 500, 389–394.

Vankova, M., Arluison, M., Leviel, V., and Tramu, G. (1992) Afferent connections of the rat substantia nigra pars lateralis with special reference to peptide-containing neurons of the amygdalo-nigral pathway. *Journal of Chemical Neuroanatomy*, 5, 39–50.

Vazdarjanova, A. and McGaugh, J.L. (1998) Basolateral amygdala is not critical for cognitive memory of contextual fear conditioning. *Proceedings of National Academy of Sciences of the United States of America* , 95, 15003–15007.

Veening, J.G. (1978a) Cortical afferents of the amygdaloid complex in the rat: an HRP study. *Neuroscience Letters*, 8, 191–195.

Veening, J.G. (1978b) Subcortical afferents of the amygdaloid complex in the rat: an HRP study. *Neuroscience Letters*, 8, 197–202.

Vertes, R.P. (1991) A PHA-L analysis of ascending projections of the dorsal raphe nucleus in the rat. *Journal of Comparative Neurology*, 313, 643–668.

Vertes, R.P., Crane, A.L., Colom, L.V., and Bland, B.H. (1995) Ascending projections of the posterior nucleus of the hypothalamus: PHA-L analysis in the rat. *Journal of Comparative Neurology*, 359, 90–116.

Wagner, C.K., Eaton, M.J., Moore, K.E., and Lookingland, K.J. (1995) Efferent projections from the region of the medial zona incerta containing A 13 dopaminergic neurons: a PHA-L anterograde tract-tracing study in the rat. *Brain Research*, 677, 229–237.

Wallace, D.M., Magnuson, D.J., and Gray, T.S. (1989) The amygdalo-brainstem pathway: selective innervation of dopaminergic, noradrenergic and adrenergic cells in the rat. *Neuroscience Letters*, 97, 252–258.

Wallace, D.M., Magnuson, D.J., and Gray, T.S. (1992) Organization of amygdaloid projections to brainstem dopaminergic, noradrenergic and adrenergic cell groups in the rat. *Brain Research Bulletin*, 28, 447–454.

Weller, K.L. and Smith, D.A. (1982) Afferent connections to the bed nucleus of the stria terminals. *Brain Research*, 232, 255–270.

Woolf, N.J. and Butcher, L.L. (1982) Cholinergic projections to the basolateral amygdala: a combined Evans blue and acetylcholinesterase analysis. *Brain Research Bulletin*, 8, 751–763.

Wright, C. and Groenewegen, H.J. (1995) Patterns of convergence and segregation in the medial nucleus accumbens of the rat: relationships of prefrontal cortical, midline thalamic and basal amygdaloid afferents. *Journal of Comparative Neurology*, 361, 383–403.

Wright, C.I. and Groenewegen, H.J. (1996) Patterns of overlap and segregation between insular cortical, intermediodorsal thalamic and basal amygdaloid afferents in the nucleus accumbens of the rat. *Neuroscience*, 73, 359–373.

Wright, C.I., Beijer, A.V.J., and Groenewegen, H.J. (1996) Basal amygdaloid complex afferents to the rat nucleus accumbens are compartmentally organized. *Journal of Neuroscience*, 16, 1877–93.

Wyss, J.M. (1981) An autoradiographic study of the efferent connections of the entorhinal cortex in the rat. *Journal of Comparative Neurology*, 199, 495–512.

Yasui, Y., Breder, C.D., Saper, C.B., and Cechetto, D.F. (1991) Autonomic responses and efferent pathways from the insular cortex in the rat. *Journal of Comparative Neurology*, 303, 355–374.

Zald, D.H. and Pardo, J.V. (1997) Emotion, olfaction and the human amygdala: amygdala activation during aversive olfactory stimulation. *Neurobiology*, 94, 4119–4124.

Zardetto-Smith, A.M. and Gray, T.S. (1990) Organization of peptidergic and catecholaminergic efferents from the nucleus of the solitary tract to the rat amygdala. *Brain Research Bulletin*, 25, 875–887.

3 Synaptic plasticity in the amygdala

Paul F. Chapman[1] and Sumantra Chattarji[2]

[1]*Cardiff School of Biosciences, Cardiff University, Cardiff, UK and*
[2]*National Centre for Biological Sciences, Tata Institute of Fundamental Research, Bangalore, India*

Summary

The amygdala clearly plays a key role in a number of important behaviours, including learning emotional and other associations. Although the amygdala promises to be an exceptionally good model system for studying the relationship between synaptic plasticity and learning, we are just beginning to explore the properties of basic synaptic physiology in the amygdala. Moreover, much of what we know is based on assumptions of similarity between the amygdala and the hippocampus. As more information accumulates, it is becoming clear that synaptic responses in the lateral and basolateral amygdala, where most investigations have been conducted, show similarity to synaptic responses in neocortical neurons. An emerging consensus also suggests that long-term potentiation (LTP) is similar, but not identical, to that of the hippocampus. Differences include dependence on *N*-methyl-D-aspartate (NMDA) receptor activation (seen in some synapses, in some subnuclei, but not in all), the type and range of tetanic stimuli sufficient to induce potentiation, and the sensitivity to deletion of genes for certain cell signalling molecules. These similarities and differences suggest that understanding the mechanisms of LTP in the amygdala is a tractable problem, and that its solution could contribute significantly to our understanding of learning, memory, and emotion.

3.1 Introduction

It is difficult to think of a mechanism for persistent memories that does not include the major features of long-term potentiation (LTP) or long-term depression (LTD). The mechanisms that account for learning and memory almost certainly must be capable of rapid activation, so that memories could be formed quickly. At the same time, they must be able to persist for what might be decades. The changes should be specific (or reasonably so) to those elements that are activated by the remembered experience. Finally, you might expect that if these mechanisms demonstrated regional specificity in the mammalian brain, they would be concentrated in the structures most strongly associated with learning and memory.

These are, indeed, the key features of LTP/LTD. Even if there are multiple mechanisms for multiple forms of LTP (and it is likely that there are), the general class or category of signalling pathways that produce LTP or LTD will give us great insight into the specific mechanisms of learning and memory. Although this is reason enough to continue studying LTP/LTD, the ultimate goal is to understand the precise relationship between these artificially induced forms of plasticity and the mechanisms of learning and memory. We have gained a tremendous amount of information about this relationship by studying the hippocampus, but it is likely that we can gain even more by understanding plasticity in the amygdala.

The advantages of investigating the function of the amygdala, and of testing amygdala-dependent behaviours, are well documented in this volume. For the purposes of developing a model system for investigating the function of LTP, the principal advantages of the amygdala are that both its input and output pathways are reasonably well defined, the nature of the sensory information that flows into it is known, and a great deal can be inferred about its function from both anatomical connections and behavioural analyses of lesion studies.

The disadvantage of physiological investigations of the amygdala can be summarized by stating that it is not the hippocampus. The amygdala is not highly laminar, making field potential observations difficult. It cannot be reproduced in multiple serial slices for *in vitro* analysis, nor can it be identified easily in neonatal brains, making it difficult to culture amygdala neurons with any degree of confidence that the cultured cells are, indeed, exclusively from the amygdala. Although there are significant similarities in the morphology of neurons between the lateral and basolateral amygdala and the neocortex or hippocampus, the heterogeneity of their distribution means that neurons selected at random for electrophysiological analysis could represent one of a variety of cell types with significant differences in physiological properties. For all these reasons, the amygdala is still underdeveloped as a model of synaptic plasticity and learning.

We intend to set the context for the more complete development of this model by first reviewing briefly the nature of long-lasting plasticity in the mammalian brain, then what is known about the physiological properties of the amygdala. Finally, we will review the current state of knowledge about plasticity in the amygdala (particularly the lateral and basolateral nuclei) and how it relates to emotional learning.

3.2 Long-term potentiation

Neuronal plasticity comes in a variety of forms. Some forms are responses to environmental experience, such as those induced by visual or somatosensory deprivation (Buonomano and Merzenich, 1998; Kossut, 1998). Others are produced by damage, as in lesion-induced sprouting or reorganization (Florence *et al.*, 1998). The most widely studied forms of synaptic plasticity, those believed to serve as the best model of learning and memory, are induced by specific patterns of electrical stimulation to synaptic afferents. By varying the pattern of stimulation and the preparation (and possibly the location in the brain), it is possible to create increases or decreases in synaptic efficacy that can last minutes, hours, days, or weeks.

In the early 1970s, Bliss, Lømo and Gardner-Medwin (Bliss and Gardner-Medwin, 1973; Bliss and Lømo, 1973) discovered that relatively brief episodes of high-frequency stimulation to the entorhinal cortical inputs to the dentate gyrus lead to long-lasting increases in the size of subsequently evoked synaptic responses. Since that time, LTP has been described in a variety of brain regions (both *in vivo* and *in vitro*) and a variety of different types of neurons. Although it appears that there are many different mechanisms for induction of LTP, and a bewildering array of intracellular second messengers, enzymes, and transcription factors that appear to be essential, there are also some consensus features that will make it possible to test hypotheses about the function of LTP (Bliss and Collingridge, 1993; Martinez and Derrick, 1996).

3.2.1 Methods of LTP induction

The signal for LTP induction typically involves postsynaptic depolarization plus presynaptic activity, and can be brought about through either high-frequency stimulation or direct depolarization plus low-frequency stimulation. The method of induction may be one of the variables that has the greatest influence over the exact set of molecular mechanisms recruited by the synapse for long-lasting enhancement. It is also the factor that is most likely to vary from one brain region or cell type to another.

The first full description of LTP (Bliss and Gardner-Medwin, 1973; Bliss and Lømo, 1973) involved stimulation of the entorhinal cortex inputs to the dentate gyrus *in vivo* at either 15 Hz for 15 s or 100 Hz for 1 s. Subsequently, both shorter duration and higher frequency tetanic stimuli have been employed. In both the perforant pathway to dentate gyrus synapses and the Schaffer collateral–commissural inputs to CA1 pyramidal neurons, the most effective stimuli mimic some of the firing properties of hippocampal neurons. High-frequency stimulus bursts (4–6 pulses per 100–400 Hz burst) presented at approximately 5 Hz produce robust, long-lasting potentiation at these synapses, though it is not yet clear whether these patterns are appropriate in other brain regions.

It is likely that the reason that patterned bursts of stimuli are effective at inducing LTP is that they produce favourable reductions in activation of inhibitory interneurons. This provides for optimal levels of the postsynaptic depolarization required for LTP induction, at least in CA1 and the dentate gyrus. Indeed, if other methods of providing sufficient depolarization can be supplied, it is possible to induce LTP with stimulation at rather low frequencies. Directly depolarizing single neurons (with current injected through the recording electrode) is sufficient to produce robust LTP when paired with afferent stimulation at 1–2 Hz. Similarly, low-frequency stimulation can produce LTP when paired with strong, high-frequency stimulation of other synapses on the same neurons. The requirement for postsynaptic depolarization endows LTP at many synapses with a property called *cooperativity* (McNaughton *et al.*, 1978) that suggests that LTP depends on the cooperative activation of a critical number of synapses. The ability to satisfy the requirement for cooperativity by stimulating two afferent pathways that converge on the same set of neurons permits LTP to be *associative*, a property that may signal a role for LTP in associative learning (Levy and Steward, 1979; Barrionuevo and Brown, 1983; Kelso and Brown, 1983; Gustaffson and

Wigström, 1986). One more property that is related to associativity is *input specificity* (Anderson *et al.*, 1977). For the most part, those synapses that are not depolarized sufficiently by tetanic stimulation do not show LTP, even if their neighbours do (but see Bonhoeffer *et al.*, 1989; Schuman and Madison, 1994).

The properties of cooperativity, associativity, and input specificity are generally believed to apply to most, if not all, forms of LTP. It is important to note, however, that most LTP experiments have been conducted in the hippocampus, and most of what we know applies to a limited set of synapses. Even so, the diversity of induction mechanisms suggests that there is no single best set of parameters for producing LTP, and that each brain region or subregion must be approached with a minimum of assumptions about how best to induce or examine LTP.

3.2.2 Mechanisms of LTP induction

Almost all forms of LTP require increases in intracellular calcium concentration in the postsynaptic neuron. Preventing the entry of calcium into neurons by blocking *N*-methyl-D-aspartate (NMDA)-type glutamate receptors (Collingridge *et al.*, 1983; Harris *et al.*, 1984) and/or voltage-gated calcium channels (Grover and Teyler, 1990), or the chelation of intracellular calcium (Lynch *et al.*, 1983) can prevent the induction of LTP. Delivery of calcium through direct activation of NMDA receptors (Kauer *et al.*, 1988), photolysis of light-sensitive calcium chelators (Malenka *et al.*, 1988), or direct activation of voltage-gated calcium channels (Wyllie *et al.*, 1994) can induce a potentiation that, while typically short lasting, resembles LTP in many key features. Beyond the requirement for calcium, however, there is no real consensus about what messengers might be necessary for LTP induction.

NMDA dependent

Collingridge *et al.* (1983) and Harris *et al.* (1984) first demonstrated that LTP of the Schaffer collateral inputs to CA1 was blocked by the glutamate receptor antagonist 5-phosphonopentanoic acid (AP5). AP5, which selectively blocks the NMDA-type glutamate receptor, had the curious property of preventing the induction of LTP without greatly reducing synaptic responses to low-frequency stimulation, or responses to exogenously applied glutamate. The discovery that the NMDA receptor was both glutamate and depolarization dependent and that the associated channel was permeable to calcium suggested that this receptor could act as an activity-dependent gateway to LTP.

NMDA dependence is one of the most prominent and persistent features of LTP at Schaffer collateral–CA1 synapses, and has been demonstrated by a range of techniques from selective antagonists to region-specific gene deletion (Tsien *et al.*, 1996). The inhibition of hippocampal LTP through blocking of NMDA receptors has also provided some of the major tests of the potential role of LTP in learning and memory (Morris *et al.*, 1986; Bannerman *et al.*, 1995). Under the circumstances, it is easy to lose sight of the fact that LTP can be induced in Schaffer–CA1 synapses in the presence of NMDA antagonists (Grover and Tyler, 1990). Moreover, at many other synapses, in the hippocampus and elsewhere in the forebrain, NMDA receptor antagonists may have little or no effect on LTP induction.

Voltage-gated calcium channel (VGCC) dependent

In many brain regions, LTP can be induced in the presence of NMDA receptor antagonists. In some of these areas, such as the mossy fibre synapses on CA3 pyramidal neurons in the hippocampus, blocking NMDA receptors seems to have no effect at all on LTP induction (Harris and Cotman, 1986; Johnston *et al.*, 1992). Although there is evidence of functional NMDA receptors that are activated by glutamate release from mossy fibres (Castillo *et al.*, 1994), blocking them with even high doses of AP5 does not affect LTP induction. In fact, associational inputs to the same CA3 pyramidal neurons do demonstrate NMDA-dependent LTP induction, clearly arguing that LTP induction mechanisms depend on the type of synapse, and not necessarily the type of neuron.

At other synapses, such as Schaffer collateral–commissural synapses in CA1, NMDA receptor antagonists can block LTP using standard tetanus parameters, but other tetani (typically higher frequency and/or more prolonged) can induce robust LTP even with NMDA receptors effectively blocked (Grover and Teyler, 1990). In these cases, LTP induction still depends on changes in intracellular calcium concentration, but the calcium influx is through voltage-gated calcium channels (VGCCs).

Finally, there are synapses, mostly those outside the hippocampus, where the relationship between NMDA-dependent and -independent synapses is not straightforward (e.g. Komatsu *et al.*, 1991). This may be because this pattern of synaptic connections within these structures is less geometrically precise and so more likely to mix synapses with primarily NMDA receptor-dependent or -independent mechanisms. It might also be because there are different types of synapses in these structures that use fundamentally different mechanisms for LTP induction than the more widely studied ones in the hippocampus. As we will describe later, the amygdala and the neocortex appear to be regions where the dependence of LTP induction on NMDA receptors is not yet fully understood.

Mechanisms of LTP maintenance

In many ways, understanding the mechanisms of LTP induction seems straightforward compared with determining how it is maintained. Preventing LTP induction by blocking NMDA receptors or VGCCs, or by chelating calcium, prevents any increases in response size and thus clearly prevents the initiation of any plasticity processes. On the other hand, some manipulations, such as blocking certain protein kinases, can lead to relatively short-term synaptic enhancements. There appear to be a number of different types of LTP that can be distinguished largely by their duration and their susceptibility to blockers of different intracellular signalling molecules thought to be critical in maintaining synaptic enhancements.

Persistent kinase activity The first class of molecule implicated in LTP maintenance were protein kinases that phosphorylate proteins at serine/threonine residues. Pharmacological inhibitors that tended to block a rather broad spectrum of serine/threonine kinases were found to shorten the duration of LTP, from more than 60 min to less than 30 min (Malinow *et al.*, 1989). This type of pharmacological experiment provided evidence that protein kinase C (PKC), calcium/calmodulin-dependent protein kinase (CaMKII), and cAMP-dependent protein kinase (PKA) were required for LTP maintenance. More recently, similar types of experiments have implicated tyrosine kinases (O'Dell *et al.*, 1991), as well as multifunctional kinases such as ERK that can phosphorylate at both tyrosine and serine/threonine (Atkins *et al.*, 1998).

Inhibitors of intracellular messengers are often difficult to work with; they typically are limited in quantity, unable to cross the blood–brain barrier and/or neuronal cell membrane, and potentially non-specific. For these reasons, experiments that defined the roles of specific protein kinases were comparatively rare until gene targeting techniques were more widely available. Although not perfect, gene targeting techniques are considerably more specific than pharmacological manipulations, since they make it possible to affect specific isoforms or subunits of an enzyme (Grant *et al.*, 1992; Silva *et al.*, 1992) or receptor (Hsia *et al.*, 1995), or a specific brain region (Mayford *et al.*, 1996; Tsien *et al.*, 1996). LTP experiments conducted in the hippocampus of mice with targeted deletions of protein kinases, for example, have confirmed some of the earlier pharmacological studies, and raised interesting questions about some others. For example, deletion of the α-isoform of CaMKII (Silva *et al.*, 1992) blocks LTP, as would be predicted by experiments with peptide inhibitors (Malenka *et al.*, 1989). On the other hand, this manipulation also eliminates short-term potentiation (as does introduction of a single point mutation that alters the dependence of αCaMKII on intracellular calcium concentration), thus blurring the distinction between 'induction' and 'maintenance' of LTP.

Protein synthesis Although LTP typically is measured for between 30 and 60 min, memory can last considerably longer than that. Reymann *et al.* (1985) were able to measure LTP in CA1 *in vitro* for a period of up to 10 h after tetanus. Based on a substantial literature on the effects of protein synthesis inhibitors on memory consolidation (e.g. Flexner and Flexner, 1966; Flood *et al.*, 1974) and on the earlier work of Stanton and Sarvey (1984), Frey *et al.* (1988) found that protein synthesis inhibitors could selectively block the late phase of LTP induced by the appropriate tetanic stimulation (repeated high-frequency stimulation with several minutes between them). Moreover, mice lacking certain activators of gene transcription (most notably the cAMP response element-binding protein, or CREB) also show deficits in long-lasting LTP in the hippocampus (Bourtchuladze *et al.*, 1994). The extent to which this type of plasticity is found in other brain regions, the nature of the stimuli required to elicit it, and its relevance to behaviour are important areas for future research.

3.3 Electrophysiological survey of the amygdala: circuits, cells, and synapses

A thorough understanding of the cellular mechanisms underlying behaviour requires a comprehensive characterization of the functional properties of the elements of the relevant neuronal network. The need for this is particularly important in the amygdala, where the difficulty of the task is compounded by the complexity of the cytoarchitecture within the structure. In other words, to explore the physiological role of the amygdala in learning and memory, we will need to characterize the properties of:

(i) The full range of postsynaptic neuron types
(ii) The presynaptic input onto any given postsynaptic neuronal type
(iii) The properties of synaptic transmission at any given type of synapse
(iv) The rules governing plasticity mechanisms at this synapse.

In the hippocampus, this information is relatively accessible and has facilitated the development of numerous biologically based network models (Kohonen, 1989; Brown and Chattarji, 1994; Rolls and Treves, 1998). To construct similarly effective models of the amygdala, neuroscientists will need to overcome several major obstacles presented by the inherent complexity of its cytoarchitecture and the rich diversity in all four aspects of the above framework. One of the major barriers has been in creating a clear roadmap of the postsynaptic neurons and how they relate to their respective afferent inputs (i.e. points i and ii above). The orderly laminar organization of the hippocampus allows one to stimulate a specific, known, replicable input pathway in a slice preparation (e.g. Schaffer collaterals) and record a well-defined synaptic response from a particular neuronal class (e.g. pyramidal neurons) in a specific part of the hippocampal circuit (e.g. area CA1). It has been difficult to demonstrate a similarly clear link between the morphology and electrophysiological properties of the various cell types in the amygdala. In spite of these problems, evidence from many different laboratories using a variety of *in vitro* and *in vivo* techniques indicates that we can begin to analyse the amygdaloid network in far greater detail at the cellular and synaptic levels (Davis *et al.*, 1994). This in turn has led to several promising results indicating that a rich diversity of synaptic plasticity mechanisms may be operating in the amygdala. In the following sections, we will first provide a brief summary of recent findings pertaining to the first three elements (cells, their inputs, and transmission between them) and then use this framework to discuss data directly related to synaptic plasticity mechanisms.

3.3.1 Diversity of cell types: electrophysiological classification of morphologically identified amygdala neurons

As described in detail elsewhere, the amygdala consists of numerous nuclei and subnuclei that have distinct connections (both within the amygdala and with other brain regions) and that may participate in discrete functions (McDonald, 1992, 1998; Pitkänen *et al.*, 1997, Chapter 2). Different investigators have grouped the amygdaloid nuclei in various ways using different criteria. On the basis of neuronal morphology, studies have revealed that one way to divide the amygdaloid nuclei is into two major groups: *cortex-like nuclei* and *non-cortex-like nuclei* (McDonald, 1992). The cortex-like amygdaloid nuclei (see Figure 3.1) contain two main cell types: (i) spiny pyramidal projection neurons that form the majority of the constituent neurons, and (ii) spine-sparse non-pyramidal neurons that are observed in far fewer numbers and function primarily as local circuit neurons. Most of the detailed studies attempting to relate electrophysiological properties to the morphology of neurons in the cortex-like nuclei have focused primarily on the lateral/basolateral amygdala. There are fewer comparable studies on the non-cortex-like nuclei and most of them have focused on the central nucleus. The principal neurons in the non-cortex-like nuclei, by definition, do not

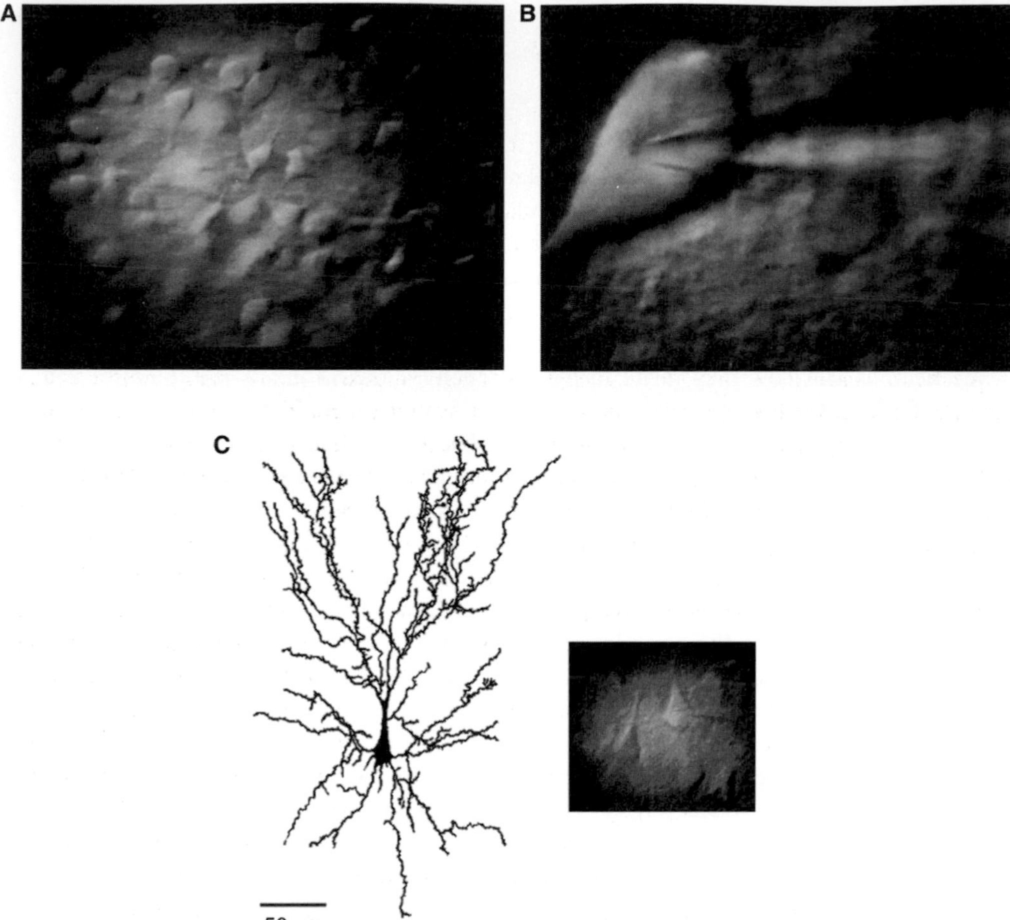

Figure 3.1 Infrared video images of neurons in living slices of basolateral amygdala. (**A**) Low-power image of neurons clustered within BLA. The image represents both the density of neurons and their relatively non-laminar arrangement. (**B**) Higher magnification permits the experimenter to apply the tip of a patch pipette to the soma of an identified neuron. The full dendritic arborization is not visible using this method, but the shape and size of the soma can give clues to the neuronal type. (**C**) The inclusion of biocytin in the recording pipette allows post-hoc reconstruction of the full dendritic structure, which can be correlated with electrophysiological properties. In this example, the pyramidal shaped neuron is a late-onset spiking cell (see Table 3.2). (S. Chattarji, unpublished data.)

have a pyramidal configuration. As in the cerebral cortex, multipolar, bitufted, and bipolar varieties of non-pyramidal cells have been observed on the basis of dendritic patterns. Similarly to neurons in the cortex-like nuclei, a majority of the non-pyramidal neurons are spine-dense while a small number are spine-sparse.

Most of the early *in vitro* studies with sharp microelectrodes used the above scheme as their starting points for characterizing the electrophysiological properties of morphologically identified neurons in the basolateral complex of the amygdala (BLA). In the first *in vitro* study describing LTP in the amygdala slice preparation, Chapman *et al.* (1990) classified BLA neurons into three categories based on their spiking properties in response to a depolarizing current step: neurons displaying a burst response (input resistance, R_N = 37 MΩ, membrane time constant, τ_0 = 27 ms), neurons that produced only a single action potential (R_N = 37 MΩ, τ_0 = 24 ms), and a third group of cells that did not fit the first two groups and responded with multiple rapidly accommodating spikes (R_N = 44 MΩ, τ_0 = 29 ms). The average resting membrane potentials for the three classes of cells studied in this report did not differ significantly.

Washburn and Moises (1992a) subsequently have studied the electrophysiological and morphological properties of BLA neurons using intracellular recordings in the amygdala slice preparation. They too grouped the BLA neurons, based on their current-evoked pattern of spike discharge, into three categories: the vast majority (~93%) of cells were identified as *pyramidal type* (R_N = 39.5 MΩ; τ_0 = 15.7 ms and *V*m = –69.5 mV); the second class of cells consisted of *late-firing neurons* (R_N = 25.8 MΩ; τ_0 = 7.3 ms and *V*m = –82.4 mV); and the third class of neurons were termed *fast-firing neurons* (R_N = 48.8 MΩ; τ_0 = 5.8 ms and *V*m = –62 mV). In one-third of the pyramidal cells studied, the accommodation response was characterized by a complete cessation of discharge following an initial burst of action potentials, whereas in the remaining two-thirds it was represented by a progressive slowing of spike discharge. A readily distinguishable feature of the late-firing neurons was the presence of a conspicuous delay in onset of spike firing in response to depolarizing current injection. No accommodation of spike discharge was observed in either the late-firing or fast-firing neurons in this study. Using intracellular labelling with Lucifer yellow, Washburn and Moises (1992a) showed the electrophysiologically identified pyramidal and late-firing BLA cells to have *pyramidal* to *stellate* cell bodies. Although having an overall pyramidal-like morphology, late-firing neurons possessed cell bodies that were smaller than those of pyramidal cells. Lucifer yellow-labelled fast-firing neurons had a non-pyramidal morphology, with somata that were spherical to multipolar in shape.

More recently, Shinnick-Gallagher and colleagues have carried out a series of detailed *in vitro* studies that have reinforced further the general pattern emerging from the earlier studies (Davis *et al.*, 1994). Rainnie *et al.* (1993) have performed intracellular current-clamp recordings from BLA neurons that conform to the morphological classification proposed by McDonald (1992). Using microelectrodes filled with biocytin, Rainnie *et al.* (1993) identified *class I pyramidal neurons* (R_N = 58.1 MΩ; τ_0 = 27.9 ms), *class I stellate neurons* (R_N = 40.1 MΩ; τ_0 = 14.5), and *class II multipolar neurons* (R_N = 58.3 MΩ; τ_0 = 19.6). The three groups did not differ significantly from each other in resting membrane potential. Rainnie *et al.* (1993) characterized the spiking properties of these three classes of neurons using two different schemes. In response to short (200 ms) depolarizing current steps, the BLA neurons displayed two distinct spiking patterns—a *burst firing pattern* with a short first interspike interval (mean 1st ISI = 6 ms) and a *regular firing pattern* with a significantly longer first ISI (91.6 ms). All the burst-firing neurons belonged to either the class I stellate or class II categories, but not to the class I pyramidal group. The majority of regular firing neurons were of the class I pyramidal type along with some class I stellate and class II neurons. Using longer (500 ms) depolarizing current steps, Rainnie *et al.* characterized the repetitive firing properties of BLA neurons into two main groups—*accommodating* and *non-accommodating*. All of the class II neurons they studied were non-accommodating; both patterns were seen in the two types of class I neuronal morphology and in the regular and burst-firing patterns.

Thus, based on electrophysiological and morphological studies using intracellular microelectrodes, it is obvious that there is significant diversity amongst amygdala neurons even within a single nuclear division. While there are a few common electrophysiological properties that emerge from these studies, there are also considerable differences between the basic membrane properties reported and the classification schemes proposed by different laboratories. As a result, a clear segregation of cell types in the BLA apparently cannot emerge based solely on passive membrane properties. However, the above data along with results from other similar studies suggest a general range of values for three commonly measured parameters for passive membrane properties (Table 3.1). In contrast to the studies in the lateral amygdala (LA)/BLA, there are very few exhaustive studies linking electrophysiological and morphological properties of the various cell types in the central nucleus (CeA) of the amygdala (Nose *et al.*, 1991; Schiess *et al.*, 1993). The available data suggest that the non-cortex-like CeA neurons are characterized by higher input resistance compared with the cortex-like LA/BLA neurons (Schiess *et al.*, 1993; Davis *et al.*, 1994).

In terms of firing characteristics, each study has adopted its own classification scheme which is often different from all the others. For example, Rainnie *et al.* (1993) have reported the presence of regular firing and burst-firing BLA neurons, but not fast-firing neurons. Washburn and Moises (1992a), on the other hand, have observed fast-firing BLA neurons,

Table 3.1 Basic passive membrane properties[a] of amygdala neurons

Membrane properties	*Amygdaloid nuclei*		
	Cortex-like		*Non-cortex-like*
	Basolateral[b]	*Lateral*[c]	*Central*[d]
Input resistance	40–60 MΩ[e]	80–93 MΩ[f]	111–133 MΩ[g]
Resting membrane potential	–62 to –70 mV[h]	–62 to –78 mV	–63 to –67 mV
Membrane time constanst (τ)	15–29 ms[i]	36–44 ms	15–23 ms

[a]Data obtained from sharp microelectrode recordings only.
[b]These values are summarized from Davis *et al.* (1994).
[c]Summary based on Sugita *et al.* (1993).
[d]Summary based on studies by Nose *et al.* (1991) and Schiess *et al.* (1993).
[e]The non-pyramidal neurons generally have higher values compared with pyramidal neurons.
[f]Non-pyramidal neurons have higher values compared with pyramidal neurons
[g]Both Nose *et al.* (1991) and Schiess *et al.* (1993) reported significantly higher values compared with BLA/LA neurons.
[h]Chapman *et al.* (1990) and Washburn and Moises (1992a) have reported more hyperpolarized values for some cell types.
[i]Washburn and Moises (1992) have reported lower values for some cell types.

but do not explicitly classify any BLA neuron as regular firing or bursting. Their pyramidal-type BLA neurons, however, do appear to display some sort of burst-firing behaviour. These pyramidal type neurons also exhibit spike frequency adaptation that is typical of the regular firing neurons observed by Rainnie *et al.* (1993). Washburn and Moises (1992a) also describe a group of BLA neurons they classify as late-firing neurons, which have not been observed by Rainnie *et al.* (1993) or Chapman *et al.* (1990). As with passive membrane properties, no clear consensus emerges based on action potential firing properties. However, there are certain basic features that emerge from all of these studies. Therefore, Table 3.2 presents a two-dimensional scheme for neuronal firing patterns that encompasses most of the salient features from the above studies.

With respect to the action potential firing patterns displayed by BLA neurons, the single most common finding from all of the previous studies appears to be the existence of two broad categories: accommodating and non-accommodating (see Figure 3.2). The other common link among all these studies seems to be the presence of pyramidal-like and clearly non-pyramidal neurons, with the former class of cells often displaying some form of spike frequency adaptation or accommodation. These basic distinguishing features are summarized in Table 3.3.

There appears to be significant overlap in the classification schemes proposed for the amygdala and those reported for neurons in the neocortex (McCormick *et al.*, 1985; Connors and Gutnick, 1990). The basic core types of responses to intracellular current injection (i.e. regular spiking, bursting, and fast spiking) are essentially identical to those previously described for neocortex. It is likely that the observation of neurons that respond with only single action potentials (Chapman *et al.*, 1990) or with late firing of either single action potentials (Washburn and Moises, 1992a) or bursts (Paré *et al.*, 1995) are either subclasses of the three main response types or represent cell types that exist in neocortex as well as cortex-like amygdala, but are relatively under-sampled in neocortex (McCormick *et al.*, 1985). Taken together, these data provide support for the contention (Swanson and Petrovich, 1998) that the lateral and basolateral nuclei of the amygdala are essentially cortical structures.

Table 3.2 Salient features of results from *in vitro* studies in BLA

Neuronal morphology	*Temporal structure of firing characteristics*			
	Fast firing	*Burst firing*	*Late firing*	*Regular firing*
Pyramidal	–	–	+ NA	+ + A, NA
Stellate	–	+ NA	+ NA	+ A
Non-pyramidal	+ + NA	+ NA	–	–

The presence and relative strength or probability of the characteristic is denoted by a plus (+) sign. The complete absence of a characteristic is denoted by a minus (–) sign. The first dimension refers to the three basic morphological categories, where the 'non-pyramidal' class includes multipolar, bipolar, and fusiform cells. The second dimension refers to the characteristics of individual action potential complexes—the responses to depolarizations that are just over threshold. Furthermore, changes in the firing frequency during a sustained depolarization are indicated by two broad categories—accommodating (A) and non-accommodating (NA). A train of spikes displays (i) non-accommodation if successive intervals do not change; and (ii) accommodation if the intervals increase. The shaded highlights indicate significant overlap in results between two or more groups.

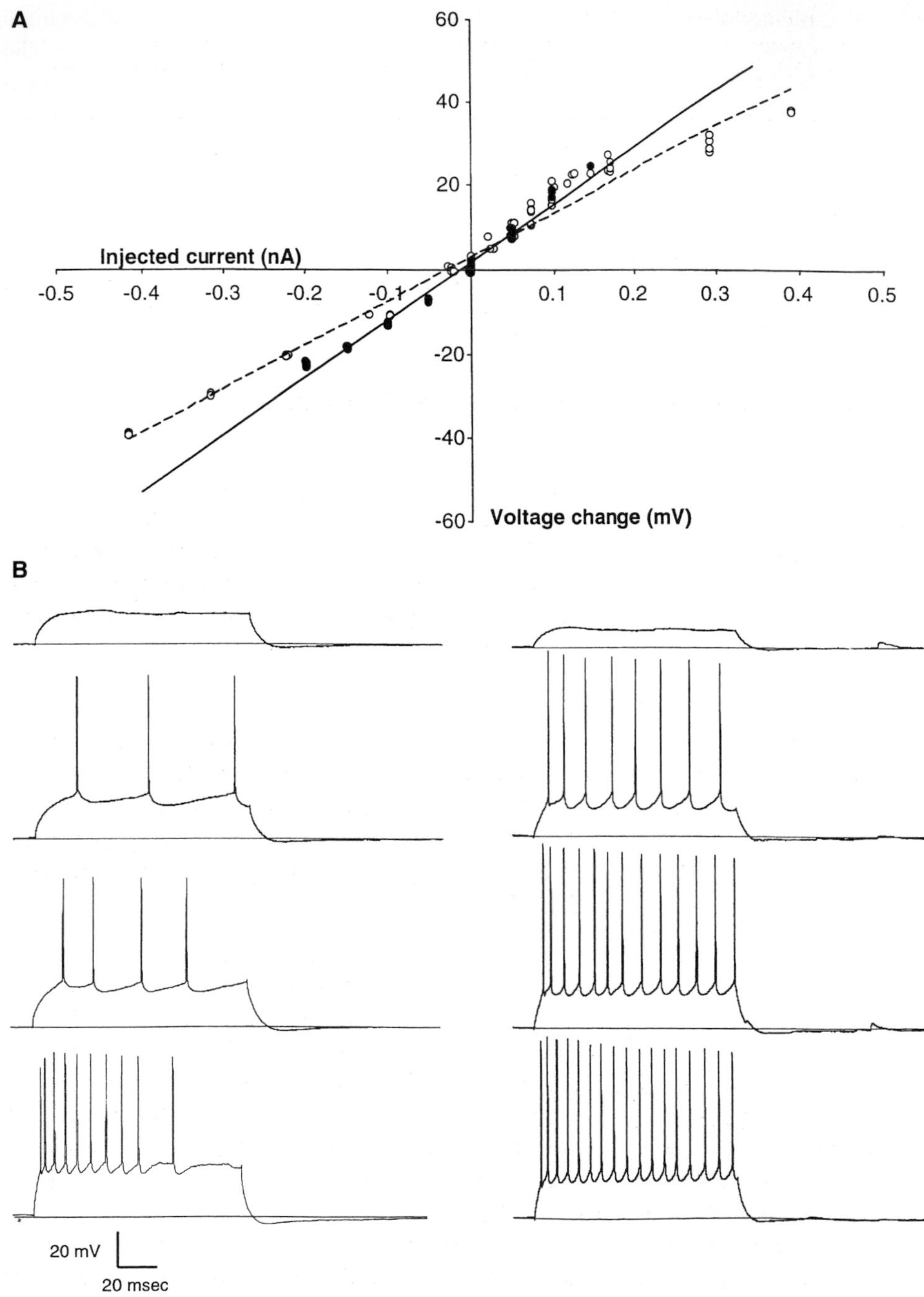

Figure 3.2 Membrane physiological properties of two representative neurons from the basolateral amygdala in horizontal slices, recorded using whole-cell current-clamp. (**A**)

Table 3.3 Distinguishing features

Cortex-like (LA/BLA)	*Non-cortex-like (CeA)*	*Between cortex-like and non-cortex-like*
R_N: Non-pyr. > pyr. Spike width: nonpyr < pyr. Firing: pyr. accomm. non-pyr. non-accomm.	AHP: present in type A cells absent in type B cells	R_N: CeA > LA/BLA

AHP, afterhyperpolarization; R_N, input resistance; pyr, pyramidal neuron; non-pyr: non-pyramidal neuron; accomm: accommodating (i.e. displays spike-frequency adaptation); non-accomm: non-accommodating (i.e. does not display spike-frequency adaptation).

3.3.2 Diversity in synaptic transmission: electrophysiological and pharmacological classification

The preceding section gives us a general scheme for classifying amygdala neurons that resembles a cortical framework. The next step towards understanding information flow and synaptic plasticity in the amygdala requires detailed knowledge of synaptic transmission to and from each of these neuronal classes. Hence, this section will summarize the basic electrophysiological and pharmacological properties of excitatory and inhibitory synaptic transmission in the amygdala.

Excitatory transmission

The early *in vitro* studies of excitatory transmission used intracellular recordings from rat brain slices. Rainnie *et al.* (1991a) used current-clamp recordings from BLA neurons to characterize postsynaptic potentials elicited through stimulation of the stria terminalis (ST) or the LA. Responses to stimulation of the ST or LA consisted of an excitatory postsynaptic potential (EPSP) followed by either a fast inhibitory postsynaptic potential (f-IPSP) only, or by a fast- and subsequent slow-IPSP (s-IPSP).

Current–voltage (IV) plot for passive membrane responses to current injection for a neuron showing spike accommodation (○) or non-accommodating regular spiking (●). The cells did not differ significantly in resting membrane potential (–65 mV for accommodating; –66 mV for non-accommodating). The input resistance, measured as the slope of a linear regression line fitted to the IV plot, indicated only a slight difference between the two, with the accommodating neuron at 104 MΩ and the non-accommodating at 137 MΩ. (**B**) Example responses of the two cells to increasing current injection steps. The accommodating cell (left traces) showed fewer action potentials per depolarization, and characteristic slowing of action potentials throughout the duration of the depolarization. The non-accommodating cell (right), in contrast, showed spiking at regular intervals for the duration of the depolarization, and increasing spike frequency with increasing depolarization. Note also the greater hyperpolarization after offset of the current step in the accommodating neuron, particularly following longer trains of action potentials. (Unpublished data from J.H. Williams and P.F Chapman.)

In normal physiological conditions at the resting membrane potential, low-frequency synaptic transmission via the ST or LA results in an EPSP consisting of dual glutamatergic components—a fast 6-cyano-7-nitroquinoxaline-2,3-dione (CNQX)-sensitive EPSP and a slow (±)-2-amino-5 phosphonovaleric acid (APV)-sensitive EPSP. Furthermore, in contrast to ST, LA stimulation evokes an f-IPSP which, when blocked by subsequent addition of bicuculline, revealed a temporally overlapping APV-sensitive slow EPSP. These data suggested that EPSP amplitude and duration are determined, in part, by the shunting of membrane conductance caused by a concomitant IPSP (e.g. see Figure 3.3). Thus, the findings by Rainnie *et al.* (1991a) are significant for subsequent studies of LTP in the amygdala for two reasons. First, unlike the hippocampal synaptic pathways, under normal physiological conditions postsynaptic NMDA receptors are activated on BLA neurons. Secondly, there is a fine balance between the presence of an f-IPSP and the full expression of the NMDA receptor-mediated synaptic component. Interestingly, both of these factors have also been shown to be important for neocortical LTP (Bear and Kirkwood, 1993).

Weisskopf and LeDoux (1999a) identified an NMDA receptor-mediated component to low-frequency stimulation of either the auditory thalamus or the external capsule. On the basis of voltage and Mg^{2+} sensitivity, however, they suggested that there are distinct populations of NMDA receptors mediating responses to thalamic input versus cortical input. They have also reported recently that the NMDA receptors activated by thalamic stimulation are not necessary for LTP induction (Weisskopf and LeDoux, 1999b). It is well to remember then that there is not a perfect correlation between the presence of NMDA receptors and the induction of CA1-like LTP.

Other *in vitro* studies (Gean and Chang, 1992) using stimulation of the ventral endopyriform nucleus also confirmed the initial findings regarding glutamate-mediated synaptic transmission in the BLA—a fast component mediated by α-amino-3-hydroxy-5-methyl-4-isoxazole proprionic acid (AMPA)/kainate receptors, and a slower component mediated by NMDA receptors. In similar studies, Sugita *et al.* (1992, 1993) have demonstrated that focal stimulation of BLA and LA evokes a glutamate-mediated EPSP in both pyramidal and non-pyramidal neurons in the lateral amygdala. Using intracellular recordings from neurons in

---

Figure 3.3 Typical synaptic responses to afferent stimulation. (**A**) Postsynaptic potentials were evoked by constant current stimulation of the external capsule in a 450 μm thick horizontal slice of the basolateral amygdala. Responses were recorded using whole-cell current-clamp, and the amplitude of the postsynaptic potential was measured at 9 ms (early peak) or 30 ms (late peak) across a range of membrane potentials from –70 to –45 mV. The current–voltage plots indicate two potentials; one excitatory (measured at the early peak) and one inhibitory (measured at the late peak). (**B**) Synaptic responses in the neuron reported in (A); the response at each holding potential is the average of 5–10 individual responses. The inhibitory postsynaptic potential appears to be mediated by $GABA_A$ receptors, as it is early, reverses at around –60 mV, and is blocked by 10 μM bicuculline (inset). In the absence of $GABA_A$-mediated inhibition, a single afferent stimulus is capable of producing a prolonged excitatory postsynaptic response, eliciting multiple action potentials.

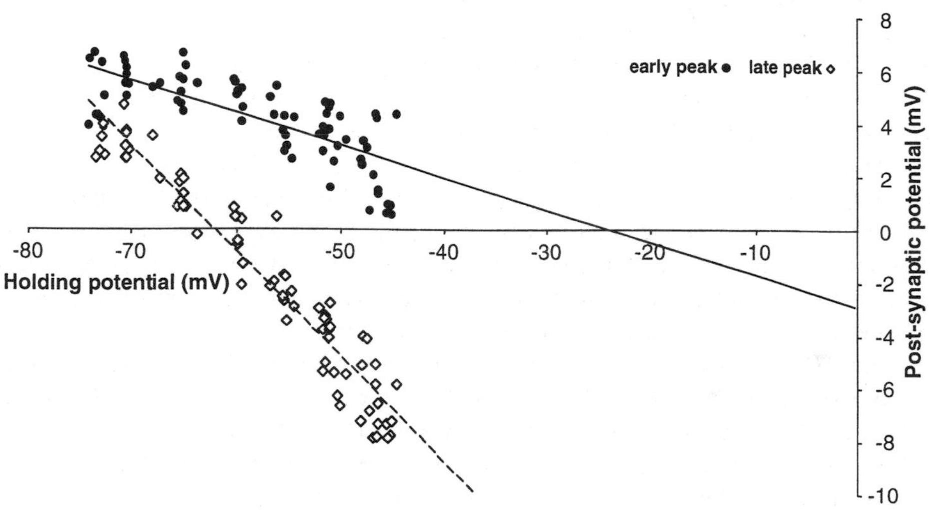
A
early peak ● late peak ◇
Holding potential (mV)
Post-synaptic potential (mV)
-80
-70
-50
-40
-30
-20
-10
8
6
4
2
0
-2
-4
-6
-8
-10

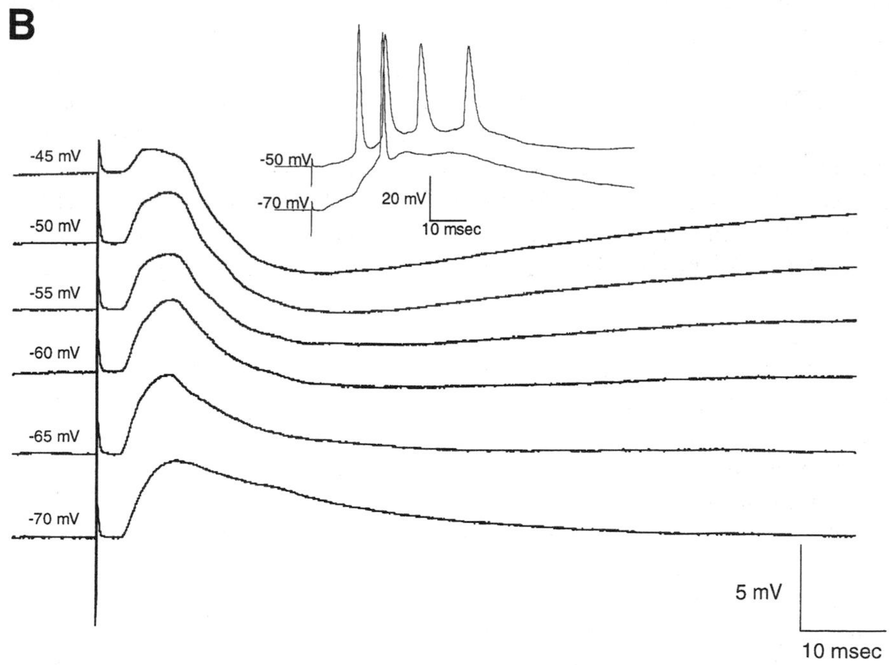
B
-45 mV
-50 mV
-55 mV
-60 mV
-65 mV
-70 mV
-50 mV
-70 mV
20 mV
10 msec
5 mV
10 msec

the CeA, Nose *et al.* (1991) have demonstrated that in the presence of bicuculline, basal nucleus stimulation evoked EPSPs mediated by both AMPA/kainate and NMDA receptors.

Inhibitory transmission

As described above, in their *in vitro* studies of excitatory synaptic transmission in BLA, Rainnie *et al.* (1991a) reported that stimulation-induced EPSPs are followed by both fast (f-IPSP) and slow IPSPs (s-IPSP). In corresponding studies (Rainnie *et al.*, 1991b), they used intracellular current-clamp recordings from BLA neurons to characterize these IPSPs evoked by stimulating either the ST or LA. The f-IPSP results from activation of γ-aminobutyric acid A ($GABA_A$) receptors, while the s-IPSP is mediated by activation of $GABA_B$ receptors. Moreover, these experiments demonstrated that the degree of expression of these two IPSPs is determined by the specific presynaptic inputs being activated—only feed-forward inhibition occurs via the ST input, whereas both feed-forward and direct inhibition occur via the LA pathway. These findings suggested that the f-IPSP probably dictates the primary state of excitability of BLA neurons, and the fast onset and short duration of the f-IPSP may also allow finely tuned control of the cellular response to excitatory inputs.

Nose *et al.* (1991) used focal, low-intensity stimulation of the dorsolateral division of the CeA to study $GABA_A$-mediated inhibitory transmission. In the same study, repetitive stimulation also revealed a slow $GABA_B$-mediated IPSP. Nose and colleagues also reported a presumed glycine-mediated IPSP following repetitive stimulation of the dorsolateral division of CeA.

Therefore, these and related studies (Washburn and Moises, 1992b; Lang and Pare, 1998) clearly indicate that GABA can have potent regulatory control over neuronal excitability in the lateral, basolateral, and central nuclei of the amygdala. Furthermore, this tight balance between excitatory and inhibitory inputs, in many respects similar to what has been observed in the neocortex, could have significant impact on the ease or difficulty with which LTP can be established as a model system in the amygdala.

3.4 LTP in the amygdala

Because of its importance in persistent, rapidly acquired forms of learning (for details, see Davis, Chapter 6; LeDoux, Chapter 7), it was natural to assume that synapses in the amygdala should demonstrate LTP, perhaps as readily as those in the hippocampus. Moreover, as surveyed above, the range of membrane and synaptic physiological response types within the neocortex-like regions of amygdala are similar to those of other brain regions that exhibit LTP. Beginning in the 1980s, several laboratories reported that LTP can be induced by a variety of stimuli in the lateral, basolateral, or medial amygdala, both *in vitro* and *in vivo*.

3.4.1 Tetanus-induced potentiation

In vivo

The first report of LTP in the amygdala came as part of a comprehensive *in vivo* study conducted by Racine *et al.* (1983). In an explicit attempt to determine whether LTP was unique to the hippocampus or distributed throughout the forebrain, Racine *et al.* stimulated eight separate forebrain sites while recording from pyriform or entorhinal cortex, CA1, CA3 and dentate gyrus, the subiculum, the septal nuclei, or the amygdala. Stimulation and recording were conducted in a chronic preparation, i.e. over a period of 3 days in unanaesthetized rats via indwelling electrodes. While not specifying which subnuclei were either stimulated or recorded from, the results illustrated that the amygdala was among the more susceptible to long-term synaptic plasticity (see Figure 3.4), ranking generally behind the hippocampal regions that Racine *et al.* examined (CA1, CA3, subiculum, and dentate gyrus), but well ahead of the other forebrain structures. While the differences were relatively small, and the relative contributions of different input pathways difficult to gauge, the results of Racine *et al.* are very consistent with subsequent experiments both *in vivo* and *in vitro*; it is possible to induce stable, long-lasting LTP in the amygdala, though it is more difficult and less dramatic than in hippocampus.

The first *in vivo* studies to address explicitly the question of whether an input pathway believed to be important for emotional learning could support LTP was conducted on inputs from the auditory thalamus to the lateral amygdala (Clugnet and LeDoux, 1990). Based

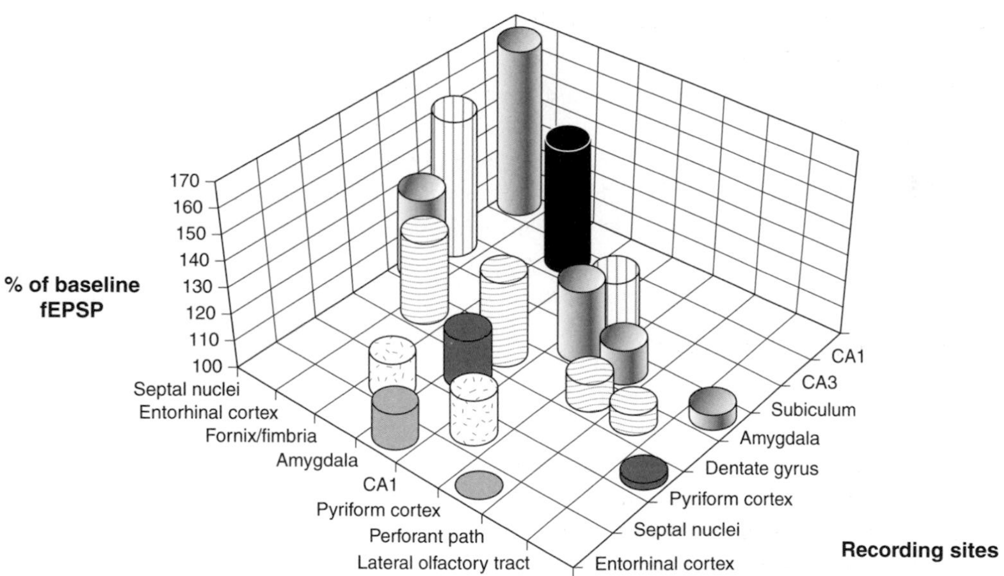

Figure 3.4 Magnitude of LTP at various sites in the limbic forebrain *in vivo*, as reported by Racine *et al.* (1983). Although not all possible sites or combinations of stimulation and recording location were attempted, the results give an overall impression that synapses in the hippocampus proper produce the greatest overall potentiation, followed by subiculum and amygdala. This impression has been confirmed essentially by subsequent *in vitro* and *in vivo* recordings.

on lesion experiments and data from anatomical tract tracing studies, LeDoux's group had determined that projections from the auditory thalamus to the LA are critical for Pavlovian fear conditioning to an acoustic stimulus (see LeDoux, Chapter 7). To begin to test the hypothesis that LTP in this pathway could constitute the synaptic mechanism of fear conditioning, Clugnet and LeDoux (1990) placed a stimulating electrode in the auditory thalamus of anaesthetized rats, and recorded presumably monosynaptic responses in the ipsilateral LA. Trains of high-frequency stimulation produced enhancement of the amplitude and slope of a short-latency positivity in the rather complex waveform elicited by auditory thalamus stimulation. LTP (defined as a >10% increase lasting at least 20 min) was evoked successfully in 10 of 20 animals in which the electrodes were positioned verifiably within the anterior thalamus and LA, though only four of these were still potentiated 50 min after tetanus. One factor in the relatively low success rate (at least compared with hippocampus) may be selection of a specific set of input fibres or target neurons, as successful LTP induction was correlated with short-latency peak responses (Clugnet and LeDoux, 1990).

The preliminary experiments conducted by Clugnet and LeDoux in attempting to determine the appropriate tetanic stimulation pattern in the auditory thalamus to LA pathway are very instructive. First, the fact that extensive experimentation on these parameters was necessary indicates the existence of significant differences between this pathway and hippocampal pathways that support LTP. Clugnet and LeDoux report that they began by using parameters taken directly from hippocampal LTP experiments; 10 trains of 10-pulse bursts in which the pulses were delivered at 400 Hz and the bursts at 3–5 s intervals. When this proved ineffective, they systematically and thoroughly varied the frequency of pulses and bursts, the duration of bursts and trains, and the monophasic nature of the stimuli until they arrived at the optimal parameters of 10-train stimuli consisting of 30 biphasic pulses delivered at 400 Hz, with the bursts delivered at 1 Hz. Whether the requirement for altered tetanization parameters arises from differences in the synaptic mechanisms of LTP, some network property (e.g. activation of inhibitory interneurons), or both still remains to be determined, though more information about the nature of basic synaptic and network properties of thalamic inputs to LA will no doubt be invaluable in this regard.

The ability to potentiate the auditory thalamus inputs to LA provided the basis for an important set of experiments that began to test the functional significance of LTP in the amygdala. Rogan and LeDoux (1995), using essentially the same protocol as Clugnet and LeDoux (1990), produced both electrically and acoustically evoked field potentials in the LA of anaesthetized rats. Although the latency of these responses differed (as the acoustic responses travelled across several brainstem and midbrain synapses before reaching the medial geniculate), the basic shape and characteristics of the two responses were similar. Using tetanus parameters very similar to those employed by Clugnet and LeDoux (1990), Rogan and LeDoux demonstrated that tetanization of the auditory thalamus to LA inputs produced enhancement of both the electrically and acoustically evoked response. This result laid the groundwork for subsequent experiments in which 'behavioural tetanization' was used to induce changes in acoustically evoked responses (see Section 3.4.4).

Maren and Fanselow (1995) also attempted to understand the synaptic basis of Pavlovian fear conditioning by inducing LTP in the amygdala, but chose to examine hippocampal inputs to the BLA. These inputs are of interest because: (i) they constitute a prominent set of BLA afferents; (ii) they are monosynaptic; (iii) they are glutamatergic and thus likely to share characteristics with other forebrain pathways that demonstrate plasticity; and, finally, (iv) they may play a role in Pavlovian fear conditioning to contextual cues (Maren and Fanselow, 1995). When rats are placed in a distinctive box and given footshocks, they later exhibit fearful behaviours when placed back in that box. This fear conditioning is disrupted by lesion to both the hippocampus and the amygdala (see Davis Chapter 6; LeDoux, Chapter 7), suggesting that information about contextual cues must be transmitted from one to the other. At some point, there should be a convergence of information about conditioned stimuli, whether they are discrete (e.g. tone or light) or diffuse (i.e. context). Maren and Fanselow (1995) offered the hypothesis that this convergence and the plasticity that may cause long-lasting changes in the response to the contextual cues result from activity in the hippocampal afferents carried through the ventral angular bundle (VAB).

After determining that the field potentials recorded in BLA following VAB stimulation were monosynaptic and mediated by excitatory amino acid receptors, Maren and Fanselow delivered tetanic stimulation that was somewhat different to that used by Clugnet and LeDoux (1990), and closer to the stimuli normally used to induce LTP in CA1. Ten bursts of 20 pulses in 200 ms were delivered at an overall frequency of 1 Hz, and this train was repeated four times over 20 min. The amplitude and slope of the presumably monosynaptic component of the evoked response was enhanced significantly over the course of 60 min, relative to pre-tetanus baseline and to two different low-frequency stimulation control groups (1 and 0.05 Hz), though it is not clear what proportion of the animals tested showed potentiation (Maren and Fanselow, 1995).

Maren and Fanselow made two additional findings of potentially great importance. First, the LTP recorded in BLA to VAB stimulation was blocked by infusion of AP5 into the BLA, indicating that induction of LTP at these synapses depends on NMDA receptors. This is important both in comparing induction mechanisms across different brain regions and in offering a potential explanation for the observation that AP5 infused into the LA/BLA can block fear conditioning (e.g. Miserendino *et al.*, 1990). Secondly, LTP was associated with a reduction in paired-pulse facilitation (PPF), implying that LTP expression in BLA might involve changes in the presynaptic terminal. This represents another unusual feature of LTP in the amygdala, as LTP in CA1 is not associated consistently with changes in PPF (Schulz *et al.*, 1994).

In vitro

Because of the complexity of the cytoarchitecture within the amygdala, the earliest attempts to induce and explain the mechanisms of LTP in the amygdala were performed on single neurons *in vitro*. This avoided the difficulty of evoking field potentials that were similar from slice to slice and the complication of interpreting the currents underlying each component of the field potential (but see Figure 3.5). Testing the ability of different cell types to support LTP is also a goal of this type of experiment, though until recently this has proven difficult due to the lack of unequivocal physiological signatures for each morphologically identified cell type (see Section 3.3).

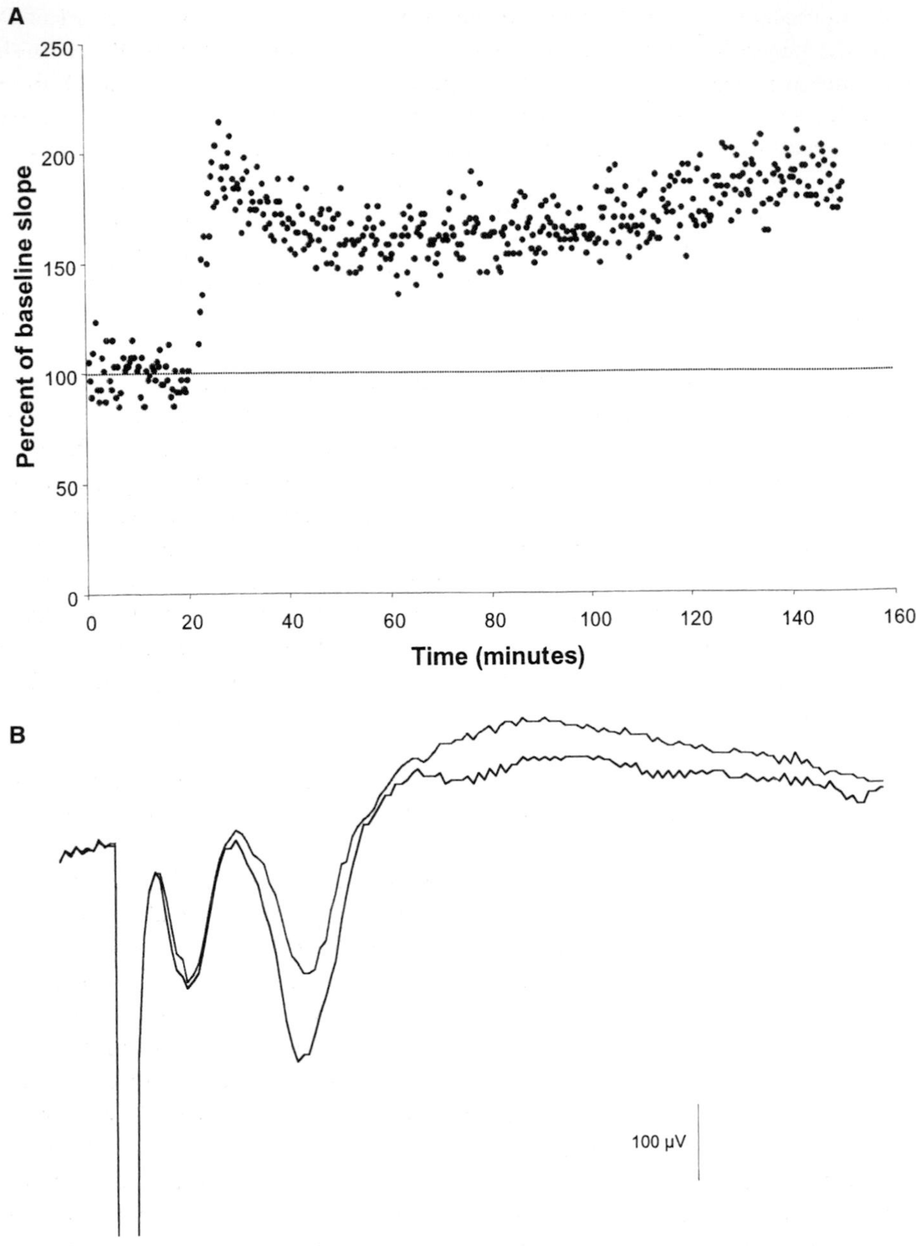

Figure 3.5 LTP in basolateral amygdala. Extracellular field potentials were recorded in basolateral amygdala in response to stimulation of the lateral amygdala of coronal slices bathed in normal cerebrospinal fluid. Following 20 min of baseline stimulation at 0.05 Hz, theta-burst stimulation was delivered, and low-frequency stimulation resumed. Potentiation developed over a 5–10 min period, and the slope and peak (not shown) of the field potential remained significantly elevated for >60 min. (M.F. Ramsay and P.F. Chapman, unpublished data.)

Presumed pyramidal/projection neurons (lateral and basolateral) Chapman *et al.* (1990) stimulated the external (extreme) capsule and recorded postsynaptic potentials and currents using intracellular sharp electrodes. They chose to stimulate the external capsule in part because it carries afferents to the amygdala from neocortical areas that may be involved in associative learning, and in part because it forms a discrete fibre pathway easily visualized with a stereomicroscope. Recordings were made 'blind' (i.e. without *a priori* knowledge of cell type) from neurons in the LA and BLA in horizontal slices. It was presumed that the majority of recordings were from large, probably pyramidal, projection neurons. Delivery of tetanic stimulation (100 Hz for 1 s) produced significant, long-lasting enhancement of the EPSP in 16 of 20 neurons, a figure comparable with that seen in hippocampal slices under similar conditions.

In an attempt to compare the induction mechanisms of LA/BLA neurons with those of hippocampal neurons, Chapman and Bellavance (1992) assessed the role of NMDA receptors in synaptic transmission and LTP in amygdala slices. Once again stimulating the external capsule and recording from LA/BLA neurons under both current-clamp and voltage-clamp conditions, they found little evidence of any NMDA-mediated response. Depolarizing neurons under voltage-clamp did not reveal a voltage-sensitive current, as would be expected of NMDA-mediated responses, nor was there a significant synaptic response after treatment of the slices with the non-NMDA antagonist CNQX. Unfortunately, the results of the LTP experiments in the study were far from unequivocal. A 50 μM concentration of DL-AP5, which is sufficient to block both NMDA receptors and LTP in hippocampal slices, did not affect LTP in amygdala. At 100 μM, DL-AP5 was effective in blocking LTP, but also significantly reduced synaptic responses, an observation that has been replicated several times (see below). It is not clear from these experiments, then, whether LTP induction is affected specifically by block of NMDA receptors, or by the effects of DL-AP5 on other glutamate receptors, or on some combination.

Although Chapman *et al.* (1990) and Chapman and Bellavance (1992) failed to find any evidence of significant NMDA responses in basolateral amygdala to stimulation of external capsule *in vitro*, it is still likely that there are functional NMDA receptors in the lateral and basolateral nuclei. Differences in the plane of section or exact stimulation site, for example, could produce differences in the ability to recruit NMDA responses in slices. Indeed, there is evidence that slow, long-latency EPSPs can be elicited *in vitro* in a minority of cells. Gean *et al.* (1993b) reported that 35% of BLA neurons exhibited late (peak latency of ~25 ms), slow (mean duration of ~125 ms) excitatory responses to relatively high-intensity stimulation of the endopyriform nucleus, located at the ventral-most extension of the external capsule. This slow EPSP was blocked by DL-AP5, enhanced by removal of Mg^{2+} from the extracellular medium, and exhibited LTP following tetanic stimulation. It is not known, however, whether these NMDA-mediated responses originate from cortical, subcortical, or, more probably, intrinsic afferents to BLA neurons, as their latency and inability to follow high-frequency stimulation indicate that they are polysynaptic responses. In another report, however, Gean *et al.* (1993a) found that tetanic stimulation of the ventral endopyriform nucleus produced LTP of the fast, early EPSP that was blocked by 50 μM DL-AP5. Although this demonstrates that NMDA receptors can contribute to LTP in the basolateral amygdala, it also suggests that stimulation of the endopyriform nucleus recruits a different set of synapses than stimulation of the external capsule.

The complexity of the relationship between NMDA receptor activation and plasticity in the BLA is also highlighted by a series of experiments by Li *et al.* (1998) into the efficacy of high-frequency and low-frequency stimulation in inducing long-lasting potentiation. Prolonged low-frequency stimulation produces LTD at many central nervous system (CNS) synapses, notably in CA1 (see Section 2.2). Surprisingly, Li *et al.* (1998) report that 900 pulses at 1 Hz produced pronounced, long-lasting (>30 min) enhancement of synaptic responses of BLA neurons to external capsule stimulation. Although AP5 blocked the enhancement that occurred *during* the 900 pulses, it did not affect the potentiation that persisted after returning to low-frequency stimulation. On the other hand, the low-frequency stimulation resulted in long-lasting reduction of synaptic responses if it was preceded by brief high-frequency stimulation. In the presence of AP5, the short-term enhancement normally produced by high-frequency stimulation was significantly reduced, but still caused subsequent low-frequency stimulation to produce depression rather than potentiation. As an additional complication, the 'switch' from potentiating to depressing effects of low-frequency stimulation could be blocked by application of a presynaptic metabotropic glutamate receptor (mGluR) antagonist. The authors suggest that high-frequency activation of external capsule–BLA synapses might sensitize presynaptic group II mGluRs so that low-frequency stimulation then activates these receptors, leading to presynaptic inhibition. In some ways, this draws a parallel to the hippocampal CA1 cell field, as LTD induced by low-frequency stimulation can also be blocked by group II mGluR antagonists (Bashir *et al.*, 1993). It also reveals a difference, as low-frequency tetanic stimulation normally does not lead to LTP in CA1. Perhaps the effect of high-frequency stimulation at 'naïve' synapses in the BLA is to make them more CA1-like! There is evidence from other experiments (described below) that there is a greater contribution of pre-synaptic plasticity in LA/BLA synapses than in CA1, and this could explain some of the differences both in the responses to low-frequency stimulation and the controversy over NMDA dependence of BLA LTP.

Inhibitory interneurons in BLA Because most single neuron recordings in amygdala slices have been performed blind, there has almost certainly been a bias towards recording from large, pyramidal-type neurons, particularly in magnocellular regions of BLA. However, persistence paid off for Mahanty and Sah (1998), who found that 44 of 596 neuron recordings using blind whole-cell techniques showed electrophysiological characteristics consistent with their being inhibitory interneurons. Using tetanus parameters that did not evoke LTP consistently in pyramidal neurons (100 stimuli at 30 Hz), Mahanty and Sah (1998) were able to obtain LTP in seven of seven interneurons. The LTP in interneurons was not affected by AP5, but was blocked by intracellular application of the calcium chelator $0_1$0'-Bis(2-aminophenyl) ethyleneglycol-N,N,N',N'-tetracetic acid (BAPTA). The dependence on intracellular calcium, lack of effect of AP5, and voltage characteristics of the excitatory postsynaptic currents (EPSCs) led the authors to suggest that LTP in interneurons is mediated by calcium-permeable AMPA (non-NMDA glutamate) receptors.

The implications of these results for network plasticity in the BLA are fascinating. Using moderately high-frequency stimulation, it is apparently quite easy to induce LTP of inhibitory neurons. Mahanty and Sah (1998) go on to demonstrate that the net effect of this is to increase inhibition of pyramidal neurons. This would not only generally reduce network excitability, but would also make it more difficult to induce LTP in pyramidal neurons, as greater inhibition reduces the reliability of LTP induction in BLA (Chapman and Bellavance, 1992). Thus, LTP in inhibitory interneurons would represent a network level metaplasticity in which the threshold for LTP induction is affected by prior experience.

3.4.2 Pharmacological and genetic manipulation of LTP

The greatest potential importance of LTP is as a mechanism for learning and memory. If we are to test the hypothesis that LTP is responsible, at least in part, for learning and memory, then we must seek to understand how LTP is induced and expressed, modified, and undone. The amygdala presents an opportunity to link LTP mechanisms to simple conditioning, provided we can learn a sufficient amount about the LTP mechanisms. Recent experiments using principally extracellular recording in amygdala slices have begun to give us insight into how LTP works in the lateral and medial amygdala and how this differs in many ways from the best understood forms of LTP.

Lateral/basolateral

There is a substantial amount of information addressing some of the more basic questions of LTP induction and expression, though most of it is from LA/BLA and much of it is conflicting. Chapman and Bellavance (1992) argued that LTP of external capsule–BLA synapses was not dependent specifically on NMDA receptor activation, an observation that was supported by Watanabe *et al.* (1995a), but disputed by Gean *et al.* (1993a) and by Maren and Fanselow (1995). Weisskopf and LeDoux recently have reported that although there are functional NMDA receptors at acoustic thalamus to LA synapses, blocking them with AP5 does not prevent the induction of LTP. LTP induction in this pathway did, however, depend on both postsynaptic depolarization and changes in intracellular calcium concentration in the LA neurons, consistent with an important role for L-type calcium channels (Weisskopf and LeDoux, 1999b).

It is not immediately clear why the results of experiments with NMDA antagonists are as inconsistent as they have been, but it is likely that differences in the input pathways contribute. In almost every case cited above, there was a significant difference in either the preparation or the site of stimulation. Chapman and Bellavance (1992) stimulated the external capsule, but in horizontal slices, while Gean *et al.* (1993a) stimulated the endopyriform nucleus in coronal slices. Maren and Fanselow (1995) very probably stimulated many of the same synapses but, by stimulating the VAB *in vivo*, it is likely that they also stimulated many others, some of which would have been NMDA dependent. Huang and Kandel (1998), stimulating external capsule in coronal slices, steered a middle course, suggesting that LTP of external capsule inputs to LA was completely blocked by AP5 under normal conditions (either weak or strong tetanic stimulation in normal extracellular media), but that the requirement for NMDA receptor activation could be overcome by blocking $GABA_A$ inhibition with picrotoxin or by pairing afferent stimulation with direct postsynaptic depolarization. They are suggesting, in other words, that LTP at external capsule–LA synapses is very much like that at synapses in CA1 in its dependence on NMDA receptors; it can be driven to NMDA-independent induction, but typically is blocked completely by NMDA antagonists.

Apart from the debate about the involvement of NMDA receptors, there have been indications that other neurotransmitters or neuromodulators can affect LTP induction in LA. Watanabe *et al.* (1995a), while demonstrating that LTP in synapses from external capsule to LA was NMDA independent, also indicated that this potentiation was affected by activation of muscarinic cholinergic receptors, as the antagonist scopolamine was able to significantly reduce long-lasting potentiation of external capsule synapses in coronal slices. This same group (Watanabe *et al.*, 1996) later demonstrated that LTP in LA was suppressed by activation of the β-adrenoceptor–cyclic AMP system. Although there is still nowhere near as wide a range of receptors implicated in LTP in amygdala as in hippocampus, the gap may be closing soon. Halbach and Albrecht (1998) indicated, using field potential recordings *in vitro*, that LA LTP is blocked by angiotensin II acting through AT1 receptors. It is likely that more such discoveries will follow.

One of the most comprehensive studies was reported recently by Huang and Kandel (1998), who conducted both whole-cell and extracellular recordings of synaptic activity and LTP in the LA, in response to external capsule stimulation. They began by addressing some of the basic features of hippocampal LTP, and reported that the LTP they recorded in LA (i) can be induced by pairing depolarization of the target neuron with low-frequency stimulation; (ii) can be blocked by AP5 (unless the slices are disinhibited or LTP is induced by pairing); and (iii) requires increases in postsynaptic calcium concentration. Huang and Kandel's results suggest that the induction of LTP in the external capsule–LA pathway depends on activation of both the presynaptic and the postsynaptic neurons. In agreement with Maren and Fanselow (1995), Huang and Kandel (1998) found that the induction of LTP in LA reduced the expression of PPF, suggesting that the *expression* of LTP might involve changes in neurotransmitter release, a presynaptic modification.

To explore further the mechanisms that might contribute to presynaptic changes, Huang and Kandel (1998) tested the contribution of the cAMP-dependent protein kinase (PKA) in the induction of LTP in external capsule synapses in LA. Previous reports from hippocampal slices had indicated that blocking PKA inhibits late-phase (protein synthesis-dependent) LTP in CA1, but blocks induction of even early-phase LTP in mossy fibre–CA3 synapses, where LTP expression is thought to be presynaptic (Abel *et al.*, 1997). The results were consistent with those of mossy fibre–CA3 LTP (Weisskopf *et al.*, 1994; Huang *et al.*, 1995) as two different PKA inhibitors blocked LTP to both single and multiple tetanus trains. Moreover, bath application of forskolin (which activates PKA by stimulating adenylyl cyclase to produce more cAMP) produced long-lasting enhancements of external capsule–LA synaptic responses. The authors suggest that this profile is similar in many respects to other synapses (e.g. mossy fibre–CA3, parallel fibre–cerebellar Purkinje cell, *Aplysia* sensory–motor neuron) that require presynaptic PKA activation for the induction of early phases of experience-dependent plasticity. Why these synapses would require both postsynaptic calcium and presynaptic PKA is a matter for future investigation.

Advances in genetic engineering have permitted the targeted disruption of proteins that previously were difficult to manipulate. This will provide additional opportunities to characterize the mechanisms underlying LTP in the amygdala, as well as to test the behavioural effects of those disruptions. While there are a multitude of studies exploring the effects of targeted gene deletions (knockouts) on hippocampal LTP and behaviour, the application of this technology to the study of LTP in the amygdala is still in its infancy. One study that has looked at both amygdala-dependent behaviour and LTP in a knockout mouse (Brambilla *et al.*, 1997) has produced yet another dissociation between the mechanisms of LTP in the hippocampus (CA1) and the amygdala.

In knocking out the gene for the calcium-responsive guanine nucleotide exchange factor RasGRF, Brambilla *et al.* expected to find deficits in hippocampal LTP and spatial learning. This prediction was based on the fact that RasGRF can be activated by calcium influx through NMDA receptors, and can (ultimately) activate the cAMP response element-binding protein (CREB) and mitogen-activated protein kinase (MAPK), both of which appear to be involved in hippocampal LTP. The behavioural and physiological tests, however, revealed no deficits in spatial learning tasks or in hippocampal LTP, induced by either theta-burst stimulation or 100 pulses at 100 Hz. On the other hand, there were significant deficits on learning tasks that are disrupted by amygdala lesions (tone–shock-mediated freezing, inhibitory avoidance, two-way active avoidance) and a deficit in LTP evoked in BLA of coronal slices by delivering theta-burst stimulation to LA. The results are consistent with the hypothesis that numerous plasticity mechanisms exist in the mammalian forebrain, and that many of these differences will be revealed by comparing mechanisms in the amygdala with those of the hippocampus.

Comparison of basolateral and medial

In fact, in searching for diverse mechanisms, it is instructive to compare LTP induction and expression mechanisms between different subnuclei of the amygdala. Although there are disappointingly few data on nuclei other than LA and BLA, what is known about LTP in the medial amygdala reflects rather striking differences from the lateral nuclei. In contrast to their findings in LA, Shindou *et al.* (1993) found that several NMDA receptor antagonists blocked LTP induction in medial amygdala. Watanabe *et al.* (1995a) replicated the results with NMDA antagonists and indicated that the muscarinic cholinergic antagonist scopolamine was capable of reducing LTP in both nuclei. The sensitivity of LTP in LA to muscarinic, but not NMDA receptors led Brambilla *et al.* (1997) to speculate that the sensitivity of these synapses to disruption of RasGRF may stem from their inability to engage NMDA receptor induced-LTP, while depending on mechanisms linked to G-protein-coupled receptors such as the muscarinic cholinergic. Watanabe *et al.* (1995b) demonstrated that inhibitors of nitric oxide synthase blocked LTP in the medial, but not lateral amygdala, and Abe *et al.* (1996) subsequently provided the complementary evidence that nitric oxide donors could facilitate LTP induction in medial, but not lateral amygdala. Perhaps the most striking differences came with tests of agonists of β-noradrenergic receptors and their effects on

LTP induction. Watanabe *et al.* (1996) showed that the β-noradrenergic agonist isoproterenol enhances LTP in the medial amygdala, but blocks it in the LA. They hypothesized that the isoproterenol effects were mediated through cAMP/PKA signalling, and found that application of forskolin enhanced potentiation in the medial amygdala, while application of Rp-adenosine-3',5'-cyclic-monophosphothioate (Rp-cAMPS) blocked medial amygdala LTP. In contrast to the results reported by Huang and Kandel (1998), Watanabe *et al.* (1996) also found that application of forskolin blocked LTP in LA, and Rp-cAMPS application blocked the LTP-suppressing effects of isoproterenol. In summary, the results from comparisons of LA and medial amygdala serve as useful reminders that we should not think of 'the amygdala' as being a single entity with a single set of rules for long-term synaptic plasticity.

3.4.3 Pharmacological induction of LTP in amygdala

Long-term plasticity at CNS synapses is induced most commonly by patterned electrical stimulation. There are, however, other methods of inducing long-lasting changes in synaptic efficacy. By applying analogues of neurotransmitters or second messengers to brain slices, we can gain insight into the biochemical pathways that can support plasticity. In amygdala, this can also be advantageous as it side-steps, to some extent, the need to identify specific synaptic inputs. In this case, one could examine (for example) all LA synapses that respond to application of β-adrenergic agonists, regardless of where the synapses are and which specific cell types might mediate the responses.

β-Adrenergic agonists

Huang *et al.* (1996) applied the β-adrenergic agonist isoproterenol to amygdala slices, and found that brief application of low concentrations produced a long-lasting enhancement of synaptic responses (recorded in single neurons) that could not be blocked with antagonists of either AMPA or NMDA receptors. Huang *et al.* argue that the effects of isoproterenol on synaptic responses are not mediated through activation of the cAMP–PKA pathway in the postsynaptic neuron. They demonstrated that inhibitors of PKA delivered through the recording pipette blocked the effects of isoproterenol on post-action potential hyperpolarization, but failed to prevent its enhancement of synaptic transmission. Extracellular application of the P/Q type VGCC antagonist Ω-agatoxin-IVA, however, was able to block the potentiating effect of isoproterenol completely. These observations, combined with the reduction of PPF by isoproterenol-induced potentiation led the authors to conclude that noradrenaline (norepinephrine) can facilitate synaptic transmission in the BLA by enhancing the function of presynaptic P/Q type VGCCs. In a more recent study, Wang *et al.* (1999) have indicated that *presynaptic* cAMP activation is critical for the induction of β-adrenoceptor-mediated potentiation. There, they report that forskolin and cAMP analogues can potentiate BLA synaptic responses, and that this enhancement can be blocked by the application of 5-HT or 5-HT_{1A} agonists. Taken together, these observations suggest that either increasing (by activating β-adrenoceptors) or by decreasing (via 5-HT_{1A} receptors) activity in the cAMP–PKA signalling pathway, can have a long-term effect on synaptic efficacy.

cAMP analogues

More direct tests of the effects of activating cAMP-dependent processes have provided results that are consistent with those obtained through activation of β-adrenergic receptors. Huang and Kandel (1998), among other manipulations (see Section 3.4.2), applied the adenylyl cyclase activator forskolin to LA in slices, and observed an LTP-like increase in the response of extracellular field potentials. Consistent with the potentiation that they recorded following tetanic stimulation of external capsule inputs to LA, this potentiation was associated with a decrease of PPF. Furthermore, the potentiation produced by forskolin occluded tetanus-induced LTP, suggesting that they are produced by similar (if not identical) synaptic mechanisms.

Huang and Gean (1995) also found that application of forskolin enhanced synaptic responses in BLA. They were interested specifically in the mechanisms by which the NMDA-mediated EPSP is enhanced. Bath application of 25 μM forskolin led to persistent enhancement of both the stimulus-evoked and pharmacologically isolated NMDA-mediated EPSP and the postsynaptic response to exogenously applied NMDA. Huang and Gean (1995) thus suggest that LTP in BLA is mediated, at least in part, by a cAMP-mediated increase in postsynaptic NMDA receptors.

Metabotropic glutamate agonists

mGluRs are known to play a role in hippocampal synaptic plasticity, and Neugenbauer *et al.* (1997) found that they are also capable of influencing plasticity in the LA. Application of 10 μM L-AP4 for approximately 14 min produced a slow-developing, long-lasting enhancement in the amplitude of EPSCs evoked by stimulation of lateral amygdala afferents. This potentiation was blocked by antagonists of group III mGluRs, but not group II antagonists. It was also blocked by prior kindling of the amygdala *in vivo*, suggesting that kindling involves a saturable presynaptic enhancement mediated by group III mGluRs. It is not clear whether this mechanism also contributes to tetanus-induced LTP.

3.4.4 Behavioural induction of LTP in amygdala

Another useful strategy for establishing the relationship between synaptic plasticity and learning is to produce LTP-like changes in synaptic transmission by activating the relevant synapses behaviourally. Two studies published sequentially in 1997 (McKernan and Shinnick-Gallagher, 1997; Rogan *et al.*, 1997) utilized this approach to understanding plasticity in LA, and both came to essentially the same conclusion; that fear conditioning induces changes in the strength of auditory thalamus–LA synapses that look very similar to the changes induced by tetanic stimulation.

In vivo

Rogan *et al.* (1997) built on the findings of Rogan and LeDoux (1995) that electrical tetanization of auditory thalamus–LA synapses enhances both electrically and acoustically evoked field potentials in LA. They implanted recording electrodes in LA, and observed the field potentials induced by a train of auditory stimuli delivered to unanaesthetized rats. They found that when the trains of auditory stimuli were delivered repeatedly immediately prior to footshock, the amplitude of the auditory-evoked potential was increased. At the same time, this paired presentation of the auditory conditioned stimulus (CS) and the footshock unconditioned stimulus (US) produced behavioural evidence of fear (i.e. complete immobility, or freezing). In contrast, control rats that had the CS and US presented in an unpaired fashion showed a high degree of freezing to the auditory stimulus, but no significant enhancement of the auditory-evoked potential.

These results are a major step forward in the attempt to explain the relationship between LTP and learning. They set the stage for additional experiments that will determine which synapses on which types of LA neurons change as a result of paired presentations of the CS and the US. It is not completely clear where the information about the footshock US enters the amygdala, onto which neurons they make synapses, or why they are required to potentiate afferent activity from the auditory thalamus. Finally, of course, we will want to know the mechanisms of learning-induced plasticity, and how they compare with more widely studied forms of synaptic plasticity.

Ex vivo

We have gained some insight into the mechanisms of fear conditioning through the work of McKernan and Shinnick-Gallagher (1997). Like Rogan *et al.* (1997), they examined the effects of fear conditioning on synaptic responses, but with the goal of investigating synaptic mechanisms of behaviourally induced plasticity. Rats were given paired presentations of auditory CS and footshock US, and conditioning was measured as enhancement by the CS of an acoustic startle response. Pseudoconditioned control animals were given unpaired presentations of the same auditory CS and footshock US. Following conditioning, the rats were killed, and coronal slices including the LA and the auditory thalamus inputs were isolated. Stimulation of presumptive thalamic afferents into the LA indicated that randomly sampled neurons in slices taken from conditioned rats showed larger evoked synaptic responses than comparable neurons in naive or pseudoconditioned slices. The enhancements were greater in the component of the EPSC mediated by AMPA receptors. Interestingly, McKernan and Shinnick-Gallagher agree with Maren and Fanselow (1995) and Huang and Kandel (1998) in that the behaviourally induced potentiation they observe in LA occludes PPF, and thus represents a change in presynaptic function. This suggests that auditory fear conditioning increases transmitter release in only those presynaptic terminals apposed to AMPA receptors, which must form a distinct population from those that contain a mixture of AMPA and NMDA receptors. This may turn out to be another unique feature of amygdala synapses.

3.5 Summary of amygdala LTP: properties and parameters

LTP in the amygdala shares many common features with the more frequently studied synapses of the hippocampus. On the other hand, there are significant differences. Some of the patterns of tetanic stimulation that reliably induce LTP in CA1 are considerably less effective in amygdala. Genetic and pharmacological modifications have different effects on LTP in not just amygdala versus hippocampus, but in medial versus LA/BLA as well. Indeed, in membrane and synaptic physiology as well as mechanisms of plasticity, there appear to be greater similarities between the amygdala and neocortex than between amygdala and hippocampus.

3.5.1 Induction parameters

Theta-burst-type stimuli tetani consisting of short (typically 4–6 pulses) high-frequency (100–250 Hz) bursts repeated at approximately 5 Hz are very effective at inducing LTP in CA1 without the need for pharmacological disinhibition. Similar theta-like protocols are also effective in inducing LTP in the LA/BLA and in sensory neocortex (M.F. Ramsay, K. Fox, and P.F. Chapman, unpublished observations), suggesting common conditions for LTP induction throughout the forebrain. The success of one single tetanisation protocol might reflect the fact that all cortical (or cortex-like) structures consist of a basic set of elements, including principle pyramidal neurons with feed-forward and feedback inhibition. The comparison of passive membrane properties, and the relative frequency with which bursting and fast-firing neurons (for example) appear in amygdala and neocortex, tends to support this contention.

Conversely, the difficulty in inducing LTP with some frequently used hippocampal tetanus parameters points out differences between hippocampus and other forebrain regions. LTP in CA1 typically is induced by using repeated trains of stimuli at 100 Hz, lasting 1 s. Mahanty and Sah (1998) indicated that stimulation patterns that would potentiate pyramidal or granule cells in hippocampus (30 Hz, 100 pulses repeated twice) readily produce LTP of inhibitory interneurons in LA/BLA but fail to elicit LTP consistently in pyramidal neurons. Li *et al.* (1998) found that 100 Hz stimulation for 1 s consistently failed to produce LTP, but did prevent the subsequent potentiation by prolonged 1 Hz stimulation. While other groups have found fairly reliable LTP using 100 Hz for approximately 1 s (e.g. Watanabe *et al.*, 1995b; Huang and Kandel, 1998), most groups that systematically have compared the efficacy of different tetanus parameters on LTP in LA or BLA (e.g. Clugnet and LeDoux, 1990; Maren and Fanselow, 1995) have found that shorter trains at somewhat higher frequency are considerably more effective. It is likely that the optimal parameters will reflect both the diversity of extrinsic inputs to the amygdala and its complex intrinsic microcircuitry. The ability to induce LTP would then depend critically on both the specific afferents stimulated and the post-synaptic neurons that respond to them.

3.5.2 Pharmacological and genetic inhibitors

LTP in the amygdala is sensitive to many of the same manipulations that affect LTP in the hippocampus. Blockade of NMDA receptors affects LTP in the LA and BLA according to some, while others find that LA/BLA LTP is blocked by VGCC antagonists, but not by NMDA antagonists. LTP in medial amygdala might be more dependent on NMDA receptor activation, but has not been tested as extensively as has LTP in the LA/BLA. Neuromodulators also seem to affect LTP in LA/BLA, particularly those that act through enhancement of the adenylyl cyclase–cAMP–PKA pathway, such as β-adrenergic receptors or group III mGluRs.

3.5.3 The functional consequences of amygdala LTP

It is tempting to think that LTP in the amygdala would have a simple effect on information processing. The most uncomplicated model would assume that information about stimuli with strong emotional content (e.g. foot shock, exposure to predators, food, or water) would activate amygdala neurons. When activity in these inputs converges with coincident activation of other inputs representing 'neutral' stimuli (e.g. simple auditory or visual stimuli), some threshold is exceeded and plasticity is induced in the neutral inputs.

The data currently available about LTP in the amygdala do not address directly the issue of convergent synaptic inputs. Most LTP experiments in amygdala have (like their counterparts in hippocampus) involved tetanic stimulation of a single pathway or administration of neuromodulators to the entire amygdala slice. Recent attempts by Weisskopf and LeDoux (1999b) to determine whether postsynaptic depolarization and low-frequency stimulation are sufficient to induce LTP in auditory thalamus–LA synapses suggest that associative or Hebbian LTP could exist in amygdala, but have not yet demonstrated either. Moreover, the identification of inputs representing stimuli with inherently strong emotional content (i.e. unconditioned stimuli) is still an outstanding problem.

We (and others) have stated frequently that one of the most attractive features of the amygdala is that it appears to be necessary for an apparently rather simple form of learning (i.e. fear conditioning). Yet this behaviour is almost certainly more complex than it appears. For example, rodents engage in a range of anticipatory behaviours in active avoidance learning. Even in Pavlovian fear conditioning, the necessity to measure freezing as an index of fear introduces variables related to exploration and habituation (Good and Honey, 1997; McNish *et al.*, 1997). Synaptic plasticity in other amygdala subnuclei activated by emotional learning must be examined in more detail, as must their basic physiological properties and the relationships among the subnuclei. The range of neuromodulators that can affect LTP in the amygdala is already impressive, and is likely to grow. The heterogeneity of cells and synaptic responses in amygdala also indicate that the relationship between plasticity and learning may be complex. On the other hand, the knowledge of anatomically distinct input pathways, identifiable cell types, and replicable effects of amygdala lesions on fear conditioning suggest that this structure still represents our best hope for understanding the relationship between synaptic plasticity and learning.

References

Abe, K., Watanabe, Y., and Saito, H. (1996) Differential role of nitric oxide in long-term potentiation in the medial and lateral amygdala. *European Journal of Pharmacology*, 297, 43–46.

Abel, T., Nguyen, P.V., Barad, M., Deuel, T.A., Kandel, E.R., and Bourtchuladze, R. (1997) Genetic demonstration of a role for PKA in the late phase of LTP and in hippocampal-based long-term memory. *Cell*, 88, 615–626.

Anderson, P., Sundberg, S.H., Sveen, O., and Wigstrom, H. (1977) Specific long-lasting potentiation of synaptic transmission in hippocampal slices. *Nature*, 266, 736–737.

Atkins, C.M., Selcher, J.C., Petraitis, J.J., Trzaskos, J.M., and Sweatt, J.D. (1998) The MAPK cascade is required for mammalian associative learning. *Nature Neuroscience*, 1, 602–609.

Bannerman, D.M., Good, M.A., Butcher, S.P., Ramsay, M., and Morris, R.G.M. (1995) Distinct components of spatial learning revealed by prior training and NMDA receptor blockade. *Nature*, 378, 182–186.

Barrionuevo, G. and Brown, T.H. (1983) Associative long-term potentiation in hippocampal slices. *Proceedings of the National Academy of Sciences of the United States of America*, 80, 7347–7351.

Bashir, Z.I., Jane, D.E., Sunter, D.C., Watkins, J.C., and Collingridge, G.L. (1993) Metabotropic glutamate receptors contribute to the induction of long-term depression in the CA1 region of the hippocampus. *European Journal of Pharmacology*, 239, 265–266.

Bear, M.F. and Kirkwood, A. (1993) Neocortical long-term potentiation. *Current Opinion in Neurobiology*, 3, 197–202.

Bliss, T.V.P. and Collingridge, G.L. (1993) A synaptic model of memory—long-term potentiation in the hippocampus. *Nature*, 361, 31–39.

Bliss, T.V.P. and Gardner-Medwin, A. (1973) Long-lasting potentiation of synaptic transmission in the dentate area of unanesthetized rabbit following stimulation of the perforant path. *Journal of Physiology*, 232, 357–374.

Bliss, T.V.P. and Lømo, T. (1973) Long-lasting potentiation of synaptic transmission in the dentate area of anesthetized rabbit following stimulation of the perforant path. *Journal of Physiology*, 232, 331–356.

Bonhoeffer, T., Staiger, V., and Aertsen, A. (1989) Synaptic plasticity in rat hippocampal slice cultures: local 'Hebbian' conjunction of pre-and postsynaptic stimulation leads to distributed synaptic enhancement. *Proceedings of the National Academy of Sciences of the United States of America*, 86, 8113–8117.

Bourtchuladze, R., Frenguelli, B., Blendy, J., Cioffi, D., Shutz, G., and Silva, A.J. (1994) Deficient long-term memory in mice with a targeted mutation of the cAMP-responsive element-binding protein. *Cell*, 79, 59–68.

Brambilla, R., Gnesutta, N., Minichiello, L., White, G.L., Roylance, A., Herron, C., Ramsey, M., Wolfer, D.P., Cestari, V., Rossi-Arnaud, C., Grant, S.G.N., Chapman, P.F., Lipp, H.-P., Sturani, E., and Klein, R. (1997) A role for the RAS signalling pathway in synaptic transmission and long-term memory. *Nature*, 390, 281–286.

Brown, T.H. and Chattarji, S. (1994) Hebbian synaptic plasticity: evolution of the contemporary concept. In *Models of Neural Networks II: Temporal Aspects of Coding and Information Processing in Biological Systems* (eds E. Domany, J.L. van Hemmen and K. Schulten), pp. 287–314. Springer Verlag, New York.

Buonomano, D.V. and Merzenich, M.M. (1998) Cortical plasticity: from synapses to maps. *Annual Review of Neuroscience*, 21, 149–186.

Castillo, P.E., Weisskopf, M.G., and Nicoll, R.A. (1994) The role of Ca^{2+} channels in hippocampal mossy fiber synaptic transmission and long-term potentiation. *Neuron*, 12, 261–269.

Chapman, P.F. and Bellavance, L.L. (1992) Induction of long-term potentiation in the basolateral amygdala does not depend on NMDA receptor activation. *Synapse*, 11, 310–318.

Chapman, P.F., Kairiss, E.W., Keenan, C.L., and Brown, T.H. (1990) Long-term synaptic potentiation in the amygdala. *Synapse*, 6, 271–278.

Clugnet, M.C. and LeDoux, J.E. (1990) Synaptic plasticity in fear conditioning circuits—induction of LTP in the lateral nucleus of the amygdala by stimulation of the medial geniculate body. *Journal of Neuroscience*, 10, 2818–2824.

Collingridge, G.L., Kehl, S.J., and McLennan, H. (1983) Excitatory amino acids in synaptic transmission in the Schaffer collateral commissural pathway of the rat hippocampus. *Journal of Physiology (London)*, 334, 33–46.

Connors, B.W. and Gutnick, M.J. (1990) Intrinsic firing patterns of diverse neocortical neurones. *Trends in Neuroscience*, 13, 99–104.

Davis, M., Rainnie, D.G., and Cassell, M. (1994) Neurotransmission in the rat amygdala related to fear and anxiety. *Trends in Neuroscience,* 17, 208–214.

Flood, J.F., Rosenzweig, M.R., Bennett, E.L., and Orme, A.E. (1974) Comparison of the effects of anisomycin on memory across six strains of mice. *Behavioural Biology*, 10, 147–160.

Flexner, L.B. and Flexner, J.B. (1966) Effect of acetoxycycloheximide and of an acetoxycycloheximide puromycin mixture on cerebral protein synthesis and memory in mice. *Proceedings of the National Academy of Sciences of the United States of America*, 55, 369–374.

Florence, S.L., Taub, H.B., and Kaas, J.H. (1998) Large scale sprouting of cortical connections after peripheral injury. *Science*, 282, 1117–1121.

Frey, U., Krug, M., Reymann, K.G., and Matthies, H. (1988) Anisomycin, an inhibitor of protein synthesis, blocks late phases of LTP phenomena in the hippocampal CA1 region *in vitro*. *Brain Research*, 452, 57–65.

Gean, P.W. and Chang, F.C. (1992) Pharmacological characterization of excitatory synaptic potentials in rat basolateral amygdaloid neurones. *Synapse*, 11, 1–9.

Gean, P.W., Chang, F.C., Huang, C.C., Lin, J.H., and Way, L.J. (1993a) Long term enhancement of EPSP and NMDA receptor mediated synaptic transmission in the amygdala. *Brain Research Bulletin*, 31, 7–11.

Gean, P.W., Chang, F.C., and Hung, C.R. (1993b) Use dependent modification of a slow NMDA receptor mediated synaptic potential in rat amygdalar slices. *Journal of Neuroscience Research*, 34, 635–641.

Good, M. and Honey, R.C. (1997) Dissociable effects of selective lesions to hippocampal subsystems on exploratory behaviour, contextual learning, and spatial learning. *Behavioral Neuroscience*, 111, 487–493.

Grant, S.G.N., O'Dell, T.J., Karl, K.A., Stein, P.L., Soriano, P., and Kandel, E.R. (1992) Impaired long-term potentiation, spatial learning, and hippocampal development in *fyn* mutant mice. *Science*, 258, 1903–1910.

Grover, L.M. and Teyler, T.J. (1990) Two components of long-term potentiation induced by different patterns of afferent activation. *Nature*, 347, 477–479.

Gustaffson, B. and Wigström, H. (1986) Hippocampal long-lasting potentiation produced by pairing single volleys and brief conditioning tetani evoked in separate afferents. *Journal of Neuroscience*, 6, 1575–1582.

Halbach, O.v.B.u. and Albrecht, D. (1998) Angiotensin II inhibits long-term potentiation within the lateral nucleus of the amygdala through AT1 receptors. *Peptides*, 19, 1031–1036.

Harris, E.W., Ganong, A.H., and Cotman, C.W. (1984) Long-term potentiation in the hippocampus involves activation of *N*-methyl-D-aspartate receptors. *Brain Research*, 323, 132–137.

Harris, E.W. and Cotman, C.W. (1986) Long-term potentiation of guinea pig mossy fiber responses is not blocked by *N*-methyl-D-aspartate antagonists. *Neuroscience Letters*, 70, 132–137.

Hsia, A.Y., Salin, P.A., Castillo, P.E., Aiba, A., Abeliovich, A., Tonegawa, S., and Nicoll, R.A. (1995) Evidence against a role for metabotropic glutamate receptors in mossy fiber LTP: the use of mutant mice and phramacological antagonists. *Neuropharmacology*, 34, 1567–1572.

Huang, C.C. and Gean, P.W. (1995) Cyclic adenosine-3',5'-monophosphate potentiates the synaptic potential mediated by NMDA receptors in the amygdala. *Journal of Neuroscience Research*, 40, 747–754.

Huang, Y.Y. and Kandel, E.R. (1998) Postsynaptic induction and PKA-dependent expression of LTP in the lateral amygdala. *Neuron*, 21, 169–178.

Huang, Y.Y., Kandel, E.R., Varshavsky, L., Brandon, E.P., Qi, M., Idzerda, R.L., McKnight, G.S., and Bourtchuladze, R. (1995) A genetic test of the effects of mutations in PKA on mossy fiber LTP and its relation to spatial and contextual learning. *Cell*, 83, 1211–1222.

Huang, C.C., Hsu, K.S., and Gean, P.W. (1996) Isoproterenol potentiates synaptic transmission primarily by enhancing presynaptic calcium influx via P- and/or Q-type calcium channels in rat amygdala. *Journal of Neuroscience*, 16, 1026–1033.

Johnston, D., Williams, S., Jaffe, D., and Gray, R. (1992) NMDA-receptor-independent long-term potentiation. *Annual Review of Physiology*, 54, 489–505.

Kauer, J., Malenka, R., and Nicoll, R. (1988) NMDA application potentiates synaptic transmission in the hippocampus. *Nature*, 334, 250–252.

Kelso, S.R. and Brown, T.H. (1986) Differential conditioning of associative synaptic enhancement in hippocampal brain slices. *Science*, 232, 85–87.

Komatsu, Y., Nakajima, S., and Toyama, K. (1991) Induction of long-term potentiation without participation of *N*-methyl-D-aspartate receptors in kitten visual cortex. *Journal of Neurophysiology*, 65, 20–32.

Kohonen T. (1989) *Self-Organization and Associative Memory*, 3rd edn. Springer Verlag, Berlin.

Kossut, M. (1998) Experience dependent changes in function and anatomy of adult barrel cortex. *Experimental Brain Research*, 123, 110–116.

Lang, E.J. and Pare, D. (1998) Synaptic responsiveness of interneurons of the cat lateral amygdaloid nucleus. *Neuroscience*, 83, 877–889.

Li, H., Weiss, S.R., Chuang, D.M., Post, R.M., and Rogawski, M.A. (1998) Bidirectional synaptic plasticity in the rat basolateral amygdala: characterization of an activity-dependent switch sensitive to the presynaptic metabotropic glutamate receptor antagonist 2S-α-ethylglutamic acid. *Journal of Neuroscience*, 18, 1662–1670.

Levy, W.B. and Steward, O. (1979) Synapses as associative memory elements in the hippocampal formation. *Brain Research*, 175, 233–245.

Lynch, G., Larson, J., Kelso, S., Barrionuevo, G., and Schottler, F. (1983) Intracellular injections of EGTA block the induction of hippocampal long-term potentiation. *Nature*, 305, 719–721.

Mahanty, N.K. and Sah, P. (1998) Calcium-permeable AMPA receptors mediate long-term potentiation in interneurons in the amygdala. *Nature*, 394, 683–687.

Malenka, R.C., Kauer, J.A., Zucker, R.S., and Nicoll, R.A. (1988) Postsynaptic calcium is sufficient for potentiation of hippocampal synaptic transmission. *Science*, 242, 81–84.

Malenka, R.C., Kauer, J.A., Perkel, D.J., Mauk, M.D., Kelly, P.T., Nicoll, R.A., and Waxham, M.N. (1989) An essential role for postsynaptic calmodulin and protein kinase activity in long-term potentiation. *Nature*, 340, 554–557.

Malinow, R., Madison, D.V., and Tsien, R.W. (1988) Persistent protein kinase activity underlying long-term potentiation. *Nature*, 335, 820–824.

Maren, S. and Fanselow, M.S. (1995) Synaptic plasticity in the basolateral amygdala induced by hippocampal formation stimulation *in vivo*. *Journal of Neuroscience*, 15, 7548–7564.

Martinez, J.L., Jr and Derrick, B.E. (1996) Long term potentiation and learning. *Annual Review of Psychology*, 47, 173–203.

Mayford, M., Bach, M.E., Huang, Y.Y., Wang, L., Hawkins, R.D., and Kandel, E.R. (1996) Control of memory formation through regulated expression of αCaMKII. *Science*, 274, 1678–1683.

McCormick, D.A., Connors, B.W., Lighthall, J.W., and Prince, D.A. (1985) Comparative electrophysiology of pyramidal and sparsely spiny stellate neurones of the neocortex. *Journal of Neurophysiology*, 54, 782–806.

McDonald, A.J. (1992) Cell types and intrinsic connections of the amygdala. In *The Amygdala: Neurobiological Aspects of Emotion, Memory, and Mental Dysfunction* (ed. J.P. Aggleton), pp 67–96. Wiley-Liss, New York.

McDonald, A.J. (1998) Cortical pathways to the mammalian amygdala. *Progress in Neurobiology*, 55, 257–332.

McKernan, M.G. and Shinnick-Gallagher, P. (1997) Fear conditioning induces a lasting potentiation of synaptic currents *in vitro*. *Nature*, 390, 607–611.

McNaughton, B.L., Douglas, R.M., and Goddard, G.V. (1978) Synaptic enhancement in fascia dentata: cooperativity among coactive afferents. *Brain Research*, 157, 277–293.

McNish, K.A., Gewirtz, J.C., and Davis, M. (1997) Evidence of contextual fear after lesions of the hippocampus: a disruption of freezing but not fear-potentiated startle. *Journal of Neuroscience*, 17, 9353–9360.

Miserendino, M.J.D., Sananes, C.B., Melia, K.R., and Davis, M. (1990) Blocking of acquisition but not expression of conditioned fear-potentiated startle by NMDA antagonists in the amygdala. *Nature*, 345, 716–718.

Morris, R.G.M., Anderson, E., Lynch, G.S., and Baudry, M. (1986) Selective impairment of learning and blockade of long-term potentiation by an *N*-methyl-D-aspartate receptor antagonist, AP5. *Nature*, 319, 774–776.

Neugebauer, V., Keele, N.B., and Shinnick-Gallagher, P. (1997) Loss of long-lasting potentiation mediated by group III mGluRs in amygdala neurons in kindling-induced epileptogenesis. *Journal of Neurophysiology*, 78, 3475–3478.

Nose, I., Higashi, H., Inokuchi, H., and Nishi, S. (1991) Synaptic responses of guinea pig and rat central amygdala neurones *in vitro*. *Journal of Neurophysiology*, 65, 1227–1241.

O'Dell, T.J., Kandel, E.R., and Grant, S.G.N. (1991) Long-term potentiation in the hippocampus is blocked by tyrosine kinase inhibitors. *Nature*, 353, 558–560.

Pitkänen, A., Savander, V., and LeDoux, J.E. (1997) Organization of intra-amygdaloid circuitries in the rat: an emerging framework for understanding functions of the amygdala. *Trends in Neuroscience*, 20, 517–523.

Racine, R.J., Milgram, N.W., and Hafner, S. (1983) Long-term potentiation phenomena in the rat limbic forebrain. *Brain Research*, 260, 217–231.

Rainnie, D.G., Asprodini, E.K., and Shinnick-Gallagher, P. (1991a) Excitatory transmission in the basolateral amygdala. *Journal of Neurophysiology*, 66, 986–998.

Rainnie, D.G., Asprodini, E.K., and Shinnick-Gallagher, P. (1991b) Inhibitory transmission in the basolateral amygdala. *Journal of Neurophysiology*, 66, 999–1009.

Rainnie, D.G., Asprodini, E.K., and Shinnick-Gallagher, P. (1993) Intracellular recordings from morphologically identified neurones of the basolateral amygdala. *Journal of Neurophysiology*, 69, 1350–1362.

Reymann, K.G., Malisch, R., Schulzeck, K., Brodemann, R., Ott, T., and Matthies, H. (1985) The duration of long term potentiation in the CA1 region of the hippocampal slice preparation. *Brain Research Bulletin*, 15, 249–255.

Rogan, M.T. and LeDoux, J.E. (1995) LTP is accompanied by commensurate enhancement of auditory-evoked responses in a fear conditioning circuit. *Neuron*, 15, 127–136.

Rogan, M.T., Staubli, U., and LeDoux, J.E. (1997) Fear conditioning induces associative long-term potentiation in the amygdala. *Nature*, 390, 604–607.

Rolls, E.T. and Treves, A. (1998) *Neural Networks and Brain Function.* Oxford University Press, New York.

Schiess, M.C., Asprodini, E.K., Rainnie, D.G., and Shinnick-Gallagher, P. (1993) The central nucleus of the rat amygdala: *in vitro* intracellular recordings. *Brain Research*, 604, 283–297.

Schulz, P.E., Cook, E.P., and Johnston, D. (1994) Changes in paired pulse facilitation suggest presynaptic involvement in long-term potentiation. *Journal of Neuroscience*, 14, 5325–5337.

Schuman, E.M. and Madison, D.V. (1994) Locally distributed synaptic potentiation in the hippocampus. *Science*, 263, 532–536.

Silva, A.J., Stevens, C.F., Tonegawa, S., and Wang, Y. (1992) Deficient hippocampal long-term potentiation in α-calcium–calmodulin kinase II mutant mice. *Science*, 257, 201–206.

Stanton, P.K. and Sarvey, J.M. (1984) Blockade of long-term potentiation in rat hippocampal CA1 region by inhibitors of protein synthesis. *Journal of Neuroscience*, 4, 3080–3088.

Sugita, S., Shen, K.Z., and North, R.A. (1992) 5-Hydroxytryptamine is a fast excitatory transmitter at 5-HT_3 receptors in rat amygdala. *Neuron*, 8, 199–203.

Sugita, S., Tanaka, E., and North, R.A. (1993) Membrane properties and synaptic potentials of three types of neurone in rat lateral amygdala. *Journal of Physiology (London)*, 460, 705–718.

Swanson, L.W. and Petrovich, G.D. (1998) What is the amygdala? *Trends in Neuroscience*, 21, 323–331.

Tsien, J.Z., Huerta, P.T., and Tonegawa, S. (1996) The essential role of hippocampal CA1 NMDA receptor dependent synaptic. *Cell*, 87, 1327–1338.

Wang, S.J., Cheng, L.L., and Gean, P.W. (1999) Cross modulation of synaptic plasticity by β-adrenergic and 5 HT_{1A} receptors in the rat basolateral amygdala. *Journal of Neuroscience*, 19, 570–577.

Washburn, M.S. and Moises, H.C. (1992a) Electrophysiological and morphological properties of rat basolateral amygdaloid neurones *in vitro*. *Journal of Neuroscience*, 12, 4066–4079.

Washburn, M.S. and Moises, H.C. (1992b) Inhibitory responses of rat basolateral amygdaloid neurones recorded *in vitro*. *Neuroscience*, 50, 811–830.

Watanabe, Y., Ikegaya, Y., Saito, H., and Abe, K. (1995a) Roles of $GABA_A$, NMDA and muscarinic receptors in induction of long-term potentiation in the medial and lateral amygdala *in vitro*. *Neuroscience Research*, 21, 317–322.

Watanabe, Y., Saito, H., and Abe, K. (1995b) Nitric oxide is involved in long-term potentiation in the medial but not lateral amygdala neuron synapses *in vitro*. *Brain Research*, 288, 233–236.

Watanabe, Y., Ikegaya, Y., Saito, H., and Abe, K. (1996) Opposite regulation by the β-adrenoceptor-cyclic AMP system of synaptic plasticity in the medial and lateral amygdala. *Neuroscience*, 71, 1031–1035.

Weisskopf, M.G., Castillo, P.E., Zalutsky, R.A., and Nicoll, R.A. (1994) Mediation of hippocampal mossy fiber long term potentiation by cyclic AMP. *Science*, 265, 1878–1882.

Weisskopf, M.G. and LeDoux, J.E. (1999a) L-type voltage-gated calcium channels mediate NMDA-independent associative long-term potentiation at thalamic input synapses to the amygdala. *Journal of Neuroscience*, 19, 10512–10519.

Weisskopf, M.G. and LeDoux, J.E. (1999b) Distinct populations of NMDA receptors at subcortical and cortical inputs to principal cells of the lateral amygdala. *Journal of Neurophysiology*, 81, 930–934.

Wyllie, D.J.A., Manabe, T., and Nicoll, R.A. (1994) A rise in postsynaptic Ca^{2+} potentiates miniature excitatory postsynaptic currents and AMPA responses in hippocampal neurons. *Neuron*, 12, 127–138.

4 Amygdala plasticity: the neurobiological implications of kindling

Susan R.B. Weiss, He Li[1], Martina Sitcoske-O'Shea, and R.M. Post

Bldg 10/3N212, NIMH/BPB, 9000 Rockville Pike, Bethesda, MD 20892 and [1]USUHS, Bethesda, Maryland, USA

Summary

In this chapter, we discuss how observations from the amygdala kindling model may offer clues about neuroplasticity in the amygdala and related limbic structures. Kindled seizures can be induced gradually and under precise experimental control, thus allowing detailed study of the emerging expression of what we believe to be a highly conserved neural plasticity. We suggest that delineation of the cellular mechanisms underlying kindling may reveal substrates of plasticity operative in non-epileptic situations ranging from normal memory formation to evolving, pathological neuropsychiatric conditions.

We begin by describing the general characteristics of amygdala kindling-induced epileptogenesis. We then discuss the long-lasting structural alterations associated with kindling and the more transient effects of amygdala stimulation on gene expression; these shorter term effects may be related to the cellular limbic reprogramming that produces the hyperexcitable kindled state and its compensatory adaptations *in vivo*. We also discuss related *in vitro* characteristics of plasticity uncovered in the electrophysiological study of amygdala slices. This paradigm reveals a readily inducible form of metaplasticity in the amygdala, in which the direction of long-term adaptation (either potentiation or inhibition) is based on the cell's prior stimulation history. Finally, we speculatively link these observations from amygdala kindling and the slice preparation to testable hypotheses concerning mechanisms underlying the development of psychopathology and potential novel therapeutic interventions for illnesses thought to involve the amygdala, including affective and anxiety disorders, recurrent depression, and post-traumatic stress disorder.

4.1 Introduction

Epilepsy has been an enigma ever since it was characterized as an organic illness by Hippocrates in the 4th century, B.C. (Penfield and Jasper, 1954). He was the first to identify seizures as a dysfunction of the brain; previous writers considered epilepsy to be caused by supernatural spirits. The word epilepsy, taken from the Greek, epilepsia, denotes a force that is outside the body which takes hold of or seizes a person's functional abilities (McDonough, 1993).

Hippocrates and his colleagues catalogued the symptoms of a seizure in graphic detail. They also recognized brief losses of consciousness without generalized convulsions as an epileptic attack. These minor seizures would be classified later as absence or petit mal seizures (Penfield and Jasper, 1954). Since then, progress has been made in distinguishing between an epileptic seizure as a symptom, and the epilepsies as a group of syndromes.

A seizure, defined as a symptom by Hughlings Jackson in 1870, arose from the 'temporary excessive discharge in an unstable tissue which spreads to a secondary discharge of healthy tissue in other areas' (Penfield and Jasper, 1954, p. 17). Two types of seizures, partial and generalized, have been characterized. Partial seizures are identified by an abnormal discharge that is localized to a specific brain region; this activity may spread to other neural areas. A partial seizure may result from a unilateral insult to the brain, e.g. a cerebral stroke confined to one hemisphere. Generalized seizures, however, have no clinically or electrographically recognizable locus of onset, e.g. petit mal, grand mal seizures (Theodore and Porter, 1995). Thus, epilepsy is a group of chronic disorders of the central nervous system (CNS) with 'various etiologies characterized by recurrent seizures due to excessive discharge of cerebral neurons' (Gastaut and Broughton, 1972, p. 75).

Recurrent seizures and excessive, abnormal electrical activity in neuronal tissue are hallmarks of all epileptic syndromes. Researchers are beginning to uncover how increased excitability affects the stability and function of neurons. In the last 15 years, data have been gathered that indicate significant losses of hippocampal CA1 and CA3 pyramidal cells in brains of patients who are undergoing resection for the treatment of intractable epilepsy (Sutula, 1993). These same lesions have been found in tissue from epileptic patients examined during autopsy (Babb *et al*., 1989; Sloviter, 1991). Moreover, a reorganization of mossy fibres from dentate granule cells also occurs in human brains subjected to repetitive seizures (Sutula *et al*., 1989). These data demonstrate that, in the hippocampus at least, neuronal remodelling is a component of human epilepsy, although the direction of causality remains undetermined.

The role of the amygdala in human epilepsy remains far less well characterized, mostly due to its more complex circuitry and the difficulty in conducting histopathological analyses of resectioned tissue from this area. Nevertheless, in those studies in which amygdala tissue from epileptic patients was examined, significant structural damage appears to have been sustained, including cell loss and gliosis (Hudson *et al*., 1993; Wolf *et al*., 1997).

While progress has been made in classifying various syndromes and in uncovering structural alterations in the brains of epileptic patients, we still do not know how excessive neuronal discharge spreads from a localized site to neighbouring and distant brain regions, and then how those regions are rendered permanently susceptible to epileptiform activation. This problem relates to fundamental issues of plasticity at the level of neural circuits or ensembles, and is amenable to study in preclinical models.

4.2 Kindling

Kindling is an experimental paradigm used to model temporal lobe epilepsy. That a full-blown seizure can be induced by a previously subconvulsant stimulus months and years after the last convulsion occurred and that triggered kindled seizures can progress to spontaneous seizures are major reasons why kindling is also considered to be a model of long-term neuronal plasticity. The kindling model has been used to study morphological, molecular, and electrophysiological changes that occur at synapses, dendrites, somata, and glia following a seizure.

Electrical kindling is the process by which a previously subconvulsive stimulus comes to induce convulsive behaviour when applied repeatedly and intermittently to selected areas of the brain (Goddard, 1967; Goddard *et al.*, 1969; Racine, 1972a,b,c). Notably, the stimulation must be of a sufficient magnitude or intensity to induce an afterdischarge (AD) in order for kindling to develop (Racine, 1972b). The AD is the focal synchronous response of the neurons being stimulated. It can be recorded on a polygraph as repetitive spike and wave activity occurring at a frequency of ≤1/s.

The development of kindling progresses through well-defined behavioural stages, concomitant with electroencephalographic (EEG) activity increasing in intensity and spread as more brain regions become activated. Goddard *et al.* (1969) were the first to identify the 'kindling effect'; however, it was Racine (1972b) who first characterized the developmental stages of the kindled seizure, which have proven to be remarkably similar across species (McNamara *et al.*, 1980; Cain, 1992). Briefly, stage I consists of intermittent behavioural arrest coupled with AD activity; stage II consists of behavioural arrest and rhythmic oral movements or head nodding; stage III occurs when the animal exhibits unilateral forelimb myoclonus, which is defined as rapid, rhythmical shaking of one forelimb, lasting 3–30 s; stage IV is defined by clonus in both forelimbs, often accompanied by the animal rearing up on its hindlegs; and stage V includes all of the above plus the loss of postural control (falling) (Racine, 1972b).

Once kindling has progressed to the point of eliciting generalized motor seizures (stage III or greater), this change in seizure susceptibility remains for the life of the animal (Goddard *et al.*, 1969; Wada *et al.*, 1974). Furthermore, if sufficient numbers of seizures are induced (usually of the order of 100 or more), spontaneous seizures may occur, indicating the development of a true epilepsy-like phenomenon (Wada *et al.*, 1974; Pinel, 1981).

Most regions of the brain are capable of being electrically stimulated to induce seizures; however, the most sensitive areas from which to elicit epileptiform activity include such limbic areas as the amygdala, the bed nucleus of the stria terminalis, the olfactory bulb, the ventral endopiriform nucleus, the 'area tempestus', and the entorhinal, piriform and perirhinal cortices (Goddard *et al.*, 1969; Piredda and Gale, 1985; Cain, 1992; McIntyre and Kelley, 1993; Loscher *et al.*, 1995).

In epilepsy, the anterior hippocampus is the structure most often damaged (Engel, 1998). Paradoxically, the hippocampus is one of the slowest structures to kindle in the brain (Goddard *et al.*, 1969; Cain, 1992). When brainstem areas (e.g. reticular formation, central grey, and ventral tegmentum) and the cerebellum are stimulated, conventional kindling does not result;

rather, the animal runs around the cage uncontrollably, exhibiting what Goddard *et al.* (1969) called a 'running fit'. However, midbrain and brainstem structures have been postulated to be important in seizure generation. When lesions are made to the midbrain and reticular formation, the limbic-kindled motor seizures are inhibited. This finding suggests that a generalized seizure may require the activation of brainstem structures; however, these areas may not be critical for early seizure development.

4.2.1 Kindling as a model of neuronal plasticity

Goddard and Douglas (1975) recognized kindling as a model of neuronal learning and memory from the outset, and, as such, a type of experience-induced plasticity. Neuronal plasticity refers to the capacity of cells to exhibit long-lasting functional alterations that occur concurrently with structural changes that result from the activity of the animal. Kandel and Jessel (1991) and Thoenen (1995) suggest that modifications in neuronal morphology, in the strengthening of pre-existing neuronal connections, and in gene expression occur following many forms of activity-dependent stimulation. Kandel and colleagues (Kandel and Jessell, 1991; Bailey and Kandel, 1993; Hawkins *et al.*, 1993) posit that the common denominator among the various manifestations of activity-dependent plasticity, e.g. habituation, sensitization, conditioning, and long-term potentiation (LTP), is a change in the efficacy of neuronal communication, which, in the long term, results from alterations in gene expression. While the methods for producing a change in an animal's actions differ, the long-lasting alterations that accompany the behavioural change are similar. These include increases in the number of synapses and in neurotransmitter release; alterations in active zones at the synapse; and new protein synthesis.

As stated previously, kindling's biggest advantage in the study of plasticity is its persistence. Elucidation of the mechanisms that contribute to the permanency of kindling is an area of intense investigation. Alterations have been found at the cellular as well as the molecular level. Most of these changes have been delineated in the hippocampus, where the cellular morphology and circuitry are easily distinguished. In general, the hippocampus appears to be a site of intense synaptic reorganization in response to many forms of environmental and physiological stimulation, including amygdaloid stimulation. However, it is likely that some of the changes described in the hippocampus may result from recruitment of and by the amygdala, and be more widespread, involving cortical and subcortical regions.

There are very few studies that directly address the question of whether distinct neuronal populations are activated by kindling of the amygdala or specific nuclei within the amygdala versus other limbic or non-limbic structures. However, there are some differences described between kindling of the amygdala and the angular bundle (the major excitatory input to the hippocampus) in the early stages of seizure development (Hosford *et al.*, 1995). Overall, irrespective of the stimulation site, there appears to be a great deal of anatomical and biochemical overlap in the structural and chemical changes produced by kindling, especially when it has progressed to the stage where generalized seizures are expressed.

The plastic changes associated with kindling occur in widely distributed circuits, mostly involving limbic and neocortical structures. Once kindled seizures have been generated, it is difficult to block their occurrence with selective lesions of the amygdala, hippocampus, or various cortical regions (Racine, 1978; Dashieff and McNamara, 1982; Savage *et al.*, 1984; Tsuru *et al.*, 1992). Similarly, while the rate of kindling development can be modulated by selective genetic mutations (Cain, 1998) or blockade of excitatory amino acid receptors (Gilbert, 1988; Gilbert and Mack, 1990; Sutula *et al.*, 1996), seizures will still develop if stimulation is continued long enough and is of a sufficient magnitude (Sutula *et al.*, 1996). Together, these data imply that no single mechanism or structure is critical to the kindling effect; rather, there may be significant redundancy in the mechanisms that are utilized during the kindling process. The corollary to this is that stimulation of a selective brain region, such as the amygdala or one of its subdivisions, is capable of reprogramming cells throughout the limbic system and cortex which are likely to be involved in a number of functions in addition to seizure generation. Thus, we suggest that the adaptive processes operative in kindling are similar in kind to those occurring in functions as diverse as embryogenesis and learning on the one hand, and addiction and certain forms of psychiatric illness on the other; we further suggest that these processes are functionally defined by and biologically enacted through the occurrence of behavioural changes resulting from repeated exposure to an appropriate conditioning stimulus, be it normal or pathological.

4.2.2 Amygdala kindling

One paradigm that is used commonly to establish amygdaloid kindling is the daily application of brief electrical stimulation to the amygdala. Within 1–2 weeks, generalized seizures emerge, which subsequently can be induced reliably even after months of no stimulation (Goddard *et al.*, 1969; Racine, 1972b). The parameters vary but typically involve high-frequency stimulation (~60–100 Hz) using biphasic square wave pulses of 1 ms duration applied for a total duration of 1 s. The stimulations must be applied intermittently, optimally at 24–48 h intervals, but necessarily more than 5 min apart in order for the stimulations to lead to a seizure (Goddard *et al.*, 1969).

The required intensity also varies depending upon which nucleus is the target of stimulation, and whether the intention is to use threshold or suprathreshold levels of current. The number of stimulations required to produce a generalized seizure following stimulation of the amygdala does not differ widely among nuclei, although the threshold for producing an AD can range from about 60 μA in the basolateral nucleus to about 350 μA in the central nucleus (Goddard *et al.*, 1969; Le Gal La Salle, 1981; Gilbert *et al.*, 1984; Mohapel *et al.*, 1995; Sitcoske *et al.*, 1995, 1997).

Since the initial description of kindling by Goddard and associates, there have been many attempts to determine whether the electrical stimulation employed leads to seizure development through neurotoxic rather than trans-synaptic (or non-synaptic) processes. Goddard *et al.* (1969) conducted extensive experiments to determine whether gliosis or oedema could be the cause of seizures. If that were the case, they reasoned, then the onset of the epileptiform activity ought to coincide with the time after surgery when these physiological responses would be most evident. No such correlation was found.

Others (Robinson *et al.*, 1975; Boast *et al.*, 1976; Brotchi *et al.*, 1978; Willimore *et al.*, 1978) have investigated the enzymatic changes that occur consequent to electrode implantation. Robinson *et al.* (1975) found changes in metabolic enzymes immediately following surgery that were restored to basal levels 3 weeks post-surgery. Thus, local enzymatic changes are an unlikely explanation for the long-term changes in brain excitability produced by kindling.

Passing current through stainless steel electrodes can deposit metallic ions in tissues surrounding the electrode tip. Goddard *et al.* (1969) and others (Racine, 1972a,b,c) investigated seizure induction with three different types of metals used to construct electrodes and four types of insulation. They concluded that platinum electrodes induced seizures at the same rate as other materials, and did not leave traces of metallic ions in the tissue.

Electrolytic lesions are produced by using large amounts of current, and by increasing the pulse duration of the stimulus (Singh and Avery, 1975). Goddard *et al.* (1969), using optimal parameters to induce kindling (1 ms pulses of 60 Hz square wave, for 1 s train duration), and light and electron microscopy to examine the tissue, found that lesions were produced at the electrode tip only when currents in excess of 1 mA were used. While lesions can be created using other parameters, Goddard was able to reach the above conclusions using only kindling conditions. Moreover, other investigators found a 'surprisingly limited amount of cell necrosis' as a result of the electrical stimulation (Racine, 1972c; Robinson *et al.*, 1975). Therefore, Goddard and others concluded that the kindling phenomenon appears to be a trans-synaptic modification of neural circuitry that evolves over time with repeated stimulation, and remains for as long as the animal survives.

More recent data have addressed the issues of cell loss, gliosis, axonal sprouting, and dysfunctional circuitry in the pathogenesis and permanence of amygdala kindling. These will be discussed in detail below. However, Goddard *et al.*'s (1969) original contention, that neuronal damage at the site of stimulation is not the cause of the spread of epileptiform activity ultimately resulting in kindling, is still supported by the data.

4.3 Kindling-induced plasticity

Kindling typically involves the repeated application of an electrical stimulus for approximately 1 s every 24 h. How this brief event could lead to such widespread and long-lasting changes in the nervous system has been one of the most intriguing aspects of the kindling model since its initial discovery by Goddard *et al.* (1969). The following discussion will focus on the reported structural, molecular, and electrophysiological alterations in the brain that have been identified in relation to the kindling process. Many of these changes are not restricted to the kindling model, and, again, bespeak the commonality or redundancy of mechanisms of plasticity within the nervous system following differing forms of stimulation.

4.3.1 Long-lasting structural changes

The structural changes that have been reported in the brains of kindled animals include synaptic reorganization, cell loss, and mossy fibre sprouting. These changes typically are observed in animals that have experienced generalized motor seizures, although sprouting has been observed following as few as five ADs (Cavazos *et al.*, 1991). Since these changes can be observed at time points of longer than 1 month after any seizure has occurred, they are thought to underlie, in part, the permanence of kindling.

However, in evaluating any kindling-induced changes in brain, it should be recognized that compensatory or anti-kindling mechanisms are also part of the kindling process. We and others have demonstrated that these compensatory mechanisms may assist anticonvulsant drug effects, stabilize seizure thresholds, and contribute to increased inhibition in some of the kindled circuits (Tuff *et al.*, 1983; de Jonge and Racine, 1987; Racine *et al.*, 1991; Post and Weiss, 1992; Weiss *et al.*, 1995). Whether these compensatory mechanisms are as long lasting as those of the primary kindling process is unclear. However, since the overall progression of kindling is towards spontaneous seizures (Pinel, 1981) and increasing behavioural disturbances (Kalynchuk *et al.*, 1997), it is likely that the pathophysiological processes are growing and enduring, while the seizure-ameliorating mechanisms may be diminishing and more transient.

Synaptic reorganization after kindling has been examined using electron microscopy. Following hippocampal kindling, Geinisman *et al.* (1991, 1998) reported increases in the number of perforations in axospinous synapses in the hippocampus, which they posit would lead to an enhancement in synaptic efficacy. Similar changes were observed during the induction phase of LTP; however, these alterations dissipated during the maintenance phase, corresponding to a decay in the synaptic enhancement. During the maintenance phase of LTP, other changes in axodendritic asymmetrical synapses were observed which were not seen after kindling. Therefore, Geinisman and associates suggested that the stabilization of the perforated axospinous synaptic connections may be related to the permanence of the kindling phenomenon. Increases in the shaft and sessile spine synapses have also been described in the hippocampus (Chang *et al.*, 1993; Hawrylak *et al.*, 1993). Within the amygdala itself, there appears to be a decrease in the number of dendritic shaft and spine synapses in the medial nucleus following kindling of the basolateral nucleus, septum, or the corpus callosum (Nishizuka *et al.*, 1991; Okada *et al.*, 1993). Since the medial nucleus is rich in GABAergic neurons, a decrease in dendritic synapses in this area could represent a loss of inhibitory tone, leading to increased seizure susceptibility.

Since Ammon's horn sclerosis is the most common form of pathology found in patients with temporal lobe epilepsy (Babb *et al.*, 1989; Gloor, 1991; Chang *et al.*, 1993; Hawrylak *et al.*, 1993), and involves cell loss and gliosis in the CA1, CA3, and hilar region, the question of whether seizures cause or are a consequence of this cell loss is of considerable clinical interest. Prolonged seizures, such as those induced by kainic acid (Nadler and Cuthbertson, 1980; Hauser, 1983) or sustained electrical stimulation (Sloviter, 1983, 1987), can lead to significant cell loss in the hippocampus and other brain areas, mimicking many of the histopathological findings in tissue from epileptic patients. However, the question of whether the brief, recurrent seizures of kindling also lead to this kind of damage has been difficult to answer conclusively.

Cavazos and Sutula (1990) first reported that kindling of the angular bundle produced cell loss in the hilar region of the hippocampus. In a more extensive follow-up study, Cavazos *et al.* (1994) reported cell loss extending beyond the hilus to the CA1 and CA3 region of the hippocampus, the medial and lateral entorhinal cortex, and the dorsal endopyriform nucleus. The locus and extent of cell loss were related directly to the number of seizures experienced by the animal. The most sensitive areas were the hilus of the dentate gyrus and CA1 region, and the most massive effects were observed after rats had experienced 150 kindled seizures (Cavazos *et al.*, 1994). In these studies, rats were kindled from several different brain regions with no differences observed based on the site of stimulation. However, few rats actually received amygdala stimulation (one per group that received three or 30 seizures, and three in the group that received 150 seizures); most were kindled by perforant path stimulation.

Some researchers have failed to demonstrate cell loss in association with kindling (Van der Zee *et al.*, 1995), and others have observed that what appears to be cell loss may actually be a decrease in cell density attributable to an increase in the volume of the hilar region produced by kindling (Bertram and Lothman, 1993; Watanabe *et al.*, 1996b; Racine *et al.*, 1998). Thus, the induction of cell loss by kindling, and particularly amygdala kindling (since few animals were examined in the study of Cavazos *et al.*, 1994), remains a debated finding. Notably, Scott *et al.* (1998) have reported that amygdala kindling can increase neurogenesis in the hippocampus. This may be another factor contributing to the disparities in the literature regarding cell loss, and may also represent another mechanism by which kindling can induce long-lasting changes in the CNS.

The most widely reported and consistently observed long-lasting (possibly permanent) structural consequence of kindling is sprouting of the dentate granule cell mossy fibre pathway into the supragranular layer of the hippocampus. Sutula and co-workers (Sutula *et al.*, 1988; Cavazos and Sutula, 1990) were the first to make this observation, using the Timm staining method, which is sensitive to the high zinc content of these fibres. Similar sprouting has also been observed in the excised hippocampus of patients with temporal lobe epilepsy (Represa *et al.*, 1989; Sutula *et al.*, 1989). Sprouting has been demonstrated to begin after the first few kindling stimulations (Cavazos *et al.*, 1991), i.e. before generalized seizures have been induced, and occurs with stimulation of various limbic regions, including the amygdala (Cavazos *et al.*, 1991, 1992; Represa and Ben-Ari, 1992; Elmer *et al.*, 1997).

Sprouting has also been demonstrated after seizures generated in non-kindling paradigms, such as with electroconvulsive shock (ECS; Burnham *et al.*, 1998). It is notable that electroconvulsive seizures can inhibit status epilepticus (Sackeim *et al.*, 1983) and amygdala kindling (Post *et al.*, 1986), and are associated with a subsequent increase, rather than decrease, in the seizure threshold (Sackeim *et al.*, 1987a,b; Weiss *et al.*, unpublished observations). Generalized kindled seizures have been shown to develop even if sprouting is inhibited through blockade of *N*-methyl-D-aspartate (NMDA) receptors (Sutula *et al.*, 1996) or deletion of the *fos* gene (Watanabe *et al.*, 1996b), or if sprouting fails to occur (e.g. in young animals; Haas *et al.*, 1998), indicating that it is not a necessary feature of kindling. In animals perfused with brain-derived neurotrophic factor (BDNF), an inhibition of hippocampal-kindled seizure development was observed; however, axonal sprouting in BDNF-treated rats was comparable with that of vehicle-treated controls, all of which did develop kindled seizures (Larmet *et al.*, 1995).

Furthermore, Elmer *et al.* (1997) have shown that rats that are slow kindlers paradoxically show a greater density of mossy fibres in the supragranular layer of the hippocampus (as measured by Timm staining) in the baseline state compared with fast kindlers. Neither group showed an increase in sprouting following the development of kindled seizures. Thus, whereas mossy fibre sprouting in the dentate gyrus has proven to be a robust and consistent example of a structural abnormality induced by kindled seizures, it does not correlate perfectly with, or appear to be necessary for, kindling to proceed (for a review of dissociations between kindling and mossy fibre sprouting, see also Corcoran *et al.*, 1998).

The activity of the aberrant synaptic connections generated by the mossy fibre sprouting is also a matter of some debate (Tauck and Nadler, 1985; Sloviter, 1992; Sutula *et al.*, 1992; Buhl *et al.*, 1996a,b). The majority of the recent work suggests that these aberrant connections lead to abnormal excitation (Tauck and Nadler, 1985; Sutula *et al.*, 1988; Cronin *et al.*, 1992), although Sloviter (1992) and others (Cronin *et al.*, 1992; Elmer *et al.*, 1997) have suggested that the mossy fibre circuits may help to restore inhibition in the dentate, particularly in response to the loss or deafferentation of inhibitory hilar neurons.

The most convincing evidence that these new synaptic contacts are functional comes from the work of Golarai and Sutula (1996). Using combined histochemical and electrophysiological methods, they were able to show a strong relationship between an abnormal inward current (with a 9–13 ms latency) and the sprouted terminals from dentate granule cells of fully kindled animals that experienced 70–120 seizures and were studied 4–5 weeks after their last seizure. They recorded from the outer stratum moleculare of the dentate gyrus and showed that this abnormal current was present following perforant path stimulation that evoked a population spike. In kindled animals that did not evidence sprouting in this area, as well as in several different control groups, the abnormal current was absent.

The asymmetric morphology of the synapses in sprouted axons suggests that they are excitatory. If they terminate on the dendrites of granule cells in the dentate gyrus, then a recurrent excitatory loop would be formed, which does not exist in normal tissue. In tissue that shows sprouting (through either kindling or kainic acid-induced seizures), the granule cells have the capacity to fire epileptic burst discharges when γ-aminobutyric acid (GABA) transmission is inhibited by bicuculline or picrotoxin (Cronin *et al.*, 1992; Sutula *et al.*, 1992). This is not normally the case, but also cannot be attributed clearly to the sprouting of the mossy fibres, since changes in NMDA receptor function (Mody *et al.*, 1988) or synaptic morphology (Geinisman *et al.*, 1988) in this region may also contribute to this effect.

The nature of the postsynaptic contacts of the sprouted terminals is not well established and may include dendrites of the granule cells, inhibitory interneurons, or both. Therefore, the ultimate effect of the abnormal synaptic connections formed by the sprouted mossy fibres is unknown. However, the data do strongly suggest that the axonal sprouting produced by kindling is physiologically relevant.

Blockade of NMDA receptors has also been shown to inhibit mossy fibre sprouting in the kindling paradigm (Sutula *et al.*, 1996). Administration of a low dose of the noncompetitive NMDA receptor blocker MK-801, which did not inhibit the AD, resulted in a slowing of kindling development and diminished mossy fibre sprouting. However, once the MK-801-treated animals developed kindled seizures, levels of sprouting comparable with controls at the same stage of seizure development were observed. This was true even though the MK-801-treated rats experienced greater numbers of and longer ADs to achieve the same seizure stage as controls. Thus, NMDA receptor activation may contribute to mossy fibre sprouting, but does not appear to be critical for this effect.

The origin of the kindling-associated mossy fibre sprouting is also is a source of some disagreement. Sutula and colleagues generally consider it to be, at least in part, a reactive process to kindling-induced cell death, while others (e.g. McNamara, 1995) view sprouting as an activity-dependent reprogramming of cellular function during the kindling process. The controversy concerning cell loss associated with kindling has already been described above. Nevertheless, it has been demonstrated that deafferentation of the dentate granule cells can lead to sprouting in certain experimental paradigms. The question of whether sprouting can occur in the absence of cell loss in fully kindled animals has been addressed in several recent papers, which have implicated c-*fos* and neurotrophic factors in kindling-induced mossy fibre sprouting.

Watanabe *et al.* (1996b) found that mice with a null mutation for the *fos* gene also demonstrate a slow rate of kindling development and a decrease in mossy fibre sprouting. A moderate inhibition of mossy fibre sprouting was also observed in mice that were heterozygous for the *fos* mutation, although their kindling development appeared normal. Van der Zee and colleagues (Van der Zee *et al.*, 1995) demonstrated that intraventricular infusion of an antibody to nerve growth factor (NGF) also slowed the development of kindling and inhibited mossy fibre sprouting in the hippocampus. In both studies, the researchers also carefully examined the kindled tissue for evidence of cell loss as a possible factor in the mossy fibre sprouting. Van der Zee *et al.* (1995) failed to find a kindling-induced loss of cells in the hilus, and the kindled *fos*-less mice showed a decrease in cell density that corresponded to an increase in hilar volume.

Thus, it appears that kindling may directly facilitate synaptic reorganization in the adult hippocampus by activating specific cellular and genetic programmes, e.g. those processes controlling immediate-early gene (IEG) expression, growth factor regulation, and receptor function. In this case, the mossy fibre sprouting may itself contribute to further epileptogenesis through the formation of recurrent excitatory synaptic connections. The latter remains to be demonstrated conclusively but, even if true, mossy fibre sprouting is still only one of no doubt many mechanisms responsible for kindling's enduring nature.

In addition to the dissociations between kindling and sprouting mentioned above, recall that in fully kindled animals, destruction of the dentate gyrus does not prevent the expression of kindled seizures. Thus, while the well-defined circuitry and architecture of the hippocampus, as well as its sensitivity to perturbations of many sorts, may make it a showcase for the observation of structural components of neuronal plasticity, the intact hippocampus nevertheless is inessential to the long-lasting changes in brain excitability attributable to kindling.

Instead, perhaps, the hippocampus is more important in the initiation of kindling-related changes in neural excitability, rather than in their ultimate expression, in the manner observed in what has been referred to as declarative or recognition memory (Mishkin and Appenzeller, 1987; Squire and Zola-Morgan, 1991). If the processes are in fact analogous, then the role of the cortical areas should be examined more intensively as potential sites of the more long-lasting modifications of kindling.

The amygdala as well may be important. Several lines of investigation indicate that the amygdala shows more persistent responses than the hippocampus, and can influence longer-lasting behavioural changes. For example, in experiments that alter stimulus–reward relationships, the amygdala is necessary for an animal to learn to modify its responses appropriately (Jones and Mishkin, 1972; Spiegler and Mishkin, 1981; Baxter and Murray, Chapter16). When extinction procedures are used, the orbitofrontal cortical input to the amygdala is required for the cells in the amygdala to change their response characteristics (Rolls, 1992). Additionally, LTP of neurons in the basolateral nucleus of the amygdala is not reversed by low-frequency stimulation, as occurs in the hippocampus (Post *et al.*, 1998). Thus, once engaged, the amygdala appears to retain information unless and until it is reprogrammed by the cortex. The circuitry between the cortex and amygdala may therefore be important in long-term neuronal plasticity, not only in traditional learning paradigms, but possibly in kindling as well. However, findings of structural alterations in the amygdala comparable with the sprouting and cell loss found in the hippocampus have not been reported. Perhaps more subtle changes occur in the amygdala, possibly in synaptic morphology or distribution. This has been demonstrated in the medial nucleus of the amygdala, as described above (Nishizuka *et al.*, 1991; Okada *et al.*, 1993), but a more comprehensive study of structure will be required in order to determine its role, if any, in long-term adaptations relevant to kindling or to learning in other paradigms.

4.3.2 Short-term molecular effects

Morgan and Curran (1989, 1991) have provided a theoretical framework from which to consider how a brief electrical kindling stimulation could lead to long-term modifications of the CNS responsible for kindling. Their now well-established view is that the expression of IEGs, which can occur rapidly in response to various kinds of cellular activity, can initiate a cascade of cellular events ultimately leading to change in the cell's phenotype and function. The term 'immediate-early gene' first was coined to describe viral genes that were transcribed quickly, transiently, and in the presence of protein inhibitors. Some characteristics of IEGs are the following:

(i) their expression is low or non-existent in quiescent cells, but they are induced within minutes following extracellular stimulation;

(ii) they are transiently expressed;

(iii) their expression is independent of new protein synthesis;

(iv) their mRNAs generally have a short half-life (Curran, 1988; Morgan and Curran, 1989; Sheng and Greenberg, 1990);

(v) they encode proteins that function as transcription factors, cytoplasm enzymes, secreted cytokines, and membrane-bound receptors (Herdegen, 1996);

(vi) IEGs that are members of the Fos family [c-*fos*, *fra-1*, *fra-2* (fos-related antigen), and *fos-B*], the Jun family (c-*jun*, *jun-B*, and *jun-D*), *NGFI-A*, *NGFI-B*, and c-*myc* (Sheng and Greenberg, 1990) form proteins, which then bind to each other as homo- or heterodimers; these can then be translocated to the nucleus to exert transcriptional effects at appropriate DNA-binding domains.

A number of researchers (Clark *et al.*, 1991; Simonato *et al.*, 1991; Teskey *et al.*, 1991; Labiner *et al.*, 1993; Chiasson *et al.*, 1995; Ebert and Loscher, 1995; Hosford *et al.*, 1995) have detected increases in mRNA expression of the immediate early genes c-*fos*, c-*jun*, *NGFI-A* (*zif 268*), *NGFI-B*, and c-*myc* following kindling. Several groups (Shin *et al.*, 1990; Clark *et al.*, 1991; Hosford *et al.*, 1995) have also found c-*fos* mRNA expression to be a function of seizure severity and AD duration when the amygdala was the site of stimulation.

During the early stages of seizure development, a unilateral elevation in c-*fos* mRNA levels, ipsilateral to the electrode site was found in the amygdala, perirhinal and entorhinal cortices, and select areas of the neocortex. When the AD duration exceeded 30 s, c-*fos* mRNA expression also occurred in the granule cell layer of the dentate gyrus and in the pyramidal cell layer of CA1 and CA3 (Clark *et al.*, 1991; Hosford *et al.*, 1995). Chiasson *et al.* (1995) found similar localization using immunostaining for the Fos protein: when the AD duration was less than 30 s, Fos immunoreactivity was observed in the piriform and perirhinal cortices and the amygdala.

During seizure stages IV and V, the pattern of c-*fos* mRNA localization was found bilaterally and in structures which were only affected unilaterally in earlier stages (Clark *et al.*, 1991; Lanaud *et al.*, 1993). Hosford *et al.* (1995) demonstrated induction of c-*fos* mRNA by a single AD of longer than 30 s duration. Expression initially occurred in the amygdaloid nuclei ipsilateral to the stimulating site; then, as seizure development progressed, expression evolved to homologous contralateral structures as well as to additional brain regions. This activational pattern, in which the spatial evolution of IEG expression progresses with the course of seizure development, was also observed with *NGFI-A* mRNA (Lanaud *et al.*, 1993; Hosford *et al.*, 1995). In contrast, this pattern of IEG induction did not occur when the site of kindling stimulation was the angular bundle. Instead, a non-progressive expression of IEGs in the hippocampus occurred during the course of kindling. In addition, no changes in c-*fos* or *NGFI-A* mRNA were observed in the amygdala even after generalized seizures emerged. Thus, there appear to be selective structures and circuits that manifest changes in gene expression during the kindling process, and the site of stimulation may be important in determining which structures are recruited.

McNamara and associates (Labiner *et al.*, 1993; McNamara, 1995) have pointed out that IEG expression is not a perfect marker of neuronal activation or even burst firing. For example, the substantia nigra, which exhibits synchronous firing during kindled seizures (Bonhaus *et al.*, 1986, 1991), does not show enhanced mRNA expression for c-*fos* or *NGFI-A*. It is possible that a different subset of IEGs are expressed in this structure, but it is also possible that certain types of activation are more likely than others to initiate changes in gene expression. McNamara (1995) has suggested that prolonged depolarization leading to increases in intracellular calcium may be critical for the induction of IEGs, and that these effects are usually mediated by glutamate neurotransmission. Available data lend support to this idea, since blockade of NMDA receptors in fully kindled animals can suppress c-*fos* expression in the dentate gyrus whilst not interfering with the seizure response, and in fact increasing the number of population action potentials in the dentate granule cells (Labiner *et al.*, 1993).

Irrespective of the mechanism of the increases in IEG expression, it is notable that these alterations occur during kindling, suggesting that transcription and translation are utilized not only during normal cellular functioning, but also during the development of a pathological condition (Kandel, 1991), such as an epileptic seizure. It is also important to remember that the changes in IEG expression are transient. They typically begin within minutes of the experimental manipulation, and disappear by 24 h. Thus, to the extent that IEGs participate in kindling-induced plasticity, it is likely to be through their initiation of a cascade of other cellular events that ultimately lead to the long-term structural changes discussed above, as well as others not yet discovered.

Growth factors provide another potential link between the brief event of a kindling stimulus and the long-term consequences related to increased excitability of the nervous system. Growth factors are synthesized in many cell types, and act in the locale where they are produced via an autocrine or paracrine action, i.e. in which the synthesizing cell stimulates itself or those surrounding it, respectively. Recently, Hans Thöenen (1995) has suggested that growth factors may also function as retrograde neuromodulators, enhancing the release of neurotransmitters from neurons that contain receptors for the secreted growth factors. However, Smith *et al.* (1997b) have also suggested that growth factors could be released in an anterograde fashion to act as neurotransmitters or neuromodulators.

Neurotrophins are one class of growth factors, comprising BDNF, NGF, neurotrophin-3 (NT-3), neurotrophin-4/5 (NT-4/5), and neurotrophin-6 (NT-6) (Persson, 1993). Levi-Montalcini and colleagues (Levi-Montalcini and Cohen, 1966; Levi-Montalcini and Angeletti, 1968) were the first to demonstrate that neurotrophic factors are involved in neuronal survival, differentiation, and growth.

A rapid increase in neurotrophic factor mRNA expression has been demonstrated following a number of different physiological events, including LTP induction (Castren *et al.*, 1993), kindling (Ernfors *et al.*, 1991), and human epilepsy (Mathern *et al.*, 1997). Hughes *et al.* (1993), and later Sano and associates (1996), demonstrated that the expression of BDNF mRNA was not diminished by the protein synthesis inhibitor cycloheximide, in primary hippocampal neurons and in animals having kainic acid seizures. Both findings are characteristic of IEGs and have led to the suggestion that growth factors may act in that capacity (Dragunow *et al.*, 1993; Lauterborn *et al.*, 1996; Sano *et al.*, 1996).

Patel and McNamara (1995) found that the application of BDNF to primary cell cultures promoted a concentration-dependent increase in the number of axonal branch points in neurons of the dentate gyrus. This is important because these data are consistent with the branching and axonal sprouting of dentate gyrus granule cells found in the hippocampi of human epileptic patients and experimentally kindled rats. In a study comparing tissue from human patients with and without hippocampal sclerosis, Mathern *et al.* (1997) found a significant increase in BDNF only in those patients diagnosed with hippocampal sclerosis. The elevation in hippocampal BDNF correlated with both increased supragranular mossy fibre sprouting and increased cell loss in Ammon's horn.

Ernfors *et al.* (1991) have found that a single AD can induce a large increase in BDNF mRNA expression in the granule cell layer of the dentate gyrus. Following a generalized amygdaloid or hippocampal seizure, BDNF mRNA was found to increase in the hippocampus, basolateral amygdaloid nucleus, and the piriform and temporal cortices (Ernfors *et al.*, 1991; Gall, 1993). Kindled seizures also elevate mRNA expression for NGF, although the time course and regional distribution differ from that of BDNF. BDNF tends to increase more quickly than NGF in regions outside of the hippocampus, and BDNF, but not NGF, is increased in the CA1 and CA3 region of the hippocampus following a kindled hippocampal seizure (Lindvall *et al.*, 1998).

The tyrosine kinase receptors that bind BDNF and NGF (trkB and trkA, respectively) have also been studied following kindled seizures. Following kindling, a rapid increase in trkB mRNA expression occurs in the same granule cells that contain BDNF (Kokaia *et al.*, 1993), while no change in trkA receptor mRNA expression has been observed (Lindvall *et al.*, 1998). NT-3 mRNA expression decreases in the hippocampus following a kindled seizure if a sufficiently long hippocampal AD is elicited (>70 s). However, trkC receptors are increased (Bengzon *et al.*, 1993). Note that although the majority of reports on neurotrophin changes rely on measurement of mRNA expression rather than protein levels, there is some confirmatory evidence using immunoassay methods for BDNF, NGF, and trkB receptors (Merlio *et al.*, 1993; Nawa *et al.*, 1993), demonstrating that the protein levels change in the same manner and regions as predicted by the mRNA data.

As with IEG expression and most other correlates of kindling, the changes reported in growth factor regulation are not unique to kindled seizures; they are also observed after seizures generated in models other than kindling (Gall and Isackson, 1989; Gall *et al.*, 1991; Isackson *et al.*, 1991; Gall, 1993), and following other forms of stimulation and injury (Lindvall *et al.*, 1994).

How these neurotrophic factors functionally affect kindling has been studied using antibody and gene knockout strategies. Deficiencies in the three growth factors NGF, BDNF, and NT-3 appear to slow the rate of kindling development (Van der Zee *et al.*, 1995; Kokaia *et al.*, 1996; Funabashi *et al.*, 1998; Lindvall *et al.*, 1998), but do not interfere with its expression or maintenance once generalized seizures have been established, although there is one conflicting report showing that intraventricular administration of BDNF can slow the rate of hippocampal kindling (Larmet *et al.*, 1995). These effects of growth factors may indicate direct modulatory actions on synaptic transmission or indirect actions related to mossy fibre sprouting, neuronal survival, or transcriptional regulation. They do suggest that growth factors may be involved importantly in the evolution of the kindling process.

Changes in mRNA expression for neurotrophins, their receptors, and IEGs all occur during kindling. These alterations are dependent on the AD and seizure duration as well as the seizure stage, and are localized to specific brain regions. Neurotrophins may play a protective role for vulnerable neuronal populations (Lindvall *et al.*, 1994), contribute to the sprouting process that accompanies kindling (Van der Zee *et al.*, 1995), or function as IEGs affecting transcription (Dragunow *et al.*, 1993). It may be that these increases in IEG and neurotrophin mRNA expression are the molecular triggers that initiate the longer-lasting structural and functional modifications in nervous system excitability that are characteristic of kindling.

The notion that IEGs initiate a biochemical cascade ultimately leading to changes in a cell's phenotype and function (Morgan and Curran, 1989, 1991) has gained general scientific acceptance; however, there are few studies that have directly linked IEG expression to changes in target genes or proteins (Chiasson *et al.*, 1997). The most convincing data so far are the observations that Fos induction following noxious stimulation leads to increases in dynorphin expression (Hunter *et al.*, 1995), and that haloperidol-induced Fos expression regulates neurotensin levels in the striatum (Merchant, 1994; Merchant and Miller, 1994).

As one of the transcriptional targets of IEG expression, peptides may also be involved in the kindling process. Amygdala kindling dramatically affects peptide levels in the brain (e.g. Smith *et al.*, 1991; Rosen *et al.*, 1992, 1994; Kubek *et al.*, 1993; Zhang *et al.*, 1996) and can induce expression in regions which normally do not contain detectable levels of either mRNA or peptide. Corticotropin-releasing hormone (CRH), for example, is found in the hilar region of the dentate gyrus of kindled animals, but is not detectable in non-kindled controls (Smith *et al.*, 1997a). Exogenous administration of peptides has been demonstrated to exert pro- (e.g. CRH) (Weiss *et al.*, 1992) or anticonvulsant (e.g. thyrotropin-releasing hormone, neuropeptide Y, and cholecystokinin) effects on pharmacologically and electrically kindled seizures (Zhang *et al.*, 1992; Kubek *et al.*, 1998; Wan *et al.*, 1998). Those peptides that are enhanced following a seizure and can exert anticonvulsant effects may be part of an endogenous compensatory system, which could limit the progression or duration of, and consequent damage produced by, seizures (Post and Weiss, 1992). However, most of the seizure-induced changes in peptide levels or mRNA expression do not persist for more than a few hours or days, suggesting that they too may contribute to, but are unlikely to mediate, the long-lasting nature of the kindling phenomena.

Kindling induces permanent changes in the behaviour and morphology of the animal. Expression of IEGs and growth factor mRNA may be molecular markers of enhanced neuronal activation however imperfect (Labiner *et al.*, 1993; McNamara, 1995), and of regions of the brain that are subject to changes in cellular function. The convergence of data indicating that the same molecules are induced in response not only to convulsions, but also to forms of stimulation as diverse as injury (Traub *et al.*, 1992; Kajander *et al.*, 1996), exposure of dark-adapted animals to light (Rusak *et al.*, 1990), and administration of drugs such as amphetamine or cocaine (e.g. Graybiel *et al.*, 1990; Moratella *et al.*, 1993, 1996), suggests that such mechanisms are probably involved in the more global processes responsible for activity-dependent plasticity.

4.3.3 Kindling-induced changes in amygdala electrophysiology

Long-lasting alterations in the electrophysiological responses of amygdala neurons have been demonstrated following kindling. The most comprehensive series of studies of these effects is the work of Shinnick-Gallagher and associates (1998), who have used an amygdala slice preparation to examine the alterations in synaptic responses in the basolateral amygdala, and the influence of excitatory and inhibitory neurotransmitters in these effects. The basolateral amygdala contains pyramidal and basket cells, which receive glutamatergic input from the stria terminalis and the lateral nucleus, and a smaller percentage of GABA-containing interneurons. To examine the properties of basolateral amygdala neurons following kindling, Shinnick-Gallagher and associates stimulated animals in the basolateral amygdala until several consecutive stage V motor seizures were induced. Slices were prepared from either the ipsilateral or contralateral amygdala at varying times after the last kindled seizure, ranging from 5 days to 6 weeks, depending upon the study.

Intracellular recording of basolateral amygdala neurons was conducted in response to stimulation of either the stria terminalis or lateral nucleus of the amygdala. Rainnie *et al.* (1992) observed spontaneous burst firing in 68% of cells from kindled slices, compared with none in controls. When they examined evoked responses, generated at a current just below that required to induce an action potential, they observed in control tissue a complex postsynaptic potential, composed of a fast excitatory postsynaptic potential (EPSP) followed by a fast and slow inhibitory postsynaptic potential (IPSP), while they found burst firing in the kindled slices. The current required to evoke a response in the kindled tissue was also less than that required in control slices (Rainnie *et al.*, 1992). Thus, neurons in the basolateral amygdala of kindled animals appear to be more excitable than those of controls.

The burst firing in the basolateral amygdala neurons was inhibited partially by blockade of NMDA receptors with (±)-2-amino-5 phosphonovaleric acid (APV), and completely inhibited by 6-cyano-7-nitroquinoxaline-2,3-dione (CNQX), which blocks α-amino-3-hydroxy-5-methyl-4 isoxazole proprionic acid (AMPA)/kainate (KA) receptors, implying that ionotropic glutamate receptors contribute to this enhanced excitability of basolateral amygdala neurons. In addition, there appeared to be impaired feed-forward GABA inhibition that was pathway specific. It was observed following stimulation of the stria terminalis but not the lateral nucleus of the amygdala, and was manifest as a loss of the IPSP response following stria terminalis stimulation (Rainnie *et al.*, 1992). This observation may be related to the earlier work of Callahan *et al.* (1991) demonstrating a decrease in GABA-immunoreactive neurons in the amygdala of kindled rats 2–6 months after their last seizure.

There also appear to be differential effects of kindling on pre- versus postsynaptic mechanisms related to the metabotropic GABA and glutamate receptors. Activation of $GABA_B$ receptors is inhibitory, although the mechanisms of this effect may differ pre- and postsynaptically. Presynaptically, $GABA_B$ receptors are thought to decrease Ca^{2+} influx and prevent the release of glutamate or GABA; postsynaptically, $GABA_B$ receptors appear to produce a hyperpolarization through actions at G-protein-linked potassium channels. In slices from kindled animals, there is a 100-fold decrease in the sensitivity of presynaptic receptors to the $GABA_B$ agonist baclofen, while at the same time there is no change in the postsynaptic sensitivity of this receptor (Asprondini *et al.*, 1992a,b). Thus, the diminished presynaptic $GABA_B$ response in kindled animals is one possible mechanism that could lead to increased excitability through enhanced glutamate neurotransmission.

Metabotropic glutamate receptors are also located pre- and postsynaptically, and fall into three general categories based on their subunit constituency and second messenger coupling: group I receptors comprise mGluR1 and 5, and are coupled to phospholipase C, which leads to increased phosphoinositide hydrolysis, Ca^{2+} mobilization, and activation of protein kinase C; group II receptors comprise mGluR2 and 3; and group III receptors comprise mGluR4, 6, 7, and 8, and are coupled to inhibition of cAMP formation. In kindled animals, Holmes *et al.* (1996) reported an increase in mGluR-mediated postsynaptic inward currents and a decrease in hyperpolarizing outward currents. These results are consistent with an up-regulation of postsynaptic mGluR1 receptors and a down-regulation of postsynaptic mGluR2 receptors, respectively, resulting in increased neuronal excitability.

Presynaptically, mGluR group II and III agonists depress synaptic transmission in basolateral amygdala neurons. Neugebauer *et al.* (1997a) observed a 30-fold increase in the sensitivity of kindled slices to group II and group III agonists. This could represent a compensatory mechanism in kindling; however, at present, there is no evidence for increased endogenous activation of this receptor in kindled slices.

Overall, there appear to be numerous changes in both excitatory and inhibitory responses of amygdala neurons in kindled animals, which persist for days to weeks after the last seizure occurrence. These have been dissected and described elegantly by Shinnick-Gallagher and her colleagues. Importantly, their observations were made days to weeks after the last kindled seizure occurred, indicating a persistence of these functional alterations in amygdala physiology. This group recently has also discovered a novel pharmacologically-induced long-lasting potentiation in slices from control animals in response to administration of an mGluRIII agonist (Neugebauer *et al.*, 1997b). This long-lasting potentiation was completely absent from slices taken from kindled animals, despite increased sensitivity to agonists at this receptor. They (Neugebauer *et al.*, 1997b) suggest that this loss of a mechanism for long-lasting potentiation could contribute to epilepsy-related impairments in memory formation or learning. Whether or not this implication is correct, it is clear that there is much to be gained by studying the physiology of the amygdala in response to seizures, and that it may have possibilities for plasticity in the adult nervous system as equally rich and complex as that already demonstrated in the hippocampus.

4.4 Synaptic plasticity and metaplasticity in the unkindled amygdala

Mechanisms of synaptic transmission and plasticity have been studied most extensively in the hippocampus but, more recently, examination of these processes has also been conducted in the amygdala (Chapman *et al.*, 1990; Rainnie *et al.*, 1991a,b, 1994; Chapman and Bellavance, 1992). Although this work is described in detail elsewhere in this volume (Chapman and Chattarji, Chapter 3), we would like to highlight several findings from our own laboratory, in collaboration with Dr M. Rogawski, indicating unique properties of plasticity in the basolateral amygdala in response to stimulation of the external capsule or the basal amygdala.

As discussed above, considerable information has been obtained regarding the pre- and postsynaptic effects of excitatory and inhibitory neurotransmitters in the amygdala following certain patterns of stimulation. In addition to the important role of AMPA and NMDA glutamate receptors in amygdala neurotransmission, recent data have also implicated the ionotropic kainate receptors in synaptic transmission in the basolateral amygdala (Bettler *et al.*, 1990; Li and Rogawski, 1998). Using selective pharmacological agents to isolate this receptor, a kainate-mediated response was demonstrated in the basolateral amygdala following stimulation of the external capsule but not the basal amygdala (Li and Rogawski, 1998). The importance of this receptor in synaptic transmission is just beginning to be recognized; however, its role in plasticity in the amygdala and other structures (e.g. hippocampal CA3 neurons; Vignes and Collingridge, 1997; Vignes *et al.*, 1997) also merits further investigation.

LTP, which typically is induced by brief high-frequency stimulation (e.g. 100 Hz for 1 s), is defined by a long-lasting enhancement of synaptic strength (Bliss and Lømo, 1973). A more recently described form of plasticity is long-term depression (LTD), which involves a decrease in synaptic strength, and typically is induced by low-frequency stimulation applied for long durations (e.g. 1 Hz for 15 min) (Dudek and Bear, 1992; Christie *et al.*, 1994; Linden, 1994; Bear and Abraham, 1996). A related form of altered synaptic responsivity is depotentiation, in which the low-frequency stimulation reverses an already present enhancement in synaptic activation (Bashir and Collingridge, 1994; O'Dell and Kandel, 1994). These forms of synaptic plasticity, especially LTP, have been well studied in the hippocampus and are thought to be cellular models of memory. LTD is less well understood than LTP, but is thought to be important in allowing neurons to alter their functional response to repeated stimulation and to reset to their basal state after LTP. However, LTD is more easily demonstrable in slices from young rather than mature animals (Bear and Malenka, 1994; Wagner and Alger, 1995), raising questions about its importance in the adult nervous system. LTP, LTD, and depotentiation largely seem to be linked to NMDA receptors (Bear and Malenka, 1994; Christie *et al.*, 1994; Linden, 1994; O'Dell and Kandel, 1994; Collingridge and Bliss, 1995), although there are exceptions (Zalutsky and Nicoll, 1990), particularly outside the hippocampus (Aroniadou *et al.*, 1993; Komatsu, 1994; Vickery *et al.*, 1997).

4.4.1 High-frequency stimulation (HFS) of the amygdala

We have found recently that when a single HFS (100 Hz for 1 s) was applied to the external capsule, an enhanced synaptic response was produced in the basolateral amygdala that persisted for approximately 10 min in 86% of the neurons tested, i.e. short-term potentiation (STP) (Li *et al.*, 1998). In the presence of the NMDA receptor antagonist APV, however, the same stimulation only induced post-tetanic potentiation, which decayed in less than 3 min. STP previously has been described in the hippocampus (Bliss and Collingridge, 1993), where it is also NMDA-receptor mediated. Interestingly, the stimulation parameters that produced STP in the amygdala would probably result in LTP in the hippocampus, while hippocampal STP appears to result from more modest levels of stimulation (Malenka, 1991; Bliss and Collingridge, 1993). Others have also reported STP in the amygdala following brief HFS (Chapman *et al.*, 1990; Chapman and Bellavance, 1992; Watanabe *et al.*, 1995, 1996a), although these authors were able to produce LTP following a single HFS if $GABA_A$ receptor inhibitors were present in the slice.

LTP in the basolateral amygdala could be induced by HFS of the external capsule, but only when a second stimulation was applied 10 min after the first (Figure 4.1; Post *et al.*, 1998). LTP has also been demonstrated in the amygdala by stimulation of other afferents (e.g. the ventral angular bundle; Maren and Fanselow, 1995) and occurs in lateral amygdala (Huang and Kandel, 1998) as well as the basolateral amygdala. In these experiments, repetitive or prolonged HFS was applied, and again the LTP response was facilitated in the presence of GABA

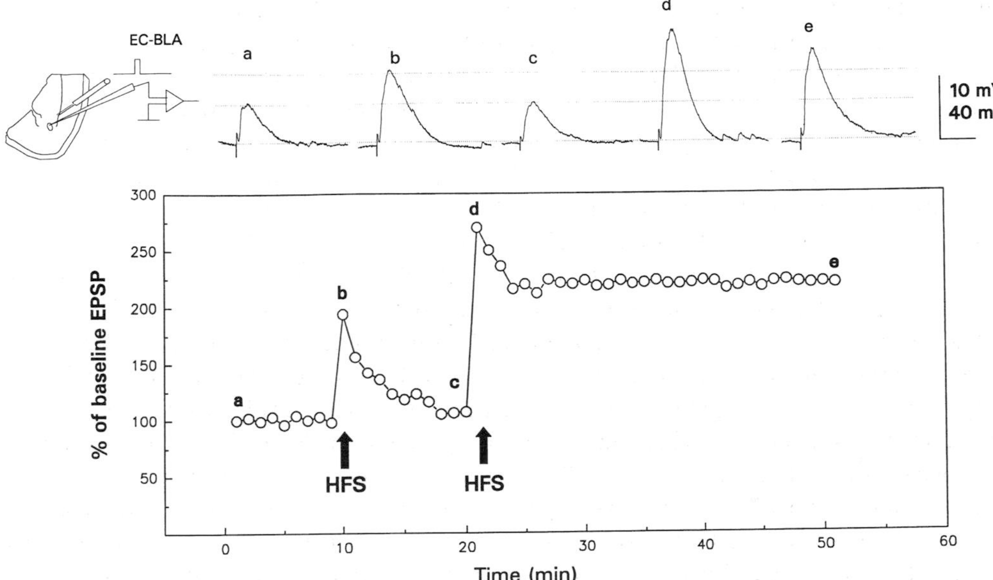

Figure 4.1 Two spaced high-frequency stimulations of the external capsule induce LTP in a basolateral amygdala (BLA) neuron. The top traces were sampled from intracellularly recorded synaptic responses in a basolateral amygdala neuron evoked by stimulation of the external capsule (EC). The preparation is illustrated schematically in the upper left portion of the figure. (a) The baseline response; (b) the response 1 min following the first high-frequency stimulation (HFS, 100 Hz for 1 s); (c) the response 10 min following the first HFS; (d) the response 1 min following the second HFS; and (e) the response 30 min following the second synaptic response. The bottom figure shows the time course of the synaptic response as a percentage of the baseline. The filled arrows indicated the timing of the HFS.

inhibitors (Huang and Kandel, 1998). Thus, the activation threshold of NMDA receptor-mediated LTP is probably influenced by inhibitory GABAergic processes in the amygdala.

4.4.2 Low-frequency stimulation (LFS) of the amygdala

Divergence in response of the amygdala and hippocampus to LFS has also been found. Using LFS parameters that generally induce LTD or depotentiation in the hippocampus (1 Hz for 15 min), we observed instead a long-term synaptic potentiation in the basolateral amygdala (Figure 4.2; Li *et al.*, 1998). Unlike conventional LTP, this LFS-induced synaptic enhancement develops slowly and monotonically in response to prolonged stimulation. There are important differences between LTP induced in the basolateral amygdala by LFS and LTP induced by more customary brief HFS. For instance, LFS-induced LTP is unaffected by NMDA receptor blockers, and is additive with STP; in contrast, HFS-induced LTP is NMDA

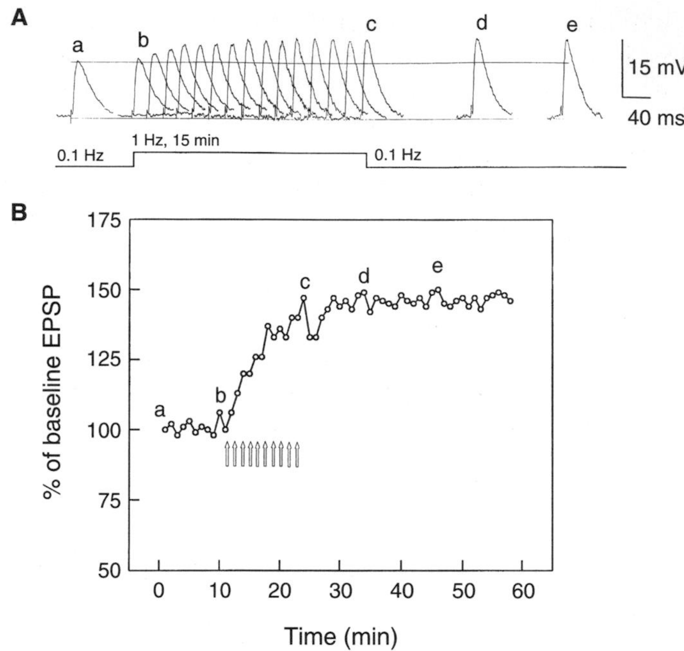

Figure 4.2 Low-frequency external capsule stimulation (LFS) induces LTP in a basolateral amygdala neuron. (**A**) Intracellularly recorded synaptic responses before, during, and after LFS (1 Hz, 15 min; 900 pulses). Traces before (a) and after (c–e) LFS are the averages of six successive responses; traces during LFS (b) are the averages of 60 responses. (**B**) Mean synaptic potential amplitudes as a percentage of the amplitude at time 0; each data point represents the average of six (during 0.1 Hz stimulation) or 60 (during LFS) successive responses. LFS was applied during the 15 min period indicated by the unfilled arrows.

receptor dependent and occludes STP. Thus, LFS-induced LTP in the basolateral amygdala may be mechanistically more similar to LTP in the CA3 region of the hippocampus (Zalutsky and Nicoll, 1990) and other brain areas where the phenomenon has also been shown to be NMDA receptor independent (Aroniadou *et al.*, 1993; Komatsu, 1994; Vickery *et al.*, 1997).

4.4.3 Metaplasticity in the amygdala

Metaplasticity is demonstrated when synaptic activation does not result immediately in an overt, enduring change in synaptic efficacy, but instead produces a persistent, latent change in the way in which a subsequent stimulation induces synaptic plasticity (Abraham and Bear, 1996). Several recent reports have documented situations where the history of synaptic activation can alter stimulation-dependent long-term synaptic plasticity (Thomas *et al.*, 1996; Manahan-Vaughan, 1998). For instance, the threshold for the induction of both LTP and LTD can be modified by prior afferent activity (Abraham and Bear, 1996). Moreover, several laboratories have reported that a tetanic stimulus which by itself does not produce a long-term enhancement in synaptic efficacy nevertheless may enable the subsequent induction of LTD in the hippocampus (Collingridge and Bliss, 1995; Wagner and Alger, 1995). The increased capacity for nuance in neuronal activity implied by this sort of modulation has led to the suggestion that metaplasticity is a higher form of synaptic plasticity.

We have observed a novel form of metaplasticity in the basolateral amygdala in which pre-treatment stimulation (priming) alters the direction of change in synaptic strength produced by low-frequency synaptic activation. In this case, with no pre-treatment stimulation, LFS of the external capsule produced a non-NMDA receptor-dependent form of LTP in the basolateral amygdala; when applied 10 min after priming with HFS (when the cell has returned to its basal status), identical LFS instead induced LTD in the basolateral amygdala (Figure 4.3; Li *et al.*, 1998). Thus, the direction of the enduring modification in synaptic strength was determined by prior synaptic activity rather than the parameters of stimulation *per se*.

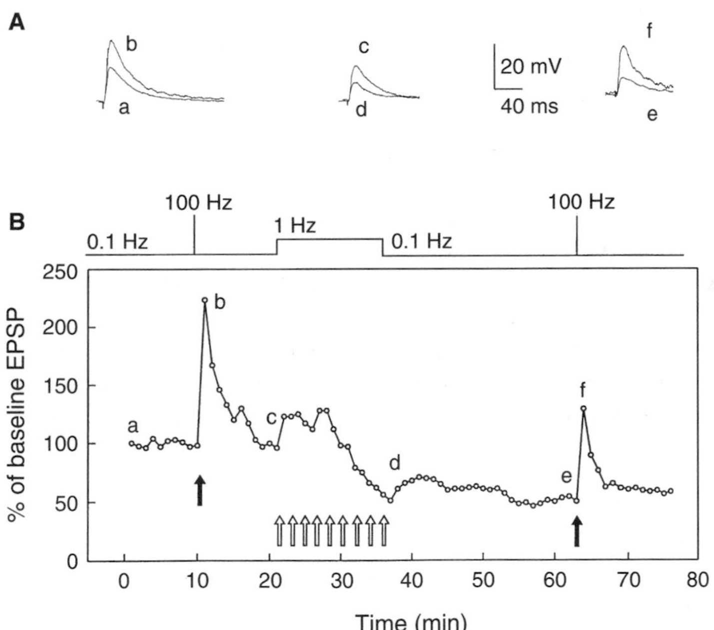

Figure 4.3 Effects of conditioning high-frequency stimulation (HFS) on the response to LFS. (**A**) Superimposed averaged synaptic responses before (a) and after (b) HFS (left); before (c) and after (d) (middle) LFS delivered 10 min after the HFS; and before (e) and after (f) a second HFS delivered 30 min after termination of the LFS. (**B**) Mean response amplitudes as a percentage of the amplitude at time 0; each data point represents the average of six (during 0.1 Hz stimulation) or 60 (during LFS) successive responses. HFS (first filled arrow) induces an initial transient potentiation. The subsequent LFS (unfilled arrows) produces a small initial facilitation and enduring synaptic depression. The depressed synaptic responses can be repotentiated transiently by HFS (second filled arrow).

This priming-dependent form of LTD is not affected by NMDA receptor blockers, but can be inhibited by an antagonist of the presynaptic type II metabotropic glutamate autoreceptors (Li *et al.*, 1998). This led us to consider whether a key event in this form of LTD is an alteration in the sensitivity of presynaptic mGluRs resulting from the prior HFS. While the presynaptic mGluRs might not contribute in a significant way to the regulation of glutamate release under unstimulated conditions, the autoreceptors after HFS might become sensitized and inhibit the release of glutamate, resulting in synaptic depression. Our data support this since an antagonist of the metabotropic type II glutamate receptor, 2S-α-ethylglutamic acid (EGLU) failed to alter the synaptic potential under basal conditions, but eliminated the enduring synaptic depression of the HFS/LFS stimulation, and in fact appeared to reveal an underlying synaptic facilitation.

Note that the metaplastic/priming-dependent LTD described above is not conventional depotentiation in as much as the stimulated cell has returned to its basal state prior to application of the LTD-inducing LFS. In addition, in contrast to LTD typically described in the hippocampus and elsewhere (Bear and Malenka, 1994; Christie *et al.*, 1994; Malenka, 1994) priming-dependent LTD is not NMDA receptor dependent, and is readily induced in slices from mature rats (>4 weeks of age). It is also the only form of LTD that we have been able to produce in the basolateral amygdala, since, unlike in the hippocampus, LFS alone, even when repeated, paradoxically induces LTP (Figure 4.2).

In the basolateral amygdala, priming with HFS stimulation appears to set the stage for a change in synaptic efficacy in either direction depending upon the subsequent stimulation pattern. A second HFS leads to LTP (Figure 4.1), while an LFS leads to LTD (Figure 4.3). This bidirectional capacity of activity-dependent synaptic plasticity adds an extraordinary level of flexibility and complexity to the ways in which LTP- and LTD-like mechanisms persistently can alter the functional strength of synaptic connections in the amygdala circuitry. The consequences of this at an organismic level are unknown; however, elucidation of the mechanisms of these effects should help us to understand the complex modulation of behaviour by the amygdala through its processing of emotional information.

4.5 Clinical implications

Given the amygdala's role in emotion and conditioned emotional responses (LeDoux, 1992; Davis, 1994; Davis *et al.*, 1994; Gallagher and Holland, 1994; Cahill *et al.*, 1995), as discussed in other chapters, the *in vitro* slice preparation may offer a unique perspective from which to examine variables involved in long-term neural adaptations in the amygdala in the direction of either potentiation or inhibition. LTP in the slice preparation thus provides a model for emotional memory formation and, potentially, its inhibition with LTD. The additional effect of metaplasticity indicates that the direction of long-term adaptation can change as a function of the cell's prior stimulation history. The slice preparation permits exploration of the physiology and molecular biology of local synaptic circuits, while the amygdala kindling paradigm allows investigation of the long-term trans-synaptic modification of excitability in pathways outside the amygdala and their biochemical, physiological, and neuroanatomical substrates. These two techniques thus help to provide complementary data about specific function and the larger context in which it operates.

The amygdala kindling model is, by definition, one that involves pathophysiological processes underlying the development of seizures and, as such, is a model of epileptogenesis. Nevertheless, embedded in this progression to a physiological and behavioural end point of generalized seizures is an underlying process of neuronal learning and memory, as originally postulated by Goddard and Douglas (1975). Moreover, Hughlings Jackson (Penfield and Jasper, 1954) believed that understanding the evolution of seizure mechanisms could provide a variety of insights into the synaptic conductivity of the brain. As such, the kindling model may be pertinent to a variety of pathophysiological processes that show increased responsivity over time, even without a seizure end point. Kindling may also mirror the progression to a full-blown behavioural syndrome from repetition of a previously subthreshold stimulation, and, ultimately, the transition from precipitated or triggered events to those occurring spontaneously, as occurs in the late behavioural and convulsive phases of amygdala-kindled seizure evolution.

This progression of symptomatology can also be obtained following repeated administration of certain pharmacological agents, including the local anaesthetics lidocaine and cocaine (Post *et al.*, 1975, 1988; Post, 1981). This can this lead not only to kindling of drug-elicited major motor seizures, but also to the emergence of spontaneous seizures (Post *et al.*, 1987). In a similar vein, cocaine-related panic attacks appear to follow a kindling-like progression in humans (Post *et al.*, 1995b). Initially, cocaine is often tolerated with a minimum of anxiety, but, with repeated administration, more anxiogenic and dysphoric components may become apparent and, in a subgroup of individuals, full-blown cocaine-related panic attacks begin to occur with each cocaine administration. In some individuals in whom this occurs often enough, spontaneous panic attacks can arise even after cocaine intake has ceased. Thus, a kindling-like progression can occur in behavioural and pathological emotional syndromes that do not involve a convulsive end point.

Similarly, a kindling-like progression appears to occur in many patients with recurrent unipolar and bipolar affective disorders (Post, 1992; Post and Weiss, 1994, 1998; Post *et al.*, 1995b). Minor traumas and psychosocial stressors may lead to the accumulation of neurobiological 'memory' traces such that with the recurrence of sufficient numbers, magnitude, or quality of stressors, the development of affective episodes may occur. Following sufficient numbers of triggered episodes, episodes may then begin to occur spontaneously as well (Kraepelin, 1921; Cutler and Post, 1982). There is considerable evidence, both for this type of stressor sensitization in the triggering of affective disorders as well as for episode sensitization wherein, like the occurrence of kindled seizure episodes, each recurrence appears to increase the likelihood that the syndrome eventually will progress to spontaneity.

Finally, in post-traumatic stress disorder (PTSD), there appear to be elements not only of LTP but also of a longer-lasting kindling-like progression. In PTSD, traumatic and horrific events (often those associated with the threat of loss of life) can leave behind permanent alterations in the form of neuronal hyperexcitability (hyperstartle), intrusive re-experiencing phenomena (flashbacks and nightmares), and withdrawal behaviours (depression and numbing) (Post *et al.*, 1995a). Considerable clinical evidence suggests that prior stressful life experiences may be vulnerability factors for the development of full-blown PTSD following the re-occurrence of a traumatic event (Bremner *et al.*, 1993; Yehuda *et al.*, 1995). In addition, trauma-related flashbacks appear to undergo a kindling-like progression, initially being triggered by environmental stimuli but often eventually occurring spontaneously. In this fashion, we would envisage that PTSD is, to some extent, a triggered or spontaneous replay of emotional memories akin to the elicited and spontaneous replay of motor events in the classical amygdala-kindled seizure paradigm (Post *et al.*, 1998).

Amygdala LTP and LTD *in vitro* preparations and kindling *in vivo* provide different models of neuronal learning and memory that may be pertinent to a variety of neuropsychiatric syndromes. To the extent that this is true, elucidation of molecular mechanisms involved in these paradigms will provide insights into ways of preventing syndrome evolution in the first place, and in reversing it once it has occurred in its full-blown form. It is of considerable interest that low-frequency (1 Hz) stimulation of the hippocampus for 10–15 min is able to depotentiate CA1 neurons that have undergone prior LTP (O'Dell and Kandel, 1994). In contrast, in the amygdala, such low-frequency stimulation is able to induce LTD in neurons subjected to prior STP, but not those in which LTP has been achieved (Li *et al.*, 1998; Post *et al.*, 1998). This suggests a relative permanence and resistance to depotentiation of the amygdala memory trace compared with that in the hippocampus. As such, ascertaining the biochemical and neurophysiological mechanisms that are sufficient to depotentiate amygdala neurons may be of particular clinical relevance for considering parameters that might depotentiate neuronal hyperexcitability in a variety of neuropsychiatric syndromes, in particular PTSD.

Similarly, the pharmacological interventions sufficient to inhibit amygdala kindling vary as a function of stage of syndrome evolution. Different agents are effective in: (i) the initial or development phase; (ii) the mid- or completed seizure phase; and (iii) the late, spontaneous stage of progression to true epilepsy (Pinel, 1983; Post and Weiss, 1988; Weiss and Post, 1998). These data suggest that similar pharmacological disjunctions may occur in the evolution of other kindling-like phenomena, and highlight the importance of exploring differential neuropharmacology of intervention as a function of stage of syndrome evolution. As noted above, the relative permanence of the kindled memory trace makes it an ideal model for exploring interventions that may depotentiate or reverse it.

The opportunity to apply brain stimulation techniques to humans is becoming increasingly feasible thanks to the availability of extracranial modes of non-convulsive brain stimulation with techniques such as repeated transcranial magnetic stimulation (rTMS). Utilization of rapid alterations in magnetic fluxes allows one to deliver relatively focal brain stimulation, not only to motor cortex to evoke topographically specific motor movements (Pascual-Leone *et al.*, 1994), but also to frontal cortex and other areas of brain that might be altered in affective and anxiety disorders (Pascual-Leone *et al.*, 1996; George *et al.*, 1997; Kirkcaldie *et al.*, 1997; McCann *et al.*, 1998).

Preliminary evidence supports the notion that high-frequency rTMS (20 Hz) over left prefrontal cortex can induce antidepressant effects in association with widespread increases in cerebral metabolism and blood flow (George *et al.*, 1996a,b). In contrast, 1 Hz rTMS appears capable of decreasing metabolism acutely and blood flow after more chronic administration; this mode of stimulation may be of importance in down-regulating hyperexcitable circuits, such as those observed in specific brain regions of PTSD patients (McCann *et al.*, 1998). Preliminary data of Kimbrell *et al.* and Speer *et al.* (unpublished observations) have suggested that depressed patients can respond positively either to high- or low-frequency rTMS stimulation, and that this might in part relate to baseline levels of neural excitability, as revealed by positron emission tomography (PET) studies of regional cerebral metabolism or blood flow. Most interestingly, 20 Hz rTMS over left frontal cortex for a period of 2 weeks was able to produce not only increases in frontal, cingulate, and striatal blood flow, but also increases in the amygdala itself; 1 Hz rTMS appeared to exert opposite effects, but to a lesser magnitude.

These data suggest the possibility that extracranial modification of neural excitability is possible not only with the convulsive stimuli of ECT, but also using non-convulsive brain stimulation with rTMS (Post *et al.*, 1997). As such, rTMS has the added potential of allowing for activity-dependent modulation of selective synapses in relation to neural circuits specifically activated by memories and behaviours induced at the time of rTMS administration. This kind of selective brain stimulation, perhaps in conjunction with pharmacological interventions, may lead to a new approach to treatment of a variety of neuropsychiatric syndromes based on modulation and, potentially, reversal of some of the long-term adaptations induced at the level of the amygdala and its synaptically related pathways. In this fashion, it is hoped that many of the preclinical findings in the *in vitro* slice preparation, and in the *in vivo* kindling model ultimately will help in the exploration of new potential therapies for a variety of psychiatric syndromes directly impacted by pathological amygdala neural adaptations and plasticities.

Acknowledgements

The authors would like to thank Drs E.L.P. Smith and T.G. Aigner for their insightful and thoughtful comments on the manuscript, and T. Postma and X.-L. Li for their help in its preparation. We also gratefully acknowledge the contribution of Ted and Vada Stanley of the Stanley foundation for their full support of Dr Li's research, and much of that of the other authors.

References

Abraham, W.C. and Bear, M.F. (1996) Metaplasticity: the plasticity of synaptic plasticity. *Trends in Neuroscience*, 19, 126–130.

Aroniadou, V.A., Maillis, A., and Stefanis, C.C. (1993) Dihydropyridine-sensitive calcium channels are involved in the induction of *N*-methyl-D-aspartate receptor-independent long-term potentiation in visual cortex of adult rats. *Neuroscience Letters*, 151, 77–80.

Asprondini, E., Rainnie, D., Anderson, A., and Shinnick-Gallagher, P. (1992a) *In vivo* kindling does not alter hyperpolarizations (AHPs) following action potential firing *in vitro* in basolateral amygdala neurons. *Brain Research*, 588, 329–334.

Asprondini, E., Rainnie, D., and Shinnick-Gallagher, P. (1992b) Epileptogenesis reduces the sensitivity of presynaptic gamma-aminobutyric acid B receptors on glutamatergic afferents in the amygdala. *Journal of Pharmacology and Experimental Therapeutics*, 262, 1011–1021.

Babb, T., Pretorius, J., Kupfer, W., and Crandall, P. (1989) Glutamate decarboxylase-immunoreactive neurons are preserved in human epileptic hippocampus. *Journal of Neuroscience*, 9, 2562–2574.

Bailey, C. and Kandel, E. (1993) Structural changes accompanying memory storage. *Annual Review of Physiology*, 55, 397–426.

Bashir, Z.I. and Collingridge, G.L. (1994) An investigation of depotentiation of long-term potentiation in the CA1 region of the hippocampus. *Experimental Brain Research*, 100, 437–443.

Bear, M.F. and Abraham, W.C. (1996) Long-term depression in hippocampus. *Annual Reviews of Neuroscience*, 19, 437–462.

Bear, M.F. and Malenka, R.C. (1994) Synaptic plasticity: LTP and LTD. *Current Opinion in Neurobiology*, 4, 389–399.

Bengzon, J., Kokaia, Z., Ernfors, P., Kokaia, M., Leanza, G., Nilsson, O.G., Persson, H., and Lindvall, O. (1993) Regulation of neurotrophin and trkA, trkB and trkC tyrosine kinase receptor messenger RNA expression in kindling. *Neuroscience*, 53, 433–446.

Bertram, E.D. and Lothman, E. (1993) Morphometric effects of intermittent kindled seizures and limbic status epilepticus in the dentate gyrus of the rat. *Brain Research*, 603, 25–31.

Bettler, B., Boulter, J., Hermans-Borgmeyer, I., O'Shea-Greenfield, A., Deneris, E., Moll, C., Borgmeyer, U., Hollmann, M., and Heinemann, S. (1990) Cloning of a novel glutamate receptor subunit, GluR5: expression in the nervous system during development. *Neuron*, 5, 583–95.

Bliss, T. and Collingridge, G. (1993) A synaptic model of memory: long-term potentiation in the hippocampus. *Nature*, 361, 31–39.

Bliss, T. and Lømo, T. (1973) Long-lasting potentiation of synaptic transmission in the dentate area of the anaesthetized rabbit following stimulation of the perforant path. *Journal of Physiology*, 232, 331–356.

Boast, C., Reid, S., Johnson, P. and Zornetzer, S. (1976) A caution to brain scientists: unsuspected hemorrhagic vascular damage resulting from mere electrode implantation. *Brain Research*, 103, 527–534.

Bonhaus, D.W., Walters, J.R., and McNamara, J.O. (1986) Activation of substantia nigra neurons: role in the propagation of seizures in kindled rats. *Journal of Neuroscience*, 6, 3024–3030.

Bonhaus, D., Russell, R., and McNamara, J. (1991) Activation of substantia nigra pars reticulata neurons: role in the initiation and behavioral expression of kindled seizures. *Brain Research*, 545, 41–48.

Bremner, J.D., Southwick, S.M., Johnson, D.R., Yehuda, R., and Charney, D.S. (1993) Childhood physical abuse and combat-related postraumatic stress disorder in Vietnam veterans. *American Journal of Psychiatry*, 150, 235–239.

Brotchi, J., Tanaka, T., and Leviel, V. (1978) Lack of activated astrocytes in kindling phenomena. *Experimental Neurology*, 58, 119–125.

Buhl, E., Otis, T., and Mody, I. (1996a) Zinc-induced collapse of augmented inhibition by GABA in a temporal lobe epilepsy model. *Science*, 271, 369–373.

Buhl, E., Szilagyi, T., Halasy, K., and Somogyi, P. (1996b) Physiological properties of anatomically identified basket and bistratified cells in the CA1 area of the rat hippocampus *in vitro*. *Hippocampus*, 6, 294–305.

Burnham, W.M., Gombos, Z., Nobrega, J., and Cottrell. (1998) Kindling-like effects of electroconvulsive shock seizures. In *Kindling 5* (eds M.E. Corcoran and S.L. Moshe), pp. 121–129. Plenum Press, New York.

Cahill, L., Babinsky, R., Markowitsch, H., and McGaugh, J. (1995) The amygdala and emotional memory [letter]. *Nature*, 377, 295–296.

Cain, D. (1992) Kindling and the amygdala. In *The Amygdala: Neurobiological Aspects of Emotion, Memory, and Mental Dysfunction* (ed. J.P. Aggleton), pp. 539–560. Wiley-Liss, New York.

Cain, D.P. (1998) Kindling in genetically altered mice: implications for the role of LTP in kindling. In *Kindling 5* (eds M.E. Corcoran and S.L. Moshe), pp. 285–298. Plenum Press, New York.

Callahan, P., Paric, J., Cunningham, K., and Shinnick-Gallagher, P. (1991) Decrease of GABA-immunoreactive neurons in the amygdala after electrical kindling in the rat. *Brain Research*, 555, 335–339.

Castren, E., Pitkanen, M., Sirvio, J., Parsadanian, A., Lindholm, D., Thoenen, H., and Riekkinen, P. (1993) The induction of LTP increases BDNF and NGF mRNA but decreases NT-3 mRNA in the dentate gyrus. *NeuroReport*, 4, 895–898.

Cavazos, J. and Sutula, T. (1990) Progressive neuronal loss induced by kindling: a possible mechanism for mossy fiber synaptic reorganization and hippocampal sclerosis. *Brain Research*, 527, 1–6.

Cavazos, J.E., Golarai, G., and Sutula, T.P. (1991) Mossy fiber synaptic reorganization induced by kindling: time course of development, progression and permanence. *Journal of Neuroscience*, 11, 2795–2803.

Cavazos, J., Golarai, G., and Sutula, T. (1992) Septotemporal variation of the supragranular projection of the mossy fiber pathway in the dentate gyrus of normal and kindled rats. *Hippocampus*, 2, 363–372.

Cavazos, J.E., Das, I., and Sutula, T.P. (1994) Neuronal loss induced in limbic pathways by kindling: evidence for induction of hippocampal sclerosis by repeated brief seizures. *Journal of Neuroscience*, 14, 3106–3121.

Chang, F., Hawrylak, N., and Greenough, W. (1993) Astrocytic and synaptic response to kindling in hippocampal subfield CA1: synaptogenesis in response to kindling *in vivo*. *Brain Research*, 603, 302–308.

Chapman, P. and Bellavance, L. (1992) Induction of long-term potentiation in the basolateral amygdala does not depend on NMDA receptor activation. *Synapse*, 11, 310–318.

Chapman, P., Kairiss, E., Keenan, C., and Brown, T. (1990) Long-term synaptic potentiation in the amygdala. *Synapse*, 6, 271–278.

Chiasson, B.J., Dennison, Z., and Robertson, H.A. (1995) Amygdala kindling and immediate-early genes. *Molecular Brain Research*, 29, 191–199.

Chiasson, B., Hong, M., and Robertson, H. (1997) Putative roles for the inducible transcription factor c-fos in the central nervous system: studies with antisense oligonucleotides. *Neurochemistry International*, 31, 459–475.

Christie, B.R., Kerr, D.S., and Abraham, W.C. (1994) Flip side of synaptic plasticity: long-term depression mechanisms in the hippocampus. *Hippocampus*, 4, 127–135.

Clark, M., Post, R.M., Weiss, S.R.B., Cain, C.J., and Nakajima, T. (1991) Regional expression of c-fos mRNA in rat brain during the evolution of amygdala kindled seizures. *Molecular Brain Research*, 11, 55–64.

Collingridge, G. and Bliss, T. (1995) Memories of NMDA receptors and LTP. *Trends in Neuroscience*, 18, 54–56.

Corcoran, M.E., Armitage, L.L., Hannesson, D.K., Jenkins, E.M., and Mohapel, P. (1998) Disssociations between kindling and mossy fiber sprouting. In *Kindling 5* (eds M.E. Corcoran and S.L. Moshe), pp. 211–224. Plenum Press, New York.

Cronin, J., Obenaus, A., Houser, C., and Dudek, F. (1992) Electrophysiology of dentate granule cells after kainate-induced synaptic reorganization of the mossy fibers. *Brain Research*, 573, 305–10.

Curran, T. (1988) The *fos* oncogene. In *The Oncogene Handbook* (eds E. Reddy, A. Skalka, and T. Curran), pp. 307–325. Elsevier, Amsterdam.

Cutler, N.R. and Post, R.M. (1982) Life course of illness in untreated manic-depressive patients. *Comprehensive Psychiatry*, 23, 101–115.

Dashieff, R.M. and McNamara, J.O. (1982) Intradentate colchicine retards the development of amygdala kindling. *Annals of Neurology*, 11, 347–352.

Davis, M. (1994) The role of the amygdala in emotional learning. *International Review of Neurobiology*, 36, 225–266.

Davis, M., Rainnie, D., and Cassell, M. (1994) Neurotransmission in the rat amygdala related to fear and anxiety. *Trends in Neuroscience*, 17, 208–214.

de Jonge, M. and Racine, R.J. (1987) The development and decay of kindling-induced increases in paired-pulse depression in the dentate gyrus. *Brain Research*, 412, 318–328.

Dragunow, M., Beilharz, E., Mason, B., Lawlor, P., Abraham, W., and Gluckman, P. (1993) Brain-derived neurotrophic factor expression after long-term potentiation. *Neuroscience Letters*, 160, 232–236.

Dudek, S.M. and Bear, M.F. (1992) Homosynaptic long-term depression in area CA1 of hippocampus and effects of *N*-methyl-D-aspartate receptor blockade. *Proceeding of the National Academy of Sciences of the United States of America*, 89, 4363–4367.

Ebert, U. and Loscher, W. (1995) Strong induction of c-fos in the piriform cortex during focal seizures evoked from different limbic brain sites. *Brain Research*, 671, 338–344.

Elmer, E., Kokaia, Z., Kokaia, M., Lindvall, O., and McIntyre, D. (1997) Mossy fibre sprouting: evidence against a facilitatory role in epileptogenesis. *NeuroReport*, 8, 1193–1196.

Engel, J. (1998) The syndrome of mesial temporal lobe epilepsy: a role for kindling. In *Kindling 5* (eds M.E. Corcoran and S.L. Moshe), pp. 469–484. Plenum Press, New York.

Ernfors, P., Bengzon, J., Kokaia, Z., Persson, H., and Lindvall, O. (1991) Increased levels of messenger RNAs for neurotrophic factors in the brain during kindling epileptogenesis. *Neuron*, 7, 165–176.

Funabashi, T., Sasaki, H., and Kimura, F. (1998) Intraventricular injection of antiserum to nerve growth factor delays the development of amygdaloid kindling. *Brain Research*, 458, 132–136.

Gall, C. (1993) Seizure-induced changes in neurotrophin expression: implications for epilepsy. *Experimental Neurology*, 124, 150–166.

Gall, C. and Isackson, P. (1989) Limbic seizures increase neuronal production of messenger RNA for nerve growth factor. *Science*, 245, 758–761.

Gall, C., Murray, K., and Isackson, P. (1991) Kainic acid-induced seizures stimulate increased expression of nerve growth factor mRNA in rat hippocampus. *Molecular Brain Research*, 9, 113–123.

Gallagher, M. and Holland, P. (1994) The amygdala complex: multiple roles in associative learning and attention. *Proceeding of the National Academy of Sciences of the United States of America*, 91, 11771–11776.

Gastaut, H. and Broughton, R. (1972) *Epileptic Seizures: Clinical and Electrographic Features, Diagnosis and Treatment*. Charles C. Thomas, Springfield, Illinois.

Geinisman, Y., deToledo-Morrell, L., and Morrell, F. (1991) Induction of long-term potentiation is associated with an increase in the number of axospinous synapses with segmented postsynaptic densities. *Brain Research*, 566, 77–88.

Geinisman, Y., Morrell, F., and de Toledo-Morrell, L. (1988) Remodeling of synaptic architecture during hippocampal 'kindling'. *Proceeding of the National Academy of Sciences of the United States of America*, 85, 3260–3264.

Geinisman, Y., Morrell, F., deToledo-Morrell, L., Persina, I., and Van der Zee, E. (1998) Comparison of synapse remodeling following hippocampal kindling and long-term potentiation. In *Kindling 5* (eds M. Corcoran and S. Moshe), pp. 179–192. Plenum Press, New York.

George, M.S., Wassermann, E.M., and Post, R.M. (1996a) Transcranial magnetic stimulation: a neuropsychiatric tool for the 21st century. *Journal of Neuropsychiatry and Clinical Neuroscience*, 8, 373–382.

George, M.S., Wassermann, E.M., Williams, W.A., Steppel, J., Pascual-Leone, A., Basser, P., Hallett, M., and Post, R.M. (1996b) Changes in mood and hormone levels after rapid-rate transcranial magnetic stimulation (rTMS) of the prefrontal cortex. *Journal of Neuropsychiatry and Clinical Neuroscience*, 8, 172–180.

George, M.S., Wassermann, E.M., Kimbrell, T.A., Little, J.T., Williams, W.E., Danielson, A.L., Greenberg, B.D., Hallett, M., and Post, R.M. (1997) Mood improvement following daily left prefrontal repetitive transcranial magnetic stimulation in patients with depression: a placebo-controlled crossover trial. *American Journal of Psychiatry*, 154, 1752–1756.

Gilbert, M.E. (1988) The NMDA-receptor antagonist, MK-801, suppresses limbic kindling and kindled seizures. *Brain Research*, 463, 90–99.

Gilbert, M.E. and Mack, C.M. (1990) The NMDA antagonist, MK-801, suppresses long-term potentiation, kindling and kindling-induced potentiation in the perforant path of the unanesthetized rat. *Brain Research*, 519, 89–96.

Gilbert, M., Gillis, B., and Cain, D. (1984) Kindling in the cortical nucleus of the amygdala. *Brain Research*, 295, 360–363.

Gloor, P. (1991) Neurobiological substrates of ictal behavioral changes. *Advances in Neurology*, 55, 1–34.

Goddard, G. (1967) Development of epileptic seizures through brain stimulation at low intensity. *Nature*, 214, 1020–1021.

Goddard, G.V. and Douglas, R.M. (1975) Does the engram of kindling model the engram of normal long term memory? *Canadian Journal of Neurological Sciences*, 2, 385–398.

Goddard, G.V., McIntyre, D.C., and Leech, C.K. (1969) A permanent change in brain function resulting from daily electrical stimulation. *Experimental Neurology*, 25, 295–330.

Golarai, G. and Sutula, T. (1996) Functional alterations in dentate gyrus after induction of long-term potentiation, kindling and mossy fiber sprouting. *Journal of Neurophysiology*, 75, 343–353.

Graybiel, A., Moratella, R., and Robertson, H. (1990) Amphetamine and cocaine induce drug-specific activation of the c-*fos* gene in striosome-matrix and limbic subdivisions of the striatum. *Proceeding of the National Academy of Sciences of the United States of America*, 87, 6912–6916.

Haas, K., Sperber, E., Benenati, B., Stanton, P., and Moshe, S. (1998) Idiosyncrasies of limbic kindling in developing rats. In *Kindling 5* (eds M. Corcoran and S. Moshe), pp. 15–26. Plenum Press, New York.

Hauser, W.A. (1983) Status epilepticus: frequency, etiology and neurological sequelae. *Advances in Neurology*, 34, 3–14.

Hawkins, R., Kandel, E., and Seigelbaum, S. (1993) Learning to modulate transmitter release: themes and variations in synaptic plasticity. *Annual Review of Neuroscience*, 6, 625–665.

Hawrylak, N., Chang, F., and Greenough, W. (1993) Astrocytic and synaptic response to kindling in hippocampal subfield CA1. II. Synaptogenesis and astrocytic process increase to *in vivo* kindling. *Brain Research*, 603, 309–316.

Herdegen, T. (1996) Jun, fos and CREB/ATF transcription factors in the brain: control of gene expression under normal and pathophysiological conditions. *Neuroscientist*, 2, 153–161.

Holmes, K., Keele, N., and Shinnick-Gallagher, P. (1996) Loss of mGluR-mediated hyperpolarizations and increase in mGluR depolarizations in basolateral amygdala neurons in kindling-induced epilepsy. *Journal of Neurophysiology*, 76, 2808–2812.

Hosford, D.A., Simonato, M., Cao, Z., Garcia-Cairasco, N., Silver, J.M., Butler, L., Shin, C., and McNamara, J.O. (1995) Differences in the anatomic distribution of immediate-early gene expression in amygdala and angular bundle kindling development. *Journal of Neuroscience*, 15, 2513–23.

Huang, Y. and Kandel, E. (1998) Postsynaptic induction and PKA-dependent expression of LTP in the lateral amygdala. *Neuron*, 21, 169–178.

Hudson, L., Munoz, D., Miller, L., McLachlan, R., Girvin, J., and Blume, W. (1993) Amygdaloid sclerosis in temporal lobe epilepsy. *Annals of Neurology*, 33, 622–631.

Hughes, P., Beilharz, E., Gluckman, P., and Dragunow, M. (1993) Brain-derived neurotrophic factor is induced as an immediate early gene following *N*-methyl-D-aspartate receptor activation. *Neuroscience*, 57, 319–328.

Hunter, J., Woodburn, V., Durieux, C., Pettersson, E., Poat, J., and Hughes, J. (1995) c-*fos* antisense oligodeoxynucleotide increases formalin-induced nociception and regulates prepordynorphin expression. *Neuroscience*, 65, 485–492.

Isackson, P.J., Huntsman, M.M., Murray, K.D., and Gall, C.M. (1991) BDNF mRNA expression is increased in adult rat forebrain after limbic seizures: temporal patterns of induction distinct from NGF. *Neuron*, 6, 937–948.

Jones, B. and Mishkin, M. (1972) Limbic lesions and the problem of stimulus–reinforcement associations. *Experimental Neurology*, 36, 362–377.

Kajander, K.C., Madsen, A.M., Iadarola, M.J., Draisci, G., and Wakisaka, S. (1996) Fos-like immunoreactivity increases in the lumbar spinal cord following a chronic constriction injury to the sciatic nerve of rat. *Neuroscience Letters*, 206, 9–12.

Kalynchuk, L., Pinel, J., Treit, D., and Kippin, T. (1997) Changes in emotional behavior produced by long-term amygdala kindling in rats. *Biological Psychiatry*, 41, 438–451.

Kandel, E.R. (1991) Cellular mechanisms of learning and the biological basis of individuality. In *Principles of Neural Science* (eds E. Kandel, J. Schwartz, and T. Jessell), pp. 1009–1031. Elsevier, New York.

Kandel, E.R. and Jessell, T.M. (1991) Early experience and the fine tuning of synaptic connections. In *Principles of Neural Science* (eds E. Kandel, J. Schwartz, and T. Jessell), pp. 945–957. Elsevier, New York.

Kirkcaldie, M.T., Pridmore, S.A., and Pascual-Leone, A. (1997) Transcranial magnetic stimulation as therapy for depression and other disorders. *Australian and New Zealand Journal of Psychiatry*, 31, 264–272.

Kokaia, Z., Bengzon, J., Metsis, M., Kokaia, M., Persson, H., and Lindvall, O. (1993) Coexpression of neurotrophins and their receptors in neurons of the central nervous system. *Proceeding of the National Academy of Sciences of the United States of America*, 90, 6711–6675.

Kokaia, M., Ferencz, I., Leanza, G., Elmer, E., Metsis, M., Kokaia, Z., Wiley, R.G., and Lindvall, O. (1996) Immunolesioning of basal forebrain cholinergic neurons facilitates hippocampal kindling and perturbs neurotrophin messenger RNA regulation erratum. *Neuroscience*, 70, 313–327.

Komatsu, Y. (1994) Plasticity of excitatory synaptic transmission in kitten visual cortex depends on voltage-dependent Ca^{2+} channels but not on NMDA receptors. *Neuroscience Research*, 20, 209–212.

Kraepelin, E. (1921) *Manic-Depressive Insanity and Paranoia*. E.S. Livingstone, Edinburgh, UK.

Kubek, M.J., Knowbach, B.S., Sharif, N.A., Burt, D.R., Buterbaugh, G.G., and Fuson, K.S. (1993) Thyrotropin-releasing hormone gene expression and receptors are differentially modified in limbic foci by seizures. *Annals of Neurology*, 33, 70–76.

Kubek, M., Liang, D., Byrd, K., and Domb, A. (1998) Prolonged seizure suppression by a single implantable polymeric-TRH microdisk preparation. *Brain Research*, 809, 189–197.

Labiner, D.M., Butler, L.S., Cao, Z., Hosford, D.A., Shin, C., and McNamara, J.O. (1993) Induction of c-fos mRNA by kindled seizures: complex relationship with neuronal burst firing. *Journal of Neuroscience*, 13, 744–751.

Lanaud, P., Maggio, R., Gale, K., and Grayson, D. (1993) Temporal and spatial patterns of expression of c-fos, zif/268, c-jun and jun-B mRNAs in rat brain following seizures evoked focally from the deep prepiriform cortex. *Experimental Neurology*, 119, 20–31.

Larmet, Y., Reibel, S., Carnahan, J., Nawa, H., Marescaux, C., and Depaulis, A. (1995) Protective effects of brain-derived neurotrophic factor on the development of hippocampal kindling in the rat. *NeuroReport*, 6, 1937–1941.

Lauterborn, J., Rivera, S., Stinis, C., Hayes, V., Isackson, P., and Gall, C. (1996) Differential effects of protein synthesis inhibition on the activity-dependent expression of BDNF transcripts: evidence for immediate-early gene responses from specific promotors. *Journal of Neuroscience*, 16, 7428–7436.

Le Gal La Salle, G. (1981) Amygdaloid kindling in the rat: regional differences and general properties. In *Kindling 2* (ed. J.A. Wada), pp. 31–48. Raven Press, New York.

LeDoux, J. (1992) Emotion and the amygdala. In *The Amygdala: Neurobiological Aspects of Emotion, Memory, and Mental Dysfunction* (ed. J.P. Aggleton), pp. 339–351. Wiley-Liss, Inc, New York.

Levi-Montalcini, R. and Angeletti, P. (1968) Nerve growth factor. *Physiological Review*, 48, 534–569.

Levi-Montalcini, R. and Cohen, S. (1966) Effects of the extract of the mouse submaxillary salivary glands on the sympathetic system of mammals. *Annals of the New York Academy of Sciences*, 85, 324–341.

Li, H. and Rogawski, M. (1998) GluR5 kainate receptor mediated synaptic transmission in rat basolateral amygdala *in vitro*. *Neuropharmacology*, 37, 1279–1286.

Li, H., Weiss, S., Chuang, D., Post, R., and Rogawski, M. (1998) Bidirectional synaptic plasticity in the rat basolateral amygdala: characterization of an activity-dependent switch sensitive to the presynaptic metabotropic glutamate receptor antagonist 2S-α-ethylglutamic acid. *Journal of Neuroscience*, 18, 1662–1670.

Linden, D.J. (1994) Long-term synaptic depression in the mammalian brain. *Neuron*, 12, 457–472.

Lindvall, O., Kokaia, Z., Bengzon, J., Elmer, E., and Kokaia, M. (1994) Neurotrophins and brain insults. *Trends in Neuroscience*, 17, 490–496.

Lindvall, O., Kokaia, Z., Elmer, E., Ferencz, I., Bengzon, J., and Kokaia, M. (1998) Neurotrophins and kindling epileptogenesis. In *Kindling 5* (eds M. Corcoran and S. Moshe), pp. 299–312. Plenum Press, New York.

Loscher, W., Ebert, T., Wahnschaffe, U., and Rundfelt, C. (1995) Susceptibility of different cell layers of the anterior and posterior part of the piriform cortex to electrical stimulation and kindling: comparison with the basolateral amygdala and 'area tempestus'. *Neuroscience*, 66, 265–276.

Malenka, R.C. (1991) Postsynaptic factors control the duration of synaptic enhancement in area CA1 of the hippocampus. *Neuron*, 6, 53–60.

Malenka, R.C. (1994) Synaptic plasticity in the hippocampus: LTP and LTD. *Cell*, 78, 535–538.

Manahan-Vaughan, D. (1998) Priming of group 2 metabotropic glutamate receptors facilitates induction of long-term depression in the dentate gyrus of freely moving rats. *Neuropharmacology*, 37, 1459–1464.

Maren, S. and Fanselow, M. (1995) Synaptic plasticity in the basolateral amygdala induced by hippocampal formation stimulation *in vivo*. *Journal of Neuroscience*, 15, 7548–7564.

Mathern, G., Babb, T., Micevych, P., Blanco, C., and Pretorius, J. (1997) Granule cell mRNA levels for BDNF, NGF and NT-3 correlate with neuron losses or supragranular mossy fiber sprouting in the chronically damaged and epileptic human hippocampus. *Molecular and Chemical Neuropathology*, 30, 53–76.

McCann, U.D., Kimbrell, T.A., Morgan, C.M., Anderson, T., Geraci, M, Benson B.E., Wassermann, E.M., Willis, M.W., and Post, R.M. (1998) Repetitive transcranial magnetic stimulation for PTSD: two case reports. *Archives of General Psychiatry*, 55, 276–279.

McDonough, J. (1993) *Stedman's Concise Medical Dictionary*. Williams & Wilkins, Baltimore, Maryland.

McIntyre, D. and Kelley, M. (1993) Are differences in dorsal hippocampal kindling related to amygdala–piriform area excitability? *Epilepsy Research*, 14, 49–61.

McNamara, J.O. (1995) Analyses of the molecular basis of kindling development. *Psychiatry and Clinical Neurosciences*, 49, S175–S178.

McNamara, J.O., Byrne, M.C., Dashieff, R.M., and Fritz, J.G. (1980) The kindling model of epilepsy: a review. *Progress in Neurobiology*, 15, 139–159.

Merchant, K. (1994) c-*fos* antisense oligonucleotide specifically attenates haloperidol-induced increases in neurotensin/neuromedin N mRNA expression in rat dorsal striatum. *Molecular and Cellular Neuroscience*, 5, 336–344.

Merchant, K. and Miller, M. (1994) Coexpression of neurotensin and c-*fos* mRNAs in rat neostriatal neurons following acute haloperidol. *Molecular Brain Research*, 23, 271–277.

Merlio, J., Ernfors, P., Kokaia, Z., Middlemas, D., Bengzon, J., Kokaia, M., Smith, M., Siesjo, B., Hunter, T., and Lindvall, O. (1993) Increased production of the TrkB protein tyrosine kinase receptor after brain insults. *Neuron*, 10, 151–64.

Mishkin, M. and Appenzeller, T. (1987) The anatomy of memory. *Scientific American*, 256, 80.

Mody, I., Stanton, P., and Heinemann, U. (1988) Activation of *N*-methyl-D-aspartate receptors parallels changes in cellular and synaptic properties of dentate gyrus granule cells after kindling. *Journal of Neurophysiology*, 59, 1033–1054.

Mohapel, P., Dufresne, C., Kelly, M., and McIntyre, D. (1995) Differential sensitivity of various temporal lobe structures in the rat to kindling and status epilepticus. *Epilepsy Research*, 800, 1–9.

Moratella, R., Vickers, E., Robertson, H., Cochran, B., and Graybiel, A. (1993) Coordinate expression of c-fos and junB induced in rat striatum by cocaine. *Journal of Neuroscience*, 13, 423–433.

Moratella, R., Ellbol, B., Vallejo, M., and Graybiel, A. (1996) Network-level changes in expression of inducible fos–jun proteins in the striatum during chronic cocaine treatment and withdrawal. *Neuron*, 17, 147–156.

Morgan, J. and Curran, T. (1989) Stumulus–transcription coupling in neurons: role of cellular immediate early genes. *Trends in Neuroscience*, 12, 459–462.

Morgan, J. and Curran, T. (1991) Stimulus–transcription coupling in the nervous system: involvement of inducible proto-oncogenes *fos* and *jun*. *Annual Review of Neuroscience*, 14, 421–451.

Nadler, J. and Cuthbertson, G. (1980) Kainic acid neurotoxicity toward the hippocampal formation: dependence on specific excitatory pathways. *Brain Research*, 195, 47–56.

Nawa, H., Bessho, Y., Carnahan, J., Nakanishi, S., and Mizuno, K. (1993) Regulation of neuropeptide expression in cultured cerebral cortical neurons by brain derived neurotrophic factor. *Journal of Neurochemistry*, 60, 772–775.

Neugebauer, V., Keele, N., and Shinnick-Gallagher, P. (1997a) Epileptogenesis *in vivo* enhances the sensitivity of inhibitory presynaptic metabotropic glutamate receptors in basolateral amygdala neurons *in vitro*. *Journal of Neuroscience*, 17, 983–995.

Neugebauer, V., Keele, N., and Shinnick-Gallagher, P. (1997b) Loss of long-lasting potentiation mediated by group III mGluRs in amygdala neurons in kindling-induced epileptogenesis. *Journal of Neurophysiology*, 78, 3475–3478.

Nishizuka, M., Okada, R., Seki, K., Arai, Y., and Iizuka, R. (1991) Loss of dendritic synapses in the medial amygdala associated with kindling. *Brain Research*, 552, 351–355.

O'Dell, T.J. and Kandel, E.R. (1994) Low-frequency stimulation erases LTP through an NMDA receptor-mediated activation of protein phosphatases. *Learning and Memory*, 1, 129–139.

Okada, R., Nishizuka, M., Reiji, I., and Yasumasa, A. (1993) Persistence of reorganized synaptic connectivity in the amygdala of kindled rats. *Brain Research Bulletin*, 31, 631–635.

Pascual-Leone, A., Rubio, B., Pallardo, F., and Catala, M.D. (1996) Rapid-rate transcranial magnetic stimulation of left dorsolateral prefrontal cortex in drug-resistant depression. *Lancet*, 348, 233–237.

Pascual-Leone, A., Valls-Sole, J., Wassermann, E.M., and Hallett, M. (1994) Responses to rapid-rate transcranial magnetic stimulation of the human motor cortex. *Brain*, 117, 847–858.

Patel, M. and McNamara, J. (1995) Selective enhancement of axonal branching of cultured dentate gyrus neurons by neurotrophic factors. *Neuroscience*, 69, 763–770.

Penfield, W. and Jasper, H. (1954) *Epilepsy and the Functional Anatomy of the Human Brain*. Little, Brown and Company, Boston.

Persson, H. (1993) Neurotrophin production in the brain. *Seminars in the Neurosciences* **5**, 227–237.

Pinel, J. (1981) Spontaneous kindled motor seizures in rats. In *Kindling 2* (ed. J. Wada), pp. 179–192. Raven Press, New York.

Pinel, J.P.J. (1983) Effects of diazepam and diphenylhydantoin on elicited and spontaneous seizures in kindled rats: a double dissociation. *Pharmacology, Biochemistry, and Behavior*, 18, 61–63.

Piredda, S. and Gale, K. (1985) A crucial epileptogenic site in deep prepiriform cortex. *Nature*, 317, 623–625.

Post, R.M. (1981) Lidocaine kindled limbic seizures: behavioral implications. In *Kindling 2* (ed. J.A. Wada), pp. 149–160. Raven Press, New York.

Post, R. (1992) Transduction of psychosocial stress into the neurobiology of recurrent affective disorder. *American Journal of Psychiatry*, 149, 999–1010.

Post, R.M. and Weiss, S.R.B. (1988) Sensitization and kindling: implications for the evolution of psychiatric symptomatology. In *Sensitization of the Nervous System* (eds P.W. Kalivas and C.D. Barnes), pp. 257–291. Telford Press, Caldwell, New Jersey.

Post, R.M. and Weiss, S.R.B. (1992) Endogenous biochemical abnormalities in affective illness: therapeutic vs. pathogenic. *Biological Psychiatry*, 32, 469–84.

Post, R. and Weiss, S. (1994) Kindling: implications for the course of treatment of affective disorders. In *Anticonvulsants in Psychiatry* (eds K. Modigh, O. Robak and P. Vestergaard), pp. 113–137. Wrightson Biomedical, Hampshire, UK.

Post, R.M. and Weiss, S.R. (1998) Sensitization and kindling phenomena in mood, anxiety and obsessive–compulsive disorders: the role of serotonergic mechanisms in illness progression. *Biological Psychiatry*, 44, 193–206.

Post, R.M., Kopanda, R.T., and Lee, A. (1975) Progressive behavioral changes during chronic lidocaine administration: relationship to kindling. *Life Sciences*, 17, 943–950.

Post, R.M., Putnam, F., Uhde, T.W., and Weiss, S.R.B. (1986) ECT as an anticonvulsant: implications for its mechanism of action in affective illness. *Annals of the New York Academy of Sciences*, 462, 376–388.

Post, R.M., Weiss, S.R.B., Pert, A., and Uhde, T.W. (1987) Chronic cocaine administration: sensitization and kindling effects. In *Cocaine: Clinical and Biobehavioral Aspects* (eds A. Raskin and S. Fisher), pp. 109–173. Oxford University Press, New York.

Post, R.M., Weiss, S.R.B., and Pert, A. (1988) Cocaine-induced behavioral sensitization and kindling: implications for the emergence of psychopathology and seizures. In *The Mesocorticolimbic Dopamine System* (eds P.W. Kalivas and C.B. Nemeroff), pp. 292–308. New York Academy of Science, New York.

Post, R., Weiss, S., and Smith, M. (1995a) Sensitization and kindling: implications for the evolving neural substrates of PTSD. In *Neurobiology and Clinical Consequences of Stress From Normal Adaptation to PTSD* (eds M. Friedman, D. Charney and A. Deutch), pp. 203–224. Raven Press, New York.

Post, R.M., Weiss, S.R., Smith, M., Rosen, J., and Frye, M. (1995b) Stress, conditioning and the temporal aspects of affective disorders. *Annals of the New York Academy of Sciences*, 771, 677–696.

Post, R.M., Kimbrell, T.A., McCann, U., Dunn, R.T., George, M.S., and Weiss, S.R. (1997) Are convulsions necessary for the antidepressive effect of electroconvulsive therapy: outcome of repeated transcranial magnetic stimulation. *Encephale*, 23 Spec. No 3, 27–35.

Post, R., Weiss, S., Li, H., Smith, M., Zhang, L., Xing, G., Osuch, E., and McCann, U. (1998) Neural plasticity and emotional memory. *Development and Psychopathology*, 10, 829–855.

Racine, R. (1972a) Modification of seizure activity by electrical stimulation. I. Afterdischarge threshold. *Electroencephalography and Clinical Neurophysiology*, 32, 269–279.

Racine, R. (1972b) Modification of seizure activity by electrical stimulation. II. Motor seizure. *Electroencephalography and Clinical Neurophysiology*, 32, 281–294.

Racine, R. (1972c) Modification of seizure activity by electrical stimulation. III. Mechanisms. *Electroencephalography and Clinical Neurophysiology*, 32, 295–299.

Racine, R. (1978) Kindling: the first decade. *Neurosurgery*, 3, 234–252.

Racine, R.J., Moore, K.A., and Evans, C. (1991) Kindling-induced potentiation in the piriform cortex. *Brain Research*, 556, 218–225.

Racine, R.J., Adams, B., Osehobo, P., Milgram, N.W., and Fahnestock, M. (1998) Neuronal growth and neuronal loss in kindling epileptogenesis. In *Kindling 5* (eds M.E. Corcoran and S.L. Moshe), pp. 193–209. Plenum Press, New York.

Rainnie, D., Asprodini, E., and Shinnick-Gallagher, P. (1991a) Excitatory transmission in the basolateral amygdala. *Journal of Neurophysiology*, 66, 986–998.

Rainnie, D., Asprodini, E., and Shinnick-Gallagher, P. (1991b) Inhibitory transmission in the basolateral amygdala. *Journal of Neurophysiology*, 66, 999–1009.

Rainnie, D., Aspirondini, E., and Shinnick-Gallagher, P. (1992) Kindling-induced long-lasting changes in synaptic transmission in the basolateral amygdala. *Journal of Neurophysiology*, 67, 443–454.

Rainnie, D., Holmes, K., and Shinnick-Gallagher, P. (1994) Activation of postsynaptic metabotropic glutamate receptors by trans-ACPD hyperpolarizes neurons of the basolateral amygdala. *Journal of Neuroscience*, 14, 7208–7220.

Represa, A. and Ben-Ari, Y. (1992) Kindling is associated with the formation of novel mossy fibre synapses in the CA3 region. *Experimental Brain Research*, 92, 69–78.

Represa, A., Robain, O., Tremblay, E., and Ben-Ari, Y. (1989) Hippocampal plasticity in childhood epilepsy. *Neuroscience Letters*, 99, 351–355.

Robinson, N., Duncan, P., Gehrt, M., Sances, A., and Evans, S. (1975) Histochemistry of trauma after electrode implantation and stimulation in the rat hippocampus. *Archives of Neurology*, 32, 98–102.

Rolls, E. (1992) Neurophysiology and functions of the primate amygdala. In *The Amygdala: Neurobiological Aspects of Emotion, Memory, and Mental Dysfunction* (ed. J.P. Aggleton), pp. 143–166. Wiley-Liss Inc, New York.

Rosen, J.B., Cain, C.J., Weiss, S.R.B., and Post, R.M. (1992) Alterations in mRNA of enkephalin, dynorphin and thyrotropin releasing hormone during amygdala kindling: an *in situ* hybridization study. *Molecular Brain Research*, 15, 247–255.

Rosen, J.B., Kim, S.-Y., and Post, R.M. (1994) Differential regional and time course increases in thyrotropin-releasing hormone, neuropeptide Y and enkephalin mRNAs following an amygdala kindled seizure. *Molecular Brain Research*, 27, 71–80.

Rusak, B., Robertson, H., Wisden, W., and Hunt, S. (1990) Light pulses that shift rhythms induce gene expression in the suprachiasmatic nucleus. *Science*, 248, 1237–1240.

Sackeim, H.A., Prohovnik, I., Decina, P., Malitz, S., and Resor, S. (1983) Anticonvulsant properties of electroconvulsive therapy: theory and case report. In *Current Problems in Epilepsy: Cerebral Blood Flow, Metabolism and Epilepsy* (eds M. Baldy-Moulinier, D.-H. Ingvar, and B.S. Meldrum), pp. 370–377. Libbey, London.

Sackeim, H., Decina, P., Prohovnik, I., and Malitz, S. (1987a) Seizure threshold in electroconvulsive therapy: effects of sex, age, electrode placement and number of treatments. *Archives of General Psychiatry*, 44, 355–360.

Sackeim, H.A., Decina, P., Portnoy, S., Neeley, P., and Malitz, S. (1987b) Studies of dosage, seizure threshold and seizure duration in ECT. *Biological Psychiatry*, 22, 249–268.

Sano, K., Nanba, H., Tabuchi, A., Tsuchiya, T., and Tsuda, M. (1996) BDNF gene can be activated by Ca^{++} signals without involvement of *de novo* AP-1 synthesis. *Biochemical and Biophysical Research Communications*, 229, 788–793.

Savage, D., Rigsbee, L., and McNamara, J.O. (1984) Knife cuts of the entorhinal cortex: effects on development of amygdaloid kindling and seizure-induced decrease in muscarinic cholinergic receptors. *Journal of Neuroscience*, 5, 408–413.

Scott, B.W., Wang, S., Burnham, W.M., De Boni, U., and Wojtowicz, J.M. (1998) Kindling-induced neurogenesis in the dentate gyrus of the rat. *Neuroscience Letters*, 248, 73–76.

Sheng, M. and Greenberg, M. (1990) The regulation and function of c-*fos* and other immediate early genes in the nervous system. *Neuron*, 4, 477–485.

Shin, C., McNamara, J.O., Morgan, J.I., Curran, T., and Cohen, D.R. (1990) Induction of c-*fos* mRNA expression by afterdischarge in the hippocampus of naive and kindled rats. *Journal of Neurochemistry*, 55, 1050–1055.

Shinnick-Gallagher, P., Keele, N., and Neugebauer, V. (1998) Long-lasting changes in the pharmacology and electrophysiology of amino acid receptors in amygdala kindled neurons. In *Kindling 5* (eds M. Corcoran and S. Moshe), pp. 75–88. Plenum Press, New York.

Simonato, M., Hosford, D., Labiner, D., Shin, C., Mansbach, H., and McNamara, J. (1991) Differential expression of immediate early genes in the hippocampus in the kindling model of epilepsy. *Molecular Brain Research*, 11, 115–124.

Singh, D. and Avery, D. (1975) *Physiological Techniques in Behavioral Research*. Wadsworth Publishing Co., New York.

Sitcoske, M.A., Rosen, J.B., Weiss, S.R.B., and Post, R.M. (1995) Electrical stimulation of discrete regions of the rat amygdala elicits differences in seizure development and response. *Society for Neuroscience Abstracts*, 21, 1973.

Sitcoske, M.A., Rosen, J.B., Post, R.M., and Weiss, S.R.B. (1997) Kindling specific rat amygdaloid nuclei affects seizure development and the induction of c-fos, NGFI-A and BDNF: a functional neuroanatomical study. *Society for Neuroscience Abstracts*, 23, 2161.

Sloviter, R. (1983) 'Epileptic' brain damage in rats induced by sustained electrical stimulation of the perforant path. I. Acute electrophysiological and light microscopic studies. *Brain Research*, 10, 675–697.

Sloviter, R. (1987) Decreased hippocampal inhibition and a selective loss of interneurons in experimental epilepsy. *Science*, 235, 73–75.

Sloviter, R. (1991) Calcium-binding protein (calbindin-D28K) and parvalbumin immunocytochemistry in the normal and epileptic human hippocampus. *Journal of Comparative Neurology*, 308, 381–396.

Sloviter, R. (1992) Possible functional consequences of synaptic reorganization in the dentate gyrus of kainate-treated rats. *Neuroscience Letters*, 137, 91–96.

Smith, M.A., Weiss, S.R.B., Abedin, T., Kim, H., Post, R.M., and Gold, P.W. (1991) Effects of amygdala kindling and electroconvulsive seizures on the expression of corticotropin releasing hormone in the rat brain. *Molecular and Cellular Neuroscience*, 2, 103–116.

Smith, M.A., Weiss, S.R., Berry, R.L., Zhang, L.X., Clark, M., Massenburg, G., and Post, R.M. (1997a) Amygdala-kindled seizures increase the expression of corticotropin-releasing factor (CRF) and CRF-binding protein in GABAergic interneurons of the dentate hilus. *Brain Research*, 745, 248–256.

Smith, M.A., Zhang, L.X., Lyons, W.E., and Mamounas, L.A. (1997b) Anterograde transport of endogenous brain-derived neurotrophic factor in hippocampal mossy fibers. *NeuroReport*, 8, 1829–1834.

Spiegler, B.J. and Mishkin, M. (1981) Evidence for the sequential participation of inferior temporal cortex and amygdala in the acquisition of stimulus-reward associations. *Behavioral Brain Research*, 3, 303–317.

Squire, L. and Zola-Morgan, S. (1991) The medial temporal lobe memory system. *Science*, 253, 1380–1386.

Sutula, T. (1993) Sprouting as an underlying cause of hyperexcitability in experimental models and in human epileptic temporal lobe. In *Epilepsy: Models, Mechanisms and Concepts* (ed. P. Schwartzkroin), pp. 304–322 Cambridge University Press, Cambridge.

Sutula, T., Xiao-Xian, H., Cavazos, J., and Scott, G. (1988) Synaptic reorganization in the hippocampus induced by abnormal functional activity. *Science*, 239, 1147–1150.

Sutula, T., Casino, G., Parada, I., and Ramirez, L. (1989) Mossy fiber synaptic reorganization in the epileptic temporal lobe. *Annals of Neurology*, 26, 321–330.

Sutula, T., Golavai, G., and Cavazos, J. (1992) Assessing the functional significance of mossy fiber sprouting. *Epilepsy Research* (suppl.) **7**, 251–259.

Sutula, T., Koch, J., Golarai, G., Watanabe, Y., and McNamara, J. (1996) NMDA receptor dependence of kindling and mossy fiber sprouting: evidence that the NMDA receptor regulates patterning of hippocampal circuits in the adult brain. *Journal of Neuroscience*, 16, 7398–7406.

Tauck, D. and Nadler, J. (1985) Evidence of functional mossy fiber sprouting in hippocampal formation of kainic acid-treated rats. *Journal of Neuroscience*, 5, 1016–1022.

Teskey, G., Atkinson, B., and Cain, D. (1991) Expression of the proto-oncogene c-*fos* following electrical kindling in the rat. *Molecular Brain Research*, 11, 1–10.

Theodore, W. and Porter, R. (1995) *Epilepsy*, 3rd edn. W.B. Saunders Co, Philadelphia.

Thoenen, H. (1995) Neurotrophins and neuronal plasticity. *Science*, 270, 595–598.

Thomas, M.J., Moody, T.D., Makhinson, M., and O'Dell, T.J. (1996) Activity-dependent beta-adrenergic modulation of low frequency stimulation induced LTP in the hippocampal CA1 region. *Neuron*, 17, 475–482.

Traub, R.J., Pechman, P., Iadarola, M.J., and Gebhart, G.F. (1992) Fos-like proteins in the lumbosacral spinal cord following noxious and non-noxious colorectal distention in the rat. *Pain*, 49, 393–403.

Tsuru, N., Kawasaki, H., Genda, S., Hara, K., Hashiguchi, H., and Ueda, Y. (1992) Effect of unilateral dentate nucleus lesions on amygdaloid kindling in rats. *Epilepsia*, 33, 213–221.

Tuff, L., Racine, R., and Adamec, R. (1983) The effects of kindling on GABA-mediated inhibition in the dentate gyrus of the rat. I. Paired-pulse depression. *Brain Research*, 277, 79–90.

Van der Zee, C., Rashid, K., Lee, K., Moore, K.-A., Stanisz, J., Diamond, J., Racine, R., and Fahnestock, M. (1995) Intraventricular administration of antibodies to nerve growth factor retards kindling and blocks mossy fiber sprouting in adult rats. *Journal of Neuroscience*, 15, 5316–5323.

Vickery, R.M., Morris, S.H., and Bindman, L.J. (1997) Metabotropic glutamate receptors are involved in long-term potentiation in isolated slices of rat medial frontal cortex. *Journal of Neurophysiology*, 78, 3039–3046.

Vignes, M. and Collingridge, G. (1997) The synaptic activation of kainate receptors. *Nature*, 388, 179–182.

Vignes, M., Bleakman, B., Lodge, D., and Collingridge, G. (1997) The synaptic activation of the GluR5 subtype of kainate receptor in area CA3 of the rat hippocampus. *Neuropharmacology*, 36, 1477–1481.

Wada, J.A., Sato, M., and Corcoran, M.E. (1974) Persistent seizure susceptibility and recurrent spontaneous seizures in kindled cats. *Epilepsia*, 15, 465–478.

Wagner, J.J. and Alger, B.E. (1995) GABAergic and developmental influences on homosynaptic LTD and depotentiation in rat hippocampus. *Journal of Neuroscience*, 15, 1577–1586.

Wan, R.-Q., Noguera, E.C., and Weiss, S.R.B. (1998) Anticonvulsant effects of intra-hippocampal injection of TRH in amygdala kindled rats. *NeuroReport*, 9, 677–682.

Watanabe, Y., Ikegaya, Y., Saito, H., and Abe, K. (1995) Roles of $GABA_A$, NMDA and muscarinic receptors in induction of long-term potentiation in the medial and lateral amygdala *in vitro*. *Neuroscience Research*, 21, 317–322.

Watanabe, Y., Ikegaya, Y., Saito, H., and Abe, K. (1996a) Opposite regulation by the beta-adrenoceptor–cyclic AMP system of synaptic plasticity in the medial and lateral amygdala *in vitro*. *Neuroscience*, 71, 1031–1035.

Watanabe, Y., Johnson, R., Butler, L., Binder, D., Spiegelman, B., Papaioannou, V., and McNamara, J. (1996b) Null mutation of c-*fos* impairs structural and functional plasticities in the kindling model of epilepsy. *Journal of Neuroscience*, 16, 3827–3836.

Weiss, S.R. and Post, R.M. (1998) Kindling: separate vs. shared mechanisms in affective disorders and epilepsy. *Neuropsychobiology*, 38, 167–180.

Weiss, S.R.B., Nierenberg, J., Lewis, R., and Post, R.M. (1992) Corticotropin-releasing hormone: potentiation of cocaine-kindled seizures and lethality. *Epilepsia*, 33, 248–254.

Weiss, S.R.B., Clark, M., Rosen, J.B., Smith, M.A., and Post, R.M. (1995) Contingent tolerance to the anticonvulsant effects of carbamazepine: relationship to loss of endogenous adaptive mechanisms. *Brain Research Reviews*, 20, 305–325.

Willimore, L., Sypert, G., Munson, J., and Hurd, R. (1978) Chronic focal epileptiform discharges induced by injection of iron into rat and cat cortex. *Science*, 200, 1501–1502.

Wolf, H., Aliashkevich, A., Blumcke, I., Wietler, O., and Zentner, J. (1997) Neuronal loss and gliosis of the amygdaloid nucleus in temporal lobe epilepsy. A quantitative analysis of 70 surgical specimens. *Acta Neuropathologica*, 93, 606–610.

Yehuda, R., Kahana, B., Schmeidler, J., Southwick, S.M., Wilson, S., and Giller, E.L. (1995) Impact of cumulative lifetime trauma and recent stress on current posttraumatic stress disorder symptoms in holocaust survivors. *American Journal of Psychiatry*, 152, 1815–1818.

Zalutsky, R. and Nicoll, R. (1990) Comparison of two forms of long-term potentiation in single hippocampal neurons. *Science*, 248, 1619–1624.

Zhang, L.X., Wu, M., and Han, J.S. (1992) Suppression of audiogenic epileptic seizures by intracerebral injection of a CCK gene vector. *NeuroReport*, 3, 700–702.

Zhang, L.X., Smith, M.A., Kim, S.Y., Rosen, J.B., Weiss, S.R., and Post, R.M. (1996) Changes in cholecystokinin mRNA expression after amygdala kindled seizures: an *in situ* hybridization study. *Brain Research. Molecular Brain Research*, 35, 278–284.

5 The amygdala: anxiety and benzodiazepines

Sandra E. File

Psychopharmacology Research Unit, Neuroscience Research Centre, GKT School of Biomedical Sciences, King's College London, UK

Summary

This chapter reviews the role of the benzodiazepine receptors in the amygdala in mediating behaviour in animal tests of anxiety. Indications of the physiological role of amygdala nuclei can be obtained from the effects of central injections of the benzodiazepine receptor antagonist, flumazenil. When benzodiazepine agonists are injected it is crucial to determine whether the effects are genuinely due to pharmacological activation of the receptors in a specific area. The use of low concentrations, injected in small volumes and an effect that is antagonised by flumazenil is the best indication that this is so. High concentrations of benzodiazepines have a local anaesthetic action and thus their effects are more those of a lesion than of receptor activation; the drug may also spread to other nuclei of the amygdala. At present, there is no strong evidence that the benzodiazepine receptors in the central nucleus play either a physiological or pharmacological role in animal tests of anxiety. However, activation of the receptors in the basolateral nucleus has anxiolytic effects in many, but not all, animal tests. These effects are dependent on the endogenous GABA tone that is generated by the particular test conditions.

5.1 Introduction

There is a growing literature implicating the amygdala in the coordination of behavioural, endocrinological, and neurochemical responses to aversive situations, including many that are considered to be animal tests of anxiety. The present chapter addresses the role of the γ-aminobutyric acid A ($GABA_A$)–benzodiazepine receptor complex in the amygdala in mediatng changes in anxiety. The benzodiazepines change behaviour in all animal tests of anxiety, and it is often assumed that one of the sites mediating this action is the amygdaloid complex. Several lines of reasoning have been advanced to support this assumption. (i) There is a particularly high density of benzodiazepine-binding sites in the amygdala, especially in the basolateral nucleus (Niehoff and Kuhar, 1983; Niehoff and Whitehouse, 1983), and recently it has been shown that very high-affinity sites are localized exclusively in limbic areas, such as the amygdala, hippocampus, and septum (Onoe *et al.*, 1996). (ii) Lesions of the amygdala block the acquisition and/or the expression of many aspects of fear responding (e.g. Davis *et al.*, 1993; Goldstein *et al.*, 1996; File *et al.*, 1998b). (iii) Electrical stimulation of the amygdala produces signs of fear and anxiety (Chapman *et al.*, 1954; Feindel and Penfield, 1954), and exposure to aversive events increases amygdaloid neuronal discharge in rats (Umemoto and Olds, 1975) and regional blood flow in humans (Zald and Pardo, 1997). (iv) Benzodiazepines suppress the firing rate of neurons in the amygdala (Chou and Wang, 1977). (v) Direct administration of benzodiazepines into the amygdala has anti-conflict or anxiolytic effects (Nagy *et al.*, 1979). The purpose of this chapter is to examine this very general conclusion in a little more detail, with regard to both the specific subnuclei of the amygdala and the particular animal test of anxiety. It will also examine the extent to which the effects of benzodiazepines, after central administration, are pharmacologically and anatomically specific.

5.1.1 Benzodiazepine binding

Whilst many stressors or aversive stimuli induce changes in benzodiazepine binding, most of the studies have focused on the cerebral cortex and hippocampus (Deutsch *et al.*, 1994). Those that have studied the amygdala have found no differences in benzodiazepine binding in Maudsley-reactive and non-reactive strains of rat, which are believed to differ in anxiety (Tamborska *et al.*, 1986), or any changes after exposure of rat pups to isolation stress (Insel *et al.*, 1989) or after forced swim stress (Medina *et al.*, 1983), exposure to cat odour (Hogg and File, 1994), or restraint stress (Farabollini *et al.*, 1997). All these stressors resulted in changes in benzodiazepine binding in other brain regions. Furthermore, the anxiolytic effect arising from kindling in the basolateral nucleus of the amygdala has been shown to be unrelated to benzodiazepine receptors in that area (Witkin *et al.*, 1988). It would therefore seem that the activation of the amygdala during aversive or stressful events does not necessarily involve the benzodiazepine receptors. This is a somewhat surprising conclusion since it would suggest that the benzodiazepine-binding sites in the amygdala do not play a physiological role in the effects of stressors. So far, only situations of inescapable stress have been studied, and it is possible that escapable stress would induce changes in benzodiazepine binding in the amygdala. However, Amat *et al.* (1998a) have found that inescapable, but not escapable, shock elevated extracellular 5-hydroxytryptamine (5-HT) in the basolateral nucleus of the amygdala, whereas the opposite pattern was found in the dorsal periaqueductal grey (Amat *et al.*, 1998b). A second explanation is that the studies did not explore specific subnuclei of the amygdaloid complex and it is quite possible that the changes are restricted to one particular nucleus, and that the type of stressor will determine which nucleus is involved. A third possibility is that binding changes do occur, but that they are restricted to a particular subunit assembly, or even that there might be an increase in one subunit, but a decrease in another. In particular, there might be changes in the very high-affinity binding site in the amygdala, identified by *in vivo* binding in a positron emission tomography (PET) study in monkeys (Onoe *et al.*, 1996). This very high-affinity site represented only about 3% of the high-affinity sites in the amygdala.

Benzodiazepine binding sites are on the $GABA_A$–chloride channel receptor complex. Benzodiazepine receptor agonists (e.g. diazepam and midazolam) act as positive allosteric modulators to enhance the action of GABA by increasing the probability of channel opening; in the absence of GABA activation, they do not open channels. The $GABA_A$ receptor complex is a pentameric structure, composed of α, β, and γ subunits; so far, six α, four β, and four γ subunits have been identified (Smith and Olsen, 1995; Sigel and Buhr, 1998). The most likely combination that expresses full receptor function has two α, two β, and one γ subunit, with the α1β2γ2 subunit the most common and one that is present in high concentrations in the amygdala. It is thought that the binding of both GABA and benzodiazepines depend on more than one subunit, with binding of GABA occurring at the interface of α and β subunits, and benzodiazepine binding at the interface of α and γ subunits. Other ligands with high affinity for the benzodiazepine-binding site act as negative allosteric modulators, i.e. they decrease channel function. These compounds are known as inverse agonists and increase anxiety in man and animals (Pellow and File, 1984). Benzodiazepine receptor antagonists (e.g. flumazenil) bind to the receptor, without any action on channel opening, and block the actions of agonists and inverse agonists. Thus, if a behavioural action is observed after flumazenil, this indicates the presence of an endogenous substance acting at the benzodiazepine receptor. An anxiogenic action of flumazenil would indicate the presence of a substance with anxiolytic actions; an anxiolytic action would indicate a substance with anxiogenic (inverse agonist) actions. The entire binding structural unit may form a single functional domain, and the partial co-localization of GABA- and benzodiazepine-binding domains to a single structural unit could explain the unique allosteric interactions between the GABA and benzodiazepine sites. Positive and negative modulation might result from different conformational changes within the unit (e.g. helical rotation). The precise nature of this change is still unknown and will only be solved when the three-dimensional structure is known.

5.1.2 Lesions

Although this review focuses on the amygdala, it is important to remember that there are many other brain regions in which the benzodiazepines have been shown to exert anxiolytic effects. Examples of important areas so far identified are the dorsal hippocampus (Gonzalez *et al.*, 1998), the lateral septum (Pesold and Treit, 1996), the dorsal and median raphe nuclei (Thiebot *et al.*, 1980; Higgins *et al.*, 1988; Gonzalez and File, 1997), and the dorsal periaqueductal grey (Russo *et al.*, 1993). Thus, the fact that systemic administration of a benzodiazepine has an anxiolytic effect, even in animals with a lesion of the amygdala, does not necessarily mean that the amygdala is not normally one of the sites for the anxiolytic action of benzodiazepines. It simply means that the benzodiazepines can act at other sites to modify behaviour in that particular test situation. It is for this reason that local infusions into the amygdala could prove especially informative.

It is also pertinent that many of the lesion studies have used lesions that extend over several different nuclei of the amygdala, but evidence is growing that specific nuclei, particularly the basolateral nucleus and the central nucleus, may play distinct roles. For example, Killcross *et al.* (1997) have found the central nucleus to play a key role in reflexive, automatic, and Pavlovian conditioned responses to aversive stimuli, and the basolateral nucleus to play a key role in voluntary or choice behaviour based on emotional events. The central nucleus has many peptide-containing neurons and reciprocal connections with the hypothalamus, whereas the phylogenetically more recent and 'cortex-like' basolateral nucleus forms part of the amygdala–hippocampal–frontal cortex circuit. These biochemical and anatomical differences between the nuclei are likely to influence the role of benzodiazepine receptors in the two nuclei.

5.1.3 Animal tests of anxiety

Since many distinct types of anxiety are recognized clinically (e.g. generalized anxiety disorder, panic disorder, post-traumatic stress disorder, specific phobia), it is quite possible that different animal tests will contain components akin to the various clinical disorders, even if there is not a precise mapping between the two. This chapter will address the question as to whether the amygdaloid benzodiazepine system plays a major role in all animal tests of anxiety. For example, studies from Treit's laboratory (Treit *et al.*, 1993; Treit and Menard, 1997) found that combined lesions of the central and basolateral nuclei were without effect on rats in the elevated plus-maze. If lesions of, or benzodiazepine administration into, the amygdala are without effect in some tests of anxiety, this provides crucial information that different brain regions are involved in different aversive states or types of anxiety. Indeed, there is considerable evidence that the dorsal hippocampus plays a major role in mediating behaviour in the social interaction, but not in the elevated plus-maze, test of anxiety (File *et al.*, 1996, 1998a; Gonzalez *et al.*, 1998) and that the dorsal raphe nucleus plays a role in only some of the animal tests of anxiety, such as the social interaction test (Higgins *et al.*, 1988; Hogg *et al.*, 1994; Picazo *et al.*, 1995; File and Gonzalez, 1996) and ultrasonic vocalizations (Schreiber and DeVry, 1993), but may be unimportant in the black–white crossing test and conditioned suppression of drinking (Carli *et al.*, 1989; Carli and Samanin, 1998). In a similar vein, Davis *et al.* (1997) have suggested that different brain regions are involved in mediating fear and anxiety, and Graeff *et al.* (1993) have suggested that there is a different neurochemical mediation of conditioned and unconditioned fear.

It is not the purpose of this chapter to provide detailed descriptions of the various animal tests of anxiety, but this section will give a brief summary of the behavioural changes in each test that are considered to indicate an anxiolytic action. Detailed experimental protocols of several of these tests can be found in File (1997). Antagonism of the pentylenetetrazole (PTZ) cue has been used as evidence that drugs are anxiolytic because they are able to antagonize the internal state generated by PTZ. PTZ is anxiogenic in several animal tests (File and Lister, 1984) and it is assumed that it generates a set of internal cues that resemble those produced by anxiety. In the Vogel punished drinking test, thirsty rats receive electric shocks as well as water reinforcement and therefore are punished for responding; an anti-conflict effect is shown by an increase in punished licking (or in the number of shocks received). In the Geller–Seifter test, there are two different schedules. In one schedule the response, usually lever pressing, results in a food reward (e.g. every 20th lever press); in the other schedule, each lever press results in both food and an electric shock. Additional cues are often provided to distinguish the two schedules. An anti-conflict effect is shown by an increase in punished responding. In the conditioned suppression of drinking, thirsty rats are trained to lick at a water spout; on one schedule they are always rewarded with water, on another each lick is both rewarded and punished by an electric shock. In both of these conflict tests, an anti-conflict action is revealed by increased responding during the punished schedule, and hence by an increase in the number of shocks received. In the conditioned burying of an electrified probe, an anxiolytic action is shown by a decrease in the active avoidance response of burying the probe and an increase in the number of shocks received (i.e. a decrease in the passive avoidance of the probe). Two other widely used ethological tests of anxiety do not use conditioned fear or electric shocks, but rely on the unconditioned responses of rats. In the social interaction test, the time that male rats spend in social investigation of another rat is suppressed by testing them in an unfamiliar test arena and/or under bright light. An anxiolytic action is shown by an increase in social interaction. In the elevated plus-maze, a rat or mouse has the choice of exploring two open elevated arms, or two that are enclosed by side walls. An anxiolytic action is indicated by an increased percentage of entries onto, and time spent on, the open arms.

5.1.4 Note on units

All the doses referred to in this chapter are for each side, and in all cases the injections were bilateral. The studies reviewed have varied in the units in which the central drug injections have been expressed. Most have used units of weight, such as micrograms, but they vary as to whether this refers to the base or the salt, and often this is not specified. With central injections, the volume of injection is also of importance and I have therefore also provided this information. Thus a dose of 10 μg injected in a volume of 1 μl will be expressed as 10 μg/μl, if it was injected in a volume of 0.5 μl it will be expressed as 10 μg/0.5 μl. Some of the studies have expressed their doses in moles and, where this has occurred, I have also provided the equivalent in grams. If doses in moles have been cited, I have provided the μg/μl equivalent as well. The actual drug concentration at the receptors is likely to be a crucial factor in determining the response to a central injection, and receptors close to the point of injection will be exposed to this concentration. The more distant the receptors, the lower the concentration will be, and the actual volume of injection will be one factor that determines the extent of the spread. At more distant sites, with a greater volume of distribution, the actual amount of drug injected will become more pertinent as this will now determine the concentration at these sites. It therefore seems that the amount of drug, drug concentration, and volume of injection are all factors that might influence the behavioural response to a central injection. If comparisons are to be made between different compounds, it is more relevant to make such comparisons in μmoles, rather than μg. In this chapter, however, no important distinctions have arisen for the different benzodiazepines used, and very many studies have used midazolam. I therefore have not translated all the doses into moles and have chosen to leave this chapter in the units cited most often in the experimental papers.

5.1.6 Methodological note on the use of high concentrations of benzodiazepines for microinjection into specific brain regions

When drugs are microinjected into specific brain regions, it is of crucial importance to establish whether their effects can be attributed to a genuine pharmacological effect in that particular area. The use of low concentrations, injected in small volumes, and the antagonism of the effects by a benzodiazepine receptor antagonist (e.g. flumazenil) would be good indicators that this is the case. Unfortunately, many of the published studies fall short of these requirements.

The use of high concentrations of benzodiazepines will, in effect, produce a chemical lesion of the area. In an excellent study, Heule *et al.* (1983) showed that midazolam injected into the central nucleus of the amygdala had anti-conflict effects in the Geller–Seifter test, but only in concentrations (24 mM) that had anaesthetic action. Indeed, the effect of midazolam was mimicked by other drugs with local anaesthetic properties. The concentration of midazolam with local anaesthetic action is equivalent to an injection of about 8 μg/μl and thus the results from experiments that have used this concentration or higher must be viewed as indicating the effects of a reversible lesion and not as the result of specific activation of benzodiazepine receptors. The use of high doses, and hence high concentrations, of benzodiazepines can also lead to 'lesion' effects, due to the precipitation in brain tissue of the drug, causing non-specific physical damage. Benzodiazepines are poorly soluble and do not dissolve in artificial cerebrospinal fluid (CSF). Only chlordiazepoxide, flurazepam, and midazolam dissolve in water or saline, the rest have to be injected as suspensions in solvents such as propylene glycol. Precipitation is most likely to occur when the drugs are injected as suspensions, and vehicles such as propylene glycol can themselves have anxiolytic effects (Petersen *et al.*, 1985), which could mask any additional effects of the drug. Finally, high doses may diffuse from their initial site of injection. Petersen *et al.* (1985) found that 10 μg of midazolam, injected in 0.5 μl, remained within the amygdala, but Heule *et al.* (1983) showed that injections of high concentrations of midazolam into the central nucleus also spread to the lateral nucleus, even with an injection volume as low as 0.2 μl.

5.2 Central nucleus

5.2.1 Effects of high doses

Bearing in mind the above comments, there are several studies in which the effects of benzodiazepine administration into the central nucleus of the amygdala are most likely to be due to lesion effects. Of course, this interpretation does not deny that the studies have shown the importance of the central nucleus in mediating anxiety, but it does seriously question the importance of the benzodiazepine receptors in this mediation.

PTZ cue

Benjamin *et al.* (1987) found that a high concentration of midazolam (16 μg/μl) produced a 50% reduction of responding on the lever associated with the PTZ cue. Vellucci *et al.* (1988) also found that a high dose of midazolam (10 μg) injected into sites just above the central and lateral nuclei antagonized the generalization of rats injected intraperitoneally (i.p.) with FG 7142, a benzodiazepine receptor inverse agonist, to the PTZ cue. Much lower doses of muscimol (12.5 and 25 ng) were able to antagonize the PTZ cue.

Vogel punished drinking and open field

High doses of diazepam (10 μg/μl) and lormetazepam (5 μg/μl) injected in polyethylene glycol had anxiolytic effects in the Vogel punished drinking test, although 40 μg of flurazepam was ineffective (Shibata *et al.*, 1989). Anxiolytic effects were also found in this test after lesions to the central nucleus (Shibata *et al.*, 1989; Yadin *et al.*, 1991). Injections of 60 nmol (20 μg) of chlordiazepoxide hydrochloride in 1 μl into the region of the central and basolateral nuclei increased the time spent in the central portion of an open field (McNamara and Skelton, 1993).

Conflict tests

In the Geller–Seifter conflict test, Shibata *et al.* (1982) found anti-conflict effects with high concentrations of midazolam (30 μg/μl), chlordiazepoxide (60 μg/μl), and diazepam (20 μg/μl). These effects are mimicked by those of lesioning the central nucleus in the Geller–Seifter (Shibata *et al.*, 1986) and conditioned suppression of drinking (Kopchia *et al.*, 1992) tests.

Elevated plus-maze and electrified probe

A high concentration of midazolam (10 μg/μl) was without effect in the elevated plus-maze and on conditioned burying of an electrified probe, but it did decrease the passive avoidance of the probe and hence increase the number of shocks taken (Pesold and Treit, 1994); a similar result was found with injections of 5 μg midazolam in 0.5 μl (Pesold and Treit, 1995). Exactly this pattern of results in the two tests was obtained from a joint lesion of the central and basolateral nuclei (Treit *et al.*, 1993; Treit and Menard, 1997).

5.2.2 Effects of lower doses

Where lower doses of benzodiazepines have been injected, at doses below those that would have a local anaesthetic action, no anxiolytic effects have been found. Thus, in the conditioned suppression of drinking test, Scheel-Kruger and Petersen (1982) found no effects of midazolam (1 μg/0.5 μl). In the Geller–Seifter conflict test, Heule *et al.* (1983) found no effect of midazolam (0.8 μg/μl), and Thomas *et al.* (1985) found no effect of chlordiazepoxide (10 μg/μl) in the conflict test or on the conditioned emotional response.

5.2.3 Effects of GABA and benzodiazepine receptor antagonists

Microinjection of receptor antagonists can provide information on the endogenous state of the $GABA_A$–benzodiazepine receptor system. Three studies provide evidence as to whether or not the endogenous $GABA_A$–benzodiazepine system is physiologically activated by exposure to the test situation. The first provides evidence that there is no endogenous GABA tone in the central nucleus when rats are tested in the social interaction test because the $GABA_A$ receptor antagonist, bicuculline, was without effect, whereas an extremely low concentration of the $GABA_A$ receptor agonist muscimol (100 pmol, or 11.4 ng, in a volume of 0.25 μl) had an anxiolytic effect (Sanders and Shekhar, 1995a). Since benzodiazepines act as modulators to enhance the effects of GABA, if there is no endogenous tone, it would be expected that injection of benzodiazepines into the central nucleus would be without effect in the social interaction test. Pesold and Treit (1995) found no effects of the benzodiazepine receptor antagonist flumazenil (15 μg/μl) in the elevated plus-maze test, on the burying of an electrified probe, or of its passive avoidance. Hence it seems that there is no endogenous benzodiazepine tone elicited by these tests. However, the results of one study do suggest that the endogenous $GABA_A$–benzodiazepine receptor system in the central nucleus may be activated when rats are exposed to the elevated plus-maze and insert a note of caution to the conclusion that the benzodiazepine receptors in this region play no role in this test. Da Cunha *et al.* (1992) found that although a low dose (10 nmol or 3 μg in 0.5 μl) of flumazenil did not change the percentage of open arm entries, it did decrease the percentage of time spent on the open arms of the elevated plus-maze, indicating there might be an anxiogenic effect. This is a potentially important finding, since it indicates that endogenous benzodiazepine receptor agonists, with an anxiolytic action, are released in this brain region by exposure to the plus-maze. If this is the case, then injections of benzodiazepines could be without effect because of the already high endogenous tone in this nucleus. Indeed, exposure to the plus-maze resulted in a decrease in the content of benzodiazepine-like molecules in the amygdala, which was interpreted as evidence for local release and subsequent metabolism of the molecules. The baseline scores in the Pesold and Treit study were higher than those in the DaCunha *et al.* study, which should have made it easier, rather than more difficult, to see an anxiogenic effect of flumazenil in the former study. One possible explanation is the use of a higher dose of flumazenil (15 μg) in the Pesold and Treit study, since at higher doses flumazenil has partial agonist properties.

5.2.4 Conclusion

At present, therefore, there is no conclusive evidence that the benzodiazepine receptors in the central nucleus play a physiological role in mediating behaviour in any of the animal tests of anxiety. There is also no evidence for a specific pharmacological action of benzodiazepines in the central nucleus having an anxiolytic effect in any animal test. The reported anxiolytic effects of the high concentrations are most probably due to a lesioning of the nucleus.

5.3 Basolateral nucleus

5.3.1 Effective doses and endogenous tone

The evidence is considerably better for a benzodiazepine site of action in the basolateral nucleus mediating anxiety in many, although not all, tests. Effective doses are much lower than those in the central nucleus, supporting the suggestion by Scheel-Kruger and Petersen (1982) that these high doses may have diffused to other areas, such as the basolateral nucleus, in order to have their effects. It also supports the possibility that the effects in the central nucleus may have been due to local anaesthetic actions (Heule *et al.*, 1983).

One reason for greater efficacy of benzodiazepines in the basolateral nucleus than in the central nucleus could be that the endogenous GABA tone elicited by the tests differs between the two nuclei. If the GABA tone is low, then few receptors are activated, and if the chloride ion channel is not opened by GABA, the benzodiazepines cannot exert any effect. Furthermore, GABA enhances benzodiazepine binding, so the benzodiazepines will be binding with lower affinity when the GABA tone is low. At the other extreme, if the endogenous GABA tone is very high, it might be difficult for benzodiazepines to enhance GABA's effects further. The sensitivity of each test situation to local administration of benzodiazepines will therefore depend on the endogenous GABA tone that each elicits in the basolateral nucleus.

5.3.2 Basolateral and lateral injection sites

Vogel punished drinking

In the Vogel punished drinking test, Petersen *et al.* (1985) found anxiolytic effects of 1 μg/0.5 μl midazolam injected into the basolateral and lateral nuclei, and this effect was antagonized by i.p. administration of flumazenil.

Conflict tests

In the conditioned suppression of drinking test, 1 μg/μl of midazolam or diazepam had significant anti-conflict effects (Scheel-Kruger and Petersen, 1982) when injected into sites extending over the basolateral and lateral nuclei. A lower dose (0.1 μg/μl) was ineffective, but a low dose of muscimol (25 ng/μl) had anti-conflict effects. The effectiveness of a low dose of muscimol suggests that the GABA tone was relatively low in this test, which would explain why 1 μg of midazolam was necessary to see an effect. Unfortunately, although bicuculline was shown to reverse the effects of both midazolam and muscimol, its effects alone were not tested.

In the Geller–Seifter conflict test, 500 ng of GABA, 1 μg of midazolam, and 10 μg of chlordiazepoxide injected in a volume of 0.5 μl into sites in the basolateral and lateral nuclei had anti-conflict effects, and those of chlordiazepoxide were antagonized by flumazenil (Hodges *et al.*, 1987). Thomas *et al.* (1985) found that 10 μg/μl of chlordiazepoxide had anti-conflict effects in the Geller–Seifter conflict test after injection into sites within the lateral region of the amygdala. The effects were greater when the rats were tested in extinction (i.e. a conditioned emotional response tested in the absence of shock, but in the presence of cues that signalled the punished schedule). Unfortunately, the effects of lower doses of chlordiazepoxide were not examined in either study, nor was there any evidence concerning the endogenous GABA tone in this test. However, another study using a similar level of food deprivation, although a different strain of rat, does provide some clues. Sanders and Shekhar (1995a) found that 2–10 pmol (1–5 ng) of bicuculline methiodide, injected in 0.25 μl, was anxiogenic in a conflict test, suggesting that this test situation elicits considerable GABA inhibitory tone.

5.3.3 Injections localized to the basolateral nucleus

More recent studies have used injections localized within the basolateral nucleus. The histological verification of such injections is extremely important and this can be helped by the use of a stain for acetylcholinesterase which allows visualization of the borders of the basolateral nucleus and thus the ability to determine more accurately the localization of the sites of injection. This stain was used by Gonzalez *et al.* (1996) and File *et al.* (1998b), but not in the other studies. Despite attempts to be accurate on the placement of needle tips, it should be remembered that however well the injection sites are localized, the use of high doses can still lead to a spread of the drug to other areas. Yet, despite the use of high doses and a relatively large injection volume, Shibata *et al.* (1982) failed to find any effects of 20 μg of diazepam, 60 μg of chlordiazepoxide, or 30 μg of midazolam injected in a volume of 1 μl into the basolateral nucleus in the Geller–Seifter conflict test. This raises the possibility that it is the lateral nucleus, rather than the basolateral nucleus, that is the more important site of action for benzodiazepine effects in the Geller–Seifter test. However, only 4–5 rats were tested with each placement in the Shibata *et al.* (1982) study, compared with 17 in the Hodges *et al.* (1987) study. Unfortunately, although Hodges *et al.* (1987) found anti-conflict effects, their injection sites also extended to the lateral nucleus and so the relative importance of the two nuclei cannot be settled at present.

Social interaction test

The social interaction test has four different test conditions that differ in the degree of anxiety that they generate. This is done by manipulating both the light level and the degree of familiarity the rats have with the test arena. These different test conditions also generate different levels of endogenous 5-HT and GABA tone. In an unspecified test condition, Sanders and Shekhar (1995a) found no effect of 250 pmol of muscimol, but anxiogenic effects of 20 pmol of bicuculline and 10 pmol of picrotoxin. This indicated that, at least in their test condition, there was a high endogenous GABA tone in the anterior portions of the basolateral nucleus. Although the cannulae were targeted at the basolateral nucleus, several of the injection sites fell in the lateral nucleus, so from this study alone it is not possible to exclude the possibility that both nuclei might have to be involved in order to obtain an anxiolytic effect. In a further study, which provided no information about the actual sites of injection, Sanders and Shekhar (1995b) found that injections of silent doses of flumazenil or bicuculline, targeted at the basolateral nucleus, were able to antagonize the anxiolytic effects of i.p. chlordiazepoxide. Using the high-light, familiar arena test condition, Gonzalez *et al.* (1996) found that 1 and 2 μg/0.5 μl of midazolam were anxiolytic. The boundaries of the basolateral nucleus were analysed with acetylcholinesterase staining, so the results suggest that it is extremely likely that this nucleus is itself an important site of action for the anxiolytic effects of benzodiazepines in this test.

Elevated plus-maze

A striking finding in the Gonzalez *et al.* (1996) study was that although there were anxiolytic responses to midazolam in the social interaction test, no effects to the same doses were found in the elevated plus-maze. This is perhaps because the amygdala does not play a major role in controlling behaviour in this test, as evidenced by the lack of effect of combined electrolytic lesions of the central and basolateral nuclei (Treit *et al.*, 1993; Treit and Menard, 1997) and the lack of effect of 5-HT_{1A} receptor agonists injected into the basolateral nucleus (Gonzalez *et al.*, 1996). Despite a relatively minor role controlling the expression of anxiety during trial 1 in the plus-maze, the basolateral nucleus does play a crucial role in the learning that takes place during the first trial in the plus-maze that leads to a change in the nature of the anxiety generated on trial 2 and to a lack of response to systemic or centrally administered benzodiazepines (File *et al.*, 1998b). The basolateral nucleus seems to play a key role in the consolidation of information, stored in other areas, that leads to phobic avoidance on trial 2 (see also Parent and McGaugh, 1994).

However, there are results which are at variance with the conclusion that the basolateral nucleus does not play an important role in controlling the response to benzodiazepines on trial 1 in the plus-maze. Pesold and Treit (1995) found that bilateral injections of 5 μg/0.5 μl midazolam into the basolateral nucleus had anxiolytic effects in the plus-maze. This was a higher dose (and concentration) than that used by Gonzalez *et al.* (1996) and, therefore, the injections may have spread to other nuclei; however, the central nucleus is unlikely to be involved since injections into this nucleus were without effect. Another difference between the two studies was that there was a lower baseline level of percentage of open arm entries in the Pesold and Treit study, indicating a higher baseline level of anxiety. It is therefore possible that benzodiazepine receptors in the basolateral nucleus can modulate behaviour in the plus-maze, but only in conditions when baseline anxiety is high and, hence, presumably, the endogenous GABA tone is low. However, this interpretation is difficult to reconcile with the absence of effect following a lesion to this area, unless other brain areas are able to compensate for the relatively minor role played by the amygdala in this test. The spread of benzodiazepines to brain areas other than the site of injection cannot be excluded and may well account for the other report of an anxiolytic effect of midazolam (1 μg/0.5 μl) in the basolateral nucleus. Green and Vale (1992) used injection cannulae at an angle of 6°, which would pass through the lateral ventricles. This means that diffusion from the needle tip upwards could have resulted in drug entering the ventricles and hence acting on quite remote areas. However, they also had very low baseline scores, indicating high anxiety, so this could also be an explanation for their findings of a positive effect of midazolam. Clearly, the issue of the role of the benzodiazepine receptors in controlling anxiety in the plus-maze needs considerable further investigation.

Electrified probe

Finally, the benzodiazepine receptors in the basolateral nucleus seem to play no role in modulating behaviour in the conditioned burying of an electrified probe. Midazolam (5 μg) was without effect, either on conditioned burying or on the passive avoidance of the probe (Pesold and Treit, 1995).

5.3.4 Conclusions

In conclusion, the basolateral and, probably, the lateral nucleus of the amygdala are sites mediating the anxiolytic actions of the benzodiazepines, which is consistent with the high density of benzodiazepine-binding sites in these areas and with the presence of very high-affinity sites. These actions are dependent on the endogenous GABA tone elicited by each test and, if this is too low or too high, the benzodiazepines will have little effect. Modulatory effects have been found in the Vogel punished drinking, the Geller–Seifter conflict, and the social interaction tests, and, in all these, the anxiolytic effects of benzodiazepines have been antagonized by flumazenil. The effects of benzodiazepines in the conditioned suppression of drinking test were antagonized by bicuculline, thus providing evidence that when the effective GABA tone in the region is modified, so too are the effects of benzodiazepines.

However, although widespread, the effects of benzodiazepines when injected into the basolateral nucleus are not universal to all tests of anxiety. They are without effect in the conditioned probe burying test and, at least in some circumstances, the elevated plus-maze. Experiments injecting GABA antagonists are needed in order to determine whether the crucial factor in determining whether benzodiazepines are effective is the endogenous GABA tone. There is no easy explanation in terms of behavioural analysis for the lack of effect of benzodiazepines in the electrified probe test. The conditioned passive avoidance of the electrified probe has strong similarities with the conditioned passive avoidance of the electrified water spout in the conditioned suppression of drinking, and some similarities with the passive avoidance in the Vogel test, although this does not involve prior conditioning. There are also similarities to the passive avoidance of the punished lever in the Geller–Seifter conflict test, although in this case punishment is through the grid floor. Furthermore, even unilateral injections of midazolam (1 μg/0.5 μl) into the basolateral nucleus have been found to impair conditioned passive avoidance in a step-down paradigm (Harris and Westbrook, 1995). The electrified probe test also provides a measure of active avoidance, the burying of the probe. Thus, simultaneously, the rat is provided with the possibility of avoiding the aversive stimulus (electrified probe) by a passive avoidance or an active avoidance response. In this respect, the electrified probe test has some elements in common with the elevated plus-maze. Rats can avoid the aversive stimulus (open arms) either by the passive avoidance response of not entering the open arms, or by the active avoidance response of entering the closed arms. Perhaps it is something in this presentation of response choice that makes the two situations less sensitive to benzodiazepine modulation in the basolateral nucleus.

5.4 Conclusions

Despite the widespread belief that the anxiolytic action of benzodiazepines is, at least in part, mediated through an action in the amygdala, we remain in considerable ignorance about many details of this. Most of the work has focused on the central and basolateral/lateral nuclei, but these may not be the only sites of importance. For example, more studies are needed in the medial nucleus, because only one anxiety test has been examined so far. Shibata *et al.* (1982) failed to find any effects of very high doses (20 μg of diazepam, 60 μg of chlordiazepoxide, and 30 μg midazolam, in 1 μl) in the Geller–Seifter conflict test. This nucleus is of importance for the anxiolytic effects of 5-HT_{1B} receptor antagonists in the social interaction and elevated plus-maze tests, but not in the Vogel punished drinking test (Duxon *et al.*, 1995, 1997). It would be most interesting to explore the effects of benzodiazepines in this nucleus in these other tests, to determine whether there is a differential role for benzodiazepine receptors in this area in different animal tests.

One report (Higgins *et al.*, 1991) suggests that a site in the amygdala, other than the basolateral nucleus, might be even more important for the anxiolytic effects of benzodiazepines. The guide cannulae were implanted well above the amygdala (calculating from lambda A +5.0, V –4.5, L ±4.5). The injection needles then extended a further 5 mm, running through the lateral ventricles to just below the posterior part of the basomedial nucleus. Since drug injections tend to track up the path of the needles, this suggests that this nucleus might be of importance to benzodiazepine action. Unfortunately, however, it is not possible to exclude the possibility that sites outside the amygdala were accessed through the ventricular system. Higgins *et al.* (1991) found anxiolytic effects of 200 ng/μl flurazepam in the high-light, unfamiliar arena test condition of the social interaction test and in the Vogel punished drinking test. These results are particularly interesting, in that such a low dose proved effective, and that higher doses (1 and 5 μg) did not.

Finally, there is a need for more extensive parametric work to determine the spread of injections from the site of injection and the effective concentration for an anxiolytic effect. At present it seems that an injection concentration of at least 6 mM midazolam might be needed. This compares with a concentration of 1–2 μM for an anxiogenic effect of 8-OH-DPAT (Gonzalez *et al.* 1996). However, in both cases, around 5–6 nmol are effective, and certainly at receptors more distant from the injection site this will be the more important factor in determining the effective concentration. Thus, although central administration of benzodiazepines confirms the amygdala as an important site of action for their anxiolytic effect, other neurotransmitters in this region, such as 5-HT, also play an important role. Endogenous neurotransmitters, such as GABA and 5-HT, play a physiological role in modulating anxiety, and the baseline levels of these transmitters will in turn influence the effects of drugs. The strategy of central administration of agonists and antagonists has proved most fruitful in understanding the neurobiology of anxiety, but considerably more work is needed to understand fully the role of the amygdala.

References

Amat, J., Matus-Amat, P., Watkins, L.R., and Maier, S.F. (1998a) Escapable and inescapable stress differentially alter extracellular levels of 5-HT in the basolateral amygdala of the rat. *Brain Research*, 812, 113–120.

Amat, J., Matus-Amat, P., Watkins, L.R., and Maier, S.F. (1998b) Escapable and inescapable stress differentially and selectively alter extracellular levels of 5-HT in the ventral hippocampus and dorsal periaqueductal gray of the rat. *Brain Research*, 797, 12–22

Benjamin, D., Emmett-Oglesby, M.W., and Lal, H. (1987) Modulation of the discriminative stimulus produced by pentylenetetrazol by centrally administered drugs. *Neuropharmacology*, 26, 1727–1731.

Carli, M. and Samanin, R. (1988) potential anxiolytic properties of 8-hydroxy-2-(di-n-propylamino)tetralin, a selective serotonin$_{1A}$ receptor agonist. *Psychopharmacology*, 94, 84–91.

Carli, M., Prontera,C., and Samanin,R. (1989) Evidence that central 5-hydroxytryptaminergic neurones are involved in the anxiolytic activity of buspirone. *British Journal of Pharmacology*, 96, 829–836.

Chapman, W.P., Schroeder, H.R., Geyer, G., Brazier, M.A.B., Fager, C., Poppeu, J.L., Solomon, H.C., and Yakolev, P.I. (1954) Physiological evidence concerning the importance of the amygdaloid nuclear region in the integration of circulating function and emotion in man. *Science,* 129, 949–950.

Chou, D.T. and Wang, S.C. (1977) Unit activity of amygdala and hippocampal neurons: effects of morphine and benzodiazepines. *Brain Research*, 126, 427–440.

Da Cunha, C., Wolfman, C., Levi de Stein, M., Ruschel, A.C., Izquierdo, I., and Medina, J.H. (1992) Anxiogenic effects of the intraamygdala injection of flumazenil, a benzodiazepine receptor antagonist. *Functional Neurology*, 7, 401–405.

Davis, M., Falls, W.A., Campeau, S., and Kim, M. (1993) Fear-potentiated startle: a neural and pharmacological analysis. *Behavioural Brain Research*, 58, 175–198.

Davis, M., Walker, D.L., and Lee, Y. (1997) Amygdala and bed nucleus of the stria terminalis: differential roles in fear and anxiety measured with the acoustic startle reflex. *Philosophical Transactions of the Royal Society of London, Series B*, 352, 1675–1687.

Deutsch, S.I., Rosse, R.B., and Mastropaolo, J. (1994) Environmental stress-induced functional modification of the central benzodiazepine binding site. *Clinical Neuropharmacology*, 17, 205–228.

Duxon, M.S., Kennett, G.A., Lightfowler, S., Blackburn, T.P., and Fone, K.C.F. (1997) Activation of 5-HT$_{2B}$ receceptors in the medial amygdala causes anxiolysis in the social interaction test in the rat. *Neuropharmacology*, 36, 601–608.

Farabollini, F., Fluck, E., Albonetti, M.E., and File, S.E. (1996) Sex differences in benzodiazepine binding in frontal cortex and amygdala of the rat 24 hours after restraint stress. *Neuroscience Letters*, 218, 177–180.

Feindel, W. and Penfield, W. (1954) Localisation of discharge in temporal lobe automatism. *Archives of Neurology and Psychiatry*, 72, 605–630.

File, S.E. (1997) Animal measures of anxiety. In *Current Protocols in Neuroscience* (eds J. Crawley, C. Gerfen, R. McKay, M.A. Rogawski, D. Sibley, and P. Skolnick), pp. 8.3.1–8.3.15. John Wiley and Sons, New York.

File, S.E. and Gonzalez, L.E. (1996) Anxiolytic effects in the plus-maze of 5-HT_{1A} receptor ligands in dorsal raphé and ventral hippocampus. *Pharmacology, Biochemistry and Behavior*, 54, 123–128.

File, S.E. and Lister, R.G. (1984) Do the reductions in social interaction produced by picrotoxin and pentylenetetrazole indicate anxiogenic actions? *Neuropharmacology*, 23, 793–796.

File, S.E., Gonzalez, L.E., and Andrews, N. (1996) Comparative study of pre- and postsynaptic 5-HT_{1A} receptor modulation of anxiety in two ethological animal tests. *Journal of Neuroscience*, 16, 4810–4815.

File, S.E., Gonzalez, L.E., and Andrews, N. (1998a) Endogenous acetylcholine in the dorsal hippocampus reduces anxiety through actions on nicotinic and $muscarinic_1$ receptors. *Behavioural Neuroscience*, 112, 352–359.

File, S.E., Gonzalez, L.E., and Gallant, R. (1998b) Role of the basolateral nucleus of the amygdala in the formation of a phobia. *Neuropsychopharmacology*, 19, 397–405.

Goldstein, L.E., Rasmusson, A.M., Bunney, B.S., and Roth, R.H. (1996) Role of the amygdala in the coordination of behavioral, neuroendocrine, and prefrontal cortical monoamine responses to psychological stress in the rat. *Journal of Neuroscience*, 16, 4787–4798.

Gonzalez, L.E. and File, S.E. (1997) A five minute experience in the elevated plus-maze alters the state of the benzodiazepine receptor in the dorsal raphe nucleus. *Journal of Neuroscience*, 17, 1505–1511.

Gonzalez, L.E., Andrews, N., and File, S.E. (1996) 5-HT_{1A} and benzodiazepine receptors in the basolateral amygdala modulate anxiety in the social interaction test, but not in the elevated plus maze. *Brain Research*, 732, 145–153.

Gonzalez, L.E., Ouagazzal, A.-M., and File, S.E. (1998) Stimulation of benzodiazepine receptors in the dorsal hippocampus and median raphe reveals different GABAergic control in two animal tests of anxiety. *European Journal of Neuroscience*, 10, 3673–3680.

Graeff, F.G., Silveira, M.C.L., Nogueira, R.L., Audi, E.A., and Oliveira, R.M.W. (1993) Role of the amygdala and periaqueductal gray in anxiety and panic. *Behavioural Brain Research*, 58, 123–131.

Green,S. and Vale,A.L. (1992) Role of amygdaloid nuclei in the anxiolytic effects of benzodiazepines in rats. *Behavioural Pharmacology*, 3, 261–264.

Harris ,J.A. and Westbrook, R.F. (1995) Effects of benzodiazepine microinjection into the amygdala or periaqueductal gray on the expression of conditioned fear and hypoalgesia in rats. *Behavioral Neuroscience*, 109, 295–304

Heule, F., Lorez, H., Cumin, R., and Haefely, W. (1983) Studies on the anticonflict effect of midazolam injected into the amygdala. *Neuroscience Letters Supplement*, 14, S164.

Higgins, G.A., Bradbury,A.J., Jones, B.J., and Oakley, N.R. (1988) Behavioural and biochemical consequences following activation of 5-HT_1-like and GABA receptors in the dorsal raphe nucleus of the rat.*Neuropharmacology*, 27, 993–1001.

Higgins, G.A., Jones, B.J., Oakley, N.R., and Tyers, M.B. (1991) Evidence that the amygdala is involved in the disinhibitory effects of 5-HT_3 receptor antagonists. *Psychopharmacology*, 104, 545–551.

Hodges, H., Green, S., and Glenn, B. (1987) Evidence that the amygdala is involved in benzodiazepine and serotonergic effects on punished responding but not on discrimination. *Psychopharmacology*, 92, 491–504.

Hogg, S. and File, S.E. (1994) Regional differences in rat and benzodiazepine binding in response to novelty and cat odour. *Neuropharmacology*, 33, 865–868.

Hogg, S., Andrew, N., and File, S.E. (1994) Contrasting behavioural effects of 8-OH-DPAT in the dorsal raphe nucleus and ventral hippocampus. *Neuropharmacology*, 33, 343–348.

Insel, T.R., Gelhard, R.E., and Miller, L.P. (1989) Rat pup isolation distress and the brain benzodiazepine receptor. *Developmental Psychobiology*, 22, 509–525.

Killcross, S., Robbins, T.W., and Everitt, B.J. (1997) Different types of fear conditioned behaviour mediated by separate nuclei within the amygdala. *Nature*, 388, 377–380.

Kopchia, K.L., Altman, H.J., and Commissaris, R.L. (1992) Effects of lesions of the central nucleus of the amygdala on anxiety-like behaviors in the rat. *Pharmacology Biochemistry and Behavior*, 43, 453–461.

McNamara, R.K. and Skelton, R.W. (1993) Effects of intracranial infusions of chlodiazepoxide on spatial learning in the Morris water maze. I. Neuroanatomical specificity. *Behavioural Brain Research*, 59, 175–191.

Medina, J.H., Novas, M.L., Wolfman, C.N.V., Levi de Stein, M., and DeTobertis, E. (1983) Benzodiazepine receptors in rat cerebral cortex and hippocampus undergo rapid and reversible changes after acute stress. *Neuroscience*, 9, 331–335.

Nagy, J., Zambo, K., and Decsi, L. (1979) Anti-anxiety action of diazepam after intra-amygdaloid application in the rat. *Neuropharmacology*, 18, 573–576.

Niehoff, D.L. and Kuhar, M.J. (1983) Benzodiazepine receptors: localisation in rat amygdala. *Journal of Neuroscience*, 3, 2091–2097.

Niehoff, D.L. and Whitehouse, P.J. (1983) Multiple benzodiazepine receptors: autoradiographic localization in normal human amygdala. *Brain Research*, 276, 237–245.

Onoe, H., Tsukada, H., Nishiyama, S., Nakanishi, S., Inoue, O., Langstrom, B. *et al.* (1996) A subclass of $GABA_A$/benzodiazepine receptor exclusively localised in the limbic system. *NeuroReport*, 8, 117–122.

Parent, M.B. and McGaugh, J. (1994) Posttraining infusion of lidocaine into the amygdala basolateral complex impairs retention of inhibitory avoidance training. *Brain Research*, 661, 97–103

Pesold, C. and Treit, D. (1994) The septum and amygdala differentially mediate the anxiolytic effects of benzodiazepines. *Brain Research*, 638, 295–301.

Pesold, C. and Treit, D. (1995) The central and basolateral amygdala differentially mediate the anxiolytic effects of benzodiazepines. *Brain Research*, 671, 213–221.

Pesold, C. and Treit, D. (1996) The neuroanatomical specificity of the anxiolytic effects of intra-septal infusions of midazolam. *Brain Research*, 710, 161–168.

Petersen, E.N., Braestrup, C., and Scheel-Kruger, J. (1985) Evidence that the anticonflict effect of midazolam in amygdala is mediated by the specific benzodiazepine receptors. *Neuroscience Letters*, 53, 285–288.

Picazo, O., Lopez-Rubalcalva, C., and Fernandez-Guasti, A. (1995) Anxiolytic effect of the 5-HT_{1A} compounds 8-hydroxy-2-(di-*n*-propylamino)tetralin and ipsapirone in the social interaction paradigm: evidence of a presynaptic action. *Brain Research Bulletin*, 37, 169–175.

Russo, A.S., Guimaraes, F.S., Deaguiar, J.C., and Graeff, F.G. (1993) Role of benzodiazepine receptors located in the dorsal periaqueductal grey of rats in anxiety. *Psychopharmacology*, 110, 198–202.

Sanders, S.K. and Shekhar, A. (1995a) Regulation of anxiety by $GABA_A$ receptors in the rat amygdala. *Pharmacology, Biochemistry, and Behavior*, 52, 701–706.

Sanders, S.K. and Shekhar, A. (1995b) Anxiolytic effects of chlordiazepoxide blocked by injection of $GABA_A$ and benzodiazepine receptor antagonists in the region of the anterior basolateral amygdala of rats. *Biological Psychiatry*, 37, 473–476.

Scheel-Kruger, J. and Petersen, E.N. (1982) Anticonflict effect of the benzodiazepines mediated by a GABAergic mechanism in the amygdala. *European Journal of Pharmacology*, 82, 115–116.

Schreiber, R. and DeVry, J. (1993) Neuronal circuits involved in the anxiolytic effects of the 5-HT_{1A} receptor agonists 8-OH-DPAT, ipsapirone and buspirone in the rat. *European Journal of Pharmacology*, 249, 341–345.

Shibata, K., Kataoka, Y., Gomita, Y., and Ueki, S. (1982) Localization of the site of the anticonflict action of benzodiazepines in the amygdaloid nucleus of rats. *Brain Research*, 234, 442–446.

Shibata, K., Kataoka, Y., Yamashita, K., and Ueki, S. (1986) An important role of the central amygdaloid nucleus and mammillary body in the mediation of conflict behavior in rats. *Brain Research*, 372, 159–162.

Shibata, S., Yamashita, K., Yamamoto, E., Ozaki, T., and Ueki, S. (1989) Effects of benzodiazepine and GABA antagonists on anticonflict effects of antianxiety drugs injected into the rat amygdala in a water-lick suppression test. *Psychopharmacology*, 98, 38–44.

Sigel,E. and Buhr,A. (1997) The benzodiazepine binding site of $GABA_A$ receptors. *Trends in Pharmacological Sciences*, 18, 425–429

Smith, G.B. and Olsen, R.W. (1995) Functional domains of $GABA_A$ receptors. *Trends in Pharmacological Sciences*, 16, 162–168

Tamborska, E., Insel, T., and Marangos, P.J. (1986) 'Peripheral' and 'central' type benzodiazepine receptors in Maudsley rats. *European Journal of Pharmacology*, 126, 281–287.

Thiebot, M.H., Jobert, A., and Soubrie, P. (1980) Chlordiazepoxide and GABA injected into raphé dorsalis release the conditioned behavioural suppression induced in rats by a conflict procedure without nociceptive component. *Neuropharmacology*, 19, 633–641.

Thomas, S.R., Lewis, M.E., and Iversen, S.D. (1985) Correlation of $[^3H]$diazepam binding density with anxiolytic locus in the amygdalaloid complex of the rat. *Brain Research*, 342, 85–90.

Tomaz, C., Dickinson-Anson, H., McGaugh, J.L., Souzasilva, M.A., Viana, M.B., and Graeff, F.G. (1993) Localization in the amygdala of the amnestic action of diazepam on emotional memory. *Behavioural Brain Research*, 58, 99–105.

Treit, D. and Menard, J. (1997) Dissociations among the anxiolytic effects of septal, hippocampal, and amygdaloid lesions. *Behavioral Neuroscience* , 111, 653–658.

Treit, D., Pesold, C., and Rotzinger, S. (1993) Dissociating the anti-fear effects of septal and amygdala lesions using two pharmacologically validated models of rat anxiety. *Behavioral Neuroscience*, 107, 770–785.

Umemoto, M. and Olds, M.E. (1975) Effects of chlordiazepoxide, diazepam and chlorpromazine on conditioned emotional behavior and conditioned neuronal activity in limbic, hypothalamic and geniculate regions. *Neuropharmacology*, 14, 413–425.

Vellucci, S.V., Martin, P.J., and Everitt, B.J. (1988) The discriminative stimulus produced by pentylenetetrazole: effects of systemic anxiolytics and anxiogenics, aggressive defeat and midazolam or muscimol infused into the amygdala. *Journal of Psychopharmacology*, 2, 80–93.

Witkin, J.M., Lee, M.A., and Walczak, D.D. (1988) Anxiolytic properties of amygdaloid kindling unrelated to benzodiazepine receptors. *Psychopharmacology*, 96, 296–301.

Yadin, E., Thomas, E., Strickland, C.E., and Grishkat, H.L. (1991) Anxiolytic effects of benzodiazepines in amygdala-lesioned rats. *Psychopharmacology*, 103, 473–479.

Zald, D.H. and Pardo, J.V. (1997) Emotion, olfaction, and the human amygdala: amygdala activation during aversive olfactory stimulation. *Proceedings of the National Academy of Sciences of the United States of America*, 94, 4119–4124.

6 The role of the amygdala in conditioned and unconditioned fear and anxiety

Michael Davis

Emory University School of Medicine, Department of Psychiatry, 1639 Pierce Drive, Atlanta, GA 30322, USA

Summary

Evidence from many different laboratories using a variety of experimental techniques and animal species indicates that the amygdala plays a crucial role in conditioned fear, anxiety, and attention. Many amygdaloid projection areas are critically involved in specific signs used to measure fear and anxiety. Electrical stimulation of the amygdala elicits a pattern of behaviours that mimic natural or conditioned fear. Lesions of the amygdala block innate or conditioned fear, as well as various measures of attention, and local infusion of drugs into the amygdala have anxiolytic or anti-stress effects in several behavioural tests. *N*-Methyl-D-aspartate (NMDA) receptors in the amygdala are important in the acquisition of conditioned fear, whereas NMDA or non-NMDA receptors are important for the expression of conditioned fear. The peptide, corticotropin-releasing hormone, appears to be especially important in fear or anxiety and may act within the amygdala, or parts of the extended amygdala, to orchestrate parts of the fear reaction.

6.1 Introduction

Fear is a hypothetical construct that is used to explain the cluster of behavioural effects that are observed and experienced when an organism faces a life-threatening situation. If suddenly confronted by a stranger holding a gun to your face, you will realize instantly that you are in danger, that you could be beaten or even killed. Your hands will sweat, your heart will pound, and your mouth will feel very dry. You will begin to tremble and feel like you cannot catch your breath. You may feel the hair standing up on the back of your neck and your mind will race, trying to decide whether to stand still, to run, or to try to take the gun out of the assailant's hand. Your senses of smell, sight, and hearing will increase and your pupils will dilate. Later, you will remember this terrible incident over and over again, seeing your assailant's face or the gun in apparently vivid detail. Returning to the place where the incident took place will revive those awful memories, often to the point where you will want to avoid that place forever. Thus fear is a complex set of behavioural reactions which include both the expression and the experience of the emotional event. Sweaty palms, increased heart rate, altered respiration, hair standing on end, and dilated pupils are part of the expression of fear. The feelings of dread, of potentially being killed, and whether to stand still or run, as well as the feeling of your heart pounding or the hair standing up on the back of your neck, are part of the experience of fear.

Very similar reactions can be seen in animals. If a cat confronts a vicious dog, the cat will assume the familiar 'halloween posture' with its back arched, hair standing on end, and teeth bared. These expressions of fear can be seen easily and measured objectively. One would also presume, based on our own experience, that the cat is experiencing a feeling of fear, of impending death and threat to survival. However, unlike humans, where it is possible to discuss the experience of fear and how it feels, such a conversation is not possible with the cat. Hence, we can only infer that the cat is feeling fearful from looking at the situation and the set of behaviours displayed by the cat.

Converging evidence now indicates that the amygdala plays a crucial role in the development and expression of conditioned fear, as well as in certain effects caused by stress which involve no obvious prior conditioning. The purpose of this chapter is to summarize data supporting the idea that the amygdala, and its many efferent projections, may represent a central fear system involved in both the expression and acquisition of conditioned and unconditioned fear.

This chapter will review how lesions or electrical stimulation of the amygdala or local infusion of drugs into the amygdala alter several components of fear and/or anxiety. These will include various autonomic and hormonal measures [heart rate, blood pressure, respiration, gastric ulcers, adrenocorticotropin (ACTH) and corticosterone release]. Measures of various motor behaviours (freezing, reflex facilitation, elevated plus-maze, social interaction, bar pressing or licking in the conflict test, high-frequency vocalization), and hypoalgesia also will be covered. It will thus update and extend previous reviews on this topic (Davis, 1992, 1997). Because most of the data have been gathered in rodents, much of the review will focus on rodents, although relevant research in other species will sometimes be included. However, it should be emphasized that it is highly probable that the brain systems that have evolved to produce the autonomic and motor effects indicative of fear, so necessary for survival, have been highly conserved across evolution.

In the interest of space and other chapters in this volume, the extensive literature on inhibitory avoidance (McGaugh *et al.*, Chapter 11); conditioned taste aversion (Lamprecht and Dudai, Chapter 9); kindling (Weiss *et al.*, Chapter 4); and positive reward (Everitt *et al.*, Chapter 10) will not be reviewed. In addition, data on recording cellular activity in the amygdala (see Chapman and Chattarji, Chapter 3; LeDoux, Chapter 7; Rolls, Chapter 13) or data from humans (see Cahill, Chapter 12; Adolphs and Tranel, Chapter 18; Dolan, Chapter 19) or monkeys (see Rolls, Chapter 13; Baxter and Murray, Chapter 16; Easton and Gaffan, Chapter 17) will not be covered. Literature on the role of the amygdala in attention will only be covered partially (see Gallagher, Chapter 8). Also, the prominent role of other brain areas, such as the central grey, in active escape responses during a state of fear (for reviews, see Graeff *et al.*, 1993, 1997; Bandler and Shipley, 1994) will not be reviewed specifically, except where noted. Finally, the very important work of Siegel and colleagues (see Siegel *et al.*, 1997) investigating the role of the amygdala in modulating aggressive behaviour in cats also will not be reviewed.

6.2 Anatomical connections between the central nucleus of the amygdala and brain areas involved in fear and anxiety

The amygdala receives highly processed sensory information primarily through its lateral and basolateral nuclei (Ottersen, 1980; Turner, 1981; VanHoesen, 1981; Amaral, 1987; LeDoux *et al.*, 1990; Burwell *et al.*, 1995; McIntyre *et al.*, 1996; for a highly comprehensive review in rats, monkeys, and cats, see McDonald, 1998). In turn, these nuclei project to the central nucleus of the amygdala (Krettek and Price, 1978b; Nitecka *et al.*, 1981; Ottersen, 1982; Roberts *et al.* 1982; Russchen, 1982; Millhouse and DeOlmos, 1983; Aggleton, 1985; Smith and Millhouse, 1985; Amaral, 1987; Nitecka and Frotscher, 1989; Pare *et al.*, 1995; Pitkänen *et al.*, 1995, 1997; Savander *et al.*, 1995; Shi, 1995), which then projects to hypothalamic and brainstem target areas that directly mediate specific signs of fear and anxiety. A great deal of evidence now indicates that the amygdala, and its many efferent projections, may represent a central fear system involved in both the expression and acquisition of conditioned fear (Gloor, 1960; Kapp *et al.*, 1984, 1990; Sarter and Markowitsch, 1985; Kapp and Pascoe, 1986; LeDoux, 1987; Gray, 1989; Davis, 1997). Figure 6.1 summarizes work done in many different laboratories indicating that the central nucleus of the amygdala has direct projections to a variety of anatomical areas that might be expected to be involved in many of the symptoms of fear or anxiety.

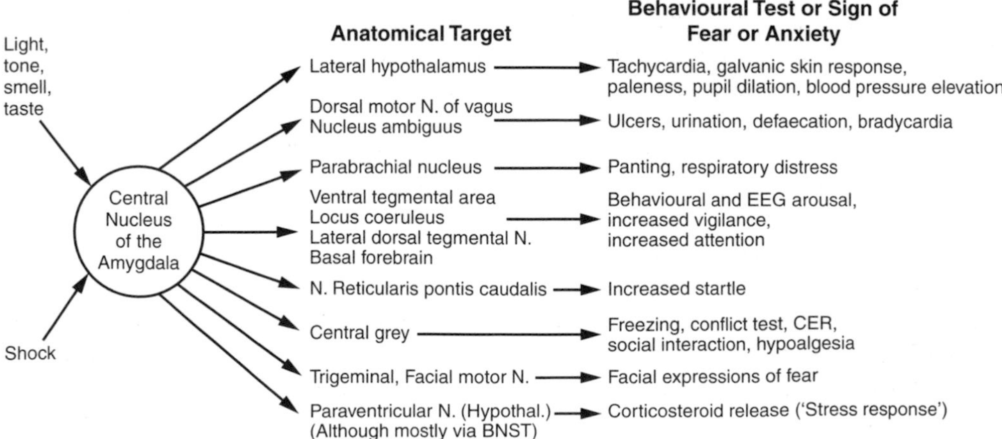

Figure 6.1 Schematic diagram of the anatomical connections of the central nucleus of the amygdala and how they relate to tests of fear or anxiety or the signs of fear and anxiety.

6.2.1 Autonomic and hormonal measures

Direct projections from the central nucleus of the amygdala to the lateral hypothalamus (Krettek and Price, 1978a; Shiosaka *et al.*, 1980; Price and Amaral, 1981) appear to be involved in activation of the sympathetic autonomic nervous system seen during fear and anxiety (LeDoux *et al.*, 1988). Direct projections to the dorsal motor nucleus of the vagus, nucleus of the solitary tract, and ventrolateral medulla (Hopkins and Holstege, 1978; Price and Amaral, 1981; Kawai *et al.*, 1982; Schwaber *et al.*, 1982; Takeuchi *et al.*, 1983; Veening *et al.*, 1984; Gray and Magnusson, 1987; Cassell and Gray, 1989; Takayama *et al.*, 1990), may be involved in amygdala modulation of heart rate and blood pressure which are known to be regulated by these brainstem nuclei. Projections of the central nucleus of the amygdala to the parabrachial nucleus (Hopkins and Holstege, 1978; Krettek and Price, 1978a; Price and Amaral, 1981; Takeuchi *et al.*, 1982; Petrovich and Swanson, 1997) may be involved in respiratory (as well as cardiovascular) changes during fear, because electrical stimulation or lesions of this nucleus alter various measures of respiration.

Although there are some direct projections of the central nucleus of the amygdala to the paraventricular nucleus of the hypothalamus (Silverman *et al.*, 1981; Tribollet and Dreifuss, 1981; Gray *et al.*, 1989; Marcilhac and Siaud, 1996a), they are very sparse (Prewitt and Herman, 1998). However, the central nucleus could affect the paraventricular nucleus via projections to the bed nucleus of the stria terminalis and preoptic area, which receive input from the amygdala (Krettek and Price, 1978a; Weller and Smith, 1982; DeOlmos *et al.*, 1985) and project to the paraventricular nucleus of the hypothalamus (Sawchenko and Swanson, 1983; Swanson *et al.*, 1983; Champagne *et al.*, 1998; Cullinan *et al.*, 1993; Moga and Saper, 1994; Prewitt and Herman, 1998). Either these direct or indirect connections may mediate the prominent neuroendocrine responses to fearful or stressful stimuli.

6.2.2 Attention and vigilance

Projections from the amygdala to the ventral tegmental area (Beckstead *et al.*, 1979; Philipson, 1979; Simon *et al.*, 1979; Wallace *et al.*, 1989, 1992) may mediate stress-induced increases in dopamine metabolites in the prefrontal cortex (Thierry *et al.*, 1976). Direct amygdaloid projections to the dendritic field of the locus coeruleus (Cedarbaum and Aghajanian, 1978; Wallace *et al.*, 1989, 1992; Van Bockstaele *et al.*, 1996, 1998; Veznedaroglu *et al.*, 1996), or indirect projections via the paragigantocellularis nucleus (Aston-Jones *et al.*, 1986), or perhaps via the ventral tegmental area (Deutch *et al.*, 1986), may mediate the response of cells in the locus coeruleus to conditioned fear stimuli (Rasmussen and Jacobs, 1986), as well as being involved in other actions of the locus coeruleus linked to fear and anxiety (Aston-Jones *et al.*, 1996; Redmond, 1977). Direct projections of the amygdala to the lateral dorsal tegmental nucleus (Hopkins and Holstege, 1978) and parabrachial nuclei (see above), which have cholinergic neurons that project to the thalamus (Pare *et al.*, 1990), may mediate increases in synaptic transmission in thalamic sensory relay neurons (Pare *et al.*, 1990; Steriade *et al.*, 1990) during states of fear. This cholinergic activation, along with increases in thalamic transmission accompanying activation of the locus coeruleus (Rogawski and Aghajanian, 1980), may thus lead to increased vigilance and superior signal detection in a state of fear or anxiety.

As emphasized by Kapp *et al.* (1992), in addition to its direct connections to the hypothalamus and brainstem, the central nucleus of the amygdala also has the potential for indirect widespread effects on the cortex via its projections to cholinergic neurons located within the sublenticular substantia innominata (Price and Amaral, 1981; Russchen *et al.*, 1985; Grove, 1988), which in turn project to the cortex. In fact, the rapid development of conditioned bradycardia during Pavlovian aversive conditioning, critically dependent on the amygdala, may simply not be a marker of an emotional state of fear, but instead a more general process reflecting an increase in attention. In the rabbit, low-voltage, fast electroencephalogram (EEG) activity, generally considered a state of cortical readiness for processing sensory information (Steriade *et al.*, 1990), is acquired during Pavlovian aversive conditioning at the same rate as conditioned bradycardia (Yehle *et al.*, 1967).

Motor behaviour

Release of noradrenaline (norepinephrine) onto motor neurons via amygdala activation of the locus coeruleus, or via amygdaloid projections to serotonin-containing raphe neurons (Magnuson and Gray, 1990), could lead to enhanced motor performance during a state of fear, because both noradrenaline and serotonin (5-HT) facilitate excitation of motor neurons (McCall and Aghajanian, 1979; White and Neuman, 1980).

Direct projections of the central nucleus of the amygdala to the nucleus reticularis pontis caudalis (Inagaki *et al.*, 1983; Rosen *et al.*, 1991; Koch and Ebert, 1993) as well as indirect projections to this nucleus via the central grey probably are involved in fear potentiation of the startle reflex (Hitchcock and Davis, 1991; Fendt *et al.*, 1994a; Yeomans and Franklin, 1994). Direct projections to the lateral tegmental field, including parts of the trigeminal and facial motor nuclei (Holstege *et al.*, 1977; Hopkins and Holstege, 1978; Post and Mai, 1980; Ruggiero *et al.*, 1982; Whalen and Kapp, 1991), may mediate some of the facial expressions of fear as well as potentiation of the eyeblink reflex (Whalen and Kapp, 1991; Canli and Brown, 1996).

The amygdala also projects to regions of the central grey (Gloor, 1978; Hopkins and Holstege, 1978; Krettek and Price, 1978a; Post and Mai, 1980; Beitz, 1982) that appear to be a critical part of a general defence system (Adams, 1979; Blanchard *et al.*, 1981; Bandler and Carrive, 1988; Bandler and Depaulis, 1988; Graeff, 1988; LeDoux *et al.*, 1988; Zhang *et al.*, 1990; Fanselow, 1991) and that have been implicated in conditioned fear in a number of behavioural tests including freezing (Liebman *et al.*, 1970; Hammer and Kapp, 1986; LeDoux *et al.*, 1988; Borszcz *et al.*, 1989; Fanselow, 1991; J.J.Kim *et al.*, 1993), sonic and ultrasonic vocalization (Yajima *et al.*, 1980, 1982; Zhang *et al.*, 1994; Borszcz, 1995; Borszcz *et al.*, 1996), and stress-induced hypoalgesia (Liebman *et al.*, 1970; Watkins and Mayer, 1982; Fanselow, 1986; Fanselow and Helmstetter, 1988; Helmstetter and Tershner, 1994; Harris, 1996; Pavlovic *et al.*, 1996b; Helmstetter *et al.*, 1998; Pavlovic and Bodnar, 1998).

6.3 Elicitation of fear responses by electrical or chemical stimulation of the amygdala

Electrical stimulation or abnormal electrical activation of the amygdala (i.e. via temporal lobe seizures) can produce a complex pattern of behavioural and autonomic changes that, taken together, highly resembles a state of fear.

6.3.1 Autonomic and hormonal measures

As outlined by Gloor (1992) 'The most common affect produced by temporal lobe epileptic discharge is fear. ... It arises 'out of the blue.' Ictal fear may range from mild anxiety to intense terror. It is frequently, but not invariably, associated with a rising epigastric sensation, palpitation, mydriasis, and pallor and may be associated with a fearful hallucination, a frightful memory flashback, or both' (p. 513). In humans, electrical stimulation of the amygdala elicits feelings of fear or anxiety as well as autonomic reactions indicative of fear (Chapman *et al.*, 1954; Gloor *et al.*, 1981). While other emotional reactions occasionally are produced, the major reaction is one of fear or apprehension.

Electrical stimulation of the central nucleus of the amygdala or chemical activation via the cholinergic agonist carbachol or the neurotransmitter glutamate produces prominent cardiovascular effects that depend on the species, site of stimulation, and state of the animal (Table 6.1). In rabbits, electrical stimulation of the central nucleus causes bradycardia, whereas in cats it produces tachycardia and increases in blood pressure. In rats, electrical or chemical stimulation of the central nucleus generally increases blood pressure and heart rate in unanaesthetized animals (but see Healy and Peck, 1997) and has the opposite effect in anaesthetized or paralysed rats. However, the exact site of chemical stimulation may be important. For example, in unanaesthetized rats, infusion of carbachol into the amygdaloid complex elicited a pressor response along with immobilization, body shaking, searching, and rearing (Ohta *et al.*, 1991; Aslan *et al.*, 1997a,b). Infusion of noradrenalinine or 5-HT had no effect. The largest pressor effect of carbachol was found after infusion into the central nucleus of the amygdala. Bradycardia was produced by infusion into the 'dorsocentral' part of the amygdala, whereas tachycardia was produced by infusion into the 'medioventral' parts of the amygdala. The pressor effects of either electrical stimulation or local infusion of carbachol into the central nucleus can be blocked by electrolytic lesions of the anteroventral third ventricle region (Tellioglu *et al.*, 1997). Electrical stimulation of the central nucleus of the amygdala also increases c-*fos* in neurons in the ventrolateral medulla which project to the nucleus of the solitary tract and in cells in the nucleus of the solitary tract which project to the ventrolateral medulla (Petrov *et al.*, 1996).

Using very small infusion cannulae, Sanders and Shekhar (1991) found increases in blood pressure and heart rate when the γ-aminobutyric acid A ($GABA_A$) antagonist bicuculline was infused into the basolateral but not the central nucleus. Equimolar concentrations of the $GABA_B$ agonist baclofen, the $GABA_B$ antagonist phaclofen, or the glycine antagonist strychnine did not have these cardiovascular effects when infused into either nucleus. Importantly, the pressor effects of blocking $GABA_A$ receptors in the amygdala were associated with

Table 6.1 Effects of electrical or chemical stimulation of the amygdala on autonomic and hormonal measures of fear and anxiety

Method	*S*	*Site*	*Effect of stimulation*	*Reference*
Elect (an)	Rb	Ce	Decrease in heart rate	Kapp *et al.* (1982); Pascoe *et al.* (1989)
Elect (an)	Rb	Ce	Decrease in heart rate, blood pressure and hindlimb vasodilatation	Cox *et al.* (1986, 1987)
Elect (un)	Rb	Ce	Decrease in heart rate	Kapp *et al.* (1990)
Elect (un)	C	Ce	Increase in blood pressure and heart rate	Heinemann *et al.* (1973); Hilton and Zbrozyna (1963)
Elect or Homo-cystate (an)	R	Ce	Decrease in blood pressure, variable heart rate effects. No effects of chemical stimulation in unanaesthetized animals	Gelsema *et al.* (1987, 1989)
Elect (an)	R	Ce	Decrease in blood pressure and heart rate	Galeno and Brody (1983); Iwata *et al.* (1987); Morgenson and Calaresu (1973)
Glutamate (an)	R	Ce	Decrease in blood pressure, heart rate. Effects reduced by infusion of GABA	Ciriello and Roder (1998)
Glutamate (an)	R	Ce	Decrease in blood pressure, heart rate, attenuated by co-infusion of NA	Roder *et al.* (1999)
Elect (un)	C	Ce	Increase in blood pressure, effect reduced in sleep	Frysinger *et al.* (1984)
Elect (un)	C	Ce	Increase in blood pressure and heart rate	Stock *et al.* (1978)
Elect or G (un)	R	Ce	Increase in blood pressure and heart rate	Galeno and Brody (1983); Iwata *et al.* (1987)
Elect or Carb (un)	R	Ce	Increase in blood pressure, blocked by cholinergic antagonists into amygdala	Aslan *et al.* (1997a,b)
Carb (un)	R	Ce	Increased blood pressure, immobilization, body shaking, searching, and rearing	Ohta *et al.* (1991)
Carb (un)	R	AC	Decrease or increase in heart rate depending on site	Ohta *et al.* (1991)
Elect or Carb (un)	R	Ce	Increase in blood pressure, blocked by lesions of the anteroventral third ventricle region	Tellioglu *et al.* (1997)
Elect (un)	R	Ce	Decrease in heart rate. Equivalent via stimulation of left or right Ce	Healy and Peck (1997)
Homocystate (an)	R	Bla only	Vasodilation in the hindlimb muscle, renal vasoconstriction and tachycardia	al Maskati and Zbrozyna (1989)
Bic (un)	R	Bla Ce	Increases in blood pressure heart rate and not locomotor activity. Bigger effect with repeated infusions	Sanders and Shekhar (1991, 1995b)
Bic (un)	R	Bla	Increases in blood pressure, heart rate. Blocked by infusion of either NMDA or non-NMDA antagonists into the amygdala)	Sajdyk and Shekhar (1997a

Table 6.1 continued

Method	*S*	*Site*	*Effect of stimulation*	*Reference*
Bic, NMDA, AMPA (un)	R	Bla	Increases in blood pressure, heart rate blocked by either NMDA or non-NMDA antagonists infused into Bla or the dorsomedial hypothalamus	Soltis *et al.* (1997, 1998)
Elect	C	AC	Increase in plasma corticosterone	Setekleiv *et al.* (1961)
Elect (un)	M	AC	Increase in plasma corticosterone	Mason (1959)
Elect (an)	R	Me	Increase in plasma corticosterone	Feldman *et al.* (1982)
Elect (an)	R	AC	Increase in plasma corticosterone	Dunn and Whitener (1986)
Elect (an)	R	Ce, Bla,L	Decrease in plasma corticosterone	Dunn and Whitener (1986)
Elect (un)	C	CM	Increase in plasma corticosterone	Matheson *et al.* (1971)
Elect (an)	R	CM	Increase in plasma corticosterone	Redgate and Fahringer (1973)
Elect (an)	R	Me	Increase in plasma corticosterone. Blocked by lesions of stria terminalis	Feldman *et al.* (1990)
Elect (an)	R	Ce	Increase in plasma corticosterone, ACTH. Blocked by systemic dexamethasone	Weidenfeld *et al.* (1997)
Elect (an)	R	Ce	Increase in c-*fos* in the supraoptic, paraventricular and arcuate nuclei of the hypothalamus	Petrov *et al.* (1994)
Elect (an)	R	Ce	Depletion of CRH in hypothalamus, increase in ACTH and corticosterone. Inhibited by depletion of catecholamines, 5-HT, prazosin, or ketanserin but not atenolol	Feldman and Weidenfeld (1998)
Glutamate (un or an)	R	VM	Increase in plasma corticosterone only in previously stressed rats	Gabr *et al.* (1995)
Elect	C	AM	Gastric ulcers	Sen and Anand (1957)
Elect (un)	R	Me	Increased gastric acid production, blocked by vagotomy	Kim *et al.* (1990)
Elect (un or an)	R	Ce	Gastric ulcers	Henke (1980b, 1988); Innes and Tansy (1980)
Elect	R	AC	Change in respiration	Anand and Dua (1956)
Elect (un)	Rb	Ce	Change in respiration	Applegate *et al.* (1983)
Elect (un)	C	Ce	Change in respiration	Harper *et al.* (1984)
Elect (st)	C	AC	Change in respiration, increase or decrease depending on site of stimulation	Bonvallet and GaryBobo (1972, 1975); GaryBobo and Bonvallet (1975)
Elect or Glutamate (an)	C	Ce	Hypoalgesia to tooth pulp stimulation measured by change in jaw muscles	Kowada *et al.* (1991, 1992)
Elect (un)	R	Ce, Bla, Me	Hypoalgesia in tail flick and formalin tests. Also decreased vocalization in tail flick test	Mena *et al.* (1995)

Table 6.1 continued

Method	*S*	*Site*	*Effect of stimulation*	*Reference*
Elect (un)	R	Ce, Me	Hypoalgesia in tail flick to heat. Blocked by systemic naloxone, methysergide, atropine,phenoxybenzamine, propranolol.	Oliveira and Prado (1998)
Elect (an)	C	Bla	Increased sweating (galvanic skin response)	Lang *et al.* (1964)

Abbreviations: AC, amygdala complex; α-CRH, α-helical corticotropin-releasing hormone; AM, 'anterior medial amygdala'; An, anaesthetized; B, bird; Bic, bicuculline; Bla, basolateral complex; C, cat; Car, carbachol; Ce, central nucleus; CM, corticomedial nucleus; CRH, corticotropin-releasing hormone; H, human; L, lateral; M, monkey; Me, medial nucleus; MG, medial geniculate; Mus, muscimol; NA, noradrenaline; PM, posteriormedial; Post, post-training; Pre, pre-training; R, rat; Rb, rabbit; S, species; St, spirally transected; TRH, thyrotropin-releasing hormone; Un, unanaesthetized; VM, 'ventromedial amygdala'.

increases in locomotor activity rather than immobilization. We have found very similar motor effects in our own laboratory (Lee and Davis, unpublished). Local infusion of NMDA or α-amino-3-hydroxy-5-methyl-4-isoxazole proprionic acid (AMPA) into the basolateral nucleus also increased blood pressure and heart rate (Soltis *et al.*, 1997). These effects, as well as those of bicuculline, could be blocked by local infusion of either NMDA or non-NMDA antagonists into the amygdala (Sajdyk and Shekhar, 1997a; Soltis *et al.*, 1997) or the dorsomedial hypothalamus (Soltis *et al.*, 1998).

Repeated infusion of initially subthreshold doses of bicuculline into the anterior basolateral nucleus led to a 'priming' effect in which increases in heart rate and blood pressure were observed after 3–5 infusions (Sanders and Shekhar, 1995b). This change in threshold lasted at least 6 weeks and could not be ascribed to mechanical damage or generalized seizure activity based on EEG measurements. It is possible, therefore, that long-term stress or prior trauma could lead to similar priming effects that would make the amygdala, or structures to which it connects, more reactive to subsequent stressors, thereby leading to certain types of psychiatric disorders. Alternatively, genetic differences in GABA tone in the amygdala could render individuals hyper-responsive to stress or anxiety [see excellent recent reviews by Adamec (1997) and Rosen and Schulkin (1998) for more on this idea].

In general, electrical stimulation of the amygdala causes an increase in plasma levels of corticosterone (Table 6.1). This seems to occur after stimulation of the medial or corticomedial nucleus and not the central nucleus (e.g. Dunn and Whitener, 1986), although electrical stimulation of the central nucleus has been shown to increase c-*fos* in the supraoptic, paraventricular, and arcuate nuclei of the hypothalamus (Petrov *et al.*, 1994), as well as plasma levels of corticosterone and ACTH (Feldman and Weidenfeld, 1998). The effect of electrical stimulation appears to depend on both noradrenaline and 5-HT in the paraventricular nucleus. Depletion of these transmitters via local infusions of 6-hydroxydopamine (6-OHDA) or 5,7-dihydroxytryptamine (5,7-DHT), or local infusion of the noradrenaline or 5-HT antagonists prazosin or ketanserin, in the paraventricular nucleus attenuated the effects of electrical stimulation (Feldman and Weidenfeld, 1998). In rats previously given chronic stress, or rats anaesthetized with urethane, infusion of glutamate into the amygdala resulted in increased plasma corticosterone as well as a release of corticotropin-releasing hormone (CRH) in the median eminence measured by *in vivo* microdialysis (Gabr *et al.*, 1995). In contrast, infusion of glutamate in non-stressed rats did not increase plasma corticosterone (Gabr *et al.*, 1995).

Amygdala stimulation can also produce gastric ulceration and increase gastric acid (Table 6.1), which can be associated with chronic fear or anxiety. It can also alter respiration (Table 6.1) a prominent symptom of fear, especially in panic disorder. Either increases or decreases in respiration can be seen, depending on the exact site of stimulation (Bonvallet and GaryBobo, 1972, 1975; GaryBobo and Bonvallet, 1975).

A small number of studies have shown that electrical stimulation of the amygdala also can produce hypoalgesia (Kowada *et al.*, 1991, 1992; Mena *et al.*, 1995; Oliveira and Prado, 1998) some of which can be attenuated by systemic naloxone, methysergide, atropine, phenoxybenzamine, or propranolol (Oliveira and Prado, 1998). In addition, electrical stimulation of the amygdala in cats produced an increase in sweating (galvanic skin response; Lang *et al.*, 1964), a prominent symptom of fear in humans.

6.3.2 Attention and vigilance

Studies in several species indicate that electrical stimulation of the central nucleus increases attention or processes associated with increased attention (Table 6.2). For example, stimulation of sites in the central nucleus that produce bradycardia (Kapp *et al.*, 1990) also produce low-voltage fast EEG activity in both rabbits (Kapp *et al.*, 1994) and rats (Dringenberg and Vanderwolf, 1996), which can be blocked by systemic administration of cholinergic antagonists (Kapp *et al.*, 1994; Dringenberg and Vanderwolf, 1996). In the cat, electrical stimulation of the dorsal amygdala, including some sites in the central nucleus, elicited EEG desynchronization which was not blocked by complete midbrain transection (Kreindler and Steriade, 1964), suggesting that it involved rostral projections from the amygdala to the basal forebrain. In fact, EEG desynchronization could be blocked by local infusion of lidocaine into the substantia innominata–ventral pallidum of the basal forebrain ipsilateral, but not contralateral, to the site of stimulation (Dringenberg and Vanderwolf, 1996). In addition, electrical stimulation of the central nucleus elicits pupillary dilation and pinna orientation (Ursin and Kaada, 1960; Applegate *et al.*, 1983), both of which would be associated with an increase in sensory processing. In fact, an attention or orienting reflex was the most common response elicited by electrical stimulation of the amygdala (Ursin and Kaada, 1960; Applegate *et al.*, 1983). These and other observations have led Kapp *et al.* (1992) to hypothesize that the central nucleus and its associated structures function, at least in part, in the acquisition of an increased state of nonspecific attention or arousal manifested in a variety of CRs which function to enhance sensory processing. This mechanism is rapidly acquired, perhaps via an inherent plasticity within the nucleus and associated structures in situations of uncertainty but of potential import; for example, when a neutral stimulus (CS) precedes either a positive or negative reinforcing, unexpected event (US)' (p. 241). Electrical stimulation of the amygdala can also activate cholinergic cells that are involved in arousal-like effects depending on the state of sleep and perhaps the species (Table 6.2).

Table 6.2 Effects of electrical stimulation of the amygdala on measures related to attention

Method	*S*	*Site*	*Effect of stimulation*	*Reference*
Elect (An or Un)	Rb	Ce	EEG arousal, blocked by cholinergic antagonists	Kapp *et al.* (1994)
Elect (An)	R	Ce	EEG arousal, blocked by cholinergic antagonists	Dringenberg and Vanderwolf (1996)
Elect (An)	C	Ce	EEG arousal, not blocked by midbrain transection but blocked by local infusion of lidocaine into the substantia innominata–ventral pallidum	Kreindler and Steriade (1964)
Elect (Un)	C	Ce	Pupillary dilation and pinna orientation	Ursin and Kaada (1960)
Elect (Un)	Rb	Ce	Pupillary dilation and pinna orientation	Applegate *et al.* (1983)
Elect (Un)	Rb	Ce	Activation of cholinergic pontogeniculo-occipital (PGO) wave generator neurons, probably indicative of increased arousal	Silvestri and Kapp (1998)
Elect (Un)	R	Ce	Increased PGO wave amplitude during REM sleep, decreased PGO wave frequency during non-REM sleep.	Deboer *et al.* (1998)

Abbreviations: see Table 6.1.

6.3.3 Motor behaviour

Table 6.3 shows that electrical or chemical stimulation of the central nucleus of the amygdala produces a cessation of ongoing behaviour, a critical component in several animal models such as freezing, the operant conflict test, the conditioned emotional response, and the social interaction test. Electrical stimulation of the amygdala also elicits jaw movements and activation of facial motor neurons, which probably mediate some of the facial expressions seen during the fear reaction. These motor effects may be indicative of a more general effect of amygdala stimulation, namely that of modulating brainstem reflexes such as the massenteric, baroreceptor nictitating membrane, eyeblink, and the startle reflex.

Viewed in this way, the pattern of behaviours seen during fear may result from activation of a single area of the brain (the amygdala), which then projects to a variety of target areas which themselves are critical for each of the specific symptoms of fear (the expression of fear), as well as the experience of fear. Moreover, it must be assumed that all of these connections are already formed in an adult organism, because electrical stimulation produces these effects in the absence of prior explicit fear conditioning. Thus, much of the complex behavioural pattern seen during a state of 'conditioned fear' has already been 'hard wired' during evolution.

In order for a formerly neutral stimulus to produce the constellation of behavioural effects used to define a state of fear or anxiety, it is only necessary for that stimulus to now activate the amygdala, which in turn will produce the complex pattern of behavioural changes by virtue of its innate connections to different brain target sites. Viewed in this way, plasticity during fear conditioning probably results from a change in synaptic inputs prior to or in the

Table 6.3 Effects of chemical or electrical stimulation of the amygdala on various motor behaviours used to measure fear or anxiety

Method	*S*	*Site*	*Effect of stimulation*	*Reference*
Elect (un)	Rb	Ce	Immobility, jaw movements	Applegate *et al.* (1983)
Elect (un)	C	Ce	Immobility, jaw movements	Kaada (1951); Ursin and Kaada (1960)
Elect (An)	R	Ce	Elicitation of jaw movements	Kaku (1984); Ohta (1984)
Carbachol	R	Ce	Immobility	Ohta *et al.* (1991)
Vasopressin	R	Ce	Immobility, seizures second infusion	Willcox *et al.* (1992)
Vasopressin	R	Ce	Immobility in rats bred for low rates of avoidance but not those bred for high avoidance rates	Roozendaal *et al.* (1992b)
Elect (An)	C	Ce	Activation of facial motoneurons	Fanardjian and Manvelyan (1987)
Elect (spinal transected)	C	AC	Facilitation and inhibition of massenteric reflex, depending on site	GaryBobo and Bonvallet (1975); Bonvallet and GaryBobo (1975)
Elect (un)	C	Ce	Modulation of baroreceptor reflex	Schlor *et al.* (1984)
Elect (an)	Rb	Ce	Facilitation of baroreceptor reflex	Pascoe *et al.* (1989)
Elect (un)	Rb	Ce	Facilitation of nictitating membrane	Whalen and Kapp (1991)
Elect (un)	R	Ce	Facilitation of the eyeblink reflex	Canli and Brown (1996)
Elect (un)	R	Ce	Facilitation of the startle reflex	Rosen and Davis (1988a,b)
Elect (un)	R	Ce	Facilitation of the startle-like responses elicited by stimulation of brainstem sites	Rosen and Davis (1990); Yeomans and Pollard (1993)
Elect (un)	R	Ce	Facilitation of tone-evoked activation of cells in the startle pathway	Koch and Ebert (1993)

Abbreviations: see Table 6.1.

amygdala (Quirk *et al.*, 1995; McKernan and Shinnick-Gallagher, 1997; Rogan *et al.*, 1997), rather than from a change in its efferent target areas. The ability to produce long-term potentiation (LTP) in the amygdala (Chapman *et al.*, 1990; Clugnet and LeDoux, 1990; Chapman and Bellavance, 1992; Gean *et al.*, 1993; Shindou *et al.*, 1993; Huang and Kandel, 1998) that can lead to an increase in responsiveness to a physiological stimulus (Rogan and LeDoux, 1995) and the finding that local infusion of NMDA antagonists into the amygdala blocks the acquisition of fear conditioning (see Table 6.13) are consistent with this hypothesis.

6.4 Effects of amygdala lesions on conditioned fear

6.4.1 Autonomic and hormonal measures (conditioned)

Patients with unilateral (LeBar *et al.*, 1995) or bilateral (Bechara *et al.*, 1995) lesions of the amygdala have been reported to have deficits in classical fear conditioning using the galvanic skin response as a measure. A large number of studies show that lesions of the amygdala, primarily the central nucleus, block the normal cardiovascular changes that develop during classical fear conditioning (Table 6.4). For example, in rabbits, a cue paired with shock leads to bradycardia that can be blocked by either chemical or mechanical lesions of the central nucleus (Kapp *et al.*, 1979; Gentile *et al.*, 1986; McCabe *et al.*, 1992; Powell *et al.*, 1997). A unilateral lesion of either the central or basolateral nucleus combined with a unilateral lesion of the contralateral prefrontal cortex causes a partial blockade, but not as great as a bilateral lesion of either the central or basolateral nucleus. Hence, the amygdala and prefrontal cortex do not act in a strictly serial fashion in these tests. Lesions of the central nucleus in rabbits also reduce tone-evoked arrhythmias following tone–shock pairings (Markgraf and Kapp, 1991). In birds, lesions of the archistriatum, believed to be homologous to the mammalian amygdala, block heart rate acceleration in response to a cue paired with a shock (Cohen, 1975). Ibotenic acid (Iwata *et al.*, 1986) or electrolytic (Sananes and Campbell, 1989) lesions of the central nucleus, or localized cooling (Zhang *et al.*, 1986) or electrolytic lesions of the lateral amygdala nucleus (LeDoux, 1990; Romanski *et al.*, 1993) also block conditioned changes in blood pressure during classical fear conditioning. Pre- or post-training electrolytic lesions of the central or basolateral nuclei alter cardiovascular and hormonal responses to a context pair with shock (Roozendaal *et al.*, 1990, a,b). Neurotoxic lesions of the central and basolateral nuclei also block conditioned increases in corticosterone release (Goldstein *et al.*, 1996). Lesions of the amygdala reduce stress-induced increases in dopamine release in the frontal cortex following mild footshock or exposure to a novel environment (Davis *et al.*, 1994) or exposure to a cue previously paired with footshock (Goldstein *et al.*, 1996).

6.4.2 Motor behaviour

Table 6.5 shows that electrolytic or chemical lesions of the central, lateral, or basolateral nuclei of the amygdala eliminate or attenuate conditioned freezing normally seen in response to a cue or context paired with shock, a dominant male rat, or during a continuous passive avoidance task. This occurs with either pre- or post-training lesions, indicating that the lesions have an effect on the expression of conditioned freezing. Chemical lesions of the basolateral nucleus produce similar effects, even when given 15 (Cousens and Otto, 1998) or 30 days after training (Maren *et al.*, 1996a), or after extensive overtraining (Maren, 1998). However, lesioned rats could partially re-acquire conditioned freezing (Maren, 1998), which was used to argue that the effects of lesions of the basolateral nucleus do not result simply from increases in locomotor activity (e.g. Vazdarjanova and McGaugh, 1998). Moreover, relearning was not influenced by the number of pre-lesion training trials as suggested by earlier studies using the startle reflex (Sananes and Davis, 1992; Kim and Davis, 1993a). Inactivation of the amygdala by direct infusion of lidocaine (Helmstetter, 1992b) or muscimol (Helmstetter and Bellgowan, 1994; Muller *et al.*, 1997) prior to testing reduced conditioned freezing. The studies by Helmstter's group found only a partial attenuation when the same doses were infused prior to training, whereas a full blockade was seen by Muller *et al.* (1997). Infusion immediately after training had no effect, suggesting that muscimol was not affecting consolidation (Muller *et al.*, 1997).

Table 6.4 Effects of lesions of the amygdala on autonomic or hormonal measures of conditioned fear or anxiety

Method	*S*	*Site*	*Effect of lesion*	*Reference*
Aspiration (Pre)	H	AC	Decreased galvanic skin response during classical fear conditioning—unilateral lesions	LeBar *et al.* (1995)
Aspiration (Pre)	H	AC	Decreased galvanic skin response during classical fear conditioning	Bechara *et al.* (1995)
Radio (Pre)	Rb	Ce	Decreased bradycardia to cue paired with shock	Gentile *et al.* (1986)
Electrolytic	Rb	Ce	Decreased bradycardia to cue paired with shock	Kapp *et al.* (1979)
Ibotenic acid (Pre)	Rb	Ce	Decreased bradycardia to cue paired with shock	McCabe *et al.* (1992)
Electrolytic (Pre)	Rb	Ce	Decreased bradycardia to cue paired with shock, bilateral bigger effect than unilateral or unilateral plus contralateral medial prefrontal	Chachich and Powell (1998); Powell *et al.* (1997)
Ibotenic acid (Pre)	Rb	Bla	Decreased bradycardia to cue paired with shock, bilateral bigger effect than unilateral or unilateral plus contralateral medial prefrontal	Powell *et al.* (1997)
Electrolytic (Post)	Rb	Ce	Decreased tone-evoked arrhythmias during digitalis administration. Tone previously paired with shock	Markgraf and Kapp (1991)
Electrolytic (Pre)	B	*	Decreased tachycardia during classical conditioning	Cohen (1975)
Cooling (Pre-testing)	Cat	Ce	Decreased bradycardia, respiratory increases and blood pressure changes to cue paired with shock	Zhang *et al.* (1986)
Electrolytic (Pre)	R	Ce	Decreased blood pressure rise to cue paired with shock	LeDoux *et al.* (1986)
Electrolytic (Pre or Post)	R	Ce or Bla	Decreased bradycardia or increased NA, prolactin,or corticosterone to context paired with shock	Roozendaal *et al.* (1990, 1991a,b); Van de Kar *et al.* (1991)
Ibotenic acid Electrolytic (MG)	R	Ce MG	Decreased blood pressure rise to cue paired with shock (Ce, unilateral, MG, contralateral)	Iwata *et al.* (1986)
Electrolytic Pre)	R	L	Decreased blood pressure rise during classical conditioning	LeDoux *et al.* (1990); Romanski *et al.*(1993)
Electrolytic (Pre training)	R pups	Ce	Decreased tachycardia to cue paired with shock	Sananes and Campbell (1989)
NMDA (Pre or Post-	R	C	Decreased secretion of corticosterone and defecation to cue paired with shock	Goldstein *et al.* (1996)
Electrolytic (Post)	R	Ce	Decreased increase in dopamine metabolites in prefrontal cortex following fear conditioning or novel stress	Davis *et al.* (1994)
NMDA (Pre- or post-	R	Bla	Decreased increase in dopamine, 5-HT, or noradrenaline metabolites in prefrontal cortex to cue paired with shock	Goldstein *et al.* (1996)

*Archistriatum, believed to be the homologue of the amygdala.
Abbreviations: see Table 6.1.

Table 6.5 Effects of lesions or chemical inactivation of the amygdala on conditioned motor behaviours used to assess fear and anxiety

Method	*S*	*Site*	*Effect of inactivation*	*Reference*
Electrolytic (Pre)	Rat	Ce	Decreased freezing to cue paired with shock	LeDoux *et al.* (1986)
Electrolytic (Pre)	R	Ce or Bla	Decreased freezing to context paired with shock	Helmstetter (1992a)
Ibotenic acid (Pre)	R	Ce and Bla	Decreased freezing to context paired with shock	Helmstetter (1992a)
Electrolytic (Post)	R	Ce	Decreased freezing to context paired with shock	McNish *et al.* (1997)
Electrolytic (Pre)	R	L	Decreased freezing to cue paired with shock	LeDoux *et al.* (1990)
Electrolytic (Pre)	R	L, Bla, and Ce	Decreased freezing to context or cue paired with shock	Phillips and LeDoux (1992)
Electrolytic (Pre)	R	Ce, L, Bla	Decreased freezing to context paired with shock tested immediately or 24 h after shock	Kim *et al.* (1993a)
Electrolytic (Post)	R	Ce	Non-significant decrease in freezing to context paired with shock	Roozendaal *et al.* (1990)
Radiofrequency	R	AC	Decreased freezing to cues paired with shock.	Blanchard and
(Pre)			Decreased shock probe avoidance	Blanchard (1972)
Electrolytic (Pre or Post)	R	Ce	Decreased freezing to shock probe, no effect on shock probe burying	Roozendaal *et al.* (1991b)
Electrolytic (Pre or Post)	R	Ce	Decreased freezing to context paired with shock	Roozendaal *et al.* (1991a)
Ibotenic acid (amygdala)	R	Ce,	Decreased freezing to cue paired with shock	Iwata *et al.* (1986)
M (medial geniculate) (Pre)	MG		(Ce, unilateral; MG, contralateral). Some damage to L and Bla	
Ibotenic acid	R	Bla	Decreased freezing during avoidance training	Lorenzini *et al.* (1991)
Electrolytic (Pre)	R	L, Bla, Ce	Decreased freezing to cue or context paired with loud noise or shock. Partial effect with unilateral lesion	LeBar and LeDoux (1996)
NMDA (Pre or Post)	R	Bla	Decreased acquisition of freezing to odour or context, or expression of both when lesions made 1 or 15 days after conditioning	Cousens and Otto (1998)
NMDA (Pre)	R	Bla	Decreased freezing to part of Y-maze where shocked. Still showed partial avoidance to this part of maze	Vazdarjanova and McGaugh (1998)

Table 6.5 continued

Method	*S*	*Site*	*Effect of inactivation*	*Reference*
NMDA (Pre and Post)	R	Bla	Decreased acquisition or expression of freezing to context or cue paired with shock even when lesions made 1 month after training	Maren *et al.* (1996a)
NMDA (Pre or Post)	R	Bla	Decreased acquisition or expression of freezing to context paired with shock even after extensive overtraining. Lesioned rats could only partially reacquire and this did not interact with level of training	Maren (1998)
Lidocaine (Pre or pre-testing, or both)	R	Ce and Bla	Decreased expression of freezing to context paired with shock. Weaker effect when inactivation given before training	Helmstetter (1992b)
Muscimol (Pre or pre-testing, or both)	R	Bla	Decreased expression of freezing to context paired with shock. Weaker effect when inactivation given before training	Helmstetter and Bellgowan (1994)
Muscimol (Pre or Post)	R	Bla	Decreased freezing when given either before testing or training but not immediately after training	Muller *et al.* (1997
NMDA (Pre or Post)	R	Bla	Decreased freezing or high-frequency vocalizations to shock or cues paired with shock	Goldstein *et al.* (1996)
Electrolytic (Pre or post defeat)	R	CM	Decreased freezing to dominant male rat following defeat, bigger effect post-lesion	Bolhuis *et al.* (1984)
Electrolytic (Pre)	R	Bla or CM	Anti-conflict effect	Poplawsky and McVeigh (1981)
Electrolytic (Pre)	Mice	AC	Anti-conflict effect and less freezing	Slotnick (1973)
Ibotenic acid (Pre)	R	Ce not Bla	Anti-conflict (licking), decreased effects of restraint stress on plus maze	Moller *et al.* (1997)
Electrolytic (Pre)	R	Ce not Bla	Anti-conflict effect	Shibata *et al.* (1986, 1989)
Electrolytic (Pre)	R	Ce or AC	Anti-conflict effect (licking) but systemic benzodiazepines still had anti-conflict effect, maybe even bigger	Kopchia *et al.* (1992); Yadin *et al.* (1991)
Quinolinic acid or 6-OHDA (Pre)	R	Bla	Decreased reduction in licking during conditioned emotional response test	Selden *et al.* (1991)
Electrolytic (Post)	Mice	AC	Decreased reduction in bar pressing during conditioned emotional response paradigm	Desmedt *et al.* (1998)
Electrolytic (Pre)	R	AC	Decreased reduction in bar-pressing during conditioned emotional response paradigm	Kellicut and Schwartzbaum (1963); Spevack *et al.* (1975)

Table 6.5 continued

Method	*S*	*Site*	*Effect of inactivation*	*Reference*
Electrolytic (Pre)	B	*	Decreased reduction in bar pressing during conditioned emotional response test	Dafters (1976)
Electrolytic (Pre)	R	Bla	Decreased avoidance of electrified water spout	Grossman *et al.* (1975); Pellegrino (1968)
NMDA (Pre)	R	AC	Decreased avoidance of water spout paired with shock but not with quinine	Cahill and McGaugh (1990)
Electrolytic (Pre)	R	Ce, Bla	Decreased avoidance of water spout paired with shock	Coover *et al.* (1992); Oakes and Coover (1997)
Electrolytic (Pre)	R	Me	Decreased avoidance of a dominant male rat conditioned by defeat	Luiten *et al.* (1985)
Ibotenic acid (Pre)	R	Ce, not Bla	Decreased disruption of bar pressing to cue paired with shock. Could still avoid shock bar.	Killcross *et al.* (1997)
Quinolinic acid (Pre)	R	Bla not Ce	Decreased avoidance of shocked bar, no reduction of disruption of bar pressing to cue paired with shock	Killcross *et al.* (1997)
Electrolytic (Post)	R	Ce	Decreased expression of fear-potentiated startle to visual or auditory conditioned stimulus	Falls and Davis (1995); Hitchcock and Davis (1986, 1987)
Electrolytic (Post)	R	Bla	Decreased expression of fear-potentiated startle to visual conditioned stimulus	Kim and Davis (1993a,b)
Electrolytic (Post)	R	Ce	Decreased expression of fear-potentiated startle to context paired with shock	McNish *et al.* (1997)
NMDA (Pre or Post)	R	Bla	Decreased expression or acquisition of fear-potentiated startle to visual conditioned stimulus	Sananes and Davis (1992)
NMDA (Post)	R	Bla	Decreased expression of fear-potentiated startle even when lesions made 1 month after training	Lee *et al.* (1996)
Ibotenic acid (Post)	R	Ce	Decreased expression of fear-potentiated startle to visual or auditory conditioned stimulus	Campeau and Davis (1995)
Electrolytic (Pre shock)	R	Ce	Decreased the increase in acoustic startle amplitude after a series of footshocks	Hitchcock *et al.* (1989)
NMDA (Pre-shock)	R	Bla	Decreased acoustic startle amplitude facilitation after a series of footshocks	Sananes and Davis (1992)
NMDA (Pre shock)	R	AC	Decreased acoustic startle amplitude facilitation after a series of footshocks	Schanbacher *et al.* (1996)
Electrolytic (Pre-testing)	R	AC	Decreased shock probe avoidance, but no effect on shock probe burying	Treit *et al.* (1993b)

Table 6.5 continued

Method	*S*	*Site*	*Effect of inactivation*	*Reference*
Electrolytic (Pre)	R	AC	Failed to block anxiolytic effects of diazepam in plus-maze	Treit *et al.* (1993b)
Lidocaine (Post)	R	Bla	Decreased normal reduction in sensitivity to benzodiazepines on trial 2 of plus-maze. Lidocaine given immediately after trial 1	File *et al.* (1998)
Electrolytic (Pre)	R	AM	Decreased place aversion after naltrexone-precipitated morphine withdrawal	Kelsey and Arnold (1994)

*Archistriatum; believed to be the homologue of the mammalian amygdala.
Abbreviations: see Table 6.1.

Lesions of the central nucleus of the amygdala counteract the normal reduction of bar pressing or licking in the operant conflict test (anti-conflict effects) and in the conditioned emotional response paradigm, and generally decrease avoidance of an electrified water spout or dominant male (Table 6.5). Killcross *et al.* (1997) looked at neurotoxic lesions of either the central or basolateral nucleus in a paradigm that measured both response suppression to a cue associated with shock and avoidance of shock in the same animals. Lesions of the central nucleus blocked response suppression but not shock avoidance, whereas lesions of the basolateral nucleus had just the opposite effect. They argued that the basolateral nucleus therefore does not relay aversive information to the central nucleus to mediate response suppression. However, the relevance of results such as these, based on a complex, operant avoidance task using pre-training lesions with multiple trials, to classical fear conditioning remains to be determined. For example, several studies show that electrolytic or chemical lesions of either the central or basolateral nuclei of the amygdala block the fear-potentiated startle effect or the increase in startle shortly after a series of footshocks (Table 6.5), which may represent a rapid form of context conditioning (Kiernan *et al.*, 1995). Animals with large amygdala lesions could relearn fear-potentiated startle after overtraining (Kim and Davis, 1993a), although animals never learned if lesions were given before any training. However, more recent studies showed that animals with total lesions of the basolateral nucleus, including its most anterior aspects, failed to relearn fear-potentiated startle (Falls and Davis, 1995). In fact, Maren (1998) noted that the animals who relearned in his study may also have had sparing of the most anterior parts of the basolateral nucleus. Hence, at least for startle and freezing, a serial circuit from the basolateral nucleus to the central nucleus seems to be involved. It would be important to know, therefore, if the Killcross *et al.* (1997) results would still occur after totally complete lesions of the basolateral nucleus, which was difficult to judge from their paper. In addition, several other issues have been raised about this particular paper, although these each have been rebutted by Killcross *et al.* (Nader and LeDoux, 1997).

Lesions of the amygdala also produce a dramatic decrease in shock probe avoidance (Treit *et al.*, 1993a) but do not affect more active kinds of anxiogenic behaviours such as open arm time in the plus-maze or burying a noxious shock probe, which are affected by lesions of the septum (Treit *et al.*, 1993a), as well as anxiolytic drugs. Furthermore, the magnitude of the anxiolytic effects after combined lesions of both structures was comparable with their magnitude after individual lesions, suggesting that the septum and amygdala independently control different fear-related behaviours. However, lesions of the amygdala can reduce the anxiogenic effects of prior stress in the plus maze (Moller *et al.*, 1997).

In a very clever experiment, reversible inactivation of the basolateral amygdala via lidocaine was used to explore why the plus-maze becomes insensitive to benzodiazepines following a single exposure to the maze (File, 1990). The hypothesis was that following exposure on trial 1 in the plus-maze, rats develop a specific phobia (fear of heights) which is then insensitive to benzodiazepines. If consolidation of the memory of trial 1 could be prevented, then rats should still be sensitive to benzodiazepines on trial 2. In fact, this is exactly was happened when lidocaine was infused into the basolateral amygdala immediately after trial 1 (File *et al.*, 1998). Now animals did show an anxiolytic effect to the benzodiazepine given prior to trial 2.

Other data indicate that the amygdala appears to be involved in some types of aversive conditioning, but this may depend on the exact unconditioned aversive stimulus that is used. For example, electrolytic lesions of the basolateral nucleus (Pellegrino, 1968), or fibre-sparing chemical lesions of most of the amygdaloid complex (Cahill and McGaugh, 1990), attenuate avoidance of thirsty rats in approaching an electrified water spout through which they previously were accustomed to receiving water. Importantly, however, these same lesioned animals did not differ from controls in the rate at which they found the water spout over successive test days or their avoidance of the water spout when quinine was added to the water (Cahill and McGaugh, 1990). This led Cahill and McGaugh to suggest that 'the degree of arousal produced by the unconditioned stimulus, and not the aversive nature *per se*, determined the level of amygdala involvement' (p. 541). Perhaps this may explain some of the apparently contradictory results concerning the effects of amygdala lesions on conditioned taste aversion (for reviews of this literature, see, for example, Dunn and Everitt, 1988; Yamamoto *et al.*, 1994; Lamprecht and Dudai, 1996, Chapter 9). Table 6.5 also shows that lesions of the amygdala attenuate aversion to a context associated with morphine withdrawal (Kelsey and Arnold, 1994).

6.4.3 Hypoalgesia

Table 6.6 shows that lesions of the amygdala block conditioned analgesia produced by re-exposure to cues associated with noxious stimulation. This effect does not seem to be due to a blockade of learning because the lesions can be made after training and still block the expression of conditioned analgesia (Helmstetter and Bellgowan, 1993).

This, along with a large literature implicating the amygdala in many other measures of fear such as active and passive avoidance (Kaada, 1972; Ursin *et al.*, 1981; Sarter and Markowitsch, 1985; McGaugh *et al.*, 1990, 1993, 1995; Poremba and Gabriel, 1997)

Table 6.6 Effects of lesions of the amygdala on conditioned analgesia

Method	*S*	*Site*	*Effect of inactivation*	*Reference*
Electrolytic (Pre)	R	Ce or Bla	Decreased hypoalgesia to context paired with shock (formalin test)	Helmstetter (1992a)
Radiofrequency (Pre)	R	Ce, L and Bla	Decreased hypoalgesia to context paired with shock (tail-flick test)	Fox and Sorenson (1994)
Electrolytic (Pre)	R	Ce and Bla	Decreased analgesia to light paired with shock (tail-flick test)	Watkins *et al.* (1993)
Ibotenic acid (Pre)	R	Ce and Bla	Decreased expression of hypoalgesia to context paired with shock (formalin test)	Helmstetter (1992a)
Electrolytic (Post)	R	AC	Decreased hypoalgesia to tone paired with shock (tail-flick test)	Helmstetter and Bellgowan (1993)

Abbreviations: see Table 6.1.

and evaluation and memory of emotionally significant sensory stimuli (Bresnahan and Routtenberg, 1972; Handwerker *et al.*, 1974; Gold *et al.*, 1975; Gallagher and Kapp, 1978, 1981; Gallagher *et al.*, 1980, 1981; Mishkin and Aggleton, 1981; Kesner, 1982; Ellis and Kesner, 1983; Bennett *et al.*, 1985; Liang *et al.*, 1985, 1986; McGaugh *et al.*, 1990), provides strong evidence for a crucial role of the amygdala in fear.

6.5 Effects of amygdala lesions on unconditioned fear

Although it is sometimes asserted that the central nucleus of the amygdala is only involved in conditioned responses, a large literature indicates that it is also important for effects that do not obviously depend on prior conditioning.

6.5.1 Autonomic and hormonal measures

Table 6.7 shows that electrolytic or chemical lesions of the central nucleus generally inhibit the increase in plasma corticosterone produced by restraint stress. Lesions of the ventroamygdalofugal pathway connecting the central nucleus to the hypothalamus attenuate the compensatory hypersecretion of ACTH that normally occurs following adrenalectomy (Allen and Allen, 1974). Lesions of the stria terminalis did not. Lesions of the amygdaloid complex inhibit adrenocortical responses following olfactory or sciatic nerve stimulation (Feldman and Conforti, 1981) or exposure to visual or auditory stimuli (Feldman *et al.*, 1994). In the latter study, lesions of the medial or central nuclei blocked these effects on the hypothalamic–pituitary axis, whereas lesions of the basal nucleus did not. However, longer periods of exposure were not affected by lesions of the amygdala (Feldman and Conforti, 1981), suggesting that other areas may act in parallel with the amygdala to activate the hypothalamus following prolonged sensory stimulation. This may explain some cases where lesions fail to affect ACTH (Prewitt and Herman, 1997). Lesions of the amygdala block some of

Table 6.7 Effects of lesions of the amygdala on autonomic or hormonal measures of unconditioned fear or anxiety

Method	*S*	*Site*	*Effect of inactivation*	*Reference*
Electrolytic	R	Ce	Decreased secretion of ACTH to immobilization stress	Beaulieu *et al.* (1986, 1987)
Ibotenic acid	R	Ce	Decreased rise in corticosterone to immobilization stress	Van de Kar *et al.* (1991)
Ibotenic acid	R	Me, not Ce	Decreased c-*fos* induction in paraventricular nucleus of hypothalamus after restraint	Dayas *et al.* (1999)
Electrolytic	R	CeL	Decreased restraint stress-induced increase in ACTH but not induced by lipopoly-sacharride injection. Lesions of CeM had no effect	Marcilhac and Siaud (1996b)
Electrolytic (Pre but not post)	R	Ce	Decreased secretion of corticosterone and prolactin to shock. No effect on adrenaline or noradrenaline	Roozendaal *et al.* (1992a)
Radiofrequency	R	**	Decreased the compensatory hypersecretion of ACTH that normally occurs following adrenalectomy	Allen and Allen (1974, 1975)
Electrolytic	R	AC	Decreased adrenocortical responses following olfactory or sciatic nerve stimulation	Feldman and Conforti (1981)
Electrolytic	R	Me, Ce	Decreased ACTH and corticosterone elicited by visual or auditory stimuli (4 min), not with 30 min exposure	Feldman and Conforti (1981); Feldman *et al.* (1994)
Electrolytic	R	Ce	No effect on acute or chronic effects of stress on corticosterone or ACTH increase or increase in c-*fos* in paraventricular nucleus	(Prewitt and Herman (1997)
Ibotenic acid	R	Ce not Bla	Decreased stress-induced decrease in renal benzodiazepine binding	Holmes and Drugan (1993)
Electrolytic	R	Ce	Decreased rise in blood pressure produced by carbachol (i.c.v.), no effect on heart rate	Ozkutlu *et al.* (1995)
Electrolytic	R	Bla not Ce	Decreased rise in blood pressure and bradycardia produced by bicuculline (i.c.v.)	Karson *et al.* (1999)
Radiofrequency	R	Ce	Decreased ulceration produced by restraint	Henke (1980a,c)
Radiofrequency	R	Ce	Decreased ulceration produced by shock stress	Henke (1981)
Electrolytic	R	Ce	Decrease gastric ulcers to water restraint	Coover *et al.* (1992)
Ibotenic acid	R	Ce	No effect on ulcers to water restraint	Coover *et al.* (1992)
Electrolytic	R	Ce	Decreased noise-elicited hypertension	Galeno *et al.* (1984)
Radiofrequency	R	Ce	Decreased CRH (i.c.v.) or noise activation of tryptophan hydroxylase	Singh *et al.* (1990, 1992)

**Ventroamygdalofugal pathway connecting Ce to the hypothalamus.
Abbreviations: see Table 6.1.

the cardiovascular effects of either carbachol or bicuculline infused intracerebroventricularly (i.c.v.). Lesions of the central nucleus significantly attenuate ulceration produced by restraint or shock stress. However, at least with respect to water restraint, gastric ulcers are reduced only by electrolytic and not chemical lesions of the rostral central nucleus (Coover *et al.*, 1992), suggesting the importance of fibres of passage. On the other hand, Van de Kar *et al.* (1991) did find that ibotenic acid lesions of the central nucleus blocked hormonal effects to immobilization stress. Lesions of the amygdala block the ability of high levels of noise, which may be an unconditioned fear stimulus (Leaton and Cranney, 1990), to produce hypertension (Galeno *et al.*, 1984) or activation of tryptophan hydroxylase (Singh *et al.*, 1990).

6.5.2 Motor behaviour

Table 6.8 shows that lesions of the amygdala are known to block several measures of innate fear in different species (Blanchard and Blanchard, 1972; Ursin *et al.*, 1981). Lesions of the cortical amygdaloid nucleus, and perhaps the central nucleus, markedly reduce emotionality in wild rats measured in terms of flight and defensive behaviours (Kemble *et al.*, 1984, 1990). Large amygdala lesions, or those that damaged the cortical, medial, and in several cases the central nucleus, dramatically increase the number of contacts a rat will make with a sedated cat (Blanchard and Blanchard, 1972). In fact, some of these lesioned animals crawl all over the cat and even nibble its ear, a behaviour never shown by the non-lesioned animals. Following lesions of the archistriatum, birds become docile and show little tendency to escape from humans (Phillips, 1964, 1968), consistent with a general taming effect of amygdala lesions reported in many species (Goddard, 1964). In rabbits, lesions of central nucleus block the unconditioned excitatory effect of a tone on the nictitating membrane reflex (Weisz *et al.*, 1992) which may be one mechanism by which the amygdala modulates eyeblink conditioning. Lesions of the amygdala also block the anxiolytic effects of buspirone in the black–white box test (Dringenberg *et al.*, 1998) or the excitatory effects of lesions of the lateral septum on the startle reflex (Melia and Davis, 1991) or other measures of 'emotionality' such as resistance to handling and being hyper-reactive to tactile stimulation (King, 1958; King and Meyer, 1958; Schwartzbaum and Gay, 1966; Kleiner *et al.*, 1967). In addition, lesions of the central nucleus can block some of the signs of naloxone-precipitated opiate withdrawal (Calvino *et al.*, 1979). NMDA-induced lesions of the central nucleus of the amygdala increased the thresholds of aversive responses to electrical stimulation of the inferior colliculus, whereas lesions of the basolateral complex decrease these thresholds (Maisonnette *et al.*, 1996).

Enhancement of the startle reflex by exposure to background noise has been reported to be attenuated by benzodiazepines (Kellogg *et al.*, 1991) but not by amygdala lesions (Schanbacher *et al.*, 1996). However, we have found that neither buspirone nor diazepam block noise-enhanced startle at doses that clearly block fear-potentiated startle (Walker and Davis, unpublished). In addition, they seem not to have effects in the plus-maze (Treit *et al.*, 1993a,b), and diazepam still had anxiolytic effects in the plus-maze in these lesioned animals (Treit *et al.*, 1993b). This is consistent with other data showing that benzodiazepines

Table 6.8 Effects of lesions of the amygdala on unconditioned motor behaviours used to assess fear and anxiety

Method	*S*	*Site*	*Effect of inactivation*	*Reference*
Electrolytic	Wild R	CO, Ce	Decrease emotionality in measured in terms of flight and defensive behaviours	Kemble *et al.* (1990, 1984)
Electrolytic	R	CO,Me Ce	Increase the number of contacts a rat will make with a sedated cat	Blanchard and Blanchard (1972)
Electrolytic	B	*	Produces docility and decreases tendency to escape from humans	Phillips (1964, 1968)
Electrolytic	Many species	AC	General taming effect	For review, see Goddard (1964)
Electrolytic	Rb	Ce	Decreased tone-enhanced excitability of the nictitating membrane response	Weisz *et al.* (1992)
Radiofrequency	R	AC	Decreased anxiolytic effect of buspirone in black–white box	Dringenberg *et al.* (1998)
Electrolytic	R	Ce	Decreased elevation in startle amplitude after lesions of lateral septum	Melia and Davis (1991)
Electrolytic	R	AC	Decreased hyper-reactivity to handling or to tactile stimulation in rats with lesions of septum	King (1958); King and Meyer (1958); Kleiner *et al.* (1967); Schwartzbaum, and Gay (1966)
Radiofrequency	R	Ce	Decreased jump withdrawal sign in morphine-dependent rats after i.p. naloxone	Calvino *et al.* (1979)
NMDA	R	Ce	Increased threshold for aversive effects elicited by electrical stimulation of inferior colliculus	Maisonnette *et al.* (1996)
NMDA	R	Bla	Decreased threshold for aversive effects elicited by electrical stimulation of inferior colliculus	Maisonnette *et al.* (1996)
NMDA	R	AC	No block of noise-enhanced startle	Schanbacher *et al.* (1996)
Electrolytic	R	AC	No effect on open arm time in plus-maze and systemic diazepam still had anxiolytic effect	Treit *et al.* (1993a)
Electrolytic	R	CM	Hyper-reactive, no effect on corticoterone	Seggie (1983)

*Archistriatum; believed to be the homologue of the mammalian amygdala.
Abbreviations: see Table 6.1.

can still act in animals with lesions of the amygdala in various tests (Yadin *et al.*, 1991; Kopchia *et al.*, 1992; Davis, 1994). It indicates that other areas can take over to mediate anxiogenic behavioural effects after amygdala lesions, and that benzodiazepines still act under these special circumstances.

6.5.3 Hypoalgesia

Table 6.9 shows that lesions of central nucleus block unconditioned analgesia to cat exposure (Fox and Sorenson, 1994), loud noise (Bellgowan and Helmstetter, 1996), or footshock (Fox and Sorenson, 1994; Werka, 1997, 1998); but see Watkins *et al.* (1993). Lesions of the central nucleus tended to blunt analgesic effects of systemic administration of flumazenil using the tail-flick test (Grijalva *et al.*, 1990). NMDA lesions of the central but not the basolateral or medial nucleus of the amygdala blocked antinociception produced by a low dose of morphine in the formalin- (Manning and Mayer, 1995a) or heat-evoked tail-flick test (Manning and Mayer, 1995b). Unilateral lesions had the same effect when formalin was infused into the paw ipsilateral to the lesion but not in the paw contralateral to the lesion (Manning, 1998), consistent with the fact that descending projections of the central nucleus

Table 6.9 Effects of lesions or chemical inactivation of the amygdala on unconditioned analgesia

Method	*S*	*Site*	*Effect of inactivation*	*Reference*
Radiofrequency	R	Ce, L and Bla	Decreased analgesia produced by exposure to cat or shock (tail-flick test)	Fox and Sorenson (1994
Electrolytic	R	L or Ce	Decreased loud noise-induced hypoalgesia (tail-flick test)	Bellgowan and Helmstetter (1996)
Electrolytic	R	Ce , Me or Co	Decreased footshock-induced analgesia (tail-flick and hot-plate tests)	Werka (1997, 1998)
Electrolytic	R	Ce and Bla	No effect on analgesia to shock (tail-flick)	Watkins *et al.* (1993)
Electrolytic	R	AC	No effect on swim stress-induced analgesia	Pavlovic *et al.* (1996a)
Electrolytic	R	Ce, not Bla	Decreased analgesic effects of systemic flumazenil (hot-plate test)	Grijalva *et al.* (1990)
NMDA	R	Ce not Bla or Me	Decreased morphine (low dose)-induced antinociception (formalin or tail flick tests)	Manning and Mayer (1995a,b)
Lidocaine	R	Ce	Decreased morphine-induced antinociception (tail-flick test)	Manning and Mayer (1995b)
Electrolytic or muscimol	R	Ce not Bla	Decreased antinociception produced by a low dose of morphine (formalin test) but only in forepaw ipsilateral to unilateral lesion or site of muscimol infusion	Manning (1998)

Abbreviations: see Table 6.1.

of the amygdala are almost exclusively ipsilateral (cf. Manning, 1998). Direct infusion of lidocaine into the central nucleus had the same effect in the tail-flick test (Manning and Mayer, 1995b).

6.6 Effects of local infusion of drugs into the amygdala on measures of fear and anxiety

Clinically, fear is regarded to be more stimulus specific than anxiety, despite very similar symptoms. Figure 6.1 suggests that spontaneous activation of the central nucleus of the amygdala would produce a state resembling fear in the absence of any obvious eliciting stimulus. In fact, fear and anxiety often precede temporal lobe epileptic seizures (Gloor, 1992; Gloor *et al.*, 1981) which are usually associated with abnormal electrical activity of the amygdala (Crandall *et al.*, 1971). An important implication of this distinction is that treatments that block conditioned fear might not necessarily block anxiety. For example, if a drug decreased transmission along a sensory pathway required for a conditioned stimulus to activate the amygdala, then that drug might be especially effective in blocking conditioned fear. However, if anxiety resulted from activation of the amygdala not involving that sensory pathway, then that drug might not be especially effective in reducing anxiety. On the other hand, drugs that act specifically in the amygdala should affect both conditioned fear and anxiety. Moreover, drugs that act at various target areas of the central nucleus of the amygdala might be expected to provide selective actions on some but not all of the somatic symptoms associated with anxiety.

6.6.1 Corticotropin-releasing hormone and the amygdala

It is also probable that certain neurotransmitters within the amygdala especially may be involved in fear and anxiety. For example, the amygdala has a high density of CRH receptors (DeSouza *et al.*, 1985) and CRH nerve endings (Uryu *et al.*, 1992), and several recent papers indicate that stress, as well as conditioned fear, can induce a release of CRH in the amygdala which results in various anxiogenic effects. Microdialysis techniques suggest that 20 min of restraint stress (Pich *et al.*, 1995) or ethanol withdrawal (Pich *et al.*, 1995) increased CRH release in the amygdala. The CRH release reached a peak 10–12 h after ethanol removal, the same time as anxiogenic-like behaviours were observed in the elevated plus-maze. CRH-like immunoreactivity was also reported to be decreased by 58% in the amygdala 48 h following chronic cocaine withdrawal, suggesting that there is an increased release and degradation of CRH at this time (Sarnyai *et al.*, 1995). In fact, again using microdialysis, withdrawal from cocaine was associated with a large increase in CRH release in the amygdala that increased steadily over the 12 h collection period, reaching a 400% increase after 12 h (Richter and Weiss, 1999). Cannabinoid withdrawal is also associated with an increase in CRH release in the amygdala (de Fonseca *et al.*, 1997). However, whether these increases in CRH release are really associated with increased anxiety has been questioned by the finding that CRH is also released within the amygdala during feeding (Merali *et al.*, 1998).

In fact, the magnitude of the CRH release during feeding was comparable with that following 20 min of restraint stress.

Individual differences in general levels of fear or anxiety may be related to differences in the amount of CRH found in the amygdala. For example, Fawn-hooded rats, a strain derived from Wistar, Long-Evans, and brown rats, show more freezing in response to stress, have an increased preference for alcohol, develop adult onset hypertension, and have elevated levels of urinary catecholamines. Compared with Wistar rats, this strain also has higher levels of CRH mRNA in the central nucleus of the amygdala (Altemus *et al*., 1995). In addition, rats that experienced prenatal stress, which can lead to high levels of anxiety, had higher CRH levels in amygdala tissue compared with non-stressed controls which was associated with a higher depolarization (KCl)-induced CRH release from amygdala tissue (Cratty *et al*., 1995).

If the amygdala is critically involved in fear and anxiety, then drugs that reduce fear or anxiety clinically may well act within the amygdala. It is noteworthy in this regard that the central nucleus of the amygdala is known to have high densities of opiate receptors (Goodman *et al*., 1980), whereas the basolateral nucleus, which projects to the central nucleus (see Introduction), has a high density of benzodiazepine receptors (Niehoff and Kuhar, 1983). A variety of measures suggest that the anxiolytic effects of both opiates and benzodiazepines may result from binding to receptors in the amygdala.

6.6.2 Autonomic and hormonal measures

Table 6.10 shows that local infusion of opiate agonists into the central nucleus of the amygdala blocks the acquisition of conditioned bradycardia in rabbits. Local infusion into the central nucleus of very low amounts of arginine-8-vasopressin increased stress-induced bradycardia and immobility responses, whereas oxytocin had an opposite effect. This effect was seen in rats bred for low rates of avoidance behaviour but not the more aggressive rats that show high avoidance rates. CRH infused into central nucleus of the amygdala increased heart rate compared with vehicle-infused animals (Wiersma *et al*., 1993). However, these cardiovascular effects depend on the strain of animals and whether they are tested under stressful on non-stressful conditions. For example, CRH increased heart rate in Roman high-avoidance rats but not low-avoidance rats measured during low stress, whereas the opposite was found when tested under stressful conditions (Wiersma *et al*., 1997b, 1998). CRH, thyrotropin-releasing hormone (TRH) or calcitonin gene related peptide (CGRP) infused into the central nucleus increased both heart rate and plasma catecholamines (Brown and Gray, 1988). These were the only 3 peptides that caused both effects compared to 13 other peptides.

Boadle-Biber *et al*. (1993) found that CRH infused into the central nucleus increased tryptophan hydroxylase activity measured in the cortex which was blocked by prior administration of α-helical CRH 9–41 into the central nucleus. Moreover, like amygdala lesions (Singh *et al*., 1990), infusion of α-helical CRH 9–41 (Boadle-Biber *et al*., 1993) or dehydroepiandrosterone, a glucocorticoid antagonist (Singh *et al*., 1994), blocked noise-induced increase in tryptophan hydroxylase after infusions aimed at the central nucleus of the amygdala. Repeated subthreshold doses of either CRH or urocortin infused into the basolateral

Table 6.10 Effects of neurotransmitters or drugs infused into the amygdala on conditioned or unconditioned autonomic measures of fear or anxiety

Substance	*S*	*Site*	*Effect of substance infused*	*Reference*
Opiate agonists	Rb	Ce	Blocked acquisition of conditioned bradycardia	Gallagher *et al.* (1981, 1982)
Vasopressin	R	Ce	Increased stress-induced bradycardia and immobility responses in rats bred for low rates of avoidance behaviour but not more aggressive rats with high avoidance rates	Roozendaal *et al.* (1992b)
Vasopressin	R	Ce	Bradycardia (low doses) or tachycardia and release of corticosterone (high dose). Tachycardia blocked by oxytocin antagonist)	Roozendaal *et al.* (1993
Oxytocin	R	Ce	Tachycardia and release of corticoterone	Roozendaal *et al.* (1993)
Oxytocin	R	Ce	Decreased stress-induced bradycardia and immobility responses	Roozendaal *et al.* (1992b)
CRH	R	Ce	Increased heart rate. Effect blocked by α-CRH into Ce	Wiersma *et al.* (1993)
CRH	R	Ce	Increased heart rate in Roman high-avoidance but not low-avoidance rats (stress free)	Wiersma *et al.* (1998)
CRH	R	Ce	No effects on heart rate in Roman high-avoidance but not low avoidance rats (stress)	Wiersma *et al.* (1997b)
CRH, TRH or CGRP	R	Ce	Increase in blood pressure, heart rate and plasma catecholamines	Brown and Gray (1988)
CRH	R	Ce	Increased tryptophan hydroxylase in cortex. Blocked by α-CRH into Ce	Boadle-Biber *et al.* (1993)
α-CRH	R	Ce	Blocked noise-elicited increase in tryptophan hydroxylase in cortex	Boadle-Biber *et al.* (1993)
Glucocorticoid antagonist	R	Ce	Blocked noise-elicited increase in tryptophan hydroxylase in cortex	Singh *et al.* (1994)
Urocortin or CRH	R	Bla	After repeated subthreshold doses, got increase in blood pressure to systemic lactate	Sajdyk *et al.* (1999a)
GABA or chlordiazepoxide	R	Ce	Decreased stress-induced gastric ulcers	Sullivan *et al.* (1989)
CRH	R	Ce	Decreased cold restraint-induced gastric mucosal lesions. Prevented by infusion of the noradrenaline neurotoxin DSP-4 or propranolol into the Ce	Ray *et al.* (1993)
Neurotensin, dopamine, apomorphine	R	Ce	Decreased stress-induced gastric ulcers	Ray and Henke (1991a); Ray *et al.* (1987, 1988a)

Table 6.10 continued

Substance	*S*	*Site*	*Effect of substance infused*	*Reference*
6-OHDA or haloperidol	R	Ce	Increased stress-induced gastric ulcers	Ray and Henke (1991a); Ray *et al.* (1987, 1988a)
TRH	R	Ce	Increased stress-induced gastric ulcers	Ray and Henke (1991b); Ray *et al.* (1988b)
TRH or physostigmine	R	Ce	Increased stress-induced gastric ulcers, blocked by muscarinic or benzodiazepine agonists	Ray *et al.* (1990)
TRH analogue	R	Ce	Increased gastric contractility, blocked by vagotomy	Morrow *et al.* (1996)
TRH	R	Ce	Produced gastric lesions and stimulated acid secretion	Hernandez *et al.* (1990)
TRH analogue	R	AC	No effect on gastric secretion, whereas large effect after infusion into dorsal vagal complex or nucleus ambiguus	Ishikawa *et al.* (1988)
Enkephalin analogue	R	Ce	Decreased stress-induced gastric ulcers, prevented by 6-OHDA or clozapine	Ray and Henke (1990, 1991b); Ray *et al.* (1988b)
Naloxone	R	Ce	Increased stress-induced gastric ulcers	Ray and Henke (1991b); Ray *et al.* (1988b)
CCK8 or CCK A agonist A-63387	R	Ce	Decreased the increase in colonic motility normally observed after intraventricular administration of CRH or exposure to a cage previously associated with shock. Not observed with CCK-B agonists	Gue *et al.* (1994)
Pirenzepine	R	Ce not Bla	Blocked increase in blood pressure and bradycardia produced by i.c.v. carbachol	Aslan *et al.* (1997a)
Neurotensin	R	Ce	Increase in heart rate, no effect on plasma catecholamines. Low dose effect blocked by local infusion of α-CRH	Wiersma *et al.* (1997d)
Prazosin	R	Ce	Decreased photic stress-induced reduction in CRH in median eminence. No effect of atenolol	Feldman and Weidenfeld (1996)
5–7 DHT or ketanserin	R	AC	Decreased photic stress-induced reduction in CRH in median eminence	Feldman *et al.* (1998)

Abbreviations: see Table 6.1.

nucleus led to increases in blood pressure and heart rate following systemic lactate infusion (Sajdyk *et al.*, 1999a). This finding provides an important animal model of human panic disorder and once again suggests that long-term changes in excitability in the amygdala may underlie certain psychiatric disorders.

Ray and colleagues have shown that GABA, dopamine, neurotensin, opiate muscarinic, or benzodiazepine receptor activation attenuate stress-induced gastric ulcers, whereas TRH or physostigmine have the opposite effect. TRH or TRH analogues can also increase gastric motility and gastric acid (Hernandez *et al.*, 1990; Morrow *et al.*, 1996); however, much lower doses can increase gastric acid secretion after infusion into either the dorsal vagal complex or nucleus ambiguus (Ishikawa *et al.*, 1988). Surprisingly, however, local infusion of CRH into the central nucleus of the amygdala attenuated cold restraint-induced gastric mucosal lesions, and these effects of CRH were prevented by infusion of the noradrenaline neurotoxin DSP-4 or propranolol into the central nucleus (Ray *et al.*, 1993). It presently is unclear how this observation relates to the general anxiogenic behavioural effects produced by local infusion of CRH into the amygdala.

Finally, Table 6.10 shows some other examples of the effects of local amygdala infusion of other receptor agonists or antagonists on autonomic measures.

6.6.3 Motor behaviours

Benzodiazepines, GABA agonists and antagonists

Table 6.11 shows that many studies have found that local infusion of benzodiazepines into the amygdala have anxiolytic effects in the operant conflict test, measures of freezing, the light–dark box measure, shock probe avoidance, or the elevated plus-maze (see also File, Chapter 5). They can also antagonize the discriminative stimulus properties of pentylenetetrazol, thought to be a anxiogenic test (Benjamin *et al.*, 1987). Infusion of diazepam into the amygdala also accelerated the rate of between-session habituation of the startle response (Young *et al.*, 1991). This is consistent with the idea that loud startle stimuli produce contextual fear conditioning which competes with the expression of long-term habituation (Borszcz *et al.*, 1989). A reduction of contextual fear conditioning via diazepam infusion into the amygdala should thus increase long-term habituation as it does after systemic administration (Young *et al.*, 1991).

The anti-conflict effect (Petersen *et al.*, 1985; Hodges *et al.*, 1987; Shibata *et al.*, 1989) or the decrease in shock probe avoidance (Pesold and Treit, 1994) can be reversed by systemic administration of the benzodiazepine antagonist flumazenil or co-administration into the amygdala of the $GABA_A$ antagonist bicuculline (Scheel-Kruger and Petersen, 1982), and mimicked by local infusion into the amygdala of GABA (Hodges *et al.*, 1987) or the $GABA_A$ agonist muscimol (Scheel-Kruger and Petersen, 1982). In general, anxiolytic effects of benzodiazepines occur after local infusion into the lateral and basolateral nuclei, the nuclei of the amygdala that have high densities of benzodiazepine receptors (Petersen and Scheel-Kruger, 1982; Scheel-Kruger and Petersen, 1982; Petersen *et al.*, 1985; Thomas *et al.*, 1985; Green and Vale, 1992) and not after local infusion into the central nucleus (Petersen and Scheel-Kruger, 1982; Scheel-Kruger and Petersen, 1982; Green and Vale, 1992), although effects

Table 6.11 Effects of neurotransmitters or drugs infused into the amygdala on motor behaviours used to measure conditioned and unconditioned fear and anxiety

Substance infused	*S*	*Site*	*Effect of substance infused*	*Reference*
Benzo-diazepines	R	Bla	Increased punished responding in operant conflict test (anti-conflict effect)	Green and Vale (1992); Petersen *et al.* (1985); Petersen and Scheel-Kruger (1982); Scheel-Kruger and Petersen (1982); Thomas *et al.* (1985)
GABA, benzo-diazepines or 5-HT	R	Bla	Increased punished responding in operant conflict test (anti-conflict effect)	Hodges *et al.* (1987)
Muscimol	R	Bla	Increased punished responding in operant conflict test (anti-conflict effect). No effect in Ce	Scheel-Kruger and Petersen (1982)
Benzo-diazepines	R	Ce	No effect in the conflict test	Green and Vale (1992); Petersen and Scheel-Kruger (1982); Scheel-Kruger and Petersen (1982)
Benzo-diazepines	R	Ce	Increased punished responding in operant conflict test (anti-conflict effect)	Shibata *et al.* (1982, 1986); Takao *et al.* (1992)
Midazolam	R	Bla	More time on open arms in plus-maze, no effect on shock probe avoidance/burying	Pesold and Treit (1995)
Midazolam	R	Ce	No effect in plus-maze or shock probe burying, decrease in probe avoidance	Pesold and Treit (1994, 1995)
Diazepam	R	Ce or Bla	Decreased freezing to footshock	Helmstetter (1993); Young *et al.* (1991)
Diazepam	R	Ce or Bla	Decreased freezing to context paired with startle stimuli. Accelerated rate of between-session habituation of the startle response due to reduction of context fear	Young *et al.* (1991)
Diazepam	Mice	AC	More time in light side in light–dark box test (anxiolytic effect)	Costall *et al.* (1989)
Midazolam	R	AC	Antagonized the discriminative stimulus properties of pentylenetetrazol, thought to be a measure of anxiety	Benjamin *et al.* (1987)
Midazolam	R	Bla	Decreased acquisition of context freezing, reinstated by formalin test which was not affected by midazolam	Harris and Westbrook (1998)
Muscimol	R	Bla	Anxiolytic effect in the social interaction test. No effect in Ce	Sanders and Shekhar (1995b)
Bicuculline, picrotoxin	R	Bla	Anxiogenic effects in the social interaction test. Repeated infusion led to sensitization	Sanders and Shekhar (1995b)

Table 6.11 continued

Substance infused	*S*	*Site*	*Effect of substance infused*	*Reference*
Bicuculline	R	Bla	Anxiogenic effects in social interaction, blocked by either NMDA or non-NMDA antagonists into the amygdala	Sajdyk and Shekhar (1997a)
Flumazenil	R	Bla	Decreased anti-conflict effect of the benzodiazepine agonist chlordiazepoxide given systemically	Hodges *et al.* (1987)
Flumazenil or bicuculline	R	Bla	Decreased the anxiolytic effect of chlordiazepoxide given systemically on the social interaction test at doses that had no anxiogenic effects by themselves	Sanders and Shekhar (1995a)
Flumazenil	R	AC	Anxiogenic effect in plus-maze	Wolterink *et al.* (1992)
α-CRH	R	Ce	Anxiolytic effect (plus-maze) in socially defeated rat	Heinrichs *et al.* (1992)
α-CRH	R	Ce	Anxiolytic effect in plus-maze during ethanol withdrawal in ethanol-dependent rats. No effect in plus-maze in non-dependent rats	Rassnick *et al.* (1993)
α-CRH	R	Ce	Decreased behavioural effects of opiate withdrawal	Heinrichs *et al.* (1995)
CRH receptor antisense	R	Ce	Anxiolytic effect in the plus-maze in rats that previously experienced defeat stress	Liebsch *et al.* (1995) Swiergiel *et al.* (1993)
α-CRH	R	Ce	Decreased duration of freezing to an initial shock treatment or to re-exposure to shock box 24 h later	
α-CRH	R	Ce	No effect on grooming and exploration activity under stress-free conditions	Wiersma *et al.* (1995)
CRH	R	Ce, not Bla	Increased grooming and exploration in animals tested under stress-free conditions (i.e. in the home cage)	Wiersma *et al.* (1995; Wiersma *et al.*, 1997c)
CRH	R	Ce	Increased defensive burying	Wiersma *et al.* (1997a)
CRH or urocortin	R	Bla	Anxiogenic effect in plus-maze, sensitization with repeated subthreshold doses. Now get behavioural and cardiovascular effects to systemic lactate	Sajdyk *et al.* (1999a)
α-CRH	R	Ce or Bla	No effect on fear-potentiated startle or startle enhanced by i.c.v. CRH	Lee and Davis (1996)
CRH	R	Ce or Bla	No effect on acoustic startle amplitude	Liang *et al.* (1992)
Carbachol	R	Ce	Immobility	Ohta *et al.* (1991)
Vasopressin	R	Ce	Immobility, seizures on second infusion	Willcox *et al.* (1992)
Vasopressin	R	Ce	Immobility in rats bred for low rates of avoidance but not those bred for high avoidance rates	Roozendaal *et al.* (1992b)

Table 6.11 continued

Substance infused	*S*	*Site*	*Effect of substance infused*	*Reference*
5-HT_3 agonist	Mice	AC	Less time in light side in light–dark box test (anxiogenic effect)	Costall *et al.* (1989)
5-HT_3 receptor antagonists	Mice	AC	More time in light side in light–dark box test (anxiolytic effect)	Costall *et al.* (1989)
5-HT_3 receptor antagonist	R	AC	Anxiogenic effect on avoidance of open arm but anxiolytic effect on escape of open arm in T-maze	Gargiulo *et al.* (1996)
5-HT_3 antagonists	R	AC	Anxiolytic in social interaction, no effect in conflict in contrast to flurazepam	Higgins *et al.* (1991)
5-HT_3 antagonist	Mice	AC	Decreased signs of withdrawal (dark–light box) following subchronic administration of diazepam, ethanol,nicotine, or cocaine	Costall *et al.* (1990)
d-AP159	R	Ce	Anxiolytic effect in the conflict test, blocked by systemic flumazenil. (d-AP159 has high affinity for 5-HT_{1A} receptors)	Takao *et al.* (1992)
5-HT	R	Bla	Anxiogenic effects in the conflict test	Hodges *et al.* (1987)
8–OH-DPAT	R	Bla	Weak anxiogenic effects in the conflict test	Hodges *et al.* (1987)
8–OH-DPAT	R	AC	Anxiolytic effect in open arm avoidance, no effect on open arm escape in T-maze	Zangrossi *et al.* (1999)
Methysergide	R	Bla	Anxiolytic effect in the conflict test	Hodges *et al.* (1987)
8-OH-DPAT, buspirone, or ipsapirone	R	PM AC	Decreased shock-induced vocalization	Schreiber and De Vry (1993)
Neuropeptide Y	R	Bla, not Ce	Anxiolytic effect in social interaction test, blocked by Y-1 antagonist	Sajdyk *et al.* (1999b)
Neuropeptide Y1 agonist	R	Ce	Anxiolytic effects in conflict test. NPY-Y2 agonist much less potent	Heilig *et al.* (1993)
Morphine	R	Ce	Anxiolytic effect in social interaction test	File and Rodgers (1979)
Naloxone	R	AC	Elicited certain signs of withdrawal (depending on site) in morphine-dependent rats (unilateral)	Calvino *et al.* (1979)
Methyl-naloxonium	R	Dorsal AC	Place aversion to context where injections given to morphine-dependent rats	Stinus *et al.* (1990)
Methyl-naloxonium	R	Dorsal AC	Weak withdrawal signs in morphine-dependent rats	Maldonado *et al.* (1992)
Clonidine, ST-91, or CNQX	R	Ce	Decreased naloxone-precipitated withdrawal signs in morphine-dependent rats	Taylor *et al.* (1998)
St-91	R	Ce	Decreased increase in startle after footshocks	Fendt *et al.* (1994b)
Yohimbine	R	Ce	Facilitation of the startle reflex	Fendt *et al.* (1994b)

Table 6.11 continued

Substance infused	*S*	*Site*	*Effect of substance infused*	*Reference*
SCH 23390	R	AC	Decreased expression of fear-potentiated startle	Lamont and Kokkinidis (1998)
SCH 23390	R	AC	Decreased acquisition and expression of freezing to tone or context. Not due to state-dependent learning.	Guarraci *et al.* (1999)
SKF 82958	R	AC	Increased acquisition and expression of freezing to tone or context. Not due to state-dependent learning.	Guarraci *et al.* (1999)
c-*fos* antisense	R	Ce	Decreased number of Fos-positive cells in rats exposed to the Vogel test. Anxiolytic effect compared with sense and random sequence oligonucleotides	Moller *et al.* (1994)
CCK analogues	R	AC	Anxiogenic effect in plus-maze but not clear because significant decrease in overall activity	Belcheva *et al.* (1994)
CCK analogues	R	Ce	No effect in plus-maze. Unilateral infusions	Huston *et al.* (1998)
NMDA	R	Ce	Facilitation of the startle reflex	Koch and Ebert (1993)
ACPD	R	Ce	Facilitation of the startle reflex, but delayed for about 4 h	Koch (1993)
Pentagastrin	R	AC	Increased acoustic startle, blocked by CCK-B antagonist that also blocked effect of pentagastrin (i.c.v.)	Frankland *et al.* (1997)
TFF peptides	R	Bla	Anxiolytic effects in plus-maze (low dose) 24 h but not 1 h after infusion. Anxiogenic effects at both time points (high dose)	Schwarzberg *et al.* (1999)
Δ9-THC	Mice	Ce	Anxiogenic-like effect in the light–dark box	Onaivi *et al.* (1995)
Pertussis toxin	R	Bla	Decreased expression of fear-potentiated startle tested 6 h after infusion, however, could have been toxic	Melia *et al.* (1992)

Abbreviations: see Table 6.1.

have been reported after infusion into the central nucleus (Shibata *et al.*, 1982, 1986; Takao *et al.*, 1992). However, in our experience, it has been very hard to differentiate effects of compounds infused into either the central or basolateral nucleus when highly lipid soluble compounds are used. More recently, however, Pesold and Treit (1995) reported that local infusion of midazolam into the basolateral nucleus had an anxiolytic effect in the plus maze, but did not impair shock probe avoidance, whereas infusion into the central nucleus impaired shock probe avoidance but did not affect plus-maze performance. This was consistent with earlier work (Green and Vale, 1992), and both of the site-specific effects of midazolam could be blocked by systemic administration of flumazenil.

Sanders and Shekhar (1995b) found that infusion of the $GABA_A$ antagonists bicuculline or picrotoxin into the anterior basolateral nucleus had anxiogenic effects in the social interaction test. These same doses had no effect when infused into the central nucleus. Conversely, infusion of the $GABA_A$ agonist muscimol into the central nucleus had an anxiolytic effect, whereas it had no effect when infused into the basolateral nucleus. These data suggest a tonic, and perhaps maximal level of GABA inhibition in the basolateral but not the central nucleus of the amygdala. Anxiogenic effects in social interaction could be blocked by local infusion of either NMDA or non-NMDA antagonists into the amygdala (Sajdyk and Shekhar, 1997a). As mentioned earlier, repeated infusion of initially subthreshold doses of bicuculline into the anterior basolateral nucleus leads to a 'priming' effect in which increases in heart rate and blood pressure were observed after 3–5 infusions (Sanders and Shekhar, 1995b). This was accompanied by anxiogenic effects in the conflict and social interaction tests.

Taken together, these results suggest that drug actions in the amygdala may be sufficient to explain both fear-reducing and anxiety-reducing effects of various drugs given systemically (see also File, Chapter 5). In fact, local infusion into the amygdala of the benzodiazepine antagonist flumazenil significantly attenuated the anti-conflict effect of the benzodiazepine agonist chlordiazepoxide given systemically (Hodges *et al.*, 1987). Similarly, Sanders and Shekhar (1995a) found that local infusion of flumazenil or bicuculline into the anterior part of the basolateral nucleus, at doses which had no anxiogenic effects by themselves, blocked the anxiolytic effect of chlordiazepoxide given systemically on the social interaction test These are very powerful experimental designs and strongly implicate the amygdala in mediating the anxiolytic effects of benzodiazepines.

Nonetheless, it should be emphasized that benzodiazepines can still have anxiolytic effects in animals with lesions of the amygdala (Yadin *et al.*, 1991; Kopchia *et al.*, 1992; Treit *et al.*, 1993b; Davis, 1994). Although these important results could be interpreted to indicate that the amygdala is not necessary for mediating anxiolytic effects of benzodiazepines, such a conclusion is difficult to reconcile with the many studies outlined above. Hence, it may be that other brain structures take over for the amygdala after it is lesioned (see Kim and Davis, 1993a), and benzodiazepine binding in these other structures accounts for the anxiolytic effects after amygdala lesions. For example, we have found that the bed nucleus of the stria terminalis can modulate the acoustic startle reflex in certain anxiogenic tests (Walker *et al.*, 1997), so that this structure might be a likely one to take over following lesions of the amygdala (see below).

Corticotropin-releasing hormone

Several studies now suggest an important role for CRH in the amygdala in mediating various anxiogenic effects in the plus-maze, as well as other tests. Local infusion of α-helical CRH 9–41 in the central nucleus attenuated the anxiogenic effect of social defeat (Heinrichs *et al.*, 1992), ethanol withdrawal in ethanol-dependent rats in the plus-maze (Rassnick *et al.*, 1993), and certain signs of opiate withdrawal (Heinrichs *et al.*, 1995). Higher doses were not effective, perhaps due to partial agonist effects of this compound. Doses effective in the plus-maze had no effect on plasma ACTH or corticosterone release, although these values returned to baseline earlier following antagonist infusion compared with control. The antagonist had no effect on overall activity or percentage time spent in open arms of the maze in rats not dependent on ethanol. Liebsch *et al.* (1995) found that local infusion into the central nucleus of the CRH receptor mRNA antisense oligonucleotide had an anxiolytic effect in the plus-maze in rats which previously experienced defeat stress. Infusion of the scrambled sequence oligonucleotide had no effect.

Using freezing as a measure, Swiergiel *et al.* (1993) found that local infusion of low doses (50 and 100 ng) of α-helical CRH 9–41 into the central nucleus reduced the duration of freezing to an initial shock treatment. A higher dose (200 ng) was not effective. This reduction in freezing by α-helical CRH 9–41 probably was not due to an alteration in sensitivity to the footshock, because infusion of the antagonist into the central nucleus immediately prior to re-exposure to the shock box 24 h later also attenuated freezing duration.

In all of the above examples, infusion of the CRH antagonists produced behavioural effects in animals which had undergone prior stress, which may be necessary to detect effects following local infusion into the amygdala. For example, although CRH infused into the central nucleus could produce increased grooming and exploration in animals tested under stress-free conditions in their home cage, local infusion of α-helical CRH9–41 had no effect on activity under these same stress-free conditions (Wiersma *et al.*, 1995). More recently, anxiogenic effects in the plus-maze were seen following repeated infusions of initially subthreshold doses of either CRH or urocortin (Sajdyk *et al.*, 1999a), suggesting that prior stress may sensitize the CRH system, leading to heightened levels of fear or anxiety.

On the other hand, enhancement of the startle reflex, either by i.c.v. infusion of CRH (CRH-enhanced startle), or by conditioned fear, does not seem to depend on activation of CRH receptors in the amygdala, at least in the central nucleus of the amygdala. Although large electrolytic lesions of the amygdala were found to block CRH-enhanced startle (Liang *et al.*, 1992), local infusion of CRH into the amygdala failed to increase startle using a large number of animals and several placements within the amygdala (Liang *et al.*, 1992). Moreover, recent experiments using fibre-sparing lesions of the central and/or basolateral nuclei of the amygdala failed to block CRH-enhanced startle (Lee and Davis, 1996). In addition, local infusion of α-helical CRH9–41 into the central nucleus of the amygdala did not block fear-potentiated startle (Lee and Davis, 1996). In contrast, neurotoxic lesions of the bed nucleus of the stria terminalis completely block CRH-enhanced startle, and direct infusion of CRH into this nucleus increases acoustic startle (Lee and Davis, 1996).

Other compounds

Infusion into the amygdala of either carbachol or vasopressin can produce immobility, although the effects of vasopressin may depend on the strain of rats (e.g. Roozendaal *et al.*, 1992b). Based on a series of observations, Deakin and Graeff (1991) hypothesized that 5-HT seems to enhance fear or anxiety in the amygdala, whereas it has the opposite effect in the dorsal central grey (Deakin and Graeff, 1991). A great deal of data support the anti-anxiety effects of 5-HT in the dorsal central grey (for a review, see Graeff *et al.*, 1993), although less direct data are available concerning the role of 5-HT in the amygdala. Local infusion of 5-HT or the 5-HT_{1A} agonist 8-hydroxy-2-(di-*n*-propylamino)tetralin (8-OH-DPAT) into the amygdala has been reported to produce anxiogenic effects in the conflict test (Hodges *et al.*, 1987; Takao *et al.*, 1992), whereas infusion of the 5-HT_2 antagonist ketanserin had an anxiolytic effect (Hodges *et al.*, 1987). On the other hand, infusion into the amygdala of the 5-HT_{1A} agonists 8-OH-DPAT, buspirone, or ipsapirone reduced shock-induced vocalization (Schreiber and De Vry, 1993). In this case, however, the 5-HT_{1A} agonists were infused into the posteromedial cortical amygdaloid nucleus rather than the basolateral nucleus (Hodges *et al.*, 1987) or the central nucleus (Takao *et al.*, 1992). Interestingly, the corticomedial nucleus, rather than the central or basolateral nuclei, was also the most effective site for morphine analgesia in the shock-induced jump response tested in freely moving rats (Rodgers, 1977, 1978) (see below). More recently, intra-amygdala infusion of either midazolam or 8-OH-DPAT impaired inhibitory avoidance of the open arms of the T-maze, said to represent conditioned fear, indicating an anxiolytic effect, but did not change escape performance from one of the open arms, said to represent unconditioned fear (Zangrossi *et al.*, 1999).

5-HT_3 receptor subtype antagonists have been reported to produce anxiolytic effects after local infusion into the amygdala (Costall *et al.*, 1989; Higgins *et al.*, 1991). Such infusions also can block some of the signs of withdrawal following subchronic administration of diazepam, ethanol, nicotine, or cocaine (Costall *et al.*, 1990), or increases in levels of dopamine or the serotonin metabolite 5-HIAA in the amygdala after activation of dopamine neurons in the ventral tegmental area (Hagan *et al.*, 1990). In addition, local infusion of a putative 5-HT_{1A} antagonist into the central nucleus has been reported to have an anti-conflict effect (Takao *et al.*, 1992). On the other hand, systemic injection of the 5-HT_3 receptor antagonist, BRL 46470A had a anxiolytic effect on inhibitory avoidance in the T-maze but an anxiogenic effect when injected into the amygdala. It had an anxiolytic action on the escape response when given either systemically or into the amygdala (Gargiulo *et al.*, 1996). These authors suggest that the contrasting results obtained with different measures of anxiety may account for the inconsistencies found in the experimental literature dealing with compounds of this nature.

Activation of neuropeptide Y1 receptors in the central nucleus has been reported to produce selective anxiolytic effects in the conflict test (Heilig *et al.*, 1993), and this effect could be blocked by prior i.c.v. administration of an antisense inhibitor of Y1 receptor expression (Heilig, 1995) which itself produced an anxiogenic effect (Wahlestedt *et al.*, 1993; Heilig, 1995). Local infusion of opiate agonists in the central nucleus was reported to have anxiolytic effects in the social interaction test (File and Rodgers, 1979). Conversely, local infusion of naloxone can elicit some signs of opiate withdrawal in morphine-dependent rats (Table 6.11), whereas local infusion of α-2 adrenergic agonists such as clonidine or ST-91 or the glutamate antagonist 6-cyano-7-nitroquinoxaline-2,3-dione (CNQX) can attenuate certain withdrawal signs after systemic naloxone (Taylor *et al.*, 1998). ST-91 also decreased shock-enhanced sensitization of the startle reflex (Fendt *et al.*, 1994b), whereas infusion of the α-2 adrenergic antagonist yohimbine caused a modest increase in baseline startle amplitude (Fendt *et al.*, 1994b).

Although dopamine is often associated with positive reward, local infusion of the dopamine D1 antagonist SCH23390 into the amygdala can block the expression of fear-potentiated startle (Lamont and Kokkinidis, 1998). The same treatment also blocks both the acquisition and expression of conditioned freezing to a context or cue, whereas local infusion of the dopamine D1 agonist SKF82958 facilitated both acquisition and expression (Guarraci *et al.*, 1999). These effects could not be accounted for by state-dependent learning.

Several studies have shown an activation of the immediate early gene c-*fos* in the amygdala following footshocks (Campeau *et al.*, 1991; Rosen *et al.*, 1998), exposure to cues previously associated with footshock (Pezzone *et al.*, 1992; Smith *et al.*, 1992; Beck and Fibiger, 1995; Campeau *et al.*, 1997; Rosen *et al.*, 1998), 15 min exposure to an elevated plus-maze (Graeff *et al.*, 1993), or the Vogel conflict test (Moller *et al.*, 1994). Bilateral infusions of c-*fos* antisense oligonucleotides into the central nucleus of the amygdala decreased the number of Fos-positive cells in rats exposed to the Vogel test and also had an anxiolytic effect compared with sense and random sequence oligonucleotides (Moller *et al.*, 1994). Finally, Table 6.11 shows that cholecystokinin (CCK) has variable effects on measures of fear or anxiety after infusion into the amygdala. However, Franklin *et al.* (1997) found that local infusion of pentagastrin increased acoustic startle and this could be blocked by local infusion of a CCK B antagonist that also blocked the effect of pentagastrin given intraventricularly. Startle amplitude also was increased by local infusion of NMDA (Koch *et al.*, 1993) as well as the metabotropic glutamate receptor agonist, *trans*-(+)-1-amino-cyclopentane-1,3, dicarboxylate (trans-ACPD) (Koch, 1993) into the central nucleus of the amygdala. Similarly to other behavioural effects after local infusion of trans-ACPD, the increase in startle was very delayed (peak effect at 4 h) and was suggested to reflect an increase in sensitization.

6.6.4 Hypoalgesia

Table 6.12 shows that infusion of morphine, mu opioid agonists, or enkephalinase inhibitors into the amygdala has antinociceptive effects, although this occasionally has not been found (Yaksh *et al.*, 1976). These analgesic effects depend on the site of infusion and the test of analgesia. Morphine and mu agonists seem to be most effective in the basolateral nucleus when the tail-flick test is carried out in anaesthetized rats (Helmstetter *et al.*, 1993, 1995). These effects appear to depend on a serial circuit from the amygdala to the central grey to the rostral ventromedial medulla because local infusion of lidocaine into these latter sites prevented the antinociceptive effects of mu agonists infused into the amygdala (Helmstetter *et al.*, 1998). Subthreshold doses of morphine, mu-selective agonists or B-endorphin into the amygdala and central grey often had synergistic effects depending on the analgesia test and the exact combination of compounds in different areas (Pavlovic and Bodnar, 1998). Furthermore, local infusion of opiate antagonists into the central grey can block antinociceptive effects of opiates infused into the amygdala (Pavlovic *et al.*, 1996b). In waking rats using jump threshold as a measure, the most sensitive placements seem to occur in the corticomedial nucleus and not in the basolateral or central nucleus (Rodgers, 1977, 1978). Morphine infused into the corticomedial nucleus also reduced open field defaecation but had no effect on tail-flick latency (Rodgers, 1978). Antinociception also occurs after injection of neurotensin (Kalivas *et al.*, 1982) into the central nucleus of the amygdala or carbachol into the central, basolateral, or medial amygdala nuclei (Klamt and Prado, 1991; Oliveira and

Table 6.12 Effects of neurotransmitters or drugs infused into the amygdala on conditioned and unconditioned analgesia

Substance infused	*S*	*Site of infusion*	*Effect of substance infused*	*Reference*
Morphine	R	Bla	Analgesic in tail-flick	(Helmstetter (1993)
Enkephalinase inhibitors	R	Ce	Antinociceptive effects in hot plate but not in tail flick	Al-Rodhan *et al.* (1990)
Morphine	R	CM not Bla or Ce	Decreased open field defecation but had no effect on tail-flick latency	Rodgers (1978)
Mu agonists	R	Bla	Analgesic in tail-flick, blocked by lidocaine in periaqueductal grey or rostral ventromedial medulla)	Helmstetter *et al.* (1995, 1998
Morphine or B-endorphin	R	Bla or Ce	Analgesia, blocked by opiate antagonists infused into central grey	Pavlovic *et al.* (1996b)
Morphine, mu-agonists, or B-endorphin	R	Bla or Ce	Synergistic analgesia with co-administration of similar compounds in the central grey depending on test and combinations of compounds	Pavlovic and Bodnar (1998)
Morphine	R	CM not Bla or Ce	Analgesic effect in jump threshold.	Rodgers (1977, 1978)
Neurotensin	R	Ce	Antinociceptive effects in hot plate, blocked by lesions of stria terminalis	Kalivas *et al.* (1982)
Carbachol	R	Ce, Bla or Me	Antinociceptive effects in tail-flick test	Klamt and Prado (1991); Oliveira and Prado (1994)
Carbachol	R	Ce	Antinociceptive effects to tooth pulp stimulation	Ahn *et al.* (1999)
Morphine (Pre, post, or both)	R	Ce not Bla	Decreased both the acquisition and expression of conditioned hypoalgesia (formalin test). Reversed by naloxone into the amygdala.	Good and Westbrook (1995)
Prepro-enkephalin	R	AC	Antinociceptive in formalin test. Over-expression via viral vector gene transfer	Kang *et al.* (1998)
Midazolam	R	Bla	Attenuation of hypoalgesia	Harris and Westbrook (1995)
Diazepam	R	Ce or Bla	Decreased shock induced analgesia (formalin test)	Helmstetter (1993)

Abbreviations: see Table 6.1.

Prado, 1994; Ahn *et al*., 1999). Unilateral local infusion of morphine into the central nucleus of the amygdala attenuated both the acquisition and expression of inhibitory avoidance and conditioned hypoalgesia measured with the formalin test (Good and Westbrook, 1995), which is sensitive to naloxone. These effects of morphine in the amygdala could be reversed by co-administration of naloxone into the amygdala, and the effects on acquisition could not be explained by state-dependent learning. Interestingly, morphine infusions did not block conditioned analgesia when rats were tested on the heated floor, a form of opiate-independent hypoalgesia. Hence, the amygdala did not seem critical for all types of conditioned analgesia. Although Good and Westbrook (1995) did not find effective sites for morphine in the basolateral amygdala, Harris and Westbrook (1995) did see an attenuation of both hypoalgesia and inhibitory avoidance after infusion of midazolam in the basolateral nucleus. Pre-proenkephalin overexpression via viral vector gene transfer in the amygdala has also been found to have an antinociceptive effect in the formalin test (Kang *et al*., 1998).

6.7 The role of excitatory amino acid receptors in the amygdala in fear-conditioning

Both NMDA-dependent (Gean *et al*., 1993) and NMDA-independent (Chapman and Bellavance, 1992) LTP can occur in amygdala brain slices or *in vivo* following tetanic stimulation of the part of the medial geniculate nucleus that projects to the lateral nucleus of the amygdala (Clugnet and LeDoux, 1990). If convergence between the conditioned stimulus and shock occurs at the amygdala, and an NMDA-dependent process is involved in the acquisition of conditioned fear, then local infusion of NMDA antagonists into the amygdala should block the acquisition of conditioned fear.

Table 6.13 shows that local infusion of the NMDA antagonist 5-phosphonopentanoic acid (AP5) into the amygdala blocks the acquisition but not the expression of fear-potentiated startle (Miserendino *et al*., 1990; Campeau *et al*., 1992) The effect did not seem to result from a decrease in sensitivity to footshock, because local infusion of AP5 into the amygdala did not alter either overall reactivity to footshock or the slope of reactivity as a function of different footshock intensities. Moreover, AP5 infused into the amygdala also blocked second-order conditioning, which at the time of infusion did not involve footshock (Gewirtz and Davis, 1997). Importantly, AP5 did not block the expression of fear-potentiated startle when infused prior to testing in rats that were conditioned drug free. In fact, in each of these studies, the level of fear-potentiated startle was slightly higher following infusion of AP5 versus its vehicle. This was statistically significant in the study by Gewirtz and Davis(1997) and indicates that AP5 blocked the ability of an auditory stimulus to serve as the reinforcement signal for second-order conditioning but not its ability to potentiate startle.

Local infusion of the AMPA/kainate antagonist CNQX into either the central or basolateral nuclei of the amygdala dose-dependently blocked the expression of fear-potentiated startle using either a visual or auditory conditioned stimulus (M.Kim *et al*., 1993; Walker and Davis, 1997). Importantly, CNQX blocked the expression of fear-potentiated startle but had no systematic effect on baseline startle after local infusion into the amygdala.

Table 6.13 Effects of glutamate antagonists infused into the amygdala on fear-potentiated startle and conditioned freezing

Drug	*S*	*Site of infusion*	*Effect*	*Reference*
AP5	R	Bla	Blocked acquisition but not expression of fear-potentiated startle, visual CS	Miserendino *et al.* (1990)
AP5	R	Bla	Blocked acquisition but not expression of fear-potentiated startle, auditory CS	Campeau *et al.* (1992)
AP5	R	Bla	Block acquisition of second-order conditioning of fear-potentiated startle. No effect on expression of first-order CS.	Gewirtz and Davis (1997)
MK-801	R	Right AC	Block increased in startle amplitude following exposure to cat when drug given during cat exposure	Adamec *et al.* (1998)
AP5	R	Bla	Blocked acquisition of conditioned freezing using context as CS. No effect in Ce	Fanselow and Kim (1994)
AP5	R	Bla	Blocked acquisition or expression of freezing to context paired with shock	Maren *et al.* (1996b)
AP5	R	Bla	Blocked acquisition or expression of freezing to context or tone paired with shock even in rats given prior fear conditioning	Lee and Kim (1998)
CNQX	R	Bla	Blocked expression of fear-potentiated startle (visual or auditory CS)	M. Kim *et al.* (1993)
NBQX	R	Bla or Ce	Blocked expression of fear-potentiated startle (visual CS)	Walker and Davis (1997)
AP5	R	Bla	Blocked facilitation of eyeblink conditioning by prior stress when given prior to stressor session. No effect in Ce	Shors and Mathew (1998)
AP5 or CNQX	R	Bla	Anxiolytic effect in social interaction test	Sajdyk and Shekhar (1997b)
MK-801	R	Left AC	Blocked increase in risk assessment, but not decrease in open arms, in plus-maze following exposure to cat when drug given during cat exposure	Adamec *et al.* (1998)
CNQX	R	Ce	Decreased naloxone-precipitated withdrawal signs in morphine-dependent rats	Taylor *et al.* (1998)

Abbreviations: see Table 6.1.

Fanselow and Kim (1994) reported that local infusion of AP5 into the basolateral nucleus of the amygdala before training blocked conditioned freezing using context as the CS. This effect was highly localized, because infusion into the immediately adjacent central nucleus had no effect. AP5 also blocked the acquisition of freezing to a tone paired with shock (Lee and Kim, 1998). Infusion of NMDA antagonists into the amygdala consistently has been found not to block conditioned fear using fear-potentiated startle as a measure, whereas infusion of AP5 does block the expression of freezing conditioned to a context (Maren *et al.*, 1996b) or an explicit cue (Lee and Kim, 1998). This could indicate that cells in the amygdala that ultimately project to target areas involved in freezing have NMDA receptors, whereas those that project to target areas involved in potentiated startle do not. These are important observations because they indicate that fear-potentiated startle and conditioned freezing do not always correlate (e.g. Hunt *et al.*, 1994; McNish *et al.*, 1997), consistent with many observations made in our own laboratory.

Walker and Davis (1997) found that local infusion of 2,3-dihydroxy-6-nitro-7-sulphamoyl-benzo(F)-quinoxaline (NBQX) into either the central or basolateral nucleus blocked fear-potentiated startle. Infusion into the bed nucleus of the stria terminalis (BNST) did not. However, in another test sensitive to anxiolytic compounds, where startle amplitude is increased following exposure to a bright light that has never been paired with shock (light-enhanced startle), NBQX had no effect when infused into the central nucleus but did after infusion into either the basolateral nucleus or the BNST. This has led to the idea that aversive information can be relayed from the basolateral nucleus to either the central nucleus or the BNST, and that the central nucleus may be more involved with phasic or conditioned information whereas the BNST may be involved in more tonic or perhaps unconditioned information (Davis and Lee, 1997). In short, the central nucleus may be more involved in stimulus-specific fear, whereas the BNST may be more involved in something more akin to anxiety. Importantly, mechanical lesions of the central nucleus would interrupt fibres coming from the basolateral nucleus to the lateral division of the BNST. Hence, it is possible that many effects that have been seen following electrolytic or radiofrequency lesions of the central nucleus may be due to interruption of the connection between the basolateral nucleus and the BNST.

Prior exposure to stress has been shown to facilitate the development of eyeblink conditioning in rats (Shors *et al.*, 1992). Local infusion of AP5 into the basolateral but not the central nucleus of the amygdala 30 min prior to application of the stressor (tailshock) prevented this facilitatory effect (Shors and Mathew, 1998). Infusion 20 min after the stressor had no effect. Finally, Table 6.13 shows that either AP5 or CNQX appears to have anxiolytic effects in the social interaction test, risk assessment in the plus-maze and, as mentioned before, can reduce certain signs of opiate withdrawal.

6.8 Are aversive memories actually stored in the amygdala?

Since the description of patient H.M., who developed profound amnesia following bilateral resection of the medial temporal lobe including the hippocampus and the amygdala (Scoville and Milner, 1957), these structures have been studied extensively for their roles in learning and memory. A prominent effect of lesions of the hippocampal formation (i.e. the hippocampus proper and its surrounding cortices) is temporally graded memory impairment for premorbid information, i.e. recent memories are selectively impaired whereas remote memories remain intact (Squire, 1992). This temporal gradient of retrograde amnesia supports the idea of a gradual consolidation or reorganization of memory over time (McGaugh, 1966; Squire, 1992) in which memory is established temporarily in the hippocampal formation at the time of learning, but then gradually is established permanently somewhere else and thus becomes independent of the hippocampal formation (Squire, 1992; Zola-Morgan and Squire, 1990) .

Regarding the amygdala, Liang *et al.* (1982) showed that retention of an inhibitory avoidance response in rats was impaired when the amygdala was lesioned 2 but not 10 days after learning. In addition, infusion of a local anaesthetic, lidocaine, or the glutamate antagonist CNQX, into the amygdala 5 min before the retention test impaired inhibitory avoidance performance in rats when the retention test was given 1–5 days, but not 12 or 21 days, after learning (Liang, 1991, personal communication, April 29, 1993). These findings suggest that the amygdala, like the hippocampal formation, plays a temporally limited role in memory processing and is not the permanent memory storage site for an avoidance response (Liang *et al.*, 1982; McGaugh, 1989).

More recent studies appear to support this conclusion. For example, Parent *et al.* (1995b) found large deficits in retention or expression of inhibitory avoidance after neurotoxic lesions of the central, basolateral, or both amygdaloid nuclei. However, because 'the retention performance of rats given footshock during training was significantly better than that of rats that were not given footshock' the authors concluded that 'amygdala lesions impair processes that influence the expression, rather than the retention, of memory' (p. 806). In another study, Parent *et al.* (1995a) found that lesions of the basolateral amygdala caused a large deficit in inhibitory avoidance retention in rats that received either one or 10 training trials. However, when the rats were then trained on a continuous multiple trial inhibitory avoidance task in the same apparatus, escape latencies on the second acquisition trial were longer in the trained lesioned rats compared with untrained lesioned rats. The authors suggest that the footshock experienced in the second learning task facilitated the expression of memory in basolateral lesioned animals. Hence, they attribute the apparent lack of memory in the retention of the inhibitory avoidance task to a retrieval failure, thus failing to support the view that the basolateral amygdala permanently mediates changes induced by prior escape learning.

It is possible that a similar process might also operate with fear-potentiated startle following extensive pre-lesion training, because even large lesions of the amygdala did not prevent relearning of fear-potentiated startle (Kim and Davis, 1993a). Moreover, the rate of relearning was quite rapid, perhaps consistent with the idea that reintroduction of footshocks facilitated the expression of the original fear memory. Similar relearning effects after amygdala lesions have been seen using conditioned freezing which did not depend on the number of initial training trials (Maren, 1998). More recent studies showed relearning after electrolytic lesions of the central nucleus (Falls and Davis, 1995). However, in a subset of rats that also had damage to anterior aspects of the basolateral nucleus, reacquisition was not found.

Reacquisition of conditioned freezing was much more disrupted (although not fully so) in animals with complete neurotoxic lesions of the basolateral complex that included the most anterior part of the basolateral nucleus (Maren, 1998).

More recently, Vazdarjanova and McGaugh (1998) found that pre-training lesions of the basolateral amygdala blocked freezing. However, these lesioned animals entered less readily and less often and spent less time in the shock arm than did the control non-shocked lesioned rats. These findings were taken to indicate that an intact basolateral amygdala 'is not essential for the formation and expression of long-term cognitive/explicit memory of contextual fear conditioning' (p. 15003). On the other hand, the shocked basolateral lesioned rats still entered more quickly and more often, and spent more time in the shock arm than the shocked, sham-lesioned rats. This seems to indicate a partial blockade of the memory for the shock arm and raises the question of lesion completeness, especially because the lesions were done prior to training (see above).

It is important to emphasize that most of the theorizing that concludes that the amygdala modulates, but does not store aversive memories, is based on procedures that involve both classical and operant conditioning. For example, inhibitory avoidance involves both conditioned fear (i.e. fear of the place where shock was received) and operant behaviour (i.e. inhibition of the natural tendency to go from a lighted area to a dark area). Initially, fear may be required to motivate the operant behaviour. Later on, the operant behaviour may not depend on an antecedent level of fear. It is conceivable, therefore, that the fear memory is actually stored in the amygdala whereas the memory of the operant response is stored elsewhere. Lesions of the amygdala shortly after training would disrupt operant performance by disrupting the fear-motivating aspect in this test. However, once the memory of the operant response (avoid that place) becomes permanently established in some other structure, lesions of the amygdala would no longer have an effect.

This line of reasoning would predict that lesions of the amygdala would always block fear memories regardless of when they were made. In order to test this, groups of rats were trained for potentiated startle and then given lesions of the amygdala or sham lesions either 6 or 30 days after training (Kim and Davis, 1993b). Lesions of the amygdala completely blocked the expression of fear-potentiated startle when given either shortly or long after training. Hence, there was no evidence of a temporal gradient of conditioned fear after amygdala lesions compared with the temporal gradients reported in some inhibitory avoidance studies. Very similar results have now been reported using fibre-sparing lesions of the basolateral amygdala (Lee *et al.*, 1996; Maren *et al.*, 1996a). These data are at least consistent with the idea that the amygdala is the actual site of storage for conditioned fear memories. Clearly, however, other interpretations are equally plausible. Thus, the amygdala may simply be an obligatory part of a neural pathway that relays the fear memory from some other structure to brainstem sites involved in freezing and startle potentiation. Alternatively, the amygdala may play an obligatory permissive role in modulating the effects of fear memories relayed from some other structure to these brainstem sites. At any rate, it is clear that conditioned fear measured in this way differs considerably from that measured with inhibitory avoidance with respect to amygdala lesions, indicating that the two paradigms are measuring different aspects of an aversive experience.

In fact, it may be impossible ever to discover whether fear memories are actually stored in the amygdala because the amygdala is so critically involved in the expression of conditioned fear. Recently, it was reported that cells recorded in amygdala slices prepared 24 h after tone–shock conditioning showed altered input–output curves to stimulation of afferent roots from the medial geniculate (McKernan and Shinnick-Gallagher, 1997). Slices from animals in which the tone and shock were paired seemed to have increased synaptic strength compared with unpaired controls. Importantly, these slices were disconnected from most of the rest of the brain so that these changes in synaptic strength could not simply reflect transmission of information from more distance structures. If these experiments can be repeated when brains are prepared many weeks after training, this could provide conclusive evidence that long-term changes following fear conditioning are actually stored in the amygdala.

Acknowledgements

Research reported in this chapter was supported by NIMH Grant MH-25642, MH-47840, Research Scientist Development Award MH-00004, Emory University, and The Woodruff Foundation.

References

Adamec, R. (1997) Transmitter systems involved in neural plasticity underlying increased anxiety and defense—implications for understanding anxiety following traumatic stress. *Neuroscience and Biobehavioral Reviews*, 21, 755–765.

Adamec, R., Burton, P., Shallow, T., and Budgell, J. (1998) Unilateral block of NMDA receptors in the amygdala prevents predator stress-induced lasting increases in anxiety-like behavior and unconditioned startle—effective hemisphere depends on the behavior. *Physiology and Behavior*, 65, 739–751.

Adams, D.B. (1979) Brain mechanisms for offense, defense and submission. *Behavioral Brain Science*, 2, 201–241.

Aggleton, J.P. (1985) A description of intra-amygdaloid connections in the old world monkeys. *Experimental Brain Research*, 57, 390–399.

Ahn, D.K., Kim, Y.S. and Park, J.S. (1999) Central-amygdaloid carbachol suppressed nociceptive jaw opening reflex in freely moving rats. *Progress in Neuropsychopharmacology and Biological Psychiatry*, 23, 685–695.

al Maskati, H. and Zbrozyna, A. (1989) Cardiovascular and motor components of the defence reaction elicited in rats by electrical and chemical stimulation in amygdala. *Journal of the Autonomic Nervous System*, 28, 127–131.

Al-Rodhan, N., Chipkin, R., and Yaksh, T.L. (1990) The antinociceptive effects of SCH-32615, a neural endopeptidase (enkephalinase) inhibitor, microinjected into the periaqueductal gray, ventral medulla and amygdala. *Brain Research*, 520, 123–130.

Allen, J.P. and Allen, C.F. (1974) Role of the amygdaloid complexes in the stress-induced release of ACTH in the rat. *Neuroendocrinology*, 15, 220–230.

Allen, J.P. and Allen, C.F. (1975) Amygdalar participation in tonic ACTH secretion in the rat. *Neuroendocrinology*, 19, 115–125.

Altemus, M., Smith, M.A., Diep, V., Aulakh, C.S., and Murphy, D.L. (1995) Increased mRNA for corticotrophin releasing hormone in the amygdala of fawn-hooded rats: a potential animal model of anxiety. *Anxiety*, 1, 251–257.

Amaral, D. (1987) Memory: anatomical organization of candidate brain regions. In *Handbook of Physiology, Section 1: Neurophysiology. Vol. 5: Higher Functions of the Brain* (ed. F. Plum), pp. 211–294. American Physiological Society, Bethesda, Maryland.

Anand, B.K. and Dua, S. (1956) Circulatory and respiratory changes induced by electrical stimulation of limbic (visceral brain). *Journal of Neurophysiology*, 19, 393–400.

Applegate, C.D., Kapp, B.S., Underwood, M.D., and McNall, C.L. (1983) Autonomic and somatomotor effects of amygdala central n. stimulation in awake rabbits. *Physiology and Behavior*, 31, 353–360.

Aslan, N., Goren, Z., Onat, F., and Oktay, S. (1997a) Carbachol-induced pressor responses and muscarinic M1 receptors in the central nucleus of amygdala in conscious rats. *European Journal of Pharmacology*, 333, 63–67.

Aslan, N., Goren, Z., Ozkutlu, U., Onat, F., and Oktay, S. (1997b) Modification of the pressor response elicited by carbachol and electrical stimulation of the amygdala by muscarinic antagonists in conscious rats. *British Journal of Pharmacology*, 121, 35–40.

Aston-Jones, G., Ennis, M., Pieribone, V.A., Nickell, W.T., and Shipley, M.T. (1986) The brain nucleus locus coeruleus: restricted afferent control of a broad efferent network. *Science*, 234, 734–737.

Aston-Jones, G., Rajkowski, J., Kubiak, P., Valentino, R.J., and Shipley, M.T. (1996) Role of the locus coeruleus in emotional activation. *Progress in Brain Research*, 107, 379–402.

Bandler, R. and Carrive, P. (1988) Integrated defence reaction elicted by excitatory amino acid microinjection in the midbrain periaqueductal grey region of the unrestrained cat. *Brain Research*, 439, 95–106.

Bandler, R. and Depaulis, A. (1988) Elicitation of intraspecific defence reactions in the rat from midbrain periaqueductal grey by microinjection of kainic acid, without neurotoxic effects. *Neuroscience Letters*, 88, 291–296.

Bandler, R. and Shipley, M.T. (1994) Columnar organization in the midbrain periaqueductal gray: modules for emotional expression? *Trends in Neurosciences*, 17, 379–389.

Beaulieu, S., DiPaolo, T., and Barden, N. (1986) Control of ACTH secretion by central nucleus of the amygdala: implication of the serotonergic system and its relevance to the glucocorticoid delayed negative feed-back mechanism. *Neuroendocrinology*, 44, 247–254.

Beaulieu, S., DiPaolo, T., Cote, J., and Barden, N. (1987) Participation of the central amygdaloid nucleus in the response of adrenocorticotropin secretion to immobilization stress: opposing roles of the noradrenergic and dopaminergic systems. *Neuroendocrinology*, 45, 37–46.

Bechara, A., Tranel, D., Damasio, H., Adolphs, R., Rockland, C., and Damasio, A.R. (1995) Double dissociation of conditioning and declarative knowledge relative to the amygdala and hippocampus in humans. *Science*, 269, 1115–1118.

Beck, C.H.M. and Fibiger, H.C. (1995) Conditioned fear-induced changes in behavior and in the expression of the immediate early gene c-*fos*: with and without diazepam pretreatment. *Journal of Neuroscience*, 15, 709–720.

Beckstead, R.M., Domesick, V.B., and Nauta, W.J.H. (1979) Efferent connections of the substantia nigra and ventral tegmental area in the rat. *Brain Research*, 175, 191–217.

Beitz, A.J. (1982) The organization of afferent projections to the midbrain periaqueductal gray of the rat. *Neuroscience*, 7, 133–159.

Belcheva, I., Belcheva, S., Petkov, V.V., and Petkov, V.D. (1994) Asymmetry in behavioral responses to cholecystokinin microinjected into rat nucleus accumbens and amygdala. *Neuropharmacology*, 33, 995–1002.

Bellgowan, P.S.F. and Helmstetter, F.J. (1996) Neural systems for the expression of hypoalgesia during nonassociative fear. *Behavioral Neuroscience*, 110, 727–736.

Benjamin, D., Emmett-Oglesby, M.W., and Lah, H. (1987) Modulation of the discriminative stimulus produced by pentylenetetrazol by centrally administered drugs. *Neuropharmacology*, 26, 1727–1731.

Bennett, C., Liang, K.C., and McGaugh, J.L. (1985) Depletion of adrenal catecholamines alters the amnestic effect of amygdala stimulation. *Behavioral Brain Research*, 15, 83–91.

Blanchard, D.C. and Blanchard, R.J. (1972) Innate and conditioned reactions to threat in rats with amygdaloid lesions. *Journal of Comparative Physiology and Psychology*, 81, 281–290.

Blanchard, D.C., Williams, G., Lee, E.M.C., and Blanchard, R.J. (1981) Taming of wild *Rattus norvegicus* by lesions of the mesencephalic central gray. *Physiology and Psychology*, 9, 157–163.

Boadle-Biber, M.C., Singh, V.B., Corley, K.C., Phan, T.H., and Dilts, R.P. (1993) Evidence that corticotropin-releasing factor within the extended amygdala mediates the activation of tryptophan hydroxylase produced by sound stress in the rat. *Brain Research*, 628, 105–114.

Bolhuis, J.J., Fitzgerald, R.E., Dijk, D.J., and Koolhaas, J.M. (1984) The corticomedial amygdala and learning in an agonistic situation. *Physiology and Behavior*, 32, 575–579.

Bonvallet, M. and GaryBobo, E. (1972) Changes in phrenic activity and heart rate elicited by localized stimulation of the amygdala and adjacent structures. *Electroencephalography and Clinical Neurophysiology*, 32, 1–16.

Bonvallet, M. and GaryBobo, E. (1975) Amygdala and masseteric reflex. II. Mechanism of the diphasic modifications of the reflex elicited from the 'Defence Reaction Area'. Role of the spinal trigeminal nucleus (pars oralis). *Electroencephalography and Clinical Neurophysiology*, 39, 341–352.

Borszcz, G.S. (1995) Increases in vocalization and motor reflex thresholds are influenced by the site of morphine microinjection: comparisons following administration into the periaqueductal gray, ventral medulla and spinal subarachnoid space. *Behavioral Neuroscience*, 109, 502–522.

Borszcz, G.S., Cranney, J., and Leaton, R.N. (1989) Influence of long-term sensitization on long-term habituation of the acoustic startle response in rats: central gray lesions, preexposure and extinction. *Journal of Experimental Psychology—Animal Behavior Processes*, 15, 54–64.

Borszcz, G.S., Johnson, C.P., and Thorp, M.V. (1996) The differential contribution of spinopetal projections to increases in vocalization and motor reflex thresholds generated by the microinjection of morphine into the periaqueductal gray. *Behavioral Neuroscience*, 110, 368–388.

Bresnahan, E. and Routtenberg, A. (1972) Memory disruption by unilateral low level, sub-seizure stimulation of the medial amygdaloid nucleus. *Physiology and Behavior*, 9, 513–525.

Brown, M.R. and Gray, T.S. (1988) Peptide injections into the amygdala of conscious rats: effects on blood pressure, heart rate and plasma catecholamines. *Regulatory Peptides*, 21, 95–106.

Burwell, R.D., Witter, M.P., and Amaral, D.G. (1995) Perirhinal and postrhinal cortices of the rat: a review of the neuroanatomical literature and comparison with findings from the monkey brain. *Hippocampus*, 5, 390–408.

Cahill, L. and McGaugh, J.L. (1990) Amygdaloid complex lesions differentially affect retention of tasks using appetitive and aversive reinforcement. *Behavioral Neuroscience*, 104, 532–543.

Calvino, B., Lagowska, J., and Ben-Ari, Y. (1979) Morphine withdrawal syndrome: differential participation of structures located within the amygdaloid complex and striatum of the rat. *Brain Research*, 177, 19–34.

Campeau, S. and Davis, M. (1995) Involvement of the central nucleus and basolateral complex of the amygdala in fear conditioning measured with fear-potentiated startle in rats trained concurrently with auditory and visual conditioned stimuli. *Journal of Neuroscience*, 15, 2301–2311.

Campeau, S., Hayward, M.D., Hope, B.T., Rosen, J.B., Nestler, E.J., and Davis, M. (1991) Induction of the c-*fos* proto-oncogene in rat amygdala during unconditioned and conditioned fear. *Brain Research*, 565, 349–352.

Campeau, S., Miserendino, M.J.D., and Davis, M. (1992) Intra-amygdala infusion of the *N*-methyl-D-aspartate receptor antagonist AP5 blocks acquisition but not expression of fear-potentiated startle to an auditory conditioned stimulus. *Behavioral Neuroscience*, 106, 569–574.

Campeau, S., Falls, W.A., Cullinan, W.E., Helmreich, D.L., Davis, M., and Watson, S.J. (1997) Elicitation and reduction of fear: behavioral and neuroendocrine indices and brain induction of the immediate-early gene c-*fos*. *Neuroscience*, 78, 1087–1104.

Canli, T. and Brown, T.H. (1996) Amygdala stimulation enhances the rat eyeblink reflex through a short-latency mechanism. *Behavioral Neuroscience*, 110, 51–59.

Cassell, M.D. and Gray, T.S. (1989) The amygdala directly innervates adrenergic (C1) neurons in the ventrolateral medulla. *Neuroscience Letters*, 97, 163–168.

Cedarbaum, J.M. and Aghajanian, G.K. (1978) Afferent projections to the rat locus coeruleus as determined by a retrograde tracing technique. *Journal of Comparative Neurology*, 178, 1–16.

Chachich, M. and Powell, D.A. (1998) Both medial prefrontal and amygdala central nucleus lesions abolish heart rate classical conditioning, but only prefrontal lesions impair reversal of eyeblink differential conditioning. *Neuroscience Letters*, 257, 151–154.

Champagne, D., Beaulieu, J., and Drolet, G. (1998) CRFergic innervation of the paraventricular nucleus of the rat hypothalamus: a tract-tracing study. *Journal of Neuroendocrinology*, 10, 119–131.

Chapman, P.F. and Bellavance, L.L. (1992) Induction of long-term potentiation in the basolateral amygdala does not depend on NMDA receptor activation. *Synapse*, 11, 310–318.

Chapman, P.F., Kairiss, E.W., Keenan, C.L., and Brown, T.H. (1990) Long-term synaptic potentiation in the amygdala. *Synapse*, 6, 271–278.

Chapman, W.P., Schroeder, H.R., Guyer, G., Brazier, M.A.B., Fager, C., Poppen, J.L., Solomon, H.C., and Yakolev, P.I. (1954) Physiological evidence concerning the importance of the amygdaloid nuclear region in the integration of circulating function and emotion in man. *Science*, 129, 949–950.

Ciriello, J. and Roder, S., (1998) GABAergic effects on the depressor responses elicited by stimulation of central nucleus of the amygdala. *American Journal of Physiology—Heart and Circulatory Physiology*, 45, H242–H247.

Clugnet, M.C. and LeDoux, J.E. (1990) Synaptic plasticity in fear conditioning circuits: induction of LTP in the lateral nucleus of the amygdala by stimulation of the medial geniculate body. *Journal of Neuroscience*, 10, 2818–2824.

Cohen, D.H. (1975) Involvement of the avian amygdala homologue (archistriatum posterior and mediale) in defensively conditioned heart rate change. *Journal of Comparative Neurology*, 160, 13–36.

Coover, G.D., Murison, R., and Jellestad, F.K. (1992) Subtotal lesions of the amygdala: the rostral central nucleus in passive avoidance and ulceration. *Physiology and Behavior*, 51, 795–803.

Costall, B., Kelly, M.E., Naylor, R.J., Onaivi, E.S., and Tyers, M.B. (1989) Neuroanatomical sites of action of 5-HT_3 receptor agonist and antagonists for alteration of aversive behaviour in the mouse. *British Journal of Pharmacology*, 96, 325–332.

Costall, B., Jones, B.J., Kelly, M.E., Naylor, R.J., Onaivi, E.S., and Tyers, M.B. (1990) Sites of action of ondasetron to inhibit withdrawal from drugs of abuse. *Pharmacology, Biochemistry, and Behavior*, 36, 97–104.

Cousens, G. and Otto, T. (1998) Both pre- and posttraining excitotoxic lesions of the basolateral amygdala abolish the expression of olfactory and contextual fear conditioning. *Behavioral Neuroscience*, 112, 1092–1103.

Cox, G., Jordan, D., Moruzz, P., Schwaber, J., Spyer, K., and Turner, S. (1986) Amygdaloid influences on brain-stem neurones in the rabbit. *Journal of Physiology*, 381, 135–148.

Cox, G.E., Jordan, D., Paton, J.F.R., Spyer, K.M., and Wood, L.M. (1987) Cardiovascular and phrenic nerve responses to stimulation of the amygdala central nucleus in the unanesthetized rabbit. *Journal of Physiology (London)*, 389, 541–556.

Crandall, P.H., Walter, R.D., and Dymond, A. (1971) The ictal electroencephalographic signal identifying limbic system seizure foci. *Proceedings of the American Association of Neurological Surgery*, 1, 1.

Cratty, M.S., Ward, H.E., Johnson, E.A., Azzaro, A.J., and Birkle, D.L. (1995) Prenatal stress increases corticotropin-releasing factor (CRF) content and release in rat amygdala minces. *Brain Research*, 675, 297–302.

Cullinan, W.E., Herman, J.P., and Watson, S.J. (1993) Ventral subicular interaction with the hypothalamic paraventricular nucleus: evidence for a relay in the bed nucleus of the stria terminalis. *Journal of Comparative Neurology*, 332, 1–20.

Dafters, R.I. (1976) Effect of medial archistriatal lesions on the conditioned emotional response and on auditory discrimination performance of the pigeon. *Physiology and Behavior*, 17, 659–665.

Davis, M. (1992) The role of the amygdala in fear and anxiety. *Annual Review of Neuroscience*, 15, 353–375.

Davis, M. (1994) The role of the amygdala in emotional learning. *International Journal of Neurobiology*, 36, 225–266.

Davis, M. (1997) Neurobiology of fear responses: the role of the amygdala. *Journal of Neuropsychiatry and Clinical Neurosciences*, 9, 382–402.

Davis, M. and Lee, Y. (1997) Fear and anxiety: possible roles of the amygdala and bed nucleus of the stria terminalis. *Cognition and Emotion*, 11, 277–306.

Davis, M., Hitchcock, J.M., Bowers, M.B., Berridge, C.W., Melia, K.R., and Roth, R.H. (1994) Stress-induced activation of prefrontal cortex dopamine turnover: blockade by lesions of the amygdala. *Brain Research*, 664, 207–210.

Dayas, C.V., Buller, K.M., and Day, T.A. (1999) Neuroendocrine responses to an emotional stressor: evidence for involvement of the medial but not the central amygdala. *European Journal of Neuroscience*, 11, 2312–2322.

de Fonseca, F.R., Carrera, M.R., Navarro, M., Koob, G.F., and Weiss, F. (1997) Activation of corticotropin-releasing factor in the limbic system during cannabinoid withdrawal. *Science*, 276, 2050–2054.

Deakin, J.W.F. and Graeff, F.G. (1991) 5-HT and mechanisms of defence. *Journal of Psychopharmacology*, 5, 305–315.

Deboer, T., Sanford, L.D., Ross, R.J., and Morrison, A.R. (1998) Effects of electrical stimulation in the amygdala on ponto-geniculo-occipital waves in rats. *Brain Research*, 793, 305–310.

DeOlmos, J., Alheid, G.F., and Beltramino, C.A. (1985) Amygdala. In *The Rat Nervous System*, Vol. 1 (ed. G. Paxinos), pp. 223–334. Academic Press, Orlando, Florida.

Desmedt, A., Garcia, R., and Jaffard, R. (1998) Differential modulation of changes in hippocampal–septal synaptic excitability by the amygdala as a function of either elemental or contextual fear conditioning in mice. *Neuroscience*, 18, 480–487.

DeSouza, E.B., Insel, T.R., Perrin, M.H., Rivier, J., Vale, W.W., and Kuhar, M.J. (1985) Corticotropin-releasing factor receptors are widely distributed within the rat central nervous system: an autoradiographic study. *Journal of Neuroscience*, 5, 3189–3203.

Deutch, A.Y., Goldstein, M., and Roth, R.H. (1986) Activation of the locus coeruleus induced by selective stimulation of the ventral tegmental area. *Brain Research*, 363, 307–314.

Dringenberg, H.C. and Vanderwolf, C.H. (1996) Cholinergic activation of the electrocorticogram: an amygdaloid activating system. *Experimental Brain Research*, 108, 285–296.

Dringenberg, H.C., Kornelsen, R.A., Pacelli, R., Petersen, K., and Vanderwolf, C.H. (1998) Effects of amygdaloid lesions, hippocampal lesions and buspirone on black–white exploration and food carrying in rats. *Behavioural Brain Research*, 96, 161–172.

Dunn, J.D. and Whitener, J. (1986) Plasma corticosterone responses to electrical stimulation of the amygdaloid complex: cytoarchitectural specificity. *Neuroendocrinology*, 42, 211–217.

Dunn, L.T. and Everitt, B.J. (1988) Double dissociations of the effects of amygdala and insular cortex lesions on conditioned taste aversion, passive avoidance and neophobia in the rat using the excitotoxin ibotenic acid. *Behavioral Neuroscience*, 102, 3–23.

Ellis, M.E. and Kesner, R.P. (1983) The noradrenergic system of the amygdala and aversive information processing. *Behavioral Neuroscience*, 97, 399–415.

Falls, W.A. and Davis, M. (1995) Lesions of the central nucleus of the amygdala block conditioned excitation, but not conditioned inhibition of fear as measured with the fear-potentiated startle effect. *Behavioral Neuroscience*, 109, 379–387.

Fanardjian, V.V. and Manvelyan, L.R. (1987) Mechanisms regulating the activity of facial nucleus motoneurons. III. Synaptic influences from the cerebral cortex and subcortical structures. *Neuroscience*, 20, 835–843.

Fanselow, M.S. (1986) Conditioned fear-induced analgesia: a competing motivational state theory of stress-analgesia. *Annals of the New York Academy of Sciences*, 102, 467.

Fanselow, M.S. (1991) The midbrain periaqueductal gray as a coordinator of action in response to fear and anxiety. In *The Midbrain Periaqueductal Gray Matter: Functional, Anatomical and Neurochemical Organization* (eds A. Depaulis and R. Bandler), pp. 151–173. Plenum Publishing Co., New York.

Fanselow, M.S. and Helmstetter, F.J. (1988) Conditioned analgesia, defensive freezing and benzodiazepines. *Behavioral Neuroscience*, 102, 233–243.

Fanselow, M.S. and Kim, J.J. (1994) Acquisition of contextual Pavlovian fear conditioning is blocked by application of an NMDA receptor antagonist D,L-2-amino-5-phosphonovaleric acid to the basolateral amygdala. *Behavioral Neuroscience*, 108, 210–212.

Feldman, S. and Conforti, N. (1981) Amygdalectomy inhibits adrenocortical responses to somatosensory and olfactory stimulation. *Neuroendocrinology*, 32, 330–334.

Feldman, S. and Weidenfeld, J. (1996) Involvement of amygdalar alpha adrenoceptors in hypothalamo-pituitary–adrenocortical responses. *NeuroReport*, 7, 3055–3057.

Feldman, S. and Weidenfeld, J. (1998) The excitatory effects of the amygdala on hypothalamo-pituitary–adrenocortical responses are mediated by hypothalamic norepinephrine, serotonin and CRF-41. *Brain Research Bulletin*, 45, 389–393.

Feldman, S., Conforti, N., and Saphier, D. (1990) The preoptic area and bed nucleus of the stria terminalis are involved in the effects of the amygdala on adrenocortical secretion. *Neuroscience*, 37, 775–779.

Feldman, S., Conforti, N., and Siegal, R.A. (1982) Adrenocortical responses following limbic stimulation in rats with hypothalamic deafferentations. *Neuroendocrinology*, 35, 205–211.

Feldman, S., Conforti, N., Itzik, A., and Weidenfeld, J. (1994) Differential effect of amygdaloid lesions on CRF-41, ACHT and corticosterone responses following neural stimuli. *Brain Research*, 658, 21–26.

Feldman, S., Newman, M.E., Gur, E., and Weidenfeld, J. (1998) Role of serotonin in the amygdala in hypothalamo-pituitary-adrenocortical responses. *NeuroReport*, 9, 2007–2009.

Fendt, M., Koch, M., and Schnitzler, H.-U. (1994a) Lesions of the central grey block sensitization and fear potentiation of the acoustic startle response in rats. *Society for Neuroscience Abstracts*, 20, 1954.

Fendt, M., Koch, M., and Schnitzler, H.U. (1994b) Amygdaloid noradrenaline is involved in the sensitization of the acoustic startle response in rats. *Pharmacology, Biochemistry, and Behavior*, 48, 307–314.

File, S.E. (1990) One-trial tolerance to the anxiolytic effects of chlordiazepoxide in the plus-maze. *Psychopharmacology*, 100, 281–282.

File, S.E. and Rodgers, R.J. (1979) Partial anxiolytic actions of morphine sulphate following microinjection into the central nucleus of the amygdala in rats. *Pharmacology, Biochemistry, and Behavior*, 11, 313–318.

File, S.E., Gonzalez, L.E., and Gallant, R. (1998) Role of the basolateral nucleus of the amygdala in the formation of a phobia. *Neuropsychopharmacology*, 19, 397–405.

Fox, R.J. and Sorenson, C.A. (1994) Bilateral lesions of the amygdala attenuate analgesia induced by diverse environmental challenges. *Brain Research*, 648, 215–221.

Frankland, P.W., Josselyn, S.A., Bradwejn, J., Vaccarino, F.J., and Yeomans, J.S. (1997) Activation of amygdala cholecystokininB receptors potentiates the acoustic startle response in the rat. *Journal of Neuroscience*, 17, 1838–1847.

Frysinger, R.C., Marks, J.D., Trelease, R.B., Schechtman, V.L., and Harper, R.M. (1984) Sleep states attenuate the pressor response to central amygdala stimulation. *Experimental Neurology*, 83, 604–617.

Gabr, R.W., Birkle, D.L., and Azzaro, A.J. (1995) Stimulation of the amygdala by glutamate facilitates corticotropin-releasing factor release from the median eminence and activation of the hypothalamic–pituitary–adrenal axis in stressed rats. *Neuroendocrinology*, 62, 333–339.

Galeno, T.M. and Brody, M.J. (1983) Hemodynamic responses to amygdaloid stimulation in spontaneously hypertensive rats. *American Journal of Physiology*, 245, 281–286.

Galeno, T.M., VanHoesen, G.W., and Brody, M.J. (1984) Central amygdaloid nucleus lesion attenuates exaggerated hemodynamic responses to noise stress in the spontaneously hypertensive rat. *Brain Research*, 291, 249–259.

Gallagher, M. and Kapp, B.S. (1978) Manipulation of opiate activity in the amygdala alters memory processes. *Life Sciences*, 23, 1973–1978.

Gallagher, M. and Kapp, B.S. (1981) Effect of phentolamine administration into the amygdala complex of rats on time-dependent memory processes. *Behavioral and Neural Biology*, 31, 90–95.

Gallagher, M., Kapp, B.S., Frysinger, R.C., and Rapp, P.R. (1980) β-Adrenergic manipulation in amygdala central n. alters rabbit heart rate conditioning. *Pharmacology, Biochemistry, and Behavior*, 12, 419–426.

Gallagher, M., Kapp, B.S., McNall, C.L., and Pascoe, J.P. (1981) Opiate effects in the amygdala central nucleus on heart rate conditioning in rabbits. *Pharmacology, Biochemistry, and Behavior*, 14, 497–505.

Gallagher, M., Kapp, B.S. and Pascoe, J.P. (1982) Enkephalin analogue effects in the amygdala central nucleus on conditioned heart rate. *Pharmacology, Biochemistry, and Behavior*, 17, 217–222.

Gargiulo, P.A., Viana, M.B., Graeff, F.G., Silva, M.A., and Tomaz, C. (1996) Effects of anxiety and memory of systemic and intra-amygdala injection of 5-HT_3 receptor antagonist BRL 46470A. *Neuropsychobiology*, 33, 189–195.

GaryBobo, E. and Bonvallet, M. (1975) Amygdala and masseteric reflex. I. Facilitation, inhibition and diphasic modifications of the reflex, induced by localized amygdaloid stimulation. *Electroencephalography and Clinical Neurophysiology*, 39, 329–339.

Gean, P.W., Chang, F.C., Huang, C.C., Lin, J.H., and Way, L.J. (1993) Long-term enhancement of EPSP and NMDA receptor-mediated synaptic transmission in the amygdala. *Brain Research Bulletin*, 31, 7–11.

Gelsema, A.J., McKitrick, D.J., and Calaresu, F.R. (1987) Cardiovascular responses to chemical and electrical stimulation of amygdala in rats. *American Journal of Physiology*, 253, 712–718.

Gelsema, A.J., Agarwal, S.K., and Calaresu, F.R. (1989) Cardiovascular responses and changes in neural activity in the rostral ventrolateral medulla elicited by electrical stimulation of the amygdala of the rat. *Journal of the Autonomic Nervous System*., 27, 91–100.

Gentile, C.G., Jarrel, T.W., Teich, A., McCabe, P.M., and Schneiderman, N. (1986) The role of amygdaloid central nucleus in the retention of differential pavlovian conditioning of bradycardia in rabbits. *Behavioral Brain Research*, 20, 263–273.

Gewirtz, J. and Davis, M. (1997) Second order fear conditioning prevented by blocking NMDA receptors in the amygdala. *Nature*, 388, 471–474.

Gloor, P. (1960) Amygdala. In *Handbook of Physiology: Section I. Neurophysiology* (ed. J. Field), pp. 1395–1420. American Physiological Society, Washington, DC.

Gloor, P. (1978) Inputs and outputs of the amygdala: what the amygdala is trying to tell the rest of the brain. In *Limbic Mechanisms: The Continuing Evolution of the Limbic System Concept* (eds K. Livingston and and K. Hornykiewicz), pp. 189–209. Plenum Press, New York.

Gloor, P. (1992) Role of the amygdala in temporal lobe epilepsy. In *The Amygdala: Neurobiological Aspects of Emotion, Memory, and Mental Dysfunction* (ed. J.P. Aggleton), pp. 505–538. Wiley-Liss, New York.

Gloor, P., Olivier, A., and Quesney, L.F. (1981) The role of the amygdala in the expression of psychic phenomena in temporal lobe seizures. In *The Amygdaloid Complex* (ed. Y. Ben-Ari), pp. 489–507. Elsevier/North Holland, New York.

Goddard, G.V. (1964) Functions of the amygdala. *Psychological Bulletin*, 62, 89–109.

Gold, P.E., Hankins, L., Edwards, R.M., Chester, J., and McGaugh, J.L. (1975) Memory inference and facilitation with post-trial amygdala stimulation: effect varies with footshock level. *Brain Research*, 86, 509–513.

Goldstein, L.E., Rasmusson, A.M., Bunney, B.S., and Roth, R.H. (1996) Role of the amygdala in the coordination of behavioral, neuroendocrine and prefrontal cortical monoamine responses to psychological stress in the rat. *Journal of Neuroscience*, 16, 4787–4798.

Good, A.J. and Westbrook, R.F. (1995) Effects of a microinjection of morphine into the amygdala on the acquisition and expression of conditioned fear and hypoalgesia in rats. *Behavioral Neuroscience*, 109, 631–641.

Goodman, R.R., Snyder, S.H., Kuhar, M.J., and Young, W.S.I. (1980) Differential of delta and mu opiate receptor localizations by light microscopic autoradiography. *Proceedings of the National Academy of Sciences of the United States of America*, 77, 2167–2174.

Graeff, F.G. (1988) Animal models of aversion. In *Selected Models of Anxiety, Depression and Psychosis*,Vol. 1 (eds P. Simon, P. Soubrie and D. Wildlocher), pp. 115–141. Karger, Basel, Switzerland.

Graeff, F.G., Silveira, M.C.L., Nogueira, R.L., Audi, E.A., and Oliveira, R.M.W. (1993) Role of the amygdala and periaqueductal gray in anxiety and panic. *Behavioral Brain Research*, 58, 123–131.

Graeff, F.G., Viana, M.B., and Mora, P.O. (1997) Dual role of 5-HT in defense and anxiety. *Neuroscience and Biobehavioral Reviews*, 21, 791–799.

Gray, T.S. (1989) Autonomic neuropeptide connections of the amygdala. In *Neuropeptides and Stress*, Vol. 1 (eds Y. Tache, J.E. Morley and M.R. Brown), pp. 92–106. Springer Verlag, New York.

Gray, T.S. and Magnusson, D.J. (1987) Neuropeptide neuronal efferents from the bed nucleus of the stria terminalis and central amygdaloid nucleus to the dorsal vagal complex in the rat. *Journal of Comparative Neurology*, 262, 365–374.

Gray, T.S., Carney, M.E., and Magnuson, D.J. (1989) Direct projections from the central amygdaloid nucleus to the hypothalamic paraventricular nucleus: possible role in stress-induced adrenocorticotropin release. *Neuroendocrinology*, 50, 433–446.

Green, S. and Vale, A.L. (1992) Role of amygdaloid nuclei in the anxiolytic effects of benzodiazepines in rats. *Behavioural Pharmacology*, 3, 261–264.

Grijalva, C.V., Levin, E.D., Morgan, M., Roland, B., and Martin, F.C. (1990) Contrasting effects of centromedial and basolateral amygdaloid lesions on stress-related responses in the rat. *Physiology and Behavior*, 48, 495–500.

Grossman, S.P., Grossman, L., and Walsh, L. (1975) Functional organization of the rat amygdala with respect to avoidance behavior. *Journal of Comparative Physiology and Psychology*, 88, 829–850.

Grove, E.A. (1988) Efferent connections of the substantia innominata in the rat. *Journal of Comparative Neurology*, 277, 347–364.

Guarraci, F.A., Frohardt, R.J., and Kapp, B.S., (1999) Amygdaloid D1 dopamine receptor involvement in Pavlovian fear conditioning. *Brain Research*, 827, 28–40.

Gue, M., Tekamp, A., Tabis, N., Junien, J.L., and Bueno, L. (1994) Cholecystokinin blockade of emotional stress- and CRF-induced colonic motor alterations in rats: role of the amygdala. *Brain Research*, 658, 232–238.

Hagan, R.M., Jones, B.J., Jordan, C.C., and Tyers, M.B. (1990) Effect of 5-HT-3 receptor antagonists on responses to selective activation of mesolimbic dopaminergic pathways in the rat. *British Journal of Pharmacology*, 99, 227–232.

Hammer, G.D. and Kapp, B.S. (1986) The effects of naloxone administered into the periaqueductal gray on shock-elicited freezing behavior in the rat. *Behavioral and Neural Biology*, 46, 189–195.

Handwerker, M.J., Gold, P.E., and McGaugh, J.L. (1974) Impairment of active avoidance learning with posttraining amygdala stimulation. *Brain Research*, 75, 324–327.

Harper, R.M., Frysinger, R.C., Trelease, R.B., and Marks, J.D. (1984) State-dependent alteration of respiratory cycle timing by stimulation of the central nucleus of the amygdala. *Brain Research*, 306, 1–8.

Harris, J.A. (1996) Descending antinociceptive mechanisms in the brainstem: their role in the animal's defensive system. *Journal of Physiology (Paris)*, 90, 15–25.

Harris, J.A. and Westbrook, R.F. (1995) Effects of benzodiazepine microinjection into the amygdala or periaqueductal gray on the expression of conditioned fear and hypoalgesia in rats. *Behavioral Neuroscience*, 109, 295–304.

Harris, J.A. and Westbrook, R.F. (1998) Benzodiazepine-induced amnesia in rats: reinstatement of conditioned performance by noxious stimulation on test. *Behavioral Neuroscience*, 112, 183–192.

Healy, B. and Peck, J. (1997) Bradycardia induced from stimulation of the left versus right central nucleus of the amygdala. *Epilepsy Research*, 28, 101–104.

Heilig, M. (1995) Antisense inhibition of neuropeptide Y (NPY)-Y1 receptor expression blocks the anxiolytic-like action of NPY in amygdala and paradoxically increases feeding. *Regulatory Peptides*, 59, 201–205.

Heilig, M., McLeod, S., Brot, M., Henrichs, S.C., Menzaghi, F., Koob, G.F., and Britton, K.T. (1993) Anxiolytic-like action of neuropeptide Y: mediation by Y1 receptors in amygdala and dissociation from food intake effects. *Neuropsychopharmacology*, 8, 357–363.

Heinemann, W., Stock, G., and Schaeffer, H. (1973) Temporal correlation of responses in blood pressure and motor reaction under electrical stimulation of limbic structures in the unanesthetized unrestrained cat. *Pflugers Archives of General Physiology*, 343, 27–40.

Heinrichs, S.C., Pich, E.M., Miczek, K.A., Britton, K.T., and Koob, G.F. (1992) Corticotropin-releasing factor antagonist reduces emotionality in socially defeated rats via direct neurotropic action. *Brain Research*, 581, 190–197.

Heinrichs, S.C., Menzaghi, F., Schulteis, G., Koob, G.F., and Stinus, L. (1995) Suppression of corticotropoin-releasing factor in the amygdala attenuates aversive consequences of morphine withdrawal. *Behavioural Pharmacology*, 6, 74–80.

Helmstetter, F.J. (1992a) The amygdala is essential for the expression of conditioned hypoalgesia. *Behavioral Neuroscience*, 106, 518–528.

Helmstetter, F.J. (1992b) Contribution of the amygdala to learning and performance of conditional fear. *Physiology and Behavior*, 51, 1271–1276.

Helmstetter, F.J. (1993) Stress-induced hypoalgesia and defensive freezing are attenuated by application of diazepam to the amygdala. *Pharmacology, Biochemistry, and Behavior*, 44, 433–438.

Helmstetter, F.J. and Bellgowan, P.S. (1993) Lesions of the amygdala block conditioned hypoalgesia on the tail flick test. *Brain Research*, 612, 253–257.

Helmstetter, F.J. and Bellgowan, P.S. (1994) Effects of muscimol applied to the basolateral amygdala on acquisition and expression of contextual fear conditioning in rats. *Behavioral Neuroscience*, 108, 1005–1009.

Helmstetter, F.J. and Tershner, S.A. (1994) Lesions of the periaqueductal gray and rostral ventromedial medulla disrupt antinociceptive but not cardiovascular aversive conditional responses. *Journal of Neuroscience*, 14, 7099–7108.

Helmstetter, F.J., Bellgowan, P.S., and Tershner, S.A. (1993) Inhibition of the tail flick reflex follwing microinjection of morphine into the amygdala. *NeuroReport*, 4, 471–474.

Helmstetter, F.J., Bellgowan, P.S.F., and Poore, L.H. (1995) Microinfusion of mu but not delta or kappa opioid agonists into the basolateral amygdala results in inhibition of the tail flick reflex in pentobarbital-anesthetized rats. *Journal of Pharmacology and Experimental Therapeutics*, 275, 381–388.

Helmstetter, F.J., Tershner, S.A., Poore, L.H., and Bellgowan, P.S.F. (1998) Antinociception following opioid stimulation of the basolateral amygdala is expressed through the periaqueductal gray and rostral ventromedial medulla. *Brain Research*, 779, 104–118.

Henke, P.G. (1980a) The amygdala and restraint ulcers in rats. *Journal of Comparative Physiology and Psychology*, 94, 313–323.

Henke, P.G. (1980b) The centromedial amygdala and gastric pathology in rats. *Physiology and Behavior*, 25, 107–112.

Henke, P.G. (1980c) Facilitation and inhibition of gastric pathology after lesions in the amygdala in rats. *Physiology and Behavior*, 25, 575–579.

Henke, P.G. (1981) Attenuation of shock-induced ulcers after lesions in the medial amygdala. *Physiology and Behavior*, 27, 143–146.

Henke, P.G. (1988) Electrophysiological activity in the central nucleus of the amygdala: emotionality and stress ulcers in rats. *Behavioral Neuroscience*, 102, 77–83.

Hernandez, D.E., Salaiz, A.B., Morin, P., and Moreira, M.A. (1990) Administration of thyrotropin-releasing hormone into the central nucleus of the amygdala induces gastric lesions in rats. *Brain Research Bullentin*, 24, 697–699.

Higgins, G.A., Jones, B.J., Oakley, N.R., and Tyers, M.B. (1991) Evidence that the amygdala is involved in the disinhibitory effects of 5-HT_3 receptor antagonists. *Psychopharmacology*, 104, 545–551.

Hilton, S.M. and Zbrozyna, A.W. (1963) Amygdaloid region for defense reactions and its efferent pathway to the brainstem. *Journal of Physiology (London)*, 165, 160–173.

Hitchcock, J.M. and Davis, M. (1986) Lesions of the amygdala, but not of the cerebellum or red nucleus, block conditioned fear as measured with the potentiated startle paradigm. *Behavioral Neuroscience*, 100, 11–22.

Hitchcock, J.M. and Davis, M. (1987) Fear-potentiated startle using an auditory conditioned stimulus: effect of lesions of the amygdala. *Physiology and Behavior*, 39, 403–408.

Hitchcock, J.M. and Davis, M. (1991) The efferent pathway of the amygdala involved in conditioned fear as measured with the fear-potentiated startle paradigm. *Behavioral Neuroscience*, 105, 826–842.

Hitchcock, J.M., Sananes, C.B., and Davis, M. (1989) Sensitization of the startle reflex by footshock: blockade by lesions of the central nucleus of the amygdala or its efferent pathway to the brainstem. *Behavioral Neuroscience*, 103, 509–518.

Hodges, H., Green, S., and Glenn, B. (1987) Evidence that the amygdala is involved in benzodiazepine and serotonergic effects on punished responding but not on discrimination. *Psychopharmacology*, 92, 491–504.

Holmes, P.V. and Drugan, R.C. (1993) Amygdaloid central nucleus lesions and cholinergic blockade attenuate the response of the renal peripheral benzodiazepine receptor to stress. *Brain Research*, 621, 1–9.

Holstege, G., Kuypers, H.G.J.M., and Dekker, J.J. (1977) The organization of the bulbar fibre connections to the trigeminal, facial and hypoglossal motor nuclei. II. An autoradiographic tracing study in cat. *Brain*, 100, 265–286.

Hopkins, D.A. and Holstege, G. (1978) Amygdaloid projections to the mesencephalon, pons and medulla oblongata in the cat. *Experimental Brain Research*, 32, 529–547.

Huang, Y.Y. and Kandel, E.R. (1998) Postsynaptic induction and PKA-dependent expression of LTP in the lateral amygdala. *Neuron*, 21, 169–178.

Hunt, P.S., Richardson, R., and Campbell, B.A. (1994) Delayed development of fear-potentiated startle in rats. *Behavioral Neuroscience*, 108, 69–80.

Huston, J.P., Schildein, S., Gerhardt, P., Privou, C., Fink, H., and Hasenohrl, R.U. (1998) Modulation of memory, reinforcement and anxiety parameters by intra-amygdala injection of cholecystokinin-fragments Boc-CCK-4 and CCK-8s. *Peptides*, 19, 27–37.

Inagaki, S., Kawai, Y., Matsuzaki, T., Shiosaka, S., and Tohyama, M. (1983) Precise terminal fields of the descending somatostatinergic neuron system from the amygdala complex of the rat. *Journal für Hirnforschung*, 24, 345–365.

Innes, D.L. and Tansy, M.F. (1980) Gastric mucosal ulceration associated with electrochemical stimulation of the limbic system. *Brain Research Bulletin*, 5, 33–36.

Ishikawa, T., Yang, H., and Tache, Y. (1988) Medullary sites of action of the TRH analogue, RX 77368, for stimulation of gastric acid secretion in the rat. *Gastroenterology*, 95, 1470–1476.

Iwata, J., LeDoux, J.E., Meeley, M.P., Arneric, S., and Reis, D.J. (1986) Intrinsic neurons in the amygdala field projected to by the medial geniculate body mediate emotional responses conditioned to acoustic stimuli. *Brain Research*, 383, 195–214.

Iwata, J., Chida, K., and LeDoux, J.E. (1987) Cardiovascular responses elicited by stimulation of neurons in the central amygdaloid nucleus in awake but not anesthetized rats resemble conditioned emotional response. *Brain Research*, 418, 183–188.

Kaada, B.R. (1951) Somatomotor, autonomic and electrophysiological responses to electrical stimulation of 'rhinencephalic' and other structures in primates, cat and dog. *Acta Psychiatrica Scandinavica*, 24, 1–285.

Kaada, B.R. (1972) Stimulation and regional ablation of the amygdaloid complex with reference to functional representations. In *The Neurobiology of the Amygdala* (ed. B.E. Eleftheriou), pp. 205–281. Plenum Press, New York.

Kaku, T. (1984) Functional differentiation of hypoglossal motoneurons during the amygdaloid or cortically induced rhythmical jaw and tongue movements in the rat. *Brain Research Bulletin*, 13, 147–154.

Kalivas, P.W., Gau, B.A., Nemeroff, C.B., and Prange, A.J. (1982) Antinociception after microinjection of neurotensin into the central amygdaloid nucleus of the rat. *Brain Research*, 243, 279–286.

Kang, W., Wilson, M.A., Bender, M.A., Glorioso, J.C., and Wilson, S.P. (1998) Herpes virus-mediated preproenkephalin gene transfer to the amygdala is antinociceptive. *Brain Research*, 792, 133–135.

Kapp, B.S. and Pascoe, J.P. (1986) Correlation aspects of learning and memory: vertebrate model systems. In *Learning and Memory: A Biological View* (eds J.L. Martinez and R.P. Kesner), pp. 399–440. Academic Press, New York.

Kapp, B.S., Frysinger, R.C., Gallagher, M., and Haselton, J.R. (1979) Amygdala central nucleus lesions: effect on heart rate conditioning in the rabbit. *Physiology and Behavior*, 23, 1109–1117.

Kapp, B.S., Gallagher, M., Underwood, M.D., McNall, C.L., and Whitehorn, D. (1982) Cardiovascular responses elicited by electrical stimulation of the amygdala central nucleus in the rabbit. *Brain Research*, 234, 251–262.

Kapp, B.S., Pascoe, J.P., and Bixler, M.A. (1984) The amygdala: a neuroanatomical systems approach to its contribution to aversive conditioning. In *The Neuropsychology of Memory* (eds N. Butters and L.S. Squire), pp. 473–488. The Guilford Press, New York.

Kapp, B.S., Wilson, A., Pascoe, J.P., Supple, W.F., and Whalen, P.J. (1990) A neuroanatomical systems analysis of conditioned bradycardia in the rabbit. In *Neurocomputation and Learning: Foundations of Adaptive Networks* (eds M. Gabriel and J. Moore), pp. 55–90. Bradford Books, New York.

Kapp, B.S., Whalen, P.J., Supple, W.F., and Pascoe, J.P. (1992) Amygdaloid contributions to conditioned arousal and sensory information processing. In *The Amygdala: Neurobiological Aspects of Emotion, Memory, and Mental Dysfunction* (ed. J.P. Aggleton), pp. 229–254) Wiley-Liss, New York.

Karson, A.B., Aker, R., Ates, N., and Onat, F. (1999) Cardiovascular effects of intracerebroventricular bicuculline in rats with absence seizures. *Epilepsy Research*, 34, 231–239.

Kawai, Y., Inagaki, S., Shiosaka, S., Senba, E., Hara, Y., Sakanaka, M., Takatsuki, K., and Tohyama, M. (1982) Long descending projections from amygdaloid somatostatin-containing neurons to the lower brainstem. *Brain Research*, 239, 603–612.

Kellicut, M.H. and Schwartzbaum, J.S. (1963) Formation of a conditioned emotional response (CER) following lesions of the amygdaloid complex in rats. *Psychological Reviews*, 12, 351–358.

Kellogg, C.K., Sullivan, A.T., Bitrain, D., and Ison, J.R. (1991) Modulation of noise-potentiated acousic startle via the benzodiazepine–gamma-aminobutyric acid receptor complex. *Behavioral Neuroscience*, 105, 640–646.

Kelsey, J.E. and Arnold, S.R. (1994) Lesions of the dorsomedial amygdala, but not the nucleus accumbens, reduce the aversiveness of morphine withdrawal in rats. *Behavioral Neuroscience*, 108, 1119–1127.

Kemble, E.D., Blanchard, D.C., Blanchard, R.J., and Takushi, R. (1984) Taming in wild rats following medial amygdaloid lesions. *Physiology and Behavior*, 32, 131–134.

Kemble, E.D., Blanchard, D.C., and Blanchard, R.J. (1990) Effects of regional amygdaloid lesions on flight and defensive behaviors of wild black rats (*Rattus rattus*). *Physiology and Behavior*, 48, 1–5.

Kesner, R.P. (1982) Brain stimulation: effects on memory. *Behavioral and Neural Biology*, 36, 315–367.

Kiernan, M.J., Westbrook, R.F., and Cranney, J. (1995) Immediate shock, passive avoidance and potentiated startle: implications for the unconditioned response to shock. *Animal Learning and Behavior*, 23, 22–30.

Killcross, S., Robbins, T.W., and Everitt, B.J. (1997) Different types of fear-conditioned behaviour mediated by separate nuclei within amygdala. *Nature*, 388, 377–380.

Kim, J.J., Rison, R.A., and Fanselow, M.S. (1993) Effects of amygdala, hippocampus and periaqueductal gray lesions on short- and long-term contextual fear. *Behavioral Neuroscience*, 107, 1093–1098.

Kim, M. and Davis, M. (1993a) Electrolytic lesions of the amygdala block acquisition and expression of fear-potentiated startle even with extensive training, but do not prevent re-acquisition. *Behavioral Neuroscience*, 107, 580–595.

Kim, M. and Davis, M. (1993b) Lack of a temporal gradient of retrograde amnesia in rats with amygdala lesions assessed with the fear-potentiated startle paradigm. *Behavioral Neuroscience*, 107, 1088–1092.

Kim, M., Jo, Y., Yoon, S., Hahn, S., Rhie, D., Kim, C., and Choi, H. (1990) Electrical stimulation of the medial amygdala facilitates gastric acid secretion in conscious rats. *Brain Research*, 524, 208–212.

Kim, M., Campeau, S., Falls, W.A., and Davis, M. (1993) Infusion of the non-NMDA receptor antagonist CNQX into the amygdala blocks the expression of fear-potentiated startle. *Behavioral and Neural Biology*, 59, 5–8.

King, F.A. (1958) Effects of septal and amygdaloid lesions on emotional behavior and conditioned avoidance in the rat. *Journal of Nervous and Mental Disorders*, 126, 57–63.

King, F.A. and Meyer, P.M. (1958) Effects of amygdaloid lesions on septal hyperemotionality in the rat. *Science*, 128, 655–656.

Klamt, J.G. and Prado, W.A. (1991) Antinociception and behavioral changes induced by carbachol microinjected into identified sites of the rat brain. *Brain Research*, 549, 9–15.

Kleiner, F.B., Meyer, P.M., and Meyer, D.R. (1967) Effects of simultaneous septal and amygdala lesions upon emotionality and retention of a black–white discrimintation. *Brain Research*, 5, 459–468.

Koch, M. (1993) Microinjections of the metabotropic glutamate receptor agonist, trans-(+)-1-amino-cyclopentane-1,3, dicarboxylate (trans-ACPD) into the amygdala increase the acoustic startle response of rats. *Brain Research*, 629, 176–179.

Koch, M. and Ebert, U. (1993) Enhancement of the acoustic startle response by stimulation of an excitatory pathway from the central amygdala/basal nucleus of Meynert to the pontine reticular formation. *Experimental Brain Research*, 93, 231–241.

Koch, M., Kungel, M., and Herbert, H. (1993) Cholinergic neurons in the pedunculopontine tegmental nucleus are involved in the mediation of prepulse inhibition of the acoustic startle response in the rat. *Experimental Brain Research*, 97, 71–82.

Kopchia, K.L., Altman, H.J., and Commissaris, R.L. (1992) Effects of lesions of the central nucleus of the amygdala on anxiety-like behaviors in the rat. *Pharmacology, Biochemistry, and Behavior*, 43, 453–461.

Kowada, K., Kawarada, K., Matsumoto, N., Ooe, M., and Suzuki, T. (1991) Inhibition of jaw-opening reflex by stimulation of the central amygdaloid nucleus in the cat. *Japanese Journal of Physiology*, 41, 513–520.

Kowada, K., Kawarada, K., and Matsumoto, N. (1992) Conditioning stimulation of the central amygdaloid nucleus inhibits the jaw-opening reflex in the cat. *Japanese Journal of Physiology*, 42, 443–458.

Kreindler, A. and Steriade, M. (1964) EEG patterns of arousal and sleep induced by stimulating various amygdaloid levels in the cat. *Archives Italienses de Biologie*, 102, 576–586.

Krettek, J.E. and Price, J.L. (1978a) Amygdaloid projections to subcortical structures within the basal forebrain and brainstem in the rat and cat. *Journal of Comparative Neurology*, 178, 225–254.

Krettek, J.E. and Price, J.L. (1978b) A description of the amygdaloid complex in the rat and cat with observations on intra-amygdaloid axonal connections. *Journal of Comparative Neurology*, 178, 255–280.

Lamont, E.W. and Kokkinidis, L. (1998) Infusion of the dopamine D1 receptor antagonist SCH 23390 into the amygdala blocks fear expression in a potentiated startle paradigm. *Brain Research*, 795, 128–136.

Lamprecht, R. and Dudai, Y. (1996) Transient expression of c-Fos in rat amygdala during training is required for encoding condtioned taste aversion memory. *Learning and Memory*, 3, 31–41.

Lang, H., Tuovinen, T., and Valleala, P. (1964) Amygdaloid afterdischarge and galvanic skin response. *Electroencephalography and Clinical Neurophysiology*, 16, 366–374.

Leaton, R.N. and Cranney, J. (1990) Potentiation of the acoustic startle response by a conditioned stimulus paired with acoustic startle stimulus in rats. *Journal of Experimental Psychology—Animal Behavior Processes*, 16, 279–287.

LeBar, K.S. and LeDoux, J.E. (1996) Partial disruption of fear conditioning in rats with unilateral amgdala damage: correspondence with unilateral temporal lobectomy in humans. *Behavioral Neuroscience*, 110, 991–997.

LeBar, K.S., LeDoux, J.E., Spencer, D.D., and Phelps, E.A. (1995) Impaired fear conditioning following unilateral temporal lobectomy in humans. *Journal of Neuroscience*, 15, 6846–6855.

LeDoux, J.E. (1987) Emotion. In *Handbook of Physiology, Section 1, Neurophysiology: Vol. 5. Higher Functions of the Brain* (ed. F. Plum), pp. 416–459. American Psychological Society, Bethesda, Maryland.

LeDoux, J.E. (1990) Information flow from sensation to emotion: plasticity in the neural computation of stimulus value. In *Learning and Computational Neuroscience* (eds M. Gabriel and J. Moore), pp. 3–51. Bradford Books/MIT Press, Cambridge, Massachusetts.

LeDoux, J.E., Sakaguchi, A., and Reis, D.J. (1986) Interruption of projections from the medial geniculate mediate emotional responses conditioned to acoustic stimuli. *Journal of Neuroscience*, 17, 615–627.

LeDoux, J.E., Iwata, J., Cicchetti, P., and Reis, D.J. (1988) Different projections of the central amygdaloid nucleus mediate autonomic and behavioral correlates of conditioned fear. *Journal of Neuroscience*, 8, 2517–2529.

LeDoux, J.E., Cicchetti, P., Xagoraris, A., and Romanski, L.M. (1990) The lateral amygdaloid nucleus: sensory interface of the amygdala in fear conditioning. *Journal of Neuroscience*, 10, 1062–1069.

Lee, H. and Kim, J. (1998) Amygdalar NMDA receptors are critical for new fear learning in previously fear-conditioned rats. *Journal of Neuroscience*, 18, 8444–8454.

Lee, Y. and Davis, M. (1996) The role of bed nucleus of the stria terminalis in CRH-enhanced startle: an animal model of anxiety. *Society for Neuroscience Abstracts*, 22, 465.

Lee, Y., Walker, D., and Davis, M. (1996) Lack of a temporal gradient of retrograde amnesia following NMDA-induced lesions of the basolateral amygdala assessed with the fear-potentiated paradigm. *Behavioral Neuroscience*, 110, 836–839.

Liang, K.C., McGaugh, J.L., Martinez, J.L., Jensen, R.A., Vasquez, B.J., and Messing, R.B. (1982) Post-training amygdaloid lesions impair retention of an inhibitory avoidance response. *Behavioral Brain Research*, 4, 237–249.

Liang, K.C., Bennett, C., and McGaugh, J.L. (1985) Peripheral epinephrine modulates the effects of post-training amygdala stimulation on memory. *Behavioral Brain Research*, 15, 93–100.

Liang, K.C., Juler, R.G., and McGaugh, J.L. (1986) Modulating effects of post-training epinephrine on memory: involvement of the amygdala noradrenergic systems. *Brain Research*, 368, 125–133.

Liang, K.C., Melia, K.R., Campeau, S., Falls, W.A., Miserendino, M.J.D., and Davis, M. (1992) Lesions of the central nucleus of the amygdala, but not of the paraventricular nucleus of the hypothalamus, block the excitatory effects of corticotropin releasing factor on the acoustic startle reflex. *Journal of Neuroscience*, 12, 2313–2320.

Liebman, J.M., Mayer, D.J., and Liebeskind, J.C. (1970) Mesencephalic central gray lesions and fear-motivated behavior in rats. *Brain Research*, 23, 353–370.

Liebsch, G., Landgraf, R., Gerstberger, R., Probst, J.C., Wotjak, C.T., Engelmann, M., Holsboer, F., and Montkowski, A. (1995) Chronic infusion of a CRH1 receptor antisense oligodeoxynucleotide into the central nucleus of the amygdala reduced anxiety-related behavior in socially defeated rats. *Regulatory Peptides*, 59, 229–239.

Lorenzini, C.A., Bucherelli, C., Giachetti, L.M., and Tassoni, G. (1991) Effects of nucleus basolateralis amygdalae neurotoxic lesions on aversive conditioning in the rat. *Physiology and Behavior*, 49, 765–770.

Luiten, P.G.M., Koolhaas, J.M., deBoer, S., and Koopmans, S.J. (1985) The cortico-medial amygdala in the central nervous system organization of agonistic behavior. *Brain Research*, 332, 282–297.

Magnuson, D.J. and Gray, T.S. (1990) Central nucleus of amygdala and bed nucleus of stria terminalis projections to serotonin or tyrosine hydroxylase immunoreactive cells in the dorsal and median raphe nucleus in the rat. *Society for Neuroscience Abstracts*, 16, 121.

Maisonnette, S.S., Kawasaki, M.C., Coimbra, N.C., and Brandao, M.L. (1996) Effects of lesions of amygdaloid nuclei and substantia nigra on aversive responses induced by electrical stimulation of the inferior colliculus. *Brain Research Bulletin*, 40, 93–98.

Maldonado, R., Stinus, L., Gold, L.H., and Koob, G.F. (1992) Role of different brain structures in the expression of the physical morphine withdrawal syndrome. *Journal of Pharmacology and Experimental Therapeutics*, 261, 669–677.

Manning, B.H. (1998) A lateralized deficit in morphine antinociception after unilateral inactivation of the central amygdala. *Journal of Neuroscience*, 18, 9453–9470.

Manning, B.H. and Mayer, D.J. (1995a) The central nucleus of the amygdala contributes to the production of morphine antinociception in the formalin test. *Pain*, 63, 141–152.

Manning, B.H. and Mayer, D.J. (1995b) The central nucleus of the amygdala contributes to the production of morphine antinociception in the rat tail-flick test. *Journal of Neuroscience*, 15, 8199–8213.

Marcilhac, A. and Siaud, P. (1996a) Identification of projections from the central nucleus of the amygdala to the paraventricular nucleus of the hypothalamus which are immunoreactive for corticotrophin-releasing hormone in the rat. *Experimental Physiology*, 82, 273–281.

Marcilhac, A. and Siaud, P. (1996b) Regulation of the adrenocorticotrophin response to stress by the central nucleus of the amygdala in rats depends upon the nature of the stressor. *Experimental Physiology*, 81, 1035–1038.

Maren, S. (1998) Overtraining does not mitigate contextual fear conditioning deficits produced by neurotoxic lesions of the basolateral amygdala. *Journal of Neuroscience*, 18, 3088–3097.

Maren, S., Aharonov, G., and Fanselow, M.S. (1996a) Retrograde abolition of conditioned fear after excitotoxic lesions in the basolateral amygdala of rats: absence of a temporal gradient. *Behavioral Neuroscience*, 110, 718–726.

Maren, S., Aharonov, G., Stote, D., and Fanselow, M. (1996b) *N*-methyl-D-aspartate receptors in the basolateral amygdala are required for both acquisition and expression of conditional fear in rats. *Behavioral Neuroscience*, 110, 1365–1374.

Markgraf, C.G. and Kapp, B.S. (1991) Lesions of the amygdaloid central nucleus block conditioned cardiac arrhythmias in the rabbit receiving digitalis. *Journal of the Autonomic Nervous System*, 34, 37–45.

Mason, J.W. (1959) Plasma 17-hydroxycorticosteroid levels during electrical stimulation of the amygdaloid complex in conscious monkeys. *American Journal of Physiology*, 196, 44–48.

Matheson, B.K., Branch, B.J., and Taylor, A.N. (1971) Effects of amygdaloid stimulation on pituitary–adrenal activity in conscious cats. *Brain Research*, 32, 151–167.

McCabe, P.M., Gentile, C.G., Markgraf, C.G., Teich, A.H., and Schneiderman, N. (1992) Ibotenic acid lesions in the amygdaloid central nucleus but not in the lateral subthalamic area prevent the acquisition of differential Pavlovian conditioning of bradycardia in rabbits. *Brain Research*, 580, 155–163.

McCall, R.B. and Aghajanian, G.K. (1979) Serotonergic facilitation of facial motoneuron excitation. *Brain Research*, 169, 11–27.

McDonald, A.J. (1998) Cortical pathways to the mammalian amygdala. *Progress in Neurobiology*, 55, 257–332.

McGaugh, J.L. (1966) Time-dependent processes in memory storage. *Science*, 153, 1351–1358.

McGaugh, J.L. (1989) Modulation of memory storage processes. In *Memory: Interdisciplinary Approaches* (eds P.R. Solomon, G.R. Goethals, C.M. Kelley, and B.R. Stephens), pp. 33–64. Springer-Verlag, New York.

McGaugh, J.L., Introini-Collison, I.B., Nagahara, A.H., Cahill, L., Brioni, J.D., and Castellano, C. (1990) Involvement of the amygdaloid complex in neuromodulatory influences on memory storage. *Neuroscience and Biobehavioral Reviews*, 14, 425–432.

McGaugh, J.L., Introini-Collison, I.B., Cahill, L., Castellano, C., Dalmaz, C., Parent, M.B., and Williams, C.L. (1993) Neuromodulatory systems and memory storage: role of the amygdala. *Behavioural Brain Research*, 58, 81–90.

McGaugh, J., Cahill, L., Parent, M.B., Mesches, M.H., Coleman-Mesches, K., and Salinas, J.A. (1995) Involvement of the amygdala in the regulation of memory storage. In *Plasticity in the Central Nervous System* (eds J. McGaugh, F. Bermudez-Rattoni and R.A. Praco-Alcala), pp. 17–40. Lawrence Erlbaum Associates, Hillsdale, New Jersey.

McIntyre, D.C., Kelly, M.E., and Staines, W.A. (1996) Efferent projections of the anterior perirhinal cortex in the rat. *Journal of Comparative Neurology*, 369, 302–318.

McKernan, M.G. and Shinnick-Gallagher, P. (1997) Fear conditioning induces a lasting potentiation of synaptic currents *in vitro*. *Nature*, 390, 607–611.

McNish, K.A., Gewirtz, J.C., and Davis, M. (1997) Evidence of contextual fear conditioning following lesions of the hippocampus: a disruption of freezing but not fear-potentiated startle. *Journal of Neuroscience*, 17, 9353–9360.

Melia, K.R. and Davis, M. (1991) Effects of septal lesions on fear-potentiated startle and on the anxiolytic effects of buspirone and diazepam. *Physiology and Behavior*, 49, 603–611.

Melia, K.R., Falls, W.A., and Davis, M. (1992) Involvement of pertussis toxin sensitive G-proteins in conditioned fear-potentiated startle: possible involvement of the amygdala. *Brain Research*, 584, 141–148.

Mena, N.B., Mathur, R., and Nayar, U. (1995) Amygdalar involvement in pain. *Indian Journal of Physiology and Pharmacology*, 39, 339–346.

Merali, Z., McIntosh, J., Kent, P., Michaud, D., and Anisman, H. (1998) Aversive and appetitive events evoke the release of corticotropin-releasing hormone and bombesin-like peptides at the central nucleus of the amygdala. *Journal of Neuroscience*, 18, 4758–4766.

Millhouse, O.E. and DeOlmos, J. (1983) Neuronal configurations in lateral and basolateral amygdala. *Neuroscience*, 10, 1269–1300.

Miserendino, M.J.D., Sananes, C.B., Melia, K.R., and Davis, M. (1990) Blocking of acquisition but not expression of conditioned fear-potentiated startle by NMDA antagonists in the amygdala. *Nature*, 345, 716–718.

Mishkin, M. and Aggleton, J. (1981) Multiple function contributions of the amygdala in the monkey. In *The Amygdaloid Complex* (ed. Y. Ben-Ari), pp. 409–420. Elsevier/North Holland, New York.

Moga, M.M. and Saper, C.B. (1994) Neuropeptide-immunoreactive neurons projecting to the paraventricular hypothalamic nucleus in the rat. *Journal of Comparative Neurology*, 346, 137–150.

Moller, C., Bing, O., and Heilig, M. (1994) c-*fos* expression in the amygdala: *in vivo* antisense modulation and role in anxiety. *Cellular and Molecular Neurobiology*, 14, 415–423.

Moller, C., Wujkybdm K, Sommer, W., Thorsell, A., and Heilig, M. (1997) Decreased experimental anxiety and voluntary ethanol consumption in rats following central but not basolateral amygdala lesions. *Brain Research*, 760, 94–101.

Morgenson, G.J. and Calaresu, F.R. (1973) Cardiovascular responses to electrical stimulation of the amygdala in the rat. *Experimental Neurology*, 39, 166–180.

Morrow, N.S., Hodgson, D.M., and Garrick, T. (1996) Microinjection of thyrotropin-releasing hormone analogue into the central nucleus of the amygdala stimulates gastric contractility in rats. *Brain Research*, 735, 141–148.

Muller, J., Corodimas, K.P., Fridel, Z., and LeDoux, J.E. (1997) Functional inactivation of the lateral and basal nuclei of the amygdala by muscimol infusion prevents fear conditioning to an explicit conditioned stimulus and to contextual stimuli. *Behavioral Neuroscience*, 111, 683–691.

Nader, K. and LeDoux, J.E. (1997) Is it time to invoke multiple fear learning systems in the amygdala? *Trends in Cognitive Neuroscience*, 1, 241–246.

Niehoff, D.L. and Kuhar, M.J. (1983) Benzodiazepine receptors: localization in rat amygdala. *Journal of Neuroscience*, 3, 2091–2097.

Nitecka, L. and Frotscher, M. (1989) Organization and synaptic interconnections of GABAergic and cholinergic elements in the rat amygdaloid nuclei: single- and double-immunolabeling studies. *Journal of Comparative Neurology*, 279, 470–488.

Nitecka, L., Amerski, L., and Narkiewicz, O. (1981) The organization of intra-amygdaloid connections: an HRP study. *Journal für Hirnforschung*, 22, 3–7.

Oakes, M.E. and Coover, G.D. (1997) Effects of small amygdala lesions on fear, but not aggression, in the rat. *Physiology and Behavior*, 61, 45–55.

Ohta, H., Watanabe, S., and Ueki, S. (1991) Cardiovascular changes induced by chemical stimulation of the amygdala in rats. *Brain Research Bulletin*, 36, 575–581.

Ohta, M. (1984) Amygdaloid and cortical facilitation or inhibition of trigmeminal motoneurons in the rat. *Brain Research*, 291, 39–48.

Oliveira, M.A. and Prado, W.A. (1994) Antinociception and behavioral manifestations induced by intracerebroventricular or intraamygdaloid administration of cholinergic agonists in the rat. *Pain*, 57, 383–391.

Oliveira, M.A. and Prado, W.A. (1998) Antinociception induced by stimulating amygdaloid nuclei in rats: changes produced by systemically administered antagonists. *Brazilian Journal of Medical and Biological Research*, 31, 681–690.

Onaivi, E.S., Chakrabarti, A., Gwebu, E.T., and Chaudhuri, G. (1995) Neurobehavioral effects of Δ9-THC and cannabinoid (CB1) receptor gene. *Behavioural Brain Research*, 72, 115–125.

Ottersen, O.P. (1980) Afferent connections to the amygdaloid complex of the rat and cat. II. Afferents from the hypothalamus and the basal telencephalon. *Journal of Comparative Neurology*, 194, 267–289.

Ottersen, O.P. (1982) Connections of the amygdala of the rat. IV. Corticoamygdaloid and intraamygdaloid connections as studied with axonal transport of horseradish peroxidase. *Journal of Comparative Neurology*, 205, 30–48.

Ozkutlu, U., Coskun, T., Onat, F., Yegen, B.C., and Oktay, S. (1995) Cardiovascular effects of centrally active cholinomimetics in conscious and anesthetized rats. *Brain Research Bulletin*, 37, 569–573.

Pare, D., Steriade, M., Deschenes, M., and Bouhassiri, D. (1990) Prolonged enhancement of anterior thalamic synaptic responsiveness by stimulation of a brain-stem cholinergic group. *Journal of Neuroscience*, 10, 20–33.

Pare, D., Smith, Y., and Pare, J.F. (1995) Intra-amygdaloid projections of the basolateral and basomedial nuclei in the cat: *Phaseolus vulgaris*-leucoagglutinin antereograde tracing at the light and electron microscopic level. *Neuroscience*, 69, 567–583.

Parent, M.B., Avila, E., and McGaugh, J.L. (1995a) Footshock facilitates the expression of aversively motivated memory in rats given post-training amygdala basolateral complex lesions. *Brain Research*, 676, 235–244.

Parent, M.B., Quirarte, G.L., Cahill, L., and McGaugh, J.L. (1995b) Spared retention of inhibitory avoidance learning after posttraining amygdala lesions. *Behavioral Neuroscience*, 109, 803–807.

Pascoe, J.P., Bradley, D.J., and Spyer, K.M. (1989) Interactive responses to stimulation of the amygdaloid central nucleus and baroreceptor afferents in the rabbit. *Journal of the Autonomic Nervous System*, 26, 157–167.

Pavlovic, Z.W. and Bodnar, R.J. (1998) Opioid supraspinal analgesic synergy between the amygdala and pariaqueductal gray in rats. *Brain Research*, 779, 158–169.

Pavlovic, Z.W., Cooper, M.L., and Bodnar, R.J. (1996a) Enhancements in swim stress-induced hypothermia, but not analgesia, following amygdala lesions in rats. *Physiology and Behavior*, 59, 77–82.

Pavlovic, Z.W., Cooper, R.J., and Bodnar, R.J. (1996b) Opioid antagonists in the periaqueductal gray inhibit morphine and B-endorphin analgesia elicited from the amygdala of rats. *Brain Research*, 741, 13–26.

Pellegrino, L. (1968) Amygdaloid lesions and behavioral inhibition in the rat. *Journal of Comparative Physiology and Psychology*, 65, 483–491.

Pesold, C. and Treit, D. (1994) The septum and amygdala differentially mediate the anxiolytic effects of benzodiazepines. *Brain Research*, 638, 295–301.

Pesold, C. and Treit, D. (1995) The central and basolateral amygdala differentially mediate the anxiolytic effects of benzodiazepines. *Brain Research*, 671, 213–221.

Petersen, E.N. and Scheel-Kruger, J. (1982) The GABAergic anticonflict effect of intraamygdaloid benzodiazepines demonstrated by a new water lick conflict paradigm. In *Behavioral Models and the Analysis of Drug Action* (eds M.Y. Spiegelstein and A. Levy), pp. 467–473. Elsevier Scientific, Amsterdam.

Petersen, E.N., Braestrup, C., and Scheel-Kruger, J. (1985) Evidence that the anticonflict effect of midazolam in amygdala is mediated by the specific benzodiazepine receptor. *Neuroscience Letters*, 53, 285–288.

Petrov, T., Jhamandas, J.H., and Krukoff, T.L. (1994) Electrical stimulation of the central nucleus of the amygdala induces *fos*-like immunoreactivity in the hypothalamus of the rat: a quantitaive study. *Molecular Brain Research*, 22, 333–340.

Petrov, T., Jhamandas, J.H., and Krukoff, T.L. (1996) Connectivity between brainstem autonomic structures and expression of c-fos following electrical stimulation of the central nucleus of the amygdala in rat. *Cell and Tissue Research*, 283, 367–374.

Petrovich, G.D. and Swanson, L.W. (1997) Projections from the lateral part of the central amygdalar nucleus to the postulated fear conditioning circuit. *Brain Research*, 763, 247–254.

Pezzone, M.A., Lee, W.-S., Hoffman, G.E., and Rabin, B.S. (1992) Induction of c-fos immunoreactivity in the rat forebrain by conditioned and unconditioned stimuli. *Brain Research*, 597, 41–50.

Philipson, O.T. (1979) Afferent projections to the ventral tegmented area of Tsai and intrafascicular nucleus. A horseradish peroxidase study in the rat. *Journal of Comparative Neurology*, 187, 117–143.

Phillips, R.E. (1964) Wildness in the Mallard duck: effects of brain lesions and stimulation on 'escape behavior' and reproduction. *Journal of Comparative Neurology*, 122, 139–156.

Phillips, R.E. (1968) Approach–withdrawal behavior of peach-faced lovebirds, *Agapornis roseicolis* and its modification by brain lesions. *Behavior*, 31, 163–184.

Phillips, R.G. and LeDoux, J.E. (1992) Differential contribution of amygdala and hippocampus to cued and contextual fear conditioning. *Behavioral Neuroscience*, 106, 274–285.

Pich, E.M., Lorang, M., Yeganeh, M., deFonseca, F.R., Raber, J., Koob, G.F., and Weiss, F. (1995) Increase of extracellular corticotropin-releasing factor-like immunoreactivity levels in the amygdala of awake rats during restraint stress and ethanol withdrawal as measured by microdialysis. *Journal of Neuroscience*, 15, 5439–5447.

Pitkänen, A., Stefanacci, L., Farb, C.R., Go, G.-G., LeDoux, J.E., and Amaral, D.G. (1995) Intrinsic connections of the rat amygdaloid complex: projections originating in the basolateral nucleus. *Journal of Comparative Neurology*, 356, 288–310.

Pitkänen, A., Savander, V., and LeDoux, J.E. (1997) Organization of intra-amygdaloid circuitries in the rat: an emerging framework for understanding functions of the amygdala. *Trends in Neuroscience*, 20, 517–523.

Poplawsky, A. and McVeigh, J.S. (1981) The effects of differential lesions of the amygdala on response suppression. *Physiology and Behavior*, 26, 617–621.

Poremba, A. and Gabriel, M. (1997) Amygdalar lesions block discriminative avoidance learning and cingulothalmaic training-induced neuronal plasticity in rabbits. *Journal of Neuroscience*, 17, 5237–5244.

Post, S. and Mai, J.K. (1980) Contribution to the amygdaloid projection field in the rat: a quantitative autoradiographic study. *Journal für Hirnforschung*, 21, 199–225.

Powell, D.A., Tebbutt, D., Chachich, M., Murphy, V., McLaughlin, J., and Buchanan, S.L. (1997) Amygdala–prefrontal interactions and conditioned bradycardia in rabbit. *Behavioral Neuroscience*, 111, 1056–1074.

Prewitt, C.M. and Herman, J.P. (1997) Hypothalamo-pituitary–adrenocortical regulation following lesions of the central nucleus of the amygdala. *Stress*, 1, 263–280.

Prewitt, C.M.F. and Herman, J.P. (1998) Anatomical interactions between the central amygdaloid nucleus and the hypothalamic paraventricular nucleus of the rat—a dual tract-tracing analysis. *Journal of Chemical Neuroanatomy*, 15, 173–185.

Price, J.L. and Amaral, D.G. (1981) An autoradiographic study of the projections of the central nucleus of the monkey amygdala. *Journal of Neuroscience*, 1, 1242–1259.

Quirk, G.J., Repa, J.C., and LeDoux, J.E. (1995) Fear conditioning enhances short-latency auditory responses of lateral amygdala neurons: parallel recordings in the freely behaving rat. *Neuron*, 15, 1029–1039.

Rasmussen, K. and Jacobs, B.L. (1986) Single unit activity of locus coeruleus in the freely moving cat. II. Conditioning and pharmacologic studies. *Brain Research*, 371, 335–344.

Rassnick, S., Heinrichs, S.C., Britton, K.T., and Koob, G.F. (1993) Microinjection of a corticotroin-releasing factor antagonist into the central nucleus of the amygdala reverses anxiogenic-like effects of ethanol withdrawal. *Brain Research*, 605, 25–32.

Ray, A. and Henke, P.G. (1990) Enkephalin–dopamine interactions in the central amygdalar nucleus during gastric stress ulcer formation in rats. *Behavioural Brain Research*, 36, 179–183.

Ray, A. and Henke, P.G. (1991a) The basolateral amygdala, dopamine and gastric stress ulcer formation in rats. *Brain Research*, 558, 335–338.

Ray, A. and Henke, P.G. (1991b) TRH–enkephalin interactions in the amygdaloid complex during gastric stress ulcer formation in rats. *Regulatory Peptides*, 35, 11–17.

Ray, A., Henke, P.G., and Sullivan, R.M. (1987) The central amygdala and immobilization stress induced gastric pathology in rats: neurotensin and dopamine. *Brain Research*, 409, 398–402.

Ray, A., Henke, P.G., and Sullivan, R.M. (1988a) Effects of intra-amygdalar dopamine agonists and antagonists on gastric stress lesions in rats. *Neuroscience Letters*, 84, 302–306.

Ray, A., Sullivan, R.M., and Henke, P.G. (1988b) Interactions of thyrotropin-releasing hormone (TRH) with neurotensin and dopamine in the central nucleus of the amygdala during stress ulcer formation in rats. *Neuroscience Letters*, 91, 95–100.

Ray, A., Henke, P.G., and Sullivan, R.M. (1990) Effects of intra-amygdalar thyrotropin releasing hormone (TRH) and its antagonism by atropine and benzodiazepines during stress ulcer formation in rats. *Pharmacology, Biochemistry, and Behavior*, 36, 597–601.

Ray, A., Henke, P.G., Gulati, K., and Sen, P. (1993) The amygdaloid complex, corticotropin releasing factor and stress-induced gastric ulcerogenesis in rats. *Brain Research*, 624, 286–290.

Redgate, E.S. and Fahringer, E.E. (1973) A comparison of the pituitary–adrenal activity elicited by electrical stimulation of preoptic, amygdaloid and hypothalamic sites in the rat brain. *Neuroendocrinology*, 12, 334–343.

Redmond, D.E., Jr (1977) Alteration in the function of the nucleus locus: a possible model for studies on anxiety. In *Animal Models in Psychiatry and Neurology* (eds I.E. Haninand and E. Usdin), pp. 292–304. Pergamon Press, Oxford, UK.

Richter, R.M. and Weiss, F. (1999) *In vivo* CRF release in rat amygdala is increased during cocaine withdrawal in self-administering rats. *Synapse*, 32, 254–261.

Roberts, G.W., Woodhams, P.L., Polak, J.M., and Crow, T.J. (1982) Distribution of neuropeptides in the limbic system of the rat: the amygdaloid complex. *Neuroscience*, 7, 99–131.

Roder, S., Rosas-Arellano, M.P., and Ciriello, J. (1999) Effect of noradrenergic inputs on the cardiovascular depressor responses to stimulation of central nucleus of the amygdala. *Brain Research*, 818, 531–535.

Rodgers, R.J. (1977) Elevation of aversive thresholds in rats by intraamygdaloid injection of morphine sulfate. *Pharmacology, Biochemistry, and Behavior*, 6, 385–390.

Rodgers, R.J. (1978) Influence of intra-amygdaloid opiate injections on shock thresholds, tail-flick latencies and open field behaviour in rats. *Brain Research*, 153, 211–216.

Rogan, M.T. and LeDoux, J.E. (1995) LTP is accompanied by commensurate enhancement of auditory-evoked responses in a fear conditioning circuit. *Neuron*, 15, 127–136.

Rogan, M.T., Staubli, U.V., and LeDoux, J.E. (1997) Fear conditioning induces associative long-term potentiation in the amygdala. *Nature*, 390, 604–607.

Rogawski, M.A. and Aghajanian, G.K. (1980) Modulation of lateral geniculate neuron excitability by noradrenaline microintophoresis or locus coeruleus stimulation. *Nature*, 287, 731–734.

Romanski, L.M., Clugnet, M.C., Bordi, F., and LeDoux, J.E. (1993) Somatosensory and auditory convergence in the lateral nucleus of the amygdala. *Behavioral Neuroscience*, 107, 444–450.

Roozendaal, B., Koolhaas, J.M., and Bohus, B. (1990) Differential effect of lesioning of the central amygdala on the bradycardiac and behavioral response of the rat in relation to conditioned social and solitary stress. *Behavioral Brain Research*, 41, 39–48.

Roozendaal, B., Koolhaas, J.M., and Bohus, B. (1991a) Attenuated cardiovascular, neuroendocrine and behavioral response after a single footshock in central amygdaloid lesioned male rats. *Physiology and Behavior*, 50, 771–775.

Roozendaal, B., Koolhaas, J.M., and Bohus, B. (1991b) Central amygdala lesions affect behavioral and autonomic balance during stress in rats. *Physiology and Behavior*, 50, 777–781.

Roozendaal, B., Koolhaas, J.M., and Bohus, B. (1992a) Central amygdaloid involvement in neuroendocrine correlates of conditioned stress responses. *Journal of Neuroendocrinology*, 4, 483–489.

Roozendaal, B., Wiersma, A., Driscoll, P., Koolhaas, J.M., and Bohus, B. (1992b) Vasopressinergic modulation of stress responses in the central amygdala of the Roman high-avoidance and low-avoidance rat. *Brain Research*, 596, 35–40.

Roozendaal, B., Schoorlemmer, G.H., Koolhaas, J.M., and Bohus, B. (1993) Cardiac, neuroendocrine and behavioral effects of central amygdaloid vasopressinergic and oxytocinergic mechanisms under stress-free conditions in rats. *Brain Research Bullentin*, 32, 573–579.

Rosen, J.B. and Davis, M. (1988a) Enhancement of acoustic startle by electrical stimulation of the amygdala. *Behavioral Neuroscience*, 102, 195–202.

Rosen, J.B. and Davis, M. (1988b) Temporal characterizations of enhancement of startle by stimulation of the amygdala. *Physiology and Behavior*, 44, 117–123.

Rosen, J.B. and Davis, M. (1990) Enhancement of electrically elicited startle by amygdaloid stimulation. *Physiology and Behavior*, 48, 343–349.

Rosen, J.B. and Schulkin, J. (1998) From normal fear to pathological anxiety. *Psychological Review*, 105, 325–350.

Rosen, J.B., Hitchcock, J.M., Sananes, C.B., Miserendino, M.J.D., and Davis, M. (1991) A direct projection from the central nucleus of the amygdala to the acoustic startle pathway: anterograde and retrograde tracing studies. *Behavioral Neuroscience*, 105, 817–825.

Rosen, J.B., Fanselow, M.S., Young, S.L., Sitcoske, M., and Maren, S. (1998) Immediate-early gene expression in the amygdala following footshock stress and contextual fear conditioning. *Brain Research*, 796, 132–142.

Ruggiero, D.A., Ross, C.A., Kumada, M., and Reis, D.J. (1982) Reevaluation of projections from the mesencephalic trigeminal nucleus to the medulla and spinal cord: new projections. A combined retrograde and anterograde horseradish peroxidase study. *Journal of Comparative Neurology*, 206, 278–292.

Russchen, F.T. (1982) Amygdalopetal projections in the cat. II. Subcortical afferent connections. A study with retrograde tracing techniques. *Journal of Comparative Neurology*, 207, 157–176.

Russchen, F.T., Amaral, D.G., and Price, J.L. (1985) The afferent connections of the substantia innominata in the monkey, *Macaca fasicularis*. *Journal of Comparative Neurology*, 242, 1–27.

Sajdyk, T.J. and Shekhar, A. (1997a) Excitatory amino acid receptor antagonists block the cardiovascular and anxiety responses elicited by γ-aminobutyric acid-a receptor blockade in the basolateral amygdala of rats. *Journal of Pharmacology and Experimental Therapeutics*, 283, 969–977.

Sajdyk, T.J. and Shekhar, A. (1997b) Excitatory amino acid receptors in the basolateral amygdala regulate anxiety responses in the social interaction test. *Brain Research*, 764, 262–264.

Sajdyk, T.J., Schober, D.A., Gehlert, D.R., and Shekhar, A. (1999a) Role of corticotropin-releasing factor and urocortin within the basolateral amygdala of rats in anxiety and panic responses. *Behavioural Brain Research*, 100, 207–215.

Sajdyk, T.J., Vandergriff, M.G., and Gehlert, D.R. (1999b) Amygdalar neuropeptide Y Y-1 receptors mediate the anxiolytic-like actions of neuropeptide Y in the social interaction test. *European Journal of Pharmacology*, 368, 143–147.

Sananes, C.B. and Campbell, B.A. (1989) Role of the central nucleus of the amygdala in olfactory heart rate conditioning. *Behavioral Neuroscience*, 103, 519–525.

Sananes, C.B. and Davis, M. (1992) *N*-Methyl-D-aspartate lesions of the lateral and basolateral nuclei of the amygdala block fear-potentiated startle and shock sensitization of startle. *Behavioral Neuroscience*, 106, 72–80.

Sanders, S.K. and Shekhar, A. (1991) Blockade of $GABA_A$ receptors in the region of the anterior basolateral amygdala of rats elicits increases in heart rate and blood pressure. *Brain Research*, 576, 101–110.

Sanders, S.K. and Shekhar, A. (1995a) Anxiolytic effects of chlordiazepoxide blocked by injection of $GABA_A$ and benzodiazepine receptor antagonists in the region of the anterior basolateral amygdala of rats. *Biological Psychiatry*, 37, 473–476.

Sanders, S.K. and Shekhar, A. (1995b) Regulation of anxiety by $GABA_A$ receptors in the rat amygdala. *Pharmacology, Biochemistry, and Behavior*, 52, 701–706.

Sarnyai, Z., Biro, E., Gardi, J., Vecsernyes, M., Julesz, J., and Telegdy, G. (1995) Brain corticotropin-releasing factor mediates 'anxiety-like' behavior induced by cocaine withdrawal in rats. *Brain Research*, 675, 89–97.

Sarter, M. and Markowitsch, H.J. (1985) Involvement of the amygdala in learning and memory: a critical review, with emphasis on anatomical relations. *Behavioral Neuroscience*, 99, 342–380.

Savander, V., Go, C.-G., LeDoux, J.E., and Pitkänen, A. (1995) Intrinsic connections of the rat amygdaloid complex: projections originating in the basal nucleus. *Journal of Comparative Neurology*, 361, 345–368.

Sawchenko, P.E. and Swanson, L.W. (1983) The organization of forebrain afferents to the paraventricular and supraoptic nucleus of the rat. *Journal of Comparative Neurology*, 218, 121–144.

Schanbacher, A., Koch, M., Pilz, P.K.D., and Schnitzler, H.U. (1996) Lesions of the amygdala do not affect the enhancement of the acoustic startle response by background noise. *Physiology and Behavior*, 60, 1341–1346.

Scheel-Kruger, J. and Petersen, E.N. (1982) Anticonflict effect of the benzodiazepines mediated by a GABAergic mechanism in the amygdala. *European Journal of Pharmacology*, 82, 115–116.

Schlor, K.H., Stumpf, H., and Stock, G. (1984) Baroreceptor reflex during arousal induced by electrical stimulation of the amygdala or by natural stimuli. *Journal of the Autonomic Nervous System*, 10, 157–165.

Schreiber, R. and De Vry, J. (1993) Neuronal circuits involved in the anxiolytic effects of the 5-HT_{1A} receptor agonists 8-OH-DPAT, ipsapirone and buspirone in the rat. *European Journal of Pharmacology*, 249, 341–351.

Schwaber, J.S., Kapp, B.S., Higgins, G.A., and Rapp, P.R. (1982) Amygdaloid basal forebrain direct connections with the nucleus of the solitary tract and the dorsal motor nucleus. *Journal of Neuroscience*, 2, 1424–1438.

Schwarzberg, H., Kalbacher, H., and Hoffmann, W. (1999) Differential behavioral effects of TFF3 into the rat amygdala. *Pharmacology, Biochemistry, and Behavior*, 62, 173–178.

Schwartzbaum, J.S. and Gay, P.E. (1966) Interacting behavioral effects of septal and amygdaloid lesions in the rat. *Journal of Comparative Physiology and Psychology*, 61, 59–65.

Scoville, W.B. and Milner, B. (1957) Loss of recent memory after bilateral hippocampal lesions. *Journal of Neurology, Neurosurgery and Psychiatry*, 20, 11–21.

Seggie, J. (1983) Corticomedial amygdala lesions, behavior, corticosterone, and prolactin: unexpected separation of effects. *Psychiatry Research*, 10, 139–150.

Selden, N.R.W., Everitt, B.J., Jarrard, L.E., and Robbins, T.W. (1991) Complementary roles for the amygdala and hippocampus in aversive conditioning to explicit and contextual cues. *Neuroscience*, 42, 335–350.

Sen, R.N. and Anand, B.K. (1957) Effect of electrical stimulation of the limbic system of brain ('visceral brain') on gastric secretory activity and ulceration. *Indian Journal of Medical Research*, 45, 515–521.

Setekleiv, J., Skaug, O.E., and Kaada, B.R. (1961) Increase of plasma 17-hydroxy-corticosteroids by cerebral cortical and amygdaloid stimulation in the cat. *Journal of Endocrinology*, 22, 119–126.

Shi, C.-J. (1995) The anatomical substrates underlying the role of the amygdala in associative learning. Dissertation, University of Iowa, Iowa City, Iowa.

Shibata, K., Kataoka, Y., Gomita, Y., and Ueki, S. (1982) Localization of the site of the anticonflict action of benzodiazepines in the amygdaloid nucleus of rats. *Brain Research*, 234, 442–446.

Shibata, K., Kataoka, Y., Yamashita, K., and Ueki, S. (1986) An important role of the central amygdaloid nucleus and mammillary body in the mediation of conflict behavior in rats. *Brain Research*, 372, 159–162.

Shibata, S., Yamashita, K., Yamamoto, E., Ozaki, T., and Ueki, S. (1989) Effect of benzodiazepine and GABA antagonists on anticonflict effects of antianxiety drugs injected into the rat amygdala in a water-lick suppression test. *Psychopharmacology*, 98, 38–44.

Shindou, T., Watanabe, S., Yamamoto, K., and Nakanishi, H. (1993) NMDA receptor-dependent formation of long-term potentiation in the rat medial amygdala neuron in an *in vitro* slice prepartation. *Brain Research Bulletin*, 31, 667–672.

Shiosaka, S., Tokyama, M., Takagi, H., Takashashi, Y., Saitoh, T., Sakumoto, H., Nakagawa, H., and Shimizu, N. (1980) Ascending and descending components of the medial forebrain bundle in the rat as demonstrated by the horseradish peroxidase–blue reaction. I. Forebrain and upper brainstem. *Experimental Brain Research*, 39, 377–388.

Shors, T.J. and Mathew, P.R. (1998) NMDA receptor antagonism in the lateral/basolateral but not central nucleus of the amygdala prevents the induction of facilitated learning in response to stress. *Learning and Memory*, 5, 220–230.

Shors, T.J., Weiss, C., and Thompson, R.F. (1992) Stress-induced facilitation of classical conditioning. *Science*, 257, 537–539.

Siegel, A., Schubert, K.L., and Shaika, M.B. (1997) Neurotransmitters regulating defensive rage behavior in the cat. *Neuroscience and Biobehavioral Reviews*, 21, 733–742.

Silverman, A.J., Hoffman, D.L., and Zimmerman, E.A. (1981) The descending afferent connections of the paraventricular nucleus of the hypothalamus (PVN). *Brain Research Bulletin*, 6, 47–61.

Silvestri, A.J. and Kapp, B.S. (1998) Amygdaloid modulation of mesopontine peribrachial neuronal activity—implications for arousal. *Behavioral Neuroscience*, 112, 571–588.

Simon, H., LeMoal, M., and Calas, A. (1979) Efferents and afferents of the ventral temental A-10 region studies after local injection of [^{3}H]leucine and horseradish peroxidase. *Brain Research*, 178, 17–40.

Singh, V.B., Onaivi, E.S., Phan, T.H., and Boadle-Biber, M.C. (1990) The increases in rat cortical and midbrain tryptophan hydroxylase activity in response to acute or repeated sound stress are blocked by bilateral lesions to the central nucleus of the amygdala. *Brain Research*, 530, 49–53.

Singh, V.B., Hao-Phan, T., Corley, K.C., and Boadle-Biber, M.C. (1992) Increase in cortical and midbrain tryptophan hydroxylase activity by intracerebroventricular administration of corticotropin releasing factor: block by adrenalectomy, by RU 38486 and by bilateral lesions to the central nucleus of the amygdala. *Neurochemistry International*, 20, 81–92.

Singh, V.B., Kalimi, M., Phan, T.H., and Boadle-Biber, M.C. (1994) Intracranial dehydroepiandrosterone blocks the activation of tryptophan hydroxylase in response to acute sound stress. *Molecular and Cellular Neurosciences*, 5, 176–181.

Slotnick, B.M. (1973) Fear behavior and passive avoidance deficits in mice with amygdala lesions. *Physiology and Behavior*, 11, 717–720.

Smith, B.S. and Millhouse, O.E. (1985) The connections between basolateral and central amygdaloid nuclei. *Neuroscience Letters*, 56, 307–309.

Smith, M.A., Banerjee, S., Gold, P.W. ,and Glowa, J. (1992) Induction of c-fos mRNA in rat brain by conditioned and unconditioned stressors. *Brain Research*, 578, 135–141.

Soltis, R.P., Cook, J.C., A.E., G., Stratton, J.M., and Flickincer, K.A., (1998) EAA receptors in the dorsomedial hypothalamic area mediate the cardiovascular response to activation of the amygdala. *American Journal of Physiology*, 275, R624–R631.

Soltis, R.P., Cook, J.C., Gregg, A.E., and Sanders, B.J. (1997) Interaction of GABA and excitatory amino acids in the basolateral amygdala: role in cardiovascular regulation. *Journal of Neuroscience*, 17, 9367–9374.

Spevack, A.A., Campbell, C.T., and Drake, L. (1975) Effect of amygdalectomy on habituation and CER in rats. *Physiology and Behavior*, 15, 199–207.

Squire, L.R. (1992) Memory and the hippocampus: a synthesis from findings with rats, monkeys and humans. *Pharmacological Reviews*, 99, 195–231.

Steriade, M., Datta, S., Pare, D., Oakson, G., and Dossi, R.C. (1990) Neuronal activities in brain-stem cholinergic nuclei related to tonic activation processes in thalamocortical systems. *Journal of Neuroscience*, 10, 2541–2559.

Stinus, L., LeMoal, M., and Koob, G.F. (1990) Nucleus accumbens and amygdala are possible substrates for the aversive stimulus effects of opiate withdrawal. *Neuroscience*, 37, 767–773.

Stock, G., Schlor, K.H., Heidt, H., and Buss, J. (1978) Psychomotor behaviour and cardiovascular patterns during stimulation of the amygdala. *Pflugers Archives of General Physiology*, 376, 177–184.

Sullivan, R.M., Henke, P.G., Ray, A., Hebert, M.A., and Trimper, J.M. (1989) The GABA/benzodiazepine receptor complex in the central amygdalar nucleus and stress ulcers in rats. *Behavioral and Neural Biology*, 51, 262–269.

Swanson, L.W., Sawchenko, P.E., Rivier, J., and Vale, W. (1983) Organization of bovine corticotropin-releasing factor immunoreactive cells and fibers in the rat brain: an immunohistochemical study. *Neuroendocrinology*, 36, 165–186.

Swiergiel, A.H., Takahashi, L.K., and Kalin, N.H. (1993) Attenuation of stress-induced behavior by antagonism of corticotropin-releasing factor in the central amygdala of the rat. *Brain Research*, 623, 229–234.

Takao, K., Nagatani, T., Kasahara, K.-I., and Hashimoto, S. (1992) Role of the central serotonergic system in the anticonflict effect of d-AP159. *Pharmacology, Biochemistry, and Behavior*, 43, 503–508.

Takayama, K., Okada, J., and Miura, M. (1990) Evidence that neurons of the central amygdaloid nucleus directly project to the site concerned with circulatory and respiratory regulation in the ventrolateral nucleus of the cat: a WGA–HRP study. *Neuroscience Letters*, 109, 241–246.

Takeuchi, Y., McLean, J.H., and Hopkins, D.A. (1982) Reciprocal connections between the amygdala and parabrachial nuclei: ultrastructural demonstration by degeneration and axonal transport of horseradish peroxidase in the cat. *Brain Research*, 239, 538–588.

Takeuchi, Y., Matsushima, S., and Hopkins, D.A. (1983) Direct amygdaloid projections to the dorsal motor nucleus of the vagus nerve: a light and electron microscopic study in the rat. *Brain Research*, 280, 143–147.

Taylor, J.R., Punch, L.J., and Elsworth, JD. (1998) A comparison of the effects of clonidine and CNQX infusion into the locus coeruleus and the amygdala on naloxone-precipitated opiate withdrawal in the rat. *Psychopharmacology*, 138, 133–142.

Tellioglu, T., Neslihan, A., Goren, Z., Onat, F., and Oktay, S. (1997) Role of the AV3V region in the pressor responses induced by amygdala stimulation. *European Journal of Pharmacology*, 336, 163–168.

Thierry, A.M., Tassin, J.P., Blanc, G., and Glowinski, J. (1976) Selective activation of the mesocortical DA system by stress. *Nature*, 263, 242–244.

Thomas, S.R., Lewis, M.E. and Iversen, S.D. (1985) Correlation of [^{3}H]diazepam binding density with anxiolytic locus in the amygdaloid complex of the rat. *Brain Research*, 342, 85–90.

Treit, D., Pesold, C., and Rotzinger, S. (1993a) Dissociating the anti-fear effects of septal and amygdaloid lesions using two pharmacologically validated models of rat anxiety. *Behavioral Neuroscience*, 107, 770–785.

Treit, D., Pesold, C., and Rotzinger, S. (1993b) Noninteractive effects of diazepam and amygdaloid lesions in two animal models of anxiety. *Behavioral Neuroscience*, 107, 1099–1105.

Tribollet, E. and Dreifuss, J.J. (1981) Localization of neurones projecting to the hypothalamic paraventricular nucleus of the rat: a horseradish peroxidase study. *Neuroscience*, 7, 1215–1328.

Turner, B.J. (1981) The cortical sequence and terminal distribution of sensory related afferents to the amygdaloid complex of the rat and monkey. In *The Amygdaloid Complex* (ed. Y. Ben-Ari), pp. 51–62. Elsevier North Holland Press, Amsterdam.

Ursin, H. and Kaada, B.R. (1960) Functional localization within the amygdaloid complex in the cat. *Electroencephalography and Clinical Neurophysiology*, 12, 109–122.

Ursin, H., Jellestad, F., and Cabrera, I.G. (1981) The amygdala, exploration and fear. In *The Amygdaloid Complex* (ed. Y. Ben-Ari), pp. 317–329. Elsevier North Holland Press, Amsterdam.

Uryu, K., Okumura, T., Shibasaki, T., and Sakanaka, M. (1992) Fine structure and possible origins of nerve fibers with corticotropin-releasing factor-like immunoreactivity in the rat central amygdaloid nucleus. *Brain Research*, 577, 175–179.

Van Bockstaele, E.J., Chan, J., and Pickel, V.M. (1996) Input from central nucleus of the amygdala efferents to pericoerulear dendrites, some of which contain tyrosine hydroxylase immunoreactivity. *Journal of Neuroscience Research*, 45, 289–302.

Van Bockstaele, E.J., Colago, E.E.O., and Valentino, R.J. (1998) Amygdaloid corticotropin-releasing factor targets locus coeruleus dendrites: substrate for the co-ordination of emotional and cognitive limbs of the stress response. *Journal of Neuroendocrinology*, 10, 743–757.

Van de Kar, L.D., Piechowski, R.A., Rittenhouse, P.A., and Gray, T.S. (1991) Amygdaloid lesions: differential effect on conditioned stress and immobilization-induced increases in cortiocosterone and renin secretion. *Neuroendocrinology*, 15, 89–95.

VanHoesen, G.W. (1981) The differential distribution, diversity and sprouting of cortical projections to the amygdala in the Rhesus monkey. In *The Amygdaloid Complex* (ed. Y. Ben-Ari), pp. 77–90. Elsevier North Holland Biomedial Press, Amsterdam.

Vazdarjanova, A. and McGaugh, J.L. (1998) Basolateral amygdala is not critical for cognitive memory of contextual fear conditioning. *Proceedings of the National Academy of Sciences of the United States of America*, 95, 15003–15007.

Veening, J.G., Swanson, L.W., and Sawchenko, P.E. (1984) The organization of projections from the central nucleus of the amygdala to brain stem sites involved in central autonomic regulation: a combined retrograde transport–immunohistochemical study. *Brain Research*, 303, 337–357.

Veznedaroglu, E., Van Bockstaele, E.J., Valentino, R.J., and Pickel, V.M. (1996) Efferent projections of the central nucleus of the amygdala (CNA) to dendrites in the peri-locus coeruleus (LC) area. *Society for Neuroscience Abstracts*, 22, 2048.

Wahlestedt, C., Pich, E.M., Koob, G., Yee, F., and Heilig, M. (1993) Modulation of anxiety and neuropeptide Y-Y1 receptors by antisense oligodeoxynucleotides. *Science*, 259, 528–531.

Walker, D.L. and Davis, M. (1997) Double dissociation between the involvement of the bed nucleus of the stria terminalis and the central nucleus of the amygdala in light-enhanced versus fear-potentiated startle. *Journal of Neuroscience*, 17, 9375–9383.

Walker, D.L., Cassella, J.V., Lee, Y., de Lima, T.C.M., and Davis, M. (1997) Opposing roles of the amygdala and dorsolateral periaqueductal gray in fear-potentiated startle. *Brain Research Bulletin*, 111, 692–702.

Wallace, D.M., Magnuson, D.J., and Gray, T.S. (1989) The amygdalo-brainstem pathway: dopamine, noradrenergic and adrenergic cells in the rat. *Neuroscience Letters*, 97, 252–258.

Wallace, D.M., Magnuson, D.J., and Gray, T.S. (1992) Organization of amygdaloid projections to brainstem dopaminergic, noradrenergic and adrenergic cell groups in the rat. *Brain Research Bulletin*, 28, 447–454.

Watkins, L.R. and Mayer, D.J. (1982) Organization of endogenous opiate and nonopiate pain control systems. *Science*, 216, 1185–1192.

Watkins, L.R., Weirtelak, E.P., and Maier, S.F. (1993) The amygdala is necessary for the expression of conditioned but not unconditioned analgesia. *Behavioral Neuroscience*, 107, 402–405.

Weidenfeld, J., Itzik, A., and Feldman, S. (1997) Effect of glucocorticoids on the adrenocortical axis responses to electrical stimulation of the amygdala and the ventral noradrenergic bundle. *Brain Research*, 754, 187–194.

Weisz, D.J., Harden, D.G., and Xiang, Z. (1992) Effects of amygdala lesions on reflex facilitation and conditioned response acquisition during nictitating membrane response conditioning in rabbit. *Behavioral Neuroscience*, 106, 262–273.

Weller, K.L. and Smith, D.A. (1982) Afferent connections to the bed nucleus of the stria terminalis. *Brain Research*, 232, 255–270.

Werka, T. (1997) The effects of the medial and cortical amygdala lesions on post-stress analgesia in rats. *Behavioral Brain Research*, 86, 59–65.

Werka, T. (1998) Involvement of the lateral and dorsolateral amygdala in conditioned stimulus modality dependent two-way avoidance performance in rats. *Acta Neurobiologiae Experimentalis*, 58, 131–147.

Whalen, P.J. and Kapp, B.S. (1991) Contributions of the amygdaloid central nucleus to the modulation of the nictitating membrane reflex in the rabbit. *Behavioral Neuroscience*, 105, 141–153.

White, S.R. and Neuman, R.S. (1980) Facilitation of spinal motoneuron excitability by 5-hydroxytryptamine and noradrenaline. *Brain Research*, 185, 1–9.

Wiersma, A., Bohus, B., and Koolhaas, J.M. (1993) Corticotropin-releasing hormone microinfusion in the central amygdala diminishes a cardiac parasympathetic outflow under stress-free conditions. *Brain Research*, 625, 219–227.

Wiersma, A., Baauw, A.D., Bohus, B., and Koolhaas, J.M. (1995) Behavioural activation produced by CRH but not α-helical CRH (CRH-receptor antagonist) when microinfused into the central nucleus of the amygdala under stress-free conditions. *Psychoneuroendocrinology*, 20, 423–432.

Wiersma, A., Bohus, B., and Koolhaas, J.M. (1997a) Corticotropin-releasing hormone microinfusion in the central amygdala enhances active behaviour responses in the conditioned burying paradigm. *Stress*, 1, 113–122.

Wiersma, A., Knollema, S., Konsman, J.P., Bohus, B., and Koolhaas, J.M. (1997b) Corticotropin-releasing hormone modulation of a conditioned stress response in the central amygdala of the Roman high-avoidance and low-avoidance rat. *Behavioral Genetics*, 27, 547–555.

Wiersma, A., Konsman, J.P., Knollema, S., Bohus, B., and Koolhaas, J.M. (1998) Differential effects of CRH infusion into the central nucleus of the amygdala in the roman high-avoidance and low-avoidance rats. *Psychoneuroendocrinology*, 23, 261–274.

Wiersma, A., Tuinstra, T., and Koolhaas, J.M. (1997c) Corticotropin-releasing hormone microinfusion into the basolateral nucleus of the amygdala does not induce any changes in cardiovascular, neuroendocrine or behavioural output in a stress-free condition. Unpublished dissertation, University of Groningen, The Netherlands.

Wiersma, A., van Oosten, S., Knollema, S., Bohus, B., and Koolhaas, J. M. (1997d) Neurotensin microinfusion in the central amygdala diminishes a cardiac parasympathetic outflow possibly via a CRH receptor mediated process, in press. Unpublished dissertation, University of Groningen, The Netherlands.

Willcox, B.J., Poulin, P., Veale, W.L., and Pittman, Q.J. (1992) Vasopressin-induced motor effects: localization of a sensitive site in the amygdala. *Brain Research*, 596, 58–64.

Wolterink, G., Van Ree, J.M., Da Cunha, C., Wolfman, C., Levi de Stein, M., Ruschel, A.C., Izquierdo, I., and Medina, J.H. (1992) Anxiogenic effects of the intraamygdala injection of flumazenil, a benzodiazepine receptor antagonist. *Functional Neurology*, 7, 401–405.

Yadin, E., Thomas, E., Strickland, C.E., and Grishkat, H.L. (1991) Anxiolytic effects of benzodiazepines in amygdala-lesioned rats. *Psychopharmacology*, 103, 473–479.

Yajima, Y., Hayashi, Y., and Yoshii, N. (1980) The midbrain central gray substance as a highly sensitive neural structure for the production of ultrasonic vocalization in the rat. *Brain Research*, 198, 446–452.

Yajima, Y., Hayashi, Y., and Yoshii, N. (1982) Ambiguus motoneurons discharging closely associated with ultrasonic vocalization in rats. *Brain Research*, 238, 445–450.

Yaksh, T.L., Yeung, J.C., and Rudy, T.A. (1976) Systematic examination in the rat of brain sites sensitive to the direct application of morphine: observation of differential effects within the periaqueductal gray. *Brain Research*, 114, 83–103.

Yamamoto, T., Shimura, T., Sako, N., Yasoshima, Y., and Sakai, N. (1994) Neural substrates for conditioned taste aversion in the rat. Behavioural Brain Research, 65, 123–137.

Yamashita, K., Kataoka, Y., Shibata, K., Ozaki, T., Miyazaki, A., Kagoshima, M., and Ueki, S. (1989) Neuroanatomical substrates regulating rat conflict behavior evidenced by brain lesioning. *Neuroscience Letters*, 104, 195–200.

Yehle, A., Dauth, G., and Schneiderman, N. (1967) Correlates of heart rate classical conditioning in curarized rabbits. *Journal of Comparative and Physiological Psychology*, 64, 98–104.

Yeomans, J.S. and Franklin, P.W. (1994) Synapses in the rostrolateral midbrain mediate 'fear' potentiation of acoustic startle and electrically evoked startle. *Society for Neuroscience Abstracts*, 20, 1753.

Yeomans, J.S. and Pollard, B.A. (1993) Amygdala efferents mediating electrically evoked startle-like responses and fear potentiation of acoustic startle. *Behavioral Neuroscience*, 107, 596–610.

Young, B.J., Helmstetter, F.J., Rabchenuk, S.A., and Leaton, R.N. (1991) Effects of systemic and intra-amygdaloid diazepam on long-term habituation of acoustic startle in rats. *Pharmacology, Biochemistry, and Behavior*, 39, 903–909.

Zangrossi, J.H., Viana, M.B., and Graeff, F.G. (1999) Anxiolytic effect of intra-amygdala injection of midazolam and 8-hydroxy-2-(di-*n*-propylamino)tetralin in the elevated T-maze. *European Journal of Pharmacology*, 369, 267–270.

Zhang, J.X., Harper, R.M., and Ni, H. (1986) Cryogenic blockade of the central nucleus of the amygdala attenuates aversively conditioned blood pressure and respiratory responses. *Brain Research*, 386, 136–145.

Zhang, S.P., Bandler, R., and Carrive, P. (1990) Flight and immobility by excitatory amino acid microinjection within distinct parts of the subtentorial midbrain periaqueductal gray of the cat. *Brain Research*, 520, 73–82.

Zhang, S.P., Davis, P. J., Bandler, R., and Carrive, P. (1994) Brain stem integration of vocalization: role of the midbrain periaqueductal gray. *Journal of Neurophsiology*, 72(3), 1337–1356.

Zola-Morgan, S. and Squire, L.S. (1990) The primate hippocampal formation: evidence for a time-limited role in memory storage. *Science*, 250, 288–290.

7 The amygdala and emotion: a view through fear

Joseph LeDoux

W.M. Keck Laboratory of Neurobiology, Center for Neural Science, New York University

Summary

While the amygdala has long been known to be involved in emotional processes, studies of fear conditioning have provided the most detailed understanding of the amygdala's role in emotion to date. In this chapter, the neural pathways and mechanisms underlying the amygdala's role in the acquisition and expression of conditioned fear are explored. The relationship of work on fear conditioning to other areas of research, such as instrumental fear learning and memory modulation, is also discussed. Although the review focuses on studies of experimental animals, recent work on the human amygdala is also considered.

7.1 Introduction

In recent years, interest in the amygdala has increased considerably within neuroscience. However, the enthusiasm has spread beyond academic fields. In 1999, the *New York Times Magazine* ran a cover story on the role of the amygdala in fear and fear disorders, and a few years earlier a monster created by surgically altering the amygdala was the topic of a Batman comic. This rising interest is, in part, attributable to the progress that has been made over the past 20 years in relating specific circuits in this region of the brain to emotional functions, and much of this work has involved studies of a behavioural procedure called conditioned fear. In this chapter, the role of the amygdala in conditioned fear will be surveyed. First, however, we will briefly examine the historical events that preceded the wave of research on conditioned fear that began in the late 1970s.

7.2 The emotional brain in a historical context

In the early years of the 20th century, the hypothalamus was identified as the centrepiece of the brain's emotional system. The basic view, as espoused by Cannon and Bard in 1929, consisted of three major points: (i) the hypothalamus evaluates the emotional relevance of environmental events; (ii) the expression of emotional responses is mediated by the discharge of impulses from the hypothalamus to the brainstem; and (iii) projections from the hypothalamus to the cortex mediate the conscious experience of emotion. The Cannon–Bard theory was reinforced in 1937 by Papez, who added additional anatomical circuits in the forebrain to the theory but retained the central role of ascending and descending connections of the hypothalamus. The Papez theory, in turn, was elaborated upon in 1949 by MacLean, who called the forebrain emotional circuits the visceral brain, and then, in 1952, renamed these circuits the limbic system.

The term limbic system is still often used to refer to the emotional circuits of the brain. However, the limbic system has come under attack both as an anatomical concept and as a theory of the emotional brain (see Brodal, 1980; Swanson, 1983; LeDoux, 1987, 1991, 1996; Kotter and Meyer, 1992). Particularly important for the present survey are two points. First, there are no widely accepted criteria for deciding what is and what is not a limbic area. Secondly, however defined, the limbic system theory does not explain how the brain makes emotions. It points to a broad area of the forebrain located roughly between the neocortex and hypothalamus, but does not account for how specific aspects of any given emotion might be mediated.

Although the amygdala was included in MacLean's limbic system theory, its reputation as a key part of the emotional brain is due in large part to a study by Klüver and Bucy (1937) on the behavioural consequences of temporal lobe lesions in primates. These researchers initially were interested in trying to understand how hallucinogenic drugs achieve their effects. In the process, they found that removal of the temporal lobe led to a strange condition which has come to be called the Klüver–Bucy syndrome. The key feature of the syndrome for our purposes was that sensory events, especially visual events, seemed to lose their emotional implications. Klüver and Bucy called this psychic blindness. The animals could see perfectly, but the objects seen became psychologically meaningless. For example, monkeys with temporal lobe lesions tried to eat inedible objects, to copulate with same-sex partners or even with members of other species, and lost their fear of snakes and people. Although a similar set of results was obtained earlier by Brown and Schafer (1888), it was Klüver and Bucy's rediscovery of this condition that left an indelible mark on the field.

The temporal lobe lesions made by Klüver and Bucy covered a lot of territory, and later studies attempted to determine which parts of the temporal lobe might be most important to the syndrome (Pribram and Bagshaw, 1953; Weiskrantz, 1956; Akert *et al.*, 1961). Particularly noteworthy was a study by Weiskrantz (1956), which pinpointed the amygdala as the culprit in producing the emotional changes.

Rather than simply observing the behavioural changes produced by the lesions, as Klüver and Bucy had done, Weiskrantz employed experimental tasks that were designed to test how emotional reactions were altered. For example, since one of the major features of the Klüver–Bucy syndrome was a loss of fear, Weiskrantz used avoidance conditioning, a task which was believed to measure fear behaviour. In avoidance conditioning, the subject learns to perform some response because that response terminates or prevents the occurrence of an aversive unconditioned stimulus (US), such as electric shock, which arouses fear. Weiskrantz found that amygdala lesions impaired avoidance conditioning and, on the basis of this and other results, proposed that amygdala lesions dissociate the affective or reinforcing properties of stimuli from their sensory representations.

In the years following Weiskrantz's publication, work on the role of the amygdala in emotion went in two directions. Some studies pursued the contribution of the amygdala to the evaluation of the reinforcing properties of sensory stimuli, mostly using instrumental learning tasks motivated by food reinforcement (Jones and Mishkin, 1972; Horel *et al.*, 1975; Mishkin and Aggleton, 1981; Aggleton and Mishkin, 1986; Everitt and Robbins, 1992; Gaffan, 1992; Ono and Nishijo, 1992; Rolls, 1992). The legacy of this work is described in other chapters in this volume. Other studies followed up on the fear-reducing effects of amygdala lesions. While the latter is the tradition we are concerned with here, the relationship between the two traditions will be discussed later in this chapter.

7.3 The amygdala and fear: Pavlovian versus instrumental conditioning

In the 1960s and, 1970s, avoidance conditioning was the main task used to examine the role of the amygdala and other brain regions in fear. However, the results were conflicting and confusing (see Goddard, 1964; Grossman, 1967; Issacson, 1982; Sarter and Markowitsch, 1985). Sometimes damage to a brain area such as the amygdala would lead to a deficit, and sometimes not.

Several factors probably account for these discrepancies. First, the kind of response measured in avoidance conditioning studies varied considerably. Sometimes it involved active behaviours (such as crossing over a barrier, moving from one place to another, or pressing a bar to prevent shock from occurring) and at other times the response was passive (no shock occurs if the animal remains where it is). It seems clear, at least in retrospect, that the brain circuits involved in these different tasks will differ because the animal is asked to do different things. This not only applies to differences between active and passive avoidance, but also to different versions of each. Secondly, the lesions were made at different times in the various studies, with some coming before and others after learning. This is especially important when it is realized that avoidance conditioning involves at least two different learning processes. Initially, cues in the environment (conditional stimuli, CSs) acquire aversive properties by virtue of their association with the aversive US. This is Pavlovian learning. Subsequently, the animal learns to perform, in the presence of the CSs, some behaviour that prevents the US from occurring. This is instrumental learning. If Pavlovian and instrumental aversive learning involve different processes, which we now believe, pre- and post-training lesions of a given area would be expected to give different results. Lesions made before training starts will prevent both Pavlovian and instrumental learning from occurring, whereas those made after learning is complete will only affect the expression of the end result of the entire learning episode, i.e. the performance of the instrumental avoidance response. Given all these variables, the mystery as to why damage to the amygdala or other brain areas might have different results in different studies is cleared up, or at least made less surprising.

In the late 1970s and early 1980s, a new wave of work on fear began that produced a very consistent picture of how the brain mediates fear. In the new studies, Pavlovian fear conditioning was studied on its own, rather than as a part of avoidance conditioning. In Pavlovian fear conditioning, an emotionally neutral CS is presented in conjunction with an aversive US. After one or several pairings, the CS acquires the capacity to elicit responses that typically occur in the presence of danger, such as defensive behaviour (freezing responses), autonomic nervous system responses (changes in blood pressure and heart rate), neuroendocrine responses (release of hormones from the pituitary and adrenal glands), etc. (Figure 7.1). The responses are not learned and are not voluntary. They are innate, species-typical responses to threats and are expressed automatically in the presence of appropriate stimuli. Fear conditioning thus allows new or learned threats automatically to activate evolutionarily tuned ways of responding to danger. The ease of establishment, rapidity of learning, long duration of the memory, and stereotyped nature of the responses all speak to the value of the simpler Pavlovian learning process over the mixed Pavlovian–instrumental process that occurs in avoidance conditioning. This does not mean that fear conditioning can tell us all we need to know about all aspects of fear. However, it is an excellent starting point.

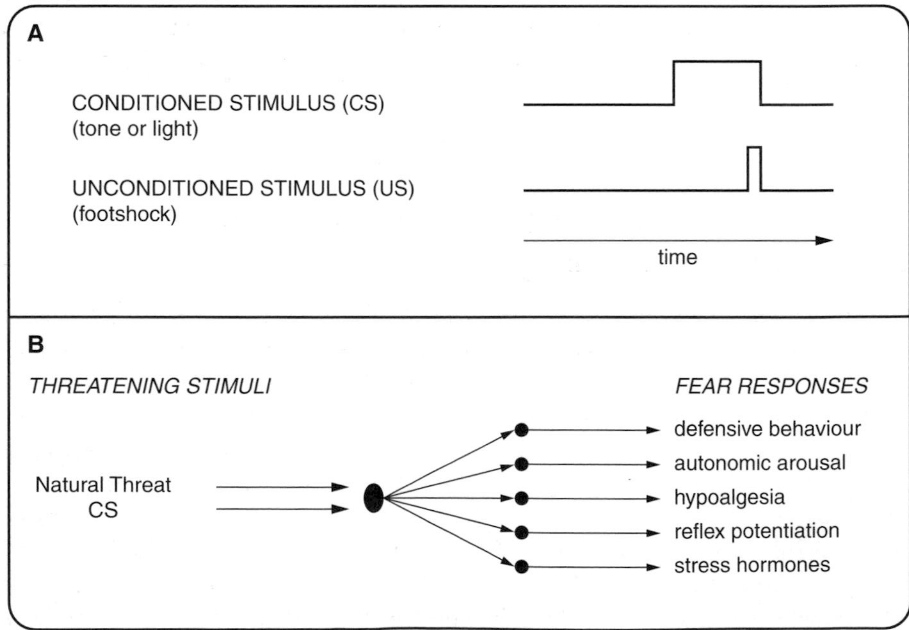

Figure 7.1 Fear conditioning involves the presentation of a noxious unconditioned stimulus (US), typically footshock, at the end of the occurrence of a relatively neutral conditioned stimulus (CS), such as a light or tone (top). After conditioning, the CS elicits a wide range of behavioural and physiological responses that characteristically occur when an animal encounters a threatening or fear-arousing stimulus (bootom). Thus, a rat that has been fear conditioned will express the same responses to a CS as to a neutral threat (i.e. a cat).

Our intent is not to malign the value of avoidance tasks. These are important in some contexts, one example being studies of the nature of emotional habits, such as the pathological habits of phobic patients who avoid normal life situations to prevent themselves from being exposed to stimuli and situations that others find innocuous. Our aim is instead to suggest that if one wants to know how threats are learned about, then the task of choice is Pavlovian fear conditioning.

7.4 Neural mechanisms underlying Pavlovian fear learning

The basic conclusion across studies of fear conditioning is that damage to the amygdala interferes with the acquisition and expression of conditioned fear (see LeDoux, 1996; Maren and Fanselow, 1996). If this were the only conclusion to emerge from the fear conditioning work over the past 20 years, it would not be very noteworthy. We already knew from the Klüver–Bucy syndrome that damage to the amygdala interferes with fear responses. By the late 1970s, there were already at least three publications that had shown that amygdala damage interferes with Pavlovian fear conditioning (Blanchard and Blanchard, 1972; Cohen, 1975; Pribram *et al.*, 1979). What the new wave of fear conditioning studies that began in the late 1970s did was to provide elaborate detail about how information about danger signals comes into the amygdala, about how signals are processed within the amygdala, about how fear responses are controlled by way of outputs of the amygdala, and about the cellular mechanisms of fear learning. Each of these topics will be discussed, as will some additional issues and controversies in the field.

7.5 Circuits into, within, and out of the amygdala involved in fear conditioning

Sensory inputs to the amygdala terminate mainly in the lateral nucleus (LA) (see Turner *et al.*, 1980; LeDoux *et al.*, 1990a; Turner and Herkenham, 1991; Amaral *et al.*, 1992; Romanski and LeDoux, 1992; Mascagni *et al.*, 1993; McDonald, 1998; Pitkänen, Chapter 2), and damage to LA interferes with fear conditioning (LeDoux *et al.*, 1990b; Campeau and Davis, 1995b). Most studies of fear conditioning have used auditory stimuli as CSs. In the following, we therefore focus on auditory fear conditioning pathways, which are summarized in Figure 7.2.

Auditory inputs to LA come from both the auditory thalamus and auditory cortex (see LeDoux *et al.*, 1990a; Romanski and LeDoux, 1993; Mascagni *et al.*, 1993; McDonald, 1998), and fear conditioning to a simple auditory CS can be mediated by either of these pathways (Romanski and LeDoux, 1992). It appears that the projection to LA from the auditory cortex is involved with a more complex auditory stimulus pattern (Jarrell *et al.*, 1987), but the exact conditions that require the cortex are poorly understood (Armony *et al.*, 1997). Although some lesion studies have questioned the ability of the thalamic pathway to mediate conditioning (Campeau and Davis, 1995a; Shi and Davis, 1998), single-unit recordings show that the cortical pathway conditions more slowly over trials than the thalamic pathway (Quirk *et al.*, 1995, 1997), thus indicating that plasticity in the amygdala occurs initially through the thalamic pathway.

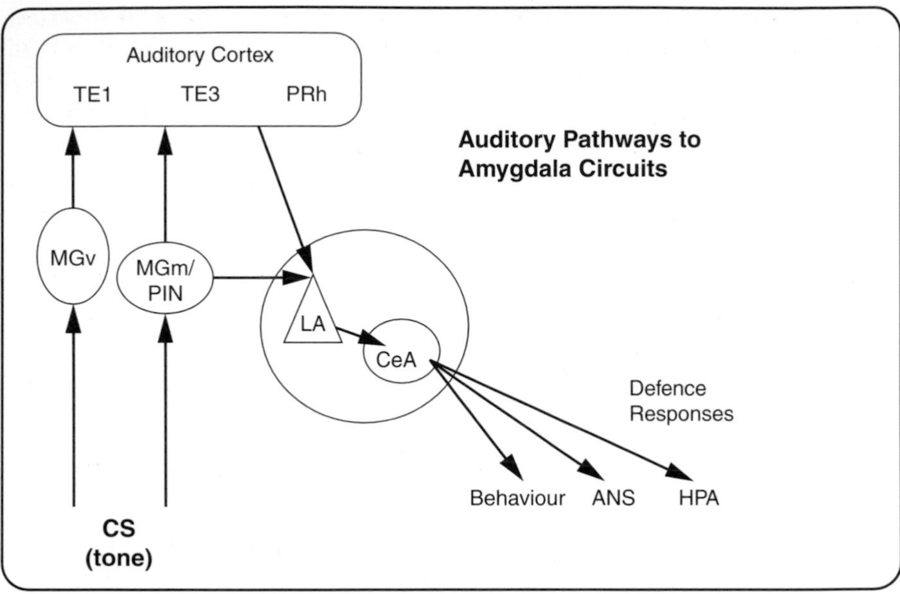

Figure 7.2 The pathways underlying fear conditioning to an acoustic CS involve auditory transmission to the lateral nucleus of the amygdala (LA) from areas in the thalamus (MGm/PIN) and cortex (TE3/PRh). LA, in turn, projects to the central nucleus of the amygdala (CeA), which controls the expression of fear responses by way of projections to brainstem areas. Abbreviations: ANS, autonomic nervous system; HPA, hypothalamic–pituitary axis; MGm/PIN, medial division of the medial geniculate body; MGv, ventral division of the medial geniculate body; TE1, primary auditory cortex; TE3, auditory association cortex; PRh, perirhinal cortex.

At present, the exact pathways involved in thalamoamygdala transmission in the primate are not well characterized. However, recent functional magnetic resonance imaging (fMRI) studies in humans have found that the human amygdala shows activity changes during conditioning that correlate with activity in the thalamus but not the cortex (Morris *et al.*, 1999). This finding suggests that the direct thalamoamygdala pathways are used in primates, but much more work is needed to determine anatomically and physiologically what these pathways are and what functional role they play. As in the rat, the clearest evidence for thalamoamygdala pathways in the primate involves the auditory system. Injections of retrograde tracers into the lateral amygdala of the monkey produces labelled cells in the peripeduncular nucleus (Jones *et al.*, 1976; Aggleton *et al.*, 1980). As suggested previously (LeDoux *et al.*, 1990b), the peripeduncular nucleus in the primate may be homologous to the posterior intralaminar nucleus in the rat, a region which receives auditory inputs from the brainstem (LeDoux *et al.*, 1985; Bordi and LeDoux, 1994) and projects to LA (LeDoux *et al.*, 1990b). There is some evidence for a decrease in the extent of subcortical versus cortical inputs to the amygdala from sensory areas in the course of evolution (Kudo *et al.*,

1986), but this conclusion was based on a fairly restrictive view of sensory thalamus (the primate peripeduncular nucleus, for example, was not included), and the issue should be re-evaluated.

Animals also exhibit fear responses when returned to the chamber in which the tone and shock were paired, or a chamber in which shocks occur alone. This is called contextual fear conditioning and requires both the amygdala and hippocampus (see Blanchard *et al.*, 1970; Phillips and LeDoux, 1992; Kim and Fanselow, 1992; Maren *et al.*, 1997; Frankland *et al.*, 1998). Areas of the ventral hippocampus (CA1 and subiculum) project to the basal and accessory basal (AB) nuclei of the amygdala (Canteras and Swanson, 1992), which are also known as the basolateral (BLA) and basomedial nuclei (Pitkanen *et al.*, 1997; Pitkänen, Chapter 2). Damage to these areas interferes with contextual conditioning (Maren and Fanselow, 1995; Majidashid *et al.*, 1996). Hippocampal projections to the BLA and AB thus seem to be involved in contextual conditioning (Figure 7.3).

The central nucleus of the amygdala (CeA) is the interface with motor systems. Damage to the CeA interferes with the expression of conditioned fear responses (Kapp *et al.*, 1979; Gentile *et al.*, 1986; Hitchcock and Davis, 1986; Iwata *et al.*, 1986; van der Kar *et al.*, 1991), while damage to areas that the CeA projects to selectively interrupts the expression of individual responses. For example, damage to the lateral hypothalamus affects blood pressure but not freezing responses, and damage to the peraqueductal grey interferes with freezing but not blood pressure responses (LeDoux *et al.*, 1988). Similarly, damage to the bed nucleus of the stria terminalis has no effect on either blood pressure or freezing responses (LeDoux *et al.*, 1988) but disrupts the conditioned release of pituitary–adrenal stress hormones (van der Kar, 1991). Because CeA receives inputs from LA, BLA, and AB (Pitkänen *et al.*, 1997), it is in a position to mediate the expression of conditioned fear responses elicited by both acoustic and contextual CSs (Figure 7.3).

The direct projection from LA to CeA seems to be sufficient for conditioning to an auditory CS, since lesions of B and AB have no effect on fear conditioning to a tone (Majidashid *et al.*, 1996). However, Killcross *et al.* (1997) recently argued that a direct projection to CeA that bypasses LA can mediate conditioning to an auditory CS. There is little evidence for direct projections to CeA from auditory processing areas: fibres from auditory areas terminate mainly in LA (see above), and auditory response latencies in LA are shorter than in CeA both before and after conditioning (see next section below). Leaving these facts aside, though, it is important to point out that the task used to rule out LA as a way station involved hundreds of training trails, whereas the tasks used to implicate LA have involved far fewer trials (see Nader and LeDoux, 1997). It is possible that the additional training trials allowed the brain to learn in a way that is not normally used when fewer trials are given. At most, a direct pathway to CeA would be an alternative rather than the main route of transmission through the amygdala.

Nevertheless, the other aspect of the Killcross study, the dissociation of the role of the CeA in reflexive fear responses from the role of the LA/BLA in instrumental fear responses, seems plausible. Indeed, we recently have found something similar (see Figure 7.4). Damage to CeA interfered with the conditioning of freezing responses to a tone CS but had no effect on conditioning the same rats to perform a response that turned the aversive CS off in a

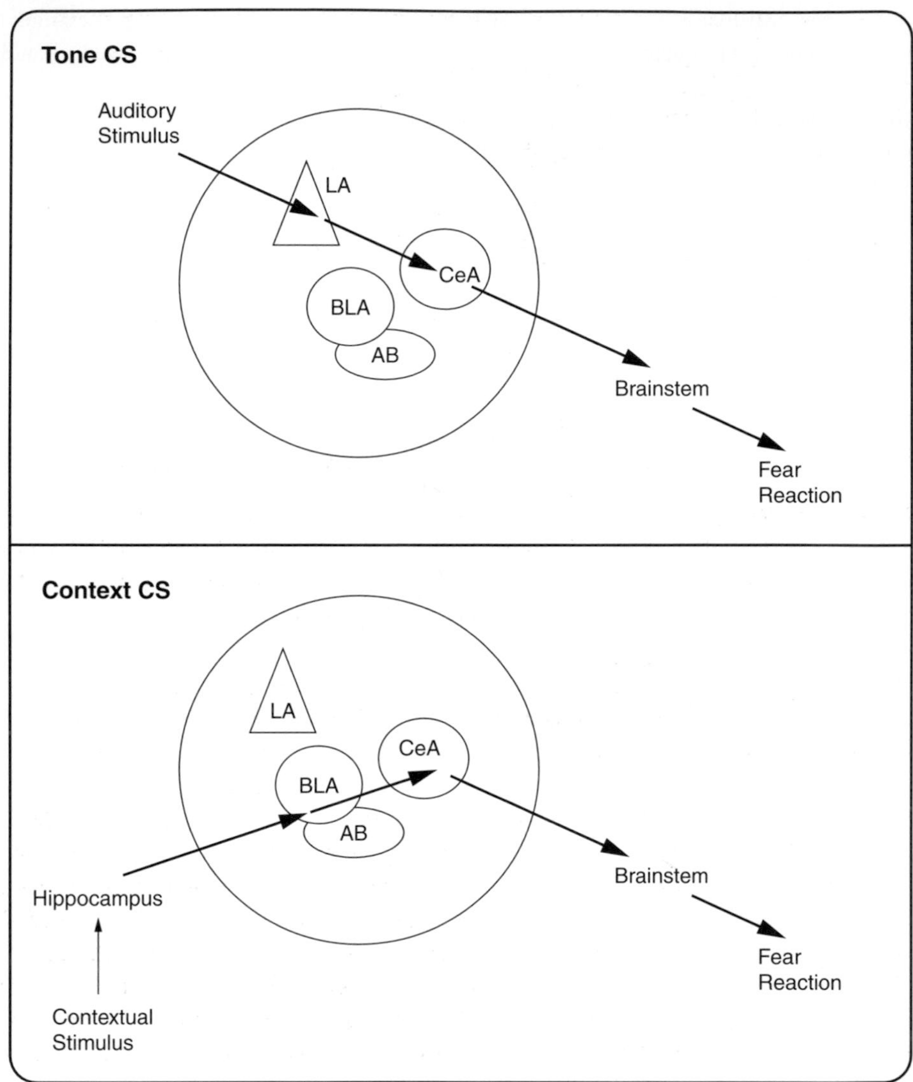

Figure 7.3 Conditioning to a tone CS involves projections from the auditory system to the lateral nucleus of the amygdala (LA) and from LA to the central nucleus (CeA). In contrast, conditioning to the apparatus and other contextual cues present when the CS and US are paired involves the representation of the context by the hippocampus and the communication between the basolateral (BLA) and accessory basal (AB) nuclei of the amygdala, which in turn project to the CeA. As for tone conditioning, CeA controls the expression of the response.

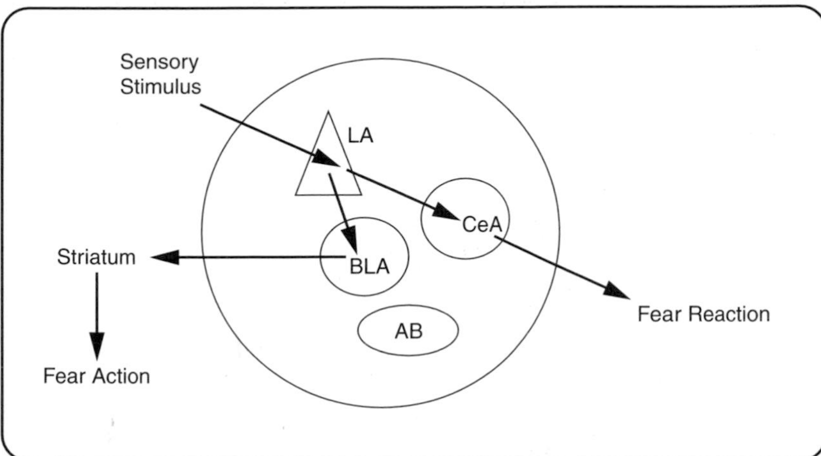

Figure 7.4 Projections from the lateral nucleus of the amygdala (LA) to the central nucleus (CeA) are involved in automatic fear reactions elicited by a CS. In contrast, emotional actions emitted in the presence of a CS and reinforced by its termination are mediated by projections from LA to BLA and from there possibly to the striatum.

new environment, whereas damage to BLA had no effect on freezing but prevented the rats from learning to perform the response that turned off the aversive CS (Amorapanth *et al.*, 2000). Further, since both responses were controlled by a tone CS, damage to the LA, which receives the tone CS from the auditory system, disrupted both responses.

In summary, different pathways within the amygdala are involved in fear conditioning depending on the nature of the CS and the learning task. For conditioning to a tone CS, projections from LA to CeA are involved, whereas for contextual conditioning, projections from the hippocampus to the BLA and/or AB, and from there to the CeA are needed. In contrast, in order to learn an instrumental fear response controlled by a tone CS, projections from LA to BLA are used. Presumably, the response is then controlled by projections from BLA to the striatum (Everitt and Robbins, 1992). Taking this logic to the next step, it might be the case that instrumental fear responses controlled by contextual stimuli might only need BLA, or BLA and AB, and the striatum.

7.6 Cellular and molecular plasticity in the amygdala related to fear conditioning

In order for conditioning to occur, pathways transmitting the CS and US have to converge in the brain. Cells in LA are responsive to nociceptive stimulation, and some of the same cells respond to auditory inputs as well (Romanski *et al.*, 1993). Thus, the substrate for conditioning (convergence of CS and US information) exists in LA. Indeed, during fear conditioning, the firing properties of cells in LA are modified (Quirk *et al.*, 1995, 1997).

Conditioned plasticity also occurs in the auditory cortex (Weinberger, 1995, 1998; Quirk *et al.*, 1997). However, the response latencies in LA within trials (<20 ms) and the rate of acquisition (1–3 trials) is best explained in terms of direct auditory thalamoamygdala transmission, rather than corticoamygdala transmission, since conditioned responses in the auditory cortex occur later both within trials and across trials (Quirk *et al.*, 1997). Plasticity in the auditory thalamus (Weinberger, 1995, 1998) could contribute to LA plasticity. Plasticity has also been observed in BLA (Maren *et al.*, 1991; Uwano *et al.*, 1995) and CeA (Pascoe and Kapp, 1985) during aversive conditioning, but the acoustic response latencies both before and after conditioning are longer than in LA. LA thus seems to be both the initial point of sensory processing and the initial site of plasticity in the amygdala.

Plasticity in the amygdala has also been studied using long-term potentiation (LTP), a physiological procedure pioneered in studies of the hippocampus (Bliss and Lømo, 1973). LTP is believed to engage the cellular mechanisms similar to those that underlie natural learning (e.g. Lynch, 1986; Bliss and Collingridge, 1993). The most extensively studied form of LTP occurs in the CA1 region of the hippocampus and involves the interaction between presynaptic glutamate and two classes of postsynaptic receptors (Nicoll and Malenka, 1995). First, glutamate binds to α-amino-3-hydroxy-5-methyl-4-isoxazole proprionic acid (AMPA) receptors and depolarizes the postsynaptic cell. The depolarization allows glutamate to bind to the *N*-methyl-D-aspartate (NMDA) class of receptors. Calcium then flows into the cell through the NMDA channel and triggers a host of intracellular events that ultimately result in gene induction and synthesis of new proteins (see Dudai, 1989; Huang *et al.*, 1996). These then help to stabilize the changes over long periods of time.

There have been a number of studies of LTP in the amygdala, mostly involving *in vitro* brain slices and pathways carrying information from the cortex to LA and BLA (Chapman *et al.*, 1990; Chapman and Bellevance, 1992; Gean *et al.*, 1993; Huang and Kandel, 1998; see Chapman and Chattarji, Chapter 3). These studies have led to mixed results regarding the possible role of NMDA receptors in corticoamygdala LTP, with some studies finding effects (Huang and Kandel, 1998) and some not (Chapman and Bellevance, 1993). Recent *in vitro* studies indicate that LTP in the thalamoamygdala pathway requires postsynaptic calcium, but the calcium does not enter through NMDA receptors (Weisskopf and LeDoux, 1999). Instead, calcium entry occurs through L-type voltage-gated calcium channels. These channels have also been implicated in a form of LTP that occurs in the hippocampus (Cavus and Teyler, 1996). It has also been shown that prior fear conditioning leads to an enhancement in synaptic responses recorded subsequently *in vitro* from amygdala slices (McKernan and Schinnick-Gallagher, 1997). The receptor mechansisms underlying this form of plasticity have not been elucidated.

LTP has also been studied *in vivo* in the thalamoamygdala pathway using recordings of extracellular field potentials (Clugnet and LeDoux, 1990; Rogan and LeDoux, 1995; Rogan *et al.*, 1997). These studies show that LTP occurs in fear processing pathways, that the processing of natural stimuli similar to those used as a CS in conditioning studies is facilitated following LTP induction, and that fear conditioning and LTP induction produce similar changes in the processing of CS-like stimuli. While exploration of mechanisms are difficult in these *in vivo* studies, they nevertheless provide some of the strongest evidence to date in any brain system of a relationship between natural learning and LTP (Barnes, 1995; Eichenbaum, 1995; Stevens, 1998). LTP has been found *in vivo* in the hippocampal–amygdala pathway, which is believed to be involved in context conditioning (Maren and Fanselow, 1995).

The fact that blockade of NMDA receptors with the drug (±)-2-amino-5 phosphonovaleric acid (APV) prevents LTP from occurring in the CA1 region of the hippocampus inspired researchers to attempt to prevent fear conditioning by infusion of APV into the amygdala. Initial studies were quite promising (Miserendino *et al.*, 1992). Infusion of APV prior to learning blocked fear conditioning, but infusion prior to testing had no effect. NMDA receptors thus seemed to be involved in the plasticity underlying learning and not in the transmission of signals through the amygdala. However, subsequently both *in vivo* (Li *et al.*, 1995, 1996; Maren and Fanselow, 1996) and *in vitro* (Weisskopf and LeDoux, 1999) studies have suggested that NMDA receptors make significant contributions to synaptic transmission in pathways that provide inputs to the amygdala. Further, several studies have found that blockade of NMDA receptors affects both the acquisition and expression of fear learning (Kim *et al.*, 1998; Maren and Fanselow, 1996), which is more consistent with the transmission than the plasticity hypothesis, but others have confirmed that acquisition could be affected independently of expression (Gewirtz and Davis, 1997).

The contribution of NMDA receptors to fear conditioning and its underlying plasticity, as opposed to synaptic transmission in amygdala circuits, remains unresolved. Given the relatively weak contribution of NMDA receptors to transmission in the cortical input, perhaps the disruption of fear learning is explained by a combination of different effects on the two pathways: blockade of transmission and plasticity in the thalamic pathway, and blockade of plasticity in the cortical pathway. It is also possible that behaviourally significant plasticity occurs downstream from LA input synapses in the amygdala, and that the effect of APV infusions is on this plasticity rather than on the plasticity at input synapses. Additional work is needed.

It is generally believed that long-term retention of the effects of learning involves intracellular cascades that are triggered by the influx of calcium during action potentials (see Dudai, 1989; Kandel, 1997). The rise in calcium then triggers several kinases and transcription factors, including calcium–calmodulin-dependent kinase II, mitogen-acivated protein kinase, cAMP-dependent kinase (PKA), protein kinase C, and cAMP response element-binding protein (CREB). These act, possibly in concert, to induce genes and initiate synthesis of new proteins. While these mechanisms have been worked out best in reduced preparations, such as studies of invertebrates or studies of LTP (see Yin *et al.*, 1994; Huang *et al.*, 1996; Kandel, 1999), many of these same intracellular signals have been implicated in fear conditioning through studies of genetically altered mice (Bourtchouladze *et al.*, 1994; Mayford *et al.*, 1996; Able *et al.*, 1997) or by infusing agents that affect the pathways in the brain (Atkins *et al.*, 1998; Bourtchouladze *et al.*, 1998; Josselyn *et al.*, 1998; Schafe *et al.*, 1999).

7.7 Memory versus modulation

In spite of a wealth of data implicating the amygdala in fear conditioning, some authors have suggested recently that the amygdala is not a site of plasticity or storage during fear conditioning (e.g. Cahill and McGaugh, 1998; Vazdarjanova and McGaugh, 1998). They argue instead that the amygdala modulates memories that are formed elsewhere. It is clear that there are multiple memory systems in the brain (see Squire, 1993; MacDonald and White, 1993; Eichenbaum, 1994), and that the amygdala does indeed modulate memories formed in other systems, such as declarative or explicit memories formed through hippocampal circuits or habit memories formed through striatal circuits (Packard *et al.*, 1994). However, evidence for a role of the amygdala in modulation should not be confused with evidence against a role in plasticity. That the amygdala is indeed important for learning is suggested by studies showing that inactivation of the amygdala during learning prevents learning from taking place (e.g. Helmstetter and Bellgowan, 1994; Muller *et al.*, 1997). Further, if the inactivation occurs immediately after training, then there is no effect on subsequent memory (Willensky *et al.*, 1999; 2000), showing that the effects of pre-training treatment are on learning and not on processes that occur after learning. The amygdala thus seems to be essential for fear learning, and does not modulate its own learning.

7.8 Fear conditioning and the human amygdala

Damage to the amygdala (Bechara *et al.*1995) or areas of temporal lobe including the amygdala (LaBar *et al.*, 1995) produces deficits in fear conditioning in humans. Further, fear conditioning leads to increases in amygdala functional activity, as measured by fMRI (Buchel *et al.*, 1998; LaBar *et al.*, 1998), and these effects also occur to subliminal stimuli (Morris *et al.*, 1998). Additionally, when the activity of the amygdala during fear conditioning is cross-correlated with the activity in other regions of the brain, the strongest relationships are seen with subcortical (thalamic and collicular) rather than cortical areas, further emphasizing the importance of the direct thalamoamygdala pathway in the human brain (Morris *et al.*, 1999). Other aspects of emotion and the human brain are reviewed in Phelps and Anderson (1997) and Davidson and Irwin (1999).

7.9 So where's the fear?

Fear and fear learning have been dealt with here without addressing the conscious experience of fear that occurs when humans are in danger. While this is more a problem about consciousness than about emotion, it is an important problem to which research on emotion may be able to contribute.

We are far from solving what consciousness is, but a number of theorists (Kihlstrom, 1987; Kosslyn and Koenig, 1992; Johnson-Laird, 1993) have proposed that it may be related to working memory (Baddeley, 1998), a serially organized mental workspace where things can be compared and contrasted and mentally manipulated. A variety of studies of humans and non-human primates point to the prefrontal cortex, especially the dorsolateral prefrontal areas—as well as the anterior cingulate and orbital cortical regions—as being involved in working memory (Goldman-Rakic, 1996; Braver *et al.*, 1997; Carter *et al.*, 1998; Fuster, 1998). Immediately present stimuli and stored representations are integrated in working memory by way of interactions between prefrontal areas, sensory processing systems (which serve as short-term memory buffers), and the long-term explicit (declarative) memory system involving the hippocampus and related areas of the temporal lobe. In the case of an affectively charged stimulus, such as a trigger of fear, the same sorts of processes will be called upon as for stimuli without emotional implications, but, in addition, working memory will become aware of the fact that the fear system of the brain has been activated. This additional information, when added to perceptual and mnemonic information about the object or event, could be the condition for the subjective experience of an emotional state of fear (LeDoux, 1996).

By way of projections to cortical areas, the amygdala can influence the operation of perceptual and short-term memory processes, as well as processes in higher order areas. Although the amygdala does not have extensive connections with the dorsolateral prefrontal cortex, it does communicate with the anterior cingulate and orbital cortex, two other components of the working memory network. However, in addition, the amygdala projects to non-specific systems involved in the regulation of cortical arousal and controls bodily responses (behavioural, autonomic, endocrine), which then provide feedback that can influence cortical processing indirectly. Thus, working memory receives a greater number of inputs, and receives inputs of a greater variety, in the presence of an emotional stimulus than in the presence of other stimuli. These extra inputs may be just what is required to add affective charge to working memory representations, and thus to turn subjective experiences into emotional experiences (Figure 7.5).

7.10 Views of the emotional brain in light of conditioned fear research: have we made progress?

It is instructive to look back on the early proposals by Cannon and Papez regarding the brain mechanisms of emotion and reconsider their contributions in light of the work that has been done since. Although the particulars have changed, the general view of how threatening stimuli incite animals to defend themselves remains somewhat the same. For example, both Cannon and Papez proposed that sensory stimuli leaving the thalamus travel both through the neocortex and to subcortical 'emotional' processing regions. Papez referred to the former as the stream of thought and the latter as the stream of feeling. For both Papez and Cannon, the hypothalamus was the key subcortical region involved in emotional processing. Its job was to send signals to the brainstem, so that emotions could be expressed as bodily responses, and to the cortex, so that emotions could be experienced as subjective states.

Contemporary research largely agrees with this general picture, painted largely on the basis of anatomical speculation in the 1920s and 1930s. However, with the accumulation of a great deal of empirical research, the amygdala has replaced the hypothalamus as the centrepiece of the subcortical networks involved in detecting and responding to threats. Thus, projections from the amygdala to the brainstem are involved in the expression of fear responses, and projections from the amygdala to the cortex are believed to contribute to the experience of fear and other cognitive aspects of emotional processing.

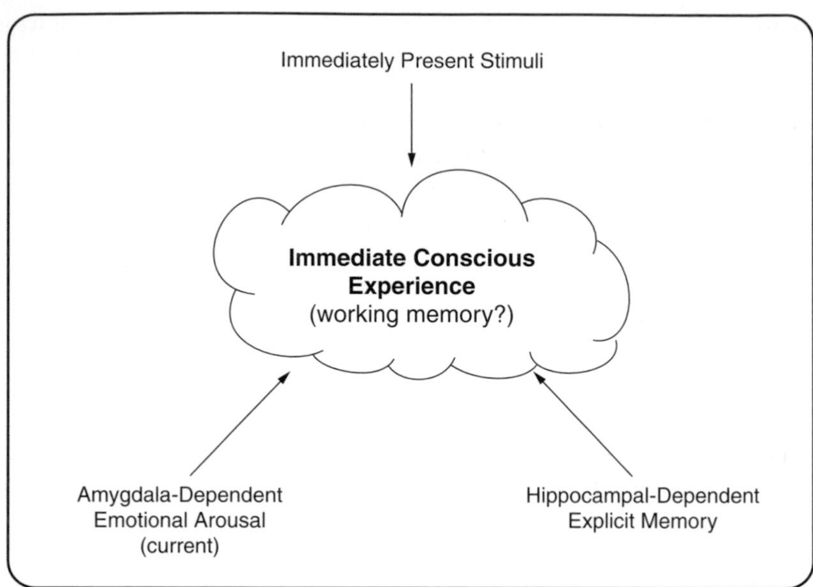

Figure 7.5 Conscious experiences are often said to reflect the contents of working memory. In this sense, a conscious emotional experience may not be that different from any other kind of conscious experience. The difference would be more in the systems that are providing inputs to working memory rather than in the mechanisms of consciousness itself. In the case of fearful experiences, or fearful feelings, the conscious emotion may be the result of some immediately present stimulus triggering long-term explicit memories and amygdala activation. The simultaneous representation in working memory of the outputs of these three, and perhaps other, systems, may be the stuff that fearful feelings are made of. Other feelings would come about similarly, but would not necessartily involve the amygdala.

Still, it would be wrong to conclude that the field has not advanced since the early days. Clearly, we now know much more about how the fear system works. In addition to pinpointing the amygdala as a key structure in the processing of danger, much has been learned about how the amygdala accomplishes its job. The anatomical inputs to and outputs from the amygdala are understood in exquisite detail, as are the internal connections that mediate processing within the amygdala. Further, the nature of physiological encoding of fear situations by neurons within the amygdala is beginning to be understood as well. We are poised now to understand the neural basis of at least a simple form of fear processing, and this will surely lay a foundation for further explorations of the neural basis of fear and fear disorders, and perhaps other emotions as well.

References

Abel, T., Nguyen, P.V., Barad, M., Deuel, T.A., Kandel, E.R., and Bourtchouladze, R. (1997) Genetic demonstration of a role for PKA in the late phase of LTP and in hippocampus-based long-term memory. *Cell*, 88, 615–626.

Aggleton, J.P. and Mishkin, M. (1986) The amygdala: sensory gateway to the emotions. In *Emotion: Theory, Research and Experience*, Vol. 3 (eds R. Plutchik and H. Kellerman), pp. 281–299. Academic Press, Orlando, Florida.

Aggleton, J.P., Burton, M.J., and Passingham, R.E. (1980) Cortical and subcortical afferents to the amygdala of the rhesus monkey (*Macaca mulatta*). *Brain Research*, 190, 347–368.

Akert, K., Gruesen, R.A., Woolsey, C.N., and Meyer, D.R. (1961) Klüver–Bucy syndrome in monkeys with neocortical ablations of temporal lobe. *Brain*, 84, 480–497.

Amaral, D.G., Price, J.L., Pitkänen, A., and Carmichael, S.T. (1992) Anatomical organization of the primate amygdaloid complex. In *The Amygdala: Neurobiological Aspects of Emotion, Memory, and Mental Dysfunction* (ed. J.P. Aggleton), pp. 1–66. Wiley-Liss, New York.

Amorapanth, P., LeDoux, J.E. and Nader, K. (2000) Different lateral amygdala outputs mediate reactions and actions elicited by a fear-arousing stimulus. *Nature Neuroscience* 3, 74–9.

Armony, J.L., Servan-Schreiber, D., Romanski, L.M., Cohen, J.D., and LeDoux, J.E. (1997) Stimulus generalization of fear responses: effects of auditory cortex lesions in a computational model and in rats. *Cerebral Cortex*, 7, 157–165.

Atkins, C.M., Selcher, J.C., Petraitis, J.J., Trzaskos, J.M., and Sweatt, J.D. (1998) The MAPK cascade is required for mammalian associative learning. *Nature Neuroscience*, 1, 602–609.

Baddeley, A. (1998) Working memory. *Comptes Rendus de l'Academie des Sciences. Serie III, Sciences de la Vie*, 321, 167–173.

Barnes, C.A. (1995) Involvement of LTP in memory: are we 'searching under the street-light? *Neuron*, 15, 751–754.

Bechara, A., Tranel, D., Damasio, H., Adolphs, R., Rockland, C., and Damasio, A.R. (1995) Double dissociation of conditioning and declarative knowledge relative to the amygdala and hippocampus in humans. *Science*, 269, 1115–1118.

Blanchard, C.D. and Blanchard, R.J. (1972) Innate and conditioned reactions to threat in rats with amygdaloid lesions. *Journal of Comparative and Physiological Psychology*, 81, 281–290.

Blanchard, R.J., Blanchard, D.C., and Fial, R.A. (1970) Hippocampal lesions in rats and their effect on activity, avoidance and aggression. *Journal of Comparative and Physiological Psychology*, 71, 92–102.

Bliss, T.V. and Collingridge, G.L. (1993) A synaptic model of memory: long-term potentiation in the hippocampus. *Nature*, 361, 31–39.

Bliss, T.V.P. and Lømo, T. (1973) Long-lasting potentiation of synaptic transmission in the dentate area of the anaesthetized rabbit following stimulation of the perforant path. *Journal of Physiology*, 232, 331–356.

Bordi, F. and LeDoux, J.E. (1994) Response properties of single units in areas of rat auditory thalamus that project to the amygdala. I. Acoustic discharge patterns and frequency receptive fields. *Experimental Brain Research*, 98, 261–274.

Bourtchuladze, R., Frenguelli, B., Blendy, J., Cioffi, D., Schutz, G., and Silva, A.J. (1994) Deficient long-term memory in mice with a targeted mutation of the cAMP-responsive element-binding protein. *Cell*, 79, 59–68.

Braver, T.S., Cohen, J.D., Jonides, J., Smith, E.E., and Noll, D.C. (1997) A parametric study of prefrontal cortex involvement in human working memory. *NeuroImage*, 5, 49–62.

Brodal, A. (1980) Changes in our view on the organization of the central nervous system. Have they significance for clinical neurology? *Tidsskr Nor Laegeforen*, 100, 1531–1534.

Brown, S. and Schafer, A. (1888) An investigation in the functions of the occipital and temporal lobes of the monkey's brain. *Philosophical Transactions of the Royal Society of London, Series B*, 179, 303–327.

Buchel, C., Morris, J., Dolan, R.J., and Friston, K.J. (1998) Brain systems mediating aversive conditioning: an event-related fMRI study. *Neuron*, 20, 947–957.

Cahill, L. and McGaugh, J.L. (1998) Mechanisms of emotional arousal and lasting declarative memory. *Trends in Neuroscience*, 21, 294–299.

Campeau, S. and Davis, M. (1995a) Involvement of subcortical and cortical afferents to the lateral nucleus of the amygdala in fear conditioning measured with fear-potentiated startle in rats trained concurrently with auditory and visual conditioned stimuli. *Journal of Neuroscience*, 15, 2312–2327.

Campeau, S. and Davis, M. (1995b) Involvement of the central nucleus and basolateral complex of the amygdala in fear conditioning measured with fear-potentiated startle in rats trained concurrently with auditory and visual conditioned stimuli. *Journal of Neuroscience*, 15, 2301–2311.

Canteras, N.S. and Swanson, L.W. (1992) Projections of the ventral subiculum to the amygdala, septum and hypothalamus: a PHAL anterograde tract-tracing study in the rat. *Journal of Comparative Neurology*, 324, 180–194.

Carter, C.S., Braver, T.S., Barch, D.M., Botvinick, M.M., Noll, D., and Cohen, J.D. (1998) Anterior cingulate cortex, error detection and the online monitoring of performance. *Science*, 280, 747–749.

Cavus, I. and Teyler, T. (1996) Two forms of long-term potentiation in area CA1 activate different signal transduction cascades. *Journal of Neurophysiology*, 76, 3038–3047.

Chapman, P.F. and Bellavance, L.L. (1992) NMDA receptor-independent LTP in the amygdala. *Synapse*, 11, 310–318.

Chapman, P.F., Kairiss, E.W., Keenan, C.L., and Brown, T.H. (1990) Long-term synaptic potentiation in the amygdala. *Synapse*, 6, 271–278.

Clugnet, M.C. and LeDoux, J.E. (1990) Synaptic plasticity in fear conditioning circuits: induction of LTP in the lateral nucleus of the amygdala by stimulation of the medial geniculate body. *Journal of Neuroscience*, 10, 2818–2824.

Davidson, R.J. and Irwin, W. (1999) The functional neuroanatomy of emotion and affective style. *Trends in Cognitive Sciences*, 3, 211–221.

Dudai, Y. (1989) *The Neurobiology of Memory*. Oxford University Press, New York.

Eichenbaum, H. (1994) The hippocampal system and declarative memory in humans and animals: experimental analysis and historical origins. In *Memory Systems* (eds D.L. Schacter and E. Tulving), pp. 147–201. MIT Press, Cambridge, Massachusetts.

Eichenbaum, H. (1995) The LTP–memory connection. *Nature*, 378, 131–132.

Everitt, B.J. and Robbins, T.W. (1992) Amygdala–ventral striatal interactions and reward-related processes. In *The Amygdala: Neurobiological Aspects of Emotion, Memory, and Mental Dysfunction* (ed. J.P. Aggleton), pp. 401–429. Wiley-Liss, New York.

Frankland, P.W., Cestari, V., Filipkowski, R.K., McDonald, R.J., and Silva, A. (1998) The dorsal hippocampus is essential for context discrimination, but not for contextual conditioning. *Behavioral Neuroscience*, 112, 863–874.

Fuster, J.M. (1998) Distributed memory for both short and long term. *Neurobiology of Learning and Memory*, 70, 268–274.

Gaffan, D. (1992) Amygdala and the memory of reward. In *The Amygdala: Neurobiological Aspects of Emotion, Memory, and Mental Dysfunction* (ed. J.P. Aggleton), pp. 471–483. Wiley-Liss, New York.

Gean, P.-W., Chang, F.-C., and Hung, C.-R. (1993) Use-dependent modification of a slow NMDA receptor-mediated synaptic potential in rat amygdalar slices. *Journal of Neuroscience Research*, 34, 635–641.

Gentile, C.G., Jarrell, T.W., Teich, A., McCabe, P.M., and Schneiderman, N. (1986) The role of amygdaloid central nucleus in the retention of differential Pavlovian conditioning of bradycardia in rabbits. *Behavioral Brain Research*, 20, 263–273.

Gewirtz, J.C. and Davis, M. (1997) Second-order fear conditioning prevented by blocking NMDA receptors in amygdala. *Nature*, 388, 471–474.

Goddard, G. (1964) Functions of the amygdala. *Psychological Review*, 62, 89–109.

Goldman-Rakic, P.S. (1996) Regional and cellular fractionation of working memory. *Proceeedings of the National Academy of Sciences of the United States of America*, 93, 13473–80.

Grossman, S.P. (1967) *A textbook of physiological psychology*, John Wiley & Sons, Inc., New York.

Helmstetter, F.J. and Bellgowan, P.S. (1994) Effects of muscimol applied to the basolateral amygdala on acquisition and expression of contextual fear conditioning in rats. *Behavioral Neuroscience*, 108, 1005–1009.

Hitchcock, J. and Davis, M. (1986) Lesions of the amygdala but not of the cerebellum or red nucleus block conditioned fear as measured with the potentiated startle paradigm. *Behavioral Neuroscience*, 100, 11–22.

Horel, J.A., Keating, E.G., and Misantone, L.J. (1975) Partial Klüver–Bucy syndrome produced by destroying temporal neocortex or amygdala. *Brain Research*, 94, 347–359.

Huang, Y.Y. and Kandel, E.R. (1998) Postsynaptic induction and PKA-dependent expression of LTP in the lateral amygdala. *Neuron*, 21, 169–178.

Huang, Y.Y., Nguyen, P.V., Abel, T., and Kandel, E.R. (1996) Long-lasting forms of synaptic potentiation in the mamalian hippocampus. *Learning and Memory*, 3, 74–85.

Isaacson, R.L. (1982) *The Limbic System*. Plenum Press, New York.

Iwata, J., LeDoux, J.E., Meeley, M.P., Arneric, S., and Reis, D.J. (1986) Intrinsic neurons in the amygdaloid field projected to by the medial geniculate body mediate emotional responses conditioned to acoustic stimuli. *Brain Research*, 383, 195–214.

Jarrell, T.W., Gentile, C.G., Romanski, L.M., McCabe, P.M., and Schneiderman, N. (1987) Involvement of cortical and thalamic auditory regions in retention of differential bradycardia conditioning to acoustic conditioned stimulii in rabbits. *Brain Research*, 412, 285–294.

Johnson-Laird, P.N. (1993) A computational analysis of consciousness. In *Consciousness in Contemporary Science* (eds A.J. Marcel and E. Bisiach), pp. 357–368. Oxford University Press, Oxford.

Jones, B. and Mishkin, M. (1972) Limbic lesions and the problem of stimulus–reinforcement associations. *Experimental Neurology*, 36, 362–377.

Jones, E.G., Burton, H., Saper, C.B., and Swanson, L.W. (1976) Midbrain, diencephalic and cortical relationships of the basal nucleus of Meynert and associated structures in primates. *Journal of Comparative Neurology*, 167, 385–420.

Josselyn, S.A., Carlezon, W.A.J., Neve, S.C.J.R., Nestler, E.J., and Davis, M. (1998) Overexpression of CREB in the amygdala facilitates the formation of long-term memory measured with fear-potentiated startle in rats. *Society for Neuroscience Abstracts*, **24**, 926.

Kandel, E.R. (1997) Genes, synapses and long-term memory. *Journal of Cellular Physiology*, 173, 124–125.

Kapp, B.S., Frysinger, R.C., Gallagher, M., and Haselton, J. (1979) Amygdala central nucleus lesions: effect on heart rate conditioning in the rabbit. *Physiologicy and Behavior*, 23, 1109–1117.

Kihlstrom, J.F. (1987) The cognitive unconscious. *Science*, 237, 1445–1452.

Killcross, S., Robbins, T.W., and Everitt, B.J. (1997) Different types of fear-conditioned behavior mediated by separate nuclei within amygdala. *Nature*, 388, 377–380.

Kim, J.J. and Fanselow, M.S. (1992) Modality-specific retrograde amnesia of fear. *Science*, 256, 675–677.

Kim, J.J., Fanselow, M.S., DeCola, J.P., and Landeira-Fernandez, J. (1998) Selective impairment of long-term but not short-term conditional fear by the *N*-methyl-D-aspartate antagonist APV. *Behavioral Neuroscience*, 106, 591–596.

Klüver, H. and Bucy, P.C. (1937) 'Psychic blindness' and other symptoms following bilateral temporal lobectomy in rhesus monkeys. *American Journal of Physiology*, 119, 352–353.

Kosslyn, S.M. and Koenig, O. (1992) *Wet Mind: The New Cognitive Neuroscience*. Macmillan, Inc., New York,

Kotter, R. and Meyer, N. (1992) The limbic system: a review of its empirical foundation. *Behavioral Brain Research*, 52, 105–127.

Kudo, M., Glendenning, K.K., Frost, S.B., and Masterson, R.S. (1986) Origin of mammalian thalamocortical projections. I. Telencephalic projection of the medial geniculate body in the opossum (*Didelphis virginiana*). *Journal of Comparative Neurology*, 245, 176–197.

LaBar, K.S., LeDoux, J.E., Spencer, D.D., and Phelps, E.A. (1995) Impaired fear conditioning following unilateral temporal lobectomy in humans. *Journal of Neuroscience*, 15, 6846–6855.

LaBar, K.S., Gatenby, J.C., Gore, J.C., LeDoux, J.E., and Phelps, E.A. (1998) Human amygdala activation during conditioned fear acquisition and extinction: a mixed-trial fMRI study. *Neuron*, 20, 937–945.

LeDoux, J.E. (1987) Emotion. In *Handbook of Physiology. 1: The Nervous System. Vol V: Higher Functions of the Brain* (ed. F. Plum), pp. 419–460. American Physiological Society, Bethesda, Maryland.

LeDoux, J.E. (1991) Emotion and the limbic system concept. *Concepts in Neuroscience*, 2, 169–199.

LeDoux, J.E. (1996) *The Emotional Brain*. Simon and Schuster, New York.

LeDoux, J.E., Ruggiero, D.A., and Reis, D.J. (1985) Projections to the subcortical forebrain from anatomically defined regions of the medial geniculate body in the rat. *Journal of Comparative Neurology*, 242, 182–213.

LeDoux, J.E., Iwata, J., Cicchetti, P., and Reis, D.J. (1988) Different projections of the central amygdaloid nucleus mediate autonomic and behavioral correlates of conditioned fear. *Journal of Neuroscience*, 8, 2517–2529.

LeDoux, J.E., Cicchetti, P., Xagoraris, A., and Romanski, L.M. (1990a) The lateral amygdaloid nucleus: sensory interface of the amygdala in fear conditioning. *Journal of Neuroscience*, 10, 1062–1069.

LeDoux, J.E., Farb, C.F., and Ruggiero, D.A. (1990b) Topographic organization of neurons in the acoustic thalamus that project to the amygdala. *Journal of Neuroscience*, 10, 1043–1054.

Li, X., Phillips, R.G. and LeDoux, J.E. (1995) NMDA and non-NMDA receptors contribute to synaptic transmission between the medial geniculate body and the lateral nucleus of the amygdala. *Experimental Brain Research*, 105, 87–100.

Li, X.F., Stutzmann, G.E., and LeDoux, J.L. (1996) Convergent but temporally separated inputs to lateral amygdala neurons from the auditory thalamus and auditory cortex use different postsynaptic receptors: *in vivo* intracellular and extracellular recordings in fear conditioning pathways. *Learning and Memory*, 3, 229–242.

Lynch, G. (1986) *Synapses, Circuits and the Beginnings of Memory*. MIT Press, Cambridge, Massachusetts,

MacLean, P.D. (1949) Psychosomatic disease and the 'visceral brain': recent developments bearing on the Papez theory of emotion. *Psychosomatoc Medicine*, 11, 338–353.

MacLean, P.D. (1952) Some psychiatric implications of physiological studies on frontotemporal portion of limbic system (visceral brain). *Electroencephalography and Clinical Neurophysiology*, 4, 407–418.

Majidishad, P., Pelli, D.G., and LeDoux, J.E. (1996) Disruption of fear conditioning to contextual stimuli but not to a tone by lesions of the accessory basal nucleus of the amygdala. *Society for Neuroscience Abstracts*, 22, 1116.

Maren, S. and Fanselow, M.S. (1995) Synaptic plasticity in the basolateral amygdala induced by hippocampal formation stimulation *in vivo. Journal of Neuroscience*, 15, 7548–7564.

Maren, S. and Fanselow, M.S. (1996) The amygdala and fear conditioning: has the nut been cracked? *Neuron*, 16, 237–240.

Maren, S., Poremba, A., and Gabriel, M. (1991) Basolateral amygdaloid multi-unit neuronal correlates of discriminative avoidance learning in rabbits. *Brain Research*, 549, 311–316.

Maren, S., Aharonov, G., and Fanselow, M.S. (1997) Neurotoxic lesions of the dorsal hippocampus and Pavlovian fear conditioning in rats. *Behavioral Brain Research*, 88, 261–74.

Mascagni, F., McDonald, A.J., and Coleman, J.R. (1993) Corticoamygdaloid and cortico-cortical projections of the rat temporal cortex: a *Phaseolus vulgaris* leucoagglutinin study. Neuroscience, 57, 697–715.

Mayford, M., Bach, M.E., Huang, Y.-Y., Wang, L., Hawkins, R.D., and Kandel, E.R. (1996) Control of memory formation through regulated expression of a CaMKII transgene. *Science*, 274, 1678–1683.

McDonald, A.J. (1998) Cortical pathways to the mammalian amygdala. *Progress in Neurobiology*, **55**, 257–332.

McDonald, R.J. and White, N.M. (1993) A triple dissociation of memory systems: hippocampus, amygdala, and dorsal striatum. *Behavioral Neuroscience*, **107**, 3–22.

McKernan, M.G. and Shinnick-Gallagher, P. (1997) Fear conditioning induces a lasting potentiation of synaptic currents *in vitro*. *Nature*, 390, 607–611.

Miserendino, M.J.D., Sananes, C.B., Melia, K.R., and Davis, M. (1990) Blocking of acquisition but not expression of conditioned fear-potentiated startle by NMDA antagonists in the amygdala. *Nature*, 345, 716–718.

Mishkin, M. and Aggleton, J. (1981) Multiple functional contributions of the amygdala in the monkey. In *The Amygdaloid Complex* (ed. Y. Ben-Ari), pp. 409–420. Elsevier/North-Holland Biomedical Press, Amsterdam.

Morris, J.S., Ohman, A., and Dolan, R.J. (1998) Conscious and unconscious emotional learning in the human amygdala. *Nature*, 393, 467–470.

Morris, J.S., Ohman, A., and Dolan, R.J. (1999) A subcortical pathway to the right amygdala mediating 'unseen' fear. *Proceeedings of the National Academy of Sciences of the United States of America*, 96, 1680–1685.

Muller, J., Corodimas, K.P., Fridel, Z., and LeDoux, J.E. (1997) Functional inactivation of the lateral and basal nuclei of the amygdala by muscimol infusion prevents fear conditioning to an explicit CS and to contextual stimuli. *Behavioral Neuroscience*, 111, 683–691.

Nader, K. and LeDoux, J.E. (1997) Is it time in invoke multiple fear learning system? *Trends in Cognitive Science*, 1, 241–244.

Nicoll, R.A. and Malenka, R.C. (1995) Contrasting properties of two forms of long-term potentiation in the hippocampus. *Nature*, 377, 115–118.

Ono, T. and Nishijo, H. (1992) Neurophysiological basis of the Klüver–Bucy syndrome: responses of monkey amygdaloid neurons to biologically significant objects. In *The Amygdala: Neurobiological Aspects of Emotion, Memory, and Mental Dysfunction* (ed. J.P. Aggleton), pp. 167–190. Wiley-Liss, New York.

Packard, M.G., Cahill, L., and McGaugh, J.L. (1994) Amygdala modulation of hippocampal-dependent and caudate nucleus-dependent memory processes. *Proceeedings of the National Academy of Sciences of the United States of America*, 91, 8477–8481.

Papez, J.W. (1937) A proposed mechanism of emotion. *Archives of Neurology and Psychiatry*, 79, 217–224.

Pascoe, J.P. and Kapp, B.S. (1985) Electrophysiological characteristics of amygdaloid central nucleus neurons during Pavlovian fear conditioning in the rabbit. *Behavioral Brain Research*, 16, 117–133.

Phelps, E.A. and Anderson, A.K. (1997) Emotional memory: what does the amygdala do? *Current Opinion in Biology*, 7, R311–R314.

Phillips, R.G. and LeDoux, J.E. (1992) Differential contribution of amygdala and hippocampus to cued and contextual fear conditioning. *Behavioral Neuroscience*, 106, 274–285.

Pitkänen, A., Savander, V., and LeDoux, J.L. (1997) Organization of intra-amygdaloid circuitries: an emerging framework for understanding functions of the amygdala. *Trends in Neuroscience*, 20, 517–523.

Pribram, K.H. and Bagshaw, M. (1953) Further analysis of the temporal lobe syndrome utilizing frontotemporal ablations. *Journal of Comparative Neurology*, 99, 347–375.

Pribram, K.H., Reitz, S., McNeil, M., and Spevack, A.A. (1979) The effect of amygdalectomy on orienting and classical conditioning in monkeys. *Pavlovian Journal of Biological Science*, 14, 203–217.

Quirk, G.J., Repa, J.C., and LeDoux, J.E. (1995) Fear conditioning enhances short-latency auditory responses of lateral amygdala neurons: parallel recordings in the freely behaving rat. *Neuron*, 15, 1029–1039.

Quirk, G.J., Armony, J.L., and LeDoux, J.E. (1997) Fear conditioning enhances different temporal components of toned-evoked spike trains in auditory cortex and lateral amygdala. *Neuron*, 19, 613–624.

Rogan, M.T. and LeDoux, J.E. (1995) LTP is accompanied by commensurate enhancement of auditory-evoked responses in a fear conditioning circuit. *Neuron*, 15, 127–136.

Rogan, M., Staubli, U., and LeDoux, J. (1997) Fear conditioning induces associative long-term potentiation in the amygdala. *Nature*, 390, 604–607.

Rolls, E.T. (1992) Neurophysiology and functions of the primate amygdala. *The amygdala: neurobiological aspects of emotion, memory, and mental dysfunction*. J.P. Aggleton. New York, Wiley-Liss, Inc.: 143–165.

Romanski, L.M. and LeDoux, J.E. (1992) Equipotentiality of thalamo-amygdala and thalamo-cortico-amygdala projections as auditory conditioned stimulus pathways. *Journal of Neuroscience*, 12, 4501–4509.

Romanski, L.M., LeDoux, J.E., Clugnet, M.C., and Bordi, F. (1993) Somatosensory and auditory convergence in the lateral nucleus of the amygdala. *Behavioral Neuroscience*, 107, 444–450.

Sarter, M.F. and Markowitsch, H.J. (1985) Involvement of the amygdala in learning and memory: a critical review, with emphasis on anatomical relations. *Behavioral Neuroscience*, 99, 342–380.

Schafe, G.E., Nadel, N.V., Sullivan, G.M., Harris, A., and LeDoux, J.E. (1999) Memory consolidation for contextual and auditory fear conditioning is dependent on protein synthesis, PKA, and MAP kinase. *Learning and Memory*, **6**, 97–110.

Shi, C. and Davis, M. (1998) Pain pathways involved in fear conditioning measured with fear potentiated startle: lesion studies. *Journal of Neuroscience*, 19, 420–430.

Squire, L.R., Knowlton, B., and Musen, G. (1993) The structure and organization of memory. *Annual Review of Psychology*, 44, 453–495.

Stevens, C.F. (1998) A million dollar question: does LTP=memory? *Neuron*, 20, 1–2.

Swanson, L.W. (1983) The hippocampus and the concept of the limbic system. In *Neurobiology of the Hippocampus* (ed. W. Seifert), pp. 3–19. Academic Press, London.

Turner, B.H. and Herkenham, M. (1991) Thalamoamygdaloid projections in the rat: a test of the amygdala's role in sensory processing. *Journal of Comparative Neurology*, 313, 295–325.

Turner, B.H., Mishkin, M., and Knapp, M. (1980) Organization of the amygdalopetal projections from modality-specific cortical association areas in the monkey. *Journal of Comparative Neurology*, 191, 515–543.

Uwano, T., Nishijo, H., Ono, T., and Tamura, R. (1995) Neuronal responsiveness to various sensory stimuli and associative learning in the rat amygdala. *Neuroscience*, 68, 339–361.

van de Kar, L.D., Piechowski, R.A., Rittenhouse, P.A., and Gray, T.S. (1991) Amygdaloid lesions: differential effect on conditioned stress and immobilization-induced increases in corticosterone and renin secretion. *Neuroendocrinology*, 54, 89–95.

Vazdarjanova, A. and McGaugh, J.L. (1998) Basolateral amygdala is not critical for cognitive memory of contextual fear conditioning. *Proceeedings of the National Academy of Sciences of the United States of America*, 95, 15003–15007.

Weinberger, N.M. (1995) Retuning the brain by fear conditioning. In *The Cognitive Neurosciences* (ed. M.S. Gazzaniga), pp. 1071–1090. MIT Press, Cambridge, Massachusetts.

Weinberger, N.M. (1998) Physiological memory in primary auditory cortex: characteristics and mechanisms. *Neurobiology of Learning Memory*, 70, 226–251.

Weiskrantz, L. (1956) Behavioral changes associated with ablation of the amygdaloid complex in monkeys. *Journal of Comparative Physiological Psychology*, 49, 381–391.

Weisskopf, M.G. and LeDoux, J.E. (1999) Distinct populations of NMDA receptors at subcortical and cortical inputs to principal cells of the lateral amygdala. *Journal of Neurophysiology*, 81, 930–934.

Wilensky, A.E., Schafe, G.E., and LeDoux, J.E. (1999) Functional inactivation of the amygdala before but not after auditory fear conditioning prevents memory formation. *Journal of Neuroscience*, E1-E5.

Wilensky, A.E., Schafe, G.E., and LeDoux, J.E. (2000) The amygdala modulates memory consolidation of fear-motivated inhibitory avoidance learning but not classical fear conditioning. *Journal of Neuroscience*, in press.

Yin, J.C., Wallach, J.S., Del Vecchio, M., Wilder, E.L., Zhou, H., Quinn, W.G., and Tully, T. (1994) Induction of a dominant negative CREB transgene specifically blocks long-term memory in Drosophila. *Cell*, **79**, 49–58.

8 The amygdala and associative learning

Michela Gallagher

Department of Psychology, Johns Hopkins University, 3400 North Charles Street, Baltimore, MD 21218, USA

Summary

The amygdala complex is composed of a heterogeneous collection of nuclei that possess widely different interconnections with other brain regions. By combining behavioural studies with a neural systems analysis, a subset of these nuclei, including the lateral, basolateral, and central nuclei, have been tied together to form a functionally unified system necessary for the acquisition and expression of conditioned fear (Davis, 1992; LeDoux, Chapter 7). This chapter considers more broadly studies of associative learning that have shown a dependence on the integrity of the amygdala complex, which include aversive and appetitive paradigms as well as both Pavlovian conditioning and instrumental learning. This review supports the perspective that the central nucleus and basolateral complex, along with their diverse interconnections with both brainstem and forebrain systems, form a largely integrated substrate for the use of associative information in the control and guidance of adaptive behaviour.

8.1 Introduction

In naturalistic settings, monkeys with amygdala damage do not survive (Kling *et al.*, 1970). Placidity and hypoemotionality have been long considered defining features of amygdala damage in humans and non-human primates (Klüver and Bucy, 1939). It is becoming apparent, however, that these negative signs are symptomatic of deficits in a remarkable range of adaptive behaviours. Specifically, a system that includes the lateral, basolateral, basomedial, and central nuclei of the amygdala complex (BLA/CeA) is important for associative learning. The schematic in Figure 8.1 shows a diagram of these cell groupings, which are perhaps best known for their role in the acquisition of classically conditioned fear (Kapp *et al.*, 1984; Davis, 1992; LeDoux, 1995). From a neuroanatomical perspective, the lateral and basolateral nuclei possess

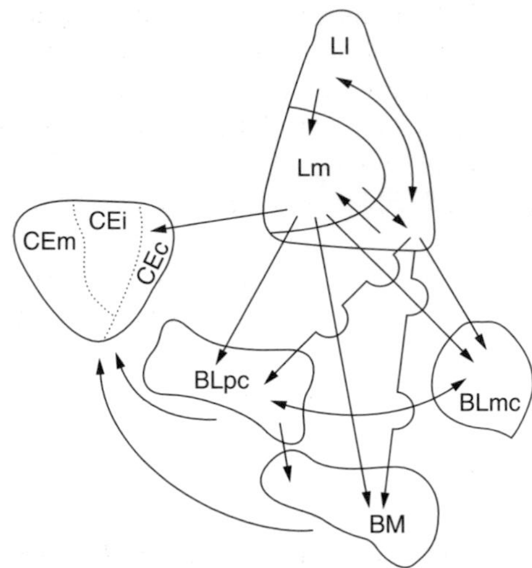

Figure 8.1 Schematic showing a group of interconnected nuclei of the amygdala complex that are implicated in associative learning. These include subdivisions of the lateral nucleus (LI and Lm), the anterior magnocellular and posterior parvocellular divisions of the basolateral nucleus (BLmc and BLpc), the basomedial nucleus (BM), and divisions of the central nucleus (Cem, Cei, and Cec).

a number of cortical-like characteristics, consistent with Johnston's (1923) determination that they are phylogenetically more recent in the evolution of vertebrates (see Alheid and Heimer, 1988; Swanson and Petrovich, 1998). By contrast, the central nucleus belongs to the phylogenetically older centromedial group of amygdala nuclei. One of the remarkable features of this circuitry is its integrative function in the evolution of adaptive behavioral systems.

This chapter will use the connectional anatomy of the BLA/CeA in considering its role in learning. The various components of this circuitry make connections with other brain regions that control a wide array of behaviours, ranging from species-typical repertoires that are critical for survival to high-level cognitive systems important for planning and decision making. In addition to allowing associative learning to influence many output/action systems, the connectional anatomy of the BLA/CeA also appears to regulate attentional processing of sensory inputs. New evidence has shown pathways through which BLA/CeA's role in attention can optimize new learning, a topic that will also be reviewed in this chapter.

8.2 Connectivity of BLA/CeA to output/action systems from brainstem to cortex

Output of the BLA/CeA system targets a remarkable array of visceromotor and somatomotor systems at all levels of the neuroaxis (reviewed in this volume, and see Amaral, 1987;

Swanson and Petrovich, 1998). Neurons originating in the amygdala central nucleus (CeA) have access to brainstem sites that directly control autonomic and somatomotor responses. Other amygdala projections originating in the posterior division of the basolateral nucleus and the basomedial nucleus terminate in medial hypothalamic regions that organize reproductive, feeding, and aggressive behaviours. At the other end of the neuroaxis, targets of the anterior division of the basolateral nucleus (BLA) include direct innervation of premotor and prefrontal cortex; the BLA also provides regulation of forebrain output via a massive widespread innervation of the striatum. Through these diverse projections, associative learning can influence behavioural control at many levels of neural processing. The following discussion will consider these outputs from a neural systems perspective that ultimately cuts across psychological categories, such as fear conditioning versus appetitive conditioning, or Pavlovian conditioning versus instrumental learning.

8.3 Connectional systems for the control of species-typical behaviour by associative learning

Much work has focused on the CeA as an output for the expression of amygdala-based learning. Neurons in the CeA project to a vast array of sites in the brainstem (Price and Amaral, 1981). Some of these sites are the origin of outputs that directly control behavioural and autonomic responses; other targets of CeA are ascending systems that innervate the forebrain, i.e. midbrain dopamine neurons (Gonzalez and Chesselet, 1990). Consistent with its connectional anatomy, CeA lesions impair both somatic and autonomic conditioned responses (Kapp *et al.*, 1979; Hitchcok and Davis, 1986; LeDoux *et al.*, 1988). The somatomotor targets of CeA in the brainstem produce freezing or control reflexive behaviours that are modulated by learning; for example, conditioned fear enhances the startle reflex via CeA projections to the pontine reticular formation (Hitchcock and Davis, 1991). The earliest behavioural studies to define clearly the contribution of the CeA in Pavolvian learning were conducted by Kapp and his associates, using aversively conditioned heart rate (Kapp *et al.*, 1979). Damage to the CeA impairs an associatively conditioned decrease in heart rate (bradycardia) that is mediated by vagal efferents. It is notable that unconditioned bradycardia, which occurs as a component of the orienting response to novel cues, is unaffected by amygdala damage. Likewise, CeA damage, which abolishes fear enhancement of startle, leaves the unconditioned startle reflex intact; the occurrence and magnitude of startle elicited by a loud noise, for example, are unaffected in rats with CeA lesions (Davis, 1986).

The role of the CeA is not confined to aversive conditioning and the expression of fear-related behaviours. For example, environmental cues associated with food elicit a conditioned insulin response (vagally mediated) that is eliminated by CeA lesions (Roozendaal *et al.*, 1990). That effect of CeA damage is, as in other cases, selective for learning because the unconditioned elevation of insulin in response to food consumption is not altered. As another example in appetitive learning, the acquisition of conditioned orienting behaviours, which occur to stimuli paired with the delivery of food, are also abolished by selective excitotoxic lesions of CeA (Gallagher *et al.*, 1990). Simple cues, such as a tone or light, that signal the delivery of food come to elicit such orienting responses. Similarly to the case of unconditioned heart rate, startle, and insulin responses, unconditioned orienting responses, e.g. rearing to initial presentation of a novel light cue, are unaffected by CeA damage. In both appetitive and aversive conditioning, therefore, the CeA provides access to output systems that can become controlled by cues on the basis of learning. It is important to note that alterations in unconditioned responses that might reflect a generalized change in arousal or might merely indicate an impairment in response systems do not occur when CeA projections to these targets are removed.

Although the expression of learning is controlled in many instances by CeA projections that directly access output systems in the brainstem, different routes to the behavioural expression of CeA-dependent learning are required in some cases. In the case of the orienting conditioned responses (CRs) observed in appetitive conditioning, the physical characteristics of the conditioned stimulus (CS) determine the topography of the CR. When a visual CS is used, rearing to the light is the characteristic CR; when a tone CS is used, rats engage in abrupt movements that do not include rearing. In order for the CR to be guided appropriately by the physical properties of the CS, integration of sensorimotor function is needed. For this purpose, the expression of conditioned behavioural orienting depends on CeA projections to nigrostriatal dopaminergic neurons, thereby engaging striatal circuitry (Han *et al.*, 1997). It is well known that damage to the nigrostriatal neurons themselves produces deficits in unconditioned orienting to sensory cues (Carli *et al.*, 1985, 1986; Fairely and Marshall, 1986). Similarly to its direct projections to output systems in the brainstem, however, the amygdala CeA engages striatal circuitry for the expression of learning while having no discernible influence on spontaneous orienting to novel unconditioned cues.

Not all amygdala-dependent functions in Pavlovian conditioning use targets of CeA; targets of BLA also appear to be involved in the behavioural expression of classical conditioning. For example, the potentiation of feeding by a CS is unaffected by CeA lesions but is diminished by damage to the basolateral region of the amygdala, as shown in Figure 8.2 (Gallagher and Holland, 1992; and unpublished observations). When rats are sated, they normally will consume more food in the presence of a Pavolvian CS that previously was conditioned by pairing it with food, relative to tests when no CS is presented (Weingarten, 1983). A dependence of CS-potentiated feeding on the BLA may reflect connectional features of this region. As noted previously, the posterior division of the basolateral nucleus projects directly to an area of the medial hypothalamus involved in the regulation of feeding. Indeed both the posterior basolateral and basomedial nuclei innervate hypothalamic regions that are separately involved in feeding, sexual, and aggressive behaviours (see Petrovich *et al.*, 1996). The ability of a CS to elicit feeding, as well as influences of conditioning on sexual behaviour and aggression, might depend on those amygdala connections, apart from CeA. By this view, the effects of learning could be brought to bear on a large range of species-typical behaviours; control by CeA and BLA on different behavioural systems or responses would reflect primarily their connectivity with different brain regions.

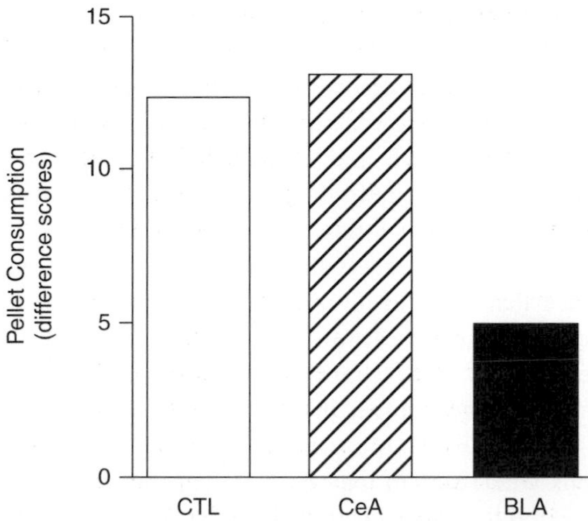

Figure 8.2 Potentiation of feeding by a conditioned stimulus. Three groups of rats were trained using standard appetitive Pavolvian procedures in which a CS (10 s duration) was followed by delivery of food pellets. After CRs were established, the rats were placed back on *ad libitum* feeding and, in addition, were given access in the home cage to the food pellets used as the US during conditioning. Two test sessions were then conducted when the rats were in this satiated condition. Twenty food pellets were made available in the original training apparatus during each of the test sessions. In one session, the cue formerly used as the CS was presented, while in the other session no CS presentations occurred. The graph shows the difference in food pellet consumption in the presence of the CS relative to the session without CS presentation. A robust potentiation of feeding occurred in the presence of the CS for the control group (CTL) and for a group that had bilateral excitotoxic lesions of the central nucleus (CeA). Lesions of the basolateral amygdala (BLA) significantly decreased this potentiation effect. It should be noted that all groups had learned to approach the food cup as a conditioned response during the original Pavlovian training.

8.4 Connectional systems for the control of voluntary behaviour on the basis of learning

Another important pathway for amygdala-dependent learning is direct innervation of the striatum. Mogenson and his associates initially drew attention to this striatal innervation as an interface between limbic processing and motor output (Mogenson *et al.*, 1984). The anterior division of the BLA provides a widespread innervation of both the dorsal and ventral striatum, i.e. the caudate and nucleus accumbens (Kelley *et al.*, 1982; Groenenwegen *et al.*, 1990; McDonald, 1991a,b). The posterior BLA and basomedial nucleus also innervate the ventral striatum, in particular the more medial portion of the nucleus accumbens (Groenenwegen *et al.*, 1990). A number of studies have shown that amygdala-based learning is dependent on these connections.

Everitt and colleagues clearly demonstrated that learning of a new instrumental response in second-order conditioning depends on BLA and its projection to ventral striatum (Everitt *et al.*, 1989, Chapter 10). In a task used in that work, rats learn to press a lever to gain presentation of a CS that had been paired with primary reward in a prior phase of training. Their research has shown that the effects of BLA damage are selective; without producing motivational deficits or sensory deficits in discriminating the CS, rats with BLA lesions are impaired when the incentive value of the Pavlovian CS is used to support instrumental behaviour. In aversive conditioning, rats with BLA damage are also impaired in learning to avoid making a response that leads to the presentation of an aversive CS (Killcross *et al.*, 1997). This instrumental avoidance learning, however, is unaffected by CeA lesions. Although rats with CeA lesions fail to suppress responding in the presence of the aversively conditioned CS, they were able to direct their actions so as to avoid further presentations of that stimulus.

The BLA connections with striatum may be more generally critical for learning whereby stimuli acquire value or reinforcing properties. This function may reflect a role for BLA in allowing neutral stimuli to gain access to primary reward systems involving the ventral striatum. A considerable number of studies have now shown that lesions of BLA, but not CeA, impair conditioning that depends on this function. These include assessments for cue preferences in choice tests (Everitt *et al.*, 1991; McDonald and White, 1993), as well as the ability of CSs to serve as reinforcers in new learning (Everitt *et al.*, 1989; Hatfield *et al.*, 1996). In addition to the case of instrumental conditioning studied by Everitt and associates, we have shown that BLA integrity is also essential for second-order Pavlovian conditioning (see Hatfield *et al.*, 1996 and Figure 8.3). Because this more general role of BLA is not shared by CeA, i.e. CeA lesions do not alter Pavlovian second-order conditioning, it is possible that such effects are mediated via the ventral striatum.

8.5 Additional connectional systems for the control of goal-directed behaviour

Interconnections of the amygdala with prefrontal cortex afford access to a further level of control over goal-directed behaviour. Associations in which cues, responses, or contextual information are linked to the incentive properties of outcomes provide an important basis for goal-directed behaviour. In this context, recent research in our laboratories has shown an important role for BLA and the orbitofrontal cortex (OFC) (Hatfield *et al.*, 1996; Schoenbaum *et al.*, 1998, 1999; Gallagher *et al.*, 1999); these areas are strongly interconnected in both rodent and primates (Krettek and Price, 1977; McDonald, 1991b).

As a model for this aspect of associative learning, we used a task in which normal performance depends on the ability of a CS to gain access to the motivational properties of an upcoming unconditioned stimulus (US). Our studies employed a procedure in which rats are first trained in standard Pavlovian conditioning, using a light CS paired with food delivery. After CRs are established to the CS, rats receive the original US (food) in another setting where it is paired with an aversive event (injection of lithium chloride). This second phase

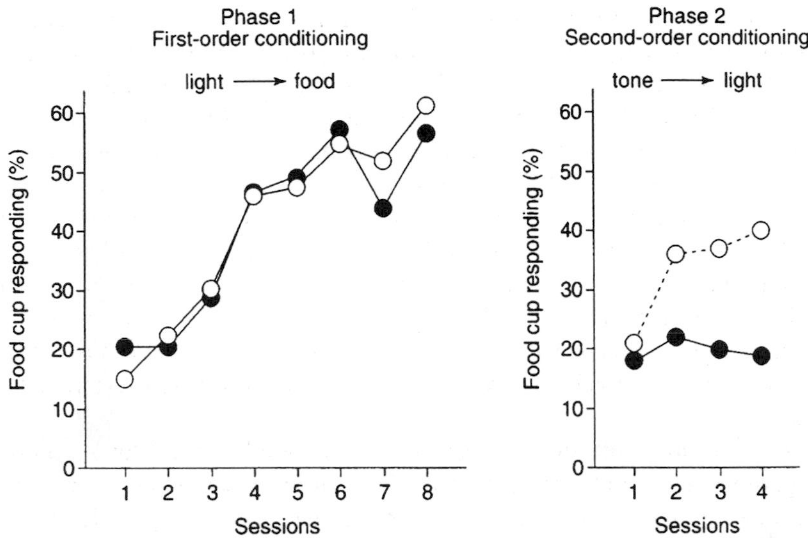

Figure 8.3 Effect of neurotoxic BLA lesions on the acquisition of Pavlovian second-order conditioning. In phase 1 of a recent experiment (Hatfield *et al.*, 1996), rats with BLA lesions (●) and control rats (○) received first-order pairings of a light conditioned stimulus (CS) and a food unconditioned stimulus (US). As a result of first-order conditioning, both groups acquired a conditioned response (CR) of approaching and entering the food cup during the light CS, prior to food delivery. In phase 2 (shown on the right), the rats received tone presentations followed by the light in the absence of food. Control rats acquired second-order food cup responses to the tone but rats with BLA lesions did not. This finding indicates that although the light acquired the ability to elicit CRs normally, it failed to acquire reinforcing value as a consequence of its first-order pairings with food in rats that had BLA lesions.

of 'US devaluation' causes normal rats subsequently to decrease their CRs on initial re-exposure to the original CS. Although the CS is absent during devaluation of the US, its earlier association with the US provides a basis for anticipating that event and its current incentive value. BLA lesions, but not CeA damage, eliminate this devaluation effect (Hatfield *et al.*, 1996). Rats with BLA lesions are unimpaired in acquisition of the CR in the initial training phase and learn the taste aversion in the second training phase. They are selectively impaired, however, in the CS test for devaluation (Figure 8.4). Recent evidence has also shown that after neurotoxic amygdala lesions, the behaviour of monkeys is similarly affected when performance depends on gaining access to a representation of reinforcement in a visual discrimination task (Malkova *et al.*, 1997; see Baxter and Murray, Chapter 16). Importantly for the current discussion, rats with neurotoxic OFC lesions resemble rats with BLA damage in failing to alter their behaviour in the presence of a CS that signals the devalued food (Gallagher *et al.*, 1999).

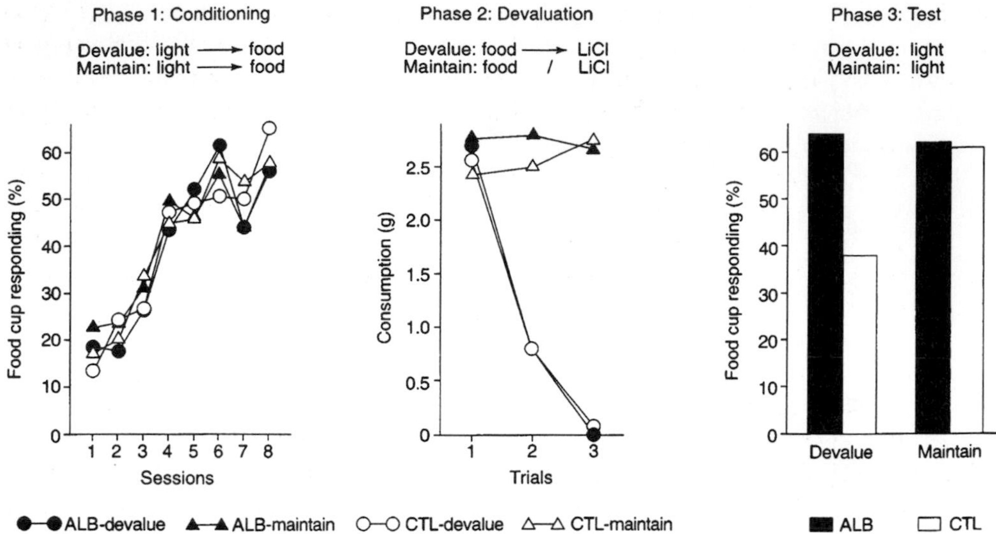

Figure 8.4 Effects of neurotoxic BLA lesions on performance in a Pavlovian reinforcer devaluation task. In phase 1 of a recent experiment (Hatfield *et al*., 1996), groups of rats with neurotoxic BLA lesions (solid symbols) or control groups (CTL, open symbols) received light–food pairings in a conditioning box. In phase 2 (middle panel), the food was devalued for one group of BLA and control rats (● and ○, respectively) by pairing presentation of the food pellets with LiCl injection. The other groups of BLA (△ and control rats and ▲) received unpaired food and LiCl, allowing the food to maintain its normal value. This phase of the experiment was conducted in the home cage. Consumption data during this phase (shown in the middle graph) revealed that pairing the food pellets with LiCl reduced consumption, i.e. produced conditioned taste aversion, whereas groups that received the unpaired procedure continued to consume the pellets. In phase 3 (data shown on the far right), a test was conducted in the conditioning box, during which the light CS was presented in the absence of US (food pellets). The group of control rats for whom the US had been devalued in phase 2 showed a spontaneous drop in CRs (approach to the food cup). Thus, in normal rats, conditioning allows the CS to gain access to a representation of the reinforcer that includes changes in its incentive value. Note that rats with BLA damage did not show the devaluation effect. Despite the normal acquisition of aversion to the food in phase 2 (middle panel), BLA rats that underwent the devaluation procedure maintained CRs in the final test.

The notion that amygdala BLA and its interconnections with OFC provide an important substrate for encoding relationships between events and the value of expected outcomes is supported further by recent neural recordings made in behaving rats. Schoenbaum *et al.* (1998) found that a substantial proportion of cells recorded in BLA and OFC exhibited expectancy-related encoding during performance of an odour-guided learning task. In particular, after rats had sampled an informative odour cue, cells fired differentially depending on whether the outcome was positive (sucrose) or negative (quinine). Approximately 36% of cells in BLA (44 of 121 neurons) and 22% of cells recorded in OFC (74 of 328 neurons) had differential activity in an interval prior to the delivery of the rewarding or aversive outcome. Evidence in that study indicated that this encoding was related prospectively to the incentive value of the impending event.

This line of research suggests that the amygdala's connectivity with prefrontal cortex brings associative information to bear on another level of behavioural control. In this case, the predictive value of cues and incentive properties of associated outcomes are encoded to guide goal-directed behaviour. These observations in rats may be relevant to understanding information processing in these regions of the primate brain. Notably, OFC is an area of prefrontal cortex in humans that is implicated in response integration and decision making (Rolls *et al.*, 1994; Duncan *et al.*, 1996; Bechara *et al.*, 1997). The role of BLA in such functions is supported by recent experimental studies of patients implicating connections between BLA and OFC in deficits displayed in choice behaviour (Bechara *et al.*, 1997).

It is intriguing to consider the relationship of BLA's contribution to the ability of a CS to gain access to reinforcer representations as measured in a US devaluation procedure, and its role in giving the CS access to putative striatal dopaminergic reward systems. In the latter case, the 'value' of the CS presumably is modified so that it can serve the role of reinforcement in higher order conditioning. In the case of devaluation, CS and US representations exist separately but are linked by association. In this context, it is interesting to note that second-order CRs are often insensitive to devaluation of the original reinforcer (Holland and Rescorla, 1975; Holland and Straub, 1979). According to a view that separate associative processes are involved in these functions, it is possible that BLA's connections with striatal and prefrontal systems are somewhat functionally segregated as well. Consistent with this idea, in the aforementioned electrophysiological recordings of neurons in BLA, cells that selectively encoded the impending US were largely separate from those that encoded the significance (value) of sampled cues. Specifically, the population of cells that fired selectively in anticipation of the trial's outcome (sucrose or quinine) did not fire differentially to the odours used to signal those outcomes. Rather, a largely separate population of BLA neurons selectively encoded odour significance when rats sampled those cues (Schoenbaum *et al.*, 1998, 1999).

In summary of this section, clearly much anatomical and behavioural justification exists for the integral importance of BLA/CeA circuitry to action systems. Through its connections, the associative functions of the amygdala are in a strategic position to influence behavioural selection, from more primitive responses organized in the brainstem to actions and decisions based on the incentive value of outcomes involving cortical systems. In considering the connectional circuitry of the BLA/CeA within a behavioural systems framework, it is also evident that its functions are not segregated easily or classified according to nuclear groups within the amygdala. For example, as described in this section, contributions of BLA/CeA nuclei cut across classification schemes based on psychological distinctions (e.g. Pavlovian or instrumental learning). As such, a high degree of integration is evident in the overall function of this circuitry, including the older central nucleus groupings of cells and the quasi-cortical components of the basolateral complex.

8.6 Connectivity of BLA/CeA to systems for regulating attention

Attentional mechanisms ultimately serve the purpose of providing for coherent control of action. In the case of attention, selection is achieved at earlier stages of information processing. Research on the neural substrates of visual attention in the primate brain, for example, increasingly has converged on the view that competitive and cooperative interactions are properties of the recurrently connected network of visual areas. Recent research has begun to show how these interactions are influenced by stimulus-driven features (bottom-up) and modulated by goal-driven factors (top-down) to give rise to selective attention (Desimone and Duncan, 1995; Behrman and Haimson, 1999). The connectional anatomy of the amygdala has prompted the suggestion that it might play a role in the top-down regulation of attention in cortical systems.

A chain of cortical processing converges on medial temporal cortex in the primate brain. Elegant anatomical studies have indicated the pattern and quantitative connectivity of cortical inputs to the perirhinal and parahippocampal cortex in the monkey (Suzuki and Amaral, 1994). More recent research has indicated a considerable homology for these systems in rat brain where cortical processing converges onto perirhinal and postrhinal areas (Burwell and Amaral, 1998a,b). These perihinal and parahippocampal/postrhinal areas provide a source of highly processed cortical information directly into the amygdala complex. Those connections are reciprocated, but a distinctive feature of amygdalocortical efferents is their wide distribution to quite early levels of the sensory processing stream. For example, in the primate visual system, amygdala efferents project to all levels of that system including primary visual cortex (V1) (Amaral *et al.*, 1992; Pitkänen, Chapter 2). This arrangement, as suggested elsewhere, would give learning and past experience access for top-down influences on selective attention in the processing of visual information. While this interesting possibility has yet to be examined experimentally, a role for the amygdala in attentional processes has begun to emerge from studies of other components of the BLA/CeA system.

8.7 Central nucleus regulation of attention

The orienting response is a simple manifestation of attention to a stimulus that can be elicited in a bottom-up manner due to the novelty or physical features (salience) of the input or as a top-down process based on 'task demands' or learned significance. As discussed in the previous section, CeA lesions abolish conditioned orienting without affecting the spontaneous orienting that is elicited by novel stimuli (Gallagher *et al.*, 1990). The orienting response traditionally has also been viewed as an adaptation for enhancing the processing of sensory inputs (Lacey and Lacey, 1974). Consistent with this view, the conditioned orienting response is normally accompanied by widespread changes in processing, from modulation of reflex pathways to cortical desynchronization of the electroencephalogram (EEG) that facilitates sensory processing (Kapp *et al.*, 1992). Such alterations in information processing during conditioning are also abolished by lesions of CeA (Whalen *et al.*, 1991).

The role of CeA in regulation of attention has been studied further using paradigms that reveal its role in the allocation of processing resources to cues (for a recent review, see Holland and Gallagher, 1999). Interestingly, the role of the CeA becomes engaged critically during learning when predictive uncertainty (or surprise) normally influences attention to cues. For example, an increase in attentional processing will occur when a consistent predictive relationship between the occurrence of two events is shifted to a less predictive relationship. That change in attention can be detected by greater facility in learning to a target cue. Figure 8.5 shows the procedures and results from one such study, in which the consistency of a light CS predicting a different tone CS was manipulated (from Holland and Gallagher, 1993a). Rats in the 'consistent' training condition received extensive exposure to the light–tone relationship. By contrast, midway through training, rats in the 'shift' condition had the light's predictive relationship to the tone degraded by omission of the tone on half the trials. This manipulation altered the ease with which new learning to the light occurred in the subsequent test phase for rats without lesions; rats with CeA lesions, however, did not show that result. Similar observations have been made in other tasks when an established expectation about the occurrence of events is violated; rats with CeA lesions do not show effects of increased attentional processing on learning (Holland and Gallagher, 1993b).

Cholinergic neurons in the basal forebrain that are regulated by CeA afferents and the basal forebrain cholinergic innervation of posterior parietal cortex (PPC) form a circuit that is critically involved in the shifts in attention described above. In the same paradigms used to study the effects of CeA damage, immunotoxic lesions of the cholinergic neurons in nucleus basalis and the substantia innominata (nBM/SI) or immuntoxic lesions of the cholinergic input to PPC produce similar impairments (Chiba *et al.*, 1995; Bucci *et al.*, 1998; Han *et al.*, 1999; crossed lesion). For example, Chiba *et al.* (1995) showed that selective removal of the cholinergic neurons in nBM/SI, similarly to CeA lesions, abolished the effect of altering an established predictive relationship between cues. That same behavioural procedure subsequently was used to test the effects of disconnecting the CeA from nBM/SI cholinergic neurons; the results of that study indicated that CeA projections to nBM/SI are essential for the enhancement of attentional processing (Han *et al.*, 1999).

In recent anatomical studies of rat PPC, it has been noted that this region of cortex may be homologous to PPC in primates (see Reep *et al.*, 1994; Bucci *et al.*, 1999). In the rat, PPC can be distinguished by a lack of input from the lateral geniculate nucleus or ventrobasal complex of the thalamus that define surrounding visual and somatosensory cortices. Instead, rat PPC receives its thalamic innervation from lateral posterior, lateral dorsal, and posterior nuclei of the thalamus, regions that probably are homologous to pulvinar/lateral posterior complex in the primate brain. The PPC in primates has been strongly implicated in the regulation of attentional processes (Heilman *et al.*, 1970; Posner *et al.*, 1984).

Selective removal of the cholinergic innervation of PPC was done in our studies of rats by injections of the cholinergic immunotoxin, 192 IgG saporin into that area (Bucci *et al.*, 1998). This selective lesion abolished the effects of altering an established predictive relationship between cues using the same task shown in Figure 8.5. Similarly to the effects of amygdala CeA lesions, removal of the cholinergic innervation of PPC also eliminated an advantage in learning normally observed in an unblocking paradigm (Bucci *et al.*, 1998).

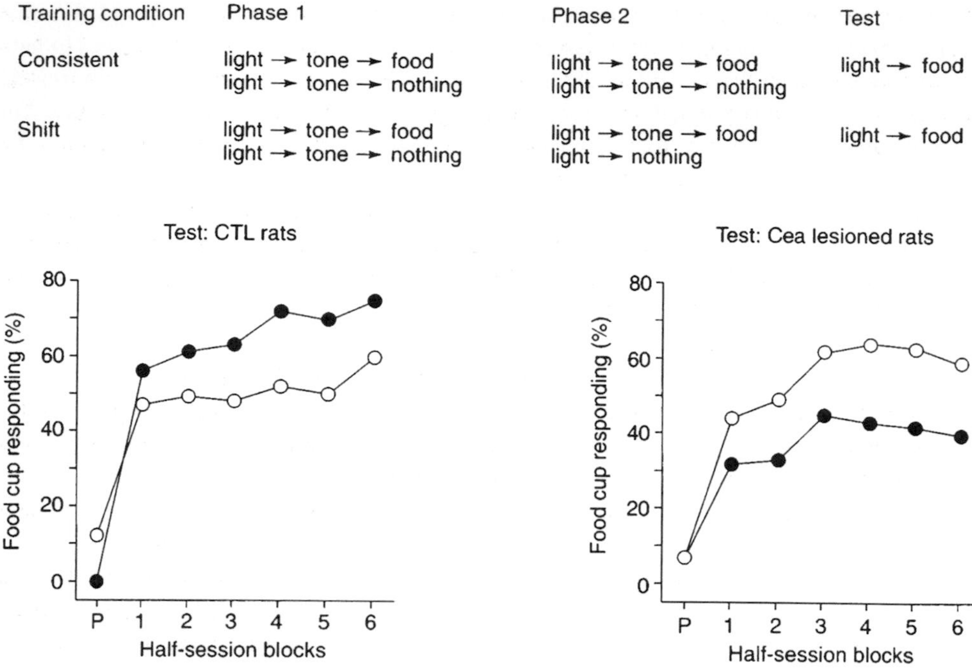

Figure 8.5 Effects of neurotoxic lesions of the amygdala central nucleus on attentional processing. The graphs show data from the final test phase (phase 3) of an extended experiment outlined at the top of the panel. In phase 1, a light was followed by a tone on every trial for all subjects in the experiment. In half of those phase 1 trials, the light–tone sequence was reinforced by food pellet delivery. In phase 2, rats in the 'consistent' condition (○) continued exposure to this same light–tone relationship. However, for rats in the 'shift' condition (●), the light's predictive relationship to the tone was changed by omitting the tone on half of the trials. Because the light was a poor temporal predictor of the food relative to the tone in phases 1 and 2, little conditioning to the light was anticipated and none was observed in those training phases. More importantly, attention to the light should decrease gradually with continued exposure in the consistent training procedure but attention should be re-engaged when the light's ability to predict the tone is shifted. We tested changes in the attentional processing of the light in the final phase of this experiment (phase 3) by pairing the light directly with food in Pavolvian conditioning sessions (shown in the graphs). To the extent that attentional processing of the light was enhanced, conditioning should occur more readily. Control rats showed that outcome; conditioning was greater in the rats that had undergone the shift in the light's relationship to the tone relative to rats in the 'consistent' procedure (compare ● with ○ in the panel on the left). In contrast, rats with CeA lesions did not show the predicted effect. Instead the experience that normally enhances attentional processing produced poorer learning. See Holland and Gallagher (1999) for a further discussion of these results. (Note that P on the abscissae refers to responding on the final block of phase 2 sessions).

It is important to note that in all of the above studies, lesions had no effect on performance when the training procedures did not encourage increased attentional processing. This was true for rats with lesions of the CeA, with removal of cholinergic neurons in the nBM/SI, as well as with selective removal of the cholinergic input to PPC. The role of this system in the regulation of attention therefore appears to be critical for adjustments in attention that are evoked by changes in the predictive relationships between events in the environment.

Other types of studies have supported a role for the basal forebrain cholinergic innervation of cortex in the regulation of attention; such studies include the use of five-choice serial reaction time and spatial pre-cueing tasks (Muir *et al.*, 1992; Voytko *et al.*, 1994; McGaughy *et al.*, 1996; Chiba *et al.*, 1999). Delimiting the role of CeA in the regulation of this ascending system is an important area for further study. For example, to date, no research has examined the effects of CeA damage on attention in the performance of tasks that do not involve new learning, such as those studied in conjuction with nBM/SI lesions. Perhaps the influence of the amygdala on the ascending cholinergic system is recruited only for the purpose of new learning, independently of a role in performance.

At the same time, little is known about what role BLA might serve in attentional processing, either by way of its efferents to sensory processing systems in posterior cortex or through its connections with prefrontal cortex. It is clear, however, that in addition to encoding the predictive value of current information and incentive value of related outcomes, the BLA/CeA system plays a more general role in tracking the expected relationships between events and detecting change.

The role of the BLA/CeA system in attentional processes may be important to incorporate into an overall understanding of this system and its role in learning. The function of BLA/CeA in learning is often cast in 'lower' level terms. For example, elegant studies of fear conditioning have suggested that the BLA/CeA system is organized to provide a fast throughput; direct routes for sensory information from thalamus provide a sketch of environmental input to elicit rapid emotional responses, such as fear (LeDoux, 1995). Such subcortical pathways undoubtedly have an adaptive function in the framework of evolution. By the same token, the BLA/CeA system's connections with cortical systems may have evolved to exploit such features. For example, the fast throughput of sensory information from thalamus could serve to influence selection of sensory processing in cortical systems by amygdalocortical efferents and could participate in the preparation for new learning via CeA. Such considerations are useful for guiding physiological and behaviour studies that will provide an understanding of the full connectional anatomy of the BLA/CeA system.

8.8 An integrative neurobiology of the BLA/CeA system

The detailed anatomy of BLA/CeA connections with other systems permits identification of the information to which this system has access and the range of functions and responses that can be influenced by its outputs. Within this neural systems framework, behavioural studies increasingly support the BLA/CeA's role in learning involving different types of associative processes, in modulation of memory functions (see McGaugh et al., Chapter 11;

Cahill, Chapter 12), and in a broader influence of learning on information processing systems. At the same time, studies of neural plasticity in BLA/CeA are permitting identification of synaptic and molecular mechanisms at sites in the amygdala that potentially can be linked to behaviour (see LeDoux, Chapter 7). Indeed, current studies of this system in Pavlovian conditioning provide one of the most promising models for linking the analysis of behaviour to underlying neural plasticity in rodents. As further research is undertaken, it will be important to maintain an integrative approach to the study of the BLA/CeA system so that its function is not viewed too narrowly through the lens of a single behavioural model, i.e. fear conditioning.

Alongside experimental research on the amygdala complex, clinical interest in this system has also evolved. Converging evidence, including studies using non-invasive neuroimaging, points to a role for the amygdala complex in a variety of neuropsychiatric conditions, including anxiety disorders and depression, schizophrenia and autism (see Drevets *et al.*, 1992; Davidson *et al.*, 1999, and the relevant chapters in this volume). Although some of these connections are compatible with a role for the amygdala in affective states, it is widely recognized that neuropsychiatric disorders such as depression and anxiety have both affective and cognitive features. Moreover, such disorders can profoundly influence a range of behavioural dispositions toward activity and action. In that context, a broader integrative perspective on the amygdala, one that encompasses how information is selected and is used to activate and guide behaviour, may not only contribute to understanding disorders of brain function, but will also allow a greater appreciation of the integration of emotional and cognitive functions.

Acknowledgements

The author thanks Anne Millman for her assistance in preparing this manuscript. Research supported by NIMH grants KO5-MH01149 and RO1-MH53667.

References

Alheid, G.F. and Heimer, L. (1988) New perspectives in basal forebrain organization of special relevance for neuropsychiatric disorders: the striatopallidal, amygdaloid, and corticopetal components of substantia innominata. *Neuroscience*, 1, 1–39.

Amaral, D.G. (1987) Memory: anatomical organization of candidate brain regions. In *Handbook of Physiology, Section 1: The Nervous System, Vol. 5* (eds V.B. Mountcastle, F. Plum and S.R. Geiger), pp. 211–294. American Physiology Society, Bethesda, Maryland.

Applegate, C.D., Frysinger, R.C., Kapp, B.S., and Gallagher, M. (1982) Multiple unit activity recorded from amygdala central nucleus during Pavlovian heart rate conditioning. *Brain Research*, 238, 457–462.

Bechara, A., Damasio, H., Tranel, D., and Damasio, A.R. (1997) Deciding advantageously before knowing the advantageous strategy. *Science*, 275, 1293–1294.

Behrman, M. and Haimson, C. (1999) The cognitive neuroscience of attention. *Current Opinion in Neurobiology*, **9**, 158–163.

Bucci, D.J., Holland, P.C., and Gallagher, M. (1998) Removal of cholinergic input to rat posterior parietal cortex disrupts incremental processing of conditioned stimuli. *Journal of Neuroscience*, 18, 8038–8046.

Bucci, D.J., Conley, M., and Gallagher, M. (1999) Thalamic and basal forebrain cholinergic connections of the rat posterior parietal cortex. *NeuroReport*, 10, 1–5.

Burwell, R.D. and Amaral, D.G. (1998a) Perirhinal and postrhinal cortices of the rat: interconnectivity and connections with the entorhinal cortex. *Journal of Comparative Neurology*, 391, 293–321.

Burwell, R.D. and Amaral, D.G. (1998b) Cortical afferents of the perirhinal, postrhinal, and entorhinal cortices of the rat. *Journal of Comparative Neurology*, 398, 179–205.

Carli, M., Evenden, J.L., and Robbins, T.W. (1985) Depletion of unilateral striatal dopamine impairs initiation of contralateral actions and not sensory attention. *Nature*, 313, 679–682.

Carli, M., Jones, G.H., and Robbins, T.W. (1989) Effects of unilateral dorsal and ventral striatal dopamine depletion on visual neglect in the rat: a neural and behavioral analysis. *Neuroscience*, 29, 309–327.

Chiba, A.A, Bucci, D.J., Holland, P.C., and Gallagher, M. (1995) Basal forebrain cholinergic lesions disrupt increments but not decrements in conditioned stimulus processing. *Journal of Neuroscience*, 15, 7315–7322.

Chiba, A.A., Bushnell, P.J., Oshiro, W.M., and Gallagher, M. (1999) Selective removal of cholinergic neurons in the basal forebrain alters cued target detection in rats. *NeuroReport*, **10**, 3119–3123.

Davidson, R.J., Abercrombie, H., Nitschke, J., and Putman, K. (1999) Regional brain function, emotion and disorders of attention. *Current Opinion in Neurobiology*, **9**, 235–239.

Davis, M. (1986) Pharmacological and anatomical analysis of fear conditioning using the fear-potentiated startle paradigm. *Behavioral Neuroscience*, 100, 814–824.

Davis, M. (1992) The role of the amygdala in conditioned fear. In *The Amygdala: Neurobiological Aspects of Emotion, Memory, and Mental Dysfunction* (ed. J.P. Aggleton), pp. 255–306. Wiley-Liss, New York.

Desimone, R. and Duncan, J. (1995) Neural mechanisms of selective visual attention. *Annual Review of Neuroscience*, 18, 193–197.

Drevets, W.C., Videen, T.O., Price, J.L., Preskorn, S.H., Carmichael, S.T., and Raichle, M.E. (1992) A functional anatomical study of unipolar depression. *Journal of Neuroscience*,12, 3628–3641.

Duncan, J., Emslie, H., and Williams, P. (1996) Intelligence and the frontal lobe: the organization of goal-directed behavior. *Cognitive Psychology*, 30, 257–303.

Everitt, B.J., Morris, K.A., O'Brien, A., Burns, L., and Robbins, T.W. (1991) The basolateral amygdala–ventral striatal system and conditioned place preference: further evidence of limbic–striatal interactions underlying reward-related processes. *Neuroscience*, 42, 1–18.

Everitt, B.J., Cador, M., and Robbins, T.W. (1989) Interactions between the amygdala and ventral striatum in stimulus–reward associations: studies using a second-order schedule of sexual reinforcement. *Neuroscience*, 30, 63–75.

Fairley, P.C. and Marshall, J.F. (1986) Dopamine in the lateral caudate–putamen of the rat is essential for somatosensory orientation. *Behavioral Neuroscience*, 100, 652–663.

Gallagher, M. and Holland, P. (1992) Understanding the function of the central nucleus: Is simple conditioning enough? *The Amygdala: Neurobiological Aspects of Emotion, Memory, and Mental Dysfunction* (ed. J.P. Aggleton), pp. 307–321. Wiley-Liss, New York.

Gallagher, M., Graham, P.W., and Holland, P.C. (1990) The amygdala central nucleus and appetitive Pavlovian conditioning: lesions impair one class of conditioned performance. *Journal of Neuroscience*, 10, 1906–1911.

Gallagher, M., McMahan, R., and Schoenbaum, G. (1999) Orbitofrontal cortex and representations of incentive value in associative learning. *Journal of Neuroscience*, **19**, 6610–6614.

Gonzales, C. and Chesselet, M.F. (1990) Amygdalonigral pathway: an anterograde study in the rat with *Phaseolus vulgaris* leucoagglutinin (PHA-L). *Journal of Comparative Neurology*, 297, 182–200.

Groenewegen, H.J., Berendse, H.W., Wolters, J.G., and Lohman, A.H.M. (1990) The anatomical relationship of the prefrontal cortex with the striatopallidal system, the thalamus, and the amygdala: evidence for a parallel organization. *Progress in Brain Research*, 85, 95–118.

Han, J.-S., McMahan, R.W., Holland, P.C., and Gallagher, M. (1997) The role of an amygdalo-nigrostriatal pathway in associative learning. *Journal of Neuroscience*, 17, 3913–3919.

Han, J.-S., Holland, P.C., and Gallagher, M. (1999) Disconnection of amygdala central nucleus and substantia innominata/nucleus basalis disrupts increments in conditioned stimulus processing. *Behavioral Neuroscience*, **113**, 143–151.

Hatfield, T., Han, J.-S., Conley, M., Gallagher, M., and Holland, P. (1996) Neurotoxic lesions of basolateral, but not central, amygdala interfere with Pavlovian second-order conditioning and reinforcer devaluation effects. *Journal of Neuroscience*, 16, 5256–5265.

Heilman, K.M., Pandya, D.N., and Geschwind, N. (1970) Trimodal inattention following parietal lobe ablations. *Transactions of the American Neurological Association*, 95, 259–261.

Hitchcock, J. and Davis, M. (1986) Lesions of the amygdala, but not the cerebellum or red nucleus, block conditioned fear as measured with the potentiated startle paradigm. *Behavioral Neuroscience*, 100, 12–22.

Hitchcock, J.M. and Davis, M. (1991) Efferent pathway of the amygdala involved in conditioned fear as measured with the fear-potentiated startle paradigm. *Behavioral Neuroscience*, 105, 826–842.

Holland, P.C. and Gallagher, M. (1993a) Effects of amygdala central nucleus lesions on blocking and unblocking. *Behavioral Neuroscience*, 107, 235–245.

Holland, P.C. and Gallagher, M. (1993b) Amygdala central nucleus lesions disrupt increments, but not decrements, in CS processing. *Behavioral Neuroscience*, 107, 246–253.

Holland, P.C. and Gallagher, M. (1999) Amygdala circuitry in attentional and representational processes. *Trends in Cognitive Science*, 3, 65–73.

Holland, P.C. and Rescorla, R.A. (1975) The effect of two ways of devaluing the unconditioned stimulus after first- and second- order conditioning. *Journal of Experimental Psychology—Animal Behavior Processes*, 1, 355–363.

Holland, P.C. and Straub, J.J. (1979) Differential effects of two ways of devaluing the unconditioned stimulus after Pavlovian appetitive conditioning. *Journal of Experimental Psychology*, 5, 65–78.

Johnston, J.B. (1923) Further contributions to the study of the evolution of the forebrain. *Journal of Comparative Neurology*, 35, 337–482.

Kapp, B.S., Frysinger, R.C. , Gallagher, M., and Haselton, J.B. (1979) Amygdala central nucleus lesions: effect on heart rate conditioning in the rabbit. *Physiology and Behavior*, 23, 1109–1117.

Kapp, B.S., Pascoe, J.P., and Bixler, M.A. (1984) The amygdala: a neuroanatomical systems approach to its contribution to aversive conditioning. In The *Neuropsychology of Memory* (eds L. Squire and N. Butters), pp. 473–428. The Guilford Press, New York.

Kapp, B.S., Whalen, P.J., Supple, W.F., and Pascoe, J.P. (1992) Amygdaloid contributions to conditioned arousal and sensory information processing. In *The Amygdala: Neurobiological Aspects of Emotion, Memory, and Mental Dysfunction* (ed. J.P. Aggleton), pp. 229–254. Wiley-Liss, New York.

Kelley, A.E., Domesick, V.B., and Nauta, W.J.H. (1982) The amygdalostriatal projection in the rat—an anatomical study by anterograde and retrograde tracing methods. *Neuroscience*, 7, 615–630.

Killcross, S., Robbins, T.W., and Everitt, B.J. (1997) Different types of fear conditioned behaviour mediated by separate nuclei within amygdala. *Nature*, 388, 377–380.

Kling, A.S., Lancaster, J., and Benitone, J. (1970) Amygdalectomy in the free ranging vervet. *Journal of Psychiatry Research*, 7,191–199.

Klüver, H. and Bucy, P.C. (1939) Preliminary analysis of the temporal lobes in monkeys. *Archives of Neurology and Psychiatry*, 42, 979–1000.

Krettek, J.E. and Price, J.L. (1977) Projections from the amygdaloid complex to the cerebral cortex and thalamus in the rat and cat. *Journal of Comparative Neurology*, 172, 687–722.

Lacey, B.C. and Lacey, J.I. (1974) Studies of heart rate and other bodily processes in sensorimotor behavior. In *Cardiovascular Psychophysiology: Current Issues in Response Mechanisms, Biofeedback and Methodology* (eds P.A. Obrist, A.H. Black, J. Brener, and L.V. DiCara), pp. 538–564. Aldine, New York.

LeDoux J.E. (1995) Emotion: clues from the brain. *Annual Review of Psychology*, 46, 209–235.

LeDoux J.E., Iwata, J., Ciccheti, P., and Reis, D.J. (1988) Different projections of the central amygdaloid nucleus mediate autonomic and behavioral correlates of conditioned fear. *Journal of Neuroscience*, 8, 2517–2529.

Malkova, L., Gaffan, D., and Murray, E.A. (1997) Excitotoxic lesions of the amygdala fail to produce impairment in visual learning for auditory secondary reinforcement but interfere with reinforcer devaluation effects in rhesus monkeys. *Journal of Neuroscience*, 17, 6011–6020.

McDonald, A.J. (1991a) Topographical organization of amygdaloid projections to the caudateputamen, nucleus accumbens, and related striatal-like areas of the rat brain. *Neuroscience*, 44, 15–33.

McDonald, A.J. (1991b) Organization of amygdaloid projections to the prefrontal cortex and associated striatum in the rat. *Neuroscience*, 44,1–14.

McDonald R.J. and White, N.M. (1993) A triple dissociation of memory systems: hippocampus, amygdala, and dorsal striatum. *Behavioral Neuroscience*, 107, 3–22.

McGaughy, J., Kaiser, T., and Sarter, M. (1996) Behavioral vigilance following infusions of 192 IgG-saporin into the basal forebrain: selectivity of the behavioral impairment and relation to cortical AChE-positive fiber density. *Behavioral Neuroscience*, 110, 247–265.

Mogenson, G., Jones, D.L., and Yim, C.Y. (1984) From motivation to action: functional interface between the limbic system and the motor system. *Progress in Neurobiology*, 14, 69–97.

Muir, J.L., Dunnett, S.B., Robbins, T.W., and Everitt, B.J. (1992) Attentional functions of the forebrain cholinergic systems: effects of intraventricular hemicholinium, physostigmine, basal forebrain lesions and intracortical grafts on a multiple choice serial reaction time task. *Experimental Brain Research*, 89, 611–622.

Petrovich, G.D., Risold, P.Y., and Swanson, L.W. (1996) Organization of projections from the basomedial nucleus of the amygdala: a PHAL study of the rat. *Journal of Comparative Neurology*, 374, 387–420.

Posner, M.I., Walker, J.A., Friedrich, F.J., and Rafal, R.D. (1984) Effects of parietal injury on covert orienting of attention. *Journal of Neuroscience*, 4, 1863–1874.

Price, J.L. and Amaral, D.G. (1981) An autoradiographic study of the projections of the central nucleus of the monkey amygdala. *Journal of Neuroscience*, 1, 1242–1259.

Reep, R.L., Chandler, H.C., King, V., and Corwin, J.V. (1994) Rat posterior parietal cortex: topography of corticocortical and thalamic connections. *Experimental Brain Research*, 100, 67–84.

Rolls, E.T., Hornak, J., Wade, D., and McGrath, J. (1994) Emotion-related learning in patients with social and emotional changes associated with frontal lobe damage. *Journal of Neurology, Neurosurgery and Psychiatry*, 57, 1518–1524.

Roozendaal, B., Oldenburger, W.P., Strubbe, J.H., Koolhaus, J.M., and Bohus, B. (1990) The central amygdala is involved in the conditioned but not in the meal-induced cephalic insulin response in the rat. *Neuroscience Letters*, 116, 210–215.

Schoenbaum, G., Chiba, A.A., and Gallagher, M. (1998) Orbitofrontal cortex and basolateral amygdala encode expected outcomes during learning. *Nature Neuroscience*, 1, 155–159.

Schoenbaum, G., Chiba, A.A., and Gallagher, M. (1999) Neural encoding in orbitofrontal cortex and basolateral amygdala during olfactory discrimination learning. *Journal of Neuroscience*, 19, 1876–1884.

Swanson, L.W. and Petrovich, G.D. (1998) What is the amygdala? *Trends in Neuroscience*, 21, 323–331.

Voytko, M.L., Olton, D.S., Richardson, R.T., Gorman, L.K., Tobin, J.R., and Price, D.L. (1994) Basal forebrain lesions in monkeys disrupt attention but not learning and memory. *Journal of Neuroscience*, 14, 167–186.

Weingarten, H.P. (1983) Conditioned cues elicit feeding in sated rats: a role for learning in meal initiation. *Science*, 220, 431–433.

Whalen, P.J. and Kapp, B.S. (1991) Contributions of the amygdaloid central nucleus to the modulation of the nictitating membrane reflex in the rabbit. *Behavioral Neuroscience*, 104, 141–153.

9 The amygdala in conditioned taste aversion: it's there, but where

Raphael Lamprecht and Yadin Dudai

Department of Neurobiology, The Weizmann Institute of Science, Rehovot 76100, Israel

Summary

Conditioned taste aversion (CTA) is a unique type of innately predisposed ('prepared') learning, in which the subject associates a tastant with malaise over long delays. Multiple studies, involving neuroanatomical lesions, cellular recordings, and molecular analysis, point to the involvement of components of the amygdaloid complex in CTA. However, the contribution of the amygdala to discrete phases in CTA behaviour and to identified operations of CTA-subserving circuits has not yet been established. It is also as yet unclear whether the amygdala is always obligatory for successful CTA in the intact animal. Based on the current data, the central (CeA) and the basolateral (BLA) amygdaloid nuclei are among the prime candidates for fulfilling a role in CTA. In the rat, the CeA is regarded by some as an autonomic-projecting motor region of the striatum, the anterior BLA as an extension of the claustrum for the temporal and frontal lobes, and the posterior BLA as a component of the central olfactory system. The involvement of CeA and BLA may hence reflect the engagement of radically different brain functions. The discrepancies concerning the role(s) of CeA and BLA in CTA may stem not only from the use of heterogeneous experimental approaches, e.g. total versus partial lesions, transient versus permanent lesions, or lesions versus correlative methods, but also from different behavioural protocols that tap different forms of learning.

9.1 Conditioned taste aversion

Farmers know, probably from the dawn of farming, that animals often learn to avoid a poisonous bait if they survive the poisoning. Common knowledge, of course, does not always penetrate academic barriers: it took John Garcia and his colleagues several distressful years to convince the referees of prominent scientific journals that conditioned taste aversion (CTA) does occur (Garcia, 1981). Also dubbed The Garcia Effect, Bait Shyness, or The Bernnaise

Sauce Effect, CTA is an association between taste and malaise. It is a type of associative learning strongly constrained by an innate predisposition ('prepared learning') to form associations between foodstuff and visceral distress. Reinforcers that act on non-visceral receptors and have less intimate association with food, such as visual cues, tones, or cutaneous pain, though very effective in classical and instrumental conditioning, are ineffective in CTA (Garcia *et al.*, 1968). CTA is optimal when the taste is encountered for the first time, and hence is primarily a novelty-dependent learning. Most importantly, CTA tolerates a very long interstimulus interval (ISI) between taste and malaise. Whereas in classical and instrumental conditioning, an ISI of more than seconds between the paired stimuli commonly renders training ineffective, CTA training tolerates an ISI of several hours. Furthermore, at least in certain CTA protocols, if the ISI is made too short, e.g. seconds only, conditioning is weak (Schafe *et al.*, 1995). It seems as though the mechanisms that subserve CTA can distinguish ingestion-induced toxicosis, naturally requiring some time before the toxins exert their action in the gut, from other types of negative reinforcers. It is this deviation from the widely accepted paradigm, namely that two stimuli must come close together in time in order to become associated in mind, that had led respectable psychologists to regard with great suspicion the early scientific reports on CTA. However, all this is now history; CTA is recognized as a *bona fide* case of memory, though of a special kind (Bures *et al.*, 1998). Furthermore, its properties, such as fast, single-trial learning, robust memory, and dissociation in time between acquisition of information about a sensory stimulus and the association of that information with a negative reinforcer, render CTA an attractive system to study acquisition, consolidation, retention, and retrieval of memory.

Figure 9. 1 A simplified flowchart of CTA-related information to and from the amygdaloid complex in the rat brain. (**A**) The flow of information from central taste processing areas into the amygdala (cortex–amygdala, Otterson, 1982; Saper, 1982; thalamus–amygdala, Turner and Herkenham, 1991; hypothalamus–amygdala, Veening, 1978; Otterson, 1980; PBN–amygdala, Norgren, 1976; Veening, 1978). (**B**) The flow of information from areas that process the perception of gastrointestinal malaise into the amygdala (NST–amygdala, Ricardo and Koh, 1978; PBN–amygdala, Saper and Loewy, 1980). (**C**) The flow of information from the amygdala to areas involved in CTA (amygdala–cortex, Saper 1982; Krettek and Price 1977; amygdala–hypothalamus, Turner and Herkenham, 1991; amygdala–PBN, Zahm *et al.*, 1999; amygdala–NST, Van der Kooy *et al.*, 1984). The connections from and to the amygdala are based on either anatomical or functional observations, or both; no attempt has been made to distinguish structural from functional evidence in this scheme. Abbreviations: ACo, anterior cortical amygdaloid nucleus; AP, area postrema; BLA, basolateral amygdaloid nucleus; BM, basomedial amygdaloid nucleus; La, lateral amygdaloid nucleus; LH, lateral hypothalamus; Me, medial amygdaloid nucleus; NST, nucleus of the solitary tract; PBN, parabrachial nucleus; Vag, vagus nerve; VPMpc, parvicellular portion of the ventroposteromedial nucleus of the thalamus; VII, IX, and X, cranial nerves. Arrows: insular cortex to and from amygdala, ——○, LH to and from amygdala, ——>, VPMpc to the amygdala, ——▷, PBN to and from the amygdala, ——►, NST to and from the amygdala, ——●. The anatomical schemes are based on Paxinos and Watson (1997).

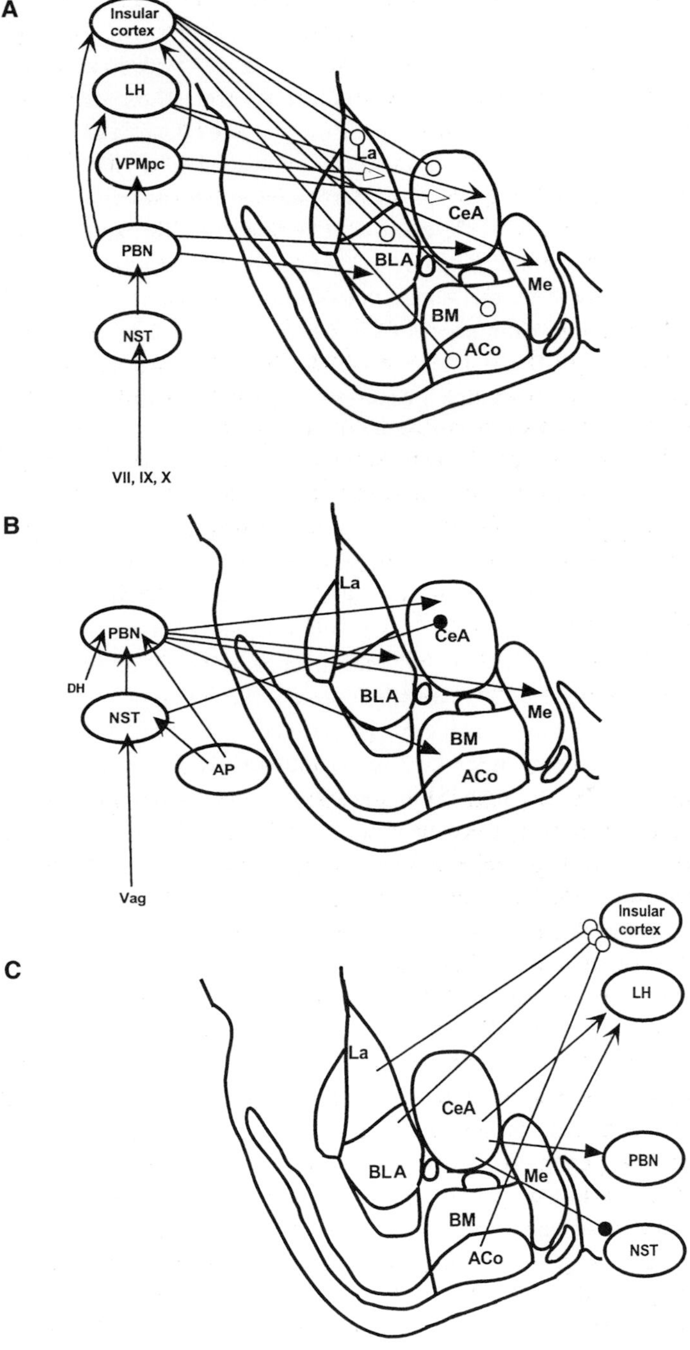
A
Insular cortex
LH
VPMpc
PBN
NST
VII, IX, X
La
CeA
BLA
Me
BM
ACo
B
PBN
DH
NST
AP
Vag
La
CeA
BLA
Me
BM
ACo
C
Insular cortex
LH
PBN
NST
La
CeA
BLA
Me
BM
ACo

The first systematic studies of CTA emerged from noticing the lingering effects of exposure to γ-irradiation on food preference (Garcia *et al.*, 1955). In the laboratory, CTA is induced by presenting an experimental animal (e.g. a rat) with a taste solution, followed 0.5–3 h later by administration of a malaise-inducing agent. The most commonly employed taste is saccharin, used by Garcia *et al.* in their early studies (Garcia *et al.*, 1966). A common malaise-inducing agent is an intraperitoneal (i.p.) injection of a LiCl solution, a procedure that induces visceral distress for 2–3 h. Odours may also be associated with toxicosis (e.g. Slotnick *et al.*, 1997), but are less tolerant than taste to long ISI, and work best when associated with taste (taste-potentiated odour aversion, TPOA; Rusiniak *et al.*, 1979). The role of amygdala in TPOA will be mentioned below only *en passant*.

Whereas the behavioural parameters of CTA have been described over the years in detail (Bures *et al.*, 1988), much less is known about brain circuits that subserve the behaviour. It is generally accepted that the central gustatory area in the insular cortex (gustatory cortex, GC) plays a role in processing and retaining internal representations of taste, although cortical lesions do not completely abolish the ability to form rudimentary taste–malaise associations: rats lacking GC lose the ability to tell the familiar from the unfamiliar, but are capable of a relatively weak CTA, similar to that formed by intact rats after conditioning to a familiar tastant (Kiefer and Braun 1977). The parabrachial nucleus is considered a candidate site for the association between taste and malaise. The amygdala, as detailed below, was implicated in multiple facets of CTA, including the acquisition of taste information, hedonic evaluation of that information, representation of the malaise-inducing stimulus, and integration, retention, and expression of CTA (Yamamoto *et al.*, 1994; Lamprecht *et al.*, 1997; Bures *et al.*, 1998). Thalamic and hypothalamic nuclei, as well as multiple diffused neuromodulatory systems, were also implicated in the circuits that subserve CTA. It is rather unlikely that the tolerance of CTA training to long ISI stems from unique molecular devices not present in other brain circuits or not recruited in other 'classical' types of associations; information gathered so far indicates that molecular mechanisms that subserve CTA learning and memory in the aforementioned areas are similar to those that subserve other forms of learning. Among these mechanisms are activation of glutamate and acetylcholine receptors and modulation of immediate-early gene expression (Lamprecht *et al.*, 1997; Rosenblum *et al.*, 1997). Probably, the tolerance to long delays results from special circuit properties, shaped in evolution to ensure avoidance of toxins (e.g. Shipley and Sanders, 1982; but see also Morris *et al.*, 1999).

In the context of the present discussion, we focus on the evidence implicating amygdala in CTA. The overall conclusion will be that amygdala indeed subserves CTA processing, learning, and memory. Considering the established role of amygdala in ingestive, emotional, and aversive learning (Chapters 7, 10), and the ingestive and aversive components in CTA, this conclusion is probably not too surprising. However, one should note at the outset that the data are not all consistent. There are multiple reasons for this current situation, and some will be outlined throughout the discussion. At this point, suffice it to note that whereas the amygdala is regarded as a collection of nuclei with different functions, not all studies addressing the role of amygdala in CTA took care to delineate precisely the individual amygdaloid nuclei affected by the experimental manipulation. The extent of damage to each specific nucleus is also a parameter occasionally neglected. Furthermore, CTA itself can be performed using a variety of protocols, ranging from multiple choice situations in freely behaving animals to forced drinking in intubated individuals. The different protocols may recruit different brain systems. The spectrum of tastes and malaise-inducing agents, which may function via a variety of neuronal mechanisms, is also rich. In addition to all this, the methods used to determine the role of amygdala vary in different studies, ranging from permanent ablations and electrolytic lesions, via transient metabolic lesions, to a search for cellular and molecular correlates. Each of these methods addresses a different physiological state (i.e. a permanently damaged brain, transiently inactivated circuits, or an intact brain), and hence may tap different amygdaloid nuclei.

9.2 The amygdala and circuits that process taste and malaise

The amygdalar complex receives taste and malaise input into multiple nuclei (Fig 9.1; Norgren *et al.*, 1989; Yamamoto *et al.*, 1994; Bures *et al.*, 1998). Taste information reaches the rostral subdivision of the nucleus of the solitary tract (NST) via three cranial nerves (VII, IX, and X). From the NST, ascending gustatory fibres project to the medial parabrachial nucleus (mPBN). Taste cells from the PBN project to the central amygdaloid nucleus (CeA) and more moderately to the basolateral amygdaloid complex (BLA) (Norgren, 1976; Veening, 1978). Taste neurons from the PBN also synapse with cells in the parvicellular portion of the ventroposteromedial nucleus of the thalamus (VPMpc) and the lateral hypothalamus (Norgren, 1976). Efferents from the VPMpc project to the central and lateral amygdaloid nuclei (Turner and Herkenham, 1991) and to the GC in the insular cortex. The posterior agranular insular cortex projects to the lateral, basolateral, cortical, basomedial, and central amygdaloid nuclei; the basolateral, central, and anterior cortical nuclei receive, in addition, projections from the ventral agranular insular cortex. The agranular insular cortex receives fibres from the lateral, basolateral, and anterior cortical amygdaloid nuclei. This was shown by anterograde and retrograde transport labelling experiments (Krettek and Price, 1977; Otterson, 1982; Saper, 1982), and by the response of GC taste neurons to CeA stimulation as well as the response of amygdala neurons to GC stimulation (Yamamoto *et al.*, 1984). Hence, the data demonstrate that taste information reaches the amygdala via multiple routes into multiple nuclei (Yamamoto *et al.*, 1984). Neurons in the central, lateral, and cortical nuclei respond to four basic taste stimuli (Azuma *et al.*, 1984; Uwano *et al.*, 1995; Nishijo *et al.*, 1998). Most amygdaloid neurons show an excitatory response with broad tuning to the taste stimuli. Such 'taste neurons' can be classified according to their 'best stimulus' properties. Across-neuron correlation between magnitudes of responses to pairs of tastants distinguished by their aversiveness or palatability suggests that processing of taste information involves computations of the hedonic valence of taste (Azuma *et al.*, 1984).

The amygdala also receives information on gastrointestinal distress. Niijima and Yamamoto (1994) reported that intraperitoneal or intraduodenal injection of LiCl activates the vagal and splanchnic nerves. The visceral information is transferred via the vagus nerve to the caudal region of the NST and by the dorsal horn to the lateral PBN (Torvik, 1956; Hylden *et al.*,

1989; Yamamoto *et al.*, 1992). It should also be added that both gustatory and visceral divisions of the NST send efferents to separate regions of the anterior PBN, whereas units in the interstitial zone in the posterior dorsomedial part of the PBN receive both taste and vagal information (Hermann *et al.*, 1983; Herman and Rogers, 1985). The PBN is hence a prime candidate for the integration of taste and malaise in CTA. Information on gastrointestinal malaise can reach the central nervous system (CNS) also via the area postrema, which is involved in emetic responses to circulating toxins, and responds to some malaise-inducing agents (e.g. c-Fos induction of the area postrema in response to LiCl i.p.; Yamamoto *et al.*, 1992). Area postrema projects to the dorsal division of the medial NST and to the lateral PBN (van der Kooy and Koda, 1983). The caudal part of the NST projects to the CeA and the lateral PBN projects to the CeA, anterior, medial, basomedial, and posterior basolateral amygdala (Ricardo and Koh, 1978; Saper and Loewy, 1980). Taken together, the aforementioned observations indicate that taste input and gastrointestinal malaise information can converge on the same amygdaloid nuclei, and suggest candidate sites for taste–malaise integration in addition to the PBN (see above).

9.3 A selection of questions

The question of whether the amygdala plays a role in CTA is too general and must be broken down into more specific elements. Ideally, one would like to have answers to the following questions:

(i) Assuming that the amygdala does play a role in CTA—is it in the perceptual processing of information presented in CTA training, in the hedonic evaluation of that information, in experience-dependent modification of the perceived information, i.e. in learning and memory, and/or, finally, in the expression of the avoidance behaviour?

(ii) Which phase(s) of learning and memory are involved (i.e. acquisition, consolidation, retention, retrieval)?

(iii) Does the amygdala itself undergo long-lasting modifications in CTA learning, or is it only involved in transient modulation of other brain structures?

(iv) Which amygdaloid nuclei are involved, and which are the loci of plasticity in these nuclei, if any?

(v) What is the interaction of specific amygdaloid nuclei with other stations in the brain circuits that acquire and retain CTA?

(vi) Are any of the roles of the amygdala in CTA indispensable for normal CTA learning and memory, and, if so, are these roles apparent only in some CTA protocols but not others, and if so, why?

Practically, these issues point to the need to distinguish processing from lasting plasticity, one phase of memory from another, and 'dispensable' functions, which take place in the normal brain and can be identified by certain cellular and molecular methods, from indispensable ones, which may be taxed by lesions. Unfortunately, we do not yet have satisfactory answers to the aforementioned questions, which at this stage could be considered merely as guidelines for future analysis. Hence, the picture on the role of amygdala in CTA is still very fragmentary. However, surveying the current data and identifying the issues may provide hints and facilitate further research.

9.4 The effect of lesions

Two basic points might be noted before briefly surveying the data on the effect of amygdalar lesions on CTA. First, most studies lesioned multiple nuclei and, in some cases, even though the attention of both the investigator and the reader was tuned to a specific nucleus, in fact, other nuclei were affected as well. Secondly, lesions are either irreversible (e.g. electrolytic or cytotoxic) or transient (e.g. metabolic). The brain is expected to treat these different types of interventions very differently. Lasting damage may lead to recruitment over time of shunts that take over the missing function, or to modifications in algorithms and computations. Furthermore, transient inhibition of a locus of processing or plasticity may result in physiological and behavioural effects which are undetected if that same locus is completely abolished and its normal role in CTA rendered obsolete, or taken over by compensating mechanisms.

The first studies on the role of amygdala in CTA involved combined bilateral electrolytic lesions which included basolateral, lateral, cortical, and basomedial amygdaloid nuclei (McGowan *et al.*, 1972; Kemble and Nagel, 1973; Rolls and Rolls, 1973; Nachman and Ashe, 1974). CTA behaviour was impaired, and the effect was larger when the lesion was made after rather than before training (Nachman and Ashe, 1974). Lesioned rats also exhibited diminished neophobic response to the novel taste, and the unfamiliarity of taste became less critical in CTA training (see also Morris *et al.*, 1999; and below). The effect was replicated with a variety of tastes (e.g. 0.1% saccharin, Bermudez-Rattoni *et al.*, 1986; Grupp *et al.*, 1976; 15% sucrose, Nachman and Ashe, 1974; 8% ethanol, Kolakowska *et al.*, 1985), as well as with different malaise-inducing agents (D-amphetamine or LiCl i.p., Grupp *et al.*, 1976; X-rays, Elkins, 1980). In some cases, large lesions in the amygdala were required to obtain an effect. Hence, only rats with more than 75% (Yamamoto and Fujimoto, 1991) or more than 90% (Morris *et al.*, 1999) cytotoxic damage to the BLA were impaired in CTA memory (see also below). Bilateral electrolytic lesions restricted to either the anterior or posterior basolateral nuclei (Fitzgerald and Burton, 1981) or the corticomedial amygdala (Aggleton *et al.*, 1981) had no effect. Lasiter and Glanzman (1985) reported that electrolytic lesion in the lateral or central amygdala was sufficient to impair CTA learning, whereas damage of the BLA was ineffective.

Other authors reported no effect whatsoever on CTA of electrolytic or cytotoxic lesions in certain locations in the amygdala. Electrolytic lesions to the CeA (Kemble *et al.*, 1979; Galaverna *et al.*, 1993) or BLA (Fitzgerald and Burton, 1981), or ibotenic acid lesions to the CeA (Touzani *et al.*, 1997) or BLA (Ferry *et al.*, 1995), had no effect on long-term CTA memory. *N*-methyl-D-aspartate (NMDA)-induced lesions (as well as infusion of an NMDA receptor antagonist) to the CeA, BLA, and lateral amygdaloid nuclei were reported not to affect CTA learning, but attenuated TPOA as well as inhibitory avoidance conditioning

(Bermudez-Rattoni and McGaugh, 1991; Hartfield and Gallagher, 1995). Microinjection of a γ-aminobutyric acid A ($GABA_A$) agonist or 6-hydroxydopamine (6-OHDA)-induced lesions to the BLA were ineffective in impairing CTA, but impaired TPOA learning (Fernandez-Ruiz *et al.*, 1993; Ferry *et al.*, 1995). Similarly, microinjection of a local anaesthetic, novocaine, into the BLA, CeA, basomedial, or lateral nuclei before the taste presentation in training did not affect CTA, but impaired TPOA when tested 3 days later. It is noteworthy that injection of novocaine immediately following the taste or just before the malaise-inducing agent actually facilitated CTA (Bermudez-Rattoni *et al.*, 1983). A heuristic conclusion from various studies (see also Bermudez-Rattoni *et al.*, 1986) is that the amygdaloid circuitry that subserves CTA is different from that which subserves TPOA, and that BLA is important in mediating the olfactory component of long-delayed toxicosis-induced aversion.

Over the years, the interest in the role of BLA in CTA has indeed come to attract much attention. One of the ideas was that it is not the BLA itself which is important, but rather fibres of passage, damaged when the amygdala is lesioned in certain protocols. The effect of a lesioned BLA on CTA, so went the argument, is hence due to the interruption of information processing in extra-amygdaloid circuits, specifically from the brainstem to cortex and *vice versa*. Indeed, Dunn and Everitt (1988) reported that rats with electrolytic lesions to their lateral nucleus, BLA, and CeA were impaired in CTA, whereas rats with ibotenate-induced lesions were not (see also Schafe *et al.*, 1998). To study the effects of the lesions on fibres passing through the amygdala, Dunn and Everitt (1988) injected a retrograde fluorescent dye into the insular cortex. They observed that in rats with ibotenic acid-induced lesions in the amygdala, the amount of stained cells in brain areas such as the lateral hypothalamus and medial parabrachial nuclei was similar to that of controls. In contrast, rats with electrolytic lesions to the amygdala showed fewer stained cells in these brain regions. Thus, the electrolytic lesion in the amygdala appeared to damage fibres of passage from cortex to other brain areas. Similarly, Lasiter and Glanzman (1985) have shown that rats with electrolytic lesions in the CeA and lateral amygdala were impaired in CTA. Anatomical analysis demonstrated that anterograde degeneration of the amygdalofugal and/or corticofugal projection to the convolution of the olfactory tubercle (medial part), subthalamic nucleus, and the PBN was correlated with deficits in CTA. However, the 'fibres of passage hypothesis' was challenged recently by Morris *et al.* (1999). In an earlier work, this group of investigators reported that the only identified fibre system that courses through the amygdala and could possibly be involved in CTA, the bidirectional PBN–insular cortex pathway, remains confined to the CeA (Frey *et al.*, 1997). They have inflicted ibotenic acid lesion confined to the BLA, hence sparing the PBN–cortical pathway. The large BLA lesion (>90%) markedly impaired CTA (Morris *et al.*, 1999). In contrast, a lesion to the CeA had no significant effect on CTA. Interestingly, when a familiar taste was used as the conditioned stimulus in CTA training, the magnitude of CTA in control rats was significantly reduced, as expected, but now the BLA-lesioned rats did not differ from the controls. Morris *et al.* (1999) concluded that the BLA is obligatory for normal CTA, that CeA is not, and that the earlier conclusions of Dunn and Everitt (1988) were due to only partial damage to the BLA by the excitotxic lesions as opposed to the electrolytic lesion which was much more extensive. Furthermore, so goes the argument, the disruption of fibres of passage seen

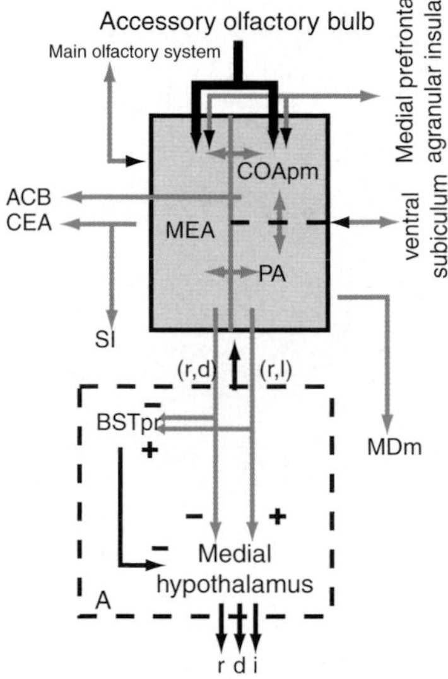

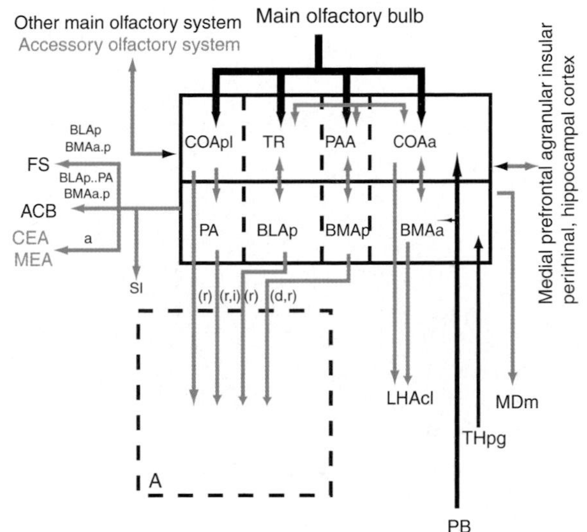

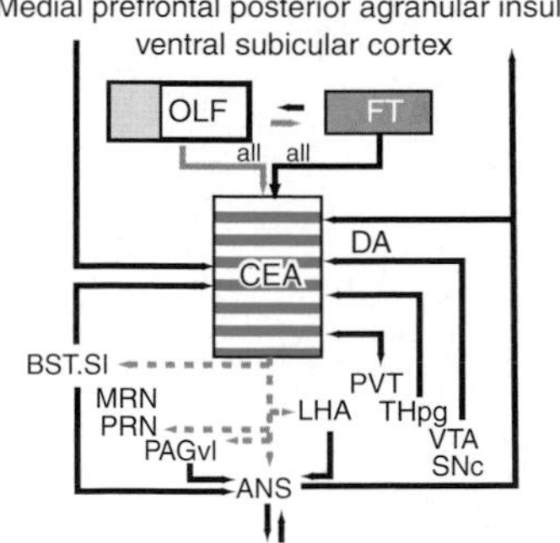

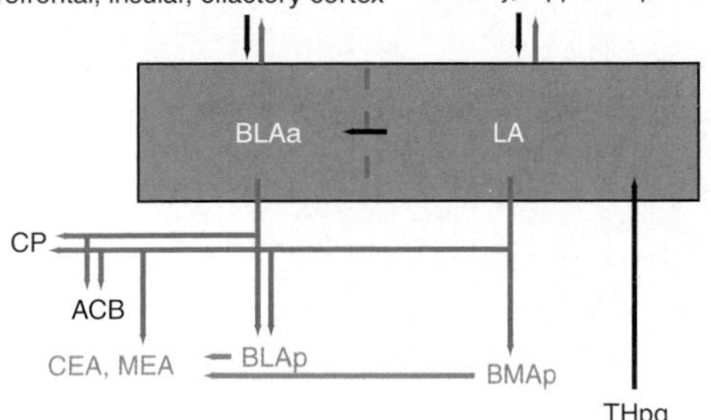

Figure 1.2 The major anatomical connections of the four functional systems associated with the amygdala as described by Swanson and Petrovich (1998). Reprinted from Trends in neuroscience, 21, 329, 1998, with permission from Elsevier Science. See pp 4 and 5 for detailed caption.

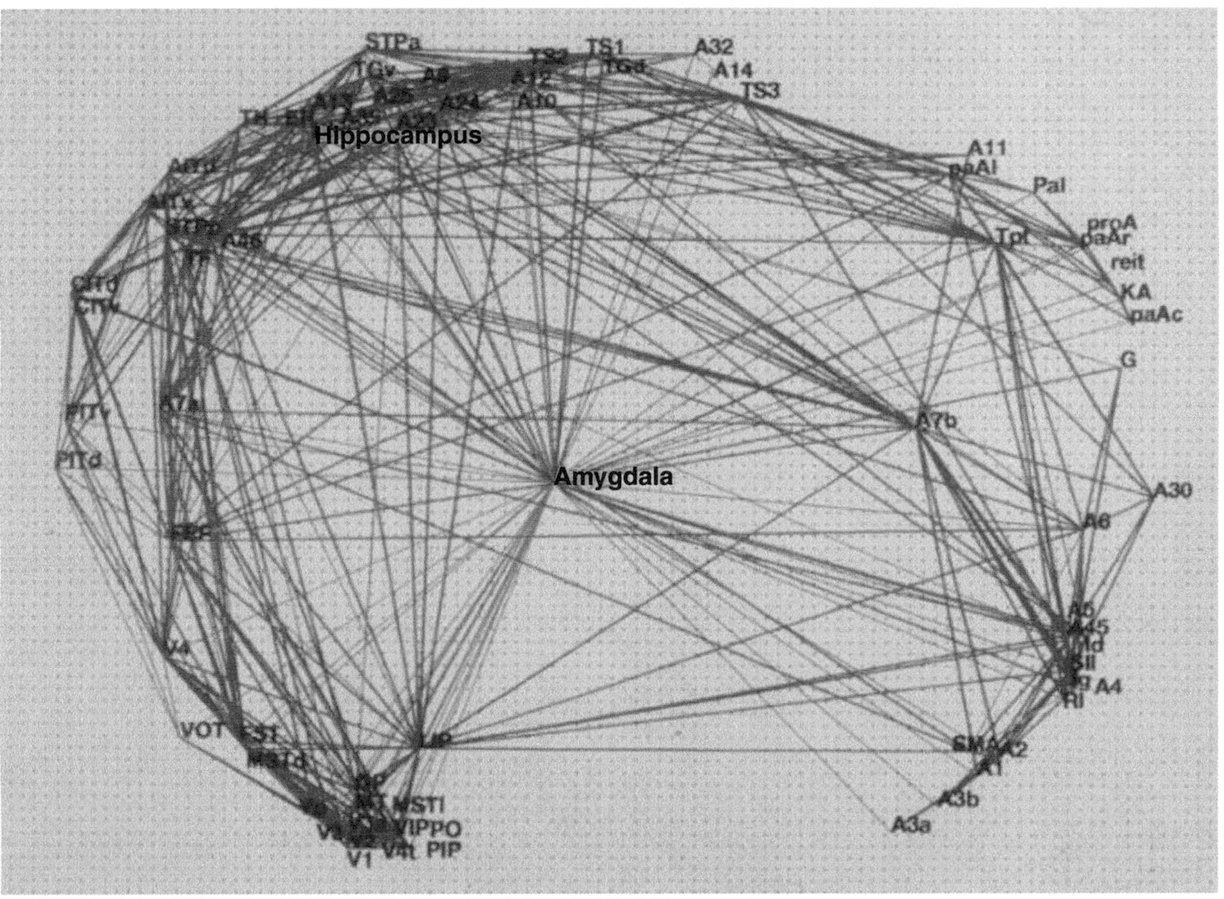

Figure 1.8 Topological organization of entire macaque cerebral cortex. A total of 758 connections between 72 areas is represented, of which 136 (18%) are one-way. Reciprocal connections are shown in red, one-way connections from left to right are in grey, and one-way connections from right to left are in blue (from Young *et al.*, 1994).

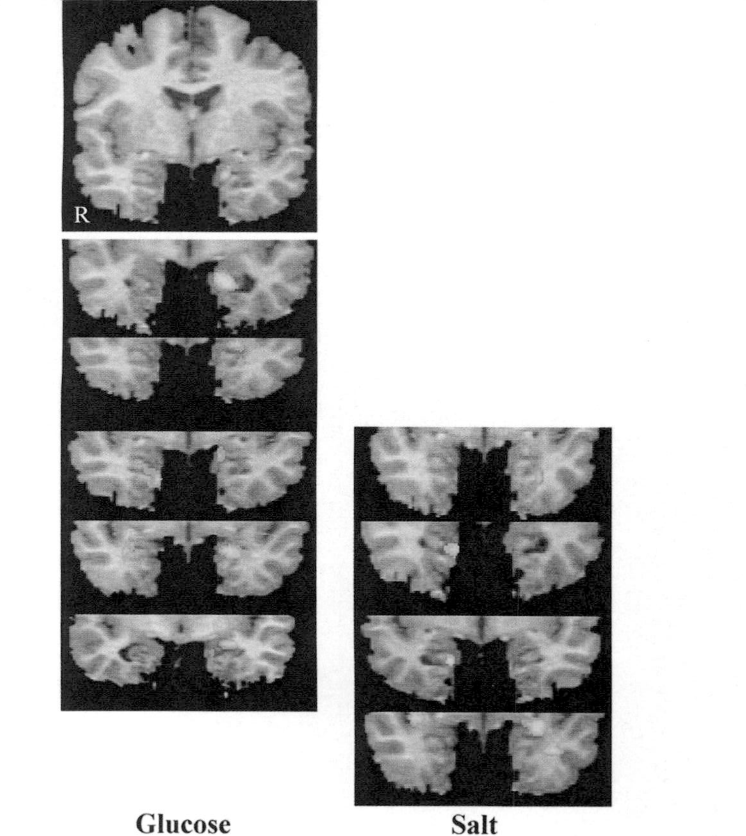

Figure 13.7 Activations produced in the human amygdala in seven subjects in an fMRI investigation by the taste of 1 M glucose versus a tasteless control solution and by 0.1 M NaCl versus a tastless control solution shown on coronal sections thresholded at P <0.025 (corrected for multiple comparisons within a region of interest). see pg 466 for detailed caption.

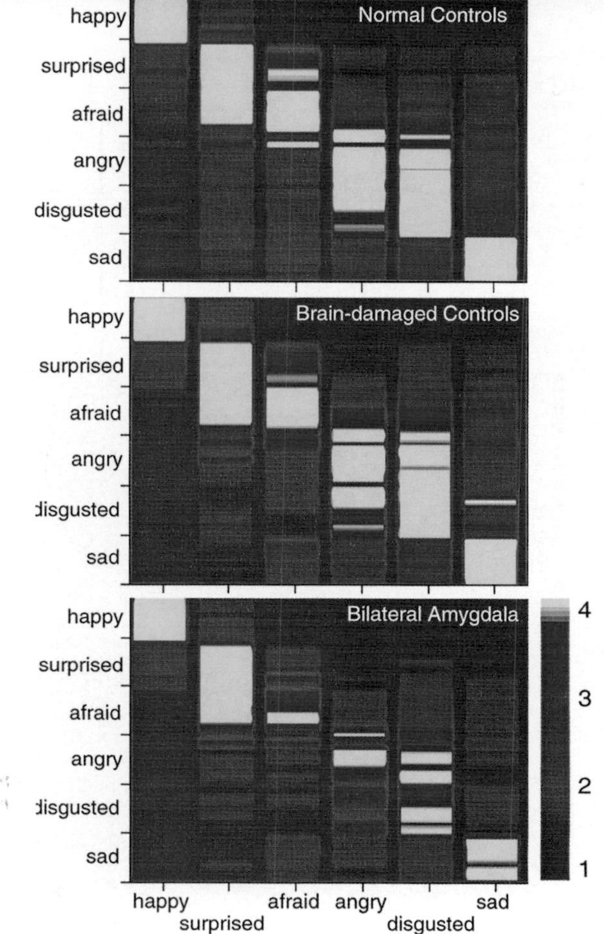

Figure 18.2 Impaired recognition of emotions from facial expressions in subjects with bilateral amygdala damage. See page 598 for detailed caption.

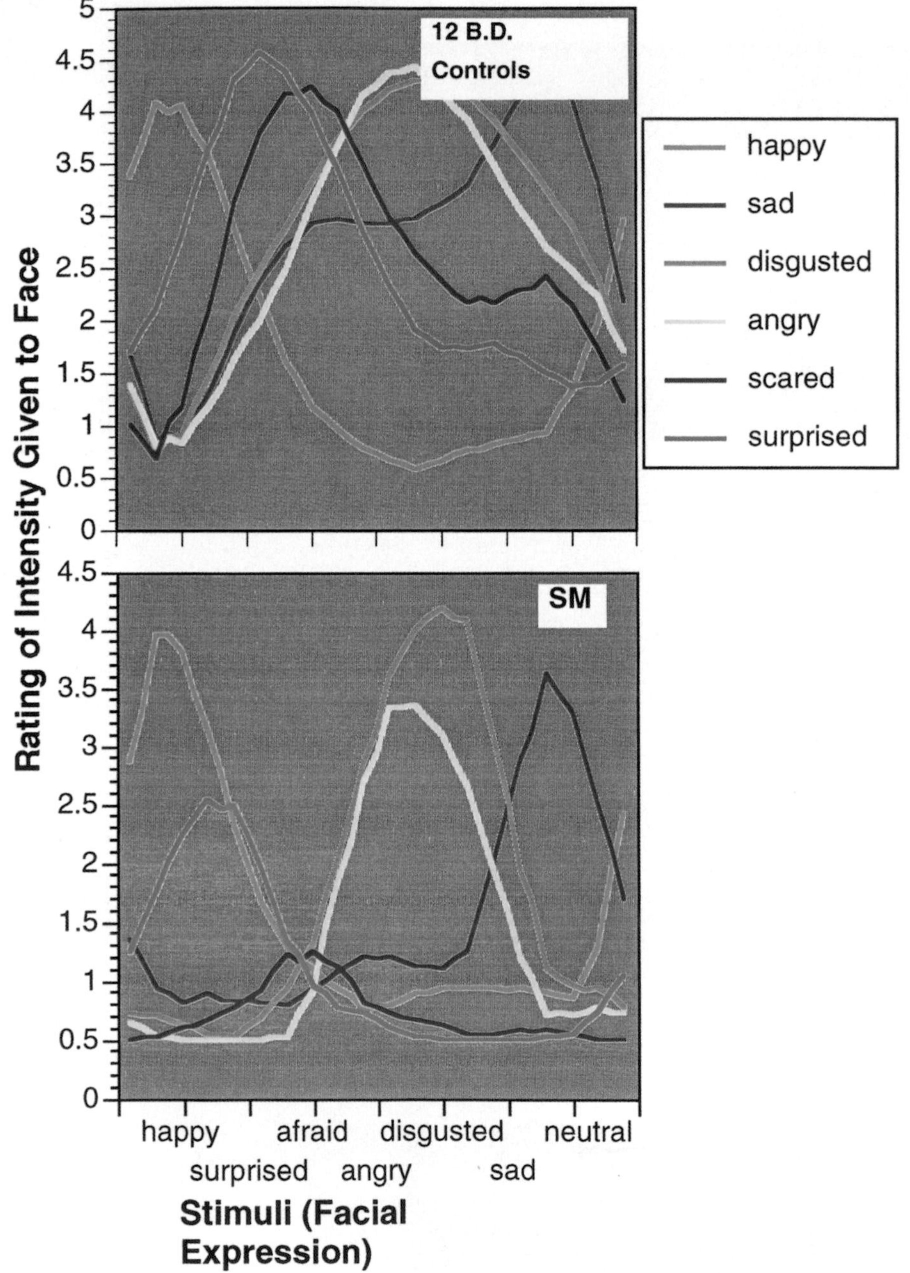

Figure 18.3 Impaired recognition of emotional facial expressions in subject S.M. (A) Impaired recognition of fear in facial expressions in S.M. See page 600 for detailed figure caption.

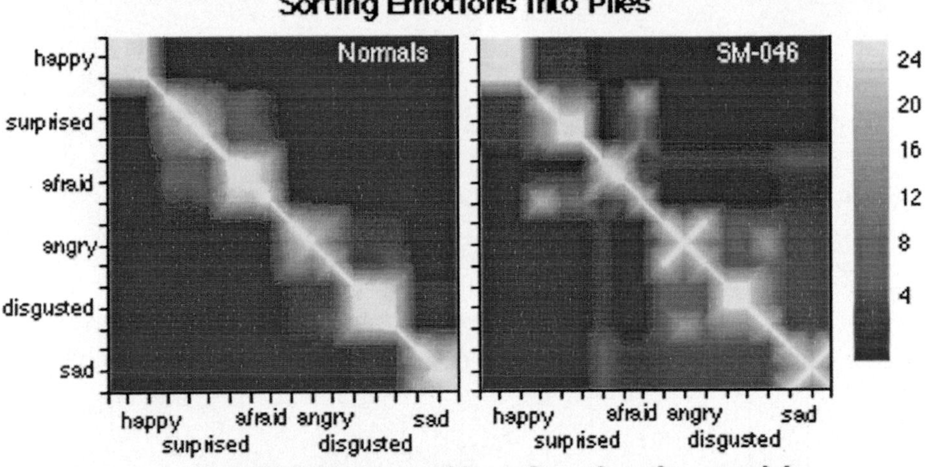

Figure 18.6 Emotion categories derived from sorting photographs of faces into piles. Normal subjects (left, n = 7) distinguished the six basic emotions, as well as superordinate categories that revealed the similarity between surprise and fear, and between anger and disgust. S.M. (right) showed an unusual structure in which she did not distinguish negative emotions normally. See p.608 for detailed caption.

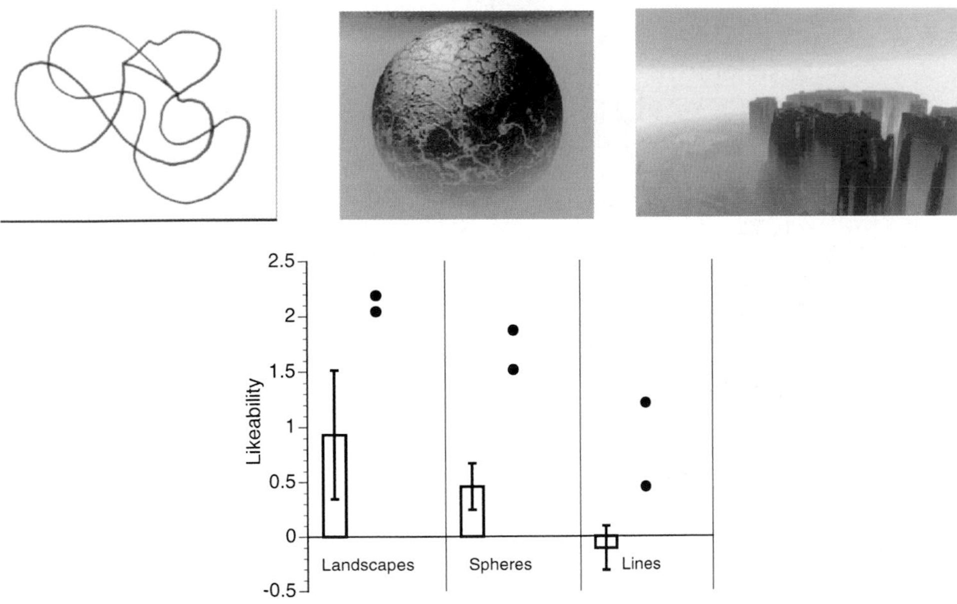

Figure 18.11 Preferences for unfamiliar visual stimuli following amygdala damage. See page p.620 for detailed caption.

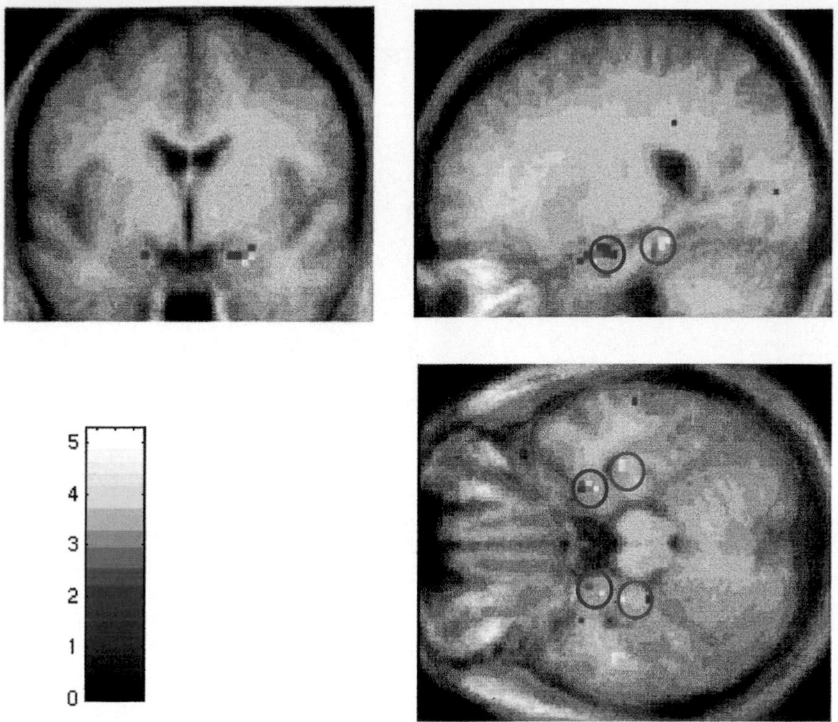

Figure 19.2 Amygdala-hippocampal neural responses during trace conditioning. See p.637 for detailed caption.

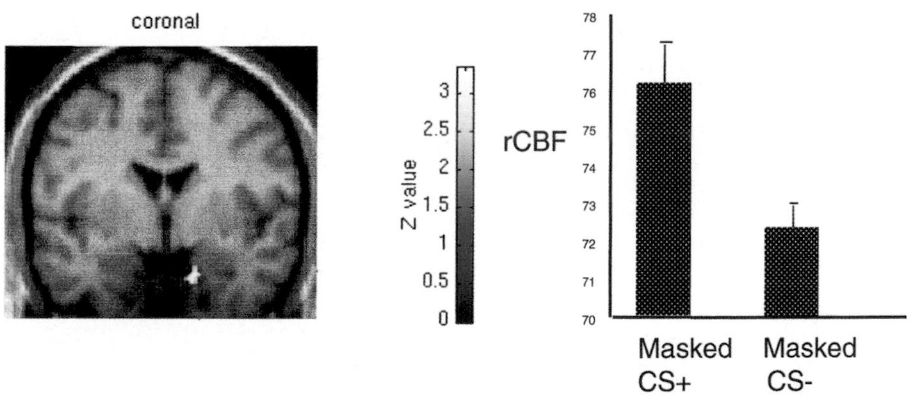

Figure 19.4 The left hand panel shows activation of the right amygdala superimposed on a coronal MRI image in a comparison of masked CS+ and masked CS- conditions. The right hand panel shows the adjusted regional cerebral blood flow (rCBF) responses in right amygdala for the same comparisons.

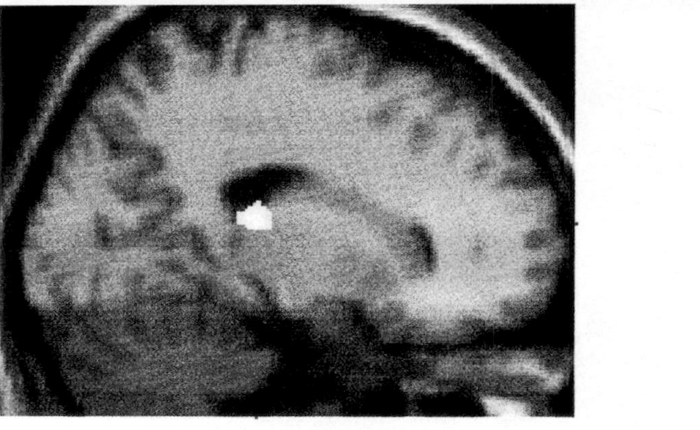

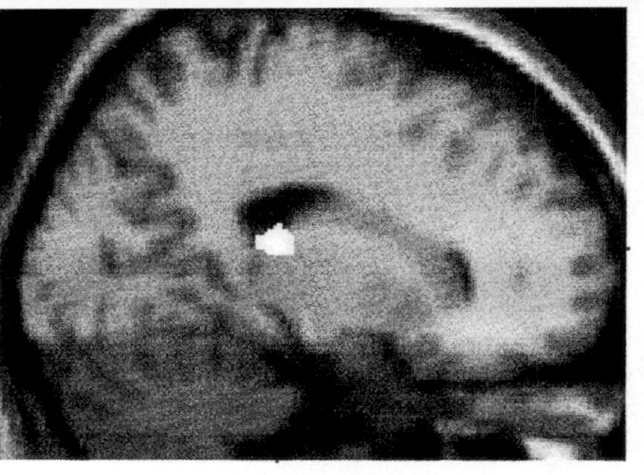

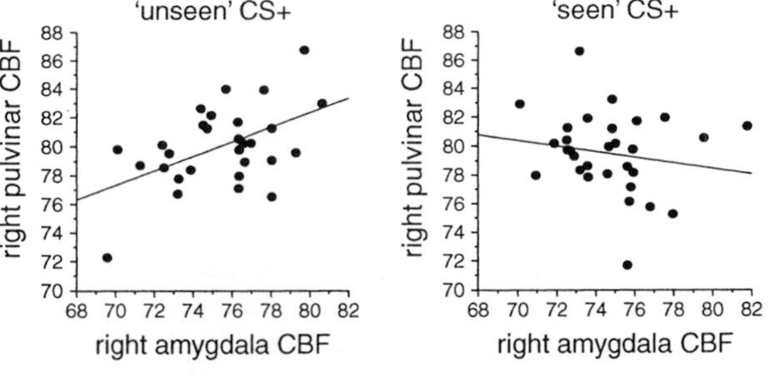

Figure 19.5 Regions which show significant covariance in reponse to activity in the right amygdala during masked CS+ compared with masked CS- presentations. The sagittal MRI sections illustrate activations in pulvinar and superior colliculus, respectively. The plots are regressions of right amygdala activity on pulvinar and superior colliculus activity for the same contrasts.

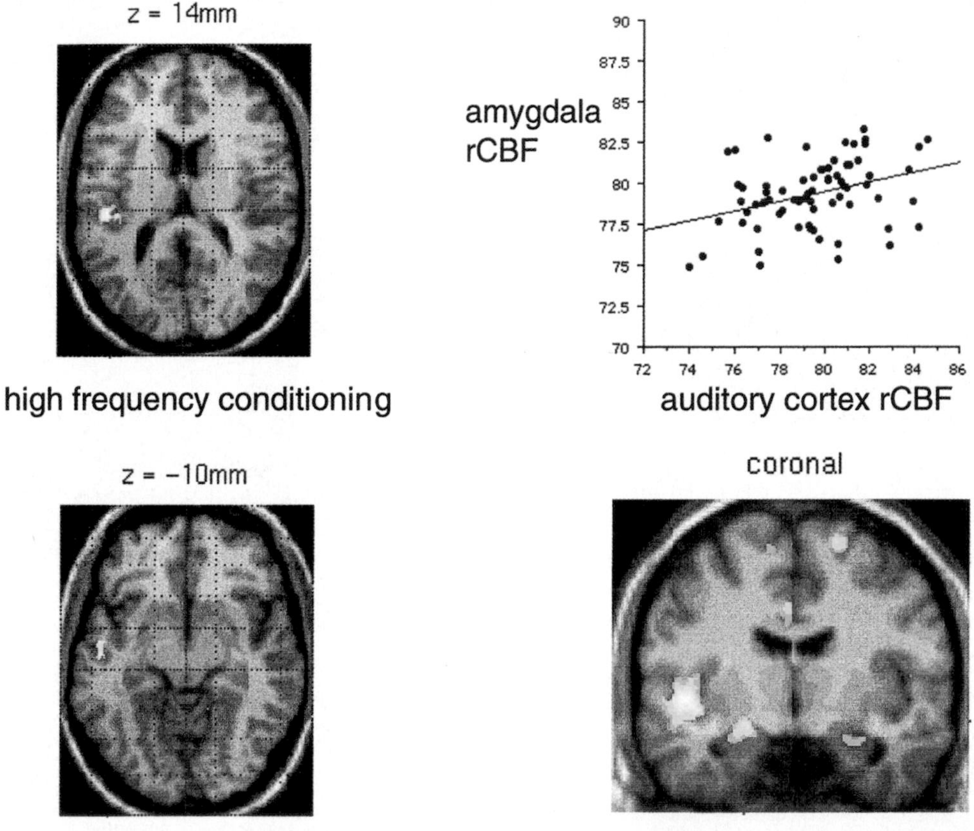

Figure 19.6 The left transverse slices through the brain illustrate auditory cortical regions which show learning-related modulation of responses as a function of conditioning to high- (left upper panel) and low- (left lower panel) frequency tones, respectively. The right lower panel shows bilateral amygdala regions which co-vary significantly in response with conditioning-related responses in auditory cortex. The plot (right upper panel) illustrates this significant co-variation in a positive regression of auditory cortex activity on activity in left amygdala.

in earlier studies was probably due to damage to the CeA rather than to the BLA. All in all, the recent data support a role for BLA in CTA and do not support the 'fibres of passage' explanation.

In addition to the irreversible lesions, transient, metabolic lesions were also used to investigate the role of amygdala in CTA, mainly in an attempt to differentiate the postulated contribution(s) of various phases of CTA learning, retention, and expression. CTA was attenuated in rats microinjected with tetrodotoxin (TTX) into the BLA and CeA 30 min before or 1.5 h (but not 6 h) after the application of the malaise-inducing agent (Gallo *et al*., 1992; Roldan and Bures, 1994). Microinjection before the beginning of training (i.e. before presentation of the taste) had no effect. Microinjection of TTX into amygdala or the GC before retrieval attenuated the expression of CTA memory, while injection of TTX to both the amygdala and the GC completely impaired CTA memory. These results were taken to suggest that the amygdala is involved with the processing of the malaise representation or its integration with the taste representation rather than with the taste representation *per se*. The data were also construed to imply that the amygdala is involved in the retrieval of taste memory and that connections between the GC and the amygdala are important for retrieval. This observation is consistent with previous studies showing that severing corticoamygdaloid connections before CTA training prevented the formation of taste memory. (The connections were cut caudally from the level of the nucleus of the lateral olfactory tract back to the ventral hippocampus, dorsoventrally from above the level of the rhinal sulcus to the base of the brain, and laterally at the extreme outer edge of the amygdala complex at the line of the BLA and lateral amygdaloid nuclei; Fitzgerald and Burton, 1983.) Severing the corticoamygdaloid connection (in the perirhinal region) after CTA training also impaired taste memory (Yamamoto *et al*., 1984). Finally, experiments using local microinjections of TTX also led to the conclusion that the processing of CTA information and its retrieval require intact ipsilateral amygdala, PBN, and GC (Bielavska and Roldan, 1996).

9.5 Cellular and molecular mechanisms

Cellular and molecular investigations of the role of amygdala in CTA cast light on potential mechanisms of CTA learning and memory, while at the same time focusing on general issues pertaining to the role of amygdala in acquisition and retention of experience-dependent internal representations. One of these questions is whether the amygdala itself stores learned information over time, or merely modulates other brain structures during learning (e.g. McGaugh *et al*., 1996; Lamprecht *et al*., 1997; Cahill *et al*., 1999; Fanselow and LeDoux, 1999). As opposed to lesions, that are performed mainly to unveil mechanisms obligatory for a certain physiological process or behaviour, cellular and molecular methods may also unveil mechanisms that are correlated with, but not obligatory for, the behaviour. The conclusions from correlative studies may hence be rather different from those obtained in lesion studies, as some mechanisms may operate in the intact brain but not in the lesioned brain, and others may still be functional but their contribution masked, due to the aberrant output of the damaged brain or the lack of sensitivity of the behavioural tests.

Several groups have reported that the responses of amygdala neurons to taste are altered following CTA to that taste. Units in the BLA, CeA, or basomedial amygdala showed no response to water and only a small sporadic response to saccharin. Unit discharge increased after LiCl injection and returned gradually to basal level within less than 2 h. When saccharin was applied again 2–4 h after CTA training, a remarkable alteration in unit discharges was elicited to saccharin and sucrose, but not to water, 0.1 mM quinine HCl, 0.1 M NaCl, or 0.01 M HCl (Yamamoto and Fujimoto, 1991; Yasoshima *et al.*, 1995). In another study (Buresova *et al.*, 1979), rats trained to avoid drinking a LiCl solution exhibited drinking-induced inhibition of unit activity in the GC, ventromedial hypothalamus, and amygdala, and excitation in the lateral hypothalamus in response to the aversive stimulus. These observations show that amygdaloid neurons participate in the retrieval of taste memory, and suggest that long-term neuronal modulations are induced in the amygdala during CTA memory formation.

Other studies have indicated that neuronal activity in amygdala can influence taste information during acquisition and retrieval of CTA (Phillips and LePiane, 1978, 1980). In these experiments, rats received a familiar taste solution (tap water) together with electrical stimulation to the BLA complex or the caudate. This was followed, 10 min later, by i.p. injection of LiCl. Aversive responses to the water while receiving the same electrical stimulation were tested in these animals 48 h later and were found to be similar to the aversion to saccharin in a saccharin–LiCl paired group. Rats that have received water without amygdalar stimulation on the training day did not develop aversion to the tap water on the test day. This effect was specific to the amygdala and was not observed following stimulation of the caudate nucleus. It was observed only when the stimulation was administrated to the amygdala during both training and testing, suggesting that the amygdala contributes to the combined representation of the taste and electrical stimulation.

Other evidence for the involvement of amygdala in the processing of the taste or taste–malaise information emerges from studies showing that electrical stimulation of the amygdala in between the taste–malaise pairing (15 min after the taste; Arthur, 1975) or within 3 h after pairing (Kesner *et al.*, 1975) disrupted CTA formation. Production of amygdala kindling following either the taste or the malaise-inducing agent also disrupted CTA (Mikulka and Freeman, 1984).

Several laboratories have investigated molecular changes that take place in the amygdala in CTA. Microinjection of NMDA antagonists, (D,L)-2-amino-5 phosphonovaleric acid (APV) or MK-801, into the amygdala during or immediately after taste presentation attenuated CTA (Yamamoto and Fujimoto, 1991; Tucci *et al.*, 1998). Tucci *et al.* (1998) measured the level of glutamate in the BLA by microdialysis. When the conditioned taste was infused into the mouth of conditioned rats, elevation of glutamate in the BLA was observed. Moreover, microinjection of glutamate into the BLA immediately after exposure to the taste induced CTA formation (Tucci *et al.*, 1998). Microinjection of 6-OHDA, a compound that depletes noradrenaline (norepinephrine), or physostigmine, an anticholinesterase, into the BLA during the onset of toxicosis impaired CTA (Ellis and Kesner, 1981; Borsini and Rolls, 1984). In addition, adrencorticotropin (ACTH) in the amygdala was suggested to mediate CTA since rats lesioned in the lateral, basolateral, basomedial, medial, central, and cortical amygdaloid nuclei combined, that received ACTH 15 min before a retrieval test, were partially rescued from CTA learning impairment (Burt *et al.*, 1980).

The role in CTA of protein kinase C (PKC), involved in signal transduction downstream of a number of neuromodulators and neurotransmiters such as acetylcholine and glutamate, was investigated. Microinjection of the PKC inhibitors H7 or polymyxin B (PMXB) disrupted CTA when injected into the amygdala between the taste and toxicosis or 30 min after CTA. It should be noted, however, that the aforementioned inhibitors are not highly specific for PKC. A less potent PKC inhibitor, HA 1004, had no effect. Injection of PMXB 4 h after CTA learning or 30 min before retrieval did not impair CTA. These results suggest that PKC is involved in the acquisition of CTA and processing of taste–malaise information, but not in the retrieval of taste memory (Bahar *et al.*, 1997; Yasoshima and Yamamoto, 1997).

Activation of second messenger cascades, such as those involving PKC, might culminate in modulation of gene expression. A prevailing hypothesis in the field of memory research is that modulation of gene expression subserves long-term memory (Davis and Squire, 1984; Goelet *et al.*, 1986; Dudai, 1989). Microinjection of anisomycin, a protein synthesis inhibitor, into an amygdala area including the CeA, under conditions that inhibit protein synthesis throughout the training trial, impaired taste memory (Lamprecht and Dudai, 1996). In contrast, anisomycin had no effect on memory when injected before retrieval. Moreover, inhibition of the cAMP response element-binding protein (CREB) or of the synthesis of c-Fos in the CeA by local microinjection of antisense oligonucleotides impaired CTA memory (Lamprecht and Dudai, 1996; Lamprecht *et al.*, 1997). CREB antisense oligonucleotides impaired long- but not short-term taste memory formation. Inhibition of the synthesis of c-Fos or CREB proteins before the test had no effect on memory retrieval. These observations suggest that modulation of gene expression in the amygdala subserves consolidation of some aspects of long-term memory of CTA.

Amygdala neurons were also shown to be responsive to gastrointestinal distress. Recording from the BLA revealed neurons that responded to LiCl i.p., these neuronal responses peaked minutes after LiCl injection and returned gradually to the basal level (Reddy and Bures, 1981; Yamamoto and Fujimoto, 1991). Injection of LiCl i.p. also induced increases in c-Fos and immediate-early genes in the CeA (Yamamoto *et al.*, 1992; Gu *et al.*, 1993; Lamprecht and Dudai, 1995). As noted above, modulation of immediate-early genes is expected to result in some long-term neuronal alterations. Taken together, the aforementioned data on the effect of inhibition of translational mechanisms suggest that in CTA, the amygdala stores information over time and does not modulate other brain structures only during learning or immediately afterwards.

As noted above, the lateral, BLA, and anterior cortical amygdaloid nuclei project to the GC, and the CeA projects to the lateral hypothalamus, PBN, and NST (Saper, 1982; Van Der Kooy *et al.*, 1984; Turner and Herkenham, 1991), areas involved in CTA formation and in ingestive behaviour (Yamamoto *et al.*, 1994; Bures *et al.*, 1998). Electrophysiological recording and immunocytochemical analysis have been employed to investigate the amygdalar influence on these structures. Neuronal responses and c-Fos levels in the NST were altered when the taste used as the conditioned taste was presented again to rats after CTA training (Chang and Scott, 1984; Houpt *et al.*, 1994; Swank and Bernstein, 1994; Schafe *et al.*, 1995; Swank *et al.*, 1995). Combined bilateral electrolytic lesions to the CeA, BLA, basomedial, and lateral amygdaloid nuclei in rats impaired CTA and abolished c-Fos induction in the NST in response to the taste. Unilateral lesion did not affect the acquisition of CTA and an increased c-Fos protein level was observed in the contralateral NST in retrieval (Schafe and Bernstein, 1996). These findings suggest that the amygdala contributes to alterations in neuronal responses observed in the NST during retrieval of CTA memory .

In still another study, investigating corticoamygdaloid connections, high-frequency stimulation in the BLA was used to induce long-term potentiation (LTP) in the granular insular cortex (Escobar *et al.*, 1998b). Microinjection of the NMDA antagonist 3-(2-carboxypiperazin-4-yl) propyl-1-phosphoric acid (CPP) into the insular cortex inhibited BLA-induced LTP. In a parallel experiment, it also disrupted CTA memory tested 4 days post-training (Escobar *et al.*, 1998a). LTP is generally considered to subserve the formation of memory (Bliss and Collingridge, 1993). The results hence raise the possibility that activation of the BLA during CTA induces some neuronal modulations in the GC that subserve long-term taste memory.

9.6 A reminder of sources of variability and some caveats

Examination of the literature on the role of the amygdaloid complex in CTA unveils marked differences in the behavioural protocols used as well as in the methodology of lesions and pharmacological interventions. This may confound the interpretation of the data. Several potential sources of variability as well as additional caveats deserve proper attention.

(i) The location of damage, its extent, and its timing often differ between studies aimed at lesioning the same nuclei, thus rendering comparisons unreliable. This may happen even between different experiments in the same study, aimed at elucidating the role of an identified amygdalar nuclear complex (e.g. see discussion in Morris *et al.*, 1999).

(ii) In pharmacological experiments, the specific ligand targeted to a given molecular target, as well as its mode and time of administration into the amygdala, may have a decisive effect on subsequent CTA. For example, Tucci *et al.* (1998) and Hartfield and Gallagher (1995) microinjected different NMDA antagonists (MK-801, an antagonist of the receptor channel, and APV, an antagonist of the glutamate-binding site) to similar locations (BLA), and obtained different results. Furthermore, acute microinjection of APV did not affect CTA; however, in another study, chronic injection of APV into the BLA did attenuate CTA (Yamamoto and Fujimoto, 1991). We must understand more about the local molecular mechanisms involved in order to account for such data.

(iii) Most importantly, different training and testing protocols may affect differentially the outcome of experiments intended to determine the role of amygdala in CTA. This, one should note, is not unique to CTA, and has been pointed out, for example, in considering the role of amygdala in fear conditioning (Killcross *et al.*, 1997; Nader and LeDoux, 1997). Schafe *et al.* (1998) observed that rats with combined ibotenic acid-induced lesions in their basolateral, lateral, and central amygdaloid nuclei, conditioned by infusion of a taste solution via oral intubation, failed to acquire CTA, whereas rats with similar lesions that were trained with bottle presentation became highly aversive. Mikulka *et al.* (1977) showed that rats with combined basolateral, cortical, basomedial, and medial amygdaloid nuclei lesions acquired taste aversion as rapidly as the control group using choice training with two bottles (30 min presentation of two bottles to the animals, one containing water, the other sucrose). In contrast, animals trained by presentation with a single bottle (one bottle of sucrose presented for 15 min followed by bottle of water for 15 min) exhibited marked retardation in CTA learning. The inclusion of all these procedures under the umbrella term of 'CTA' is convenient indeed, but may mask significantly different behavioural states and learning processes. Furthermore, the different procedures may also blur the contribution of sensory input in addition to taste, e.g. odour, in the processing of which the amygdala may play a decisive role. The type and dose of the gastrointestinal malaise associated with the taste is also expected to affect the contribution of the amygdala to CTA. For example, BLA was reported to be involved in CTA produced by i.p. injection of LiCl, which causes upper gastrointestinal malaise, but not by consumption of lactose, which induces lower gastrointestinal malaise (Simbayi *et al.*, 1986; Simbayi, 1987).

(iv) Furthermore, the CTA training protocol inherently engulfs multiple types of learning. It starts with 'incidental learning', i.e. the acquisition of information about an unfamiliar taste in the absence of a specific exogenous reinforcer; it proceeds with an association between an internal representation of taste and a negative reinforcer. The retrieval, at least the first time it is practised, contrasts a manifestation of a decrease in neophobia with an increase in avoidance due to the acquired aversion. It is unlikely that all these types of experience-dependent representational and behavioural modification will be subserved by a single common circuit, and it is unrealistic to assume that the weight of the various components will remain the same when the training and testing protocols are modified. Moreover, note that based on the current data, the central (CeA) and the basolateral (BLA) amygdaloid nuclei are among the prime candidates for fulfilling a role in CTA; yet, at least in the rat, the CeA is suggested to be an autonomic-projecting motor region of the striatum, the anterior BLA an extension of the claustrum for the temporal and frontal lobes, and the posterior BLA a component of the central olfactory system (Swanson and Petrovich, 1998). The involvement of CeA and BLA hence may reflect the engagement of radically different brain functions. It is likely, therefore, that some discrepancies concerning the role(s) of CeA and BLA in CTA stem not only from the use of heterogeneous anatomical, cellular, and molecular tools to probe the role of the amygdala, but also from different behavioural protocols that tap different forms of behaviour and learning.

(v) In addition, the remarkable survival value of CTA has probably led in evolution to the existence of multiple neuronal 'backups' that can sustain the behavioural modification. It is therefore unlikely to find a single nucleus that will abolish CTA completely. Hence, lack of a marked effect of a lesion does not imply that the lesioned site is not involved in CTA *in vivo*, and only very substantial lesions might produce an effect (e.g. in BLA). Similarly, sites that show CTA-correlated activity and plasticity (e.g. CeA) may not necessarily produce an effect when lesioned.

9.7 Concluding remarks

Detailed answers to the questions posed in Section 9.3 are not yet available. One currently can offer only general and mostly heuristic statements concerning the role of amygdala in CTA. It is plausible to conclude, despite discrepancies stemming from various sources some of which are listed above, that multiple nuclei in that complex, highly differentiated region dubbed 'amygdala' do subserve representational and behavioural modifications in CTA. The position of the amygdaloid complex in circuits that subserve ingestive as well as aversive behaviours predicts *a priori* a role in information processing in CTA, but the data currently show that the amygdalar complex does more: not only does it process the information but it also undergoes plastic changes in the course of CTA learning and memory. Molecular studies show that the CeA is clearly engaged in CTA in the intact rat, and that an area concentrated on the CeA (possibly including adjacent tissue) is indispensable for CTA acquisition but not for retrieval. This implies that sensory, motor, and motivational processing are unaffected, but memory formation is (Lamprecht *et al.*, 1997). Furthermore, the region centering upon the CeA appears to be involved in plasticity and in retention of CTA information over time, as reasoned from the obligatory role of protein synthesis and gene expression (Lamprecht *et al.*, 1997). The CeA, on the other hand, may not be indispensable under certain protocols in the chronically lesioned rat. In contrast, at least a small intact portion of the BLA is indispensable for CTA in the chronically lesioned rat. The BLA may also be involved in subtle olfactory components of CTA, and in the neophobic elements of the training experience. Other nuclei, e.g. lateral, are possibly also subserving CTA. The detailed amygdalar circuits involved in CTA processing, learning, and memory and in expression of the aversive behaviour have not yet been identified, and cellular models are unavailable as yet. CTA is hence still far from the situation which applies to another amygdala-subserved conditioning, classical fear conditioning, in which detailed circuit models have been proposed.

Research on CTA is related to multiple, intriguing issues in memory research, e.g. the mechanisms of incidental learning, of long-delayed associations, of innately constrained ('prepared') learning, the role of amygdala in modulation of learning and in storage of memory, and cortical control of implicit, visceral learning. Over the years, CTA was investigated extensively as a behavioural phenomenon, but most of its neuronal substrates are as yet a *terra incognita*. It seems that research on the neurobiology of CTA now enters a new era. In it, the role of components of the amygdaloid complex will be better understood. This is due to multiple developments. First, the potential pitfalls and caveats (e.g. see Sections 9.1 and 9.6) are now better appreciated. Secondly, several majority-vote conclusions can now be extracted more confidently from the accumulated combined research of several laboratories. Thirdly, much information becomes available from other amygdala-dependent learning systems, e.g. fear conditioning, and these data reflect on potential mechanisms of amygdala involvement in CTA. Fourthly, 'classical' methods, such as cytotoxic and pharmacological lesions, are now improved. Finally, novel methodologies can now be recruited, including neurogenetics (preferably involving the use of conditional mutants) and functional magnetic resonance imaging (Neduva, Degani, and Dudai, unpublished). For example, one now encounters more and more reference to CTA in papers dealing with knockout mice, as part of the battery of tests used to characterize mutants, as well as in other publications in molecular neurobiology. A better understanding of the role in CTA of identified brain regions, including amygdalar nuclei and circuits, is therefore practically inescapable.

Acknowledgements

We thank K. Nader and G.E. Schafe for valuable comments. The work in the authors' laboratory mentioned in this review was supported by a grant from the Reich Foundation and by the Dominic Institute for Brain Research, Rehovot.

References

Aggleton, J.P., Petrides, M., and Iversen, S.D. (1981) Differential effects of amygdaloid lesions on conditioned taste aversion learning by rats. *Physiology and Behavior*, 27, 397–400.

Arthur, J.B. (1975) Taste aversion learning is impaired by interpolated amygdaloid stimulation but not by posttraining amygdaloid stimulation. *Behavioral Biology*, 13, 369–376.

Azuma, S., Yamamoto, T., and Kawamura, Y. (1984) Studies on gustatory responses of amygdaloid neurons in rats. *Experimental Brain Research*, 56, 12–22.

Bahar, A., Hazvi, S., Lamprecht, R., Ofen, N., and Dudai, Y. (1997) Molecular mechanisms of conditioned taste aversion memory in the rat insular cortex: potential involvement of protein kinase C. *Society for Neuroscience Abstracts*, 823.1.

Bermudez-Rattoni, F., and McGaugh, J.L. (1991) Insular cortex and amygdala lesions differentially affect acquisition on inhibitory avoidance and conditioned taste aversion. *Brain Research*, 549, 165–170.

Bermudez-Rattoni, F., Rusiniak, K.W., and Garcia, J. (1983) Flavor–illness aversions: potentiation of odor by taste is disrupted by application of novocaine into amygdala. *Behavioral and Neural Biology*, 37, 61–75.

Bermudez-Rattoni, F., Grijalva, C.V., Kiefer, S.W., and Garcia, J. (1986) Flavor–illness aversions: the role of the amygdala in the acquisition of taste-potentiated odor aversions. *Physiology and Behavior*, 38, 503–508.

Bielavska, E and Roldan, G. (1996) Ipsilateral connections between the gustatory cortex, amygdala and parabrachial nucleus are necessary for acquisition and retrieval of conditioned taste in rats. *Behavioural Brain Research*, 81, 25–31.

Bliss, T.V. and Collingridge, G.L. (1993) A synaptic model of memory: long-term potentiation in the hippocampus. *Nature*, 361, 31–39.

Borsini, F. and Rolls, E.T. (1984) Role of noradrenaline and serotonin in basolateral region of the amygdala in food preferences and learned taste aversions in the rat. *Physiology and Behavior*, 33, 37–43.

Bures, J., Bermudez-Rattoni, F., and Yamamoto, T. (1998) *Conditioned Taste Aversion: Memory of a Special Kind*. Oxford University Press, Oxford.

Bures, J., Buresova, O., and Krivanek, J. (1988) *Brain and Behavior: Paradigms for Research in Neural Mechanisms*. Wiley, New York.

Buresova, O., Aleksanyan, Z.A., and Bures, J. (1979) Electrophysiological analysis of retrieval of conditioned taste aversion in rats. Unit activity changes in critical brain regions. *Physiologia Bohemoslovaca*, 28, 525–536.

Burt, G.S. and Smotherman, W.P. (1980) Amygdalectomy induced deficits in conditioned taste aversion: possible pituitary–adrenal involvement. *Physiology and Behavior*, 24, 651–655.

Cahill, L., Weinberger, N.M. , Roozendaal, B., and McGaugh, J.L. (1999) Is the amygdala a locus of 'conditioned fear'? Some questions and caveats. *Neuron*, 23, 227–228.

Chang, F.C. and Scott, T.R. (1984) Conditioned taste aversions modify neural responses in the rat nucleus tractus solitarius. *Journal of Neuroscience*, 4, 1850–1862.

Davis, H.P. and Squire, L.R. (1984) Protein synthesis and memory. *Psychological Bulletin*, 96, 518–559.

Dudai, Y. (1989) *The Neurobiology of Memory. Concepts, Findings, Trends*. Oxford University Press, Oxford.

Dunn, L.T. and Everitt, B.J. (1988) Double dissociation of the effects of amygdala and insular cortex lesions on conditioned taste aversion, passive avoidance, and neophobia in the rat using excitotoxin ibotenic acid. *Behavioral Neuroscience*, 102, 3–23.

Elkins, R.L. (1980) Attenuation of X-ray-induced taste aversions by olfactory-bulb or amygdaloid lesions. *Physiology and Behavior*, 24, 515–521.

Ellis, M.E. and Kesner, R.P. (1981) Physostigmine and norepinephrine: effects of injection into amygdala on taste association. *Physiology and Behavior*, 27, 203–209.

Escobar, M.L., Alcocer, I., and Chao, V. (1998a) The NMDA receptor antagonist CPP impairs conditioned taste aversion and insular cortex long-term potentiation *in vivo*. *Brain Research*, 812, 246–251.

Escobar, M.L., Chao, V., and Bermudez-Rattoni, F. (1998b) *In vivo* long-term potentiation in the insular cortex: NMDA receptor dependence. *Brain Research*, 779, 314–319.

Fanselow, M.S. and LeDoux, J.E. (1999) Why we think plasticity underlying pavlovian fear conditioning occurs in the basolateral amygdala. *Neuron*, 23, 229–232.

Fernandez-Ruiz, J., Miranda, M.I., Bermudez-Rattoni, F., and Drucker-Colin, R. (1993) Effects of catecholaminergic depletion of the amygdala and insular cortex on the potentiation of odor by taste aversion. *Behavioral and Neural Biology*, 60, 189–191.

Ferry, B., Sander, G., and Di Scala, G. (1995) Neuroanatomical and functional specificity of the basolateral amygdaloid nucleus in taste-potentiated odor aversion. *Neurobiology of Learning and Memory*, 64, 169–180.

Fitzgerald, R.E. and Burton, M.J. (1981) Effects of small basolateral amygdala lesions on ingestion in the rat. *Physiology and Behavior*, 27, 431–437.

Fitzgerald, R.E. and Burton, M.J. (1983) Neophobia and conditioned taste aversion deficits in the rat produced by undercutting temporal cortex. *Physiology and Behavior*, 30, 203–206.

Frey, S., Morris, R., and Petrides, M. (1997) A neuroanatomical method to assess the integrity of fibers of passage following ibotenate-induced damage to the central nervous system. *Neuroscience Research*, 28, 285–288.

Galaverna, O.G., Seeley, R.J,. Berridge, K.C., Grill, H.J., Epstein, A.N., and Schulkin, J. (1993) Lesions of the central nucleus of the amygdala. I: Effects on taste reactivity, taste aversion and sodium appetite. *Behavioural Brain Research*, 59, 11–17.

Gallo, M., Roldan, G., and Bures, J. (1992) Differential involvement of gustatory insular cortex and amygdala in the acquisition and retrieval of conditioned taste aversion in rats. *Behavioural Brain Research*, 52, 91–97.

Garcia, J. (1981) Tilting at the paper mills of academe. *American Psychologist*, 36, 149–158.

Garcia, J., Kimmeldorf, D.J., and Koelling, R.A. (1955) Conditioned aversion to saccharin resulting from exposure to gamma radiation. *Science*, 122, 157–158.

Garcia, J., Ervin, F.R., and Koeling, R.A. (1966) Learning with prolonged delay of reinforcement. *Psychonomic Science*, 5, 121–122.

Garcia, J., McGowan, B.K., Ervin, F.R., and Koelling, R.A. (1968) Cues: their relative effectiveness as a function of the reinforcer. *Science*, 160, 794–795.

Goelet, P., Castellucci, V.F., Schacher, S., and Kandel, E.R. (1986) The long and the short of long-term memory—a molecular framework. *Nature*, 322, 419–422.

Grupp, L.A., Linseman, A., and Cappel, H. (1976) Effects of amygdala lesions on taste aversions produced by amphetamine and LiCl. *Pharmacology, Biochemistry, and Behavior*, 4, 451–544.

Gu, Y., Gonzalez, M.F., Chin, D.Y., and Deutsch, J.A. (1993) Expression of c-*fos* in brain subcortical structures in response to nauseant lithium chloride and osmotic pressure in rats. *Neuroscience Letters*, 157, 49–52.

Hartfield, T. and Gallagher, M. (1995) Taste-potentiated odor conditioning: impairment produced by infusion of an *N*-methyl-D-aspartate antagonist into basolateral amygdala. *Behavioral Neuroscience*, 109, 663–668.

Hermann, G.E. and Rogers, R.C. (1985) Convergence of vagal and gustatory afferent input within the parabrachial nucleus of the rat. *Journal of the Autonomic Nervous System*, 13, 1–17.

Hermann, G.E., Kohlerman, N.J., and Rogers, R.C. (1983) Hepatic–vagal and gustatory afferent interactions in the brainstem of the rat. *Journal of the Autonomic Nervous System*, 9, 477–495.

Houpt, T.A., Philopena, J.M., Wessel, T.C., Joh, T.H., and Smith, G.P. (1994) Increased c-*fos* expression in nucleus of the solitary tract correlated with conditioned taste aversion to sucrose in rats. *Neuroscience Letters*, 172, 1–5.

Hylden, J.L., Anton, F., and Nahin, R.L. (1989) Spinal lamina I projection neurons in the rat: collateral innervation of parabrachial area and thalamus. *Neuroscience*, 28, 27–37.

Kemble, E.D. and Nagel, J.A. (1973) Failure to form a learned taste aversion in rats with amygdaloid lesions. *Bulletin of the Psychonomic Society*, 2, 155–166.

Kemble, E.D., Studelska, D.R., and Schmidt, M.K. (1979) Effects of central amygdaloid nucleus lesions on ingestion, taste reactivity, exploration taste aversion. *Physiology and Behavior*, 22, 789–793.

Kesner, R.P., Berman, R.F., Burton, B., and Hankins, W.G. (1975) Effects of electrical stimulation of amygdala upon neophobia and taste aversion. *Behavioral Biology*, 13, 349–358.

Kiefer, S.W. and Braun, J.J. (1977) Absence of differential associative responses to novel and familiar taste stimuli in rats lacking gustatory cortex. *Journal of Comparative and Physiological Psychology*, 91, 498–507.

Killcross, S., Robbins, T.W., and Everitt, B.J. (1997) Different types of fear-conditioned behaviour mediated by separate nuclei within amygdala. *Nature*, 388, 377–380.

Kolakowska. L, Laurue-Achagiotis, C., and Le Magnen, J. (1985) Effects of amygdaloid lesions on ethanol intake in rats. *Pharmacology, Biochemistry, and Behavior*, 23, 333–338.

Krettek, J.E. and Price, J.L. (1977) Projections from the amygdaloid complex to the cerebral cortex and thalamus in the rat and cat. *Journal of Comparative Neurology*, 172, 687–722.

Lamprecht, R. and Dudai, Y. (1995) Differential modulation of brain immediate early genes by intraperitoneal LiCl. *NeuroReport*, 29, 289–293.

Lamprecht, R. and Dudai, Y. (1996) Transient expression of c-Fos in rat amygdala during training is required for encoding conditioned taste aversion memory. *Learning and Memory*, 3, 31–41.

Lamprecht, R., Hazvi, S., and Dudai, Y. (1997) cAMP response element-binding protein in the amygdala is required for long- but not short-term conditioned taste aversion memory. *Journal of Neuroscience*, 17, 8443–8450.

Lasiter, P.S. and Glanzman, D.L. (1985) Cortical substrates of taste aversion learning: involvement of dorsolateral amygdaloid nuclei and temporal neocortex in taste aversion learning. *Behavioral Neuroscience*, 99, 257–276.

McGaugh, J.L., Cahill, L., and Roozendaal, B. (1996) Involvement of the amygdala in memory storage: interaction with other brain systems. *Proceedings of the National Academy of Sciences of the United States of America*, 93, 13508–13514.

McGowan, B.K., Hankins, W.G. and Garcia, J. (1972) Limbic lesions and control of the internal and external environment. *Behavioral Biology*, 7, 841–852.

Mikulka, P.J. and Freeman, F.G. (1984) The effect of amygdala-kindled seizures on the acquisition of taste and odor aversions. *Physiology and Behavior*, 32, 967–972.

Mikulka, P.J., Freeman, F.G., and Lindstorm, P. (1977) The effect of training technique and amygdala lesions on the acquisition and retention of taste aversion. *Behavioral Biology*, 19, 509–517.

Morris, R., Frey, S., Kasambira ,T., and Petrides, M. (1999) Ibotenic acid lesions of the basolateral, but not the central, amygdala interfere with conditioned taste aversion: evidence from a combined behavioral and anatomical tract-tracing investigation. *Behavioral Neuroscience*, 113, 291–302.

Nachman, M. and Ashe, J.H. (1974) Effects of basolateral amygdala lesions on neophobia, learned taste aversions, and sodium appetite in rats. *Journal of Comparative and Physiological Psychology*, 87, 622–643.

Nader, K. and LeDoux, J.E. (1997) Is it time to invoke multiple fear learning systems in the amygdala? *Trends in Cognitive Science*, 1, 241–244.

Niijima, A. and Yamamoto, T. (1994) The effects of lithium chloride on the activity of the afferent nerve fibers from the abdominal visceral organs in the rat. *Brain Research Bulletin*, 35, 141–145.

Nishijo, H., Uwano, T., Tamura, R., and Ono, T. (1998) Gustatory and multimodal neuronal responses in the amygdala during licking and discrimination of sensory stimuli in awake rats. *Journal of Neurophysiology*, 79, 21–36.

Norgren, R. (1976) Taste pathways to hypothalamus and amygdala. *Journal of Comparative Neurology*, 166, 17–30.

Norgren, R., Nishijo, H., and Travers, S.P. (1989) Taste responses from the entire gustatory apparatus. *Annals of the New York Academy of Sciences*, 575, 246–263.

Ottersen, O.P. (1980) Afferent connections to the amygdaloid complex of the rat and cat. II. Afferents from the hypothalamus and the basal telencephalon. *Comparative Neurology*, 194, 267–289.

Ottersen, O.L. (1982) Connections of the amygdala of the rat. IV. Corticoamygdaloid and intraamygdaloid connections as studies with axonal transport of horseradish peroxidase. *Journal of Comparative Neurology*, 205, 30–48.

Paxinos, G. and Watson, C (1997) *The Rat Brain in Stereotaxic Coordinates*. Academic Press, San Diego.

Phillips, A.G. and LePiane, F.G. (1978) Electrical stimulation of the amygdala as a conditioned stimulus in a bait-shyness paradigm. *Science*, 201, 536–538.

Phillips, A.G. and LePiane, F.G. (1980) Disruption of conditioned taste aversion in the rat by stimulation of amygdala: a conditioned effect, not amnesia. *Journal of Comparative and Physiological Psychology*, 94, 664–674.

Reddy, M.M. and Bures, J. (1981) Unit activity changes elicited in amygdala and neocortex of anaesthetized rats by intraperitoneal injection of lithium chloride. *Neuroscience Letters*, 22, 169–172.

Ricardo, J.A. and Koh E.T. (1978) Anatomical evidence of projections from the nucleus of the solitary tract to the hypothalamus, amygdala, and other forebrain structures in the rat. *Brain Research*, 153, 1–26.

Roldan, G, and Bures, J. (1994) Tetrodotoxin blockade of amygdala overlapping with poisoning impairs acquisition of conditioned taste aversion in rats. *Behavioural Brain Research*, 65, 213–219.

Rolls, E.T. and Rolls, B.J. (1973) Altered food preference after lesions in the basolateral region of the amygdala in the rat. *Journal of Comparative and Physiological Psychology*, 83, 248–259.

Rosenblum, K., Berman, D.E., Hazvi, S., Lamprecht, R., and Dudai, Y. (1997) NMDA receptor and the tyrosine phosphorylation of its 2B subunit in taste learning in the rat insular cortex. *Journal of Neuroscience*, 17, 5129–5135.

Rusiniak, K.W., Hankins, W.G., Garcia, J., and Brett, L.P. (1979) Flavor–illness aversions: potentiation of odor by taste in rats. *Behavioral and Neural Biology*, 25, 1–17.

Saper, C.B. (1982) Convergence of autonomic and limbic connections in the insular cortex of the rat. *Journal of Comparative Neurology*, 210, 163–173.

Saper, C.B. and Loewy, A.D. (1980) Efferent connections of the parabrachial nucleus in the rat. *Brain Research*, 197, 291–317.

Schafe, G.E. and Bernstein, I.L. (1996) Forebrain contribution to induction of a brainstem correlate of conditioned taste aversion: I. The amygdala. *Brain Research*, 741, 109–116.

Schafe, G.E., Seeley, R.J., and Bernstein, I.L. (1995a) Forebrain contribution to the induction of a cellular correlate of conditioned taste-aversion in the nucleus of the solitary tract. *Journal of Neuroscience*, 15, 6789–6796.

Schafe, G.E., Sollars, S.I., and Bernstein, I.L. (1995b) The CS–US interval and taste aversion learning: a brief look. *Behavioral Neuroscience*, 109, 799–802.

Schafe, G.E., Thiele, T.E., and Bernstein, I.L. (1998) Conditioning methods dramatically alter the role of amygdala in taste aversion learning. *Learning and Memory*, 5, 481–492.

Shipley, T. and Sanders, M.S. (1982) Special senses are really special: evidence for a reciprocal, bilateral pathway between insular cortex and nucleus parabrachialis. *Brain Research Bulletin*, 8, 493–501.

Simbayi, L.C. (1987) Effects of anterior basolateral amygdala lesions on taste aversions produced by high and low oral doses of LiCl and lactose in the rat. *Behavioural Brain Research*, 25, 131–142.

Simbayi, L.C., Boakes, R.A., and Burton M.J. (1986) Effects of basolateral amygdala lesions on taste aversions produced by lactose and lithium chloride in the rat. *Behavioral Neuroscience*, 100, 455–465.

Slotnick, B.M., Westbrook, F., and Darling, F.M.C (1997) What the rat's nose tells the rat's mouth: long delay aversion conditioning with aqueous odors and potentiation of taste by odors. *Animal Learning and Behavior*, 25, 357–369.

Swank, M.W. and Bernstein, I.L. (1994) c-Fos induction in response to a conditioned stimulus after single trial taste aversion learning. *Brain Research*, 636, 202–208.

Swank, M.W., Schafe, G.E., and Bernstein, I.L. (1995) c-Fos induction in response to taste stimuli previously paired with amphetamine or LiCl during taste aversion learning. *Brain Research*, 673, 251–261.

Swanson, L.W. and Petrovich, G.D. (1998) What is the amygdala? *Trends in Neuroscience*, 21, 323–331.

Torvik, A. (1956) Afferent connections to the sensory trigeminal nuclei, the nucleus of the solitary tract and adjacent structures: an experimental study of the rat. *Journal of Comparative Neurology*, 106, 51–141.

Touzani, K., Taghzouti, K., and Velley, L. (1997) Increase of aversive value of taste stimuli following ibotenic acid lesion of the central amygdaloid nucleus in the rat. *Behavioural Brain Research*, 88, 133–142.

Tucci, S., Rada, P., and Hernandez, L. (1998) Role of glutamate in the amygdala and lateral hypothalamus in conditioned taste aversion. *Brain Research*, 813, 44–49.

Turner, B.H. and Herkenham, M. (1991) Thalamoamygdaloid projections in the rat: a test of the amygdala role in sensory processing. *Journal of Comparative Neurology*, 313, 295–325.

Uwano, T., Nishijo, H., Ono, T., and Tamura, R. (1995) Neuronal responsiveness to various sensory stimuli, and associative learning in the rat. *Neuroscience*, 68, 339–361.

Van der Kooy, D. and Koda, L.Y. (1983) Organization of the projections of a circumventricular organ: the area postrema in the rat. *Journal of Comparative Neurology*, 219, 328–338.

Van der Kooy, D., Koda, L.Y., McGinty, J.F., Gerfen, C.R., and Bloom, F.E. (1984) The organization of projections from the cortex, amygdala, and hypothalamus to the nucleus of the solitary tract in rat. *Journal of Comparative Neurology*, 224, 1–24.

Veening, J.G. (1978) Subcortical afferents of the amygdaloid complex in the rat: an HRP study. *Neuroscience Letters*, 8, 197–202.

Yamamoto, T., Azuma, S., and Kawamura, Y. (1984) Functional relations between the cortical gustatory area and the amygdala: electrophysiological and behavioral studies in the rats. *Experimental Brain Research*, 56, 23–31.

Yamamoto, T. and Fujimoto, Y. (1991) Brain mechanisms in taste aversion learning in the rat. *Brain Research Bulletin*, 27, 403–406.

Yamamoto, T., Shimura, T., Sako, N., Azuma, S., Bai, W.Z., and Wakisaka, S. (1992) c-fos expression in the rat brain after intraperitoneal injection of lithium chloride. *NeuroReport*, 3, 1049–1052.

Yamamoto, T., Shimura, T., Sako, N., Yasoshima, Y., and Sakai, N. (1994) Neural substrates for conditioned taste aversion in the rat. *Behavioural Brain Research*, 65, 123–137.

Yasoshima, Y. and Yamamoto, T. (1997) Rat gustatory memory requires protein kinase C activity in the amygdala and cortical gustatory cortex. *NeuroReport*, 8, 1363–1367.

Yasoshima, Y., Shimura, T., and Yamamoto, T. (1995) Single unit responses of the amygdala after conditioned taste aversion in conscious rats. *NeuroReport*, 6, 2424–2428.

Zahm, D.S., Jensen, S.L., Williams, E.S., and Martin, J.R. (1999) Direct comparison of projections from the central amygdaloid region and nucleus accumbens shell. *European Journal of Neuroscience*, 11, 1119–1126.

10 Differential involvement of amygdala subsystems in appetitive conditioning and drug addiction

Barry J. Everitt, Rudolf N. Cardinal, Jeremy Hall, John A. Parkinson, and Trevor W. Robbins

Department of Experimental Psychology, University of Cambridge, Downing Street, Cambridge CB2 3EB, UK

Summary

We review data from appetitive conditioning studies using measures of Pavlovian approach behaviour and measures of the effects of Pavlovian conditioned stimuli on instrumental behaviour, including the Pavlovian-to-instrumental transfer effect and conditioned reinforcement. These studies consistently demonstrate double dissociations of function between the basolateral area and the central nucleus of the amygdala. Moreover, these data show marked parallels with data derived from studies of aversive (fear) conditioning, and are consistent with the idea that these subsystems of the amygdala use different associative representations formed during conditioning, as part of a larger limbic corticostriatal circuit. We suggest that the basolateral amygdala is required for a conditioned stimulus to gain access to the current value of the specific unconditioned stimulus with which it has been paired, while the central nucleus is responsible for conditioned motivational responses using a simpler stimulus–response representation. Though these systems normally operate together, they modulate ongoing behaviour in distinct ways. We illustrate this by considering the contributions of both systems to the process of drug addiction, using second-order schedules of intravenous drug self-administration.

10.1 Introduction

In this chapter, we will review data from our own and other studies which demonstrate that the amygdala is critically involved in distinct associative processes in appetitive settings and that the pattern of results indicates marked parallels with the mass of data derived from similar investigations of aversively motivated learning. Indeed, prevailing theories of amygdala function have for some years been based predominantly on the results of studies of conditioned fear (Davis, 1992a,b; LeDoux, 1996; Maren and Fanselow, 1996; Fendt *et al.*, 1999). Thus, the lateral nucleus of the amygdala is generally regarded as the primary, even unique, site for the convergence and association of aversive conditioned and unconditioned stimuli, thereby providing the locus of Pavlovian fear conditioning (Clugnet and LeDoux, 1990; LeDoux *et al.*, 1990; Davis, 1992a; Fendt *et al.*, 1999). Via its projections to the central amygdaloid nucleus (CeA), the lateral amygdaloid associative mechanism gains access to the neural controllers of autonomic, neuroendocrine, and reflexive behavioural components of integrated emotional responses (LeDoux *et al.*, 1988; Davis, 1992a). This lateral-to-central flow of information is the basis of the dominant model of information processing within the amygdala, which identifies the lateral amygdala as the only locus of fear conditioning.

However, some data do not conform to this model. For example, although it has been shown that conditioned freezing may be impaired following basolateral amygdala lesions, other indices suggest a persistence of conditioned fear in the same subjects (Selden *et al.*, 1991; Killcross *et al.*, 1997a; Vazdarjanova *et al.*, 1998). We have reported that Pavlovian conditioned suppression can be established in rats with excitotoxic lesions of the basolateral area (lateral and basal magnocellular nuclei) of the amygdala (BLA), whereas their instrumental (voluntary) avoidance behaviour is impaired (Killcross *et al.*, 1997a). Moreover, rats with specific lesions of the CeA show impaired Pavlovian conditioned suppression, but preserved instrumental avoidance behaviour (Killcross *et al.*, 1997a). This double dissociation of different forms of fear conditioning within the amygdala and the persistence of Pavlovian fear conditioning in rats in which the BLA had been destroyed suggest a more complex pattern of functional interaction between the CeA and BLA. In particular, it must be considered that these nuclear domains of the amygdala and their associated cortical and subcortical circuitries subserve distinct aspects of emotional processing and do so in a way that does not conform to the prevailing, lateral-to-central model of information transfer within the amygdala. We will argue that this is not only the case for fear conditioning, but applies equally to appetitive conditioning. For example, discrete excitotoxic lesions of the BLA impair the way in which stimuli endowed with positive affect can support goal-directed instrumental behaviour (conditioned reinforcement) and also impair second-order Pavlovian conditioning and the re-evaluation of affective value in the neural representations of food rewards (Everitt and Robbins, 1992; Gallagher *et al.*, 1994; Everitt *et al.*, 1999; Holland and Gallagher, 1999). Whilst lesions of the CeA do not significantly impair conditioned reinforcement, they do disrupt other forms of appetitive Pavlovian conditioning (Everitt *et al.*, 1999; Parkinson *et al.*, 2000b).

In fact, contemporary studies of the organization and connections of the amygdala provide some basis for entertaining more complex forms of processing within its component nuclei. While it is clearly the case that sensory thalamic nuclei, high-order sensory cortices, and association cortex project richly to the lateral and basal nuclei and that these in turn project heavily onto the CeA, it is equally clear that parallel high-order sensory projections arrive directly at the CeA, especially its lateral subdivision (McDonald, 1998). Thus, the lateral/capsular division of the CeA may provide a gateway of sensory convergence lateral/capsular parallels that provided by the lateral nucleus (McDonald, 1998). The efferent projections of the BLA and CeA also provide clear evidence of segregation, as well as convergence. The CeA is well known to project to neuroendocrine and autonomic domains of the hypothalamus and brainstem, thereby providing a route for the BLA to access these sites. However, the BLA has independent projections to the ventral striatum and prefrontal, especially orbitofrontal, cortex. Such connections give the BLA access to higher order response mechanisms than those provided by the downstream projections, as we have argued previously and demonstrated experimentally (Everitt and Robbins, 1992; Everitt *et al.*, 1999).

Two other features of amygdala anatomy should also be borne in mind. The first concerns the concept of the extended amygdala, whereby the central and medial nuclei of the amygdala are seen to be extended not only into the bed nucleus of the stria terminalis, but, more controversially, through the basal forebrain (the subcommissural extended amygdala), incorporating the interstitial nucleus of the posterior limb of the anterior commissure (IPAC) to encroach upon the shell of the nucleus accumbens (NAcc) (Alheid *et al.*, 1988; De Olmos *et al.*, 1999). The NAcc shell is thus seen as a complex mix of striatal neurons and CeA neurons, sharing with the CeA a variety of histochemical features and connections. Notable among the commonalities in the afferent connections of the CeA and the NAcc shell are a rich dopaminergic innervation arising from the ventral tegmental area (VTA) and projections from the BLA (Alheid *et al.*, 1988). However, an alternative view of the CeA and its relationship to the striatum has been put forward by Swanson and Petrovich (1998), who suggest that the CeA is a specialized autonomic-projecting region of the striatum. The second feature concerns the marked projections from the CeA to the monoaminergic and cholinergic neurons of the isodendritic core, including the noradrenergic locus coeruleus, the dopaminergic substantia nigra and VTA, the serotoninergic raphé nuclei, and the cholinergic nucleus basalis magnocellularis (Price *et al.*, 1987; Amaral *et al.*, 1992; Davis, 1992a; Gallagher and Holland, 1994; Holland and Gallagher, 1999). Increasingly, these connections are seen as providing a mechanism for the CeA to influence attentional, response-activating, rewarding, and other arousal processes mediated by these diffuse projections to the forebrain (Everitt *et al.*, 1999; Holland and Gallagher, 1999).

10.2 Appetitive Pavlovian conditioning and conditional reinforcement

In the experiments to be described, we have used three procedures to assess associative mechanisms that impact on reflexive and voluntary behavioural responses. These are: (i) Pavlovian approach behaviour, a measure of the tendency of animals to approach stimuli that have acquired motivational salience through their predictive (Pavlovian) association with a primary reward (Tomie *et al.*, 1989); (ii) the ability of an appetitive Pavlovian conditioned stimulus (CS) to exert a direct effect on the vigour of instrumental behaviour (the so-called Pavlovian-to-instrumental transfer effect; Dickinson, 1994); and (iii) conditioned reinforcement, the process by which a predictive CS is able to reinforce instrumental behaviour (Mackintosh, 1974). Although we have studied these processes in isolation in order to explore their neuroanatomical bases, they will usually occur together in the integrated expression of behaviour by animals in naturalistic settings. We will illustrate this by reference to some of the associative mechanisms underlying drug-seeking behaviour that may be important determinants of the persistence of drug-taking habits in humans. We will suggest that dissociable amygdala subsystems involving central and basolateral parts of the amygdala operate in parallel, as well as in series, to subserve different behavioural processes in integrated forms of behaviour.

10.2.1 Appetitive Pavlovian conditioning: autoshaping

Whilst in aversive conditioning experiments, Pavlovian conditioned responses are readily elicited and quantified (e.g. freezing, startle), this is not so straightforward in appetitive settings. In the present experiments, we have focused on an 'autoshaping' task, in order to provide a relatively easily measurable appetitive Pavlovian conditioned response (approach behaviour) and to minimize the contributions of other learning mechanisms to the process by which environmental stimuli are associated with primary reward, thereby gaining motivational salience (Hearst and Jenkins, 1974; Tomie *et al.*, 1989; Tomie, 1996). The apparatus, procedure, and theoretical basis of this task have been discussed elsewhere (Bussey *et al.*, 1997). Briefly, a visual stimulus (CS+) is presented on a VDU which is then followed by the delivery of food in a *different* spatial location, non-contingently with respect to the animal's behaviour. A second stimulus (CS–) is also presented, but never followed by food. Over training, animals develop a discriminated conditioned response of approaching the CS predictive of food before returning to the food hopper to retrieve the primary reward. This preparatory approach behaviour is deemed to be under the control of Pavlovian mechanisms as it lacks the behavioural flexibility of instrumental, goal-directed actions (Williams and Williams, 1969) and has been described as a form of sign tracking, by which such stimuli capture attention and elicit automatic responses that are likely to bring animals into direct contact with primary goals (Hearst and Jenkins, 1974).

Quite different consequences of inactivating the CeA and BLA were observed on this task (Parkinson *et al.*, 2000b). Bilateral excitotoxic lesions of the BLA had no effect on the acquisition of autoshaping; lesioned subjects came progressively to approach the CS+ and eliminate their approaches to the CS–. In contrast, bilateral lesions of the CeA greatly impaired autoshaping such that lesioned animals did not increase their approaches to the CS+ (Figure 10.1). These results clearly indicate that Pavlovian associations between an environmental stimulus and primary reinforcement can be established in the absence of the BLA, as we have also found for Pavlovian conditioned suppression.

There is perhaps a tendency to assume that the amygdala alone is involved in associations between environmental stimuli and reinforcing events, especially in studies of aversive conditioning. However, not only is it clear that some forms of fear-motivated learning, such as aversive eyeblink conditioning, develop normally in the absence of a functioning amygdala, depending more on cerebellar circuitry (Lavond *et al.*, 1993), but also that it is increasingly possible to define a more widely dispersed neural network involved in such associative functions. For example, it is well established that the anterior, but not posterior, cingulate cortex is critically important for the formation of stimulus–reinforcer associations. Indeed, we have shown previously that lesions of the anterior cingulate cortex profoundly

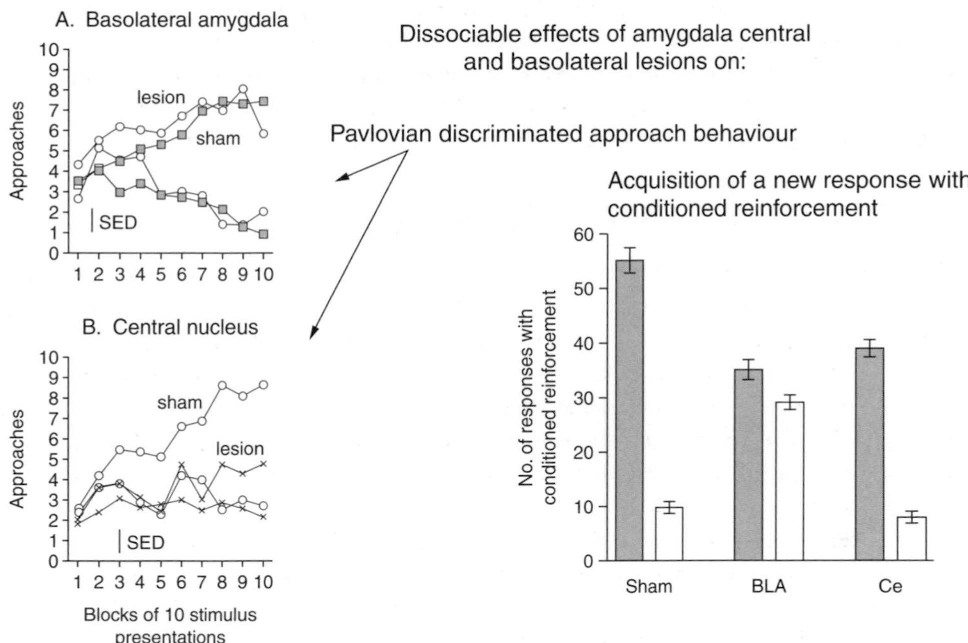

Figure 10.1 The effects of lesions of the CeA and BLA on Pavlovian approach behaviour measured in an autoshaping task (left panels) and the acquisition of a new response with conditioned reinforcement (right panel). (A) and (B) show the acquisition of autoshaping in (**A**) BLA-lesioned and control subjects and (**B**) CeA-lesioned and control subjects. It can be seen that, over 10 blocks of 10 trials, control subjects come selectively to approach the CS+ (which is paired with food reward) and to withhold approaches to the CS–. Rats with BLA lesions are unimpaired (A), whereas rats with CeA lesions do not acquire discriminated approach to the CS+ over the 10 blocks of trials (B). The right panel shows the effects of lesions of the CeA and BLA on the acquisition of a new response with conditioned reinforcement. A CS previously associated with sucrose in a Pavlovian stage is then presented contingent upon responding on one of two levers, the CRf lever (shaded bars); responding on the second lever (open bars) has no programmed consequence. No sucrose is available at this stage and the conditioned reinforcing properties of the CS are assessed by its ability to support the learning of this new instrumental response. Control subjects respond selectively upon the CRf lever, as do rats with lesions of the CeA. However, rats with BLA lesions are impaired in acquisition, i.e. they do not respond selectively on the lever that produces the conditioned reinforcer. The data have been taken from Burns *et al.* (1993) Robledo *et al.* (1996) and Parkinson *et al.*, 2000b. Thus, in this figure, the double dissociation of the effects of CeA and BLA lesions on discriminated approach and conditioned reinforcement is shown.

impair the acquisition of autoshaping (Bussey *et al.*, 1997), while Gabriel and colleagues have demonstrated electrophysiologically and in lesion studies, the involvement of the same area of cortex early in the course of aversive conditioning (Gabriel, 1990; Freeman *et al.*, 1996). Moreover, the integrity of specific areas of the ventral striatum also appears to be required in order for Pavlovian approach behaviour to develop. Thus, while selective excitotoxic lesions of the NAcc shell were without effect on autoshaping, lesions of the NAcc core profoundly disrupted its acquisition (Parkinson *et al.*, 2000a). In addition, lesions of the pedunculopontine nucleus, a major output target of the ventral striatum, profoundly impair autoshaping (Inglis *et al.*, 2000), confirming the involvement of the ventral striatopallidal system in this form of conditioning.

Since our own tract-tracing experiments confirmed that the anterior cingulate cortex is a major source of projections to the NAcc core, we investigated the possible functional relationship between the two structures by making a 'disconnection lesion' (a unilateral lesion of the anterior cingulate cortex and a contralateral, unilateral lesion of the NAcc core) and assessing the effects on autoshaping. The disconnection lesion disrupted autoshaping as effectively as bilateral lesions of either structure alone (Parkinson *et al.*, 2000a). This provides strong evidence for a functional connection between the anterior cingulate cortex and NAcc core, but leaves open the issue concerning the relationship between the CeA and this limbic corticostriatal circuit. This is a critical issue because our data together indicate that each of these structures is necessary, but not sufficient, for autoshaping to develop. Since there is no obvious direct connection between the CeA and this cingulate cortex–NAcc core circuit, the answer may involve regulation of the dopaminergic innervation of the NAcc by the CeA.

There are substantial projections from the CeA to the VTA and substantia nigra that we have confirmed recently by anterograde and retrograde tract-tracing studies (Fudge and Haber, 2000; Hall, Parkinson, and Everitt, unpublished observations). It has been shown in very different kinds of studies that manipulations of the CeA can influence dorsal and ventral striatal dopamine function. For example, dopaminergic lesions of the CeA or infusions of dopamine receptor antagonists into the amygdala both affect levels of extracellular dopamine in the NAcc and also cocaine self-administration (which depends upon the integrity of the mesolimbic dopamine system) (Louilot *et al.*, 1985; Simon *et al.*, 1988; McGregor and Roberts, 1993; Caine *et al.*, 1995; Hurd *et al.*, 1997). Moreover, a disconnection lesion of the CeA and the dopaminergic innervation of the dorsolateral striatum has been shown to impair the acquisition of a conditioned orienting response (Han *et al.*, 1997). Consistent with this notion of a link between the CeA and the mesolimbic dopamine system, we have shown in our recent studies (Parkinson *et al.*, 1998) that 6-hydroxydopamine-induced dopamine depletion from the NAcc abolishes the acquisition of autoshaping.

Taken together, these results suggest a distributed neural network underlying Pavlovian approach behaviour that involves the anterior cingulate cortex, NAcc core, CeA, and mesolimbic dopamine system (Figure 10.2). The anterior cingulate cortex may be of primary importance in this network, projecting as it does both to the NAcc core and to the CeA, the latter projections have been suggested to be the route via which the anterior cingulate cortex influences autonomic responses (Vogt, 1985). The elements of this network have comple-

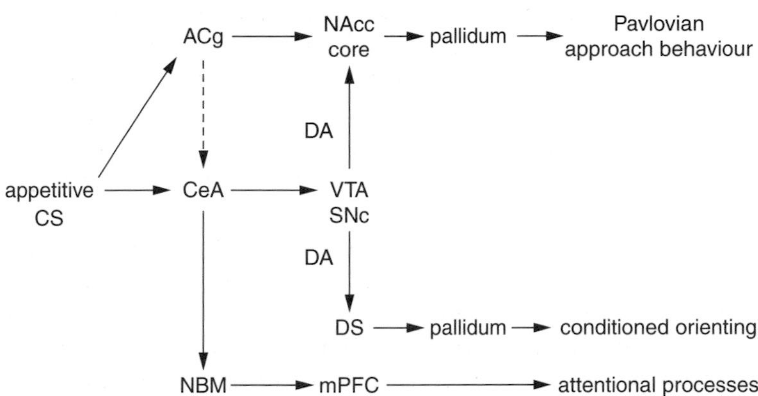

Figure 10.2 A schematic diagram of the neural network underlying aspects of Pavlovian conditioned approach based upon our own data discussed in the text and also data from Gallagher, Holland, and co-workers (Gallagher and Holland, 1994; Holland and Gallagher, 1999). The anterior cingulate cortex (ACg), NAcc core, CeA, and the dopaminergic innervation of the NAcc are all necessary, but not sufficient, to support the development of Pavlovian approach behaviour. We hypothesize that the anterior cingulate cortex and NAcc core are part of a corticostriatal loop that subserves conditioning *per se*, i.e. subserves informational processes that give direction to approach behaviour. We also hypothesize that there is a relationship between the CeA and ventral tegmental area (VTA) dopamine neurons innervating the NAcc that is also engaged by appetitive CSs to activate or 'energize' Pavlovian approach response tendencies via brainstem locomotor regions (see text for details). In separate, but related experiments, Gallagher, Holland, and colleagues have shown that the CeA is critical for conditioned orienting responses, which depend upon interactions of the CeA with the nigrostriatal dopamine system, and for attentional processes which depend upon interactions with the cholinergic nucleus basalis magnocellularis (NBM). (Figure reproduced from Everitt *et al.*, 1999, with permission.) Abbreviations: DA, dopamine; SNc, substantia nigra pars compacta; DS, dorsal stratum; mPFC, medial prefrontal cortex

mentary patterns of connectivity that allow them to mediate the component processes underlying an integrated response to appetitive stimuli. We hypothesize that the anterior cingulate cortex–NAcc core system mediates Pavlovian associative processes and give direction to Pavlovian approach responses (Everitt *et al.*, 1999; Parkinson *et al.*, 2000a). But, clearly, information about appetitive stimuli also impinges on the CeA from a variety of sources (including the anterior cingulate cortex, high-order sensory cortices, BLA, and thalamus), enabling the CeA, through its differentiated outputs, to orchestrate not only autonomic and endocrine responses but also different forms of arousal processes dependent upon the chemically defined systems of the reticular core of the brain (Davis, 1992a; Everitt *et al.*, 1999).

Projections from the CeA to the mesolimbic dopaminergic neurons in the VTA, for example, may regulate behavioural activation, thereby invigorating approach responses, while also enhancing the coupling of the anterior cingulate cortex–NAcc core circuit that provides direction to those responses (Everitt *et al.*, 1999; Parkinson *et al.*, in press). In addition, and perhaps especially early in conditioning, the CeA will engage attentional mechanisms through interactions with the basal forebrain cholinergic system (Han *et al.*, 2000), and also orienting responses through interactions with the nigrostriatal dopaminergic system innervating the dorsolateral caudate–putamen (Han *et al.*, 1997).

A clearer understanding of these processes requires experiments designed to explore the specificity of the effects of manipulating each of the components of this network on the development of the Pavlovian approach response. For example, it is uncertain whether impairments in autoshaping reflect disruption of the associative process *per se* or the orchestration and coupling of response mechanisms. Prevailing data would implicate the anterior cingulate cortex in the former and the NAcc core with its dopaminergic innervation in the latter. However, the CeA may have more complex functions that transcend associative, output, attentional, and arousal processes. Traditionally, functions of the CeA have been constrained by its perceived role as simply being subordinate to the lateral and basal nuclei of the amygdala and by its projections to neuroendocrine, autonomic, and primitive motor domains of the hypothalamus and brainstem (LeDoux, 1996; Fendt and Fanselow, 1999). Increasingly, however, more diverse afferents to the CeA have been demonstrated (McDonald, 1998), while its efferents to the neurochemically defined diffuse projection systems of the isodendritic core (arousal systems) have to be taken into account in order to understand the coordinating and integrative functions of this component of the amygdaloid nuclear complex. These latter projections bring the entire forebrain under the modulatory control of the CeA (Figure 10.3).

10.2.2 Pavlovian-to-instrumental transfer

The key demonstration of the motivational impact of Pavlovian CSs on instrumental behaviour comes from an experiment by Lovibond (1983). Rabbits were trained to lift a lever for delivery of a sugar solution directly into the mouth. The lever was then removed in a second, Pavlovian stage in which a 10 s stimulus was repeatedly paired with the sugar solution. In the final stage, presenting the Pavlovian CS while the animal was performing the instrumental task resulted in a marked elevation of responding—an effect of the CS which is also modulated by the animal's motivational state. While there has been some debate about the precise mechanisms underlying this so-called Pavlovian-to-instrumental transfer effect (Dickinson, 1994), it is generally assumed that the Pavlovian CS exerts a general motivational or activational influence on goal-directed instrumental behaviour. The procedure we have used in the experiment reported here was essentially that described by Balleine (1994). Briefly, animals were first trained to associate presentations of a 2 min auditory stimulus (CS) with delivery of food pellets into a hopper. During training, animals came to approach the food hopper preferentially during the CS period. After this Pavlovian conditioning, the animals were trained to lever press for the same food reward in the absence of the CS. Finally, in the test phase, the ability of the CS to enhance lever pressing in extinction was

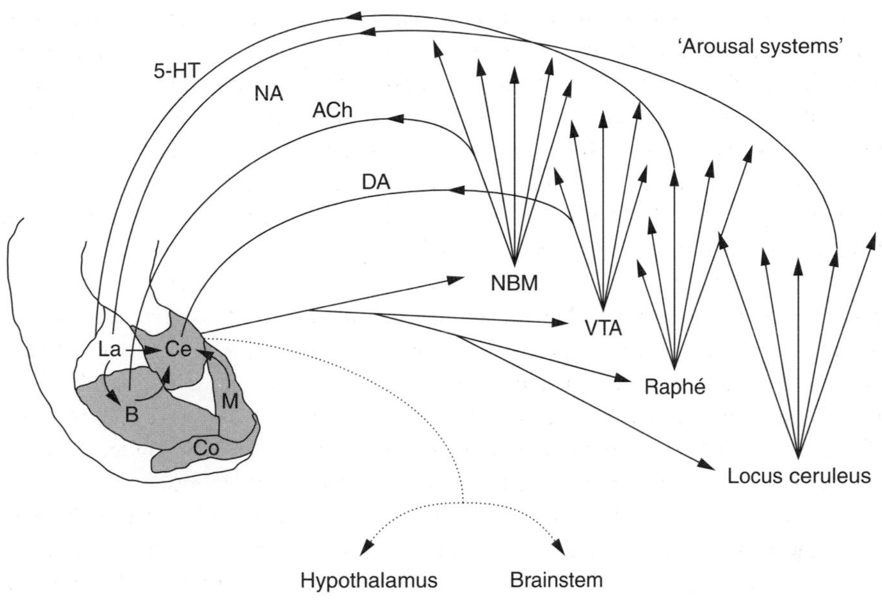

Figure 10.3 A schematic illustrating some of the outputs of the CeA. Projections to autonomic, neuroendocrine, and primitive motor domains of the hypothalamus and brainstem are well known (see text). The CeA also has rich projections to the chemically defined systems of the isodendritic core, namely the nucleus basalis in the basal forebrain (cholinergic), ventral tegmental area/substantia nigra (dopaminergic), midbrain raphé nuclei (serotoninergic), and pontine locus coeruleus (noradrenergic). Through these routes, the CeA is able to bring widespread areas of the forebrain under its control, thereby influencing component arousal processes including motor activation and attention.

assessed, compared to equivalent periods of baseline responding and responding during a control stimulus (one explicitly not paired with food).

Bilateral excitotoxic lesions of the BLA had no effect on this Pavlovian-to-instrumental transfer procedure. However, selective bilateral lesions of the CeA completely blocked the ability of the CS to enhance lever pressing in the test phase (Figure 10.4; Hall, Parkinson, Connor, Dickinson, and Everitt, unpublished). This result directly parallels the dissociation of effects of CeA and BLA lesions on Pavlovian approach behaviour and leads us to speculate that the neural basis of this effect of the CS to invigorate instrumental behaviour again depends upon interactions between the CeA and the mesolimbic dopamine system. Some evidence in support of this speculation comes from the observation that the dopamine receptor antagonist, pimozide, also blocks the Pavlovian-to-instrumental transfer effect, thereby indicating that a dopaminergic mechanism mediates this motivational influence of a Pavlovian CS (Smith *et al.*, 1998).

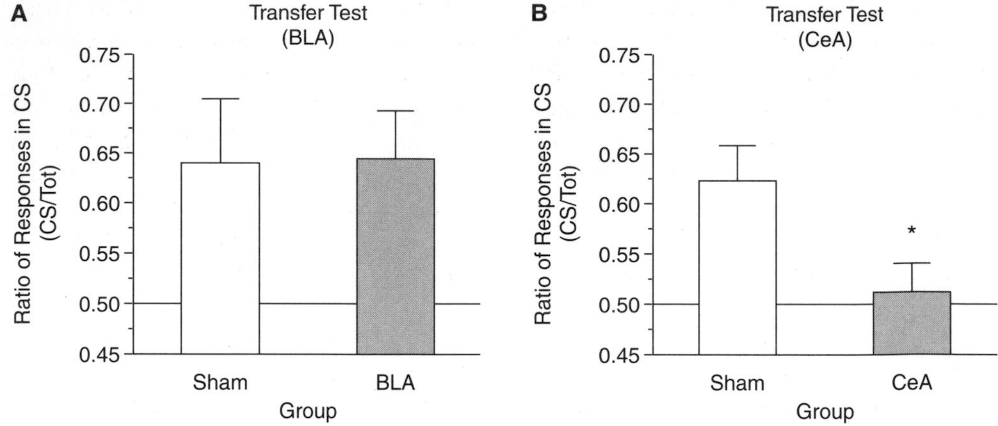

Figure 10.4 Pavlovian-to-instrumental transfer in animals with lesions of the BLA (**A**) and CeA (**B**). Subjects were trained to associate a CS with food reinforcement and were then trained to lever press for the same reinforcer. In normal subjects, presentation of the food-associated CS enhances pressing in a test session—the Pavlovian-to-instrumental transfer effect. Control subjects in both experiments showed this enhancement of lever pressing during the presentation of the Pavlovian CS at test, illustrated here as the ratio of lever responses during the CS presentation to the total responses during both the CS and inter-stimulus interval. Rats with lesions of the BLA also showed normal Pavlovian-to-instrumental transfer. However, rats with lesions of the CeA failed to enhance their lever responding during the CS, showing a ratio of responding equivalent to that expected by chance performance (represented by the horizontal line on the graph). This suggests that the CeA, but not the BLA, is part of a neural system required to mediate the excitatory effects of Pavlovian stimuli on instrumental behaviour.

10.2.3 Conditioned reinforcement

Appetitive Pavlovian CSs not only elicit behavioural arousal and approach responses but, by acquiring some of the properties of a goal, they gain motivational salience and thereby control over instrumental—or voluntary—behaviour acting as conditioned reinforcers (Mackintosh, 1974; Robbins, 1978; Everitt and Robbins, 1992). We have studied this using a procedure that isolates the conditioned reinforcement process. Briefly, there are two phases to the procedure. First, rather as in the autoshaping procedure, a neutral stimulus (light, sound, or a compound of both) is paired with primary reward (we have used water in thirsty subjects, sucrose in hungry subjects, or intravenous cocaine) and the development of Pavlovian conditioning is assessed by measuring discriminated approach to the CS. In the second phase, which is carried out in extinction, thereby removing any influence of primary reinforcement, two novel levers enter the testing chamber; responding on one of them (CRf lever) results in presentation of the light CS. Responding on the second lever (NCRf lever) has no programmed consequence. The acquired motivational properties of the CS to serve as a conditioned reinforcer is therefore assessed by its ability to reinforce the acquisition of this novel and arbitrary response. An important aspect of this process is that the control over behaviour by a conditioned reinforcer (CRf) is amplified powerfully by psychomotor stimulants, and this effect has been shown to depend critically upon the dopaminergic innervation of the NAcc (Taylor and Robbins, 1984, 1986; Robbins *et al.*, 1989). However, even in the face of extensive dopamine depletion from the NAcc, or general dopamine receptor blockade, rats still acquire a new response with conditioned reinforcement (Taylor and Robbins, 1986; Robbins *et al.*, 1989; Wolterink *et al.*, 1993). That is, the mesolimbic dopamine system does not mediate conditioned reinforcement, but only its potentiation by stimulant drugs. Thus, information about conditioned reinforcers must be derived from another source, presumably one that interacts with the NAcc where its impact can be gain amplified by increases in dopamine transmission (Everitt and Robbins, 1992; Robbins *et al.*, 1989). A wealth of neuroanatomical data emphasize the limbic cortices as the primary sources of information processed within the NAcc, most notably the BLA, hippocampal formation (via the subiculum), and the prelimbic and anterior cingulate cortices (Kelley and Domesick, 1982; Kelley *et al.*, 1982; Mogenson *et al.*, 1984; Groenewegen *et al.*, 1996; De Olmos and Heimer, 1999). We reviewed much of our data on the differential contributions of these sources of afferents to the NAcc on conditioned reinforcement and its dopaminergic modulation previously (Everitt and Robbins, 1992). These data will be summarized briefly here and more recent findings emphasized.

As can be seen in Figure 10.1, rats with selective BLA lesions are impaired in their acquisition of a new response, failing to respond selectively on the CRf lever (Cador *et al.*, 1989; Burns *et al.*, 1993). Thus although BLA lesions were without major effects on appetitive Pavlovian conditioning (see above), the control over behaviour by the CS was attenuated and, as a consequence, 'gain-amplifying' effects on conditioned reinforcement of intra-NAcc infusions of D-amphetamine were also greatly reduced. These results are consistent with a burgeoning literature that shows marked effects of BLA lesions on the control over instrumental behaviour by Pavlovian CSs using a variety of behavioural procedures, including so-called conditioned place—or cue—preference, a superficially simple task that in fact embodies both Pavlovian approach behaviour and instrumental response contingencies (Everitt *et al.*, 1989, 1991; Hiroi and White, 1991).

In contrast, lesions of the ventral subiculum, a major outflow structure of the hippocampal formation, did not affect conditioned reinforcement itself (lesioned subjects still responded selectively on the CRf lever), but the potentiative effects of intra-accumbens amphetamine on the control over behaviour by the conditioned reinforcer *were* abolished, as were the locomotor stimulant effects of amphetamine (Burns *et al.*, 1993). Neither prelimbic nor anterior cingulate cortex lesions had any effect on responding with conditioned reinforcement (Burns *et al.*, 1993; Cardinal, Robbins, and Everitt, unpublished).

Thus, while the BLA and ventral subicular afferents to the NAcc are both essential for conditioned reinforcement and its potentiation by the mesolimbic dopamine system, their involvements are dissociable: (i) the BLA is part of the mechanism whereby Pavlovian CSs control instrumental behaviour as conditioned reinforcers, providing the substrate for the potentiative effects of stimulant drugs on conditioned reinforcement that are expressed in the NAcc; and (ii) the ventral subicular outflow from the hippocampal formation to the NAcc is essential for the potentiation of locomotor activity and conditioned reinforcement by stimulant drugs, but does not mediate informational aspects of the conditioned reinforcement process itself. We have hypothesized that the contribution of ventral subicular processes to this potentiation may be to provide the contextual background upon which the enhancement of locomotor activity presumably depends (Burns *et al.*, 1993; Everitt *et al.*, 1999). Additionally, psychomotor stimulation provides a mechanism by which the effects of conditioned reinforcers are 'gain-amplified' (Figure 10.5).

More recently, we have assessed the consequences of manipulating the CeA on conditioned reinforcement and its potentiation by increased NAcc dopamine. Excitotoxic lesions of the CeA did not impair responding with conditioned reinforcement (Figure 10.1) but completely abolished the effects of intra-NAcc infusions of D-amphetamine (Robledo *et al.*, 1996). This again demonstrates an intimate relationship between the CeA and the mesolimbic dopaminergic innervation of the NAcc, in this case specifically the shell (see below), so far as the potentiation by stimulants of responding with conditioned reinforcement is concerned. Selective excitotoxic lesions of the shell abolished the effects of intra-accumbens amphetamine (and significantly attenuated the locomotor stimulant effects of systemic amphetamine), but did not interfere with the control over instrumental behaviour by the conditioned reinforcer (Parkinson *et al.*, 1999). These effects of shell lesions are similar to those of ventral subiculum lesions, an observation that is of interest in the context of the strong preferential glutamatergic projection from the ventral subiculum to that part of the NAcc shell (septal pole) which was lesioned in these experiments (Kelley and Domesick, 1982).

The effects of excitotoxic NAcc core lesions were more complex. First, unlike shell lesions, core lesions retarded the re-attainment of criterion levels of Pavlovian discriminated approach preceding the acquisition of a new response (Parkinson *et al.*, 1999). These data suggest that the NAcc core is involved not only in learning, but also in the expression, of the discriminated approach response—perhaps indicating a difference in NAcc core and amygdala involvement in this behaviour. Secondly, although NAcc core lesions did not significantly affect the acquisition of responding with conditioned reinforcement under saline conditions, the interaction between intra-NAcc D-amphetamine and responding with conditioned reinforcement was affected by lesions of the NAcc core, in that there was a loss of selectivity in the potentiation of responding (Parkinson *et al.*, 1999). Subjects with lesions of the BLA showed similar impairments, including a loss of control over responding for the CRf under control conditions (Burns *et al.*, 1993). We have previously reported similar effects of manipulations of the NAcc and BLA, leading us to suggest that the integrity of the BLA is critical for stimulus–reward information to gain influence over voluntary behaviour (Everitt and Robbins, 1992; Everitt *et al.*, 1999). Thus, information reaching the NAcc concerned with the nature and direction of behaviour depends upon the BLA, presumably via its projections to both the core and shell, and may be 'gain-amplified' by dopamine transmission in the shell in a way that is critically dependent on the shell's glutamatergic inputs arising from the ventral subiculum (Figure 10.5).

Furthermore, in animals with NAcc shell lesions and an intact NAcc core, we observed that intra-NAcc infusions of D-amphetamine dose-dependently increased magazine approach during the acquisition of a new response with conditioned reinforcement, suggesting that the

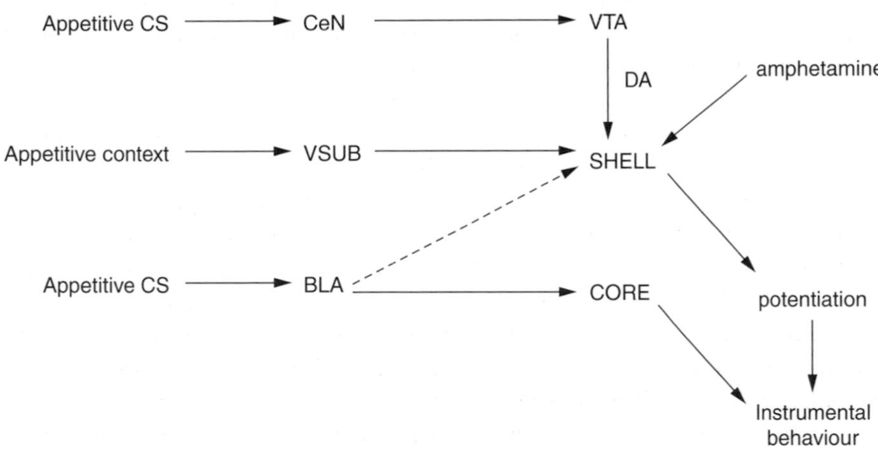

Figure 10.5 A schematic diagram of the neural network underlying conditioned reinforcement and its potentiation by intra-accumbens D-amphetamine based on the data presented (Taylor and Robbins, 1984, 1986; Cador, 1989; Burns, 1993; Robledo *et al.*, 1996; Everitt *et al.*, 1999; Parkinson *et al.*, 1999; Taylor *et al.*, 1986). The conditioned reinforcement process, whereby a Pavlovian CS+ supports the acquisition of a new response as a conditioned reinforcer (see Figure 10.1), depends upon the integrity of the BLA and NAcc core (CORE); there are rich projections from the BLA to this area of the NAcc. Lesions of either BLA or NAcc core do not directly affect the potentiative effects of D-amphetamine, other than by reducing the conditioned reinforcement effect itself. In contrast, the NAcc shell (SHELL) and CeA appear to be critical substrates for the potentiative effect of D-amphetamine on CRf, but not the control over instrumental behaviour by the CS in its role as a conditioned reinforcer. We hypothesize that the commonality in effects of NAcc shell and CeA lesions, supportive of the 'extended amygdala' concept, depends upon regulatory influences of the CeA on the dopaminergic innervation of the NAcc shell via projections to the VTA dopamine cell bodies. The ventral subiculum is also critical for the effects of intra-NAcc D-amphetamine on conditioned reinforcement. We hypothesize that this influence of the ventral subiculum depends upon its known projections to the caudomedial NAcc shell. Whilst the BLA and CeA appear to be concerned particularly with discrete CS processing, we further hypothesize, based on neuropsychological data, that the ventral subiculum provides contextual information upon which the CRf potentiation effect is based. Clearly, then, there is an interaction between the BLA and ventral subiculum in determining the control over behaviour by a conditioned reinforcer and its potentiation by increasing dopaminergic activity in the NAcc shell, and this interaction may be subserved by convergent projections onto NAcc shell neurons. (Figure reproduced from Everitt *et al.*, 1999, with permission.)

dopaminergic innervation of the NAcc core may also modulate the vigour of Pavlovian responses (Parkinson *et al.*, 1999a).

It is intriguing that both the CeA and NAcc shell, often considered as a functional continuum, the 'extended amygdala', mediate the important property of psychostimulant drugs to potentiate the impact of conditioned reinforcers. Consistent with our arguments above, we consider that the CeA (via its projections to the VTA) regulates the dopaminergic system innervating both the NAcc shell, mediating stimulant drug effects on instrumental behaviour and locomotor activity, and the NAcc core, mediating effects on Pavlovian approach behaviour. It is difficult to postulate another mechanism by which damage to the CeA can so effectively prevent the conditioned reinforcement potentiation that follows intra-accumbens infusions of D-amphetamine (Everitt *et al.*, 1999).

Previously, when discussing interactions between the amygdala and ventral striatum, our attention has been focused on glutamatergic projections from the BLA directly to the NAcc core and shell and dopaminergic modulation of this corticostriatal loop at that site (Everitt and Robbins, 1992; Everitt *et al.*, 1999), much as envisaged by Mogenson *et al.* (1984). However, it is now clear that interactions between amygdala and NAcc are more complex in that the CeA is also able to modulate ventral and dorsal striatal processing, not via direct projections, but by influencing the activity of the mesolimbic and nigrostriatal dopaminergic pathways. Moreover, dopaminergic mechanisms within the CeA and BLA also influence subcomponents of Pavlovian conditioning in a dissociable way. Thus, pre-trial infusions of 7-hydroxy-DPAT 7-OHDPAT into the BLA, but not the CeA, impaired acquisition of a new instrumental response with conditioned reinforcement, whereas Pavlovian approach behaviour, measured in the same task, was impaired by CeA, but not BLA, infusions of the drug (Hitchcott *et al.*, 1997a; Hitchcott and Phillips, 1998). These dissociations in associative functions of subregions of the amygdala following dopaminergic manipulations support the evidence and hypotheses derived from lesion studies reviewed above.

10.3 Associate representations in the amygdala

10.3.1 Dissociable processes within the amygdala

The results of our experiments summarized so far emphasize the importance of the amygdala in associative processes engaged during appetitive behaviour. Although initial studies of amygdala function, involving gross aspiration techniques that destroyed much of the temporal lobe, also revealed effects in appetitive settings (Klüver and Bucy, 1939; Weiskrantz, 1956; Henke *et al.*, 1972; Gaffan, 1992), more recent studies of the amygdala both in animals and in humans have been dominated by fear conditioning, perhaps at the cost of minimizing the more general importance of this collection of temporal lobe nuclei in associative processes. Indeed, our recent data indicate marked parallels in the effects of CeA and BLA lesions on both appetitive and aversive conditioning. Thus, lesions of the CeA impair both appetitive Pavlovian approach responses and Pavlovian conditioned suppression, whereas BLA lesions were without effect on these measures. In contrast, BLA lesions have been shown to impair the acquisition of instrumental, or voluntary, responses with both appetitive and aversive conditioned reinforcement, whereas CeA lesions were without effect. These dissociations of CeA and BLA function have also been demonstrated clearly by Gallagher, Holland, and co-workers in appetitive paradigms by studying the effects of selective excitotoxic lesions of these subdivisions of the amygdala (Gallagher *et al.*, 1990; Gallagher and Holland, 1992; Holland and Gallagher, 1999), but this distinctive pattern of results does not only depend on the use of lesions. For example, as indicated above, Phillips and co-workers have demonstrated striking differences in the effects of dopaminergic manipulations of the BLA and CeA on instrumental and Pavlovian conditioned responses, respectively (Hitchcott *et al.*, 1997a,b; Hitchcott and Phillips, 1998).

Clearly, these sets of data do not sit comfortably with the notion that associations are formed and stored exclusively within the BLA and that this processing is an antecedent of subsequent response production orchestrated by the CeA. Subjects with lesions or other forms of inactivation of the BLA should not, according to this scheme, be able to form associations between environmental stimuli and reinforcing events, and hence they should be unable subsequently to mount adaptive behavioural responses in the presence of such predictive cues. The explanations for these discrepancies in the data, if they are indeed discrepancies, should be considered.

One possibility that has been suggested to explain the preservation of some forms of fear conditioning in rats with BLA lesions is that the lesions themselves are 'not complete' (see Davis, Chapter 6). Excitotoxic lesions of the BLA such as we have made are never 'complete' in every subject, as lesion schematics make clear by showing the smallest and largest lesions (e.g. Killcross *et al.*, 1997b). However, in many subjects, we have seen no neuronal survival within the lateral and basal magnocellular nuclei at any anterior–posterior level and such subjects showed preserved classical fear conditioning. This total neuronal loss from the BLA has been confirmed in a recent study (Hall and Everitt, unpublished observations) in which the neuron-specific antibody NeuN was used to demonstrate cell loss immunocytochemically: following quinolinic acid-induced BLA lesions, no BLA neurons survived in the lateral and basal magnocellular nuclei. To dwell on this point, however, is also to miss the wider importance and interpretation of the *double dissociation* of the effects of CeA and BLA lesions: Pavlovian conditioned suppression *was preserved* in BLA-lesioned rats that showed marked impairments in conditioned punishment. Even if a tiny population of neurons were preserved in the BLA (which in many cases they were not), this is a dramatic result. It should also be emphasized that in interpreting these effects we have never asserted either (i) that serial information transfer from lateral to central amygdala does not underlie fear conditioning—clearly it does (e.g. freezing and fear-potentiated startle)—or (ii) that the CeA is a site of CS–US *association*; whether it is or not remains to be shown, but the CeA is clearly required for some forms of fear conditioning. We return to a possibly more interesting resolution of these issues below.

A second possibility that we have raised previously concerns differences in the conditioning procedures used. In the great majority of conditioned fear paradigms, very few (1–5) pairings of CS and shock are used, whereas in our own fear conditioning studies (Killcross *et al.*, 1997a), there were many pairings of CS and US. Similarly, in the autoshaping procedure, there were many pairings of ingestive reward and the CS. This has led to the suggestion that extended training somehow recruits otherwise redundant neural mechanisms to support learning—a suggestion based in part upon the assumption that small numbers of CS–US pairings represent the critical test of fear conditioning (Nader and LeDoux, 1997; Fendt *et al.*, 1999). While it is clearly the case that such associations can and do form in one trial and that it is adaptive to learn the value of danger signals rapidly, repeated pairings of CS and US, whether appetitive or aversive, are very likely to occur in naturalistic circumstances and learning in these circumstances is itself adaptive, allowing initial associations to be modified by subsequent experience. We find it difficult to accept the notion that Pavlovian associations formed over multiple trials recruit otherwise redundant neural mechanisms (Killcross *et al.*, 1997b).

Another issue of significance in this debate concerns the nature of the measures of conditioned fear. As has been argued elsewhere (Killcross *et al.*, 1997a; Cahill *et al.*, 1999), it is important to distinguish the effects of a neural manipulation, such as a lesion, on mnemonic versus non-mnemonic processes, perhaps especially the preserved ability of a subject to make the response that subsequently provides the measure of conditioning. In the case of conditioned freezing or fear-potentiated startle, there are few, if any, demonstrations that BLA manipulations impair the conditioned responses of freezing or startle without also affecting unconditioned freezing or startle. Indeed, Davis and colleagues have provided evidence that the BLA is critical for unconditioned freezing and fear-potentiated startle (Davis, 1997; Walker and Davis, 1997). Although we have shown recently that rats with excitotoxic lesions of the BLA can, with over training, develop a freezing response to contextual cues (Hall and Everitt, in preparation), this result violates the generally held rule that rats cannot acquire conditioned fear responses to contextual cues without an intact BLA, a belief held even though we previously and clearly have demonstrated contextual fear in BLA-, but not in hippocampal-lesioned rats (Selden *et al.*, 1991).

Inherent in the debate about associative processes in the amygdala is the notion that associations are formed exclusively in the lateral amygdala via the convergent activation of pathways conveying information about the CS and US (Clugnet and LeDoux, 1990; Maren, 1996; McKernan *et al.*, 1997). However, it is also clear that structures extraneous to the amygdala also participate in Pavlovian associative processes, including the anterior cingulate cortex, the NAcc core, and the hippocampus itself (Gabriel *et al.*, 1991; Bussey *et al.*, 1997; Maren *et al.*, 1997; Cahill *et al.*, 1999; Parkinson *et al.*, 2000a). These data derive from lesion and electrophysiological approaches and include aversive and appetitive tasks. Moreover, the lateral capsular division of the CeA is also in receipt of thalamic, cortical, and subcortical afferents, suggesting that the ingredients of associative learning exist within this component of the amygdala (McDonald, 1998), even though associative long-term potentiation (LTP) has not been demonstrated there to date as it has within the lateral nucleus (Clugnet *et al.*, 1990; Maren, 1996; McKernan and Shinnick-Gallagher, 1997). However, neurons in the CeA do respond to both conditioned and unconditioned fear stimuli (Pascoe and Kapp, 1985b) and undergo plastic changes during fear conditioning (Applegate *et al.*, 1982; Pascoe and Kapp, 1985a). It should also be noted that there is also evidence of plasticity within structures afferent to the amygdala, most notably in the thalamic medial geniculate nucleus, during auditory fear conditioning (Cahill *et al.*, 1999).

10.3.2 What representations are formed during conditioning?

It is timely to consider the existing results at face value and consider what explanations can best accommodate the main body of data. The lack of effect of BLA lesions on Pavlovian conditioning in some of our own, as well as in other, studies is perhaps at first sight surprising, as there are many demonstrations, again including our own, that BLA lesions can impair appetitive and aversive Pavlovian conditioning. For example, the integrity of the BLA has been shown to be critical for the acquisition of appetitive conditioned place preferences (Everitt *et al.*, 1991; Hiroi *et al.*, 1991). It must be appreciated that although conditioned place preferences and aversions provide useful measures of associations between environmental stimuli and reinforcement, the nature of the precise learning mechanisms operating during their acquisition and performance is ambiguous, being consistent with the involvement of the BLA in either Pavlovian or instrumental behaviour (Everitt and Robbins, 1992; McAlonan *et al.*, 1993; McDonald and White, 1993). However, when considering Pavlovian procedures unconfounded by conditioned instrumental performance, as above, it is increasingly clear that the BLA is not always critical for this form of learning. Thus, results with the autoshaping paradigm used in the studies summarized here, as well as those assessing conditioned suppression, indicate a general role for the CeA in Pavlovian conditioned responding. However, when considering conditioned freezing and fear-potentiated startle, both BLA and CeA lesions are effective in disrupting conditioning.

Perhaps one way of disentangling these issues is to consider the nature of the representations underlying Pavlovian conditioning, and associative learning in general. Associations are generally believed to be represented in the brain by altering the 'weights' of unidirectional synapses. As synaptic weights can only change on the basis of information available to the neurons involved, the association of representations A and B in Figure 10.6 can only occur at points where information about these two representations converge, no matter what mechanisms exist to supervise and use the association. Such associations may be used for different purposes, for example as a representation of a higher order property of stimuli (a 'feature detector'), or for commanding behavioural responses directly.

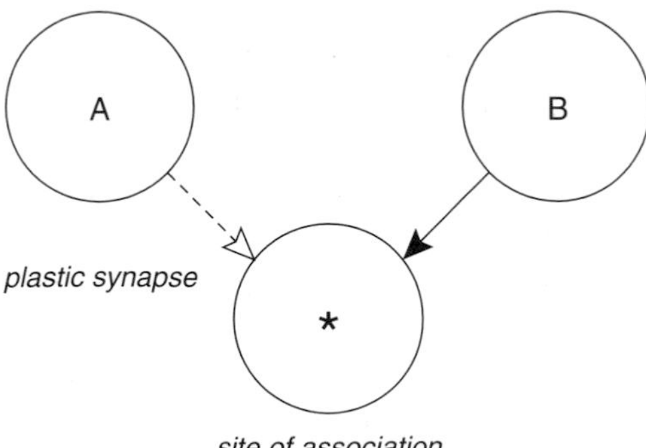

Figure 10. 6 Simple associative representations. Plastic synapses change their weight on the basis of locally available information, requiring convergence of information about the representations to be associated.

In Pavlovian conditioning, there is the potential for several associations to form, as illustrated in Figure 10.7. Lesions that remove a representation of either the CS, the US, or the response would have obvious consequences not only for conditioned, but also for unconditioned responding (sites A, B, and D in Figure 10.7). Lesions of site C, representing a central motivational state (such as fear), might not impair primitive unconditioned responses, yet could impair conditioned responses that were based on the elicitation of fear. Again, however, any properties of the unconditioned response to the US that depended on this hypothesized 'fear' state would be lost.

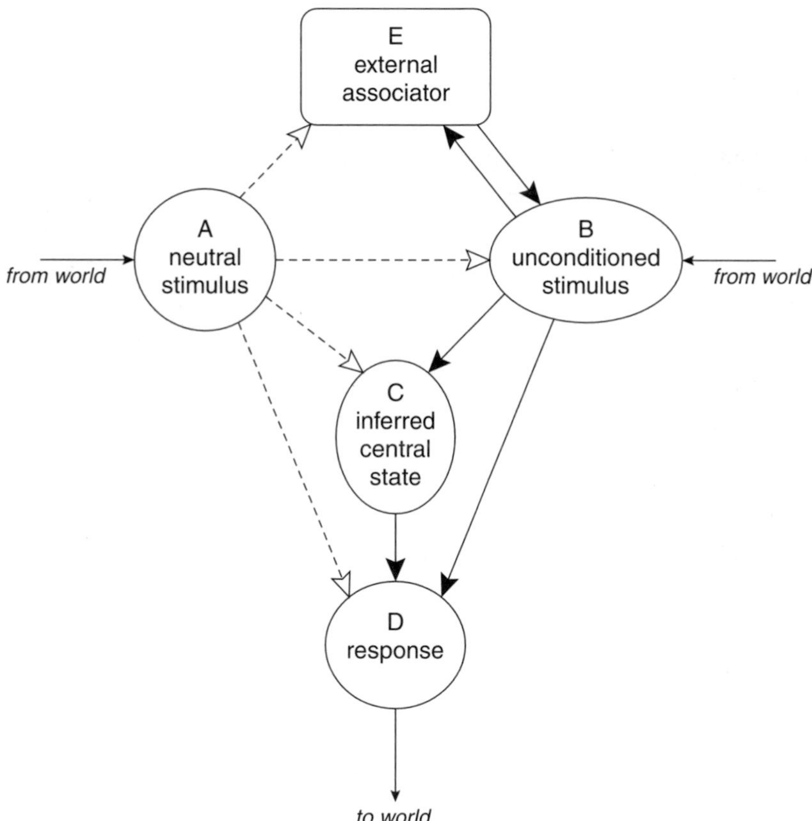

Figure 10.7 From a theoretical perspective, Pavlovian conditioning has the potential to create associations between a conditioned stimulus (CS) and representations of the unconditioned stimulus (US), central states such as fear, and unconditioned responses. Only a single response is shown; distinctions between different kinds of response are discussed in the text and shown in later figures. Bidirectional communication also allows representations to be associated in 'third-party' sites (E) (Damasio and Damasio, 1993; Fuster, 1995). Note that lesions of such a site might prevent conditioning without impairing any form of unconditioned response, as would selectively *disconnecting* the CS from a representation involved in responding.

Experimental analysis of Pavlovian conditioning has shown that CS–US pairings may cause the CS to elicit at least three of these representations in the brain (Mackintosh, 1983; Gewirtz and Davis, 1998). The first and simplest of these is that the CS may become directly associated with the *unconditioned response* (UR), forming a simple stimulus–response association.

The second is a representation of *affect*, as demonstrated by the phenomenon of trans-reinforcer blocking, in which a CS paired with shock can block conditioning to a CS paired with the absence of an otherwise expected food reward (Dickinson and Dearing, 1979). These two reinforcers share no common properties other than their aversiveness and, therefore, the blocking effect must depend upon an association between the CS and affect. Affective states can therefore be independent of the specific reinforcer and response. This concept has been widely used in theories of learning (Konorski, 1948, 1967; Dickinson and Dearing, 1979) and is illustrated in Figure 10.8. Associations between the stimulus and an affective state appear to be critical in second-order conditioning (S_1–US followed by S_2–S_1); unlike a first-order conditioned response (CR), a second-order CR is relatively insensitive to post-training changes in the value of the US (implying that it does not depend on S_2–US associations) and the response to S_2 may differ from the response to S_1 or the US (implying that it does not depend on S_2–R associations).

The third form of representation is *specific to the US*. If a CS is paired with a desirable food and the food subsequently is devalued by pairing it with LiCl, such that the food now

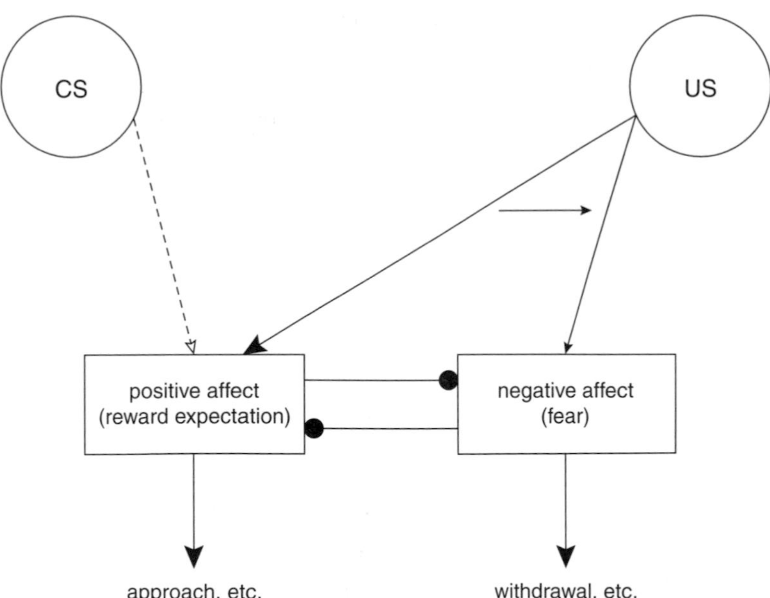

Figure 10. 8 Conditioning to affective states leaves the response independent of the current value of the US. The CS associates with the affective state elicited by the US during conditioning, but if the US subsequently alters its value, the conditioned response (CR) will not alter.

becomes aversive and elicits appropriate responses, the reaction to the first-order CS changes in normal animals (Mackintosh, 1983). Therefore, the CS cannot have been associated with an abstract 'positive affect' representation, but must have been associated with that particular reinforcer. The association must be specific to the US because the reaction to a second CS that predicted a different food does not alter, and its connections with valence information must be modifiable and *downstream* of the CS–US association.

Further evidence that a CS becomes associated with a relatively specific representation of the properties of a reinforcer is provided by studies of cued instrumental discrimination (Trapold, 1970). Rats acquired an instrumental discrimination between two levers paired with different appetitive reinforcers more rapidly if the discriminative cues had been paired with the same reinforcers (same condition) in a previous Pavlovian stage than when the outcome was switched between stages (different condition). A rigorous demonstration of the formation of associations between the *specific sensory properties* of stimuli comes from sensory preconditioning, the process by which neutral stimuli are paired in the form S_2–S_1, after which S_1–US conditioning causes a CR to occur to S_2. Thus, in the first stage, associations form between representations that have no motivational component. Taken together, these procedures demonstrate that animals are able to encode the relationship between a CS and specific sensory properties of the US and, furthermore, that they can relate this sensory representation to the affective valence of the reinforcer.

10.3.4 Nature of representations in different regions of the amygdala

Basolateral amygdala

A great deal of evidence has accumulated showing that rats with BLA lesions can acquire first-order conditioned responses, but that these responses are insensitive to reinforcer revaluation. For example, rats with BLA lesions acquired normal food cup responding to a CS paired with food, and showed normal acquisition of an aversion to that food when it subsequently was paired with LiCl, but failed spontaneously to adjust their responding (orienting and food cup approach) to the CS after the food was devalued (Hatfield *et al.*, 1996). The most parsimonious explanation is that the conditioned responses learned by these rats were a result of direct associations between the CS and the response. They lacked the ability to use the CS to access the value of a specific US and use that representation to alter their response. Holland and Gallagher define this ability as 'mediated performance': the ability to respond based on a CS-activated representation of the US (Holland and Gallagher, 1999).

The idea that BLA-lesioned animals cannot use a CS to gain access to the current value of its specific US has great explanatory power. Second-order conditioning requires that the second-order stimulus becomes associated with the affective value that is called up by the first-order CS (as discussed above); BLA-lesioned rats cannot acquire second-order conditioning (Hatfield *et al.*, 1996), cannot acquire responding under second-order instrumental schedules (Everitt *et al.*, 1989; Whitelaw *et al.*, 1996), or use a first-order CS as a conditioned reinforcer (Cador *et al.*, 1989; Burns *et al.*, 1993) (see Table 10.1). Clearly, the responses which still occur to the first-order CS do not support second-order conditioning,

Table 10.1 Summary of some of the effects of BLA and CeA lesions on different forms of association and the behavioural procedures used to demonstrate them.

Association type	*Lesion*	*Behaviour sensitive to lesion*
CS–UR	CeA	Acquisition of autoshaping
		Acquisition of conditioned orienting
		Conditioned salivation
		Pavlovian-to-instrumental transfer
CS–US	BLA	Second-order Pavlovian responding
		Second-order instrumental responding
		Conditioned reinforcement
		Conditioned place or cue preference/avoidance
		Conditioned freezing[a]
		Conditioned startle[a]

[a]Note that these behaviours are also sensitive to lesions of the CeA.

while the effects on reward devaluation demonstrate that the deficit in BLA-lesioned animals is not restricted to second-order conditioning *per se*. Specific modulation of instrumental choice behaviour by a CS also requires that the subject utilizes the motivational value of a particular US; in this capability, too, BLA-lesioned animals are impaired (Killcross, 1998; Killcross *et al.*, 1997a).

The formation of an association between a CS and the affective value of a US also accounts for responses such as conditioned freezing, which cannot be accounted for readily in terms of a CS–UR association. Thus, the conditioned freezing response does not resemble the UR to shock, which is characterized by agitation, jumping, vocalization, and escape, but instead represents an adaptive response to danger. At the time of conditioning, therefore, there is no freezing response occurring to which a CS–UR association can be formed. In addition, freezing is a US-specific conditioned response: while freezing occurs to a CS for shock, it does not occur to a CS for the omission of expected food, even though both signal aversive events (as discussed above). It seems plausible to suggest, therefore, that the BLA is critical for the acquisition of conditioned freezing because it subserves the formation of an association between the CS and a neural representation of the affective properties of the US (Bolles and Fanselow, 1980). Similarly, fear-potentiated startle may reflect the potentiation of a reflexive startle response by an affective representation retrieved by the CS, and is thereby sensitive to BLA lesions.

Central nucleus

Even though it receives neuronal afferents appropriate to support them, there is no direct evidence to suggest that the CeA is itself a site of CS–US associations; it might receive an already-associated input. However, it is clear from the data discussed above that animals lacking a BLA can form some kinds of association, the conditioned expression of which is sensitive to CeA, but not BLA, lesions. The simplest analysis at present seems to be that the CeA does form simple CS–UR ('sensorimotor') associations, which do not depend upon a specific US, i.e. they are independent of the identity and current motivational value of the US and are also unable to support second-order conditioning. We suggest that the responses subserved by CeA-dependent associations include particularly the modulation of reflexes organized within the brainstem, including some that conventionally might be regarded as 'affective', such as conditioned suppression, conditioned orienting, and Pavlovian-to-instrumental transfer. These are all disrupted by CeA lesions (see Table 10.1). Responses such as conditioned suppression may influence instrumental behaviour non-specifically, but are insufficient to modulate multiple instrumental behaviours differentially, as assessed in choice tasks (Killcross *et al.*, 1997a). This is not to deny the role of CeA-dependent associations in discriminated approach as assessed by autoshaping. Indeed, autoshaping is a capability to which the BLA does not seem to contribute (Everitt *et al.*, 1999).

This view of amygdala function is illustrated speculatively in Figure 10.9. When a CS comes to predict an appetitive US, it may form associations with sensory and motivational representations of that US (links 1 and 2), with central affective states (3), and with unconditioned responses at some level (4). When the US is devalued, its motivational representation is redirected selectively in some way to an aversive state (not shown), so it is through links 1 or 2 that the changed response to a first-order CS occurs. It should be noted that while affective states are illustrated as 'centres', very little is known of the neuronal mechanism by which valence might be encoded: such information might just as easily be carried as a temporal or chemical code and be multiply represented, rather than existing in distinct spatial loci. Indeed, it has been argued convincingly that the orbitofrontal cortex provides an important site for the representation of affective valence (Schoenbaum *et al.*, 1998, 1999; Rolls, 1999).

10.3.5 Unresolved issues

It is at present unclear whether the BLA is involved in representing specific sensory information about USs, required for S–S associations. Each sensory modality projects to a region of sensory cortex, a reason to question *a priori* whether the BLA is required, and rats can learn stimulus discrimination tasks in the absence of the BLA (Schwartzbaum, 1965; Sarter and Markowitsch, 1985; Burns *et al.*, 1999). If the BLA is involved, it would therefore have to be as an 'independent associator' (E in Figure 10.7). According to this scenario, BLA-lesioned animals make unconditioned responses and learn simple CS–UR associations, including 'emotional' responses, but the CS would convey no information about the identity of the US. Alternatively, the US-specific representation involving the BLA might be purely affective; in this alternative scenario, BLA-lesioned animals can learn CS–UR associations and CS–US (sensory) associations, but cannot learn CS–US (affective) associations, and the sensory representation they can activate is without affective valence. One crucial test will be to see if BLA lesions impair sensory preconditioning.

Similarly, it is unclear whether the BLA holds US-specific representations which excite general appetitive/aversive states in another structure, or itself contains this 'affective processor', or contains both. It is clearly difficult to distinguish whether BLA-lesioned animals

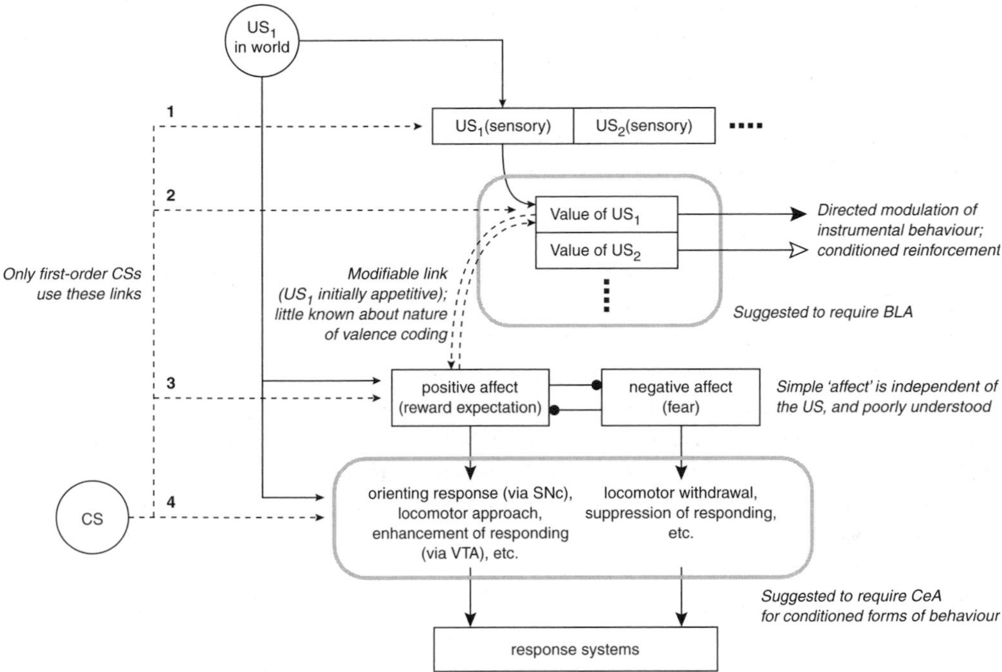

Figure 10.9 Schematic of representations that may be involved in Pavlovian conditioning, emphasizing the hypothesized role of amygdaloid subregions. The BLA is required for a CS to gain access to the current value of its specific US. In the figure, the CS has been associated with US_1, initially appetitive, while an unrelated US_2 maintains a separate value (connections not shown for clarity). As discussed in the text, the precise nature of the information encoded in the BLA is uncertain; here, it is illustrated as binding US-specific sensory information to an affective value. The BLA may use this information to control CeA function but also to modulate specific instrumental (choice) behaviour, as in conditioned reinforcement tasks; the nucleus accumbens and prefrontal cortex are key targets of this information. In contrast, the CeA is required for CS–UR learning, particularly when the response involves modulation of hypothalamic and brainstem functions.

lack affective states that may take part in associations, or merely cannot call them up via a CS; however, transreinforcer blocking and performance (but not acquisition) of second-order conditioning are two phenomena that appear to depend on simple affect.

In summary, it remains uncertain whether the BLA (i) encodes or retrieves the specific sensory properties of a US; (ii) encodes or retrieves the affective nature of a US; or (iii) is required for *coupling* the sensory and affective properties of a US. Therefore, determining the subtleties of processing subserved by the BLA is important and will require further experiments.

10.4 Dissociable amygdala subsystems and drug addiction

The dissociations demonstrated in our studies between CeA and BLA function may reflect the more recent evolutionary development of lateral and basal nuclei of the amygdaloid complex and the ability of the BLA to modify more primitive processes organized within the CeA (Swanson and Mogenson, 1998). Although sharing some afferent connections, the BLA and CeA also show marked differences in terms of their afferents, but especially in their efferent connections. In particular, the distributed outputs of the CeA allow it to orchestrate autonomic, endocrine, and behavioural responses that characterize integrated patterns of emotional behaviour (Krettek and Price, 1978; Swanson *et al.*, 1981; LeDoux *et al.*, 1988; Davis, 1992a; Zahm *et al.*, 1999). These patterns are measured most frequently in studies of fear conditioning in terms of increased heart rate, increased adrenal hormone secretion, and responses such as freezing or startle (LeDoux *et al.*, 1988; Davis, 1992a), but they are evident in appetitive situations as well, and include not only approach and orientation responses, but also ingestive reflexes such as salivation and possibly other responses of the cephalic phase (Lagowska and Fonberg, 1975; Parkinson *et al.*, 2000a; Roozendaal *et al.*, 1990). These responses orchestrated by the CeA depend upon downstream projections primarily to the hypothalamus and brainstem (Swanson *et al.*, 1981). The phylogenetically more recently developed BLA can recruit this response output mechanism via its rich projections to the CeA. However, in addition, via its unique projections to the orbital prefrontal cortex and ventral striatum (Amaral *et al.*, 1992), the BLA may also influence more flexible responses, including goal-directed instrumental behaviour, perhaps at the same time overriding reflexive responses engendered by simple CS–UR mechanisms within the CeA.

We have also highlighted here what we consider to be a key aspect of CeA function, which is to influence ascending arousal systems through its projections to the brainstem monoaminergic and basal forebrain cholinergic neurons of the isodendritic core. These connections may not only influence attentional and plastic processes through cholinergic projections to the cortex, as demonstrated in elegant experiments by Gallagher and Holland (Gallagher and Holland, 1994; Holland and Gallagher, 1999), but also invigorate conditioned orienting or approach responses via ascending dopaminergic projections to the striatum (Han *et al.*, 1997; Everitt *et al.*, 1999). Our demonstration that the NAcc core and its dopaminergic innervation are critical substrates of appetitive Pavlovian approach behaviour (Everitt *et al.*, 1999; Parkinson *et al.*, 2000a), together with the marked impact of a CeA–dorsal striatal dopaminergic disconnection on conditioned orienting (Han *et al.*, 1997), provides a neuroanatomical basis for the integrated functioning of the CeA, nucleus accumbens, and dorsal striatum via the projections from the CeA to midbrain dopamine neurons.

The amygdaloid complex may therefore affect emotional processes by several mechanisms that have evolved through an organism's need to respond adaptively to affective events in its environment. The CeA increasingly is seen as having a quite complex set of functions, which might conveniently be thought of as providing at least two of these mechanisms. (i) To coordinate specific autonomic, endocrine, and reflexive behavioural responses to cues of emotional significance; this depends upon hypothalamic and brainstem projections. (ii) To energize more general processes, such as the vigour of behavioural responses (activation), enhancing attention, and signalling reward, all of which depend upon projections to the isodendritic core. Both (i) and (ii) are, of course, components of the unconditioned response to the US, being consistent with a postulated involvement of the CeA in CS–UR representations. However, Holland and co-workers (Holland, 1984; Holland and Gallagher, 1999) have argued that motor responses directed towards the US, rather than the CS, have a separate neural basis and one that appears to be independent of the amygdala. A similar conclusion has been reached concerning aversive eyeblink conditioning, which also survives lesions of either central or basolateral parts of the amygdala (Lavond *et al.*, 1993). A third function of the amygdala depends upon the BLA, which subserves more complex representations of the affective value or specific sensory attribution of conditioned stimuli, enabling goal-directed actions to be influenced via its projections to the prefrontal cortex and ventral striatum, as well as recruiting the diverse processes regulated by the CeA that will also impact on the vigour of such actions.

10.4.1 Implications for addiction and drug dependence

Associative conditioning clearly comprises several distinct mechanisms, some of which we have shown to depend upon dissociable regions of the amygdala, thereby allowing this structure to influence the complex processes underlying emotional behaviour. While we have been focusing on the involvement of the amygdala in learning involving appetitive and aversive natural stimuli, it is plausible that the mechanisms we have identified may also apply to other reinforcers, such as drugs of abuse. Several theorists have argued strongly that different forms of conditioning contribute to the persistence of compulsive drug use in humans (Wikler, 1965; Stewart *et al.*, 1984; Childress *et al.*, 1992; O'Brien *et al.*, 1992a,b; Robinson and Berridge, 1993; Everitt, 1996; Di Chiara, 1998; Everitt *et al.*, 1999; Robbins and Everitt, 1999). Wikler, in his two-factor theory of addiction, argued that the Pavlovian association of specific environments with opiate withdrawal provided the basis for the phenomenon of conditioned withdrawal (Wikler, 1965). According to this theory, drug-abstinent (detoxified) individuals, even those who have been abstinent for a relatively long time, experience a conditioned withdrawal syndrome sufficient to induce drug craving and relapse to heroin self-administration upon entering an environment previously paired with opiate withdrawal. There are both clinical and experimental demonstrations of this phenomenon (Goldberg and Schuster, 1967; Childress *et al.*, 1988), which has also been proposed to explain why veterans of the Vietnam war, many of whom were dependent upon heroin while in Vietnam, did not relapse in any numbers to heroin abuse on their return to the USA because of the change in context, i.e. because the heroin withdrawal-associated environmental cues were no longer present to precipitate conditioned withdrawal and thereby relapse to heroin abuse (Robins *et al.*, 1975). Other conditioning theories have emphasized the association of environmental stimuli with the positive reinforcing effects of abused drugs, especially cocaine, but also opiates (Stewart *et al.*, 1984; Robinson and Berridge, 1993; Di Chiara, 1998). While specific drug-associate cues sometimes result in conditioned 'highs', in which the ritual of intravenous injection of vehicle alone is sufficient to induce some of the responses usually only seen to the injected drug (O'Brien *et al.*, 1986), such cues are also well known to induce drug craving in former cocaine-dependent subjects and to be a major contributory factor in the maintenance and reinstatement of a drug-taking habit (Gawin, 1991; O'Brien and McLellan, 1996). In a variant of conditioned positive reinforcement theories of addiction, Robinson and Berridge (1993) have argued that the attribution of what they term 'incentive salience' to environmental cues associated with drug effects imbues the cues with the power to induce 'drug wanting'.

In our own experiments, some of which are reviewed here, we have demonstrated that amphetamine and other stimulant drugs clearly exaggerate the motivational effects of CSs by increasing dopamine transmission in the ventral striatum. Indeed, this may be a major component of the reinforcing effects of such drugs. Since this effect of amphetamine depends upon associative information derived from the amygdala, we see the importance of trying to understand the ways in which associative learning, which might be seen as maladaptive, could lead to the progressive development of the complex syndrome of drug addiction (Robbins and Everitt, 1999). Such maladaptive learning might, then, result in the establishment of compulsive drug use, in which drug-associated cues powerfully induce drug craving and relapse to drug-seeking behaviour following abstinence (Gawin, 1991; O'Brien and McLellan, 1996). Thus, for example, the simple associative influence exerted by the CeA over ascending arousal systems may provide a key mechanism underlying the increased salience, attractiveness, and motivational properties of drug-associated cues. Operating in parallel, by mediating representations of the CS–US (drug) association, the BLA may impact upon processes of conditioned reinforcement whereby drug cues can support and direct instrumental acts having the goal of procuring drugs such as cocaine for self-administration. Relapse to drug addiction precipitated by exposure to drug-associated cues can also be seen as part of the vicious circle of cocaine addiction, which is completed by the effect of the self-administered drug to boost further the dopaminergic processes within the CeA and NAcc that support conditioning to environmental stimuli while simultaneously enhancing their impact on craving and drug-seeking behaviour (Phillips and Fibiger, 1990; Everitt *et al.*, 1999).

In order to test this hypothesis, we have successfully developed a second-order schedule of intravenous (i.v.) cocaine reinforcement to investigate the neural and pharmacological basis of cue-controlled cocaine-seeking behaviour in rats (Whitelaw *et al.*, 1996; Weissenborn *et al.*, 1997; Arroyo *et al.*, 1998; Pilla *et al.*, 1999). Rats are trained to self-administer cocaine, which is always paired with a discrete light CS. Subsequently, the CS supports responding for a protracted period prior to the i.v. drug infusion, providing a measure of drug-seeking behaviour that is not affected by pharmacological effects of the self-administered drug. The importance of contingent presentations of the cocaine-associated cue in maintaining responding has been demonstrated by the finding that responding decreases to about 40% of the control level following the omission of the CS during each of three daily sessions (despite the fact that i.v. cocaine is still self-administered at the end of each of five daily fixed intervals of responding). Responding is re-established promptly at baseline levels following re-introduction of the CS (Arroyo *et al.*, 1998). Presentations of the cocaine cue following extinction of responding are also able to reinstate drug-seeking behaviour, a model of cue-induced relapse (Arroyo *et al.*, 1998).

Rats with bilateral excitotoxic lesions of the BLA could not acquire adequate levels of responding under a second-order schedule of cocaine reinforcement (Whitelaw *et al.*, 1996). Thus, the acquisition of drug-seeking behaviour that depends upon presentation of drug-associated cues requires the integrity of this part of the amygdaloid complex, as does the acquisition of a new response with conditioned reinforcement. However, BLA lesions did not impair the acquisition of i.v. cocaine self-administration *per se*, indicating that the primary rewarding effects of cocaine do not depend upon the BLA (Whitelaw *et al.*, 1996). Only when responding depended upon presentation of the drug CS was the impact of BLA lesions revealed, consistent with the hypothesis that the BLA is essential for the CS to elicit the affective representation of the primary reinforcer (in this case, cocaine) and consistent with other data reviewed above for appetitive conditioning in general (Cador *et al.*, 1989; Everitt *et al.*, 1989; Burns *et al.*, 1993; Hatfield *et al.*, 1996; Whitelaw *et al.*, 1996). Moreover, cocaine-associated cues are ineffective in reinstating cocaine self-administration in rats with bilateral BLA lesions (Meil and See, 1997), further emphasizing the importance of this structure in mediating the effects of the drug-associated CS on drug-taking behaviour. Taken together, these data strongly suggest that the BLA is part of the neural mechanism through which drug-associated CSs can control instrumental behaviour, presumably by interacting directly or indirectly with the ventral striatum, a primary site for the rewarding effects of cocaine and amphetamine (Everitt *et al.*, 1999). Interestingly, rats responding at high rates for heroin under a second-order schedule of reinforcement do not depend critically on contingent presentations of heroin-associated cues and are relatively not affected by CS omission in the way in which rats responding for cocaine are (Alderson *et al.*, 2000). Lesions of the BLA identical to those that prevented the acquisition of cue-controlled cocaine-seeking behaviour were without effect on the acquisition of this form of heroin-seeking behaviour, further emphasizing the importance of the BLA only for behaviour under the control of CSs associated with the self-administered drug (Alderson, Robbins, and Everitt, in press).

Thus, the involvement of the amygdala in the complex processes underlying addictive behaviour appears to be quite specific. In addition to the demonstrations summarized above showing that the BLA is important for cue-controlled cocaine-seeking behaviour, reinstatement of cocaine self-administration following extinction, and for conditioned reinforcement, it has been shown additionally that a conditioned place preference for an environment paired with cocaine also depends upon the BLA (Brown and Fibiger, 1993) and that exposure to a cocaine-paired environment induces the expression of c-*fos* in the amygdala, among other limbic cortical structures (Brown *et al.*, 1992). However, other responses are not affected by BLA lesions, for example: (i) conditioned locomotor activity induced by exposing rats to an environment in which they repeatedly had received injections of cocaine; (ii) the unconditioned locomotor response to cocaine (Brown *et al.*, 1993) or amphetamine (Burns *et al.*, 1993; Robledo *et al.*, 1996); and (iii) the sensitization of locomotor activity to stimulant drugs, which instead depends upon glutamatergic projections from the prefrontal cortex to the VTA (Pierce and Kalivas, 1997; Pierce *et al.*, 1998; Wolf, 1998; Kalivas and Nakamura, 1999). Thus, BLA lesions only attenuate the acquisition of appetitive behavioural responses that are in large measure under the control of discrete drug-paired stimuli.

Apparently quite different, non-associative influences on cocaine self-administration are seen following dopaminergic manipulations of the amygdala. While 6-hydroxydopamine-induced lesions of the amygdala have only minor effects on cocaine self-administration (McGregor *et al.*, 1994), infusions of dopamine D1 receptor antagonists into the amygdala both increase cocaine self-administration (McGregor and Roberts, 1993; Caine *et al.*, 1995; Hurd *et al.*, 1997) and simultaneously increase dopamine levels in the NAcc (Hurd *et al.*, 1997). These effects of manipulating dopamine transmission in the amygdala are generally similar to those following identical manipulations of dopamine transmission in the NAcc (McGregor and Roberts, 1993; Caine *et al.*, 1995; Hurd *et al.*, 1997) except that infusions of a D1 receptor antagonist into the NAcc also increased the break point for cocaine self-administration under a progressive ratio schedule, whereas intra-amygdala infusions did not (McGregor and Roberts, 1993). It seems likely that these effects of dopaminergic treatments in the amygdala are mediated indirectly by the CeA (which receives the richest dopaminergic innervation among amygdala subregions) via its midbrain projections which can regulate the activity of mesolimbic dopamine neurons and hence dopamine levels in the NAcc. Such interactions may be considered within the conceptual framework of the extended amygdala, which has been strongly implicated in mediating the reinforcing effects of drugs of abuse (Koob, 1999), or may reflect the influence of the CeA upon ascending dopaminergic transmission (Schulteis *et al.*, 2000).

In studies parallel to those on associative processes influencing cocaine self-administration, we have also shown that the BLA is important in mediating the depressant effects on appetitive behaviour of stimuli associated with heroin withdrawal (Everitt *et al.*, 1993). In these experiments, rats were trained to lever press at high rates for food on a fixed interval schedule. They were then made opiate dependent by implanting them subcutaneously with morphine pellets, and their baseline level of responding for food was re-established. Subsequently, acute withdrawal was precipitated on four occasions by injection of low doses of the opiate antagonist, naloxone, in the presence of a distinctive visual/auditory CS. Following these four conditioning trials, the rats were again allowed to respond for food and the effects on responding of presentations of the withdrawal-associated CS were measured. The marked suppression of responding induced by the withdrawal-associated CS in control rats was not observed in rats that had received excitotoxic lesions of the BLA prior to conditioning, even though these lesions did not alter the unconditioned withdrawal precipitated by naloxone in dependent rats. These results are again consistent with the hypothesis that the BLA is essential for retrieval by the CS of the affective representation of the primary reinforcer, in this case the aversive state of withdrawal. They also emphasize that the associative mechanisms subserved by the amygdala are independent of the positive or negative affective valence of the reinforcer.

Functional imaging studies of human cocaine and heroin abusers have demonstrated that exposure to cocaine cues, including the paraphernalia associated with drug self-administration and videos of drug use, results in significant activation of medial temporal lobe structures, which is at least partly attributable to the amygdala (Grant *et al.*, 1996; Childress *et al.*, 1999). It is perhaps important to note that these same studies reveal the activation of a cortical network on exposure to drug cues that includes the anterior cingulate, orbitofrontal and dorsolateral prefrontal cortices, but not the striatum. The latter is, however, strongly affected by self-administered cocaine and other dopaminergic drugs (Breiter *et al.*, 1996; Volkow *et al.*, 1996, 1997a,b), frequently in a way that is correlated with indices of craving. As in animal experimental studies, these data suggest that the neural mechanisms mediating the primary reinforcing effects of abused drugs can be dissociated from those mediating conditioned reinforcement and the impact of drug-conditioned cues on drug craving. This realization suggests that pharmacological or other interference with the mechanisms by which drug cues induce craving and drug-seeking behaviour might present a therapeutic target for drugs having utility in the treatment of this aspect of cocaine addiction. Indeed, we have shown that a dopamine D3 receptor partial agonist, BP 897, which has no primary rewarding effects, selectively reduces cocaine cue-dependent responding under a second-order schedule of cocaine self-administration in rats (Pilla *et al.*, 1999). It remains to be seen whether such a compound is able to diminish the propensity of drug-associated cues to induce relapse to drug taking in otherwise abstinent cocaine or other drug abusers.

10.5 Conclusion

The results presented here, taken together with a growing literature, support the notion that functionally dissociable amygdala subsystems are involved in associative processes underlying both appetitive and aversive emotional behaviour. We have suggested that apparent discrepancies in the larger database can be resolved around the hypothesis that the CeA and its associated circuitry underlies simple conditioned motivational influences on behaviour, whereas the BLA provides a more complex representational role in emotionally charged decisions and voluntary behaviour. This analysis of amygdala function has wide-ranging implications for understanding the neural basis of emotional behaviour and its disorders, highlighted here by considering the importance of associative processes to the development and persistence of addiction to drugs.

Acknowledgements

The research summarized here was supported by an MRC Programme Grant No. G9537855 to B.J.E. and T.W.R.

References

Alderson, H.L., Robbins, T.W., and Everitt, B.J. (2000) Heroin self-administration under a second-order schedule of reinforcement: acquisition and maintenance of heroin-seeking behaviour in rats. *Psychopharmacology*, DOI10.1007/5002130000429.

Alderson, H.L., Robbins, T.W., and Everitt, B.J. The effects of excitotoxic lesions of the basolateral amygdala on the acquisition of heroin-seeking behaviour in rats. *Psychopharmacology*, in press.

Alheid, G.F. and Heimer, L. (1988) New perspectives in basal forebrain organization of special relevance for neuropsychiatric disorders: the striatopallidal, amygdaloid and corticopetal components of the substantia innominata. *Neuroscience*, 27, 1–39.

Amaral, D.G., Price, J.L., Pitkänen, A., and Carmichael, S.T. (1992) Anatomical organization of the primate amygdaloid complex. In *The Amygdala: Neurobiological Aspects of Emotion, Memory, and Mental Dysfunction* (ed. J.P. Aggleton), pp. 1–66. Wiley-Liss, New York.

Applegate, C.D., Frysinger, R.C., Kapp, B.S., and Gallagher, M. (1982) Multiple unit activity recorded from the amygdala central nucleus during Pavlovian heart rate conditioning in the rabbit. *Brain Research*, 238, 457–462.

Arroyo, M., Markou, A., Robbins, T.W., and Everitt, B.J. (1998) Acquisition, maintenance and reinstatement of intravenous cocaine self-administration under a second-order schedule of reinforcement in rats: effects of conditioned cues and continuous access to cocaine. *Psychopharmacology (Berlin)*, 140, 331–344.

Balleine, B. (1994) Asymmetrical interactions between thirst and hunger in Pavlovian-instrumental transfer. *Quarterly Journal of Experimental Psychology*, 47B, 211–231.

Bolles, R.C. and Fanselow, M.S. (1980) A perceptual–defensive–recuperative model of fear and pain. *Behavioral Brain Sciences*, 3, 291–323.

Breiter, H., Gollub, R., Weisskoff, R., Kennedy, D., Kanto, H., Gastfriend, D., Berke, J., Riorden, J., Mathew, T., Makris, N., Guimaraes, A., Rosen, B., and Hyman, S. (1996) Activation of human brain reward circuitry by cocaine observed using fMRI. *Society for Neuroscience Abstracts*, 22, 758.6.

Brown, E.E. and Fibiger, H.C. (1993) Differential effects of excitotoxic lesions of the amygdala on cocaine-induced conditioned locomotion and conditioned place preference. *Psychopharmacology*, 113, 123–130.

Brown, E.E., Robertson, G.S., and Fibiger, H.C. (1992) Evidence for conditional neuronal activation following exposure to a cocaine-paired environment: role of forebrain limbic structures. *Journal of Neuroscience*, 12, 4112–4121.

Burns, L.H., Everitt, B.J., and Robbins, T.W. (1999) Effects of excitotoxic lesions of the basolateral amygdala on conditional discrimination learning with primary and conditioned reinforcement. *Behavioural Brain Research*, 100, 123–133.

Burns, L.H., Robbins, T.W., and Everitt, B.J. (1993) Differential effects of excitotoxic lesions of the basolateral amygdala, ventral subiculum and medial prefrontal cortex on responding with conditioned reinforcement and locomotor activity potentiated by intra-accumbens infusions of D-amphetamine. *Behavioural Brain Research*, 55, 167–183.

Bussey, T.J., Everitt, B.J., and Robbins, T.W. (1997) Dissociable effects of cingulate and medial frontal cortex lesions on stimulus–reward learning using a novel Pavlovian autoshaping procedure for the rat: implications for the neurobiology of emotion. *Behavioral Neuroscience*, 111, 908–919.

Cador, M., Robbins, T.W., and Everitt, B.J. (1989) Involvement of the amygdala in stimulus–reward associations: interaction with the ventral striatum. *Neuroscience*, 30, 77–86.

Cahill, L., Weinberger, N.M., Roozendaal, B., and McGaugh, J.L. (1999) Is the amygdala a locus of 'conditioned fear'? Some questions and caveats. *Neuron*, 23, 227–228.

Caine, S.B., Heinrichs, S.C., Coffin, V.L., and Koob, G.F. (1995) Effects of the dopamine D-1 antagonist SCH 23390 microinjected into the accumbens, amygdala or striatum on cocaine self-administration in the rat. *Brain Research*, 692, 47–56.

Childress, A.R., Ehrman, R., Roohsenow, D.J., Robbins, S.J., and O'Brien, C.P. (1992) Classically conditioned factors in drug dependence. In *Substance Abuse: A Comprehensive Text Book* (eds W. Lowinson, P. Luiz, R.B. Millman, and J.G. Langard), pp. 56–69. Williams and Wilkins. Baltimore.

Childress, A.R., McLellan, A.T., Ehrman, R., and O'Brien, C.P. (1988) Classically conditioned responses in opioid and cocaine dependence: a role in relapse? *NIDA Research Monographs*, 84, 25–43.

Childress, A.R., McElgin, W., Mozley, P.D., and Obrien, C.P. (1999) Limbic activation during cue-induced craving for cocaine and for natural rewards. *Biological Psychiatry*, 45, 170.

Clugnet, M.-C. and LeDoux, J.E. (1990) Synaptic plasticity in fear conditioning circuits: induction of LTP in the lateral nucleus of the amygdala by stimulation of the medial geniculate body. *Journal of Neuroscience*, 10, 2818–2824.

Damasio, A.R. and Damasio, H. (1993) Cortical systems underlying knowledge retrieval: evidence from human lesion studies. In *Exploring Brain Functions: Models in Neuroscience* (eds T.A. Poggio and D.A. Glaser), pp. 233–248. John Wiley and Sons, Chichester, UK.

Davis, M. (1992a) The role of the amygdala in conditioned fear. In *The Amygdala: Neurobiological Aspects of Emotion, Memory, and Mental Dysfunction* (ed. J.P. Aggleton), pp. 255–306. Wiley-Liss, New York.

Davis, M. (1992b) The role of the amygdala in fear and anxiety. *Annual Review of Neuroscience*, 15, 353–75.

Davis, M. (1997) Neurobiology of fear responses: the role of the amygdala. *Journal of Neuropsychiatry and Clinical Neuroscience*, 9, 382–402.

De Olmos, J.S. and Heimer, L. (1999) The concepts of the ventral striatopallidal system and extended amygdala. *Annals of the New York Academy of Sciences*, 877, 1–32.

Di Chiara, G. (1998) A motivational learning hypothesis of the role of mesolimbic dopamine in compulsive drug use. *Journal of Psychopharmacology*, 12, 54–67.

Dickinson, A. (1994) Instrumental conditioning. In *Animal Learning and Cognition* (ed. N.J. Mackintosh), pp. 45–78. Academic Press, London.

Dickinson, A. and Dearing, M.F. (1979) Appetitive–aversive interactions and inhibitory processes. In *Mechanisms of Learning and Motivation* (eds A. Dickinson and R.A. Boakes), pp. 203–231. Erlbaum, Hillsdale, New Jersey.

Everitt, B.J. (1996) Drug cues and craving, actions and habits: the search for a neuropsychological basis of addiction. *Medical Research Council News*, Summer, 11–15.

Everitt, B.J. and Robbins, T.W. (1992) Amygdala–ventral striatal interactions and reward-related processes. In *The Amygdala: Neurobiological Aspects of Emotion, Memory, and Mental Dysfunction* (ed. J.P. Aggleton), pp. 401–430. Wiley-Liss, New York.

Everitt, B.J., Cador, M., and Robbins, T.W. (1989) Interactions between the amygdala and ventral striatum in stimulus–reward associations: studies using a second-order schedule of sexual reinforcement. *Neuroscience*, 30, 63–75.

Everitt, B.J., Morris, K.A., O'Brien, A., and Robbins, T.W. (1991) The basolateral amygdala–ventral striatal system and conditioned place preference: further evidence of limbic–striatal interactions underlying reward-related processes. *Neuroscience*, 42, 1–18.

Everitt, B.J., Parkinson, J.A., Olmstead, M.C., Arroyo, M., Robledo, P., and Robbins, T.W. (1999) Associative processes in addiction and reward: the role of amygdala–ventral striatal subsystems. *Annals of the New York Academy of Sciences*, 877, 412–438.

Fendt, M. and Fanselow, M.S. (1999) The neuroanatomical and neurochemical basis of conditioned fear. *Neuroscience and Biobehavioral Reviews*, 23, 743–760.

Freeman, J.H., Cuppernell, C., Flannery, K., and Gabriel, M. (1996) Limbic thalamic, cingulate cortical and hippocampal neuronal correlates of discriminative approach learning in rabbits. *Behavioural Brain Research*, 80, 123–136.

Fudge, J.L., and Haber, S.N. (2000) The central nucleus of the amygdala projection to dopamine subpopulations in primates. *Neuroscience*, **97**, 479–494.

Fuster, J.M. (1995) *Memory in the Cerebral Cortex: An Empirical Approach to Neural Networks in the Human and Nonhuman Primate*. MIT Press, Cambridge, Massachusetts.

Gabriel, M. (1990) Functions of anterior and posterior cingulate cortex during avoidance-learning in rabbits. *Progress in Brain Research*, 85, 467–483.

Gabriel, M., Vogt, B.A., Kubota, Y., Poremba, A., and Kang, E. (1991) Training-stage related neuronal plasticity in limbic thalamus and cingulate cortex during learning—a possible key to mnemonic retrieval. *Behavioural Brain Research*, 46, 175–185.

Gaffan, D. (1992) Amygdala and the memory of reward. In *The Amygdala: Neurobiological Aspects of Emotion, Memory, and Mental Dysfunction* (ed. J.P. Aggleton), pp. 471–484. Wiley-Liss, New York.

Gallagher, M. and Holland, P.C. (1992) Understanding the functions of the central nucleus: is simple conditioning enough? In *The Amygdala: Neurobiological Aspects of Emotion, Memory, and Mental Dysfunction* (ed. J.P. Aggleton), pp. 307–322. Wiley-Liss, New York.

Gallagher, M. and Holland, P.C. (1994) The amygdala complex: multiple roles in associative learning and attention. *Proceedings of the National Academy of Sciences of the United States of America*, 91, 11771–11776.

Gallagher, M., Graham, P.W., and Holland, P.C. (1990) The amygdala central nucleus and appetitive Pavlovian conditioning: lesions impair one class of conditioned behaviour. *Journal of Neuroscience*, 10, 1906–1911.

Gawin, F.H. (1991) Cocaine addiction: psychology and neurophysiology. *Science*, 251, 1580–1586.

Gewirtz, J.C. and Davis, M. (1998) Application of Pavlovian higher-order conditioning to the analysis of the neural substrates of fear conditioning. *Neuropharmacology*, 37, 453–459.

Goldberg, S.R. and Schuster, C.R. (1967) Conditioned suppression by a stimulus associated with nalorphine in post morphine-dependent monkeys. *Journal of the Experimental Analysis of Behavior*, 10, 235–242.

Grant, S., London, E.D., Newlin, D.B., Villemagne, V.L., Xiang, L., Contoreggi, C., Phillips, R.L., Kimes, A.S., and Margolin, A. (1996) Activation of memory circuits during cue-elicited cocaine craving. *Proceedings of the National Academy of Sciences of the United States of America*, 93, 12040–12045.

Groenewegen, H.J., Wright, C.I., and Beijer, A.V.J. (1996) The nucleus accumbens: gateway for limbic structures to reach the motor system? *Progress in Brain Research*, 107, 485–511.

Han, J.S., McMahan, R.W., Holland, P., and Gallagher, M. (1997) The role of an amygdalo-nigrostriatal pathway in associative learning. *Journal of Neuroscience*, 17, 3913–3919.

Han, J.S., Holland, P.C., and Gallagher, M. (2000) Disconnection of amygdala central nucleus and substantia innominata/nucleus basalis disrupts increments in conditioned stimulus processing. *Behavioral Neuroscience*, **113**, 143–151.

Hatfield, T., Han, J.S., Conley, M., Gallagher, M., and Holland, P. (1996) Neurotoxic lesions of basolateral, but not central, amygdala interfere with Pavlovian second-order conditioning and reinforcer devaluation effects. *Journal of Neuroscience*, 16, 5256–5265.

Hearst, E. and Jenkins, H.M. (1974) *Sign Tracking: The Stimulus–Reinforcer Relation and Directed Action*. Monograph of the Psychonomic Society.

Henke, P.G., Allen, J.D., and Davison, C. (1972) Effects of lesions in the amygdala on behavioral contrast. *Physiology and Behavior*, 8, 173–176.

Hiroi, N. and White, N.M. (1991) The lateral nucleus of the amygdala mediates expression of the amphetamine-produced conditioned place preference. *Journal of Neuroscience*, 11, 2107–2116.

Hitchcott, P.K. and Phillips, G.D. (1998) Double dissociation of the behavioural effects of R (+) 7-OH-DPAT infusions in the central and basolateral amygdala nuclei upon Pavlovian and instrumental conditioned appetitive behaviours. *Psychopharmacology*, 140, 458–69.

Hitchcott, P.K., Bonardi, C.M.T., and Phillips, G.D. (1997a) Enhanced stimulus–reward learning by intra-amygdala administration of a D-3 dopamine receptor agonist. *Psychopharmacology*, 133, 240–248.

Hitchcott, P.K., Harmer, C.J., and Phillips, G.D. (1997b) Enhanced acquisition of discriminative approach following intra-amygdala D-amphetamine. *Psychopharmacology*, 132, 237–246.

Holland, P.C. (1984) The origins of Pavlovian conditioned behavior. In *The Psychology of Learning and Motivation* (ed. G. Bower), pp. 129–173. Prentice-Hall, New York.

Holland, P.C. and Gallagher, M. (1999) Amygdala circuitry in attentional and representational processes. *Trends in Cognitive Sciences*, 3, 65–73.

Hurd, Y.L., McGregor, A., and Ponten, M. (1997) *In vivo* amygdala dopamine levels modulate cocaine self-administration behaviour in the rat: D1 dopamine receptor involvement. *European Journal of Neuroscience*, 9, 2541–2548.

Inglis, W.L., Olmstead, M.C., and Robbins, T.W. (2000) Pedunculopontine tegmental nucleus lesions impair stimulus–reward learning in autoshaping and conditioned reinforcement paradigms. *Behavioral Neuroscience*, 114, 285–294.

Kalivas, P.W. and Nakamura, M. (1999) Neural systems for behavioral activation and reward. *Current Opinion in Neurobiology*, 9, 223–227.

Kelley, A.E. and Domesick, V.B. (1982) The distribution of the projection from the hippocampal formation to the nucleus accumbens in the rat: an anterograde- and retrograde-horseradish peroxidase study. *Neuroscience*, 7, 2321–2335.

Kelley, A.E., Domesick, V.B., and Nauta, W.J.H. (1982) The amygdalostriatal projection in the rat—an anatomical study by anterograde and retrograde tracing methods. *Neuroscience*, 7, 615–630.

Killcross, A.S. (1998) Dissociable effects of excitotoxic lesions of amygdala sub-nuclei on appetitive conditioning. *Journal of Psychopharmacology*, 12, A4.

Killcross, S., Robbins, T.W., and Everitt, B.J. (1997a) Different types of fear-conditioned behaviour mediated by separate nuclei within amygdala. *Nature*, 388, 377–380.

Killcross, S., Robbins, T.W., and Everitt, B.J. (1997b) Is it time to invoke multiple fear systems in the amygdala?: A reply to Nader and LeDoux. *Trends in Cognitive Sciences*, 1, 244–247.

Klüver, H. and Bucy, P.C. (1939) Preliminary analysis of functions of the temporal lobes in monkeys. *Archives of Neurology and Psychiatry*, 8, 2153–2163.

Konorski, J. (1948) *Conditioned Reflexes and Neuron Organization*. Cambridge University Press, Cambridge, UK.

Konorski, J. (1967) *Integrative Activity of the Brain*. University of Chicago Press, Chicago, Illinois.

Koob, G.F. (1999) The role of the striatopallidal and extended amygdala systems in drug addiction. *Annals of the New York Academy of Sciences*, 877, 445–460.

Krettek, J.E. and Price, J.L. (1978) Amygdaloid projections to subcortical structures within the basal forebrain and brainstem in the rat and cat. *Journal of Comparative Neurology*, 178, 225–253.

Lagowska, J. and Fonberg, E. (1975) Salivary reactions in dogs with dorsomedial amygdalar lesions. *Acta Neurobiologiae Experimentalis*, 35, 17–26.

Lavond, D.G., Kim, J.J., and Thompson, R.F. (1993) Mammalian brain substrates of aversive classical conditioning. *Annual Reviews of Psychology*, 44, 317–342.

LeDoux, J. (1996) *The Emotional Brain*. Simon and Schuster, New York.

LeDoux, J.E., Iwata, J., Cicchetti, P., and Reid, D.J. (1988) Different projections of the central amygdaloid nucleus mediate autonomic and behavioral correlates of conditioned fear. *Journal of Neuroscience*, 8, 2517–2529.

LeDoux, J.E., Cicchetti, P., Xagoraris, A., and Romanski, L.M. (1990) The lateral amygdaloid nucleus: sensory interface of the amygdala in fear conditioning. *Journal of Neuroscience*, 10, 1062–1069.

Louilot, A., Simon, H., Taghzouti, K., and Le Moal, M. (1985) Modulation of dopaminergic activity in the nucleus accumbens following facilitation or blockade of the dopaminergic transmission in the amygdala: a study by *in vivo* differential pulse voltammetry. *Brain Research*, 346, 141–145.

Lovibond, P.F. (1983) Facilitation of instrumental behavior by a Pavlovian appetitive conditioned stimulus. *Journal of Experimental Psychology: Animal Behavior Processes*, 9, 225–247.

Mackintosh, N.J. (1974) *The Psychology of Animal Learning*. Academic Press, London.

Mackintosh, N.J. (1983) *Conditioning and Associative Learning*. Oxford University Press, Oxford.

Maren, S. (1996) Synaptic transmission and plasticity in the amygdala—an emerging physiology of fear conditioning circuits. *Molecular Neurobiology*, 13, 1–22.

Maren, S. and Fanselow, M.S. (1996) The amygdala and fear conditioning: has the nut been cracked? *Neuron*, 16, 237–240.

Maren, S., Aharonov, G., and Fanselow, M.S. (1997) Neurotoxic lesions of the dorsal hippocampus and Pavlovian fear conditioning in rats. *Behavioural Brain Research*, 88, 261–274.

McAlonan, G.M., Robbins, T.W., and Everitt, B.J. (1993) Effects of medial dorsal thalamic and ventral pallidal lesions on the acquisition of a conditioned place preference: further evidence for the involvement of the ventral striatopallidal system in reward-related processes. *Neuroscience*, 52, 605–620.

McDonald, A.J. (1998) Cortical pathways to the mammalian amygdala. *Progress in Neurobiology*, 55, 257–332.

McDonald, R.J. and White, N.M. (1993) A triple dissociation of memory systems: hippocampus, amygdala and dorsal striatum. *Behavioral Neuroscience*, 107, 3–22.

McGregor, A. and Roberts, D.C.S. (1993) Dopaminergic antagonism within the nucleus accumbens or the amygdala produces differential effects on intravenous cocaine self-administration under fixed and progressive ratio schedules of reinforcement. *Brain Research*, 624, 245–252.

McGregor, A., Baker, G., and Roberts, D.C.S. (1994) Effect of 6-hydroxydopamine lesions of the amygdala on intravenous cocaine self-administration under a progressive ratio schedule of reinforcement. *Brain Research*, 646, 273–278.

McKernan, M. and Shinnick-Gallagher, P. (1997) Fear conditioning induces a lasting potentiation of synaptic currents *in vitro*. *Nature*, 390, 604–607.

Meil, W.M. and See, R.E. (1997) Lesions of the basolateral amygdala abolish the ability of drug associated cues to reinstate responding during withdrawal from self-administered cocaine. *Behavioural Brain Research*, 88, 139–148.

Mogenson, G., Jones, D.L., and Yim, C.Y. (1984) From motivation to action: functional interface between the limbic system and the motor system. *Progress in Neurobiology*, 14, 69–97.

Nader, K. and LeDoux, J. (1997) Is it time to invoke multiple fear systems in the amygdala? *Trends in Cognitive Sciences*, 1, 241–243.

O'Brien, C.P. and McLellan, A.T. (1996) Myths about the treatment of addiction. *Lancet*, 347, 237–240.

O'Brien, C.P., Ehrman, R.N., and Ternes, J.W. (1986) Classical conditioning in human opioid dependence. In *Behavioral Analysis of Drug Dependence* (eds S.R. Goldberg and I.P. Stolerman), pp. 329–356. Academic Press, London.

O'Brien, C.P., Childress, A.R., McLellan, A.T., and Ehrman, R. (1992a) Classical conditioning in drug-dependent humans. *Annals of the New York Academy of Sciences*, 654, 400–415.

O'Brien, C.P., Childress, A.R., McLellan, A.T., and Ehrman, R. (1992b) A learning model of addiction. *Research Publications of the Association for Research on Nervous and Mental Diseases*, 70, 157–177.

Parkinson, J.A., Dally, J.W., Bamford, A., Fehrent, B., Robbins, T.W., and Everitt, B.J. (1998) Effects of 6-OHDA lesions of the rat nucleus accumbens on appetitive Pavlovian conditioning. *Journal of Psychopharmacology*, **12**, Supplement A, A8.

Parkinson, J.A., Olmstead, M.C., Burns, L.H., Robbins, T.W., and Everitt, B.J. (1999) Dissociation in effects of lesions of the nucleus accumbens core and shell on appetitive Pavlovian approach behavior and the potentiation of conditioned reinforcement and locomotor activity by D-amphetamine. *Journal of Neuroscience*, 19, 2401–2411.

Parkinson, J.A., Willoughby, P.J., Robbins, T.W., and Everitt, B.J. (2000a) Disconnection of the anterior cingulate cortex and nucleus accumbens core impairs Pavlovian approach behavior: further evidence for limbic cortico-ventral striatopallidal systems. *Behavioral Neuroscience*, 114, 42–63.

Parkinson, J.P., Robbins, T.W., and Everitt, B.J. (2000b) Dissociable roles of the central and basolateral amygdala in appetitive emotional learning. *European Journal of Neuroscience*, **12**, 405–413.

Parkinson, J.A., Cardinal, R.N., and Everitt, B.J. Limbic cortico-ventral striatal systems underlying appetitive conditioning. *Progress in Brain Research*, **126**, (eds Uylings, H.B.M., Van Eden, C.G., De Bruin, J.P.C., Feenstra, M.G.P., and Pennartz, C.M.A.). In press.

Pascoe, J.P. and Kapp, B.S. (1985a) Electrophysiological characteristics of amygdaloid central nucleus neurons during pavlovian fear conditioning in the rabbit. *Behavioral Brain Research*, 16, 117–133.

Pascoe, J.P. and Kapp, B.S. (1985b) Electrophysiological characteristics of amygdaloid central nucleus neurons in the awake rabbit. *Brain Research Bulletin*, 14, 331–338.

Phillips, A.G. and Fibiger, H.C. (1990) Role of reward and enhancement of conditioned reward in persistence of responding for cocaine. *Behavioural Pharmacology*, 1, 269–282.

Pierce, R.C. and Kalivas, P.W. (1997) A circuitry model of the expression of behavioral sensitization to amphetamine-like psychostimulants. *Brain Research Reviews*, 25, 192–216.

Pierce, R.C., Reeder, D.C., Hicks, J., Morgan, Z.R., and Kalivas, P.W. (1998) Ibotenic acid lesions of the dorsal prefrontal cortex disrupt the expression of behavioral sensitization to cocaine. *Neuroscience*, 82, 1103–1114.

Pilla, M., Perachon, S., Sautel, F., Garrido, F., Mann, A., Wermuth, C.G., Schwartz, J.-C., Everitt, B.J., and Sokoloff, P. (1999) Selective inhibition of cocaine-seeking behaviour by a partial dopamine D3 receptor agonist. *Nature*, 400, 371–375.

Price, J.L., Russchen, F.T., and Amaral, D. (1987) The limbic region. II. The amygdaloid complex. In *Handbook of Chemical Neuroanatomy, Volume 5: Integrated Systems of the CNS, Part 1* (eds A. Björklund, T. Hökfelt, and L.W. Swanson), pp. 279–388. Elsevier, Amsterdam.

Robbins, T.W. (1978) The acquisition of responding with conditioned reinforcement: effects of pipradrol, methylphenidate, D-amphetamine and nomifensine. *Psychopharmacology*, 58, 79–87.

Robbins, T.W. and Everitt, B.J. (1999) Drug addiction: bad habits add up. *Nature*, 398, 567–570.

Robbins, T.W., Cador, M., Taylor, J.R., and Everitt, B.J. (1989) Limbic–striatal interactions in reward-related processes. *Neuroscience and Biobehavioral Reviews*, 13, 155–162.

Robins, L.N., Helzer, J.E., and Davis, D.H. (1975) Narcotic use in southeast Asia and afterwards. *Archives of General Psychiatry*, 32, 955–961.

Robinson, T.E. and Berridge, K.C. (1993) The neural basis of drug craving—an incentive–sensitization theory of addiction. *Brain Research Reviews*, 18, 247–291.

Robledo, P., Robbins, T.W., and Everitt, B.J. (1996) Effects of excitotoxic lesions of the central amygdaloid nucleus on the potentiation of reward-related stimuli by intra-accumbens amphetamine. *Behavioral Neuroscience*, 110, 981–990.

Rolls, E.T. (1999) *The Brain and Emotion*. Oxford University Press, Oxford.

Roozendaal, B., Oldenburger, W.P., Strubbe, J.H., Koolhaas, J.M., and Bohus, B. (1990) The central amygdala is involved in the conditioned but not in the meal-induced cephalic insulin response in the rat. *Neuroscience Letters*, 116, 210–215.

Sarter, M. and Markowitsch, H. (1985) Involvement of the amygdala in learning and memory: a critical review with emphasis on anatomical relations. *Behavioral Neuroscience*, 99, 342–380.

Schoenbaum, G., Chiba, A.A., and Gallagher, M. (1998) Orbitofrontal cortex and basolateral amygdala encode expected outcomes during learning. *Nature Neuroscience*, 1, 155–159.

Schoenbaum, G., Chiba, A.A., and Gallagher, M. (1999) Neural encoding in orbitofrontal cortex and basolateral amygdala during olfactory discrimination learning. *Journal of Neuroscience*, 19, 1876–1884.

Schulteis, G., Ahmed, S.H., Morse, A.C., Koob, G.F., and Everitt, B.J. (2000) Conditioning and opiate withdrawal. *Nature*, **405**, 1013–1014.

Schwartzbaum, J.S. (1965) Discrimination behavior after amygdalectomy in monkeys: visual and somesthetic learning and perceptual capacity. *Journal of Comparative and Physiological Psychology*, 60, 314–319.

Selden, N.R.W., Everitt, B.J., Jarrard, L.E., and Robbins, T.W. (1991) Complementary roles for the amygdala and hippocampus in aversive conditioning to explicit and contextual cues. *Neuroscienc*e, 42, 335–350.

Simon, H., Taghzouti, K., Gozlan, H., Studler, J.M., Louilot, A., Herve, D., Glowinski, J., Tassin, J.P., and Le Moal, M. (1988) Lesion of dopaminergic terminals in the amygdala produces enhanced locomotor response to D-amphetamine and opposite changes in dopaminergic activity in prefrontal cortex and nucleus accumbens. *Brain Research*, 447, 335–340.

Smith, J.W. and Dickinson, A. (1998) The dopamine antagonist, pimozide, abolishes Pavlovian–instrumental transfer. *Journal of Psychopharmacology*, 12, A6.

Stewart, J., de Wit, H., and Eikelboom, R. (1984) The role of unconditioned and conditioned drug effects in the self administration of opiates and stimulants. *Psychological Reviews*, 91, 251–268.

Swanson, L.W. and Mogenson, G.J. (1981) Neural mechanisms for the functional coupling of autonomic, endocrine and somatomotor responses in adaptive behavior. *Brain Research Reviews*, 3, 1–34.

Swanson, L.W. and Petrovich, G.D. (1998) What is the amygdala? *Trends in Neurosciences*, 21, 323–331.

Taylor, J.R. and Robbins, T.W. (1984) Enhanced behavioural control by conditioned reinforcers following microinjections of D-amphetamine into the nucleus accumbens. *Psychopharmacology*, 84, 405–412.

Taylor, J.R. and Robbins, T.W. (1986) 6-Hydroxydopamine lesions of the nucleus accumbens, but not of the caudate nucleus, attenuate enhanced responding with reward-related stimuli produced by intra-accumbens D-amphetamine. *Psychopharmacology*, 90, 390–397.

Tomie, A. (1996) Locating reward cue at response manipulandum (CAM) induces symptoms of drug abuse. *Neuroscience and Biobehavioural Reviews*, 20, 505–535.

Tomie, A., Brooks, W., and Zito, B. (1989) Sign-tracking: the search for reward. In *Contemporary Learning Theories—Pavlovian Conditioning and the Status of Traditional Learning Theory* (eds S.B. Klein and R.R. Mowrer), pp. 191–226. Lawrence Erlbaum Associates. Hillsdale, New Jersey.

Trapold, M.A. (1970) Are expectancies based upon different positive reinforcing events discriminably different? *Learning and Motivation*, 1, 129–140.

Vazdarjanova, A. and McGaugh, J.L. (1998) Basolateral amygdala is not critical for cognitive memory of contextual fear conditioning. *Proceedings of the National Academy of Sciences of the United States of America*, 95, 15003–15007.

Vogt, B.A. (1985) Cingulate cortex. In *Cerebral Cortex* (eds E.G. Jones and A. Peters), pp. 89–149. Plenum Press, New York.

Volkow, N.D., Ding, Y.-S., Fowler, J.S., and Wang, G.-J. (1996) Cocaine addiction: hypothesis derived from imaging studies with PET. *Journal of Addictive Diseases*, 15, 55–71.

Volkow, N.D., Wang, G.J., Fischman, M.W., Foltin, R.W., Fowler, J.S., Abumrad, N.N., Vitkun, S., Logan, J., Gatley, S.J., Pappas, N., Hitzemann, R., and Shea, C.E. (1997a) Relationship between subjective effects of cocaine and dopamine transporter occupancy. *Nature*, 386, 827–830.

Volkow, N.D., Wang, G.J., Fowler, J.S., Logan, J., Gatley, S.J., Hitzemann, R., Chen, A.D., Dewey, S.L., and Pappas, N. (1997b) Decreased striatal dopaminergic responsiveness in detoxified cocaine-dependent subjects. *Nature*, 386, 830–833.

Walker, D.L. and Davis, M. (1997) Double dissociation between the involvement of the bed nucleus of the stria terminalis and the central nucleus of the amygdala in startle increases produced by conditioned versus unconditioned fear. *Journal of Neuroscience*, 17, 9375–9383.

Weiskrantz, L. (1956) Behavioral changes associated with ablation of the amygdaloid complex in monkeys. *Journal of Comparative and Physiological Psychology*, 49, 381–391.

Weissenborn, R., Robbins, T.W., and Everitt, B.J. (1997) Effects of medial prefrontal or anterior cingulate cortex lesions on responding for cocaine under fixed-ratio and second-order schedules of reinforcement in rats. *Psychopharmacology*, 134, 242–257.

Whitelaw, R.B., Markou, A., Robbins, T.W., and Everitt, B.J. (1996) Excitotoxic lesions of the basolateral amygdala impair the acquisition of cocaine-seeking behaviour under a second-order schedule of reinforcement. *Psychopharmacology*, 127, 213–224.

Wikler, A. (1965) Conditioning factors in opiate addiction and relapse. In *Narcotics* (eds D.I. Willner and G.G. Kassenbaum), pp. 7–21. McGraw-Hill, New York.

Williams, D.R. and Williams, H. (1969) Auto-maintenance in the pigeon: sustained pecking despite contingent non-reinforcement. *Journal of the Experimental Analysis of Behavior*, 12, 511–520.

Wolf, M.E. (1998) The role of excitatory amino acids in behavioral sensitization to psychomotor stimulants. *Progress in Neurobiology*, 54, 679–720.

Wolterink, G., Phillips, G., Cador, M., DonselaarWolterink, I., Robbins, T.W., and Everitt, B.J. (1993) Relative roles of ventral striatal D1 and D2 dopamine receptors in responding with conditioned reinforcement. *Psychopharmacology*, 110, 355–364.

Zahm, D.S., Jensen, S.L., Williams, E.S., and Martin, I.J.R. (1999) Direct comparison of projections from the central amygdaloid region and nucleus accumbens shell. *European Journal of Neuroscience*, 11, 1119–1126.

11 Amygdala: role in modulation of memory storage

James L. McGaugh, Barbara Ferry, Almira Vazdarjanova, and Benno Roozendaal

Center for the Neurobiology of Learning and Memory and Department of Neurobiology and Behavior, University of California, Irvine, CA 92697-3800, USA

Summary

This chapter reviews evidence from studies investigating the involvement of the amygdala in modulating the consolidation of long-term explicit/declarative memory. Extensive findings from animal experiments indicate that drugs of several classes, as well as the adrenal stress hormones adrenaline and corticosterone, modulate memory storage when administered post-training and that such effects critically involve activation of the basolateral amygdala (BLA). Lesions of the BLA block such modulatory influences on memory storage. Further, memory storage is modulated by post-training infusions of adrenergic and glucocorticoid agonists and antagonists administered selectively into the BLA. The memory-modulatory influences involve activation of β-adrenoceptors within the BLA and subsequent activation of other brain regions through projections mediated, primarily if not exclusively, by the stria terminalis. As lesions of the BLA do not prevent the learning or retention of the tasks used in these experiments, it is clear that this brain region is not essential for the learning and is not a likely neural locus of the explicit/declarative memory of the training experiences. Rather, our findings suggest that the BLA modulates the consolidation of explicit/declarative memory in other brain regions and that such modulation serves to ensure that the significance of experiences influences their remembrance.

11.1 Introduction

Interest in the role of the amygdala in learning and memory began over 60 years ago when Klüver and Bucy (1937) reported findings suggesting that damage to the temporal lobe of monkeys, including damage to the amygdala, produced disturbances attributable, at least in part, to disruption of memory processes. Subsequently, findings from many laboratories suggested that the amygdala may be involved in mediating the effects of reward and punishment, by enabling the learning of associations among stimuli or perhaps by serving as a locus of neural changes underlying emotionally influenced learning (Weiskrantz, 1956; Jones and Mishkin, 1972; Davis, 1992, Chapter 6; LeDoux, 1992, Chapter 7; McDonald and White 1993). There is now general agreement that the amygdala is involved in the learning of emotionally arousing information. Considerable evidence suggests, however, that lasting explicit/declarative memory for emotionally arousing information is stored in other brain regions and that activation of the amygdala modulates the storage of memory in those brain regions (McGaugh *et al.*, 1984, 1992, 1996; Weinberger *et al.*, 1990; Weinberger, 1995; Cahill and McGaugh, 1998; Cahill, Chapter 12). This chapter focuses on research addressing this issue in experiments with animals. Studies examining this issue in experiments with human subjects are reviewed by Cahill (Chapter 12).

11.2 Amygdala stimulation and modulation of memory storage

Much current research investigating the role of the amygdala in learning and memory has its origin in Goddard's finding (1964) that, in rats, electrical stimulation of the amygdala shortly after aversive training induced retrograde amnesia. Subsequent studies reported that post-training amygdala stimulation produced retrograde amnesia for training in a variety of aversively motivated learning tasks (Kesner and Doty, 1968; Gold *et al.*, 1974; Kesner and Wilburn, 1974; McGaugh and Gold, 1976).

One interpretation of such findings is that electrical stimulation disrupts memory storage processes localized within the amygdala. However, several findings challenge this interpretation. First, post-training electrical stimulation of the amygdala can either enhance or impair retention depending on the training conditions and stimulation intensity (Gold *et al.*, 1975). Furthermore, amygdala stimulation that induces retrograde amnesia in intact rats enhances memory in adrenally demedullated rats. However, as is shown in Table 11.1, the same stimulation induces amnesia in adrenally demedullated rats if adrenaline (epinephrine) is administered systemically prior to the stimulation (Liang *et al.*, 1985). These findings, together with other findings discussed below, indicate that peripheral adrenaline modulates amygdala activity. Secondly, lesions of the stria terminalis, a major amygdala pathway, and infusions of the opioid peptidergic antagonist naloxone into the bed nucleus of the stria terminalis block the amnesic effects of amygdala stimulation (Liang and McGaugh, 1983; Liang *et al.*, 1983). Such findings suggest that the effects of amygdala stimulation on memory storage are not due solely to alterations in neural activity induced at the site of stimulation. Rather, they suggest that stimulation-induced alterations in amygdala activity modulate memory storage processes occurring in other brain regions, especially, perhaps, those brain regions influenced either directly or indirectly via the stria terminalis pathway. These findings are consistent with Gerard's (1961) suggestion that, '. . . the amygdala (acts) directly on cortical neurones to alter . . . their responsiveness to the discrete impulses that reach the cortex . . .

Table 11.1 Adrenaline modulates the effects of post-training electrical stimulation of the amygdala on consolidation of memory for inhibitory avoidance and active avoidance training

Systemic injections before or after post-training electrical stimulation of the amygdala	*Memory on 24 h retention test*	
	Adrenal intact	*Adrenal demedullated*
Saline	Impaired	Enhanced
Adrenaline before stimulation	Impaired	Impaired
Adrenaline after stimulation		No effect

From Liang *et al.* (1985)

. . . these deep nuclei could easily modify the ease and completeness of experience fixation even if the nuclei were not themselves the loci of engrams.' (p. 30). We address this issue more extensively later in this chapter.

The use of post-training treatments to alter brain functioning shortly after training has provided a highly effective technique for examining the effects of various treatments, including drugs and hormones, on memory consolidation (McGaugh, 1966, 1989a; McGaugh and Herz, 1972; McGaugh and Gold, 1989). With the use of this paradigm, brain functioning is altered experimentally only after learning and, thus, the treatments do not influence acquisition or directly affect subsequent retention performance. Findings from our laboratory first reported several decades ago indicated that post-training injections of stimulant drugs enhance long-term memory when administered shortly after training (Breen and McGaugh, 1961; McGaugh, 1966, 1968, 1973, 1989a; McGaugh and Herz, 1972). Such findings strongly support the hypothesis that the drugs enhance memory by modulating the consolidation of recently acquired information. Additionally, as is discussed below, there is now considerable evidence indicating that such drug effects on memory consolidation are mediated by influences involving the amygdaloid complex.

11.3 Hormonal modulation of memory storage

Hormones of the adrenal medulla and adrenal cortex are released during and immediately after stressful stimulation of the kinds used in aversively motivated learning tasks (McCarty and Gold, 1981; McGaugh and Gold, 1989). Extensive findings indicate that adrenal stress hormones modulate memory storage and that the modulation is mediated by influences involving the amygdaloid complex (Gold and McGaugh, 1975; McGaugh, 1983a,b; McGaugh and Gold, 1989; McGaugh *et al.*, 1984, 1996; Roozendaal, 2000).

To our knowledge, Gerard (1961) was the first to suggest that the adrenal medullary hormone adrenaline might have enhancing effects on memory storage comparable with those of stimulant drugs. Gerard proposed that as, '. . . epinephrine . . . is released in vivid emotional experiences, such an intense adventure should be highly memorable.' (p. 30). In support of this suggestion, Gold and van Buskirk (1975) found that systemic post-training injections of adrenaline administered to rats enhance long-term retention of inhibitory avoidance. As with stimulant drugs, the memory enhancement was greatest when the injections were administered shortly after training. These findings, which have been confirmed by experiments using many different types of training tasks, support the hypothesis that endogenously released adrenaline modulates memory storage (Izquierdo and Diaz, 1985; Sternberg *et al.*, 1985; Introini-Collison and McGaugh, 1986a; Liang *et al.*, 1986; Liang, 2000; Williams, 2000).

Adrenocortical hormones are also involved in modulating memory storage (for reviews, see de Kloet, 1991; Bohus, 1994; McEwen and Sapolsky, 1995; Lupien and McEwen, 1997; Roozendaal, 2000). As with adrenaline, post-training administration of moderate doses of glucocorticoids induces dose- and time-dependent modulation of memory storage (Cottrell and Nakajima, 1977; Sandi and Rose, 1994; Roozendaal and McGaugh, 1996a). The memory-modulating effects of glucocorticoids appear to involve selective activation of glucocorticoid receptors (Oitzl and de Kloet, 1992; Roozendaal *et al.*, 1996; Lupien and McEwen, 1997). Such findings strongly suggest that glucocorticoids released by emotionally arousing experiences enhance the consolidation of the memory for the experiences (Roozendaal *et al.*, 1997; Roozendaal, 2000).

The dose–response curves obtained with memory-enhancing drugs and hormones are generally in the form of an inverted U. Memory enhancement generally is found with low to moderate doses and either no effect or memory impairment is found with high doses. The memory impairment, like the memory enhancement, appears to be due to effects on memory consolidation. Available evidence indicates that the memory-enhancing and memory-impairing effects are permanent and are not due to state dependency (e.g. Introini-Collison and McGaugh, 1986b; Castellano and McGaugh, 1989a,b). It is not known whether high levels of stress-released endogenous stress hormones can induce retrograde amnesia. Although available evidence suggests that they do not, this issue is worthy of further study.

11.4 Amygdala mediation of neuromodulatory influences on memory storage

As briefly noted above, findings of many studies indicate that the amygdala is critically involved in mediating adrenaline and glucocorticoid effects on memory. Although these adrenal hormones differ in the routes by which they influence the amygdala, they have remarkably similar effects on memory consolidation. Furthermore, as is discussed below, activation of noradrenaline (NA) release in the amygdala appears to be an essential step in mediating the effects of peripheral adrenaline as well as those of glucocorticoids on memory storage.

The idea that emotional activation may influence memory storage has a long history (Conway, 1995). As indicated above, Gerard (1961) suggested that release of adrenaline may play a role. Kety (1972) subsequently suggested that NA release in the brain may regulate memory consolidation. As Kety put it, 'If the emotional state accompanying the . . . outcome of behaviors could produce generalized intracerebral release of a trophic neurogenic substance, an additional adaptation might be subserved, i.e., the transcription into a more permanent form of the present and immediately preceding states of neuronal activation where the outcome had been significant to the organism (p. 71). This hypothesis would predict that drugs which release or enhance noradrenaline in the brain would favor consolidation and facilitate memory (p. 74).' Gold and van Buskirk's finding (1978) that adrenaline and footshock induce the release of NA in the forebrain of rats provided evidence consistent with Gerard's and Kety's suggestions. More specifically, recent evidence now indicates that NA release within the amygdala is of critical importance in enabling neuromodulatory influences on memory storage.

As discussed above, our interest in investigating the amygdala as a brain site involved in mediating adrenaline effects on memory was guided by evidence that: (i) electrical stimulation of the amygdala modulates memory storage (McGaugh and Gold, 1976); (ii) adrenal demedullation alters the memory-modulating effects of electrical stimulation of the amygdala (Liang *et al.*, 1985); and (iii) lesions of the amygdala or the stria terminalis block adrenaline effects on memory storage (Liang and McGaugh, 1983; Cahill and McGaugh, 1991). The findings that post-training intra-amygdala infusions of the β-adrenoceptor antagonist propranolol block adrenaline effects on memory storage (Liang *et al.*, 1986) and that post-training infusions of NA or the β-adrenoceptor agonist clenbuterol into the amygdala produce dose-dependent enhancement of memory storage (Liang *et al.*, 1986, 1990, 1995; Introini-Collison *et al.*, 1991, 1996; Ferry and McGaugh, 1999; Hatfield and McGaugh, 1999) provide strong support for the hypothesis that the amygdala plays a critical role in memory consolidation. As these amygdala influences are blocked by lesions of the stria terminalis, they are probably due to activation of amygdala efferents (Liang *et al.*, 1990; Introini-Collison *et al.*, 1991). Post-training infusions of β-adrenoceptor antagonists impair retention and block the memory-enhancing effects of NA administered into the amygdala concurrently (Liang *et al.*, 1986, 1995; Salinas *et al.*, 1997; Hatfield and McGaugh, 1999). Additionally, intra-amygdala infusions of the noradrenergic neurotoxin DSP4 impair memory for inhibitory avoidance training and the impairment is attenuated by post-training intra-amygdala infusions of NA (Liang, 1998). The finding that peripherally administered adrenaline does not attenuate the memory impairment induced by DSP4 indicates that peripheral adrenaline does not directly activate adrenoceptors in the amygdala (Liang, 1998, in press). Direct activation would not, of course, be expected as adrenaline passes the blood–brain barrier poorly, if at all (Weil-Malherbe *et al.*, 1959).

This evidence of a critical role for adrenoceptor activation in the amygdala suggests that footshock stimulation similar to that typically used in inhibitory avoidance training should induce the release of NA in the amygdala. The results of experiments using *in vivo* microdialysis and high-performance liquid chromatography (HPLC) strongly support this implication (Galvez *et al.*, 1996). As is shown in Figure 11.1, NA is released in the amygdala following footshock stimulation and the amount released varies directly with the intensity of stimulation (Quirarte *et al.*, 1998). Furthermore, peripheral injections of adrenaline activate the release of NA in the amygdala (Williams *et al.*, 1998; Williams, 2000). The finding that the opioid peptidergic antagonist naloxone potentiates NA release induced by footshock (Quirarte *et al.*, 1998) is consistent with evidence that intra-amygdala infusions of β-adrenoceptor antagonists block naloxone-induced enhancement of memory storage (McGaugh *et al.*, 1988; Introini-Collison *et al.*, 1989). Additionally, the findings that the GABAergic antagonist bicuculline

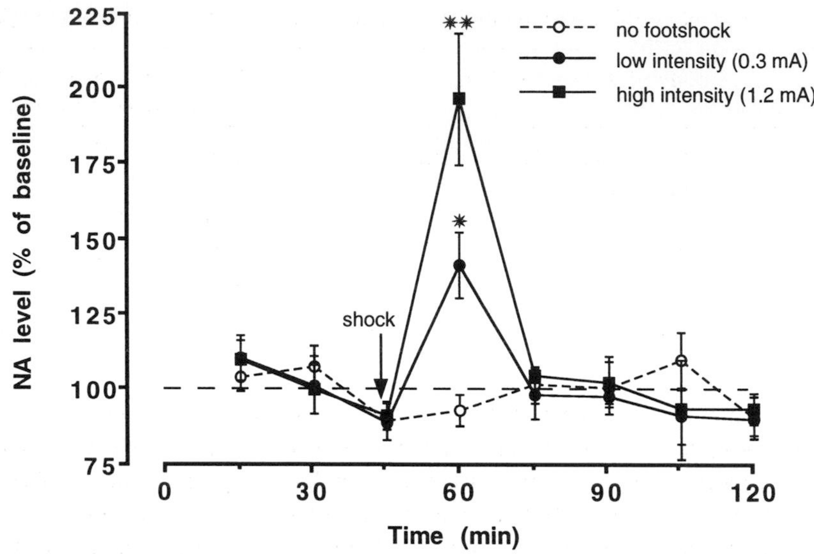

Figure 11.1 Effects of low- and high-intensity footshock on noradrenaline release in the amygdala assessed by *in vivo* microdialysis and HPLC. Noradrenaline levels are expressed as the mean (±SEM) of basal levels prior to footshock. *P <0.05; **P <0.01 as compared with the no footshock group. (From Quirarte *et al.*, 1998, with permission.)

enhances NA release and that the GABAergic agonist muscimol impairs NA release (Hatfield *et al.*, 1999) are consistent with extensive evidence that GABAergic agonists and antagonists impair and enhance memory storage, respectively (Breen and McGaugh, 1961; Castellano and McGaugh, 1990; Ammassari-Teule *et al.*, 1991), (see Table 11.2).

In the periphery, β-adrenoceptors are located on vagal afferents that project to the nucleus of the solitary tract located in the brainstem (Schreurs *et al.*, 1986). Projections from the nucleus of the solitary tract are known to release NA within the amygdala (Ricardo and Koh, 1978). As adrenaline does not readily pass the blood–brain barrier, it seems likely that adrenaline effects on memory storage are initiated by activation of peripheral β-adrenoceptors on vagal afferents. In support of this hypothesis, inactivation of the nucleus of the solitary tract with lidocaine blocks adrenaline effects on memory storage (Williams and McGaugh, 1993). Additionally, in humans as well as in rats, post-training electrical stimulation of vagal afferents enhances memory storage (Clark *et al.*, 1995, 1999; Jensen, in press). Considered together, these findings thus provide strong support for the hypothesis that adrenaline effects on memory involve noradrenergic projections from the nucleus of the solitary tract to the amygdala. Noradrenergic projections from the locus coeruleus also influence memory storage (Liang and Chiang, 1994). Post-training infusions of the α_2-adrenoceptor agonist clonidine into the locus coeruleus impaired inhibitory avoidance retention, and NA infused into the amygdala attenuated the memory impairment. Furthermore, a low and otherwise ineffective dose of clonidine infused into the locus coeruleus blocked the effects of

Table 11.2 Treatment effects on memory storage and amygdala noradrenaline release

Treatment	*Effect on memory storage*	*Effect on amygdala noradrenaline release*
Footshock	Varies directly with FS intensity	Increases
Adrenaline	Enhances	Increases
Picrotoxin	Enhances	Increases
Muscimol	Impairs	Decreases
Naloxone	Enhances	Increases
β-Endorphin	Impairs	Decreases

systemically administered adrenaline on memory. Additionally, intra-locus coeruleus infusions of the α_2-adrenoceptor antagonist yohimbine enhanced retention and the enhancement was attenuated by intra-amygdala infusions of propranolol (Liang and Chiang, 1994). It seems likely that the locus coeruleus effects on memory are influenced by activation of the nucleus of the solitary tract as this latter nucleus projects to the nucleus paragigantocellularis which is known to provide the major excitatory afferents to the locus coeruleus.

In an extensive series of experiments, Gold and his colleagues (Gold, 1988, 1995) have found that post-training administration of glucose enhances memory consolidation. As it is well established that adrenaline induces the release of glucose, Gold has proposed that adrenaline effects on memory may be due, at least in part, to the effects of glucose on neuronal functioning. Because glucose readily passes the blood–brain barrier, it might be that glucose directly activates critical neuronal systems in the amygdala. In support of this view, Ragozzino and Gold (1994) reported that glucose infused into the amygdala after inhibitory avoidance training blocked the memory-impairing effects of morphine infused into the amygdala prior to training. However, unlike the effects of adrenoceptor agonists, glucose infused into the amygdala post-training did not attenuate the memory-impairing effects of the β-adrenoceptor antagonist propranolol administered prior to training (McNay and Gold, 1998). Such findings suggest that although glucose can influence amygdala functioning in memory, glucose effects on memory for aversive training seem not to be mediated by noradrenergic influences within the amygdala.

Other recent findings from our laboratory indicate that the amygdala is involved in mediating glucocorticoid influences on memory storage (Roozendaal, 2000). Lesions of the stria terminalis or of the amygdala block the memory-enhancing effects of post-training systemic injections of the synthetic glucocorticoid dexamethasone (Roozendaal and McGaugh, 1996a,b). Furthermore, as is discussed below, post-training infusions of glucocorticoids into specific amygdala nuclei modulate memory storage (Roozendaal and McGaugh, 1997a). These glucocorticoid effects, like those of adrenaline, involve noradrenergic activation in the amygdala.

Noradrenergic activation in the amygdala is also critical for other neuromodulatory influences on memory storage. As noted above, post-training systemic injections of opioid peptides and opiates generally impair memory storage and opiate antagonists enhance memory storage

(Izquierdo and Diaz, 1983; McGaugh, 1989b; McGaugh *et al.*, 1993). GABAergic antagonists and agonists administered post-training enhance and impair retention, respectively (Brioni and McGaugh, 1988; Brioni *et al.*, 1989). As we found with adrenergic and glucocorticoid influences, lesions of the amygdala or stria terminalis block opioid peptidergic and GABAergic influences on memory storage (McGaugh *et al.*, 1986; Ammassari-Teule *et al.*, 1991). Additionally, and perhaps most importantly, intra-amygdala infusions of the β-adrenoceptor antagonist propranolol block opioid peptidergic and GABAergic influences on memory storage (McGaugh *et al.*, 1988; Introini-Collison *et al.*, 1989). Furthermore, in experiments using both inhibitory avoidance and water maze spatial tasks, intra-amygdala infusions of the β-adrenoceptor agonist clenbuterol blocked the memory-impairing effects of β-endorphin administered concurrently (Introini-Collison *et al.*, 1995). These neuromodulatory interactions within the amygdala, as well as those discussed below, are summarized schematically in Figure 11.2.

Although many of our experiments have used inhibitory avoidance training, experiments using other training tasks have yielded highly similar findings. Several experiments examined

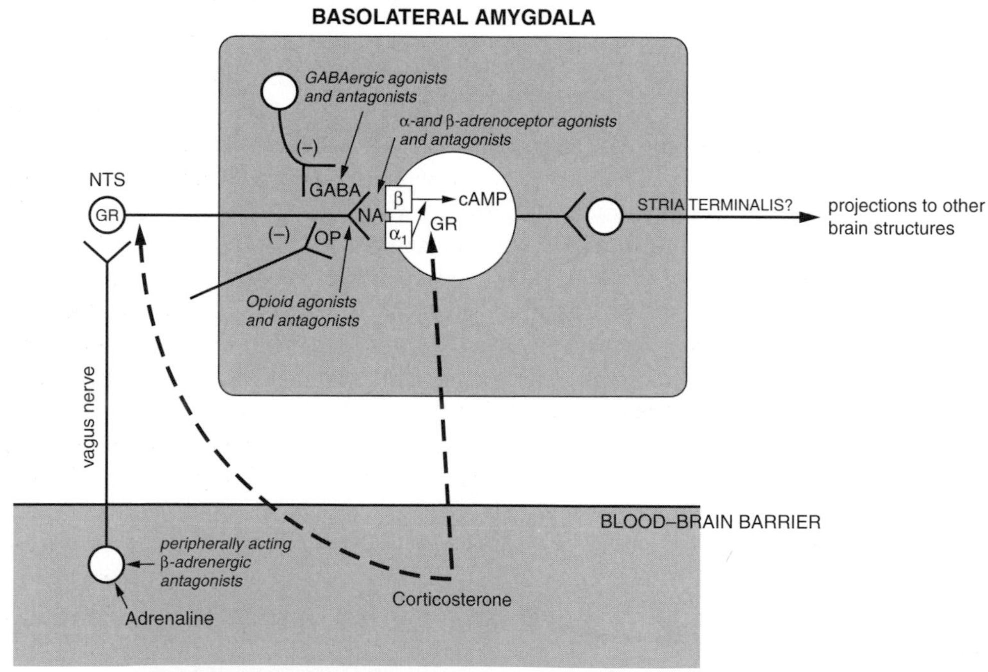

Figure 11.2 Schematic summarizing the interactions of neuromodulatory influences in the basolateral amygdala on memory storage as suggested by the findings of our experiments. (Abbreviations: α_1 = α_1-adrenoceptor; β = β-adrenoceptor; cAMP = cyclic 3'5'adenosine monophosphate; GR = glucocorticoid receptor; NA = noradrenaline; NTS = nucleus of the solitary tract; OP = opioids.)

the involvement of the amygdala in memory for a change in reward magnitude (CRM). Rats were first trained for several days to run in a straight alley for a large reward (10 pellets of food) and the reward was then reduced to one pellet. Slower running speeds seen on the following day indicated that the rats remembered the reduction in reward magnitude. As with other types of training, post-training administration of drugs influence memory for CRM. Post-training systemic administration of the peripherally acting drug, 4-hydroxyamphetamine enhanced memory (Salinas *et al.*, 1996), whereas the GABAergic agonist muscimol impaired memory (Salinas and McGaugh, 1995). More importantly, other findings indicate that memory for CRM involves the amygdala. Post-training intra-amygdala infusions of muscimol, lidocaine, or propranolol impaired memory for CRM (Salinas *et al.*, 1993, 1997; Salinas and McGaugh, 1995). Additionally, post-training intra-amygdala infusions of the GABAergic antagonist bicuculline enhanced memory for an increase in reward magnitude (Salinas and McGaugh, 1996). These latter findings provide additional evidence that amygdala influences on memory storage are not restricted to the learning of aversive information.

11.5 Selective involvement of the basolateral nucleus

Considerable evidence suggests that two of the amygdala nuclei, the basolateral (BLA) and central (CeA) nuclei, are most critically involved in aversively based learning (Davis, 1992; LeDoux, 1995; Killcross *et al.*, 1997). However, the findings of a series of experiments (see Table 11.3) indicate that one of these nuclei, the BLA, is involved selectively in modulating memory storage. Studies investigating the effects of benzodiazepines (BZDs) on memory provided the initial evidence suggesting a selective involvement of the BLA. It is well established that the memory-impairing effects of BZDs involve potentiation of GABAergic mechanisms in the amygdala (Izquierdo *et al.*, 1990a,b). Selective lesions of the BLA block BZD-induced amnesia (Tomaz *et al.*, 1992) and infusions of a BZD selectively into the BLA induce amnesia (de Souza-Silva and Tomaz, 1995). Furthermore, post-training intra-amygdala infusions of the BZD antagonist flumazenil enhance memory when administered selectively into the BLA (Da Cunha *et al.*, 1999).

Studies of the effects of post-training inactivation of amygdala nuclei with lidocaine provide additional evidence that the BLA is involved selectively in modulating memory storage. Lidocaine infused into the BLA immediately after inhibitory avoidance training impairs retention, whereas infusions into the CeA are ineffective (Parent and McGaugh, 1994). Post-training infusions of lidocaine into the BLA also impair memory for contextual fear conditioning (Vazdarjanova and McGaugh, 1999). Post-training infusions of clenbuterol into the BLA enhance inhibitory avoidance retention (Ferry and McGaugh, 1999). Noradrenergic influences on memory storage for spatial training in a water maze also selectively involve the BLA. Post-training infusions of NA into the BLA enhance spatial memory, whereas infusions of propranolol into the BLA impair spatial memory (Hatfield and McGaugh, 1999).

Glucocorticoid influences on memory storage also selectively involve the BLA. As is shown in Figure 11.3A, lesions of the amygdala restricted selectively to the BLA block the memory-enhancing effects of post-training systemic injections of the synthetic glucocorticoid

Table 11.3 Selective involvement of the basolateral amygdala in memory modulation

Amygdala treatment	*Task*	*Basolateral nucleus*	*Central nucleus*	*Reference*
Infusion of lidocaine, post-training	IA	Impairs memory	No effect	Parent and McGaugh (1994)
	CFC	Impairs memory	Not tested	Vazdarjanova and McGaugh (1999)
Infusion of glucocorticoid receptor agonist, post-training,	IA	Enhances memory	No effect	Roozendaal and McGaugh
or antagonist, pre-training	WM	Impairs memory	No effect	(1997a)
Infusion of diazepam, pre-training	IA	Impairs memory	No effect	Tomaz *et al.* (1993)
Infusion of benzodiazepine antagonist, post-training	IA	Enhances memory	No effect	DaCunha *et al.* (1999)
Infusion of muscarinic cholinergic agonist, post-training	CFC	Enhances memory	Not tested	Vazdarjanova and McGaugh (1999)
Infusion of noradrenaline or	WM	Enhances memory	No effect	Hatfield and McGaugh
β-adrenoceptor antagonist, post-training		Impairs memory	No effect	(1999)
Infusion of β-adrenoceptor agonist, post-training	IA	Enhances memory	Not tested	Ferry and McGaugh (1999)
Infusion of α_1-adrenoceptor agonist, post-training	IA	Enhances memory	Not tested	Ferry *et al.* (1999a)
Infusion of α_1-adrenoceptor agonist; β-adrenoceptor antagonist	IA	Blocks enhancement	Not tested	Ferry *et al.* (1999a)
or β-adrenoceptor agonist; α_1-adrenoceptor antagonist		Attenuates enhancement	Not tested	Ferry *et al.* (1999b)
Infusion of β-adrenoceptor antagonist, pre-training; systemic glucocorticoid, post-training	IA	Blocks enhancement	No effect	Quirarte *et al.* (1997a)
Infusion of muscarinic cholinergic antagonist; systemic glucocorticoid, post-training	IA	Blocks enhancement	Not tested	Power *et al.* (in press)
Lesions of AC nuclei; adrenalectomy	WM	Blocks impairment	No effect	Roozendaal *et al.* (1996)
Lesions of AC nuclei; post-training systemic glucocorticoid	IA	Blocks enhancement	No effect	Roozendaal and McGaugh (1996a)
Lesions of AC nuclei; pre-training systemic diazepam	IA	Blocks impairment	No effect	Tomaz *et al.* (1992)
Lesions of AC nuclei; infusion of glucocorticoid receptor	IA	Blocks enhancement	No effect	Roozendaal and McGaugh
agonist or antagonist into hippocampus	WM	Blocks impairment	No effect	(1997b)

IA = inhibitory avoidance, CFC = contextual fear conditioning, WM = water maze, AC = amygdaloid complex.

dexamethasone (Roozendaal and McGaugh, 1996a). Furthermore, post-training infusions of the specific glucocorticoid receptor agonist RU 28362 enhance retention when administered selectively into the BLA (Figure 11.3B) (Roozendaal and McGaugh, 1997a). Selective lesions of the BLA also block glucocorticoid effects on memory for water maze spatial learning (Roozendaal *et al.*, 1996). Adrenalectomy several days prior to training impaired memory

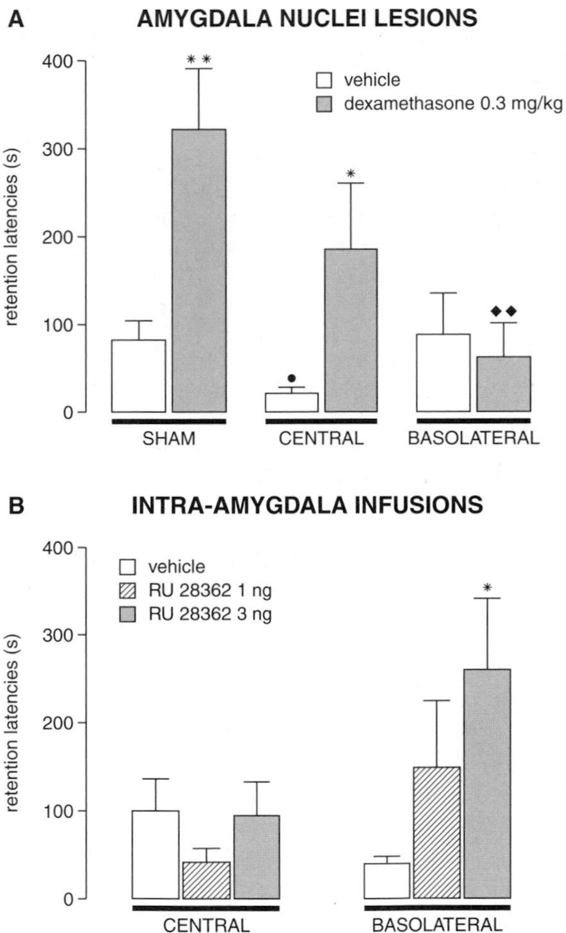

Figure 11.3 Step-through latencies (mean ± SEM) for a 48 h inhibitory avoidance test. (**A**) Rats with sham lesions, or lesions of either the central or basolateral nucleus of the amygdala had been treated with dexamethasone (0.3 mg/kg, s.c.) or vehicle immediately after training. (**B**) Rats received post-training infusions of the glucocorticoid receptor agonist RU 28362 (1.0 or 3.0 ng in 0.2 μl) into the central or basolateral nucleus. $^*P < 0.05$; $^{**}P < 0.01$ as compared with the corresponding vehicle group; $\bullet P < 0.05$ as compared with the corresponding sham lesion–vehicle group; $\blacklozenge\blacklozenge P < 0.01$ as compared with the corresponding sham lesion–dexamethasone group. (From Roozendaal and McGaugh, 1996a, 1997a, with permission.)

in this task, and immediate post-training dexamethasone attenuated the impairment. Additionally, BLA lesions block the effect of both adrenalectomy and glucocorticoids on memory storage. In contrast, lesions of the CeA impair acquisition and retention performance but do not block the glucocorticoid-induced modulation of memory storage (Roozendaal and McGaugh, 1996a; Roozendaal *et al.*, 1996).

Glucocorticoid influences on memory storage depend critically on activation of β-adrenergic mechanisms in the BLA. β-Adrenoceptor antagonists infused selectively into the BLA block the memory-enhancing effects of post-training systemic dexamethasone (Figure 11.4) (Quirarte *et al.*, 1997a). Glucocorticoid effects on memory storage also appear to depend on activation of glucocorticoid receptors in the ascending noradrenergic cell groups in the brainstem that are known to have high densities of glucocorticoid receptors (Harfstrand *et al.*, 1986). As discussed above, noradrenergic projections from the nucleus of the solitary tract (as well as the locus coeruleus) activate the amygdala. We recently found that post-training infusions of the glucocorticoid receptor agonist RU 28362 into the nucleus of the solitary tract enhanced memory for inhibitory avoidance training (Roozendaal *et al.*, 1999). Moreover, and most importantly, infusions of the β-adrenoceptor antagonist atenolol into the BLA blocked the memory enhancement. Other findings (Figure 11.5) provide further evidence that the BLA is a locus of interaction between glucocorticoids and noradrenergic activation affecting memory storage. Infusions of a glucocorticoid receptor antagonist into the BLA attenuated the memory-enhancing effect of clenbuterol infused into the BLA concurrently (Quirarte *et al.*, 1997b). Glucocorticoid receptor activation in the BLA thus appears to influence the effectiveness of β-adrenoceptor stimulation in modulating memory storage. Evidence

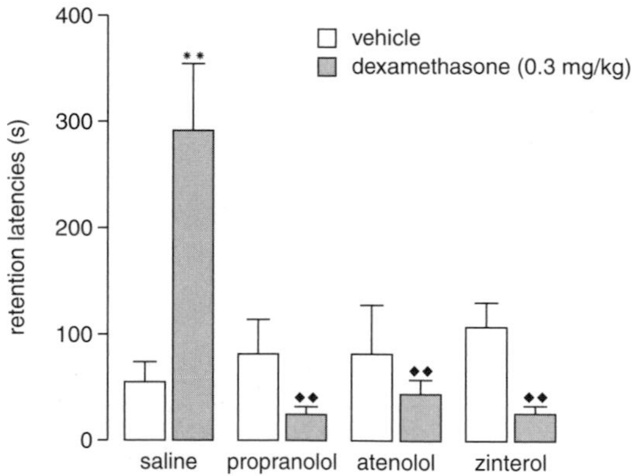

Figure 11.4 Step-through latencies (mean ± SEM) for a 48 h inhibitory avoidance test. Effects of pre-training infusions of either the non-specific β-adrenoceptor antagonist propranolol (0.5 μg in 0.2 μl), the β_1-adrenoceptor antagonist atenolol (0.5 μg in 0.2 μl), or the β_2-adrenoceptor antagonist zinterol (0.5 μg in 0.2 μl) into the basolateral amygdala and immediate post-training injections of dexamethasone (0.3 mg/kg, s.c.). $^{**}P < 0.01$ as compared with the corresponding vehicle group; ◆◆$P < 0.01$ as compared with the corresponding saline–dexamethasone group. (From Quirarte *et al.*, 1997a, with permission.)

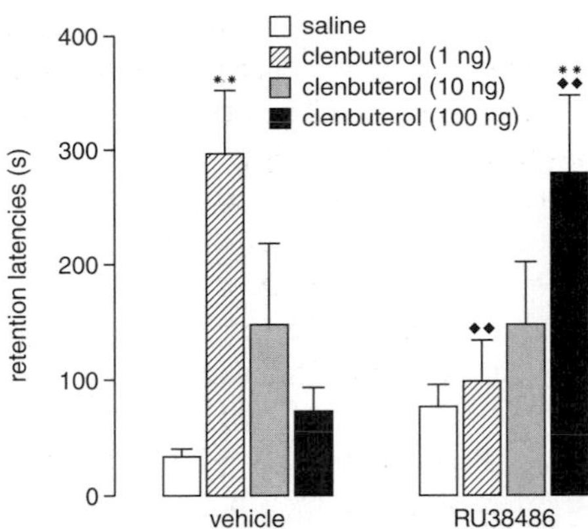

Figure 11.5 Step-through latencies (mean ± SEM) for a 48 h inhibitory avoidance test. Effects of pre-training infusions of the specific glucocorticoid receptor antagonist RU 38486 (1.0 ng in 0.2 μl) into the basolateral amygdala and immediate post-training infusions of the β-adrenoceptor agonist clenbuterol (1, 10, or 100 ng in 0.2 μl) into the basolateral amygdala. $^{**}P < 0.01$ as compared with the corresponding saline group; ◆◆$P < 0.01$ as compared with the corresponding vehicle–clenbuterol group. (From Quirarte *et al.*, 1997b, with permission.).

that glucocorticoids interact with the noradrenergic system in regulating memory storage is consistent with evidence from biochemical studies examining such interactions in other brain regions (McEwen, 1987).

11.6 α- and β-adrenergic interactions in the BLA

Although our research has focused primarily on the involvement of β-adrenergic activation within the BLA in memory storage, recent findings from our laboratory indicate that α-adrenoceptors within the BLA, in a close interaction with β-adrenergic mechanisms, are also involved in regulating memory storage processes. The amygdala contains a high density of α-adrenoceptor subtypes (Unnerstal *et al.*, 1984; Zilles *et al.*, 1993). Post-training intra-BLA infusions of low doses of the non-selective α-adrenoceptor agonist phexylephrine did not significantly affect inhibitory avoidance retention (Ferry *et al.*, 1999a). However, post-training intra-BLA infusions of phenylephrine together with the presynaptic α_2-adrenoceptor antagonist yohimbine enhanced retention, whereas infusions of the selective α_1-adrenoceptors antagonist prazosin impaired retention. These findings suggest that activation of α_1-adrenoceptor enhances memory storage and that activation of presynaptic α_2-adrenoceptors impairs memory storage. This hypothesis is consistent with evidence that activation of presynaptic α_2-adrenoceptors blocks NA release (Langer, 1974; Starke, 1979).

The α_1-adrenergic influence on memory appears to be mediated by an interaction with β-adrenoceptors within the BLA. As is shown in Figure 11.6, post-training intra-BLA infusions of the β-adrenoceptor antagonist atenolol blocked the memory enhancement induced by selective activation of α_1-adrenoceptors (Ferry *et al.*, 1999a). Additionally, intra-BLA infusions of the α_1-adrenoceptor antagonist prazosin shifted the dose–response memory-enhancing effects of the β-adrenoceptor agonist clenbuterol to the right when both drugs were infused together post-training (Figure 11.7A) (Ferry *et al.*, 1999b). These results suggest that α_1-adrenergic activity in the BLA facilitates the effects of β-adrenergic activation on memory formation. Previously, Liang and his colleagues (Liang *et al.*, 1995) reported that infusions of the synthetic cAMP analogue 8-bromo-cAMP administered into the amygdala post-training enhanced inhibitory avoidance retention. In our studies, we found that infusions of 8-bromo-cAMP administered selectively into the BLA enhanced retention in a manner similar to that found with clenbuterol. However, as is shown in Figure 11.7B, prazosin did not shift the dose–response effects induced by 8-bromo-cAMP (Ferry *et al.*, 1999b). These findings are consistent with pharmacological evidence suggesting that β-adrenoceptors modulate memory storage by a direct coupling to adenylate cyclase. α_1-Adrenoceptors may act indirectly on this process by influencing the β-adrenergic-induced synthesis of cAMP (Perkins and Moore, 1973; Schultz and Daly, 1973; Leblanc and Ciaranello, 1984).

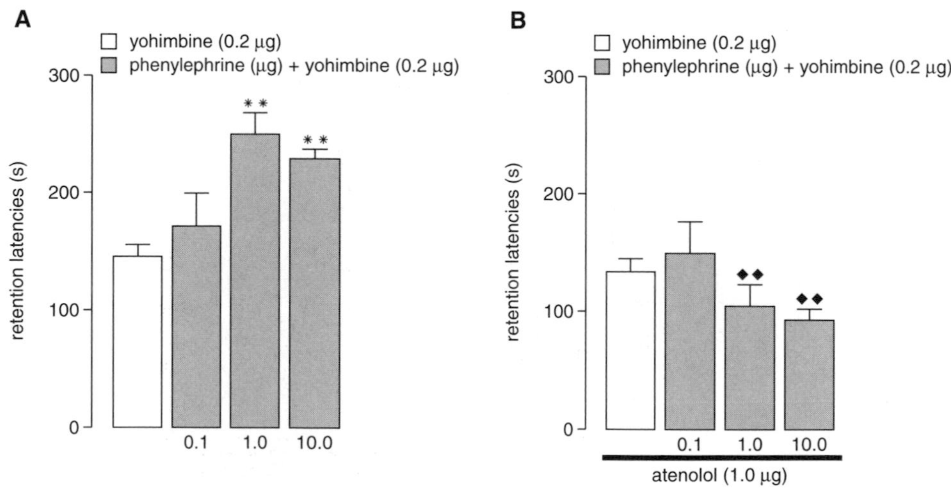

Figure 11.6 Step-through latencies (mean ± SEM) for a 48 h inhibitory avoidance test. Effects of immediate post-training infusions of the non-specific α-adrenoceptor agonist phenylephrine (0.1–10 μg) + the specific α_2-adrenoceptor antagonist yohimbine (0.2 μg in 0.2 μl) into the basolateral amygdala alone (**A**) or together with the β_1-adrenoceptor antagonist atenolol (1.0 μg) (**B**). $**P < 0.01$ as compared with the corresponding yohimbine group; ◆◆$P < 0.01$ as compared with the corresponding phenylephrine + yohimbine group. (From Ferry *et al.*, 1999a, with permission.)

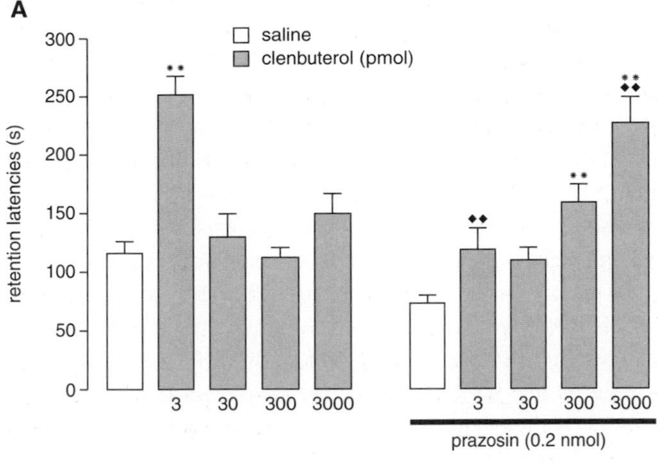

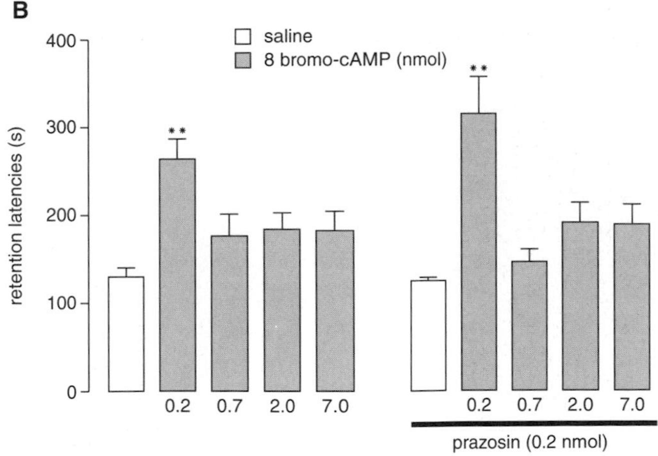

Figure 11.7 Step-through latencies (mean ± SEM) for a 48 h inhibitory avoidance test. Effects of immediate post-training infusions of the α_1-adrenoceptor antagonist prazosin (0.2 nmol in 0.2 μl) into the basolateral amygdala on the dose–response effects of the concurrently administered β-adrenoceptor agonist clenbuterol (**A**) or the synthetic cAMP analogue 8-bromo-cAMP (**B**). $**P<0.01$ as compared with the corresponding saline group; ◆◆$P<0.01$ as compared with the corresponding clenbuterol group. (From Ferry *et al.*, 1999b, with permission.)

11.7 Amygdala interactions with other brain systems in modulating memory storage

The findings reviewed above strongly support the hypothesis that the BLA is a critical locus of interactions of neuromodulatory systems influencing memory storage. However, the findings do not reveal the brain site(s) at which amygdala activity modulates memory storage. Evidence from many studies has suggested that neural changes mediating fear conditioning may be located at least partly within the amygdala (Davis, 1992, Chapter 6; LeDoux, 1995, Chapter 7). However, there is also substantial evidence suggesting that the amygdala is not a unique site of fear-based memory (Cahill *et al.*, 1999) and that the amygdala has a time-limited role in modulating memory storage in other brain regions (McGaugh *et al.*, 1996). A recent study examining c-*fos* expression induced by olfactory discrimination training and retention testing (Hess *et al.*, 1997) reported that c-*fos* was activated selectively in the BLA by the training and not by the retention testing. Quirk and colleagues (1997) recorded changes in unit activity in the lateral amygdala and auditory cortex of rats induced by fear conditioning and extinction, and reported that conditioned changes in cell firing in the auditory cortex generally occurred after changes recorded in the amygdala. Futhermore, the amygdala units extinguished relatively rapidly whereas the cortical units persisted in responding during the extinction. Additionally, Weinberger (1995, 1998) has shown that fear conditioning induced by pairing tones with footshock rapidly induces long-lasting changes in tone-specific receptive fields in the auditory cortex. Activation of muscarinic cholinergic receptors in the cortex plays a critical role in the conditioning-induced retuning. Weinberger has proposed that the cholinergic influences result from activation of the nucleus basalis by projections from the amygdala (Weinberger *et al.*, 1990). Other recent findings (Bianchin *et al.*, 1999) indicate that immediate post-training intra-amygdala infusions of many compounds, including NA and picrotoxin as well as the *N*-methyl-D-aspartate (NMDA) antagonist 2-amino-5-phosphonopentanoate (AP5) and the muscarinic cholinergic receptor antagonist scopolamine, did not affect memory tested 90 min after training but influenced memory tested 24 h after training. These findings clearly indicate that the amygdala is not involved in short-term memory and are consistent with the hypothesis that the amygdala modulates long-term memory storage in other brain regions. These findings are also consistent with extensive evidence indicating that different brain regions participate in memory storage at different times after training (Izquierdo *et al.*, 1992, 1997; Izquierdo and Medina, 1997).

Other evidence supporting the hypothesis that the amygdala is not a unique locus of aversive learning includes the findings indicating that amygdala lesions induced after training do not block memory for footshock-motivated escape training (Parent *et al.*, 1992, 1994, 1995; Parent and McGaugh, 1994). In one of several experiments investigating this issue (Parent *et al.*, 1995), rats were first given either one or 10 training trials in which they escaped from a footshock by running from one compartment to a safe compartment in a straight alley. They then received sham or excitotoxically induced BLA lesions 1 week later. Approximately 2 weeks after the escape training, they were placed in the safe compartment of the alley and received a footshock each time they entered the shock compartment (i.e. inhibitory avoidance training). Figure 11.8 shows the number of shocks received by each group in reaching a criterion of remaining in the safe compartment for 100 consecutive seconds. For both the sham-lesioned controls and the BLA-lesioned group, animals given prior escape training made fewer entries into the shock compartment; those given 10 escape training trials made the fewest entries. Additionally, for both prior escape training groups (one or 10 trials), BLA-lesioned rats made slightly more entries. However, as such an increased number of entries was also seen in the non-shocked BLA-lesioned group, this difference was very probably due to an effect of the BLA lesions on locomotor activity. This interpretation is supported by the finding that the BLA-lesioned rats were also significantly more active than controls in a locomotor activity test. It is important to note that in this experiment, the animals first learned to move quickly to escape from footshock. The memory of the training was then tested by training them in the same apparatus to cease moving (i.e. inhibitory avoidance). In both sham- and BLA-lesioned rats, increased amounts of escape training resulted in more rapid learning of the inhibitory avoidance response. Clearly, the BLA lesions did not block the memory of the escape training and did not prevent the learning of the inhibitory avoidance response. The findings thus indicate that the explicit/declarative memory of the shock compartment formed during the escape training survived the BLA lesions and strongly suggest that such information enabled the animals' rapid learning to avoid entering the shock compartment during the inhibitory avoidance training.

Although amygdala lesions typically impair the expression of conditioned fear as assessed by 'freezing' behaviour (LeDoux, 1995) or fear-potentiated startle (Davis, 1992), overtraining of fear conditioning attenuates the lesion-induced freezing deficit (Maren, 1998) and enables

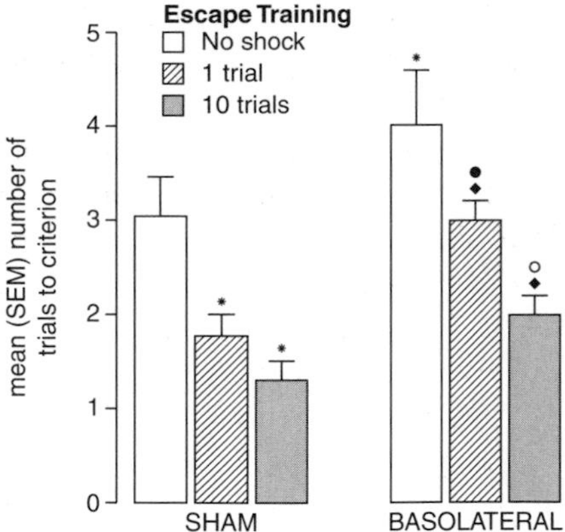

Figure 11.8 Basolateral amygdala lesions induced after escape training in a two-compartment alley do not block memory as assessed by subsequent training (inhibitory avoidance) to avoid entering the shock compartment. Mean (±SEM) entries of the shock compartment to reach criterion of remaining in the safe compartment for 100 consecutive seconds. **P* <0.05 versus sham–no shock; ●*P* <0.05 versus sham one trial; ◆*P* <0.05 versus BLA-lesioned–no shock; ○*P* <0.05 versus BLA-lesioned one trial. (From Parent *et al.*, 1995, with permission.)

reacquisition of fear-potentiated startle (Kim and Davis, 1993). It is, of course, essential to distinguish the effects of amygdala lesions on performance of the response used as an index of fear from effects on learning of the significance of the cues inducing the fear (Cahill *et al.*, 1999). We addressed this issue in a recent experiment (Vazdarjanova and McGaugh, 1998). BLA-lesioned and sham-lesioned control rats were given a series of unsignalled footshocks in one arm of a Y-maze. One day later, the rats were placed in one of the other 'safe' arms and several measures of behaviour were recorded for 8 min (see Figure 11.9). As was expected (see Figure 11.9A), the lesions significantly impaired freezing. However, the lesions attenuated but did not block the animals' memory of the place in the Y-maze where they had received footshock. In comparison with BLA-lesioned animals not given footshock on the previous day, both the BLA-lesioned rats and the sham-lesioned controls that had received footshock had long entrance latencies to enter the shock arm (Figure 11.9B) and spent significantly less time in the arm where they received the footshock (Figure 11.9C). These findings indicate that although an intact BLA may be essential for enabling the expression of freezing, an intact BLA is clearly not required for expressing explicit/declarative memory of contextual fear conditioning.

The finding of an experiment examining conditioned neuroendocrine responses provides further evidence that the amygdala is not a unique locus of memory for fear conditioning

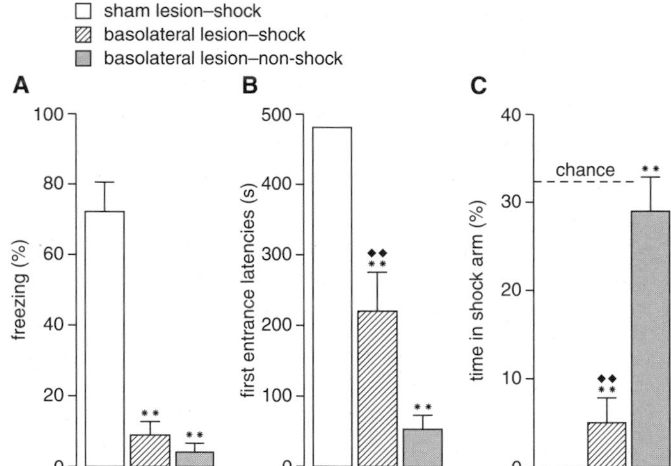

Figure 11.9 Effects of basolateral amygdala lesions on several measures of retention 24 h after context footshock pairing in a three-arm maze. (**A**) Percentage of total time (mean ± SEM) rats spent in freezing behaviour. (**B**) First entrance latency (mean ± SEM) to enter the former shock arm. (**C**) Percentage of total time (mean ± SEM) rats spent in the former shock arm. The dotted line depicts the level of change. $**P < 0.01$ as compared with the sham-lesion–shock group; ◆◆$P < 0.01$ as compared between the basolateral nucleus lesion–non-shock and basolateral nucleus lesion–shock groups. (From Vazdarjanova and McGaugh, 1998, with permission.)

(Roozendaal *et al.*, 1992). Lesions of the amygdala induced 1 day after training blocked rats' subsequent freezing behaviour but did not block the expression of conditioned neuroendocrine responses. Additionally, in a study using two strains of rats that differ in their response to shock stimulation, post-training intra-amygdala infusions of NA enhanced memory of the aversive experience (mild shock delivered through a probe inserted into the cage). However, rats of the two strains differed in the behaviour expressing memory of the experience. Post-training NA infusions enhanced freezing in the strain of rats that normally displayed freezing but enhanced another natural defensive response (i.e. burying and biting of the probe) typically displayed by rats of the other strain (Roozendaal *et al.*, 1993). Such findings indicate that the amygdala has a comparable time-limited role in regulating memory storage for contextual fear conditioning and inhibitory avoidance learning. Further, they suggest that although these two types of training differ in procedures used and retention responses measured, they have common underlying cognitive and neural bases. That is perhaps not a surprising conclusion because when animals are given a single aversive stimulus such as a footshock, they are highly likely to be making some kind of response. This is explicit in the case of one-trial inhibitory avoidance training and less explicit for contextual fear conditioning. Thus the delivery of the footshock is contingent on a response even though that response may not be one of interest to or noted by the investigator. The aversive stimulus is also, of course, administered in a particular stimulus context. Thus, for one-trial aversive training, both response-contingent (i.e. instrumental conditioning) and response-non-contingent (i.e. Pavlovian contextual conditioning) learning could occur concurrently. From another perspective, it has been suggested that contextual fear conditioning can be induced with just a single footshock and that such learning occurs too quickly to enable instrumental learning (Fanselow, 1980). From this perspective, one-trial inhibitory avoidance training, in which animals receive only one brief footshock (after leaving a safe compartment and entering the shock compartment), should also not be considered as instrumental learning. In any case, contextual fear conditioning and one-trial inhibitory avoidance training (which was used extensively in the studies reviewed in this chapter) both induce explicit/declarative memory for the aversive training experience; given an opportunity, rats given a footshock subsequently will avoid the place where they received the footshock.

Recent studies of the effects of post-training intra-BLA infusions of drugs on memory for contextual fear conditioning provide additional evidence that the BLA has a time-limited role in modulating the consolidation of fear-based memory (Vazdarjanova and McGaugh, 1999). Rats were given a series of footshocks in an arm of a Y-maze as in the study summarized above (Vazdarjanova and McGaugh, 1998). Immediately after training, they received intra-BLA infusions of a control solution, lidocaine, or the muscarinic receptor agonist oxotremorine. Previous findings of studies using inhibitory avoidance training indicate that lidocaine infusions impair retention and oxotremorine infusions enhance memory (Parent and McGaugh, 1994; Introini-Collison *et al.*, 1996). On the day following the contextual fear conditioning in the shock arm of the maze, the rats were placed in one of the 'safe' arms and allowed access to all arms. As indicated by several response measures, time spent freezing, latency to enter the shock arm, and time spent in the shock arm, the post-training lidocaine infusions impaired memory and the oxotremorine infusions enhanced memory

(Vazdarjanova and McGaugh, 1999). These findings provide further evidence that post-training manipulations of the BLA produce comparable effects on memory for contextual fear conditioning and inhibitory avoidance training. For both types of training, the rats learn and remember that footshock is experienced in a particular context (i.e. a place in the apparatus).

As the amygdala is known to project directly or indirectly to many brain regions, it is not surprising that many findings suggest that amygdala activation regulates memory consolidation occurring in other brain regions. As was noted above (see Figure 11.2), lesions of the stria terminalis block drug and hormone effects on memory. Thus, as the stria terminalis seems to be critically involved in enabling amygdala regulation of memory storage, studies investigating brain regions activated directly or indirectly by amygdala efferents mediated by the stria terminalis may provide important clues to the brain regions involved in consolidating memories.

The amygdala sends direct projections to the striatum via the stria terminalis. Evidence that NMDA infused into the amygdala induces the expression of the proto-oncogene c-*fos* in the caudate nucleus as well as the dentate gyrus of the dorsal hippocampus indicates that the amygdala is functionally connected with both of these brain structures (Packard *et al.*, 1995). Findings of many 'double-dissociation' studies support the view that the caudate nucleus and hippocampus mediate different forms of memory (Packard and McGaugh, 1992, 1996; McDonald and White, 1993). Hippocampal lesions selectively impair spatial learning (Olton *et al.*, 1979; Morris *et al.*, 1982; Moser *et al.*, 1993), whereas caudate lesions selectively impair visually cued learning in a water maze (Packard and McGaugh, 1992).

Evidence from several experiments indicates that the amygdala modulates memory storage for both hippocampal- and caudate nucleus-dependent learning tasks (Packard *et al.*, 1994; Packard and Teather, 1998). As is shown in Table 11.4, unilateral infusions of amphetamine administered into the dorsal hippocampus immediately after a single training session enhanced memory for spatial, but not for cued training in the water maze. Conversely, amphetamine infused into the caudate nucleus after training enhanced memory for the cued, but not the spatial training. However, and most importantly, amphetamine infused into the amygdala post-training enhanced memory storage for both types of training. Additionally, inactivation of the amygdala prior to the retention tests did not block the enhanced retention induced by the post-training intra-amygdala infusions of amphetamine (Packard *et al.*, 1994). This finding clearly indicates that the amygdala is not the locus of memory processes enhanced by the intra-amygdala amphetamine infusions.

In other experiments examining the effects of post-training intra-amygdala infusions of amphetamine, Packard and Teather (1998) found that infusions of lidocaine into the hippocampus prior to retention testing selectively blocked the enhanced memory for spatial training, whereas infusions of lidocaine into the caudate selectively blocked the enhanced memory for cued training. Also, in confirmation of our previous findings (Packard *et al.*, 1994), lidocaine infused into the amygdala prior to the retention test did not block amphetamine-induced memory enhancement in either task. These findings provide further evidence that the amygdala-induced memory enhancement is not mediated by lasting neural changes within the amygdala.

Table 11.4 Amygdala modulation of hippocampal-dependent and caudate nucleus-dependent memory processes

	Retention	
	Spatial task	*Cued task*
Post-training infusions		
D-amphetamine, hippocampus[a]	Enhanced	No effect
D-amphetamine, caudate nucleus[a]	No Effect	Enhanced
D-amphetamine, amygdala[a]	Enhanced	Enhanced
D-amphetamine, amygdala + lidocaine, hippocampus[b]	Enhancement blocked	Enhanced
D-amphetamine, amygdala + lidocaine, caudate nucleus[b]	Enhanced	Enhancement blocked
Post-training and pre-testing infusions		
Post: D-amphetamine, hippocampus Pre: lidocaine, hippocampus[b]	Enhancement blocked	(not tested)
Post: D-amphetamine, caudate nucleus Pre: lidocaine, caudate nucleus[b]	(not tested)	Enhancement blocked
Post: D-amphetamine, amygdala Pre: lidocaine, amygdala[a]	Enhanced	Enhanced

[a]Packard *et al.* (1994); Packard and Teather (1998).
[b]Packard and Teather (1998).

Other recent findings from our laboratory provide additional evidence that inputs from the BLA influence the processing of hippocampally dependent memory. In this study, post-training intra-hippocampal infusions of a glucocorticoid receptor agonist administered directly into the dorsal hippocampus enhanced retention of inhibitory avoidance training. However, the memory enhancement was blocked completely in animals with selective BLA lesions (Roozendaal and McGaugh, 1997b). Consistent with previous studies indicating the importance of noradrenergic activation in BLA in memory storage modulation, intra-BLA infusions of the β-adrenoceptor antagonist atenolol also blocked the memory enhancement induced by post-training glucocorticoid administration into the hippocampus (Roozendaal *et al.*, 1999). Furthermore, the memory-enhancing effects of the unilateral intra-hippocampal infusions of the glucocorticoid were blocked only by treatments affecting the ipsilateral BLA. Infusions of atenolol into the contralateral BLA did not block the memory enhancement. There is some evidence suggesting that the BLA affects hippocampal functioning via the BLA–nucleus accumbens pathway. The nucleus accumbens receives projections from both the BLA and the hippocampus (O'Donnell and Grace, 1995). As discussed above, lesions of the stria terminalis, which carries projections from the BLA to the nucleus accumbens, have effects that are highly comparable with those induced by amygdala or selective BLA lesions. Moreover, excitotoxic lesions of the nucleus accumbens also block the memory-modulating effects of post-training systemic injections of dexamethasone (Setlow *et al.*, 2000). Other findings indicate that the medial prefrontal cortex is also involved in memory storage and that the amygdala and medial prefrontal cortex interact in modulating memory storage but are differentially involved at different post-training stages of memory storage (Izquierdo *et al.*, 1997; Liang, in press).

11.7 Concluding comments

The findings summarized in this chapter leave little doubt that the amygdala is involved in the consolidation of emotionally arousing experiences. Although we have focused on experiments using aversive experiences, our hypothesis is that the involvement of the amygdala is not restricted to aversively motivated learning. Our findings also indicate that the BLA is the region of the amygdala that is critical for mediating the effects of stress-activated neuromodulatory influences on memory storage. Although lesions of the BLA do not block learning or memory storage, they do block the memory-modulating effects of adrenaline and glucocorticoids, as well as those of drugs affecting several other systems. Additionally, our findings indicate that NA release within the amygdala is critical for mediating neuromodulatory influences on memory storage. Finally, the evidence reviewed in this chapter strongly suggests that the amygdala influences memory storage by modulating storage processes in brain regions activated by the amygdala. The findings indicate that the amygdala influences memory processes that involve the caudate nucleus and the hippocampus and are mediated by pathways in the stria terminals projecting to the nucleus accumbens. Additionally, there is evidence suggesting that the amygdala may modulate information processing within the hippocampal formation via projections to the entorhinal cortex, hippocampus subiculum, and parasubiculum (Pikkarainen *et al.*, 1999).

Finally, although the findings reviewed in this chapter are based on experimental studies using animals, highly comparable findings are emerging from studies of human subjects. Recent studies investigating the effects of β-adrenoceptor antagonists and lesions of the amygdala, as well as amygdala activation assessed by brain imaging provide extensive evidence that the effect of emotional arousal on long-term explicit/declarative memory in human subjects involves β-adrenoceptor activation as well as activation of the amygdaloid complex (Cahill *et al.*, 1994, 1995, 1996; Cahill and McGaugh, 1998; Cahill, Chapter 12). These findings, like those of the animal studies reviewed in this chapter, provide strong support for our hypothesis that the amygdala has a critical time-limited role in modulating memory storage processes in other regions of the brain. Future exploration of amygdala projections to other brain regions, including further exploration of cortical regions, will in all likelihood reveal that the amygdala has widespread influences on memory processes throughout many brain regions. The evidence indicating that the amygdala modulates the storage of different forms of memory and, in particular, influences the formation of explicit/declarative memory would seem to require the hypothesized widespread modulation of brain processes involved in memory storage.

Acknowledgements

Supported by a Ralph W. and Leona Gerard Family Trust Fellowship (B.F. and B.R.), a Schneiderman Graduate Fellowship (A.V.), and USPHS Grant MH 12526 (J.L.M.)

References

Ammassari-Teule, M., Pavone, F., Castellano, C., and McGaugh, J.L. (1991) Amygdala and dorsal hippocampus lesions block the effects of GABAergic drugs on memory storage. *Brain Research*, 551, 104–109.

Bianchin, M., Mello e Souza, T., Medina, J.H., and Izquierdo, I. (1999) The amygdala is involved in the modulation of long-term memory, but not in working or short-term memory. *Neurobiology of Learning and Memory*, 71, 127–131.

Bohus, B. (1994) Humoral modulation of memory processes. Physiological significance of brain and peripheral mechanisms. In *The Memory System of the Brain* (ed. J. Delacour), Vol. 4, pp. 337–364. Advanced Series of Neuroscience, World Scientific, New Jersey.

Breen, R.A. and McGaugh, J.L. (1961) Facilitation of maze learning with posttrial injections of picrotoxin. *Journal of Comparative and Physiological Psychology*, 54, 498–501.

Brioni, J.D. and McGaugh, J.L. (1988) Posttraining administration of GABAergic antagonists enhance retention of aversively motivated tasks. *Psychopharmacology*, 96, 505–510.

Brioni, J.D., Nagahara, A.H., and McGaugh, J.L. (1989) Involvement of the amygdala GABAergic system in the modulation of memory storage. *Brain Research*, 487, 105–112.

Cahill, L. and McGaugh, J.L. (1991) NMDA-induced lesions of the amygdaloid complex block the retention enhancing effect of posttraining epinephrine. *Psychobiology*, 19, 206–210.

Cahill, L. and McGaugh, J.L. (1998) Mechanisms of emotional arousal and lasting declarative memory. *Trends in Neuroscience*, 21, 294–299.

Cahill, L., Prins, B., Weber, M., and McGaugh, J.L. (1994) Beta-adrenergic activation and memory for emotional events. *Nature*, 371, 702–704.

Cahill, L., Babinsky, R., Markowitsch, H., and McGaugh, J.L. (1995) The amygdala and emotional memory. *Nature*, 377, 295–296.

Cahill, L., Haier, R., Fallon, J., Alkire, M., Tang, C., Keator, D., Wu, J., and McGaugh, J.L. (1996) Amygdala activity at encoding correlated with long-term, free recall of emotional information. *Proceedings, National Academy of Sciences of the United States of America*, 93, 8016–8021.

Cahill, L., Weinberger, N.M., Roozendaal, B., and McGaugh, J.L. (1999) Is 'conditioned fear' stored in the amygdala? Some questions and caveats. *Neuron*, **23**, 227–228.

Castellano, C. and McGaugh, J.L. (1989a) Retention enhancement with posttraining picrotoxin: lack of state dependency. *Behavioral and Neural Biology*, 51, 165–170.

Castellano, C. and McGaugh, J.L. (1989b) Effect of morphine on one-trial inhibitory avoidance in mice: lack of state dependency. *Psychobiology*, 17, 89–92.

Castellano, C. and McGaugh, J.L. (1990) Effects of post-training bicuculline and muscimol on retention: lack of state dependency. *Behavioral and Neural Biology*, 54, 156–164.

Clark, K.B., Krahl, S.E, Smith, D.C., and Jensen, R.A. (1995) Post-training unilateral vagal stimulation enhances retention performance in the rat. *Neurobiology of Learning and Memory*, 63, 213–216.

Clark, K.B., Naritoku, D.K., Smith, D.C., Browning, R.A., and Jensen, R.A. (1999) Enhanced recognition memory following vagus nerve stimulation in human subjects. *Nature Neuroscience*, 2, 94–98.

Conway, M. (1995) *Flashbulb Memories*. Lawrence Erlbaum Associates, Hillsdale, New Jersey.

Cottrell, G.A. and Nakajima, S. (1977) Effects of corticosteroids in the hippocampus on passive avoidance behavior in the rat. *Pharmacology, Biochemistry, and Behavior*, 7, 277–280.

Da Cunha, C., Roozendaal, B., Vazdarjanova, A., and McGaugh, J.L. (1999) Microinfusions of flumazenil into the basolateral but not the central nucleus of the amygdala enhance memory consolidation in rats. *Neurobiology of Learning and Memory*, **72**, 1–7.

Davis, M. (1992) The role of the amygdala in conditioned fear. In *The Amygdala: Neurobiological Aspects of Emotion, Memory, and Mental Dysfunction* (ed. J.P. Aggleton), pp. 255–306. Wiley-Liss, New York.

de Kloet, E.R. (1991) Brain corticosteroid receptor balance and homeostatic control. *Frontiers of Neuroendocrinology*, 12, 95–164.

de Souza-Silva, M.A. and Tomaz, C. (1995) Amnesia after diazepam infusion into basolateral but not central amygdala of *Rattus norvegicus. Neuropsychobiology*, 32, 31–36.

Fanselow, M.S. (1980) Conditioned and unconditional components of post-shock freezing. *Pavlovian Journal of Biological Sciences*, 15, 177–182.

Ferry, B. and McGaugh, J.L. (1999) Clenbuterol administration into the basolateral amygdala post-training enhances retention in an inhibitory avoidance task. *Neurobiology of Learning and Memory*.

Ferry, B., Roozendaal, B., and McGaugh, J.L. (1999a) Involvement of α1-adrenergic receptors in the basolateral amygdala in modulation of memory storage. *European Journal of Pharmacology*, 372, 9–16.

Ferry, B., Roozendaal, B., and McGaugh,J.L. (1999b) Basolateral amygdala noradrenergic influences on memory storage are mediated by an interaction between β- and α1-adrenoceptors. *Journal of Neuroscience*, **19**, 5119–5123.

Galvez, R., Mesches, M., and McGaugh, J.L. (1996) Norepinephrine release in the amygdala in response to footshock stimulation. *Neurobiology of Learning and Memory*, 66, 253–257.

Gerard, R.W. (1961) The fixation of experience. *In Brain Mechanisms and Learning* (consulting eds A. Fessard, R.W. Gerard, and J. Konorski,), pp. 21–35. Charles C. Thomas, Springfield, Illinois.

Goddard, G.V. (1964) Amygdaloid stimulation and learning in the rat. *Journal of Comparative and Physiological Psychology*, 58, 23–30.

Gold, P.E. (1988) Plasma glucose regulation of memory storage processes. In *Cellular Mechanisms of Conditioning and Behavioral Plasticity* (eds C.D. Woody, D.L. Alkon, and J.L. McGaugh), pp. 329–341. Plenum Press, New York.

Gold, P.E. (1995) Modulation of emotional and non-emotional memories: same pharmacological systems, different neuroanatomical systems. In *Brain and Memory: Modulation and Mediation of Neuroplasticity* (eds J.L. McGaugh, N.M. Weinberger, and G. Lynch), pp. 41–74. Oxford University Press, New York.

Gold, P.E. and McGaugh, J.L. (1975) A single-trace, two process view of memory storage processes. In *Short-term Memory* (eds D. Deutsch and J.A. Deutsch), pp. 355–378. Academic Press, New York.

Gold, P.E. and van Buskirk, R. (1975) Facilitation of time-dependent memory processes with posttrial epinephrine injections. *Behavioral Biology*, 13, 145–153.

Gold, P. and van Buskirk, R. (1978) Posttraining brain norepinephrine concentrations: correlation with retention performance of avoidance training with peripheral epinephrine modulation of memory processing. *Behavioral Biology*, 23, 509–520.

Gold, P.E., Zornetzer, S.F., and McGaugh, J.L. (1974) Electrical stimulation of the brain: effects on memory storage. In *Advances in Psychobiology* (eds G. Newton and A. Riesen), Vol. 2, pp. 193–224. Wiley Interscience, New York.

Gold, P.E., Hankins, L., Edwards, R.M., Chester, J., and McGaugh, J.L. (1975) Memory interference and facilitation with posttrial amygdala stimulation: effect on memory varies with footshock level. *Brain Research*, 86, 509–513.

Harfstrand, A., Fuxe, K., Cintra, A., Agnati, L., Mzini, L., Wikstrom, A.C., Okret, S., Yu, Z.Y., Goldstein, M., Steinbusch, H., Verhofstad, A., and Gustafsson, J.-A. (1986) Glucocorticoid receptor immunoreactivity in monoaminergic neurons of rat brain. *Proceedings of the National Academy of Sciences of the United States of America*, 83, 9779–9783.

Hatfield, T. and McGaugh, J.L. (1999) Norepinephrine infused into the basolateral amygdala posttraining enhances retention in a spatial water maze task. *Neurobiology of Learning and Memory*, 71, 232–239.

Hatfield, T., Spanis, C., and McGaugh, J.L. (1999) Response of amygdalar norepinephrine to footshock and GABAergic drugs using *in vivo* microdialysis and HPLC. *Brain Research*, **835**, 340–345.

Hess, U.S., Gall, C.M., Granger, R., and Lynch, G. (1997) Differential patterns of c-*fos* mRNA expression in amygdala during successive stages of odor discrimination learning. *Learning and Memory*, 4, 262–283.

Introini-Collison, I.B. and McGaugh, J.L. (1986a) Interaction of adrenergic, cholinergic and opioid systems in modulation of memory storage. *Society for Neuroscience Abstracts*, 12, 710.

Introini-Collison, I.B. and McGaugh, J.L. (1986b) Epinephrine modulates long-term retention of an aversively-motivated discrimination. *Behavioral and Neural Biology*, 45, 358–365.

Introini-Collison, I.B., Nagahara, A.H., and McGaugh, J.L. (1989) Memory-enhancement with intra-amygdala posttraining naloxone is blocked by concurrent administration of propranolol. *Brain Research*, 476, 94–101.

Introini-Collison, I.B., Miyazaki, B., and McGaugh, J.L. (1991) Involvement of the amygdala in the memory-enhancing effects of clenbuterol. *Psychopharmacology*, 104, 541–544.

Introini-Collison, I.B., Ford, L., and McGaugh, J.L. (1995) Memory impairment induced by intra-amygdala β-endorphin is mediated by noradrenergic influences. *Neurobiology of Learning and Memory*, 63, 200–205.

Introini-Collison, I.B., Dalmaz, C., and McGaugh, J.L. (1996) Amygdala β-noradreneric influences on memory storage involve cholinergic activation. *Neurobiology of Learning and Memory*, 65, 57–64.

Izquierdo, I. and Diaz, R.D. (1983) Effect of ACTH, epinephrine, β-endorphin, naloxone, and of the combination of naloxone or β-endorphin with ACTH or epinephrine on memory consolidation. *Psychoneuroendocrinology*, 8, 81–87.

Izquierdo, I. and Diaz, R.D. (1985) Influence on memory of posttraining or pre-test injections of ACTH, vasopressin, epinephrine or β-endorphin and their interaction with naloxone. *Psychoneuroendocrinology*, 10, 165–172.

Izquierdo, I. and Medina, J.H. (1997) Memory formation: the sequence of biochemical events in the hippocampus and its connection to activity in other brain structures. *Neurobiology of Learning and Memory*, 68, 285–316.

Izquierdo, I., DaCunha, C., Huang, C. H., Walz, R., Wolfman, C., and Medina, J. H. (1990a) Post-training down regulation of memory consolidation by a GABA-A mechanism in the amygdala modulated by endogenous benzodiazepines. *Behavioral and Neural Biology*, 54, 105–109.

Izquierdo, I., DaCunha, C., and Medina, J. (1990b) Endogenous benzodiazepine modulation of memory processes. *Neuroscience and Biobehavioral Review*, 14, 419–424.

Izquierdo, I., Da Cunha, C., Rosat, R., Jerusalinsky, D., Ferreira, M.B.C., and Medina, J.H. (1992) Neurotransmitter receptors involved in memory processing by the amygdala, medial septum and hippocampus of rats. *Behavioral and Neural Biology*, 58, 16–25.

Izquierdo, I., Quillfeldt, J.A., Zanatta, M.S., Quevedo, J., Schaeffer, E., Schmitz, P.K., and Medina, J.H. (1997) Sequential role of hippocampus and amygdala, entorhinal cortex and parietal cortex in formation and retrieval of memory for inhibitory avoidance in rats. *European Journal of Neuroscience*, 9, 786–793.

Jensen, R.A. (2000) Neural pathways mediating modulation of learning and memory by peripheral factors. In *Four Decades of Memory: A Festschrift Honoring James L. McGaugh* (eds P.E. Gold and W.T. Greenough), American Psychological Association, Washington, DC, in press.

Jones, B. and Mishkin, M. (1972) Limbic lesions and the problem of stimulus–reinforcement associations. *Experimental Neurology*, 36, 362–377.

Kesner, R.P. and Doty, R.W. (1968) Amnesia produced in cats by local seizure activity initiated from the amygdala. *Experimental Neurology*, 21, 58–68.

Kesner, R.P. and Wilburn, M. (1974) A review of electrical stimulation of the brain in the context of learning and retention. *Behavioral Biology*, 10, 259–293.

Kety, S. (1972) Brain catecholamines, affective states and memory. In *The Chemistry of Mood, Motivation and Memory* (ed. J.L. McGaugh), pp. 65–80. Plenum Press, New York.

Killcross, S., Robbins, T.W., and Everitt, B.J. (1997) Different types of fear-conditioned behaviour mediated by separate nuclei within amygdala. *Nature*, 388, 377–380.

Kim, M. and Davis, M. (1993) Electrolytic lesions of the amygdala block acquisition and expression of fear-potentiated startle even with extensive training but do not prevent reacquisition. *Behavioral Neuroscience*, 7, 580–595.

Klüver, H. and Bucy, P.C. (1937) 'Psychic blindness' and other symptoms following bilateral temporal lobectomy in rhesus monkeys. *American Journal of Physiology*, 119, 352–353.

Leblanc, G.G. and Ciaranello, R.D. (1984) α-Noradrenergic potentiation of neurotransmitter-stimulated cAMP production in rat striatal slices. *Brain Research*, 293, 57–65.

LeDoux, J.E. (1992) Emotion and the amygdala. In *The Amygdala: Neurobiological Aspects of Emotion, Memory, and Mental Dysfunction* (ed. J.P. Aggleton), pp. 339–352. Wiley-Liss, New York.

LeDoux, J.E. (1995) Emotion: clues from the brain. *Annual Review of Psychology*, 46, 209–235.

Langer, S.Z. (1974) Presynaptic regulation of catecholamine release. *Biochemical Pharmacology*, 23, 1793–1800.

Liang, K.C. (1998) Pretraining infusion of DSP-4 into the amygdala impaired retention in the inhibitory avoidance task: involvement of norepinephrine but not serotonin in memory facilitation. *Chinese Journal of Physiology*, 41, 223–233.

Liang, K.C. and Chiang, T.-C. (1994) Locus coeruleus infusion of clonidine impaired retention and attenuated memory enhancing effects of epinephrine. *Society for Neuroscience Abstracts*, 20, 153.

Liang, K.C. and McGaugh, J.L. (1983) Lesions of the stria terminalis attenuate the enhancing effect of posttraining epinephrine on retention of an inhibitory avoidance response. *Behavioural Brain Research*, 9, 49–58.

Liang, K.C., Messing, R.B., and McGaugh, J.L. (1983) Naloxone attenuates amnesia caused by amygdaloid stimulation: the involvement of a central opioid system. *Brain Research*, 271, 41–49.

Liang, K.C., Bennett, C., and McGaugh, J.L. (1985) Peripheral epinephrine modulates the effects of posttraining amygdala stimulation on memory. *Behavioural Brain Research*, 15, 93–100.

Liang, K.C., Juler, R., and McGaugh, J.L. (1986) Modulating effects of posttraining epinephrine on memory: involvement of the amygdala noradrenergic system. *Brain Research*, 368, 125–133.

Liang, K.C., McGaugh, J.L., and Yao, H. (1990) Involvement of amygdala pathways in the influence of posttraining amygdala norepinephrine and peripheral epinephrine on memory storage. *Brain Research*, 508, 225–233.

Liang, K., Chen, L., and Huang, T.-E. (1995) The role of amygdala norepinephrine in memory formation, involvement in the memory enhancing effect of peripheral epinephrine. *Chinese Journal of Physiology*, 38, 81–91.

Liang, K.C. (2000) Epinephrine modulation of memory: amygdala activation and regulation of long-term storage. In *Four Decades of Memory: A Festschrift Honoring James L. McGaugh* (eds P.E. Gold and W.T. Greenough), American Psychological Association, Washington, DC, in press.

Lupien, S.J. and McEwen, B.S. (1997) The acute effects of corticosteroids on cognition: integration of animal and human model studies. *Brain Research Review*, 24, 1–27.

Maren, S. (1998) Overtraining does not mitigate contextual fear conditioning deficits produced by neurotoxic lesions of the basolateral amygdala. *Journal of Neuroscience*, 18, 3088–3097.

McCarty, R. and Gold, P.E. (1981) Plasma catecholamines: effects of footshock level and hormonal modulators of memory storage. *Hormones and Behavior*, 15, 168–182.

McDonald, R.J. and White, N.M. (1993) A triple dissociation of memory systems: hippocampus, amygdala and dorsal striatum. *Behavioral Neuroscience*, 107, 3–22.

McEwen, B.S. (1987) Glucocorticoid–biogenic amine interactions in relation to mood and behavior. *Biochemical Pharmacology*, 36, 1755–1763.

McEwen, B.S. and Sapolsky, R.M. (1995) Stress and cognitive function. *Current Opinion in Neurobiology*, 5, 205–216.

McGaugh, J.L. (1966) Time-dependent processes in memory storage. *Science*, 153, 1351–1358.

McGaugh, J.L. (1968) Drug facilitation of memory and learning. In *Psychopharmacology: A Review of Progress* (PHS publication 1836), pp. 891–904. US Government Printing Office, Washington, DC.

McGaugh, J.L. (1973) Drug facilitation of learning and memory. *Annual Review of Pharmacology*, 13, 229–241.

McGaugh, J.L. (1983a) Hormonal influences on memory. *Annual Review of Psychology*, 34, 297–323.

McGaugh, J.L. (1983b) Preserving the presence of the past: hormonal influences on memory storage. *American Psychologist*, 38, 161–174.

McGaugh, J.L. (1989a) Dissociating learning and performance: drug and hormone enhancement of memory storage. *Brain Research Bulletin*, 23, 339–345.

McGaugh, J.L. (1989b) Involvement of hormonal and neuromodulatory systems in the regulation of memory storage. *Annual Review of Neuroscience*, 12, 255–287.

McGaugh, J.L. and Gold, P.E. (1976) Modulation of memory by electrical stimulation of the brain. In *Neural Mechanisms of Learning and Memory* (eds M.R. Rosenzweig and E.L. Bennett), pp. 549–560. MIT Press, Cambridge, Massachusetts.

McGaugh, J.L. and Gold, P.E. (1989) Hormonal modulation of memory. In *Psychoendocrinology* (eds R.B. Brush and S. Levine), pp. 305–339. Academic Press, New York.

McGaugh, J. L. and Herz, M.J. (1972) *Memory Consolidation*. Albion, San Francisco.

McGaugh, J.L., Liang, K.C., Bennett, C., and Sternberg, D.B. (1984) Adrenergic influences on memory storage: interaction of peripheral and central systems. In *Neurobiology of Learning and Memory* (eds G. Lynch, J.L. McGaugh, and N.M. Weinberger), pp. 313–333. The Guilford Press, New York.

McGaugh, J.L., Introini-Collison, I.B., Juler, R.G., and Izquierdo, I. (1986) Stria terminalis lesions attenuate the effects of posttraining naloxone and β-endorphin on retention. *Behavioral Neuroscience*, 100, 839–844.

McGaugh, J.L., Introini-Collison, I.B., and Nagahara, A.H. (1988) Memory-enhancing effects of posttraining naloxone: involvement of β-noradrenergic influences in the amygdaloid complex. *Brain Research*, 446, 37–49.

McGaugh, J.L., Introini-Collison, I.B., Cahill, L., Kim, M., and Liang, K.C. (1992) Involvement of the amygdala in neuromodulatory influences on memory storage. In *The Amygdala: Neurobiological Aspects of Emotion, Memory, and Mental Dysfunction* (ed. J.P. Aggleton), pp. 431–451. Wiley-Liss, New York.

McGaugh, J.L., Introini-Collison, I., and Castellano, C. (1993) Involvement of opioid peptides in learning and memory. In *Handbook of Experimental Pharmacology, Opioids, Part I and II* (eds A. Herz, H. Akil, and E.J. Simon), pp. 419–477. Springer-Verlag, Heidelberg.

McGaugh, J.L., Cahill, L., and Roozendaal, B. (1996) Involvement of the amygdala in memory storage: interaction with other brain systems. *Proceedings of the National Academy of Sciences of the United States of America*, 93, 13508–13514.

McNay, E.C. and Gold, P.E. (1998) Memory modulation across neural systems: intra-amygdala glucose reverses deficits caused by intraseptal morphine on a spatial task but not on an aversive task. *Journal of Neuroscience*, 18, 3853–3858.

Morris, R.G.M., Garrud, P., Rawlins, J.N.P., and O'Keefe, J. (1982) Place navigation impaired in rats with hippocampal lesions. *Nature*, 297, 681–683.

Moser, E., Moser, M.-B., and Andersen, P. (1993) Spatial learning impairment parallels the magnitude of dorsal hippocampal lesions, but is hardly present following ventral lesions. *Journal of Neuroscience*, 13, 3916–3925.

O'Donnell, P. and Grace, A.A. (1995) Synaptic interactions among excitatory afferents to nucleus accumbens neurons: hippocampal gating of prefrontal cortical input. *Journal of Neuroscience*, 15, 3622–3639.

Oitzl, M.S. and de Kloet, E.R. (1992) Selective corticosteroid antagonist modulate specific aspects of spatial orientation learning. *Behavioral Neuroscience*, 106, 62–71.

Olton, D.S., Becker, J.T., and Handelman, G.E. (1979) Hippocampus, space, and memory. *Behavioral and Brain Sciences*, 2, 313–365.

Packard, M.G. and McGaugh, J.L. (1992) Double dissociation of fornix and caudate nucleus lesions on acquisition of two water maze tasks, further evidence for multiple memory systems. *Behavioral Neuroscience*, 106, 439–446.

Packard, M.G. and McGaugh, J.L. (1996) Inactivation of hippocampus or caudate nucleus with lidocaine differentially affects expression of place and response learning. *Neurobiology of Learning and Memory*, 65, 65–72.

Packard, M.G. and Teather, L. (1998) Amygdala modulation of multiple memory systems: hippocampus and caudate–putamen. *Neurobiology of Learning and Memory*, 69, 163–203.

Packard, M.G., Cahill, L., and McGaugh, J.L. (1994) Amygdala modulation of hippocampal-dependent and caudate nucleus-dependent memory processes. *Proceedings of the National Academy of Sciences of the United States of America*, 91, 8477–8481.

Packard, M.G., Williams, C., Cahill, L., and McGaugh, J.L. (1995) The anatomy of a memory modulatory system: from periphery to brain. In *Neurobehavioral Plasticity, Learning, Development and Response to Brain Insults* (eds N. Spear, L. Spear, and M. Woodruff), pp. 149–184. Lawrence Erlbaum Associates, Hillsdale, New Jersey.

Parent, M. and McGaugh, J.L. (1994) Posttraining infusion of lidocaine into the amygdala basolateral complex impairs retention of inhibitory avoidance training. *Brain Research*, 661, 97–103.

Parent, M., Tomaz, C., and McGaugh, J.L. (1992) Increased training in an aversively motivated task attenuates the memory impairing effects of posttraining *N*-methyl-D-aspartic acid-induced amygdala lesions. *Behavioral Neuroscience*, 106, 791–799.

Parent, M., West, M., and McGaugh, J.L. (1994) Memory of rats with amygdala lesions induced 30 days after footshock-motivated escape training reflects degree of original training. *Behavioral Neuroscience*, 6, 1080–1087.

Parent, M., Avila, E., and McGaugh, J.L. (1995) Footshock facilitates the expression of aversively motivated memory in rats given post-training amygdala basolateral complex lesions. *Brain Research*, 676, 235–244.

Perkins, J.P. and Moore, M.M. (1973) Characterization of the adrenergic receptors mediating a rise in cyclic 3',5'-adenosine monophosphate in rat cerebral cortex. *Journal of Pharmacology and Experimental Therapeutics*, 185, 371–378.

Pikkarainen, M., Ronko, S., Savander, V., Insausti, R., and Pitkanen, A. (1999) Projections from the lateral, basal, and accessory basal nuclei of the amygdala to the hippocampal formation in rat. *Journal of Comparative Neurology*, 403, 229–260.

Power, A., Roozendaal, B. and McGaugh, J.L. (in press) Glucocorticoid enhancement of memory consolidation in the rat involves cholinergic activation in the basolateral amygdala. *European Journal of Neuroscience*.

Quirarte, G.L., Roozendaal, B., and McGaugh, J.L. (1997a) Glucocorticoid enhancement of memory storage involves noradrenergic activation in the basolateral amygdala. *Proceedings of the National Academy of Sciences of the United States of America*, 94, 14048–14053.

Quirarte, G.L., Roozendaal, B., and McGaugh, J.L. (1997b) Glucocorticoid receptor antagonist infused into the basolateral amygdala inhibits the memory enhancing effects of the noradrenergic agonist infused clenbuterol. *Society for Neuroscience Abstracts*, 1314.

Quirarte, G.L., Galvez, R., Roozendaal, B., and McGaugh, J.L. (1998) Norepinephrine release in the amygdala in response to footshock and opioid peptidergic drugs. *Brain Research*, 808, 134–140.

Quirk, G.J., Armony, J.L., and LeDoux, J.E. (1997) Fear conditioning enhances different temporal components of tone-evoked spike trains in auditory cortex and lateral amygdala. *Neuron*, 19, 613–624.

Ragozzino, M.E. and Gold, P.E. (1994) Task-dependent effects of intra-amygdala morphine injections: attentuation by intra-amygdala glucose injections. *Journal of Neuroscience*, 14, 7478–7485.

Ricardo, J. and Koh, E. (1978) Anatomical evidence of direct projections from the nucleus of the solitary tract to the hypothalamus, amygdala, and other forebrain structures in the rat. *Brain Research*, 153, 1–26.

Roozendaal, B. (2000) Glucocorticoids and the regulation of memory consolidation, *Psychoneuroendocrinology*, **25**, 213–238.

Roozendaal, B. and McGaugh, J.L. (1996a) Amygdaloid nuclei lesions differentially affect glucocorticoid-induced memory enhancement in an inhibitory avoidance task. *Neurobiology of Learning and Memory*, 65, 1–8.

Roozendaal, B. and McGaugh, J.L. (1996b) The memory-modulatory effects of glucocorticoids depend on an intact stria terminalis. *Brain Research*, 709, 243–250.

Roozendaal, B. and McGaugh, J.L. (1997a) Glucocorticoid receptor agonist and antagonist administration into the basolateral but not central amygdala modulates memory storage. *Neurobiology of Learning and Memory*, 67, 176–179.

Roozendaal, B. and McGaugh, J.L. (1997b) Basolateral amygdala lesions block the memory-enhancing effect of glucocorticoid administration in the dorsal hippocampus of rats. *European Journal of Neuroscience*, 9, 76–83.

Roozendaal, B., Koolhaas, J.M., and Bohus, B. (1992) Central amygdaloid involvement in neuroendocrine correlates of conditioned stress response. *Journal of Neuroendocrinology*, 4, 483–489.

Roozendaal, B., Koolhaas, J.M., and Bohus, B. (1993) Posttraining norepinephrine infusion into the central amygdala differentially enhances later retention in Roman high-avoidance and low-avoidance rats. *Behavioral Neuroscience*, 7, 575–579.

Roozendaal, B., Portillo-Marquez, G., and McGaugh, J.L. (1996) Basolateral amygdala lesions block glucocorticoid-induced modulation of memory for spatial learning. *Behavioral Neuroscience*, 110, 1074–1083.

Roozendaal, B., Quirarte, G.L., and McGaugh, J.L. (1997) Stress-activated hormonal systems and the regulation of memory storage. *Annals of the New York Academy of Sciences*, 821, 247–258.

Roozendaal, B., Williams, C.L., and McGaugh, J.L. (1999b) Glucocorticoid receptor activation of noradrenergic neurons within the rat nucleus of the solitary tract facilitates memory consolidation: involvement of the basolateral amygdala. *European Journal of Neuroscience*, 11, 1317–1323.

Roozendaal, B., Nguyen, B.T., Power, A.E., and McGaugh, J.L. (1999a) Basolateral amygdala noradrenergic influence on the memory-enhancing effect of glucocorticoid receptor activation into the hippocampus, *Proceedings of the National Academy of Science*, **96**, 11642–11647.

Salinas, J. and McGaugh, J.L. (1995) Muscimol induces retrograde amnesia for changes in reward magnitude. *Neurobiology of Learning and Memory*, 63, 277–285.

Salinas, J. and McGaugh, J.L. (1996) The amygdala modulates memory for changes in reward magnitude, involvement of the amygdaloid GABAergic system. *Behavioural Brain Research*, 80, 87–98.

Salinas, J., Packard, M.G., and McGaugh, J.L. (1993) Amygdala modulates memory for changes in reward magnitude, reversible post-training inactivation with lidocaine attenuates the response to a reduction reward. *Behavioural Brain Research*, 59, 153–159.

Salinas, J.A., Williams, C.L., and McGaugh, J.L. (1996) Peripheral posttraining administration of 4-OH amphetamine enhances retention of a reduction in reward magnitude. *Neurobiology of Learning and Memory*, 65, 192–195.

Salinas, J., Introini-Collison, I.B., Dalmaz, C., and McGaugh, J.L. (1997) Posttraining intra-amygdala infusion of oxotremorine and propranolol modulate storage of memory for reduction in reward magnitude. *Neurobiology of Learning and Memory*, 68, 51–59.

Sandi, C. and Rose, S.P.R. (1994) Corticosterone enhances long-term retention in one-day-old chicks trained in a weak passive avoidance learning paradigm. *Brain Research*, 647, 106–112.

Schultz J. and Daly, J.W. (1973) Accumulation of cyclic adenosine 3′,5′-monophosphate in cerebral cortical slices from rat and mouse: stimulatory effect of α- and β-adrenergic agents and adenosine. *Journal of Neurochemistry*, 21, 1319–1326.

Schreurs, J., Seelig, T. and Schulman, H. (1986) β_2-Adrenergic receptors on peripheral nerves. *Journal of Neurochemistry*, 46, 294–296.

Setlow, B., Roozendaal, B., and McGaugh, J.L. (2000) Involvement of a basolateral amygdala complex–nucleus accumbens pathway in glucocorticoid-induced modulation of memory storage, *European Journal of Neuroscience*, 12, 367–375.

Starke, K. (1979) Presynaptic regulation of catecholamines release in the central nervous system. In *The Release of Catecholamines from Adrenergic Neurons* (ed. D.M. Paton), pp. 143–183. Pergamon Press, New York.

Sternberg, D.B., Isaacs, K., Gold, P.E., and McGaugh, J.L. (1985) Epinephrine facilitation of appetitive learning: attenuation with adrenergic receptor antagonists. *Behavioral and Neural Biology*, 44, 447–453.

Tomaz, C., Dickinson-Anson, H., and McGaugh, J.L. (1992) Basolateral amygdala lesions block diazepam-induced anterograde amnesia in an inhibitory avoidance task. *Proceedings of the National Academy of Sciences of the United States of America*, 89, 3615–3619.

Tomaz, C., Dickinson-Anson, H., McGaugh, J.L., Souza-Silva, M.A., Viana, M.B., and Graeff, F.G. (1993) Localization in the amygdala of the amnestic action of diazepam on emotional memory. *Behavioral Brain Research*, 58, 99–105.

Unnerstal, J.R., Kopajtic, T.A., and Kuhar, M.J. (1984) Distribution of α_2-agonist binding sites in the rat and human central nervous system: analysis of some functional, anatomic correlates of the pharmacological effects of clonidine and related adrenergic agents. *Brain Research*, 319, 69–101.

Vazdarjanova, A. and McGaugh, J. L. (1998) Basolateral amygdala is not a critical locus for memory of contextual fear conditioning. *Proceedings of the National Academy of Sciences of the United States of America*, 95, 15003–15007.

Vazdarjanova, A. and McGaugh, J.L. (1999) Basolateral amygdala is involved in modulating consolidation of memory for classical fear conditioning. *Journal of Neuroscience*, **19**, 6615–6622.

Weil-Malherbe, H., Axelrod, J., and Tomchick, R. (1959) Blood–brain barrier for adrenaline. *Science*, 129, 1226–1228.

Weinberger, N.M. (1995) Retuning the brain by fear conditioning. In *The Cognitive Neurosciences* (ed. M.S. Gazzaniga), pp. 1071–1089. MIT Press, Cambridge, Massachusetts.

Weinberger, N.M. (1998) Tuning the brain by learning and by stimulation of the nucleus basalis. *Trends in Cognitive Sciences*, 2, 271–273.

Weinberger, N.M., Ashe, J.H., Diamond, D.M., Metherate, R., McKenna, T.M., and Bakin, J.S. (1990) Retuning auditory cortex by learning: a preliminary model of receptive field plasticity. *Concepts in Neuroscience*, 1, 91–132.

Weiskrantz, L. (1956) Behavioral changes associated with ablation of the amygdaloid complex in monkeys. *Journal of Comparative Physiology and Psychology*, 49, 381–391.

Williams, C.L. (2000) Brainstem contributions to memory formation. In *Four Decades of Memory: A Festschrift Honoring James L. McGaugh* (eds P.E. Gold and W.T. Greenough), American Psychological Association, Washington, DC, in press.

Williams, C.L. and McGaugh, J.L. (1993) Reversible lesions of the nucleus of the solitary tract attenuate the memory-modulating effects of posttraining epinephrine. *Behavioral Neuroscience*, 107, 1–8.

Williams, C.L., Men, D., Clayton, E.C., and Gold, P.E. (1998) Norepinephrine release in the amygdala following systemic injection of epinephrine or escapable footshock: contribution of the nucleus of the solitary tract. *Behavioral Neuroscience*, 112, 1414–1422.

Zilles, K., Qu, M., and Schleicher, A. (1993) Regional distribution and heterogeneity of α-adrenoceptors in the rat and human central nervous system. *Journal für Hirnforshung*, 2, 123–132.

12 Modulation of long-term memory storage in humans by emotional arousal: adrenergic activation and the amygdala

Larry Cahill

Department of Neurobiology and Behavior, and Center for the Neurobiology of Learning and Memory, University of California, Irvine, CA 92697-3800, USA

Summary

Anchored in an extensive literature involving infra-human subjects, a rapidly growing number of studies involving human subjects confirms the theory that the sympathetic nervous system and the amygdala are crucial for the modulation of long-term memory storage for emotionally arousing events. Several studies indicate adrenergic participation in memory for emotional events in humans. Amygdala participation is indicated by converging evidence from neuropsychological and brain imaging studies. Substantial evidence from both infra-human and human subject studies suggests that the degree of emotional arousal involved in a learning situation, rather than its pleasant/unpleasant nature, determines the degree of amygdala engagement in learning. Although evidence for amygdala participation in long-term memory storage for emotionally arousing events in humans is strong, evidence for its participation in memory retrieval, or for its participation in the production of emotion *per se*, currently is less clear. The chapter closes with a novel, testable proposal regarding a mechanism by which this system may modulate long-term memory storage.

12.1 Introduction

> 'Excitement may be the successor of other emotions. When fear is relieved by the sudden disappearance of a menace, as when one has killed a rattlesnake faced suddenly in the mountains, there is no instant calm. The alarm is gone, but the waters continue to be troubled as after a squall.'
> George Stratton, 1928

An emotionally arousing experience such as that described by Stratton would likely be well remembered. Abundant experimental and anecdotal evidence suggests that, in general, such an experience would be recalled more accurately, more easily, and for a longer time than would a more mundane experience. Why? This chapter addresses some potential neurobiological mechanisms by which emotional arousal sculpts the contents of long-term memory.

Most neurobiological investigations of memory focus on potential mechanisms by which the brain stores information—the 'memory trace.' The research focused on here begins with the assumption that the brain must also possess the means to 'weight', or modulate, the actual information storage mechanisms in general proportion to the importance of the information being stored (Gold and McGaugh, 1975). Without modulatory mechanisms, the brain would be unable to distinquish the important from the trivial in long-term memory.

There appear to be, at minimum, two interacting neurobiological components mediating the modulatory actions of emotional arousal on memory: the adrenergic system and the amygdala (especially the basolateral nucleus). Findings from a large variety of investigations involving both human and animal subjects converge on this view. The primary aim of this chapter is to summarize the key findings from studies involving human subjects addressing this view. However, because research with infra-human animals provides the foundation on which these views rest, I first describe some of the most relevant animal research. I close by proposing a novel mechanism by which an interacting adrenergic hormone/amygdala-based system may modulate long-term memory for emotionally arousing events. A central feature of the proposal is anticipated in the above quote by Stratton: post-event ruminative processes.

12.2 Understanding memory formation for emotionally stressful events: the foundation in animal research

Extensive animal research provides a theoretical framework for understanding the neurobiological underpinnings of emotionally influenced memory. An interaction between endogenous stress hormones activated by emotional experiences and the amygdala appears critical. Additionally, adrenal medullary and cortical hormones appear to interact in modulating memory formation. Since this research is reviewed in detail elsewhere (McGaugh *et al.*, 1984, 1996, Chapter 11), only some key points are highlighted here.

There are many demonstrations that post-learning systemic administration of adrenergic agonists [such as adrenaline (epinephrine)] can enhance memory formation in animals. Somewhat surprisingly, therefore, there are no unequivocal demonstrations in the literature that post-learning systemic administration of adrenergic antagonists impairs memory. The hypothesis that adrenergic activation modulates memory consolidation predicts that, under appropriate conditions, post-learning systemic administration of adrenergic antagonists will impair memory. However, disruption of a modulatory influence will not necessarily be apparent in all conditions; rather, its detection will depend on the experimental conditions, such as drug dose, degree of arousal produced by the learning situation, and the strength of the memory involved.

With these considerations in mind, we recently examined the effect of post-learning adrenergic blockade on memory formation in rats (Cahill *et al.*, in press). Rats received six training trials in a task known to produce substantial adrenergic activation ('Morris' spatial water maze training). Immediately after training, they received a systemic injection of either saline or the $\beta_1\beta_2$-adrenergic antagonist propranolol (5 mg/kg). Memory for the location of the platform was tested 24 h later. The results revealed a significant impairment of retention by propranolol. Furthermore, as may be expected from a modulatory treatment, the memory impairing effect was not apparent in all rats. Propranolol strongly impaired memory in those rats that exhibited good learning during the acquisition session, yet had no effect in rats that exhibited poor learning during acquisition. These findings provide important additional support for the hypothesis that post-learning adrenergic activation modulates memory for emotionally arousing events. Further, they help to explain why previous investigations (which did not examine drug–degree of learning interactions) may have failed to find memory impairments with systemic administration of adrenergic-blocking drugs.

Adrenergic stress hormones interact with the amygdala to influence memory (McGaugh *et al.*, Chapter 11). Lesions of amygdala circuitry [in particular the basolateral nucleus (BLA) and stria terminalis] block the memory-modulating effects of systemically administered hormones. Indeed, it is a remarkably consistent finding that basolateral amygdala or stria terminalis lesions block both memory-enhancing and memory-impairing effects of virtually every drug and hormone tested to date (McGaugh *et al.*, 1996, Chapter 11).

If a primary function of the amygdala is to interact with endogenous stress hormones to influence memory storage, then impairing effects of amygdala lesions on memory should be most evident for relatively arousing (i.e. sympathetic nervous system-activating) learning situations. This implication has been tested (Cahill and McGaugh, 1990). In one experiment, rats were trained over four successive days to find water at one end of a Y-maze. One-trial appetitively motivated learning was evident in the decreased latencies to locate the water between training days 1 and 2 (see Figure 12.1). On day 3, rats received a footshock when they began to drink. One-trial aversively motivated learning was evident in the increased latencies to drink between days 3 and 4. Excitotoxin-induced amygdala lesions made before training had no effect on the presumably less arousing one-trial appetitive learning, but significantly impaired the more highly arousing, one-trial aversive learning. In another experiment, rats received a milder aversive stimulus (quinine solution) when attempting to drink on day 3. Amygdala lesions in this case affected neither the appetitively nor aversively motivated training (see Figure 12.2). On the basis of findings such as these, Cahill and McGaugh (1990) concluded that '*the degree of arousal produced by the unconditioned stimulus, and not the aversive nature* per se*, determines the level of amygdala involvement*' in a learning situation. By this hypothesis, sufficiently emotionally arousing (i.e. sympathetic nervous system-activating) learning situations should engage amygdala participation in memory formation, independently of whether the particular emotions involved are positive or negative. This prediction is now supported by studies of humans with selective amygdala damage, as well as human brain imaging experiments (discussed below).

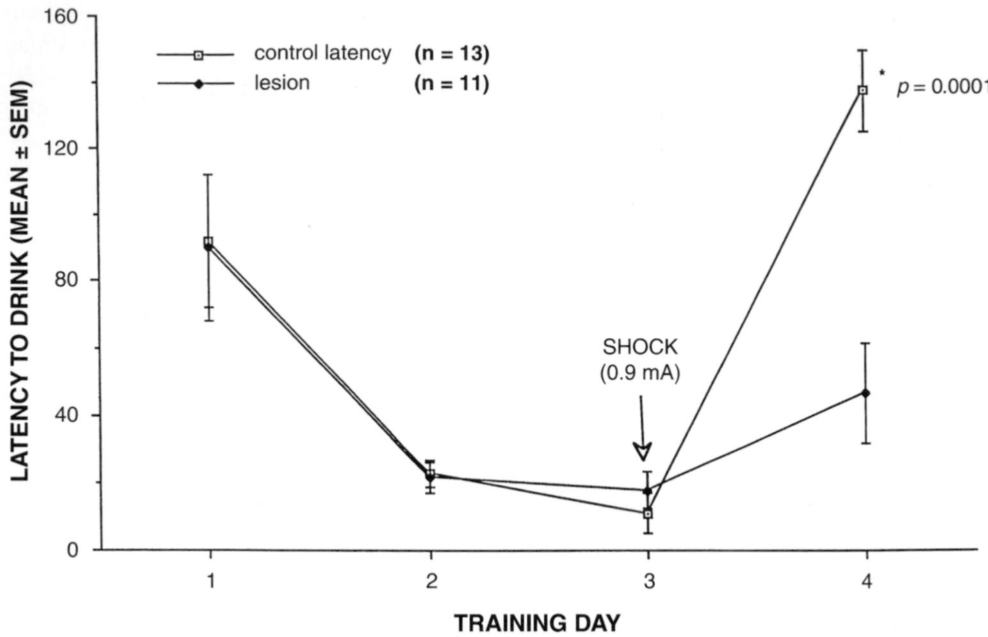

Figure 12.1 Amygdala lesions do not block acquisition of a simple, appetitively motivated task (learning to find a water reward) which is seen in the decreased latencies to find water in a Y-maze between training days 1 and 2. Lesions significantly impaired retention of one-trial aversive learning with a highly arousing stimulus (footshock), seen in the increased latencies to drink between days 3 and 4. (From Cahill and McGaugh, 1990, with permission.)

12.3 Neural mechanisms of explicit memory for emotionally arousing events in humans

In recent years, several experiments involving human subjects have provided strong converging evidence for the 'memory modulation' framework derived from animal research. There now is clear evidence from these studies that adrenergic activation and the amygdala are important for enhanced long-term memory associated with emotionally arousing events in humans.

12.3.1 Role of the adrenergic system

Several studies indicate that activation of the adrenergic system in humans is required for the enhancing effect of arousal (either emotionally or physically induced) on memory. For example, propranolol attenuates the enhanced long-term memory associated with emotionally arousing information without affecting memory for more emotionally neutral information (Cahill *et al.*, 1994; Nielson and Jensen, 1994; van Stegeren *et al.*, 1998). Because of the selectivity for emotionally salient information, the impairing effect of propranolol

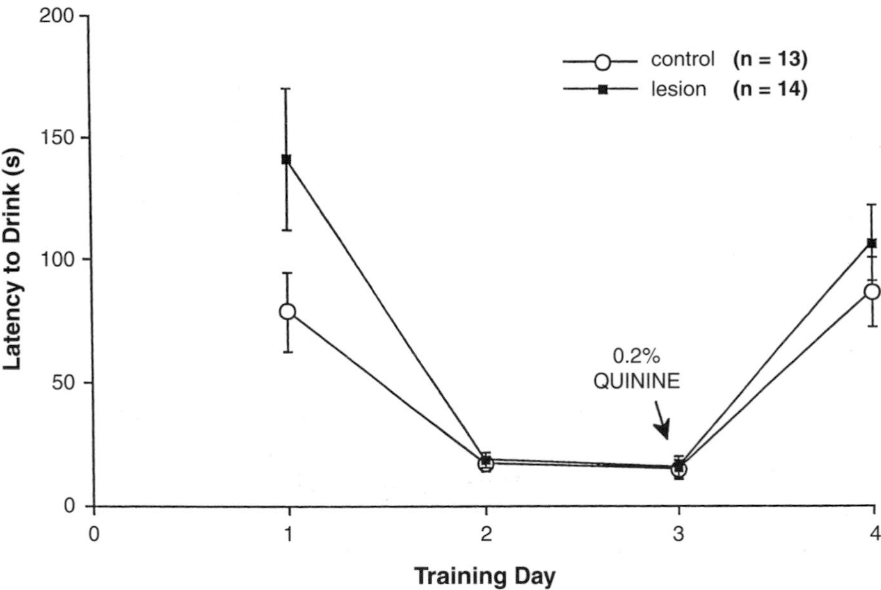

Figure 12.2 Amygdala lesions do not significantly affect either one-trial appetitive learning (decreased latencies between days 1 and 2) or one-trial aversively motivated learning (increased latencies between days 3 and 4) when a relatively mild aversive stimulus (quinine) is used. (From Cahill and McGaugh, 1990, with permission.)

cannot easily be attributed to potential effects of the drug on either attention, sedation, or the emotional reactions to the material (Cahill *et al.*, 1994).

van Stegeren and colleagues (1998) investigated whether the impairing effect of propranolol on memory for emotionally arousing material was due to actions at central or peripheral receptors. Subjects in this study received either a placebo or propranolol before viewing either a relatively emotionally arousing story, or a closely matched but more emotionally neutral story. An additional group received nadolol (a peripherally acting $\beta_1\beta_2$-adrenergic blocker) at a dose producing heart rate and blood pressure effects comparable with those produced by propranolol. Recall of the stories was tested 1 week later. As expected, propranolol selectively impaired memory of the emotional story. In contrast, nadolol had no effect on memory for either the emotionally arousing or neutral stories, strongly suggesting that propranolol acted via central receptors to impair memory for the emotional story. It should be emphasized, however, that the findings of van Stegeren *et al.* (1998) leave open the possibility, suggested by animal research, that an influence of peripheral adrenergic blockade on emotionally influenced memory would be detected in other, perhaps more highly arousing learning situations in humans.

Additional evidence is refining our understanding of adrenergic involvement in memory for emotional events in humans. O'Carroll and colleagues (1999) examined the effects of a more selective adrenergic blockade than that produced by propranolol, as well as the effects of adrenergic stimulation on memory. Subjects in this study received either a placebo, metoprolol (a β_1-receptor antagonist), or yohimbine (which stimulates noradrenergic activity via blockade of the α_2-adrenergic autoreceptor) before viewing an emotionally arousing story. Retention of the story information was tested 1 week later. The results indicated that metoprolol impaired, and yohimbine enhanced retention relative to placebo controls. These findings therefore suggest that blockade of β_1-receptors alone impairs memory for emotionally arousing material. Further, they suggest that adrenergic stimulation can enhance memory for emotional material.

Importantly, in another parallel with animal research, adrenergic stimulation can act in a retrograde manner to enhance memory in humans. Soetens and colleagues (1995) reported the first evidence of retrograde memory enhancement with a drug injection in humans. Subjects in this study learned lists of words, and immediately after received an intramuscular injection of either amphetamine or vehicle. Retention of the words was tested after varying intervals. The results revealed a clear enhancing effect of the amphetamine injections on long-term memory for the words. These findings therefore support the view that post-learning adrenergic stimulation enhances memory consolidation.

Findings from another recent study (Cahill and Alkire, submitted) suggest that administration of an endogenous catecholamine hormone, adrenaline, can also enhance memory consolidation. Subjects viewed a series of 21 slides. Immediately after, they received a 3 min intravenous infusion of either saline or adrenaline. Retention of the slides was assessed in a surprise free recall test 1 week later. The results revealed a selective, but significant effect of the adrenaline infusions: adrenaline produced a dose-dependent enhancement of memory for the initial slides in the series. Although in need of confirmation in other experimental situations, these findings provide the first suggestion in human subjects that a physiological dose of adrenaline given immediately after learning can produce retrograde memory enhancement. Consequently, they provide additional support in human subjects for the view that enhanced memory associated with emotionally arousing events depends, at least in part, on adrenergic system activation induced by the emotional arousal.

Two potential clinical effects of this proposed 'memory-modulating' system are worth considering. First, overactivation of this normally adaptive system may underlie the formation of the excessively strong ('intrusive') memories characteristic of post-traumatic stress disorder (PTSD; Pitman, 1989). If so, then appropriate treatment with β-blocking drugs as soon as possible after a person has experienced an emotional trauma should reduce or prevent the development of PTSD (Cahill, 1997). Several clinical trials to test this important implication are underway. Secondly, it has long been known that amygdala stimulation can produce retrograde amnesia (McGaugh *et al.*, 1984, 1996, Chapter 11). Thus, it is also possible that overactivation of an amygdala-based memory-modulating system could produce retrograde amnesia, as is sometimes seen in persons experiencing an extremely stressful event. This possibility will of course be much more difficult to examine clinically.

12.3.2 The amygdala's role in emotionally influenced, long-term memory

Paralleling research with adrenergic manipulations, research investigating the amygdala's role in memory also suggests a selective role for this structure in emotionally influenced, long-term memory. These include studies of patients with selective amygdala damage, and human brain imaging investigations.

Beginning with the famous study of Scoville and Milner (1957), a role for the amygdala in explicit memory was questioned. They examined memory in 10 patients, including some with relatively selective amygdala damage (e.g. patient I.S.), and concluded that 'removal of the amygdala bilaterally does not appear to cause memory impairment.' However, the tests employed involved short-term memory, and/or memory for non-emotionally arousing material. Negative findings such as these (see also Bechara *et al.*, 1995) fit well with the 'memory modulation' view of amygdala function, which predicts that amygdala activity should not be critical for short-term memory, or for long-term memory of non-emotionally arousing events or material. Instead, by this view, amygdala activity should be required for the enhanced long-term memory associated with emotional arousal (Cahill and McGaugh, 1990, 1998; McGaugh *et al.*, 1984, 1996, Chapter 11).

Several studies involving subjects with discrete amygdala lesions provide evidence that the amygdala is involved specifically with enhanced explicit memory associated with emotionally arousing material. In the first of these studies, Babinsky and colleagues (1993) reported deficits in memory for emotional material in a rare patient with damage confined almost exclusively to her amygdala. Others report that enhanced long-term memory associated with an emotionally arousing story is impaired in patients with selective (Cahill *et al.*, 1995) or nearly selective (Adolphs *et al.*, 1997) amygdala damage. The story used in these latter investigations was shown previously to be sensitive to adrenergic blockade (Cahill *et al.*, 1994); thus these studies provide additional, indirect evidence for an interaction between the adrenergic system and the amygdala in emotionally influenced memory. Finally, amnesic subjects with intact amygdalae show relatively intact enhancement of memory for emotional material despite their overall impaired memory performance, further implicating the amygdala in the effect of emotion on memory (Hamann *et al.*, 1997a).

Several studies suggest that the emotional reactions (both cognitive and physiological) of patients with amygdala damage to emotionally provocative stimuli are not significantly different from those of controls (Cahill *et al.*, 1995; Adolphs *et al.*, 1997; Hamann *et al.*, 1997b) even though long-term memory for emotional material is impaired. One subject even spontaneously described to the experimenters her strong negative emotional reaction to a particular aversive stimulus, yet failed to demonstrate enhanced recall of that stimulus as seen in control subjects (Adolphs *et al.*, 1997). Other evidence suggests that electrodermal responses to emotionally stressful events are intact in humans with amygdala damage (Bechara *et al.*, 1995). On the basis of findings such as these [and positron emission tomography (PET) findings discussed below], Cahill and colleagues (1996) proposed that amygdala activity in humans 'may be more important for the translation of an emotional reaction into heightened recall than it is for the generation of an emotional reaction *per se*.' A recent study of electrodermal reactions to emotional stimuli in a patient with bilateral amygdala damage provides additional support for this proposal (Hamann *et al.*, 1999a).

A study of memory in Alzheimer's disease (AD) patients provides striking new evidence consistent with the 'memory modulation' view of amygdala function. Mori and colleagues (1999) studied memory of AD patients who had experienced a highly emotional event, the

Kobe earthquake. Using magnetic resonance imaging (MRI), they measured the volume of the amygdala in the patients. They found that amygdala volume correlated significantly with retention of the personal events experienced during the earthquake, and not with retention of semantic knowledge of the earthquake (such as its size on the Richter scale). These findings suggest that the modulatory role for the amygdala in emotionally influenced long-term memory is very a robust phenomenon.

12.2.3 Brain imaging studies

Brain imaging studies provide convergent evidence with neuropsychological data and animal research in suggesting a selective role for the amygdala in enhanced long-term memory for emotionally arousing events. In the first of these studies, subjects received two PET scans: one while viewing a series of relatively emotionally arousing films, another while viewing a series of relatively emotionally neutral films (Cahill *et al.*, 1996). Memory for the films was tested in a surprise free recall test 3 weeks later. Activity in the right amygdala correlated very highly ($r = 0.93$) with the number emotional films recalled 3 weeks later, but not with recall of the neutral films (see Figure 12.3).

Another PET study both confirms this amygdala finding and provides strong additional evidence for the 'memory modulation' view of amygdala function. This view, as described earlier, predicts that the degree of arousal involved in an emotional learning situation, and not the pleasant/unpleasant nature of the emotion, should be the key determinant of amygdala participation in memory storage (Cahill and McGaugh, 1990, 1998). Hamann and colleagues (1999b) used PET to study cerebral blood flow while subjects viewed either pleasant or unpleasant arousing pictures. Amygdala activity while viewing either the pleasant or unpleasant pictures correlated very highly with memory for the pictures 1 month later. Amygdala activity while viewing emotionally neutral pictures (including pictures of novel, but not emotionally arousing objects) did not correlate with recall. That the arousing dimension of the pictures was essential to amygdala engagement in memory is suggested by the fact that removal of the most clearly arousing pleasant slides (erotic scenes) eliminated the correlation between amygdala activity and memory for pleasant slides (S. Hamann, personal communication, 1999). A recent functional MRI (fMRI) investigation demonstrating amygdala responsiveness to erotic scenes (Labar *et al.*, 1998a) provides still more evidence supporting the view that amygdala's participation in a learning situation depends most critically on the degree of arousal induced by the stimuli, rather than their pleasant or unpleasant nature (Cahill and McGaugh, 1990).

Other aspects of the findings of Hamann *et al.* (1999b) fit very well with the 'memory modulation' framework of amygdala function. For example, amygdala activity in no instance correlated with short-term memory of the pictures. Additionally, although activity of both the left and right amygdala correlated with recall of arousing material, the degree appeared greater on the right for negative slides. This finding fits well with those of Cahill *et al.* (1996), who used emotionally negative material, and may help to explain why the effect was unilateral in that study. They also suggest that differences in left versus right amygdala participation in memory for emotionally arousing events may relate to their pleasant/unpleasant nature.

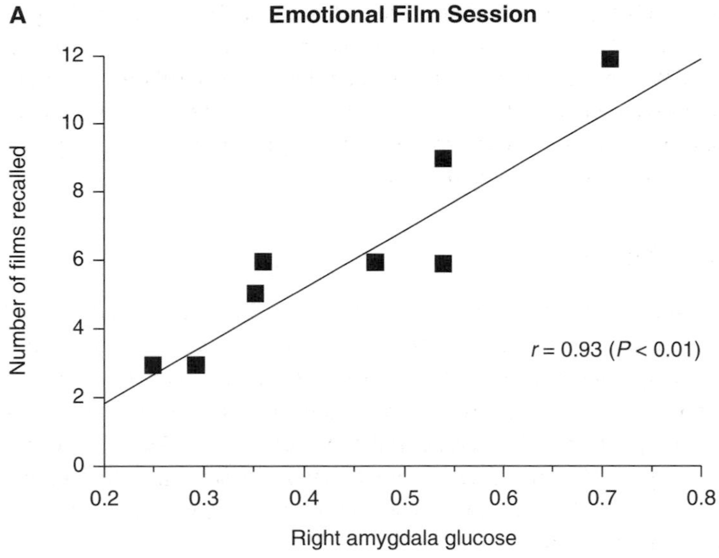

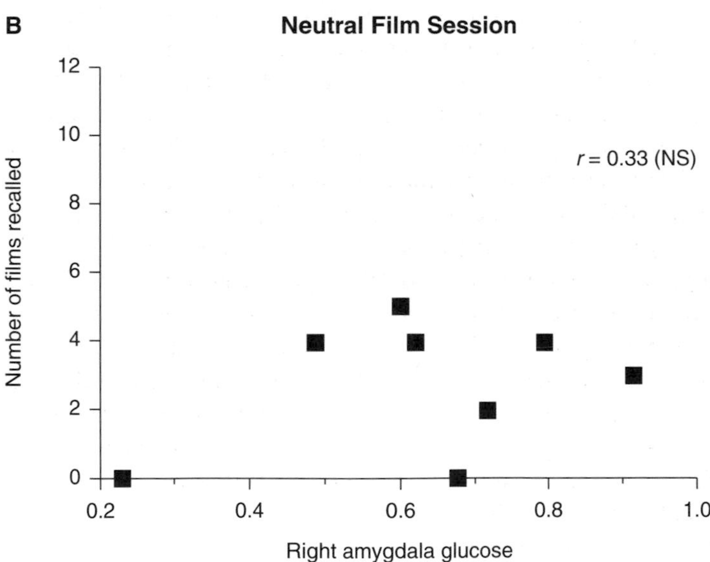

Figure 12.3 (**A**) Amygdala activity while watching a series of emotionally arousing films correlated very highly with long-term (3 week) recall of the films. (**B**) Amygdala activity in the same subjects while viewing a series of relatively emotionally neutral films did not correlate significantly with recall. (From Cahill *et al.*, 1996, with permission.)

Activation of the left amygdala appears to be produced consistently by any of a variety of aversive stimuli used in human brain imaging studies (Cahill and McGaugh, 1998). However, no compelling explanation exists at present for such asymmetries in amygdala function. The issue of laterality of amygdala function in relation to emotion and memory is clearly an important area for future research (Canli *et al.*, 1998; Davidson and Irwin, 1999).

Two studies involving fMRI further confirm amygdala participation in memory storage for emotional material in humans. Canli and colleagues (1999) reported that amygdala activity in response to emotionally negative pictures correlated with long-term (2–14 months) retention of the pictures. Also, in an individual-trial fMRI study conducted in collaboration with these investigators, we have found evidence that increasing the degree of arousal induced by emotional pictures increases the degree to which amygdala activity is correlated with long-term recall of the pictures (Canli *et al.*, 2000).

Thus, evidence from several human brain imaging studies, including both PET and fMRI investigations, converges with both neuropsychological data and findings from animal research to support the view that the amygdala is involved preferentially with long-term storage of explicit memory for emotionally arousing events (Cahill and McGaugh, 1990, 1998; McGaugh *et al.*, Chapter 11), although its role in the production of emotional responses *per se* in humans is less clear (Cahill *et al.*, 1996; Cahill and McGaugh, 1998).

Finally, a report by Whalen and colleagues (1998) indicates that the human amygdala can be activated by briefly presented stimuli (fearful faces) that are 'masked' by other stimuli (neutral faces), and thus are not perceived consciously. These findings clearly weaken the link between amygdala activity and the production of emotional responses *per se*, since robust amygdala activation occurred in the complete absence of any perceived emotional experience by the subjects. It is not clear, however, how they relate to amygdala participation in explicit memory formation. If the amygdala response indicates activation of a memory-modulating mechanism for explicit memory, then the masking stimuli perceived during amygdala activation should be better recalled, at least in some conditions, than those perceived in the absence of amygdala activation. This possibility has not been examined.

12.3.4 Candidate sites of modulation

Evidence from animal subject studies suggests that the amygdala affects memory by influencing memory storage processes in other brain regions (McGaugh *et al.*, 1984, 1996, Chapter 11). Although this issue has not as yet been examined systematically with brain imaging techniques, some clues as to potential brain regions with which the amygdala functions to affect memory are offered by imaging studies to date. For instance, activity of the cholinergic basal forebrain region (the 'substantia innominata') correlated significantly with recall of emotional but not neutral films in the report of Cahill *et al.* (1996) discussed above. Another investigation reported that activity of the amygdala covaried with that of the basal forebrain during acquisition of aversively motivated classical conditioning (Morris *et al.*, 1998). Several authors have proposed that the amygdala may influence cortical processing via the cholinergic basal forebrain (Weinberger *et al.*, 1990; Kapp *et al.*, 1992; Rolls, 1992;

Gutierrez *et al.*, 1997), and these findings regarding the substantia innominata fit well with this view. I return to this idea in the closing section of this chapter.

Animal research implicates the hippocampal region as a potential site of modulation by the amygdala (Packard *et al.*, 1994; Packard and Teather, 1998). In the PET study reported by Cahill *et al.* (1996), activity of the parahippocampal cortex correlated with memory of both the neutral and emotional films. The finding that parahippocampal cortex activity during encoding correlates generally with long-term memory for either emotional or neutral material has been confirmed by both PET (Alkire *et al.*, 1998) and fMRI (Brewer *et al.*, 1998; Wagner *et al.*, 1998) studies. Data suggesting coincident amygdala and hippocampal region activation during emotionally arousing events (Cahill *et al.*, 1996; Hamann *et al.*, 1999b) are consistent with—although certainly do not prove—the idea that the amygdala affects memory via influences on the hippocampal region.

Other brain regions are likely candidates through which the amygdala may function to modulate memory. One example is the orbitofrontal cortex, which has strong connections to the amygdala (Porrino *et al.*, 1981). Several studies have reported coincident orbitofrontal and amygdala activations during emotionally arousing learning situations (Cahill *et al.*, 1996; Zald and Pardo, 1996; Morris *et al.*, 1997). Another example is the retrosplenial cortex, which is among the cortical regions activated most consistently by emotionally salient stimuli, and which is involved with explicit memory formation (Maddock, 1999). Interestingly, the retrosplenial cortex is also among the cortical regions activated most consistently in rats (as assessed with c-Fos immunochemistry) by pharmacological stimulation of the amygdala (L. Cahill, unpublished findings).

Studies examining the covariance of amygdala activity with other brain regions in the context of emotionally arousing versus emotionally neutral learning situations should help to identify a network of structures through which the amygdala modulates memory. Some studies along these lines have been reported. For example, a PET investigation of aversive auditory classical conditioning found that activity in regions of the auditory cortex positively covaried with activity in the amygdala (as well as the basal forebrain and orbitofrontal cortex) during conditioning (Morris *et al.*, 1998). Covariance analyses such as this, especially when combined with converging evidence from neuropsychological studies, neuropharmacological studies, and animal research, will probably be a powerful tool for examining amygdala functions in memory in humans.

12.3.5 Amygdala participation in acquisition, retrieval, or both?

Understanding the amygdala's role in memory will require understanding whether, and to what degree, it is necessary for acquisition versus retrieval processes. The imaging studies discussed above clearly implicate the amygdala in encoding/consolidation processes, but do not address its role in retrieval processes. Other studies report evidence consistent with amygdala participation in encoding/consolidation, but not retrieval processes. Two fMRI studies of amygdala involvement in aversive classical conditioning reported that the amygdala was active in response to a conditioned stimulus during learning of a conditioned association, but not once the association was learned (Büchel *et al.*, 1998; LaBar *et al.*, 1998b). A PET investigation reported amygdala activation while subjects initially viewed emotional pictures, but not when retrieval of the pictures was tested later (Taylor *et al.*, 1998). Similarly, viewing (and presumably forming memories of) emotionally arousing films has been reported to activate the amygdala (assessed with PET), although retrieval of previously experienced emotional events did not (Reiman *et al.*, 1997), findings again consistent with a primary, if not selective, amygdala role in acquisition of memory for emotional events.

Others reports indicate amygdala activation during retrieval of emotional events. For example, Fink and colleagues (1996) reported unilateral amygdala (and temporal lobe) activation in subjects retrieving emotionally laden autobiographical memories. Others report amygdala activation in persons with PTSD when they recall the distressful event that caused their disorder (Rauch *et al.*, 1996). Findings such as these are consistent with amygdala participation in retrieval of memory for emotional events. However, when considering evidence of amygdala participation in retrieval, it is essential to distinguish between retrieval *with or without concomitant emotional arousal*. The reason is that, according to the 'memory modulation' hypothesis, the amygdala should influence memory storage processes whenever a situation is sufficiently emotionally arousing—independently of whether the arousal is produced by an external or internal event (such a memory which induces an emotional response (Cahill and McGaugh, 1998). Indeed, Fink *et al.* (1996) reported that their subjects probably experienced substantial emotional arousal during retrieval. Similarly, retrieval of traumatic events in PTSD patients generally is very emotionally stressful. Thus, amygdala activation during retrieval occurring with a concomitant emotional response may reflect amygdala participation in memory storage, rather than retrieval processes. To help to clarify this issue, future studies should be designed to determine whether concomitant emotional arousal is critical to amygdala activation at the time of retrieval.

12.3.6 The role of the vagus

In addition to implicating stress hormone activation and the amygdala, animal research implicates vagal nerve function in emotionally influenced memory (Clark *et al.*, 1998). Adrenaline, which does not cross the blood–brain barrier, is thought to influence memory via stimulation of the vagus nerve (McGaugh *et al.*, 1996, Chapter 11). A role for the vagus nerve in memory of humans subjects is suggested by a recent study by Clark and colleagues (1999), who studied memory for words in subjects given vagal nerve stimulation immediately after exposure to the words. Vagal nerve stimulation dose-dependently increased word recognition as compared with word recognition in the same subjects when stimulation was not given. These findings thus converge with animal research in suggesting a mechanism by which peripheral hormones such as adrenaline, which do not cross the blood–brain barrier, influence central memory storage processes.

12.3.7 Is a 'memory-modulating' amygdala mechanism necessary?

It has been suggested that it is not necessary to posit the existence of a 'special mechanism' such as amygdala modulation of memory to account for enhanced memory associated with emotion. For example, Neisser and colleagues (1996), who investigated memory in persons who experienced a powerful earthquake, propose that narrative rehearsal is the most likely explanation for the exceptionally strong and long-lasting memory they observed. It is a reasonable proposal *a priori*, since we do tend to talk more about (and thus rehearse) emotionally significant experiences compared with emotionally neutral experiences. We examined this proposal experimentally (Guy and Cahill, 1999). Narrative rehearsal (discussing the films) was manipulated in subjects after they had viewed a series of relatively emotionally arousing and relatively emotionally neutral films. The films were those for which we have evidence of an amygdala influence on their storage in memory (Cahill *et al.*, 1996). Memory for the films was tested about 1 week later. The results revealed a significant advantage for the emotional versus neutral films in memory, irrespective of the degree of narrative rehearsal engaged in by the subjects. Retention of the emotional films was significantly better than retention of the neutral films even in subjects who did not rehearse the films at all. These findings therefore argue strongly against the view that narrative rehearsal is a sufficient explanation of enhanced memory associated with emotional arousal, and provide indirect evidence for amygdala modulation of memory for emotional material. They leave open, however, the possibility (discussed next) that post-event ruminative processes influence memory for emotional events.

12.4 Modulation of memory by modulation of reverberation?

Strong converging evidence from many levels of investigation suggests that peripheral stress activation (in particular adrenergic activation) and the amygdala (in particular the BLA) interact to influence long-term memory consolidation for emotionally stressful events (Cahill and McGaugh, 1990, 1998; McGaugh *et al.*, 1984, 1996, Chapter 11). In this closing section, I propose a novel, testable mechanism by which these effects may occur.

The hypothesized mechanism, presented schematically in Figure 12.4, is summarized as follows: the BLA facilitates consolidation of cortical memory storage processes via activation of the cholinergic basal forebrain, and by interaction with peripheral adrenergic feedback. Modulation of long-term memory storage occurs, at least in part, via modulation of the duration of reverberatory activity in cortical–subcortical loops. The hypothesis requires synthesis of many lines of research, including anatomical, physiological, pharmacological, and behavioural studies. No single aspect of the mechanism is entirely new, and some aspects admittedly are speculative. I also do not suggest that it is the only mechanism by which the amygdala may influence memory. Still, it is hoped that this synthetic effort will, at minimum, have heuristic value for those attempting to make sense of the extremely large and diverse body of information (accumulating for >40 years) relevant to understanding amygdala functions in memory.

I begin with consideration of a commonly observed reaction to emotionally stressful events: post-event, ruminative memory processes. The phenomenon often is observed anecdotally. William James (1890), for example, noted that ‘When we have been exposed to an unusual

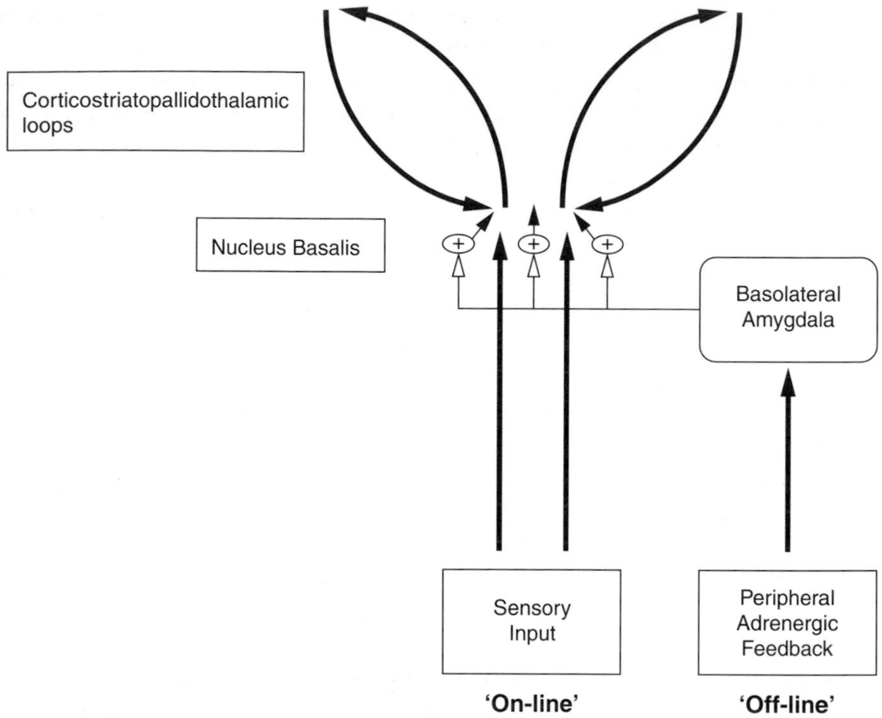

Figure 12.4 A mechanism by which the basolateral amygdala, interacting with peripheral stress hormone feedback, may influence memory consolidation for emotionally arousing events.

stimulus . . . a nervous process is set up which results in the haunting of consciousness by the impression for a long time afterwards.' A few studies document ruminative processes in memory after emotionally stressful events. For example, a study of persons involved in the horrible collapse of two skywalks at the Hyatt Regency Hotel in Kansas City on July 17, 1981, which killed over 100 people and injured hundreds more, found that nearly 90% kept remembering the disaster repeatedly and intrusively in the following weeks (Wilkinson, 1983). It seems a reasonable assumption that understanding neural mechanisms underlying post-event rumination after emotionally arousing events will also be central to understanding memory formation for the events.

Studies of amygdala participation in memory demonstrate its influence on post-event, memory consolidation processes (McGaugh *et al.*, 1984, 1996, Chapter 11). The BLA and the stria terminalis (a major afferent/efferent amygdala pathway) appear essential for these effects. As mentioned earlier, lesions of either the BLA or stria terminalis block memory modulation produced by post-learning administration of peripheral drugs and hormones. Thus the BLA and stria terminalis interact with peripheral nervous system activity to influence post-event consolidation processes. Additionally, strong evidence suggests that the BLA influences memory storage processes occurring elsewhere in the brain (McGaugh *et al.*, 1996,

Chapter 11). An explanation of memory for emotionally stressful events will probably require incorporation of these well-supported principles.

BLA modulation of post-event memory processes in other brain regions is especially interesting in light of a well-established, but largely unknown aspect of its function. In the 1950s, Kaada and colleagues discovered that stimulation of the amygdala, in particular the basolateral regions, produces a 'response indistinguishable from the arousal or orienting reaction induced by brain stem reticular activation and is associated with cortical desynchronization' (Kaada, 1972). Similar behavioural effects, with accompanying changes in the cortical electroencephalogram (EEG), have also been observed in humans following amygdala stimulation (Halgren, 1992). Clear evidence, however, dissociates cortical arousal induced by amygdala versus 'reticular formation' stimulation. First, unlike brainstem 'reticular' lesions, amygdala lesions do not affect the direct cortical EEG activation induced by sensory input, such as a tail-pinch (Kaada, 1972; Dringenberg and Vanderwolf, 1996). Secondly, amygdala-induced cortical activation does not require the integrity of the 'reticular formation' (Kaada, 1972; Dringenberg and Vanderwolf, 1996). Finally, the arousal response produced by amygdala stimulation is blocked by lesions of the stria terminalis, which also block the memory-modulating effects of amygdala stimulation (Kaada, 1972; McGaugh *et al.*, 1984, Chapter 11). Collectively, these observations suggest that whereas the brainstem 'reticular' arousal systems function in a relatively stimulus-linked, 'on-line' fashion, the BLA influences cortical arousal in a less directly stimulus-linked, 'off-line' manner.

Cortical activation by the BLA appears to require the cholinergic basal forebrain. The amygdala is one of the principal sources of afferents to the basal forebrain cholinergic nuclei (Russchen *et al.*, 1985). Activation of cortical EEG activity by BLA stimulation is blocked both by systemic administration of the cholinergic antagonist scopolamine, and by infusions of a local anaesthetic (lidocaine) into the cholinergic basal forebrain (Dringenberg and Vanderwolf, 1996). Of particular relevance to the present proposal, direct stimulation of the basal forebrain has been shown to enhance the duration of an EEG response evoked by somatosensory stimulation (Dykes, 1997). Recall also that activity of the basal forebrain ('substantia innominata'), like the amygdala, correlated with memory for emotionally arousing, but not emotionally neutral films in the PET scan study of Cahill *et al.* (1996).

The evidence presented so far supports several components of the present hypothesis (Figure 12.4). First, post-event ('off-line') ruminative processes are probably important in understanding the effect of emotional arousal on long-term memory. Secondly, the BLA and stria terminalis interact with peripheral hormone feedback to influence post-event memory consolidation. Thirdly, the BLA region influences cortical activity, and does so in a manner that is both (i) not directly stimulus linked, and (ii) dependent on both the stria terminalis and the cholinergic basal forebrain. Fourthly, the cholinergic basal forebrain is both (i) capable of modulating the duration of cortical activation evoked by a stimulus and (ii) particularly important for memory of emotionally arousing events.

Interestingly, amygdala stimulation also produces behavioural effects with a delayed, post-event temporal characteristic. This characteristic is best seen by contrast with the effects of hypothalamic stimulation. Stimulation of either hypothalamic or amygdalar sites has long been known to produce any of a variety of emotional reactions (e.g. vocalizations, autonomic responses). Emotional reactions induced by hypothalamic stimulation generally begin rapidly upon stimulation, and disappear rapidly following termination of the stimulation (Zbrozyna, 1972). In contrast, emotional reactions after amygdala stimulation generally appear gradually after stimulation onset, and dissipate slowly after termination of the stimulation. These features of amygdala reactivity, among others, prompted Zbrozyna (1972) to suggest that the amygdala may be part of a 'system of self reverberating circuits which are capable of sustaining their excitatory state.' (p. 599). This intriguing feature of amygdala function—its apparent connection to the duration of an emotional reaction—can also be inferred from anecdotal evidence from human case studies. Emotional changes resulting from amygdala stimulation in humans have been reported to persist for hours after the stimulation (Mark *et al.*, 1972). In contrast, rapidly fading emotional reactions have been reported in some patients with amygdala damage (e.g. Corkin, 1984), although the duration of emotional reactions in amygdala patients has not, to my knowledge, been examined systematically.

The most speculative part of the present proposal concerns the manner in which a BLA-based system can influence post-event ruminative processes and memory consolidation. A well-accepted architectural principle of the brain is the existence of multiple, topographically organized corticostriatopallidal (CSP) systems (Fallon *et al.*, 1983) that interface with thalamic projections to the cortex to form re-entrant circuits, or 'loops' (Alexander *et al.*, 1986; Fallon and Loughlin, 1987; Groenewegen *et al.*, 1996). The concept of 'reverberatory circuits' as a neural basis for short-term memory can be dated at least to Hebb (1949), and remains a viable concept today (Sakurai, 1998). The 'CSP loops' (Fallon and Loughlin, 1987) may be a mechanism by which information is held in the short term. The BLA, interacting with a relatively 'slow' peripheral adrenergic feedback response, could then influence the rate of decay of reverberatory activity in these loops via the basal forebrain. An analogous idea regarding BLA function was suggested by Fallon and colleagues (1983), who noted that the BLA, because of its unique anatomical connections with both cortical and endocrine systems, 'must interface with the time environment of both the brain (milliseconds) and the hormonal–circulatory systems (seconds, hours, days)' and can therefore 'impose a longer time constant on neuronal events' (p. 116). A BLA mechanism, activated by an emotionally stressful event, and presumably in proportion to the degree of the emotional arousal, could potentiate consolidation into long-term memory of information held in, or dependent on, the CSP loops.

No hypothesis, no matter how much information it can incorporate, is useful unless it is testable. There are many ways in which the present proposal can be tested. For example, the rate of decay of a cortical activation (e.g. a cellular or EEG response) produced by a stimulus should be modulated (lengthened or shortened) by appropriate BLA stimulation. Further, it should be possible to relate the influence of the BLA on the rate of decay of cortical activation to retention of the stimuli that induced the activation. In humans, it should be possible to relate both the adrenergic system (with pharmacological manipulations) and amygdala/basal forebrain activity (with brain imaging) to the degree of post-event ruminative processes, EEG activation, and long-term memory after subjects view emotionally arousing versus emotionally neutral arousing material.

12.5 Concluding remarks

From a synthesis of over 40 years of research into amygdala participation in memory, the outlines of a neurobiological explanation of how emotional arousal influences memory can be seen. While no doubt an incomplete explanation, the interaction of peripheral stress hormone feedback and the BLA seems to be a critical influence on memory for emotional events. Human subject investigations that address such unresolved issues as laterality of function, amygdala subnuclei functions, and the pharmacology of memory modulation, and that continue to be educated by animal research, will no doubt further clarify the outlines.

Acknowledgements

I thank Dr James Fallon for his expertise and advice regarding anatomical issues, and my long-time collaborator and mentor, Dr James L. McGaugh for his friendship and constant support of my research efforts. Some of the research discussed in this article was supported by NIMH Grant MH57508-02 to L.C.

References

Adolphs, R., Cahill, L., Schul, R., and Babinsky, R. (1997) Impaired declarative memory for emotional stimuli following bilateral amygdala damage in humans. *Learning and Memory*, 4, 291–300.

Alexander, G., DeLong, M., and Strick, P. (1986) Parallel organization of functionally segregated circuits linking basal ganglia and cortex. *Annual Review of Neuroscience*, 9, 357–381.

Alkire, M., Haier, R., Fallon, J., and Cahill, L. (1998) Hippocampal, but not amygdala, activity at encoding correlates with long-term, free recall of non-emotional information. *Proceedings of the National Academy of Sciences of the United States of America*, 95, 14506–14510.

Babinsky, R., Calabrese, P., Durwen, H.F., Markowitsch, H.J., Brechtelsbauer, D., Heuser, L., and Gehlen, W. (1993) The possible contribution of the amygdala to memory. *Behavioral Neurology*, 6, 167–170.

Bechara, A., Tranel, D., Damasio, H., Adolphs, R., Rockland, C., and Damasio, A. (1995) Double dissociation of conditioning and declarative knowledge relative to the amygdala and hippocampus in humans. *Science*, 269, 1115–1118.

Brewer J.B., Zhao Z., Desmond J.E., Glover G.H., and Gabrieli J.D. (1998) Making memories: brain activity that predicts how well visual experience will be remembered. *Science*, 281, 1185–1187.

Büchel, C., Morris, J., Dolan, R.J., and Friston, K.J. (1998) Brain systems mediating aversive conditioning: an event-related fMRI study. *Neuron*, 20, 947–957.

Cahill, L. (1997) The neurobiology of emotionally influenced memory: implications for the treatment of traumatic memory. *Annals of the New York Academy of Sciences*, 821, 238–246.

Cahill, L., Babinsky, R., Markowitsch, H., and McGaugh, J.L. (1995) The amygdala and emotional memory. *Nature*, 377, 295–296.

Cahill, L., Haier, R., Fallon, J., Alkire, M., Tang, C., Keator, D., Wu, J., and McGaugh, J.L. (1996) Amygdala activity at encoding correlated with long-term, free recall of emotional information. *Proceedings of the National Academy of Sciences of the United States of America*, 93, 8016–8021.

Cahill, L. and McGaugh, J.L. (1990) Amygdaloid complex lesions differentially affect retention of tasks using appetitive and aversive reinforcement. *Behavioral Neuroscience*, 104, 532–543.

Cahill, L. and McGaugh J.L. (1998) Mechanisms of emotional arousal and lasting declarative memory. *Trends in Neuroscience*, 21, 294–299.

Cahill, L., Pham, C., and Setlow, B. (in press) Impaired memory consolidation in rats produced with β-adrenergic blockade. *Neurobiology of Learning and Memory*.

Cahill, L., Prins, B., Weber, M., and McGaugh, J.L. (1994) β-Adrenergic activation and memory for emotional events. *Nature*, 371, 702–704.

Canli, T., Brewer, J., Zhao, Z., Gabrieli, J.D.E., and Cahill, L. (2000) Event-related activation in the human amygdala associates with later memory for individual emotional experience. *Journal of Neuroscience*, in press.

Canli, T., Desmond, J.E., Zhao, Z., Glover, G., and Gabrieli, J.D.E. (1998) Hemispheric asymmetry for emotional stimuli detected with fMRI. *NeuroReport*, 9, 3233–3239.

Canli, T., Zhao, Z., Desmond, J., Glover, G., and Gabrieli, J.D.E. (1999) fMRI identifies a network of structures correlated with retention of positive and negative emotional memory. *Psychobiology*, 27: 441–452.

Clark, K., Naritoku, D., Smith, D., Browning, R., and Jensen, R. (1999) Enhanced recognition memory following vagus nerve stimulation in human subjects. *Nature Neuroscience*, 2, 94–98.

Clark, K.B., Smith, D.C., Hassert, D.L., Browning R.A., Naritoku, D.K., and Jensen, R.A. (1998) Posttraining electrical stimulation of vagal afferents with concomitant vagal efferent inactivation enhances memory storage processes in the rat. *Neurobiology of Learning and Memory*, 70, 364–373.

Corkin, S. (1984) Lasting consequences of bilateral medial temporal lobectomy: clinical course and experimental findings in H.M. *Seminars in Neurology*, 4, 249–259.

Davidson, R.J. and Irwin, W. (1999) The functional neuroanatomy of emotion and affective style. *Trends in Cognitive Sciences*, 3, 11–21.

Dringenberg, H., and Vanderwolf, C. (1996) Cholinergic activation of the electrocorticogram: an amygdaloid activating system. *Experimental Brain Research*, 108, 285–296.

Dykes, R.W. (1997) Mechanisms controlling neuronal plasticity in somatosensory cortex. *Canadian Journal of Physiology and Pharmacology*, 75, 535–545.

Fallon, J. and Loughlin, S. (1987) Monoamine innervation of cerebral cortex and a theory of the role of monoamines in cerebral cortex and basal ganglia. In *Cerebral Cortex, Volume 6, Further Aspects of Cortical Function, Including Hippocampus* (eds E.G. Jones and A. Peters), pp. 41–109. Plenum Press, New York.

Fallon, J., Loughlin, S., and Ribak, C. (1983) The islands of Calleja complex of rat basal forebrain. III. Histochemical evidence of a striatopallidal system. *Journal of Comparative Neurology*, 218, 91–120.

Fink, G., Markowitsch, H., Reinkemeier, M., Bruckbauer, T., Kessler, J., and Heiss, W. (1996) Cerebral representation of one's own past: neural networks involved in autobiographical memory. *Journal of Neuroscience*, 16, 4275–82.

Gold, P.E. and McGaugh, J.L. (1975) A single-trace, two process view of memory storage processes. In *Short-term Memory* (eds J. Deutsch and D. Deutsch), pp. 355–378. Academic Press, New York.

Groenewegen, H.J., Wright, C.I., and Beijer, A. (1996) The nucleus accumbens: gateway for limbic structures to reach the motor system? *Progress in Brain Research*, 107, 485–511.

Gutierrez, H., Miranda, M.I., and Bermudez-Rattoni, F. (1997) Learning impairment and cholinergic deafferentation after cortical nerve growth factor deprivation. *Journal of Neuroscience*, 17, 3796–3803.

Guy, S. and Cahill, L. (1999) Role of overt rehearsal in enhanced conscious memory for emotional events. *Consciousness and Cognition*, 8, 114–122.

Halgren, E. (1992) Emotional neurophysiology of the amygdala within the context of human cognition. In *The Amygdala: Neurobiological Aspects of Emotion, Memory, and Mental Dysfunction* (ed. J.P. Aggleton), pp. 191–228. Wiley-Liss, New York.

Hamann, S., Cahill, L., McGaugh, J.L., and Squire, L. (1997a) Intact enhancement of declarative memory by emotional arousal in amnesia. *Learning and Memory*, 4, 301–309.

Hamann, S.B., Cahill, L., and Squire, L.R. (1997b) Emotional perception and memory in amnesia. *Neuropsychology*, 11, 1–10.

Hamann, S.B., Lee, G., and Adolphs, R. (1999a) Impaired declarative emotional memory but intact emotional responses following human bilateral amygdalectomy. *Society for Neuroscience Abstracts*, **25**, 99.

Hamann, S., Elt, T., Grafton, S., and Kilts, C. (1999b) Amygdala activity related to enhanced memory for pleasant and unpleasant aversive stimuli. *Nature Neuroscience*, 2, 289–293.

Hebb, D.O. (1949) *The Organization of Behavior—A Neuropsychological Theory*. Wiley, New York.

James, W. (1890) *Principles of Psychology*. H. Holt & Co, New York.

Kaada, B.R. (1972) Stimulation and regional ablation of the amygdaloid complex with reference to functional representations. In *The Neurobiology of the Amygdala* (ed. B. Eleftheriou), pp. 205–282. Plenum Press, New York.

Kapp, B.S., Whalen, P.J., Supple, W.F., and Pascoe, J.P. (1992) Amygdaloid contributions to conditioned arousal and sensory information processing. In *The Amygdala: neurobiological aspects of emotion, memory and mental dysfunction* (ed. J.P.Aggleton), pp. 229–254. Plenum Press, New York.

LaBar, K.S., Gatenby, J.C., Gore, J.C., and Phelps, E.A (1998a) Role of the amygdala in emotional picture evaluation as revealed by fMRI. *Journal of Cognitive Neuroscience*, Supplement S: 108.

LaBar, K.S., Gatenby, J.C., Gore, J.C., LeDoux, J.E., and Phelps, E.A. (1998b) Human amygdala activation during conditioned fear acquisition and extinction: a mixed-trial fMRI study. *Neuron*, 20, 937–945.

Maddock, R.J. (1999) The retrosplenial cortex and emotion? New insights from functional neuroimaging of the human brain. *Trends in Neuroscience*, 22: 310–316.

Mark, V.H., Ervin, F.R., and Sweet, W.H. (1972) Deep temporal lobe stimulation in man. In *The Neurobiology of the Amygdala* (ed. B. Eleftheriou), pp. 485–510. Plenum Press, New York.

McGaugh, J.L., Liang, K.C., Bennett, C., and Sternberg, D.B. (1984) Adrenergic influences on memory storage: interaction of peripheral and central systems. In *Neurobiology of Learning and Memory* (eds G. Lynch, J.L. McGaugh, and N.M. Weinberger), pp. 313–332. The Guilford Press. New York.

McGaugh, J.L., Cahill, L., and Roozendaal, B. (1996) Involvement of the amygdala in memory storage: interaction with other brain systems. *Proceedings of the National Academy of Sciences of the United States of America*, 93, 13508–13514.

Morris, J.S., Friston, K.J., and Dolan, R.J. (1997) Neural responses to salient visual stimuli. *Proceedings of the Royal Society of London, Series B*, 264, 769–775

Morris, J.S., Friston, K.J., and Dolan, R.J. (1998) Experience-dependent modulation of tonotopic neural responses in human auditory cortex. *Proceedings of the Royal Society of London, Series B*, 265, 649–657.

Mori, E., Ikeda, M., Hirono, N., Kitagaki, H., Imamura,T., and Shimomura, T. (1999) Amygdalar volume and emotional memory in Alzheimer's disease. *American Journal of Psychiatry*, 156, 216–222.

Neisser, U., Winograd, E., Shreiber, C., Palmer, S., and Weldon, M. (1996) Remembering the earthquake: direct experience vs. hearing the news. *Memory*, 4, 337–357.

Nielson, K.A. and Jensen, R. (1994) Beta-adrenergic receptor antagonist antihypertensive medications impair arousal-induced modulation of working memory in elderly humans. *Behavioral and Neural Biology*, 62, 190–200.

O'Carroll, R.E., Drysdale, E., Cahill, L., Shajahan, P., and Ebmeier, KP (1999) Stimulation of the noradrenergic system enhances and blockade reduces memory for emotional material in man. *Psychological Medicine*, **29**, 1083–1088.

Packard, M. and Teather, L. (1998) Amygdala modulation of multiple memory systems: hippocampus and caudate–putamen. *Neurobiology of Learning and Memory*, 69, 163–203.

Packard, M., Cahill, L., and McGaugh, J.L. (1994) Amygdala modulation of hippocampal-dependent and caudate nucleus-dependent memory processes. *Proceedings of the National Academy of Sciences of the United States of America*, 91, 8477–8481.

Pitman, R.K. (1989) Post-traumatic stress disorder, hormones, and memory [editorial]. *Biological Psychiatry*, 26, 221–3.

Porrino, L.J., Crane, A.M., and Goldman-Rakic, P.S. (1981) Direct and indirect pathways from the amygdala to the frontal lobe in rhesus monkeys. *Journal of Comparative Neurology*, 198, 121–36.

Rauch, S.L., vander Kolk, B.A., Fisler, R.E., Alpert, N.M., Orr, S.P., Savage, C.R., Fischman, A.J., Jenike, M.A., and Pitman, R.K. (1996) A symptom provocation study of posttraumatic stress disorder using positron emission tomography and script-driven imagery. *Archives of General Psychiatry*, 53, 380–387.

Reiman, E.M., Lane, R.D., Ahern, G.L., Schwartz, G.E., Davidson, R.J., Friston, K.J., Yun, L.S., and Chen, K. (1997) Neuroanatomical correlates of externally and internally generated human emotion. *American Journal of Psychiatry*, 154, 918–25.

Rolls, E.T. (1992) Neurophysiology and functions of the primate amygdala. In *The Amygdala: Neurobiological Aspects of Emotion, Memory, and Mental Dysfunction* (ed. J.P. Aggleton), pp. 143–166. Wiley-Liss, New York.

Russchen, F.T., Amaral, D.G., and Price, J.L. (1985) The afferent connections of the substantia innominata in the monkey, *Macaca fascicularis. Journal of Comparative Neurology*, 242, 1–27.

Sakurai, Y. (1998) Cell-assembly coding in several memory processes. *Neurobiology of Learning and Memory*, 70, 212–225.

Scoville, W.B. and Milner, B. (1957) Loss of recent memory after bilateral hippocampal lesions. *Journal of Neurology, Neurosurgery, and Psychiatry*, 20, 11–21.

Soetens, E., Casaer, S., D'Hooge, R., and Hueting, J.E. (1995) Effect of amphetamine on long-term retention of verbal material. *Psychopharmacology*, 119, 155–62.

Stratton, G.M. (1928) Excitement as undifferentiated emotion. In *Feelings and Emotions: The Wittenberg Symposium* (ed. M. Reymert), pp. 220 Clark University Press, Worchester.

Taylor, S., Liberzon, M., Decker, L., Minoshima, S., and Koeppe, R. (1998) The effect of emotional content on visual recognition memory: a PET activation study. *Neuroimage*, 8, 188–197.

van Stegeren, A., Everaerd, W. , Cahill., L., McGaugh, J.L., and Goeren, L., (1998) Memory for emotional events: differential effects of centrally versus peripherally acting beta-blocking agents. *Psychopharmacology*, 138, 305–310.

Wagner, A.D., Schacter, D.L., Rotte, M., Koutstaal, W., Maril, A., Dale, A.M., Rosen, B.R., and Buckner, R.L. (1998) Building memories: remembering and forgetting of verbal experiences as predicted by brain activity. *Science*, 281, 1188–91.

Weinberger, N.M., Ashe, J.H., Metherate, R., McKenna, T., Diamond, D., and Bakin, J. (1990) Retuning auditory cortex by learning: a preliminary model of receptive field plasticity. *Concepts in Neuroscience*, 1, 91–132.

Whalen, P.J., Rauch, S.L., Etcoff, N.L., McInernet, S.C., Lee, M.B., and Jenike, M.A. (1998) Masked presentations of emotional facial expressions modulate amygdala activity without explicit knowledge. *Journal of Neuroscience*, 18, 411–418.

Wilkinson, C. (1983) Aftermath of a disaster: the collapse of the Hyatt Regency Hotel skywalks. *American Journal of Psychiatry*, 140, 1134–1139.

Zald, D.H., and Pardo, J.V. (1997) Emotion, olfaction, and the human amygdala: amygdala activation during aversive olfactory stimulation. *Proceedings of the National Academy of Sciences of the United States of America*, 94, 4119–4124.

Zbrozyna, A.W. (1972) The organization of the defence reaction elicited from amygdala and its connections. In *The Neurobiology of the Amygdala* (ed. B. Eleftheriou), pp. 597–608. Plenum Press, New York.

13 Neurophysiology and functions of the primate amygdala, and the neural basis of emotion

Edmund T. Rolls

University of Oxford, Department of Experimental Psychology, South Parks Road, Oxford, UK

Summary

Four main groups of neurons in the primate amygdala are described. One group responds to stimuli which are primary (unlearned) reinforcers, such as taste. Both rewarding and aversive tastes are represented neuronally in macaques and, correspondingly, functional magnetic resonance imaging (fMRI) investigations in humans show that the amygdala can be activated by both pleasant and unpleasant tastes.

The second group of amygdala neurons responds to visual stimuli which previously have been paired with primary reinforcers such as taste. These neurons respond to the reward-related visual stimulus in a visual discrimination task being performed for taste, and to the sight of some foods. By responding differently to the sight of different reinforcers, these neurons provide evidence about which reinforcer is available. However, these neurons may not reverse rapidly (in a few trials) the visual stimulus to which they respond when the reinforcement contingencies reverse in a visual discrimination task. Neurons which do reverse their responses rapidly are found in the primate orbitofrontal cortex. It is therefore suggested that although these amygdala neurons play a role in the learned associations between visual stimuli and primary reinforcers, the orbitofrontal cortex, which develops greatly in primates, becomes important when such associations have to be adjusted rapidly during repeated learning. This group of amygdala neurons also responds to relatively novel stimuli, which are found reinforcing in that they are approached and inspected. It is suggested that this population of amygdala neurons implements the positively reinforcing effects produced by novel stimuli.

The third group of amygdala neurons responds to novel stimuli but not to familiar stimuli in a recognition memory task. These neurons do not respond on the basis of the previous association of a visual stimulus with primary reinforcement (as shown in a visual discrimination task). Although the amygdala is not implicated in recognition memory, these neurons may be part of a mechanism that enables the second group of amygdala neurons to respond to both rewarding and relatively new stimuli.

The fourth group of amygdala neurons responds to faces, and may be involved in social and emotional responses to faces, which are disrupted by damage to the amygdala. These neurons may receive their inputs from the inferior temporal cortex and from the cortex in the superior temporal sulcus, in which neurons are also found that respond to faces, and in which the encoding of information is in a form which could be suitable as an input to an associative memory in the amygdala.

In so far as emotions can be defined as states produced by reinforcing stimuli, then the amygdala and orbitofrontal cortex are seen to be important for emotions, in that they are involved respectively in the elicitation of learned emotional responses, and in the correction or adjustment of these emotional responses as the reinforcing value of environmental stimuli alters. The face-selective neurons in both these brain regions may be involved in social and emotional responses to faces, which can act as primary (e.g. face expression) and secondary reinforcers. It is also proposed that in addition to its role in emotional responses to stimuli previously paired with primary reinforcers, the amygdala is also involved in emotional and approach responses to relatively novel stimuli, a function which may be implemented by the second group of amygdala neurons described here which respond to relatively novel visual stimuli as well as to visual stimuli paired on previous occasions with reward. In that the amygdala contains different neurons that respond to both rewards and punishers, it is unlikely to play a special role in any one emotion, but is instead likely to implement a similar function for many emotions.

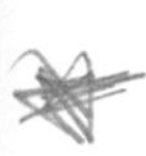

Some of the outputs of the amygdala are directed to the hypothalamus, which not only provides one route for these reinforcing environmental events to produce autonomic responses, but is also implicated in the utilization of such stimuli in motivational responses such as feeding and drinking, and in emotional behaviour. Another output of the amygdala which may enable it to influence behaviour is directed to the striatum. A third output of the amygdala consists of backprojections to some of the cortical regions from which it receives inputs. It is suggested that these latter projections are important in the effects which mood states have on cognitive processing, and in memory consolidation in emotional circumstances.

13.1 Introduction

To understand how the primate amygdala operates, it is necessary to know what information is represented in it, and in the brain regions from which it receives inputs and to which it sends outputs. This provides an understanding of how the amygdala operates at the systems level of brain function, and in particular how it transforms the inputs it receives, and what effects the results of its computations have on output regions. To understand what information is represented in the amygdala and connected regions, and how it is represented and transformed from brain region to brain region, it is necessary to analyse the responses of single neurons and groups of single neurons, as it is at this level that information is being transmitted between the computing elements of the brain, the neurons (Rolls and Treves, 1998). It is therefore the aim of this chapter to consider the functions of the primate amygdala in the light particularly of the responsiveness of single neurons in the amygdala. Neuronal activity in the amygdala is most relevant to understanding the functions of the amygdala if it is recorded while the amygdala is functioning normally during behaviour, and in test situations for which the amygdala is required. The neurophysiology must thus proceed closely with lesion studies to assess the functions of the amygdala, as shown by behavioural deficits produced by amygdala damage. Because lesion and anatomical connectivity studies are important in setting the context for neurophysiological studies of the amygdala, anatomical and lesion studies which provide indications of the functions performed by the primate amygdala are considered briefly. Particular attention is paid to research in non-human primates. Part of the reason for this is that the developments in primates in the structure and connections of neural systems connected to the amygdala (such as the temporal lobe cortical areas and the orbitofrontal cortex) make studies in primates particularly important for understanding amygdala function in humans, including its role in emotion and emotional disorders.

13.1.1 Systems level connections

The amygdala is a subcortical region in the anterior part of the temporal lobe. It receives massive projections in the primate from the overlying temporal lobe cortex (see Amaral *et al.*, 1992). These come in the monkey to overlapping but partly separate regions of the lateral and basal amygdala from the inferior temporal visual cortex, the superior temporal auditory cortex, the cortex of the temporal pole, and the cortex in the superior temporal sulcus. Thus the amygdala receives inputs from temporal lobe association cortex, but not from earlier stages of cortical visual information processing. It also receives projections from the orbitofrontal cortex. Subcortical inputs to the amygdala include projections from the midline thalamic nuclei, the subiculum, and CA1 parts of the hippocampal formation, the hypothalamus, and substantia innominata, and from olfactory structures. Although there are some inputs from early on in some sensory pathways, for example auditory inputs from the medial geniculate nucleus (LeDoux, 1995, 1996), this route is unlikely to be involved in most emotions, for which cortical analysis of the stimulus is likely to be required (Rolls, 1999a, 2000a). The outputs of the amygdala include the well-known projections to the hypothalamus, from the lateral amygdala via the ventral amygdalofugal pathway to the lateral hypothalamus, and from the medial amygdala, which is relatively small in the primate, via the stria terminalis to the medial hypothalamus. The ventral amygdalofugal pathway contains some long descending fibres that project to the autonomic centres in the medulla oblongata, and provide a route for cortically processed signals to reach the brainstem. A further interesting output of the amygdala is to the ventral striatum (Heimer *et al.*, 1982) including the nucleus accumbens, because via this route information processed in the amygdala could gain access to the basal ganglia and thus influence motor output. The amygdala also projects to the medial part of the mediodorsal nucleus of the thalamus, which projects to the orbitofrontal cortex and provides the amygdala with another output. In addition, the amygdala has direct projections back to many areas of the temporal, orbitofrontal, and insular cortices from which it receives inputs (see Amaral *et al.*, 1992). It is suggested elsewhere (Rolls, 1989, 1992a, 1999a; Rolls and Treves, 1998) that the functions of these backprojections include the guidance of information representation and storage in the neocortex (when this is performed by reinforcing stimuli), and recall. Another interesting set of output pathways of the amygdala projects to the entorhinal cortex, which provides the major input to the hippocampus and dentate gyrus, and to the ventral subiculum, which provides a major output of the hippocampus (Price, 1981; Amaral *et al.*, 1992).

These anatomical connections of the amygdala indicate that it is placed to receive highly processed information from the cortex and to influence motor systems, autonomic systems, some of the cortical areas from which it receives inputs, and other limbic areas. The functions mediated through these connections will now be considered, using information available from the effects of damage to the amygdala and from the activity of neurons in the amygdala.

13.1.2 Effects of lesions of the amygdala

Bilateral removal of the amygdala in monkeys produces striking behavioural changes which include tameness, a lack of emotional responsiveness, excessive examination of objects, often with the mouth, and eating of previously rejected items such as meat (Weiskrantz, 1956). These behavioural changes comprise much of the Klüver–Bucy syndrome which is produced in monkeys by bilateral anterior temporal lobectomy (Klüver and Bucy, 1939). In analyses of the bases of these behavioural changes, it has been observed that there are deficits in some types of learning. For example, Weiskrantz (1956) found that bilateral ablation of the amygdala in the monkey produced a deficit on learning an active avoidance task. The monkeys failed to learn to make a response when a light signalled that shock would follow unless the response was made. He was perhaps the first to suggest that these monkeys had difficulty in forming associations between stimuli and reinforcement, when he suggested that 'the effect of amygdalectomy is to make it difficult for reinforcing stimuli, whether positive or negative, to become established or to be recognized as such' (Weiskrantz, 1956). In this avoidance task, associations between a stimulus and negative reinforcement were impaired. Evidence soon became available that associations between stimuli and positive reinforcement (reward) were also impaired in, for example, serial reversals of a visual discrimination made to obtain food (Jones and Mishkin, 1972) and other tasks. In this task, the monkey must learn that food is under one of two objects and, after he has learned this, he must then relearn (reverse) the association as the food is then placed under the other object. Jones and Mishkin (1972) showed that the stages of this task which are particularly affected by damage to this region are those when the monkeys are responding at chance to the two visual stimuli or are starting to respond more to the currently rewarded stimuli. In contrast, the stage when the monkeys are continuing to make perseverative responses to the previously rewarded visual stimulus was impaired by lesions of the orbitofrontal cortex. They thus argued that the difficulty produced by this anterior temporal lobe damage is in learning to associate stimuli with reinforcement, in this case with food reward. Further evidence for this is that amygdalectomized monkeys were impaired on a test in which they had to remember, on the basis of a single presentation, whether or not a trial-unique object had been paired with reward (Mishkin and Aggleton, 1981; Spiegler and Mishkin, 1981), and in other reward-related learning tasks (see, for example, Gaffan, 1992).

Lesion studies are subject to the criticism that the effects of a lesion could be due to inadvertent damage to other brain structures or pathways close to the intended lesion site. For this reason, many of the older lesion studies are being repeated and extended with lesions in which instead of an ablation (removal) or electrolytic lesion (which can damage axons passing through a brain region), a neurotoxin is used to damage cells in a localized region, but leave intact fibres of passage (see Baxter and Murray, Chapter 16). Using such lesions (made with ibotenic acid) in monkeys, Malkova *et al.* (1997) showed that amygdala lesions did not impair visual discrimination learning when the reinforcer was an auditory secondary reinforcer learned as being positively reinforcing preoperatively. This was in contrast to an earlier study by Gaffan and Harrison (1987; see also Gaffan, 1992) using aspiration lesions. In the study by Malkova *et al.* (1997), the animals with amygdala lesions were somewhat slower to learn a visual discrimination task for food reward, and made more errors, but with the small numbers of animals (the numbers in the groups were 3 and 4), the difference did not reach statistical significance. It would be interesting to test non-human primates when the association to be learned is directly between a visual stimulus and a primary reinforcer such as taste. It is this type of association learning, between a previously neutral visual or auditory stimulus and a primary (unlearned) reinforcer such as a rewarding or punishing taste or touch, that the amygdala and orbitofrontal cortex are hypothesized to implement (see Rolls, 1992a, 1999a, 2000a; Rolls and Treves, 1998). Part of the basis for this hypothesis is that anatomically the amygdala and orbitofrontal cortex are brain regions where pathways from high-order visual and auditory cortical areas converge, and that neurophysiologically single neurons in these regions can be activated by primary reinforcers, or by potential secondary reinforcers (visual and auditory stimuli), or show convergence between both, and moreover show evidence of altering their responses during visual-to-primary reinforcer association learning (see below, and Rolls *et al.*, 1996; Rolls, 1999a, 2000a,b). In most non-human primate studies, the reward being given is usually solid food (typically a pellet of laboratory chow), which is seen before it is tasted, and for which the food delivery mechanism makes a noise. These factors mean that the reward for which the animal is working includes secondary reinforcing components, the sight and sound. When the association to be learned is a purely sensory–sensory (e.g. visual-to-visual or visual-to-auditory) association where neither is a primary reinforcer, cortical areas where these particular sensory signals converge, such as the rhinal cortex, may be able to learn these associations. However, the hypothesis that would be particularly useful to see tested in non-human primate lesion studies is that associations of sensory stimuli to primary reinforcers depend on the amygdala. (For the orbitofrontal cortex, there is already evidence showing this, see Baylis and Gaffan, 1991.) Many of the studies that interfere with amygdala neuronal activity in rats are indeed consistent with this hypothesis, that it is associations of sensory stimuli with primary reinforcers including painful stimuli that are dependent on the amygdala (see Everitt and Robbins, 1992; LeDoux, 1992, 1995).

Consistent with this hypothesis that the amygdala is involved in learning associations with primary reinforcers and therefore in emotion (see Rolls, 1999a, and below), in the investigation by Malkova *et al.* (1997) in macaques it was shown that amygdala lesions made with ibotenic acid did impair the processing of reward-related stimuli, in that when the reward value of one set of foods was reduced by feeding it to satiety (i.e. sensory-specific satiety, see Rolls, 1999a), the monkeys still chose the visual stimuli associated with the foods with which they had been satiated. Further evidence that neurotoxic lesions of the amygdala in primates affect behaviour to stimuli learned as being reward-related as well as punishment-related is that monkeys with neurotoxic lesions of the amygdala showed abnormal patterns of food choice, picking up and eating foods not normally eaten such as meat, and picking up and placing in their mouths inedible objects (Murray *et al.*, 1996). Further, Meunier *et al.* (1996) (see Baxter and Murray, Chapter 16) showed that macaques with neurotoxic amygdala lesions showed altered emotional behaviour, including reduced fear and aggressiveness, increased submission, and excessive manual and tactile exploration. These symptoms produced by selective amygdala lesions are classical Klüver–Bucy symptoms. None of these effects is ascribable to rhinal cortex damage (see Baxter and Murray, Chapter 16). Thus, in primates, there is evidence that selective amygdala lesions impair some types of behaviour to learned reward-related stimuli as well as to learned punishment-related stimuli, thus including stimuli that normally elicit emotional behaviour. However, we should not conclude that the amygdala is the only brain structure involved in this type of learning as, especially when rapid stimulus–reinforcement association learning is performed in primates, the orbitofrontal cortex is involved, as discussed below and by Rolls (1999a, 2000b).

Although Easton and Gaffan (Chapter 17) revise the previous view of Gaffan (1992) that the amygdala is involved in stimulus–reinforcement association learning, the evidence they discuss (part of it based in the neurotoxic amygdala lesion studies described above) is also directed to stimulus–stimulus (e.g. visual-to-visual) rather than stimulus-to-primary-reinforcer association learning. Their view that basal forebrain neurons are important in stimulus–reinforcement association learning is consistent with the neurophysiological evidence that basal forebrain neurons can be activated by primary reinforcers such as tastes; by secondary reinforcers such as the sight of food; by both; reverse their responses during stimulus-to-primary reinforcer learning; and reflect reward and even sensory-specific satiety in that their responses are modulated by hunger and sensory-specific satiety (Burton *et al.*, 1976; Mora *et al.*, 1976; Rolls *et al.*, 1976, 1979, 1980, 1986; Wilson and Rolls, 1990a,c; see Rolls, 1999a). The signals that activate these basal forebrain neurons are probably actually received from the orbitofrontal cortex and amygdala (Rolls, 1999a). However, although these neurons probably project to many cortical areas including the inferior temporal cortex, the suggestion is not that they provide the reward or unconditioned stimulus that enables cortical neurons to respond to visual stimuli associated with rewards (as implied by Easton and Gaffan, Chapter 17), because inferior temporal cortex neurons do not respond to visual stimuli based on the association of visual stimuli with reward or punishment (Rolls *et al.*, 1977). Instead, Rolls (1992a, 1999a; see also Rolls and Treves, 1998) has suggested that one function of the basal forebrain neurons is via their cortical terminals to facilitate learning in the cerebral cortex, enabling whatever type of learning is implemented in a cortical area to take place better at times when basal forebrain neurons are active, consistent with the evidence that acetylcholine is involved in cortical long-term potentiation (Bear and Singer, 1989).

Further evidence linking the amygdala to reinforcement mechanisms is that monkeys will work in order to obtain electrical stimulation of the amygdala, and that single neurons in the amygdala are activated by brain-stimulation reward of a number of different sites (Rolls, 1975; Rolls *et al.*, 1980; see Rolls, 1999a).

Jones and Mishkin (1972) elaborated the hypothesis that many of the symptoms of the Klüver–Bucy syndrome, including the emotional changes, could be a result of this type of deficit in learning stimulus–reinforcement associations. For example, the tameness, the hypoemotionality, the increased orality, and the altered responses to food would arise because of damage to the normal mechanism by which stimuli become associated with reward or punishment. Other evidence is also consistent with the hypothesis that there is a close relationship between the learning deficit and the symptoms of the Klüver–Bucy syndrome. For example, in a study of subtotal lesions of the amygdala, Aggleton and Passingham (1981) found hypoemotionality only in those monkeys in which the lesions produced a serial reversal learning deficit.

The amygdala is well placed anatomically for such stimulus–reinforcement association learning, as not only does it receive highly processed inputs about visual and auditory stimuli from the temporal lobe cortex, but it also receives inputs about primary reinforcers from the taste cortex (directly from the primary cortex in the rostral insula and via the secondary gustatory cortex in the orbitofrontal cortex; see Baylis *et al.*, 1994), somatosensory cortex (via the insula in the primate; Mesulam and Mufson, 1982), and from the olfactory and visceral systems (see Amaral *et al.*, 1992), so that a variety of well-processed stimuli and information about primary reinforcers should have access to the amygdala. This type of anatomical convergence is appropriate for a system implicated in stimulus–reinforcement association formation, in which it may be necessary to learn associations in a pattern associator between previously neutral stimuli and primary (unlearned) reinforcers (see Rolls and Treves, 1998; Rolls, 1999a). Moreover, the outputs of the amygdala include connections to the autonomic centres of the brainstem and the hypothalamus through which the autonomic changes in emotion to learned stimuli could be elicited; to the ventral striatum and the central grey of the brainstem through which behaviour to learned reinforcing stimuli could be elicited; and to the basal forebrain magnocellular neurons and back to the cerebral cortex through which effects of emotional state on memory could be produced. In line with this, LeDoux *et al.* (1988) were able to show in rats that lesions of the lateral hypothalamus (which receives inputs from the central nucleus of the amygdala) blocked conditioned heart rate (autonomic) responses but not the conditioned behavioural emotional response of freezing to an aversive conditioned stimulus. In contrast, lesions of the central grey (which also receives from the central nucleus of the amygdala) blocked the conditioned freezing but not the conditioned autonomic response to the aversive conditioned stimulus. Further, Cador *et al.* (1989) obtained evidence consistent with the hypothesis that the learned incentive (conditioned reinforcing) effects of previously neutral stimuli paired with rewards are mediated by the amygdala acting through the ventral striatum, in that amphetamine injections into the ventral striatum enhanced the effects of a conditioned reinforcing stimulus only if the amygdala was intact.

Although much evidence is thus consistent with the hypothesis that the amygdala is involved in responses made to stimuli associated with reinforcement, there is evidence that it may also be involved to some extent in behavioural responses made to novel, as opposed to familiar, stimuli, in a different type of memory. It has been found, for example, that the alteration in responses to foods in rats with damage to the amygdala is due in part to decreased neophobia, i.e. the rats accept new foods more quickly (Rolls and Rolls, 1973; see also Dunn and Everitt, 1988; Wilson and Rolls, 1993). However, the suggestion that the amygdala lesions affect recognition memory *per se* has now been shown to be incorrect, with such effects now ascribed to damage to the perirhinal cortex (Zola-Morgan *et al.*, 1989; Baxter and Murray, Chapter 16).

13.2 Neurophysiology of the primate amygdala

13.2.1 Visual stimulus–reinforcement associations and the responses of amygdala neurons in primates

In tests of whether amygdala neurons in primates responded on the basis of the association of stimuli with primary reinforcement, Sanghera *et al.* (1979) showed that 19.5% of their sample of neurons with visual responses tended to respond on the basis of whether the stimuli were reinforcing in, for example, a visual discrimination task. Although these neurons responded, for example, to the visual stimulus in the visual discrimination task which indicated that (unseen) taste reward was available, and responded to some other positively reinforcing stimuli such as some foods, they did not respond to all visual stimuli that were positively reinforcing. This is an indication that they convey information about which reinforcer was given, not just that any reward was given. Knowledge of which reward is available is important for selecting which goals in the environment should be selected for action given the current need states (see Rolls, 1999a,b). The observation that some of these neurons responded to one or more stimuli which were not positively reinforcing (Sanghera *et al.*, 1979; Rolls, 1981) may now be understood by the more recent finding that some amygdala neurons that respond to rewarding visual stimuli also respond to relatively novel visual stimuli (and hence may make the novel stimuli somewhat rewarding), as now described. In a more recent study, Wilson and Rolls (2000) in recordings from 659 amygdala neurons showed that 17 from a sample of 165 amygdala neurons with visual responses had responses that occurred differentially to the visual stimulus in a visual discrimination task that indicated that the monkey could lick to obtain the taste of food, compared with the other visual stimulus which indicated that a lick should not be made otherwise a taste of aversive saline would be delivered (see an example in Figure 13.1). Of these neurons, 16 responded significantly more to the reward-related than to the punishment-related visual stimulus, and one neuron responded more to the aversive stimulus, as shown in Figure 13.2. The neurons did not fire just in relation to movements being made, in that they did not respond differentially in a recognition memory task described below in which lick responses were made to familiar but not to novel visual stimuli. The mean differential response latency was 203 ms (range

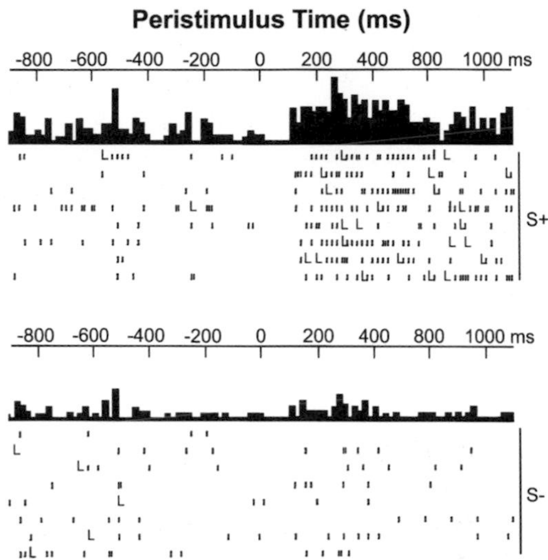

Figure 13.1 Responses of a primate amygdala neuron in a visual discrimination task. Each tic represents the occurrence of an action potential; each row of tics represents the firing of the neuron on a single trial to the presentation of the S+ visual stimulus (which indicated that a lick could be made to obtain a taste of fruit juice) or of the S– visual stimulus (which indicated that a lick should not be made or that aversive saline would be delivered). Presentations of the S+ and S– occurred in pseudorandom order but are grouped for clarity. The L indicates the occurrence of the lick response. The scale at the right of the histogram represents a firing rate of 100 spikes/s. Bin width = 10 ms.

90–380 ms), compared with the behavioural response latencies of 250–400 ms. (Some of these neurons had earlier non-differential responses to reward- and punishment-related visual stimuli, with a mean latency for the non-differential response of 131 ms.) The mean spontaneous firing rate of these differential neurons was 15 spikes/s (range 3–46 spikes/s). These neurons are found in the lateral, basal, and central nuclei of the amygdala (Sanghera *et al.*, 1979; Wilson and Rolls, 2000). In addition, in the sample of visual neurons studied by Wilson and Rolls (2000), six neurons had responses that were selective for foods, providing further evidence that the identity of the particular reinforcer being seen is encoded by some amygdala neurons. The results show clearly that some primate amygdala neurons have responses to visual stimuli that signify reward (and other neurons have responses to visual stimuli that signify punishment). Primate amygdala neurons do not code only for punishment-related visual stimuli that produce fear.

Another way of investigating the coding of reinforcement valence by neurons is to reverse the reinforcers obtained to two visual stimuli in a visual discrimination task. Sanghera *et al.* (1979) found that eight of nine neurons tested in the reversal of a visual discrimination (in which the visual stimulus associated with food reward delivery becomes associated with aversive saline delivery and vice versa) did not reverse their responses (and for the remaining

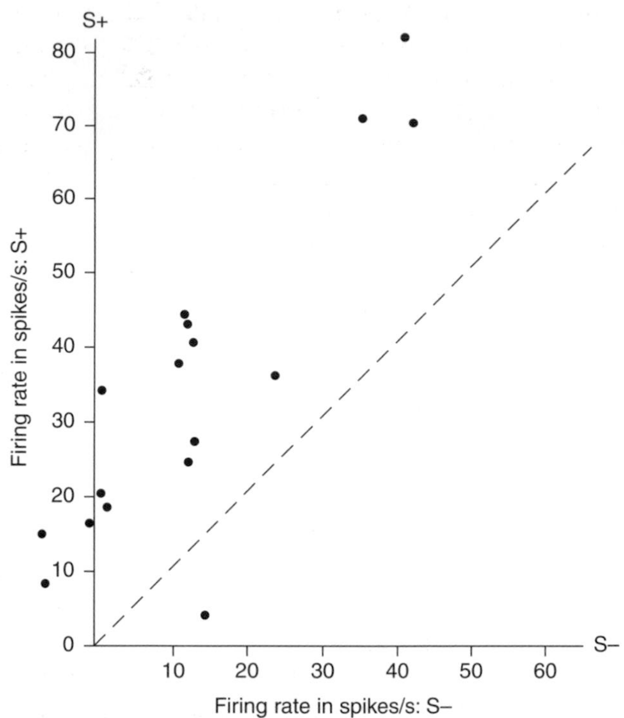

Figure 13.2 Responses of amygdala neurons that responded more in a visual discrimination task to the reward-related visual stimulus (S+) than to the saline-related visual stimulus (S–). In the task, the macaque monkeys made lick responses to obtain fruit juice when the S+ was the discriminandum, and had to withhold lick responses when the S– was the discriminandum in order to avoid the taste of saline. Each point shows the responses of one neuron to the S+ and to the S– measured in a 0.5 s period starting 100 ms after the visual stimulus was shown. Most of the points lie above the dashed line drawn at 45°, showing that most of these neurons responded more to the S+ than to the S–. (After Wilson and Rolls, 2000)

neuron the evidence was not clear). Wilson and Rolls (2000) tested two further amygdala neurons with visual responses in reversal, and found that the responses of the neurons were not altered during reversal. They also showed that the same two neurons did not rapidly acquire differential responses to two stimuli, one of which was made the positive discriminative stimulus and the other the negative discriminative stimulus. Thus these amygdaloid neurons did not alter their responses flexibly and rapidly when the reinforcement value of a visual stimulus was altered, although such neurons are found in the orbitofrontal cortex (Thorpe *et al.*, 1983; Rolls *et al.*, 1996) and basal forebrain (Mora *et al.*, 1976; Rolls *et al.*, 1976; Wilson and Rolls, 1990a,b,c; Rolls, 1999a).

Neurons with responses which are probably similar to these have also been described by Ono *et al.* (1980) and by Nishijo *et al.* (1988a,b) (see also Ono and Nishijo, 1992). Although the amygdaloid neurons studied by Sanghera *et al.* (1979) had a preference for reinforcing stimuli, they did not alter their responses flexibly and rapidly when the reinforcement value of a visual stimulus was altered during reversal. On the other hand, Nishijo *et al.* (1988a) have tested four amygdala neurons in a rather simpler re-learning situation in which salt was added to a piece of food such as watermelon, and the neurons' responses to the sight of the watermelon diminished. This was an extinction rather than a reversal test, and it was not clear whether in extinction with repeated trials the monkeys continued to fixate the piece of food once salt had been added to it. The advantage of the visual discrimination task studied by Sanghera *et al.* (1979) and Wilson and Rolls (2000) is that the monkey must fixate the visual stimuli on every trial in the random trial sequence, to determine whether the visual stimulus currently associated with reward is being shown. It will be of interest in further studies to investigate whether in extinction, evidence can be found for a rapid decrease in the responses to visual stimuli formerly associated with reward when reward is no longer given, even when fixation of the stimuli is adequate.

13.2.2 Responses of these amygdala neurons to novel stimuli that are reinforcing

Wilson and Rolls (2000) extended the finding of Sanghera *et al.* (1979) that there is a population of neurons in the primate amygdala which discriminates between reward- and punishment-associated visual stimuli in a visual discrimination task, by comparing the responses of these neurons in the visual discrimination task with their responses in a recognition memory task in which a rule was used to determine whether a behavioural response should be made to a visual stimulus. This is in contrast to the visual discrimination task, in which the reward value of a stimulus is based on previous association of the visual stimulus with a primary reinforcer, the taste of food. In the recognition memory task, the monkey used the rule that lick responses to (trial-unique) novel stimuli were associated with the delivery of saline, and lick responses to the same stimulus when shown a second time as 'familiar' were rewarded. Several trials separated the novel and familiar presentations of each stimulus, and each stimulus was shown only twice per day. In this running recognition memory task, the majority (12/14 analysed) of these neurons responded equally well to novel and familiar stimuli even though these stimuli differentially signalled aversive saline or juice reward. Thus these amygdala neurons did not reflect the reinforcement value of visual stimuli when this was determined by a rule ('respond to familiar stimuli'), but did respond differentially when the reinforcement value of the visual stimuli was determined by a previous association with a primary reinforcer (the taste of food in the visual discrimination task). Expressed in another way, this shows that these amygdala neurons do not respond to all visual stimuli which signify reward, for example when reward value is computed on the basis of a rule, but do respond to rewarding stimuli when this is based on a previous association between the visual stimulus and a primary reinforcer.

A second interesting finding of this study was that these amygdaloid neurons responded to the S+ (the visual discriminative stimulus associated with fruit juice reward delivery) in the visual discrimination task and to both the novel and familiar visual stimuli in the recognition memory task (see Figure 13.3), but did not respond to the S– (the discriminative visual stimulus which indicated that the monkey should not lick or salt solution would be obtained) in the visual discrimination task. It is suggested that the lack of response to the S– was because it had been presented on many occasions without reinforcement, so that the monkey had no tendency to explore or approach it further. In contrast, the novel and familiar stimuli in the trial-unique recognition task had not been seen before the novel presentation, and for only 1.5 s on the familiar presentation and, with this limited degree of exposure, the monkeys were likely to still be interested in the stimuli, and to wish to explore them further (Humphrey, 1972). The S+ stimuli still elicited approach because of their previous association with primary reinforcement. The hypothesis proposed is that the responses of these amygdala neurons reflected the tendency of the monkeys to explore and/or approach the relatively novel stimuli. According to this hypothesis, the deficit in visual discrimination learning that can occur in monkeys after amygdala lesions occurs in part because the normal habituation to a familiar and unrewarded object does not occur without the amygdala, so that the lesioned monkeys are more likely than normal monkeys to choose the S–. This tendency to explore and select repeatedly even familiar but not rewarded objects is a feature of the Klüver–Bucy syndrome. The hypothesis is also that the reward value which relatively novel visual stimuli have, leading to their exploration and thus discovery of whether these novel stimuli are associated with primary reinforcers (an important function in genetic

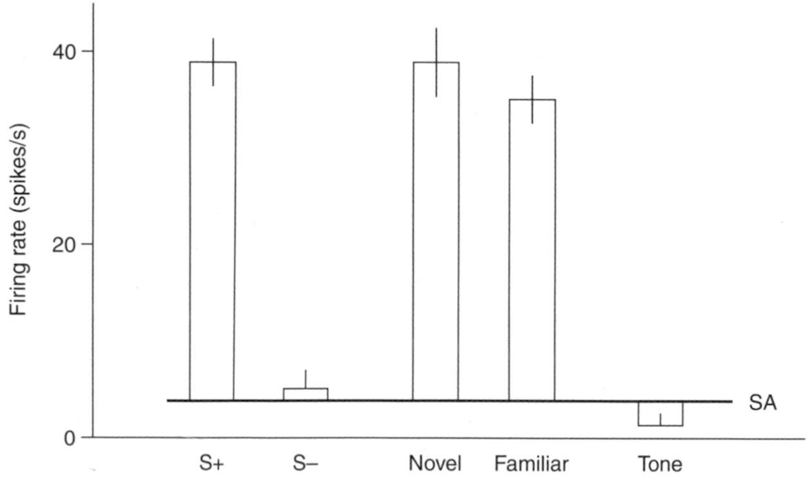

Figure 13.3 This macaque amygdala neuron responded to the sight of a stimulus associated with food reward (S+), but not to a visual stimulus associated with aversive saline (S–) in a visual discrimination task. The same neuron responded to visual stimuli while they were relatively novel, including here on the first (Novel) and second (Familiar) presentations of new stimuli. The neuron did not respond to the tone which indicated the start of a trial. SA, spontaneous firing rate of the neuron. The mean responses and the SEM to the different stimuli are shown. (After Wilson and Rolls, 2000; and Rolls, 1999a, Figure 4.13a.)

evolution; see Chapter 10 in Rolls, 1999a,), is implemented by these response properties of these amygdala neurons. A possible neural mechanism to implement this is that these amygdala neurons receive inputs from visual stimuli by synapses which normally habituate with a time course of several presentations of a stimulus unless that stimulus is associated with a positive primary reinforcer, when the postsynaptic activity produced by the primary reinforcer in association with the presynaptic firing produced by the visual stimulus would lead those synapses to strengthen rather than habituate by a process of homosynaptic long-term depression (see Rolls and Treves, 1998). Although these experiments (Wilson and Rolls, 2000) were performed with positive reinforcers, it is suggested that an analogous function is performed by the amygdala in filtering out stimuli sometimes associated with punishment from those not associated with reinforcement. The functions of this type of processing may be to influence the interest shown in a stimulus, whether it is approached or avoided, whether an affective response occurs to it, and whether a representation of the stimulus is made or maintained via an action mediated through either the basal forebrain nucleus of Meynert or the backprojections to the cerebral cortex (Rolls, 1989, 1990, 1992a, 1999a; Rolls and Treves, 1998).

13.2.3 Responses of amygdala neurons to novel visual stimuli

Although the effects of large amygdala lesions on recognition memory can be ascribed to damage to the overlying entorhinal and perirhinal cortices (Zola-Morgan *et al.*, 1989), some aspect of whether stimuli have been seen before does influence the reward-related amygdala neurons described above, in that at least some of them respond to relatively novel stimuli, for at least a number of presentations until they become very familiar and are found not to be associated with reinforcement (Wilson and Rolls, 2000). Moreover, there are neurons in the overlying inferior temporal cortex which projects to the amygdala that respond more to novel than to familiar stimuli (Baylis and Rolls, 1987; Wilson *et al.*, 1990). Both of these lines of evidence suggest that some aspect of whether visual stimuli are novel or familiar is represented in the amygdala. To investigate this further, Wilson and Rolls (1993) recorded the responses of 659 amygdala neurons in monkeys performing recognition memory and visual discrimination tasks. In the running or serial recognition memory task, trial-unique stimuli were shown twice, once as novel, and after a varied number of intervening trials used to assess the memory span of the neurons, as familiar. The macaques had not to lick to the novel presentation of a stimulus otherwise a taste of aversive saline would be obtained, but could lick to the stimulus when it appeared later as familiar to obtain fruit juice reward. The intertrial interval was 6 s.

Three groups of neurons showed memory-like activity. One group (n = 10) responded maximally to novel stimuli and significantly less so to the same stimuli when they were familiar. The largest differential response to novel and familiar presentations of the same stimuli occurred when there were no other stimuli intervening between the novel and the familiar presentations of a given stimulus, and the differential response became smaller as the number of intervening stimuli increased (see example in Figure 13.4). The number of intervening trials over which the response to a familiar stimulus had increased to be similar

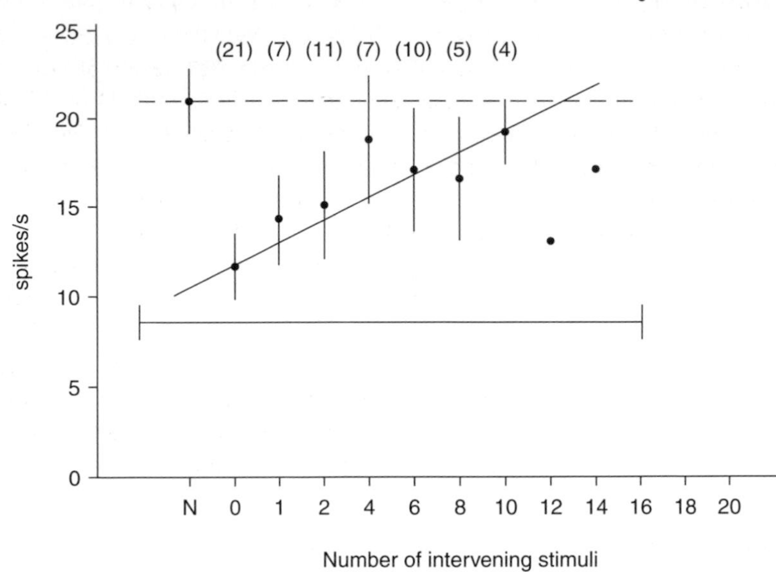

Figure 13.4 Responses of an amygdala neuron to visual stimuli when they were novel (N), but not when they were familiar with no other stimuli intervening between the novel and familiar presentations of the visual stimuli (0 intervening stimuli). The neuronal responses gradually became like that to novel stimuli when a number of other stimuli intervened between the novel and familiar presentations of a stimulus. The neuronal responses shown are the mean ± SEM to different stimuli when novel (N) and when shown again as familiar after different numbers of intervening stimuli, recorded in a 500 ms period starting 100 ms after the visual stimuli were shown. The horizontal line shows the spontaneous firing rate ± the SEM (After Wilson and Rolls, 1993.)

to that to a novel stimulus was defined as the memory span. Of the five neurons for which this analysis was done, the average memory span was estimated to be five intervening trials (range = 2–10 intervening trials), a time period of approximately 80 s for the neuron with the most robust 'memory span'. Wilson and Rolls (1993) ensured that the different reinforcement values of novel and familiar stimuli in the recognition memory task were not responsible for the differential responses to the same stimulus when it was novel as compared with when it was familiar. This was done by recording the activity of these neurons during the performance of the visual discrimination task, in which the S+ and the S– differed in their reinforcement value but were equally familiar. In almost all cases, the response to novel stimuli was significantly greater than it was to familiar stimuli or to the S+ and S–. Thus the novelty of the stimuli, but not their differential reinforcement value, was the basis of the neuronal responses to novel stimuli. These neurons were found in part of the dorsal amygdala, and in part of the basal nucleus (see Wilson and Rolls, 1993).

The two other groups of neurons responded to certain classes of visual stimuli, but included some neurons with memory-related activity in that their responses were greater to novel than to familiar visual stimuli. One such group of neurons ($n = 6$) with responses which occurred to some foods included four neurons which responded more to a food when it had not been seen recently, and three neurons that responded more to novel than to familiar non-food visual stimuli. The third group of neurons ($n = 10$) responded to faces, and for two of these neurons the response to a novel face decreased as it became familiar.

These findings indicate that there is a small proportion of neurons in the primate amygdala which respond in recognition memory and similar tasks with information about the recency with which a visual stimulus has been seen. The memory spans of these neurons are up to 10 intervening stimuli. These neurons could contribute to the behavioural activation which is produced by novel stimuli, perhaps acting via ventral forebrain neurons (see Wilson and Rolls, 1990b). The activity of these neurons may also be related to amygdala processing of novel stimuli which leads to such stimuli becoming intrinsically rewarding, as shown by the behavioural tendency to approach such novel stimuli.

13.2.4 Neuronal responses in the primate amygdala to faces

Another interesting group of neurons in the amygdala responds primarily to faces (Rolls, 1981; Leonard *et al.*, 1985; Wilson and Rolls, 1993). Each of these neurons responds to some but not all of a set of faces, and thus across an ensemble conveys information about the identity of the face (see Figure 13.5). These neurons are found especially in the basal accessory nucleus of the amygdala (see Figure 13.6 and Leonard *et al.*, 1985), a part of the amygdala that develops markedly in primates (Amaral *et al.*, 1992; see Barton and Aggleton, Chapter 14). It will be of interest to investigate whether some of these amygdala face neurons respond on the basis of facial expression. Some neurons in the monkey amygdala do respond to stimuli which arise between conspecifics during social interactions (Brothers *et al.*, 1990; Brothers and Ring, 1993). Amygdala neurons that respond to faces have now also been found in humans (Fried *et al.*, 1997; Dolan, Chapter 19). It is probable that the amygdala neurons responsive to faces receive their inputs from groups of neurons in the temporal lobe visual cortex that respond to faces (Perrett *et al.*, 1982; Rolls, 1992b, 1997b) and, consistent with this, the response latencies of the amygdala neurons tend to be longer than those of neurons in the cortex in the superior temporal sulcus (Rolls, 1984; Leonard *et al.*, 1985). In the temporal visual cortex, one group of neurons found especially in the ventral lip of the cortex forming the superior temporal sulcus responds to face identity, while a separate population of cells in the cortex in the superior temporal sulcus conveys information about facial expression (Baylis *et al.*, 1987; Hasselmo *et al.*, 1989a). This latter group of neurons in the cortex in the depths of the superior temporal sulcus is in an area where some neurons respond only to moving stimuli (Baylis *et al.*, 1987), and some of these neurons are tuned to respond only to moving faces or heads (Hasselmo *et al.*, 1989b). The neurons that respond to moving heads or faces encode properties of the stimulus such as ‘head turning from either left or right profile to frontal view’, ‘head rotating away from frontal view’, ‘eyes closing or averting’, and ‘lips moving’ (see Hasselmo *et al.*, 1989b). Both groups of temporal

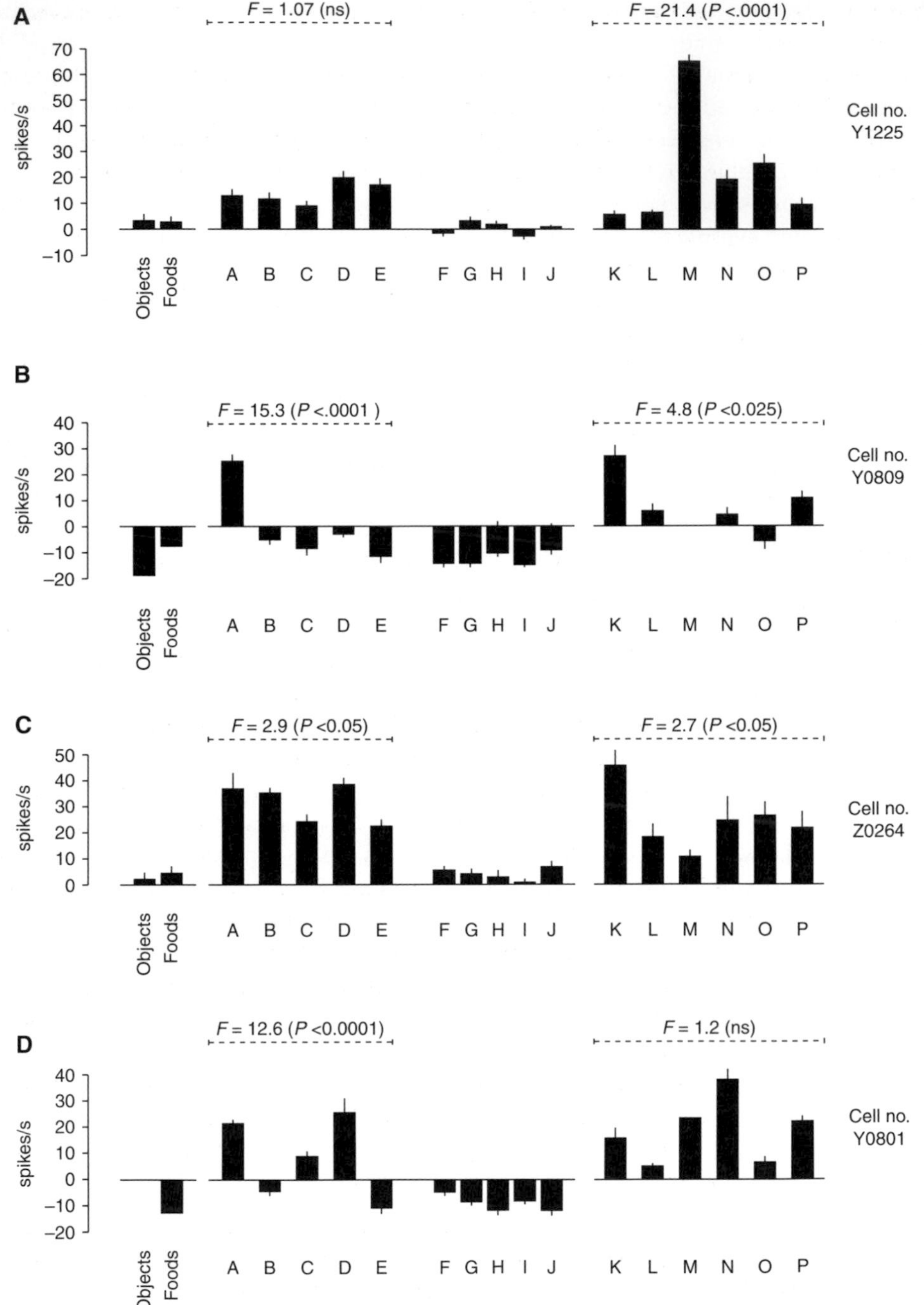

Figure 13.5 The responses of four cells (a–d) in the amygdala to a variety of monkey and human face stimuli (A–E and K–P), and to non-face stimuli (F–J, objects and foods). Each

cortex neurons responding to faces probably provide inputs to the amygdaloid neurons that respond to faces.

The representation of face identity in the primate amygdala (Leonard *et al.*, 1985) may allow the identity of individuals providing reinforcers to be learned in the amygdala by stimulus–reinforcement association with information about primary reinforcers received from, for example, the somatosensory system (via the insula; Mesulam and Mufson, 1982), or the gustatory system (via, for example, the orbitofrontal cortex). Face expression, and head and face movement may be represented in the amygdala because it provides information which may itself be a primary reinforcer, useful in social interactions and as the primary reinforcer in stimulus–reinforcer association learning (see Rolls, 1999a). For example, a threat face expression, or a head turning to stare, is a negative reinforcer in primate social interactions. One output from the amygdala for this information is probably via the ventral striatum, as a small population of neurons has been found in the primate ventral striatum with responses selective for faces (Williams *et al.*, 1993).

It has been suggested that this is part of a system that has evolved for the rapid and reliable identification of individuals from their faces, because of the importance of this in primate social behaviour (Rolls, 1981, 1984, 1992b,c, 1999a; Perrett and Rolls, 1983; Leonard *et al.*, 1985). The part of this system in the amygdala may be particularly involved in emotional and social responses to faces. Indeed, it is suggested that the tameness of the Klüver–Bucy syndrome, and the inability of amygdalectomized monkeys to interact normally in a social group (Kling and Steklis, 1976), arises because of damage to this system specialized for processing faces (Rolls, 1981, 1984, 1992a,b, 1999a, 2000b).

In relation to the neurons in the macaque amygdala with responses selective for faces and social interactions (Leonard *et al.*, 1985; Brothers and Ring, 1993; Wilson and Rolls, 1993), it is interesting that impairments in face expression identification have now been found in humans with amygdala damage, as described below (see also Adolphs and Tranel, Chapter 18).

The temporal cortex visual cells that respond to the identity of faces and objects found in regions such as areas TEa, TEm, and TPO (Baylis *et al.*, 1987; Booth and Rolls, 1998) which project into the amygdala have response properties which would enable them to provide useful inputs to a stimulus–reinforcer associative learning mechanism in the amygdala (see Rolls, 1992b, 1999a; Wallis and Rolls, 1997; Rolls and Treves, 1998). These cortical neurons represent information about which face is being seen by the profile of firing across a subpopulation of neurons (Baylis *et al.*, 1985; Rolls and Tovee, 1995; Rolls *et al.*, 1997b), i.e. ensemble encoding rather than 'grandmother cell' encoding is used. It has been shown that the information represented by the firing rates of different members of the ensemble is independent (at least for up to, for example, 14 neurons which can allow identification of which of 20 faces was presented for 0.5 s with ~70% accuracy), so that the number of faces that can be

---

bar represents the mean response above baseline with the standard error calculated over 4–10 presentations. The F ratio for an analysis of variance calculated over the face sets indicates that the units shown range from very selective between faces (Y0809) to relatively non-selective (Z0264). Some stimuli for cells Y0801 and Y0809 produced inhibition below the spontaneous firing rate. (From Leonard *et al.*, 1985, with permission.)

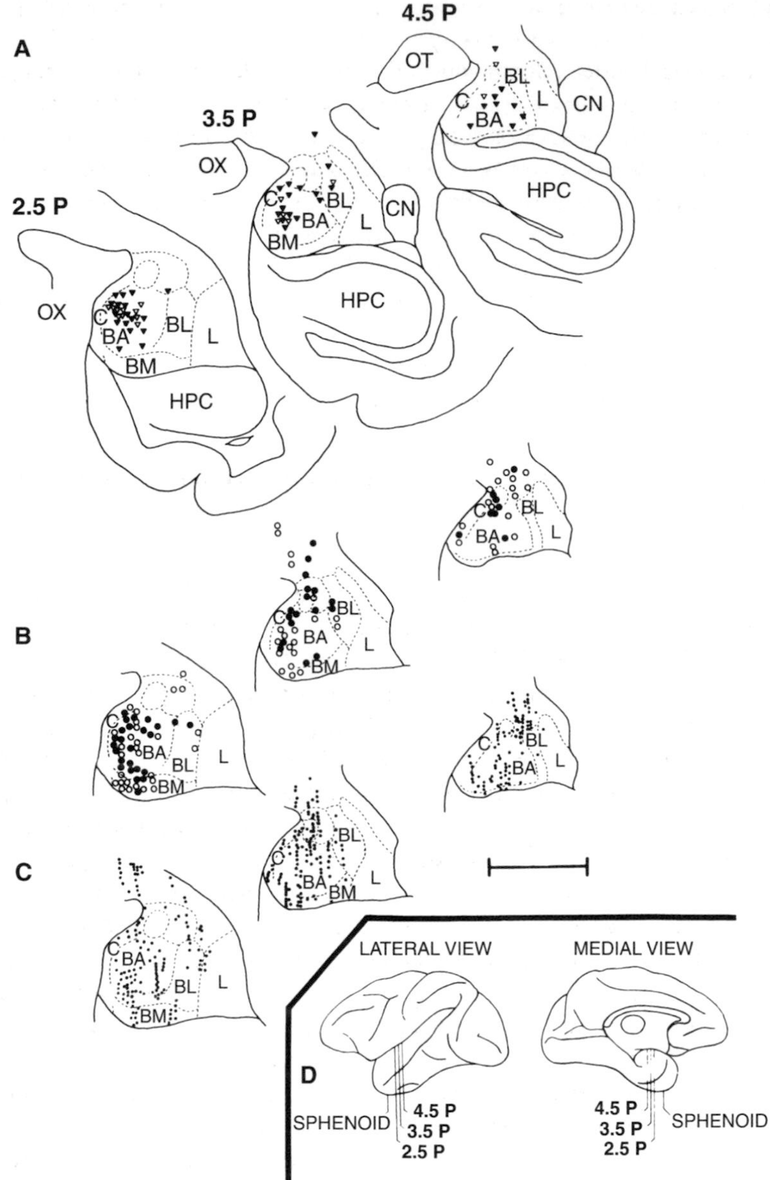

Figure 13.6 (**A**) The distribution of neurons responsive to faces in the amygdala of four monkeys. The cells are plotted on three coronal sections at different distances (in mm) posterior (P) to the sphenoid (see inset): ▲, cells selective for faces; △, cells responding to face and hands. (**B**) Other responsive neurons: ●, cells with other visual responses; ○, cells responding to cues, movement, or arousal. (**C**) The locations of non-responsive cells. Abbreviations: BA, basal accessory nucleus of the amygdala; BL, basolateral nucleus of the

represented increases exponentially with the number of neurons in the ensemble (Abbott *et al.*, 1996; Rolls *et al.*, 1997a). This form of sparse yet distributed encoding, also found for objects in the temporal visual cortex (Booth and Rolls, 1998), is ideal as an input to a pattern association memory such as one for stimulus–reinforcer association learning, because it allows very high capacity and at the same time generalization to similar instances of the same stimulus (Rolls and Treves, 1998; Rolls, 1999a). The representation of faces and objects which is built in temporal cortical areas shows considerable size, contrast, spatial frequency, translation, and view invariance (Rolls and Baylis, 1986; Hasselmo *et al.*, 1989b; Rolls, 1992b; Tovee *et al.*, 1994; Wallis and Rolls, 1997; Booth and Rolls, 1998). This invariance also makes it ideal as an input to a stimulus–reinforcer association learning network in, for example, the amygdala and orbitofrontal cortex, because it means that what is learned to one view (and size, etc.) of a stimulus generalizes correctly to other views (etc.) of the same stimulus (see Rolls and Treves, 1998), a feature that is biologically very useful (Rolls, 1999a, 2000c).

13.2.5 Taste, olfactory, somatosensory, and auditory responses of primate amygdala neurons

Sanghera *et al.* (1979) described taste responses in some amygdala neurons in macaques, and Wilson and Rolls (1993, 2000) found more. Nishijo *et al.* (1988a,b) found ingestion-related amygdala neurons, at least some of which were probably taste related. Scott *et al.* (1993) analysed the responses of 35 taste neurons in the macaque amygdala. Although individual neurons were quite broadly tuned to different tastes, the population as a whole clearly discriminated between the tastes sweet, salt (NaCl), and umami (monosodium glutamate, protein taste; see Rolls, 1997a; Rolls *et al.*, 1998). To test whether the representation of taste in the primate amygdala may encode its reward value, Yan and Scott (1996) fed monkeys to satiety to determine whether decreasing the reward value of the taste to zero in this way decreased to zero the responses of primate amygdala sweet taste neurons, as has been found for orbitofrontal cortex neurons (Rolls *et al.*, 1989). Yan and Scott found that only a partial reduction of the responses of amygdala neurons was produced by feeding to satiety (by an average of 62%). The implication is that amygdala neurons in primates can respond differently to rewarding and punishing stimuli, but reflect less completely than do orbitofrontal cortex neurons the reward value when it changes rapidly, as during feeding to satiety, or, as described above for visual neurons, in visual discrimination reversal.

In an fMRI study in humans, Francis *et al.* (1999) found activation of the human amygdala by the taste of glucose. Extending this study, O'Doherty *et al.* (1999, 2000) showed that the human amygdala was as much activated by the affectively pleasant taste of glucose as by the affectively negative taste of NaCl, and thus provided evidence that the human amygdala is not especially involved in processing aversive as compared with rewarding stimuli (see Figure 13.7).

---

amygdala; BM, basomedial nucleus of the amygdala; C, cortical nucleus of the amygdala; CN, tail of the caudate nucleus; HPC, hippocampus; L, lateral nucleus of the amygdala; OT, optic tract; OX, optic chiasm. (From Leonard *et al.*, 1985, with permission.)

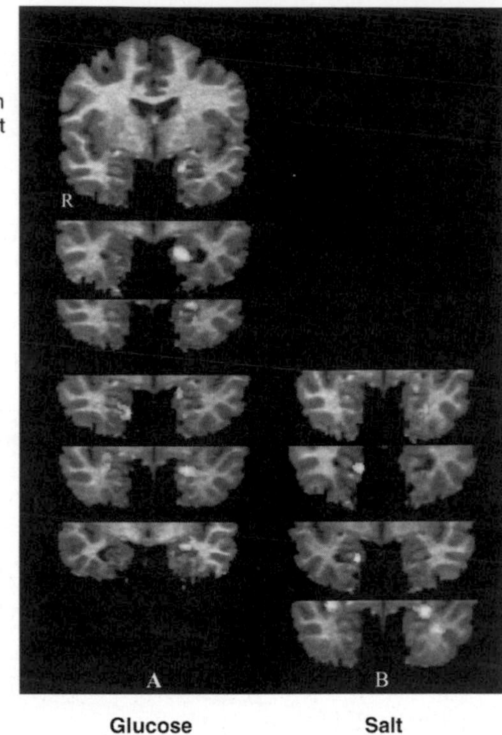

Figure 13.7 Activations produced in the human amygdala in seven subjects in an fMRI investigation by the taste of 1 M glucose versus a tasteless control solution and by 0.1 M NaCl versus a tasteless control solution shown on coronal sections thresholded at $P < 0.025$ (corrected for multiple comparisons within a region of interest). Each row has data for one subject in both conditions for the sections where activations significant at this criterion were found. The top left image shows for the glucose condition the median of the voxels with significant activation across the five subjects. (The location was not sufficiently similarly located in the different subjects for the taste of salt for a median image to be produced.) The activations shown were calculated from the difference in voxel intensity over the 8 s period during which the activation for each brain region was maximal, from that measured during the control OFF period with 0.5 ml of tasteless solution delivered into the mouth. (After O'Doherty *et al.*, 1999, 2000.) See also colour plate section.

Somatosensory responses have also been found in the monkey amygdala, to, for example, oral stimuli or touch to the limbs (Sanghera *et al.*, 1979; Leonard *et al.*, 1985). Although these neurons could well encode the primary reinforcing value of tactile stimuli, this has not been studied as directly as it has for primate orbitofrontal cortex neurons that respond, for example, to the texture of food in the mouth (Rolls *et al.*, 1999). Olfactory responses have also been found in the primate amygdala (Sanghera *et al.*, 1979), and the anterior cortical nucleus of the amygdala, and the periamygdaloid cortex, receive direct connections from the olfactory bulb (Carmichael *et al.*, 1994). Auditory stimuli can also activate some amygdala neurons, and, in some cases, the neuronal responses may discriminate between reward- and punishment-related auditory stimuli (Nishijo *et al.*, 1988a,b; Wilson and Rolls, 2000).

13.3 Comparisons of the responses of neurons in the primate amygdala and orbitofrontal cortex

Although as described above some visual neurons in the primate amygdala do respond to rewarding visual stimuli, and others to punishment-associated visual stimuli in a visual discrimination task, they did not reverse their responses to visual stimuli in the same complete and rapid way (in one or two trials) that reversal occurs in neurons in the primate orbitofrontal cortex (Thorpe *et al.*, 1983; Rolls *et al.*, 1996) and in a region to which it projects, the basal forebrain (Wilson and Rolls, 1990a,c; Rolls, 1999a). On the basis of these findings, it is suggested that the orbitofrontal cortex is more involved than the amygdala in the rapid readjustments of behavioural responses made to stimuli when their reinforcement value is changing repeatedly, as in discrimination reversal tasks (Thorpe *et al.*, 1983; Rolls, 1999a). The ability to alter responses flexibly to stimuli based on their changing reinforcement associations is important in motivated behaviour (such as feeding) and in emotional behaviour, and it is this flexibility which it is suggested that the orbitofrontal cortex adds to a more basic capacity that the amygdala implements for stimulus–reinforcement learning (Rolls, 1986, 1990, 1999a). Consistent with this, in another situation in which the reward value of visual stimuli alters rapidly, when a food is fed to satiety and becomes no longer rewarding, the responses of orbitofrontal cortex neurons (Critchley and Rolls, 1996a) and basal forebrain neurons (Rolls *et al.*, 1986) also decrease to very low values. This function may also be implemented in the human orbitofrontal cortex, because ventral frontal lobe damage does impair visual discrimination reversal and extinction in humans (Rolls *et al.*, 1994). With respect to learning associations of faces with reinforcers, and using face expression as a reinforcing signal, it is now known that there are face-selective neurons in the primate orbitofrontal cortex (Booth *et al.*, 1998; Rolls, 1999a), and ventral frontal lobe damage in humans does impair the identification of face expression but not of face identity (Hornak *et al.*, 1996).

Although the amygdala does receive taste inputs, the primate orbitofrontal cortex is now known to contain the secondary taste cortex, in that it receives massive projections from the primary taste cortex and not from the thalamic taste nucleus, VPMpc (Baylis *et al.*, 1994). The responses of taste neurons in the orbitofrontal cortex do encode the reward value of food, in that their responses decrease to zero when the monkey is fed to satiety, and in fact implement sensory-specific satiety (Rolls *et al.*, 1989), neither of which is reflected in the responses of neurons in the primary taste cortex (see Rolls, 1997a, 1999a). In primates (in contrast to rodents), the brainstem taste pathways do not have connections which directly access subcortical structures such as the amygdala, but instead the projections are via the taste thalamus and primary taste cortex (Norgren, 1984). This implies that cortical processing of taste is relatively more important in primates, and the beautiful elaboration of the representation of taste in the primate orbitofrontal cortex may be partly to enable direct linking by rapid cortical learning of associative connections between invariant representations of the sight of objects (reaching the orbitofrontal cortex via corticocortical connections from the inferior temporal visual cortex), and primary reinforcers such as taste. The primate orbitofrontal cortex also contains secondary (area 13a) and tertiary olfactory cortical areas (Carmichael *et al.*, 1994), and some neurons in the orbitofrontal cortex respond to the reward value of odours in that their responses are greatly decreased by feeding to satiety (Critchley and Rolls, 1996a). Moreover, the responses of approximately 40% of orbitofrontal cortex olfactory neurons are shaped by (slow) olfactory-to-taste association learning to build representations of flavour (Critchley and Rolls, 1996b; Rolls *et al.*, 1996). Thus again the orbitofrontal cortex, which develops greatly in primates, may overshadow some of the functions of the primate amygdala, to which it certainly is connected.

The primate orbitofrontal cortex also has a representation of the affective value of somatosensory stimuli, including in monkeys of the texture of food (Rolls *et al.*, 1999), and in humans of both the positively affective (Francis *et al.*, 1999) and the negatively affective (O'Doherty *et al.*, in preparation) aspects of touch.

The concept that is proposed is as follows. Whereas the amygdala is evolutionarily old (and is present in, for example, the reptile brain), the orbitofrontal cortex is much newer, and has expanded greatly in primates. The primate orbitofrontal cortex, which receives inputs of the same general type as the amygdala, partly because of the great development of other cortical areas and the importance of corticocortical general connection schemes and the power of cortical processing and learning, may then perform some of the functions originally performed by the amygdala, particularly when rapid learning is required.

13.4 The role of the amygdala in emotion

The evidence described above implicates the amygdala in the learning of associations between stimuli and reinforcement, in social behaviour, and in emotion. How may its roles in these functions be related? It has been proposed that emotions are states elicited by reinforcing stimuli (Weiskrantz, 1968; Rolls, 1990, 1999a, 2000a). The reinforcers can be primary (unlearned), or learned by stimulus–reward and stimulus–punisher association learning. Given that the amygdala is implicated in stimulus–reinforcer association learning, this suggests that a function of the amygdala in emotion, and in social behaviour, is to perform emotional (stimulus–reinforcer association) learning. To perform this function, the amygdala would need to have neurons that are activated by primary reinforcers, and examples of these are the taste and somatosensory inputs in the primate described here. The amygdala would also need to receive input from previously neutral, e.g. visual, stimuli, which as described here in primates is the case. It would also need to have associative modifiability in the connections between neurons that respond to such to-be-conditioned stimuli and primary reinforcers, for which there is evidence from studies in rats (Davis, 1992, 1994; LeDoux, 1995, 1996). The primate neurons that respond to faces may be important in these functions in two ways.

First, they may convey information of a primary reinforcing nature, for example, a threat expression on a face. Secondly, by conveying information about face identity, face-selective amygdala neurons may be important in learned emotional responses to the faces of particular individuals, via the process of face-to-primary reinforcer association learning. This analysis provides a theoretical basis for understanding how the amygdala is involved in emotion.

The theory described above about the role of the amygdala in emotion, based largely on research in non-human primates, has been followed up by studies in humans which are producing generally consistent results. One type of evidence comes from the effects of brain damage, which though rarely restricted just to the amygdala, and almost never bilateral, does provide some consistent evidence (Aggleton, 1992; Adolphs and Tranel, Chapter 18). For example, in some patients, alterations in feeding behaviour and emotion might occur after damage to the amygdala (see Aggleton, 1992; Halgren, 1992). In relation to neurons in the macaque amygdala with responses selective for faces and social interactions (Leonard *et al.*, 1985; Brothers and Ring, 1993), Young *et al.* (1995, 1996) have described in patient D.R., who has bilateral damage to or disconnection of the amygdala, an impairment of face–expression matching and naming, but not of matching face identity or in discrimination. This patient is also impaired at detecting whether someone is gazing at the patient, another important social signal (Perrett *et al.*, 1985). The same patient is also impaired in the auditory recognition of fear and anger (Scott *et al.*, 1997). Adolphs *et al.* (1994) also found face expression but not face identity impairments in a patient (S.M.) with bilateral damage to the amygdala. A similar impairment was not found in patients with unilateral amygdala damage (Adolphs *et al.*, 1995). The bilateral amygdala patient S.M. was especially impaired at recognizing the face expression of fear, and also rated expressions of fear, anger, and surprise as less intense than did control subjects.

For comparison, in a much more extensive series of patients, it has been shown that damage to the orbitofrontal cortex can produce face expression deficits in the absence of face identification deficits, and that some patients with orbitofrontal cortex damage are impaired in the auditory identification of emotional sounds (Hornak *et al.*, 1996). Interestingly, the visual face expression and auditory vocal expression impairments are partly dissociable in these orbitofrontal patients, indicating partially separate processing systems in the orbitofrontal cortex, and indicating that a general emotional impairment produced by these lesions is not the simple explanation of the alterations in face and voice expression processing after damage to the orbitofrontal cortex. Indeed the most consistent change after orbitofrontal cortex damage in our series of patients (Rolls *et al.*, 1994; Hornak *et al.*, 1996; Rolls, 1999b) was an alteration in face expression decoding.

Functional brain imaging studies have also shown activation of the amygdala by face expression (see Dolan, Chapter, 19). For example, Morris *et al.* (1996) found more activation of the left amygdala by face expressions of fear than of happiness in a positron emission tomography (PET) study. They also reported that the activation increased as the intensity of the fear expression increased, and decreased as the intensity of the happy expression increased.

However, although in studies of the effects of amygdala damage in humans greater impairments have been reported to face expressions of fear than to some other expressions (Adolphs *et al.*, 1994; Scott *et al.*, 1997), and in functional brain imaging studies greater activation may be found to certain classes of emotion-provoking stimuli, e.g. to stimuli that provoke fear compared with those that produce happiness (Morris *et al.*, 1996), it is most unlikely that the amygdala is specialized for the decoding of only certain classes of emotional stimulus, such as fear. (Fear conditioning has been a model system used in rats; see LeDoux, 1992, 1994, 1995, 1996.) However, in contrast to the view that the amygdala may be particularly involved in behavioural responses to aversive stimuli, it is quite clear from single-neuron neurophysiological studies in non-human primates that different neurons are activated by different classes of both rewarding and punishing stimuli (Sanghera *et al.*, 1979; Ono and Nishijo, 1992; Rolls, 1992c; Wilson and Rolls, 1993, 2000) and by a wide range of different face stimuli (Leonard *et al.*, 1985). Also, lesions of the macaque amygdala impair the learning of both stimulus–reward and stimulus–punisher associations (see above). Amygdala lesions with ibotenic acid impair the processing of reward-related stimuli, in that when the reward value of a set of foods was reduced by feeding it to satiety (i.e. sensory-specific satiety), the monkeys still chose the visual stimuli associated with the foods with which they had been satiated (Malkova *et al.*, 1997). Further, electrical stimulation of the macaque and human amygdala at some sites is rewarding and humans report pleasure from stimulation at such sites (Rolls, 1975; Rolls *et al.*, 1980; Sem-Jacobsen, 1968, 1976; Halgren, 1992). Thus any differences in the magnitude of effects between different classes of emotional stimuli which appear in human functional brain imaging studies (Morris *et al.*, 1996) or even after amygdala damage (Adolphs *et al.*, 1994; Scott *et al.*, 1997) should not be taken as showing that the human amygdala is involved in only some emotions, but instead may reflect differences in the efficacy of the stimuli in leading to strong emotional reactions, or differences in the magnitude *per se* of different emotions, making some effects more apparent for some emotions than others. Additional factors are that some expressions are much more identifiable than others. For example, we (Hornak *et al.*, 1996; Rolls, 1999b) found that happy faces were easier to identify than other face expressions in the Ekman set, and that the orbitofrontal patients we studied were not impaired on identifying the (easy) happy face expression, but showed deficits primarily on the more difficult set of other expressions (fear, surprise, anger, sadness, etc.). Another factor in imaging studies in which the human subjects may be slightly apprehensive is that happy expressions may produce some relaxation in the situation, whereas expressions of fear may do the opposite, and this could contribute to the results found. Thus Rolls (1999a, 2000a) suggests caution in interpreting human studies as showing that the amygdala (or orbitofrontal cortex) is involved only in certain emotions. It is much more likely that both are involved in emotions produced to positively as well as to negatively reinforcing stimuli. Consistent with this, in a recent fMRI study, we have found that the human amygdala is activated just as much by affectively positive taste stimuli (glucose) and by affectively negative taste stimuli (salt) (O'Doherty *et al.*, 1999, 2000, see Figure 13.7).

All these findings indicate that the amygdala is involved in both positive and negative emotions (i.e. emotions produced by positive and negative reinforcers), by representing primary reinforcers, and by performing stimulus–reinforcer association learning. However, in primates performing these functions, the amygdala appears to be somewhat overshadowed by the orbitofrontal cortex, as described above.

Finally, although Le Doux's (1992, 1994, 1995, 1996) model of emotional learning emphasizes subcortical inputs (from, for example, the medial geniculate nucleus) to the amygdala for conditioned reinforcers, this can apply only to very simple auditory stimuli (such as pure tones). In contrast, a visual stimulus normally will need to be analysed to the object level (to the level, for example, of face identity, which requires cortical processing) before the representation is appropriate for input to a stimulus–reinforcement evaluation system such as the amygdala or orbitofrontal cortex. Similarly, it is typically to complex auditory stimuli (such as a particular person's voice, perhaps making a particular statement) that emotional responses are elicited. The point here is that emotions are usually elicited to environmental stimuli analysed to the object level (including other organisms), and not to retinal arrays of spots, or pure tones. Thus cortical processing to the object level is required in most normal emotional situations, and these cortical object representations are projected to reach multimodal areas such as the amygdala and orbitofrontal cortex where the reinforcement label is attached using stimulus–reinforcer pattern association learning to the primary reinforcers represented in these areas (Rolls, 1999a). Thus while LeDoux's (1996, Chapter 7) approach to emotion focuses mainly on fear responses to simple stimuli such as tones which are implemented considerably by subcortical processing, Rolls (1999a) considers how in primates (including humans), most stimuli, which happen to be complex and require cortical processing, produce a wide range of emotions. In doing this, Rolls (1999a) addresses the functions in emotion of the highly developed temporal and orbitofrontal cortical areas of primates, including humans, areas which are much less developed in rodents, and which in primates provide major inputs to the amygdala.

Acknowledgements

The author has worked on some of the research described here with G.C. Baylis, L.Baylis, R.Bowtell, A.Browning, M.J. Burton, S.Francis, M.E. Hasselmo, C.M. Leonard, F.McGlone, F. Mora, J. O'Doherty, D.I. Perrett, M.K. Sanghera, T.R. Scott, S.J. Thorpe, A. Treves, and F.A.W. Wilson, and their collaboration is sincerely acknowledged. Some of the research described was supported by the Medical Research Council, grants PG8513790 and PG9826105.

References

Abbott, L.F., Rolls, E.T., and Tovee, M.J. (1996) Representational capacity of face coding in monkeys. *Cerebral Cortex*, 6, 498–505.

Adolphs, R., Tranel, D., Damasio, H., and Damasio, A. (1994) Impaired recognition of emotion in facial expressions following bilateral damage to the human amygdala. *Nature*, 372, 669–672.

Adolphs, R., Tranel, D., Damasio, H., and Damasio, A.R. (1995) Fear and the human amygdala. *Journal of Neuroscience*, 15, 5879–5891.

Aggleton, J.P. (1992) The functional effects of amygdala lesions in humans: a comparison with findings from monkeys. In *The Amygdala: Neurobiological Aspects of Emotion, Memory, and Mental Dysfunction* (ed. J.P. Aggleton), pp. 485–503. Wiley-Liss, New York.

Aggleton, J.P. and Passingham, R.E. (1981) Syndrome produced by lesions of the amygdala in monkeys (*Macaca mulatta*). *Journal of Comparative and Physiological Psychology*, 95, 961–977.

Amaral, D.G., Price, J.L., Pitkanen, A., and Carmichael, S.T. (1992) Anatomical organization of the primate amygdaloid complex. In *The Amygdala: Neurobiological Aspects of Emotion, Memory, and Mental Dysfunction* (ed. J.P. Aggleton), pp. 1–66. Wiley-Liss, New York.

Baylis, G.C. and Rolls, E.T. (1987) Responses of neurons in the inferior temporal cortex in short-term and serial recognition tasks. *Experimental Brain Research*, 65, 614–622.

Baylis, G.C., Rolls, E.T., and Leonard, C.M. (1985) Selectivity between faces in the responses of a population of neurons in the cortex in the superior temporal sulcus of the monkey. *Brain Research*, 342, 91–102.

Baylis, G.C., Rolls, E.T., and Leonard, C.M. (1987) Functional subdivisions of the temporal lobe neocortex. *Journal of Neuroscience*, 7, 330–342.

Baylis, L.L. and Gaffan, D. (1991) Amygdalectomy and ventromedial prefrontal ablation produce similar deficits in food choice and in simple object discrimination learning for an unseen reward. *Experimental Brain Research*, 86, 617–622.

Baylis, L.L., Rolls, E.T., and Baylis, G.C. (1994) Afferent connections of the orbitofrontal cortex taste area of the primate. *Neuroscience*, 64, 801–812.

Bear, M.F. and Singer, W. (1986) Modulation of visual cortical plasticity by acetylcholine and noradrenaline. *Nature*, 320, 172–176.

Booth, M.C.A. and Rolls, E.T. (1998) View-invariant representations of familiar objects by neurons in the inferior temporal visual cortex. *Cerebral Cortex*, 8, 510–523.

Booth, M.C.A., Rolls, E.T., Critchley, H.D., Browning, A.S. and Hernandi, I. (1998) Face-selective neurons in the primate orbitofrontal cortex. *Society for Neuroscience Abstracts*, **24**, 898.

Brothers, L. and Ring, B. (1993) Mesial temporal neurons in the macaque monkey with responses selective for aspects of socal stimuli. *Behavioural Brain Research*, 57, 53–61.

Brothers, L., Ring, B., and Kling, A. (1990) Response of neurons in the macaque amygdala to complex social stimuli. *Behavioural Brain Research*, 41, 199–213.

Burton, M.J., Rolls, E.T., and Mora, F. (1976) Effects of hunger on the responses of neurones in the lateral hypothalamus to the sight and taste of food. *Experimental Neurology*, 51, 668–677.

Cador, M., Robbins, T.W., and Everitt, B.J. (1989) Involvement of the amygdala in stimulus–reward associations: interaction with the ventral striatum. *Neuroscience*, 30, 77–86.

Carmichael, S.T., Clugnet, M.-C., and Price, J.L. (1994) Central olfactory connections in the macaque monkey. *Journal of Comparative Neurology*, 346, 403–434.

Critchley, H.D. and Rolls, E.T. (1996a) Hunger and satiety modify the responses of olfactory and visual neurons in the primate orbitofrontal cortex. *Journal of Neurophysiology*, 75, 1673–1686.

Critchley, H.D. and Rolls, E.T. (1996b) Olfactory neuronal responses in the primate orbitofrontal cortex: analysis in an olfactory discrimination task. *Journal of Neurophysiology*, 75, 1659–1672.

Davis, M. (1994) The role of the amygdala in emotional learning. *International Review of Neurobiology*, 36, 225–266.

Davis, M. (1992) The role of the amygdala in conditioned fear. In *The Amygdala: Neurobiological Aspects of Emotion, Memory, and Mental Dysfunction* (ed. J.P. Aggleton), pp. 255–305. Wiley-Liss, New York.

Dunn, L.T. and Everitt, B.J. (1988) Double dissociations of the effects of amygdala and insular cortex lesions on conditioned taste aversion, passive avoidance, and neophobia in the rat using the excitotoxin ibotenic acid. *Behavioral Neuroscience*, 102, 3–23.

Everitt, B.J. and Robbins, T.W. (1992) Amygdala–ventral striatal interactions and reward-related processes. In *The Amygdala: Neurobiological Aspects of Emotion, Memory, and Mental Dysfunction* (ed. J.P. Aggleton), pp. 401–429. Wiley-Liss, New York.

Francis, S., Rolls, E.T., Bowtell, R., McGlone, F., O'Doherty, J., Browning, A., Clare, S., and Smith, E. (1999) The representation of the pleasantness of touch in the human brain, and its relation to taste and olfactory areas. *NeuroReport*, 10, 453–459.

Fried, I., MacDonald, K.A., and Wilson, C.L. (1997) Single neuron activity in human hippocampus and amygdala during recognition of faces and objects. *Neuron*, 18, 753–765.

Gaffan, D. (1992) Amygdala and the memory of reward. In *The Amygdala: Neurobiological Aspects of Emotion, Memory, and Mental Dysfunction* (ed. J.P. Aggleton), pp. 471–483. Wiley-Liss, New York.

Gaffan, D. and Harrison, S. (1987) Amygdalectomy and disconnection in visual learning for auditory secondary reinforcement by monkeys. *Journal of Neuroscience*, 7, 2285–2292.

Halgren, E. (1992) Emotional neurophysiology of the amygdala within the context of human cognition. In *The Amygdala: Neurobiological Aspects of Emotion, Memory, and Mental Dysfunction* (ed. J.P. Aggleton), pp. 191–228. Wiley-Liss, New York.

Hasselmo, M.E., Rolls, E.T., and Baylis, G.C. (1989a) The role of expression and identity in the face-selective responses of neurons in the temporal visual cortex of the monkey. *Behavioural Brain Research*, 32, 203–218.

Hasselmo, M.E., Rolls, E.T., Baylis, G.C., and Nalwa, V. (1989b) Object-centred encoding by face-selective neurons in the cortex in the superior temporal sulcus of the the monkey. *Experimental Brain Research*, 75, 417–429.

Heimer, L., Switzer, R.D., and Van Hoesen, G.W. (1982) Ventral striatum and ventral pallidum. Components of the motor system? *Trends in Neurosciences*, 5, 83–87.

Hornak, J., Rolls, E.T., and Wade, D. (1996) Face and voice expression identification in patients with emotional and behavioural changes following ventral frontal lobe damage. *Neuropsychologia*, 34, 247–261.

Humphrey, N.K. (1972) 'Interest' and 'pleasure': two determinants of a monkey's visual preferences. *Perception*, 3, 105–114.

Jones, B. and Mishkin, M. (1972) Limbic lesions and the problem of stimulus–reinforcement associations. *Experimental Neurology*, 36, 362–377.

Kling, A. and Steklis, H.D. (1976) A neural substrate for affiliative behavior in nonhuman primates. *Brain, Behavior and Evolution*, 13, 216–238.

Klüver, H. and Bucy, P.C. (1939) Preliminary analysis of functions of the temporal lobes in monkeys. *Archives of Neurology and Psychiatry*, 42, 979–1000.

LeDoux, J.E. (1992) Emotion and the amygdala. In *The Amygdala: Neurobiological Aspects of Emotion, Memory, and Mental Dysfunction* (ed. J.P. Aggleton), pp. 339–351. Wiley-Liss, New York.

LeDoux, J.E. (1994) Emotion, memory and the brain. *Scientific American*, 270, 32–39.

LeDoux, J.E. (1995) Emotion: clues from the brain. *Annual Review of Psychology*, 46, 209–235.

LeDoux, J.E. (1996) *The Emotional Brain*. Simon and Schuster, New York.

LeDoux, J.E., Iwata, J., Cicchetti, P., and Reis, D.J. (1988) Different projections of the central amygdaloid nucleus mediate autonomic and behavioral correlates of conditioned fear. *Journal of Neuroscience*, 8, 2517–2529.

Leonard, C.M., Rolls, E.T., Wilson, F.A.W., and Baylis, G.C. (1985) Neurons in the amygdala of the monkey with responses selective for faces. *Behavioural Brain Research*, 15, 159–176.

Malkova, L., Gaffan, D., and Murray, E.A. (1997) Excitotoxic lesions of the amygdala fail to produce impairment in visual learning for auditory secondary reinforcement but interfere with reinforcer devaluation effects in rhesus monkeys. *Journal of Neuroscience*, 17, 6011–6020.

Mesulam, M.-M. and Mufson, E.J. (1982) Insula of the old world monkey. III Efferent cortical output and comments on function. *Journal of Comparative Neurology*, 212, 38–52.

Meunier, M., Bachevalier, J., Murray, E.A., Malkova, L., and Mishkin, M. (1996) Effects of aspiration vs. neurotoxic lesions of the amygdala on emotional reactivity in rhesus monkeys. *Society for Neuroscience Abstracts*, 22, 1867.

Mishkin, M. and Aggleton, J. (1981) Multiple functional contributions of the amygdala in the monkey. In *The Amygdaloid Complex* (ed. Y. Ben-Ari), pp. 409–420. Elsevier, Amsterdam.

Mora, F., Rolls, E.T., and Burton, M.J. (1976) Modulation during learning of the responses of neurones in the lateral hypothalamus to the sight of food. *Experimental Neurology*, 53, 508–519.

Morris, J.S., Frith, C.D., Perrett, D.I., Rowland, D., Young, A.W., Calder, A.J., and Dolan, R.J. (1996) A differential neural response in the human amygdala to fearful and happy facial expressions. *Nature*, 383, 812–815.

Murray, E.A., Gaffan, E.A., and Flint, R.W. (1996) Anterior rhinal cortex and amygdala: dissociation of their contributions to memory and food preference in rhesus monkeys. *Behavioral Neuroscience*, 110, 30–42.

Nishijo, H., Ono, T., and Nishino, H. (1988a) Single neuron responses in amygdala of alert monkey during complex sensory stimulation with affective significance. *Journal of Neuroscience*, 8, 3570–3583.

Nishijo, H., Ono, T., and Nishino, H. (1988b) Topographic distribution of modality-specific amygdalar neurons in alert monkey. *Journal of Neuroscience*, 8, 3556–69.

Norgren, R. (1984) Central neural mechanisms of taste. In *Handbook of Physiology—The Nervous System III. Sensory Processes 1* (ed. I. Darien-Smith), pp. 1087–1128. American Physiological Society, Washington, DC.

O'Doherty, J., Rolls, E.T., Francis, S., McGlone, F., and Bowtell, R. (1999) Areas of the orbitofrontal cortex and amygdala activated by pleasant and unpleasant taste. *Society for Neuroscience Abstracts*, 25, 2149.

O'Doherty, J., Rolls, E.T., Francis, S., McGlone, F., and Bowtell, R. (2000) The representation of pleasant and aversive taste in the human brain.

Ono, T. and Nishijo, H. (1992) Neurophysiological basis of the Klüver–Bucy syndrome: responses of monkey amygdaloid neurons to biologically significant objects. In *The Amygdala: Neurobiological Aspects of Emotion, Memory, and Mental Dysfunction* (ed. J.P. Aggleton), pp. 167–190. Wiley-Liss, New York.

Ono, T., Nishino, H., Sasaki, K., Fukuda, M., and Muramoto, K. (1980) Role of the lateral hypothalamus and amygdala in feeding behavior. *Brain Research Bulletin*, 5, 143–149.

Perrett, D.I. and Rolls, E.T. (1983) Neural mechanisms underlying the visual analysis of faces. In *Advances in Vertebrate Neuroethology* (eds J.-P. Ewert, R.R. Capranica, and D.J. Ingle), pp. 543–566. Plenum Press, New York.

Perrett, D.I., Rolls, E.T., and Caan, W. (1982) Visual neurons responsive to faces in the monkey temporal cortex. *Experimental Brain Research*, 47, 329–342.

Perrett, D.I., Smith, P.A., Potter, D.D., Mistlin, A.J., Head, A.S., Milner, A.D., and Jeeves, M.A. (1985) Visual cells in the temporal cortex sensitive to face view and gaze direction. *Proceedings of the Royal Society of London, Series B*, 223, 293–317.

Price, J.L. (1981) The efferent projections of the amygdaloid complex in the rat, cat and monkey. In *The Amygdaloid Complex* (ed. Y. Ben-Ari), pp. 121–132. Elsevier, Amsterdam.

Rolls, E.T. (1975) *The Brain and Reward*. Pergamon, Oxford.

Rolls, E.T. (1981) Responses of amygdaloid neurons in the primate. In *The Amygdaloid Complex* (ed. Y. Ben-Ari), pp. 383–393. Elsevier, Amsterdam.

Rolls, E.T. (1984) Neurons in the cortex of the temporal lobe and in the amygdala of the monkey with responses selective for faces. *Human Neurobiology*, 3, 209–222.

Rolls, E.T. (1986) Neural systems involved in emotion in primates. In *Emotion: Theory, Research, and Experience. Vol. 3. Biological Foundations of Emotion* (eds R. Plutchik and H. Kellerman), pp. 125–143. Academic Press, New York.

Rolls, E.T. (1989) Functions of neuronal networks in the hippocampus and neocortex in memory. In *Neural Models of Plasticity: Experimental and Theoretical Approaches* (eds J.H. Byrne and W.O. Berry), pp. 240–265. Academic Press, San Diego.

Rolls, E.T. (1990) A theory of emotion, and its application to understanding the neural basis of emotion. *Cognition and Emotion*, 4, 161–190.

Rolls, E. T. (1992a) Neurophysiology and functions of the primate amygdala. In *The Amygdala: Neurobiological Aspects of Emotion, Memory, and Mental Dysfunction* (ed. J.P. Aggleton), pp. 143–165. Wiley-Liss, New York.

Rolls, E.T. (1992b) Neurophysiological mechanisms underlying face processing within and beyond the temporal cortical visual areas. *Philosophical Transactions of the Royal Society of London, Series B*, 335, 11–21.

Rolls, E.T. (1992c) The processing of face information in the primate temporal lobe. In *Processing Images of Faces* (eds V. Bruce and M. Burton), pp. 41–68. Ablex, Norwood, New Jersey.

Rolls, E.T. (1997a) Taste and olfactory processing in the brain and its relation to the control of eating. *Critical Reviews in Neurobiology*, 11, 263–287.

Rolls, E.T. (1997b) A neurophysiological and computational approach to the functions of the temporal lobe cortical visual areas in invariant object recognition. In *Computational and Psychophysical Mechanisms of Visual Coding* (eds M. Jenkin and L. Harris), pp. 184–220. Cambridge University Press, Cambridge.

Rolls, E.T. (1999a) *The Brain and Emotion*. Oxford University Press, Oxford.

Rolls, E.T. (2000b) The orbitofrontal cortex and reward. *Cerebral Cortex*, **10**, 284–294.

Rolls, E.T. (1999c) The functions of the orbitofrontal cortex. *Neurocase*, 5, 301–312.

Rolls, E. T. (2000b) Précis of the brain and emotion. *Behavioral and Brain Sciences*, **23**, 177–233.

Rolls, E.T., Judge, S.J. and Sanghera, M. (1977) Activity of neurones in the inferotemporal cortex of the alert monkey. *Brain Research*, **130**, 229–238.

Rolls, E.T., (2000c) Functions of the primate temporal lobe cortical visual areas in invariant visual object and face recognition. *Neuron*, in press.

Rolls, E.T. and Baylis, G.C. (1986) Size and contrast have only small effects on the responses to faces of neurons in the cortex of the superior temporal sulcus of the monkey. *Experimental Brain Research*, 65, 38–48.

Rolls, E.T. and Rolls, B.J. (1973) Altered food preferences after lesions in the basolateral region of the amygdala in the rat. *Journal of Comparative and Physiological Psychology*, 83, 248–259.

Rolls, E.T. and Tovee, M.J. (1995) Sparseness of the neuronal representation of stimuli in the primate temporal visual cortex. *Journal of Neurophysiology*, 73, 713–726.

Rolls, E.T. and Treves, A. (1998) *Neural Networks and Brain Function*. Oxford University Press, Oxford.

Rolls, E.T., Burton, M.J., and Mora, F. (1976) Hypothalamic neuronal responses associated with the sight of food. *Brain Research*, 111, 53–66.

Rolls, E.T., Sanghera, M.K., and Roper-Hall, A. (1979) The latency of activation of neurons in the lateral hypothalamus and substantia innominata during feeding in the monkey. *Brain Research*, 164, 121–135.

Rolls, E.T., Burton, M.J., and Mora, F. (1980) Neurophysiological analysis of brain-stimulation reward in the monkey. *Brain Research*, 194, 339–357.

Rolls, E.T., Murzi, E., Yaxley, S., Thorpe, S.J., and Simpson, S.J. (1986) Sensory-specific satiety: food-specific reduction in responsiveness of ventral forebrain neurons after feeding in the monkey. *Brain Research*, 368, 79–86.

Rolls, E.T., Sienkiewicz, Z.J., and Yaxley, S. (1989) Hunger modulates the responses to gustatory stimuli of single neurons in the caudolateral orbitofrontal cortex of the macaque monkey. *European Journal of Neuroscience*, **1**, 53–60.

Rolls, E.T., Hornak, J., Wade, D., and McGrath, J. (1994) Emotion-related learning in patients with social and emotional changes associated with frontal lobe damage. *Journal of Neurology, Neurosurgery and Psychiatry*, 57, 1518–1524.

Rolls, E.T., Critchley, H.D., Mason, R., and Wakeman, E.A. (1996) Orbitofrontal cortex neurons: role in olfactory and visual association learning. *Journal of Neurophysiology*, 75, 1970–1981.

Rolls, E.T., Treves, A., and Tovee, M.J. (1997a) The representational capacity of the distributed encoding of information provided by populations of neurons in the primate temporal visual cortex. *Experimental Brain Research*, 114, 177–185.

Rolls, E.T., Treves, A., Tovee, M.J., and Panzeri, S. (1997b) Information in the neuronal representation of individual stimuli in the primate temporal visual cortex. *Journal of Computational Neuroscience*, 4, 309–333.

Rolls, E.T., Critchley, H.D., Browning, A., and Hernadi, I. (1998) The neurophysiology of taste and olfaction in primates, and umami flavor. *Annals of the New York Academy of Sciences*, 855, 426–437.

Rolls, E.T., Critchley, H.D., Browning, A.S., Hernadi, A., and Lenard, L. (1999) Responses to the sensory properties of fat of neurons in the primate orbitofrontal cortex. *Journal of Neuroscience*, 19, 1532–1540.

Sanghera, M.K., Rolls, E.T., and Roper-Hall, A. (1979) Visual responses of neurons in the dorsolateral amygdala of the alert monkey. *Experimental Neurology*, 63, 610–626.

Scott, S.K., Young, A.W., Calder, A.J., Hellawell, D.J., Aggleton, J.P., and Johnson, M. (1997) Impaired auditory recognition of fear and anger following bilateral amygdala lesions. *Nature*, 385, 254–257.

Scott, T.R., Karadi, Z., Oomura, Y., Nishino, H., Plata-Salaman, C.R., Lenard, L., Giza, B.K., and Ao, S. (1993) Gustatory neural coding in the amygdala of the alert monkey. *Journal of Neurophysiology*, 69, 1810–1820.

Sem-Jacobsen, C.W. (1968) *Depth-Electrographic Stimulation of the Human Brain and Behavior: From Fourteen Years of Studies and Treatment of Parkinson's Disease and Mental Disorders with Implanted Electrodes*. C.C. Thomas, Springfield, Illinois.

Sem-Jacobsen, C.W. (1976) Electrical stimulation and self-stimulation in man with chronic implanted electrodes. Interpretation and pitfalls of results. In *Brain-Stimulation Reward* (eds A. Wauquier and E.T. Rolls), pp. 505–520. North-Holland, Amsterdam.

Spiegler, B.J. and Mishkin, M. (1981) Evidence for the sequential participation of inferior temporal cortex and amygdala in the acquisition of stimulus–reward associations. *Behavioural Brain Research*, 3, 303–317.

Thorpe, S.J., Rolls, E.T., and Maddison, S. (1983) Neuronal activity in the orbitofrontal cortex of the behaving monkey. *Experimental Brain Research*, 49, 93–115.

Tovee, M.J., Rolls, E.T., and Azzopardi, P. (1994) Translation invariance in the responses to faces of single neurons in the temporal visual cortical areas of the alert macaque. *Journal of Neurophysiology*, 72, 1049–60.

Wallis, G. and Rolls, E.T. (1997) Invariant face and object recognition in the visual system. *Progress in Neurobiology*, 51, 167–194.

Weiskrantz, L. (1956) Behavioral changes associated with ablation of the amygdaloid complex in monkeys. *Journal of Comparative and Physiological Psychology*, 49, 381–391.

Weiskrantz, L. (1968) Emotion. In *Analysis of Behavioural Change* (ed. L. Weiskrantz), pp. 50–90. Harper and Row, New York.

Williams, G.V., Rolls, E.T., Leonard, C.M., and Stern, C. (1993) Neuronal responses in the ventral striatum of the behaving macaque. *Behavioural Brain Research*, 55, 243–252.

Wilson, F.A.W. and Rolls, E.T. (1990a) Neuronal responses related to reinforcement in the primate basal forebrain. Brain Research, 502, 213–231.

Wilson, F.A.W. and Rolls, E.T. (1990b) Neuronal responses related to the novelty and familiarity of visual stimuli in the substantia innominata, diagonal band of Broca and periventricular region of the primate. *Experimental Brain Research*, 80, 104–120.

Wilson, F.A.W. and Rolls, E.T. (1990c) Learning and memory are reflected in the responses of reinforcement-related neurons in the primate basal forebrain. *Journal of Neuroscience*, 10, 1254–1267.

Wilson, F.A.W. and Rolls, E.T. (1993) The effects of stimulus novelty and familiarity on neuronal activity in the amygdala of monkeys performing recognition memory tasks. *Experimental Brain Research*, 93, 367–382.

Wilson, F.A.W. and Rolls, E.T. (2000) The primate amygdala and reinforcement: a dissociation between rule-based and associatively-mediated memory revealed in amygdala neuronal activity.

Wilson, F.A.W., Riches, I.P., and Brown, M.W. (1990) Hippocampus and medial temporal cortex: neuronal responses related to behavioural responses during the performance of memory tasks by primates. *Behavioral Brain Research*, 40, 7–28.

Yan, J. and Scott, T.R. (1996) The effect of satiety on responses of gustatory neurons in the amygdala of alert cynomolgus macaques. *Brain Research*, 740, 193–200.

Young, A.W., Aggleton, J.P., Hellawell, D.J., Johnson, M., Broks, P., and Hanley, J.R. (1995) Face processing impairments after amygdalotomy. *Brain*, 118, 15–24.

Young, A.W., Hellawell, D.J., Van de Wal, C., and Johnson, M. (1996) Facial expression processing after amygdalotomy. *Neuropsychologia*, 34, 31–39.

Zola-Morgan, S., Squire, L.R., and Amaral, D.G. (1989) Lesions of the amygdala that spare adjacent cortical regions do not impair memory or exacerbate the impairment following lesions of the hippocampal formation. *Journal of Neuroscience*, 9, 1922–1936.

14 Primate evolution and the amygdala

Robert A. Barton[1] and John P. Aggleton[2]

[1]*Evolutionary Anthropology Research Group, Department of Anthropology, University of Durham, 43 Old Elvet, Durham DH1 3HN and* [2]*School of Psychology, Cardiff University, Park Place, Cardiff CF10 3YG, UK*

Summary

We studied the evolution of the amygdala using data on the volume of amygdaloid components and of related brain structures in 83 species of primates and insectivores (Stephan *et al.*, 1987, 1991). We found a pattern indicative of both mosaic evolution, in which each component evolved separately with its own specific inputs and outputs, and coordinated evolution, in which the separate components evolved together. The corticobasolateral group of nuclei and the neocortex show the same pattern of size differences across taxonomic groups, with both being particularly expanded in the haplorhine primates (monkeys, apes, and tarsiers), which are mostly diurnal and gregarious. The centromedial amygdala shows no such taxonomic differences, indicating a degree of mosaic evolution of the amygdala. However, using a comparative method designed to detect correlated evolution, we found that amygdaloid components correlated most strongly with each other, rather than with other brain structures, emphasizing the functional and connectional integrity of the amygdala. Reflecting this, evolutionary changes in the size of both amygdaloid components correlated positively with changes in the size of the palaeocortex (principally olfactory cortex), pointing to the role of the amygdala in olfactorily-guided behaviour. Once the effects of palaeocortex size were partialled out, the size of the corticobasolateral group also correlated with neocortex size, perhaps reflecting the expansion and elaboration of the connections between temporal cortex and amygdala which are involved in the emotional modulation of visual stimuli in monkeys. In support of this idea, corticobasolateral amygdala correlated with parvocellular layers of the lateral geniculate nucleus, which project indirectly to the sociovisual processing areas of temporal cortex. Both neocortex size and corticobasolateral amygdala size correlate positively with social group size, lending further weight to the hypothesized link between the conjoint expansion of these structures and specialization for processing social information. Thus the primate amygdala has evolved with both its olfactory connections and its visual connections. Each may reflect the elaboration of mechanisms for processing social, and perhaps also sexual, information, with olfactory and visual modalities being emphasized differently according to the ecological factors operating in each lineage.

14.1 Introduction

Brains are products of natural selection. Their structure and mechanisms are evolutionary adaptations for particular lifestyles. Neuroscientists, however, have tended to neglect the evolutionary context of the systems they study. One consequence of this neglect is that species differences in the organization and functions of particular neural systems tend to be ignored or played down. This is a pity, because there is considerable evidence that brains have been fine tuned by natural selection for particular lifestyles (e.g. Sherry *et al.*, 1989; deVoogd *et al.*, 1993; Barton *et al.*, 1995). Evolved differences must therefore be taken into account in interpreting experimental results from different species. This does not mean only that species differences are an inconvenient confounding variable. Studying the evolution of a neural system, e.g. how its separate components have co-evolved and what ecological factors such evolution correlates with, potentially illuminates how it is organized and how it functions within particular species.

The original notion of the limbic system tended to imply that, as an evolutionarily ancient brain system, its structure and functions must be primitive compared with the more highly elaborated and advanced neocortex (MacLean, 1970). We now understand that this conception is too simplistic, both as applied to specific limbic structures such as the amygdala, and as a general view of brain evolution. As brains evolved, new functions were built onto, integrated with, and transformed existing systems (Damasio, 1994). Emotional and cognitive systems evolved together, and are not really dissociable. They are aspects of the unified process that underlies adaptive behaviour:

> 'Emotion is not just running away from a bear. It can be set off by the most sophisticated information processing the mind is capable of . . . And the emotions help to connive intricate plots for escape, revenge, ambition, and courtship'.
> Pinker (1998, p. 382)

This idea of a close integration between cognitive and emotional evolution suggests that comparative neuroanatomy might reveal something more interesting than a conserved limbic system beneath an elaborated neocortex. The neocortex is widely held to have been the focus of mammalian brain evolution; it is the structure that shows most marked interspecific variation in size, and in the number of functionally distinct areas (Crick, 1990; Finlay and Darlington, 1995; Kaas, 1995; Allman, 1999). The brains of anthropoids are 2–3 times larger, relative to body size, than in the average mammal (Passingham, 1982), and this overall size difference is predominantly a function of neocortical expansion. Anthropoid species that have particularly large brains also have particularly expanded neocortices (Barton, 2000). Nevertheless, the neocortex is unlikely to have evolved in isolation, without modification of its connections with other structures, including the amygdala. It is not too surprising then that the amygdala of monkeys has a distinctive pattern of cortical connections. Meta-analyses of connectivity by Young *et al.* (1994, p. 247) show that the macaque amygdala 'makes very widespread output projections, connecting with all but 8 of the cortical areas', whereas in cats 'the amygdala connects with relatively few areas outside the fronto-limbic complex'. One of the issues we address in this chapter is the relevance of the profuse corticoamygdaloid connections in anthropoid primates for understanding how and why their brains are specialized.

Pinker's example of social conniving quoted above may be particularly apt in the context of corticoamygdaloid evolution in primates. Social interaction in large and complex groups is what anthropoids, including ourselves, do pre-eminently well (deWaal, 1982; Cheney and Seyfarth, 1990; Harcourt and DeWaal, 1992). As such, it is to be expected that anthropoid brains evolved to facilitate such skills. It has been suggested repeatedly that the evolution of large brains in primates reflects the cognitive demands of competitive and cooperative social relationships (e.g. Humphrey, 1976; Whiten and Byrne, 1997). One reason for suggesting this is that the processing of social information in such groups is likely to be computationally and neurally highly demanding (Barton and Dunbar, 1997). First, social information is multifaceted, consisting of a diverse array of sensory input that must be integrated: auditory, tactile, olfactory, and, in diurnal species, especially visual (Allman, 1987; Brothers, 1990). During a polyadic (multi-individual) social interaction, a monkey must, as a minimum requirement for appropriate action, monitor and rapidly coordinate information on the identity and social attributes (e.g. dominance rank) of the other individuals, who may be numerous. Secondly, social interactions and relationships are in a constant state of flux, demanding continuous on-line processing of the dynamically and rapidly varying 'dispositions and intentions' of conspecifics, as revealed by facial expressions, for example (Brothers, 1990). Individuals also take into account the past actions of particular individuals, not just in the previous seconds, but also in the previous hours, days, and weeks (Cheney and Seyfarth, 1990). Managing social interactions and relationships is crucial to the individual's reproductive success (Strum, 1987; Dunbar, 1988). In sum, the individual is confronted by, and must process, a constant stream of complex social information. In accord with the idea that such social information processing is computationally demanding, neocortical expansion correlates positively with social group size (Sawaguchi and Kudo, 1990; Dunbar, 1992; Barton, 1996).

Anthropoid primates, then, have enlarged neocortices and extensive corticoamygdaloid connections. These traits may be associated with an increased emphasis on the processing of emotionally modulated social information in the context of more complex social lives. Both physiological and neuropsychological data support this idea. For example, the amygdala of monkeys contains neurons responsive to faces (Rolls, Chapter 13), reflecting its afferents from the inferotemporal cortex and superior temporal sulcus, where 'face cells' are also found (Leonard *et al.*, 1985; Brothers *et al.*, 1990; Rolls, Chapter 13). Furthermore, pathology in the human amygdala can produce selective deficits in the ability to identify emotional facial expressions. These deficits are most consistent for the identification of fearful faces (Adolphs and Tranel, Chapter 18). These findings give rise to several questions, which we address in the rest of this chapter. First, has the amygdala undergone expansion along with the neocortex during primate evolution? Secondly, if so, was this expansion restricted to certain functional components of the amygdala? Thirdly, with which other brain structures do amygdaloid components show the strongest evolutionary relationships, and do these relationships reflect the specific connections and functions of those components? Finally, what social or ecological factors are associated with evolutionary differences in the size of amygdaloid components? The answers to these questions may reveal much about the specialization of the primate brain for processing emotionally significant information.

14.2 The comparative method and evolutionary neuroanatomy

The purpose of the comparative method is to reveal facts about evolution (Harvey and Pagel, 1991). Comparisons amongst extant or fossil species can be used: (i) to study the phylogenetic distribution of character states; (ii) to show how related traits have evolved together; or (iii) to identify the selection pressures associated with the evolution of the traits. All three types of study have been carried out on neuroanatomical traits. Studies of the phylogenetic distribution of neuroanatomical character states focus on discrete traits, such as the presence or absence of specific brain structures or connections (e.g. Krubitzer, 1998). They have been used in two ways: to inform inferences about the phylogenetic relationships among species (e.g. Kaas and Preuss, 1993; Joffe and Dunbar, 1998) and to reconstruct the evolutionary history of the brain in particular lineages (Allman, 1982; Kaas, 1995; Butler and Hodos, 1996; Krubitzer, 1998). Neither of these is our aim here. Instead, we apply uses (ii) and (iii) of the comparative method to neuroanatomical data. Specifically, we are interested in using comparisons of a quantitative neural trait that indexes functionality (information processing capacity) to show how anatomically and functionally linked brain structures have co-evolved, and to investigate the selection pressures associated with such evolution. In order to do this, methods are required that use phylogenetic information to map evolutionary changes in one trait onto evolutionary changes in another (see Section 14.2.2).

14.2.1 Measures of information processing capacity

We use volume as an index of information-processing capacity. This is reasonable, as processing capacity is a function of the number of neurons in a network (Foldiak and Young, 1995; Barton and Dunbar, 1997), which in turn correlates with volume (Jerison, 1991; Barton, 1998). Direct evidence shows that brain structure size correlates with behaviour (Hampton and Shettleworth, 1996). There are of course aspects of functionality other than capacity, which should be measured in different ways. For example, impulse transmission speed may be important and, for this, axon diameter and myelination are the most direct measures. In fact, both the number and size of neurons potentially affect the volume of a structure, such that we cannot, without studies beyond the scope of this one, be certain about which aspects of functionality are indexed by volume in particular cases. We can, however, be confident that natural selection would not tolerate variation in the amount of neural tissue within a particular system if it bestowed no functional advantage, as neural tissue is metabolically expensive (Martin, 1996). Also, if two separate structures show closely correlated evolutionary changes in size, this is very likely to reflect strong antomical and functional connections between them.

The volumetric data we use here were produced by Stephan and co-workers (Stephan *et al.*, 1981, 1987, 1991), who provide details of the species, samples, and methods. We are interested primarily in the primate data, since this can be related to what is known about the connections and physiology of the relevant structures in monkeys. We also include insectivores as a comparison group, to highlight the specializations of primates. Mean volumes of all major brain structures are available for 39 insectivore species and 44 primate species.

Data for *Homo sapiens* are not included in the statistical analyses, but they are superimposed on the graphs for the purposes of comparison.

The data for the amygdala consist of total amygdala volume and volumes of components that were readily delimitable across species: the central–medial group of nuclei (consisting of the central and medial nuclei and the anterior amygdaloid area) and the corticobasolateral group (combining cortical, basal, and lateral nuclei). These groups are referred to hereafter as CM and CBL, respectively. The advantage of this grouping is that it separates all those amygdalar nuclei that are cortex-like (CBL) from those that are non-cortex-like (CM), as defined by the cell types within each nucleus (McDonald, 1992). There are, however, some drawbacks with these groupings. As noted by Stephan *et al.* (1987), it has been conventional to group the cortical nucleus with the central and medial nuclei, rather than the basolateral group (Humphrey, 1936). A recent connectional analysis by Emery (1997) supports this closer affinity of the cortical nucleus for the central and medial nuclei, while other evidence points to the unique status of the central nucleus (Swanson and Petrovich, 1998) which is set apart from other amygdaloid nuclei by its prominent brainstem connections (Amaral, 1992; Pitkänen, Chapter 2). While the groupings used here may not be ideal, the cortical nucleus is a relatively small component of the CBL, and so evolutionary changes in CBL size are probably driven primarily by changes in the more homogenous basolateral component. Nevertheless, this ambiguity needs to be born in mind when discussing the results.

Within the CBL grouping, Stephan *et al.* (1987) also measured a subcomponent, the magnocellular part of the basal nucleus. This subcomponent is referred to hereafter as MB. This region is of interest as the basal nucleus is the principal source of projections from the amygdala to tne neocortex (Amaral and Price, 1984; Amaral *et al.*, 1992). This leaves the logical possibility of calculating the volume of the CBL minus its MB component. Because this residual CBL component consists mainly of the lateral nucleus and accesory basal nucleus, we effectively are left with the regions that receive direct inputs from visual and auditory association cortex (Turner *et al.*, 1980) and which are densely interconnected (Aggleton, 1985). This component is abbreviated to LAB. A listing and definition of the components analysed is given in Table 14.1 for ready reference. Finally, Stephan *et al.* (1987) also measured the nucleus of the lateral olfactory tract, but since this structure is absent from most anthropoid primates we do not consider it in our analyses.

14.2.2 Analysis

Allometric considerations

Many biological traits, including brain size and the size of specific brain components, scale with body size, often in a non-linear fashion. The study of such scaling is termed allometry. It is generally accepted that any analysis of interspecific variation in a quantitative anatomical trait must take allometry into acount. It is usual to plot values of the trait against body size on a log–log plot, since this tends to linearize allometric relationships, making them suitable for conventional regression analysis. Commonly, the effects of size are removed by fitting a regression line and calculating residuals for each data point (see Figure 14.1). Residual brain size values are referred to commonly as 'encephalization' or 'relative brain

Table 14.1 Amygdala and other brain components for which comparative data are available

Structure	*Volume measurement includes*
Amygdala	Whole amygdala
Central–medial nuclear group (**CM**)	Central and medial nuclei, anterior amygdaloid area
Corticobasolateral nuclear group (**CBL**)	Lateral, basal, and cortical nuclei
Magnocellular basal (**MB**)	Magnocellular part of basal nucleus
Residual portion of CBL (**LAB**)	Lateral and cortical nucleus and non-magnocellular part of basal nucleus
Palaeocortex[a]	Olfactory cortices (piriform cortex, olfactory tubercle, anterior olfactory nucleus)
Neocortex	Neocortex
Lateral geniculate nucleus (**LGN**)	
Parvocellular	Layers 2–6
Magnocellular	Layers 1–2

The subdivisions were defined and measured in primate and insectivore species by Stephan *et al.* (1981, 1987), except for the LGN subdivisions, provided by Shulz (1967). Abreviations used in the text for amygdaloid components are given in bold.

[a]Palaeocortex volumes were derived from volumes of the piriform lobe and amygdala given by Stephan *et al.* (1981, 1987, 1991). These authors state that the piriform lobe consists of palaeocortex plus amygdala. Hence, palaeocortical volume was calculated by subtracting amygdala volume from piriform lobe volume. Direct measurements of palaeocortex volume were made by Stephan *et al.* for some of the species, and these measurements are almost identical to our estimates derived by subtraction. Stephan *et al.* (1991) included part of the substantia inominata in palaeocortex, but this constituted only 2–3% of total palaeocortical volume.

size' (e.g. Jerison, 1973; Harvey and Krebs, 1990). This approach has been applied by Stephan *et al.* (1987) to the analysis of individual brain structures such as the amygdala. However, this does not allow global differences in relative brain size, wherein all or most brain structures have evolved together, to be differentiated from more specific neural adaptations, wherein certain structures have evolved independently of the whole. This is not just a theoretical problem, since there is evidence that both evolutionary processes have been involved in mammalian brain evolution (Finlay and Darlington, 1995; Barton, 1998). For example, although only some brain structures are markedly bigger relative to body size in primates than in insectivores, most, including even the relatively conserved medulla, show at least slight differences (Barton, 2000). In order to evaluate taxonomic differences in amygdala size that are independent of such generalized brain size differences, and which therefore reflect specific specializations for amygdala functions, we use the medulla as our main control variable. Since medulla size is very highly correlated with body size, this effectively removes body size and general brain size effects simultaneously. We also, however, assess how much difference it makes to results when body size itself is used as the control variable, and incorporate body weight in multiple regressions where appropriate.

General phylogenetic trends and grade shifts

Examination of allometric plots often reveals that different taxonomic groups cluster around regression lines that have similar slopes—perhaps because of some fundamental scaling

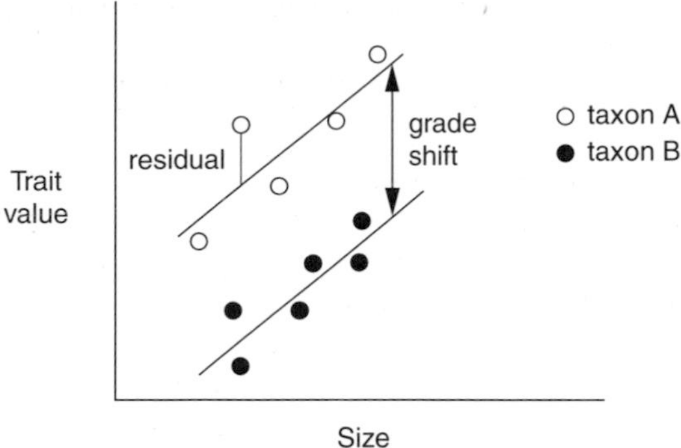

Figure 14.1 Illustration of the analysis of residual variation and grade shifts in allometric plots. The dependent variable, a continuously varying trait such as brain size, is plotted against some measure of size, typically body weight. Residual values for the data points provide a measure of the dependent variable after taking scaling into account. Where members of different taxonomic groups cluster around regression lines with similar slopes but different elevations (intercepts), they are said to occupy distinct 'grades'.

constraint—but different elevations. Such taxonomic differences in elevation are termed grade shifts (Martin, 1990; and see Figure 14.1). Primates, for example, have brains that are large for their body size in comparison with other mammalian taxa. In order to evaluate the extent to which primates are specialized for information processing involving the amygdala, we begin by examining broad differences in amygdala volume among orders and sub-orders. Although similar data are available for bats (Baron *et al.*, 1996), we focus on comparisons between insectivores and primate sub-orders because bats are in some respects highly specialized. Insectivores, on the other hand, are considered to represent a more generalized mammalian condition and are closer in morphology and behaviour to the ancestors of primates (Eisenberg, 1981). This should not be taken to mean that extant primates evolved directly from the insectivores (they did not), and it should be born in mind that comparisons with different mammalian orders might lead to slightly different inferences about what sets primates apart.

Within the primate orders, two distinct sub-orders are recognized: the haplorhini (monkeys, apes, and tarsiers) and the strepsirhini (lemurs and lorises). This differs from the older classification into prosimians and anthropoids, as tarsiers are now placed with the monkeys and apes. Although tarsiers bear superficial resemblances to other small-bodied nocturnal primates, they share a number of derived morphological features with anthropoids (Martin, 1990). Nevertheless, we occasionally refer to anthropoids as a separate group, as tarsier behaviour and ecology are quite distinct.

Correlated evolution and the method of independent contrasts

In recent years, methodological developments have clarified the objectives of comparative studies (see Harvey and Pagel, 1991). For many studies, the objective is to reveal adaptive associations amongst traits, or between traits and features of the environment. In the past, individual species often were treated as though they represent independent data points in statistical analyses. This presents a problem, which has been dealt with extensively elsewhere (see, for example, Felsenstein, 1985; Harvey and Pagel, 1991; Purvis and Rambaut, 1995). Briefly, hypothesizing an adaptive association between two character states, such as brain size and an aspect of lifestyle, implies that they have tended to evolve together. Valid statistical tests for such correlated evolution must be based on *independent evolutionary events*. It is not sufficient to calculate correlations across species values, because species share traits through common descent as well as through independent evolution. A hypothetical example is given in Figure 14.2. Here, a statistical test for an association between activity timing (nocturnal versus diurnal habits) and amygdala size might give a significant result, because the average amygdala size in the diurnal species is greater than in the nocturnal species. A closer look, however, would reveal no convincing evidence for an adaptive association: in only one of three comparisons between lineages differing in activity timing has the diurnal lineage evolved a larger amygdala. It is these evolutionarily independent comparisons, or contrasts, that must provide the data for valid statistical tesis of adaptive associations. Within primates, for example, the two sub-orders, the strepsirhinii and haplorhinii, differ in an array of features. Strepsirhines have smaller brains, lower metabolic rates, shorter gestations, a different type of placentation, smaller neonates, and tend to be more nocturnal and less gregarious (Martin, 1990). A non-phylogenetic analysis of any of these traits would risk finding spurious correlations between them as a result of the gross differences between the two taxonomic groups. The gross differences are of interest in themselves, in revealing something about how the taxa have become specialized differently. However, an analysis designed to test for the more general case of consistently correlated evolution among traits should be based on phylogenetically independent contrasts.

We used the CAIC computer package (Purvis and Rambaut, 1995), which implements Felsenstein's (1985) method of independent contrasts, with modifications by Pagel (1992) and Purvis (Purvis and Rambaut, 1995). The program computes standardized contrasts in trait values between pairs of taxa at each node of the phylogeny. These contrast values can then be analysed using methods such as regression, allowing analysis of correlated evolutionary change in the traits. The primate phylogeny used in analyses, including branch lengths, was taken from Purvis (1995). The insectivore phylogeny was taken from Barton *et al.* (1995). Where tests are to be made between quantitative brain traits and categorical variables (such as nocturnal versus diurnal habits), contrasts normally should be calculated only between nodes on the phylogeny where an evolutionary transition in the categorical variable has occurred (Purvis and Rambaut, 1995). Correlated evolution of the continuous variable and the categorical variable is indicated by a set of contrasts whose mean differs significantly from zero.

14.3 Evolution of amygdala size

14.3.1 Grade shifts in amygdala size

Graphs plotting the volume of amygdaloid components against medulla volume in primates and insectivores are shown in Figure 14.3 (gross subdivisions of the amygdala) and Figure

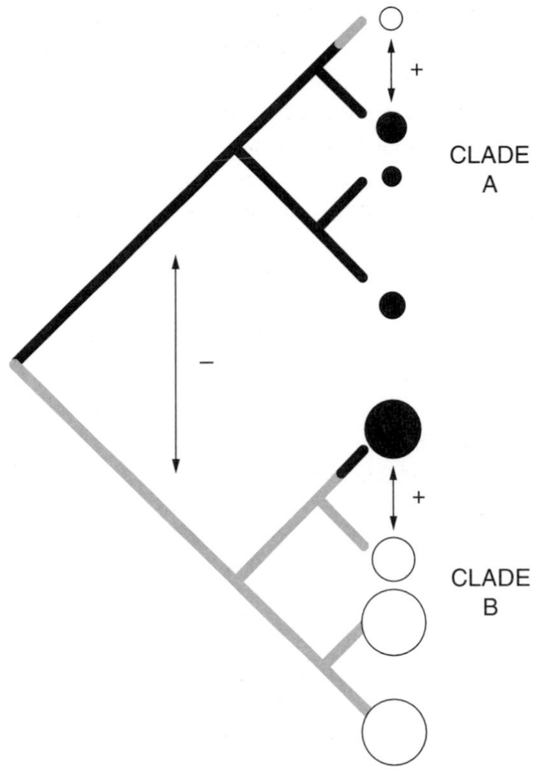

Figure 14.2 Hypothetical comparative analysis of amygdala size in relation to activity timing. The size of the circle represents amygdala size. Nocturnal species are represented by filled circles, diurnal species by open circles. The average amygdala size of nocturnal species is less than that of diurnal species. However, this average difference is a product of only one evolutionary event, the divergence between the two major taxonomic groups. A difference in amygdala size evolved at the divergence of clades A and B. There is no evidence in this hypothetical case that amygdala size and activity timing have evolved together consistently. The shading on the branches of the phylogeny indicates the inferred state at each point in the evolutionary radiation of the group, black for nocturnal, hatched for diurnal. In this data set, we can infer three evolutionary transitions in activity timing (shown by the arrows), where we can assess the evolutionary effects on amygdala size: larger amygdalae in nocturnal lineages are indicated by a + sign, and smaller amygdalae in nocturnal lineages by a – sign. In only one of these three comparisons (the comparison between the wholly nocturnal parts of clade A and wholly diurnal parts of clade B) is amygdala size greater in the diurnal taxon. Two out of three phylogenetic comparisons show the reverse. Hence, an analysis that did not take phylogeny into account could even give a statistical relationship between two variables that was the opposite of a real evolutionary relationship.

14.4 (MB and LAB components of the CBL). Visual inspection suggests that the CBL but not CM exhibits taxonomic grade shifts in relative size. This can be tested by analysis of variance (ANOVA) on the residuals from the common regression slope. The latter must either be calculated as the within-grade slope or by using independent contrasts, since to calculate a slope across grades would conflate grade shifts with allometric scaling and yield phylogenetically biased residuals. We report results using the mean within-grade slope, but slopes calculated by independent contrasts are similar and do not affect the results substantially. This analysis showed no significant variation among taxonomic groups for the CM

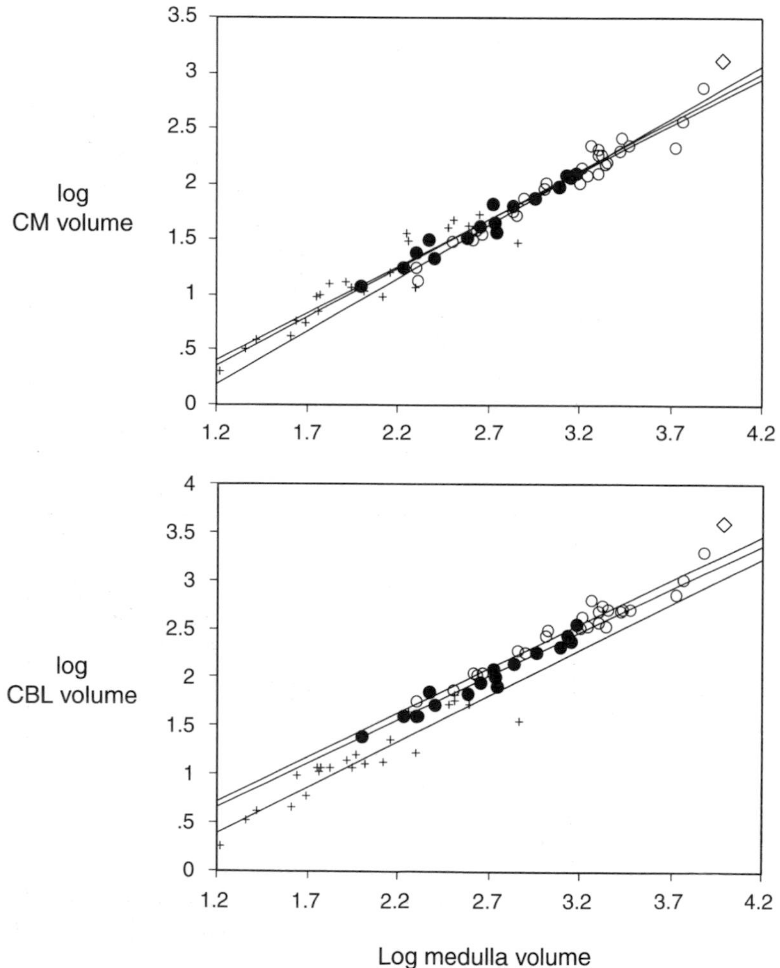

Figure 14.3 Taxonomic differences in the volume of centromedial (CM) and corticobasolateral (CBL) amygdala relative to volume of the medulla. Variables were log-transformed and lines fitted by least-squares regression. ○, haplorhine primates; ●, strepsirhine primates; + insectivores; ◇ humans.

($F = 0.7$, df = 2,65, $P = 0.48$), but significant variation for the CBL ($F = 45.8$, df = 2,65, $P < 0.0001$). Bonferroni/Dunn *post-hoc* tests on the latter reveal that all the taxonomic differences are significant (insectivores versus strepsirhines, mean difference = 0.22, $P < 0.0001$; insectivores versus haplorhines, mean difference = 0.30, $P < 0.0001$; strepsirhines versus haplorhines, mean difference = 0.07, $P = 0.04$). These differences appear to be a function primarily of differences in the size of the LAB rather than MB (Figure 14.4). However, ANOVA on the residuals does indicate significant heterogeneity amongst the MB means ($F = 7.9$, df = 2,65, $P = 0.0008$). *Post-hoc* tests show that this is attributable to significant differences between haplorhine primates and the other two groups (haplorhines versus

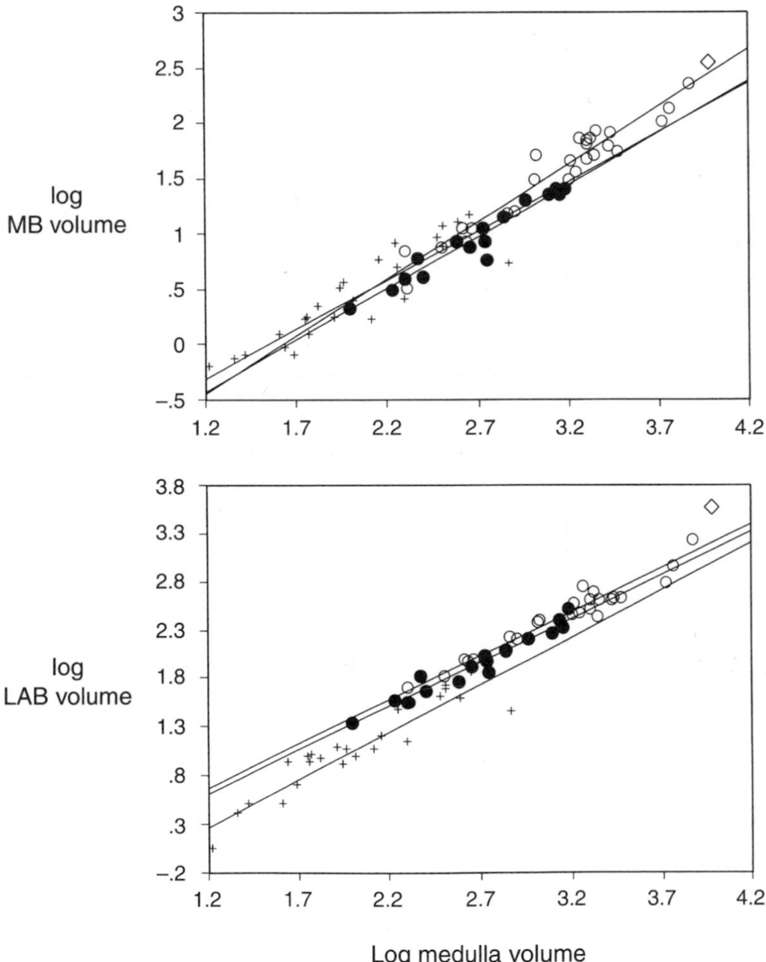

Figure 14.4 Taxonomic differences in the volume of corticobasolateral amygdala components relative to volume of the medulla. See Table 14.1 for definition of each component. Other details as for Figure 14.3.

insectivores, mean difference = 0.09, $P = 0.03$; haplorhines versus strepsirhines, mean difference = 0.18, $P = 0.0002$). The strepsirhine–insectivore difference is non-significant, though only just (mean difference = 0.08, $P = 0.06$). The heterogeneity of means is more marked for the LAB ($F = 59.5$, df = 2,65, $P < 0.0001$). Also, in contrast to the results for the MB, the significant differences are between insectivores and both of the primate taxa (insectivores versus haplorhines, mean difference = 0.32, $P < 0.0001$; insectivores versus strepsirhines, mean difference = 0.27, $P < 0.0001$; haplorhines versus strepsirhines, mean difference = 0.06, $P = 0.15$).

In summary, separate components of the amygdala show evolutionary dissociations. The relative size of the CBL is significantly greater in primates than in insectivores, and, amongst primates, is bigger in haplorhines (monkeys, apes, and tarsiers) than in strepsirhines (lemurs and lorises). The differences in CBL size are partly attributable to the MB component, which is enlarged in haplorhine primates, but shows no difference between strepsirhines and insectivores, and partly to the LAB component, which is larger in both primate taxa than in insectivores. The CM, on the other hand, shows no grade differences.

Evidently the CBL has been the focus of evolutionary change in the primate amygdala, supporting the conclusions of the allometric analysis by Stephan *et al.* (1987) which used body weight as the control variable. We find that, when body size instead of medulla size is used as the allometric control variable, the main difference is that the CM is significantly larger in both primate groups than in insectivores. This difference, however, reflects a global difference in brain size relative to body size, as explained above (Section 14.2.2), and is therefore not indicative of any specialized expansion of the CM in primates.

Figures 14.3 and 14.4 show that the human amygdala is enlarged compared with the non-human amygdala, even when the general enlargement of the human brain (as indexed by medulla size) is taken into account. All of the components, with the possible exception of the MB, show this enlargement, although the difference is smaller for the CM than for the CBL and MB. Indeed, CM residuals for several insectivores are as great as for the human data point.

A striking similarity is apparent between the grade shifts in CBL size and those in the size of the neocortex (Figure 14.5). In the case of both structures, insectivores, strepsirhines, and haplorhines are ranked in ascending order, even after removing the effects of general brain size differences. The similarity in the taxonomic patterns exhibited by these two structures reflects their connectivity (as also pointed out by Stephan *et al.*, 1987). These two highly interconnected structures seem to have co-evolved. In the next section, we assess further such co-evolutionary relationships using the method of independent contrasts to detect correlated evolution.

14.3.2 Correlated evolution of amygdala and other brain regions

The evidence that the analysis of grade shifts provides for the CBL and neocortex having evolved together boils down to two evolutionary events: the divergence between the lineages leading to insectivores and primates, and the divergence between the two primate sub-orders. How general is the evolutionary link between these two structures, and what other brain

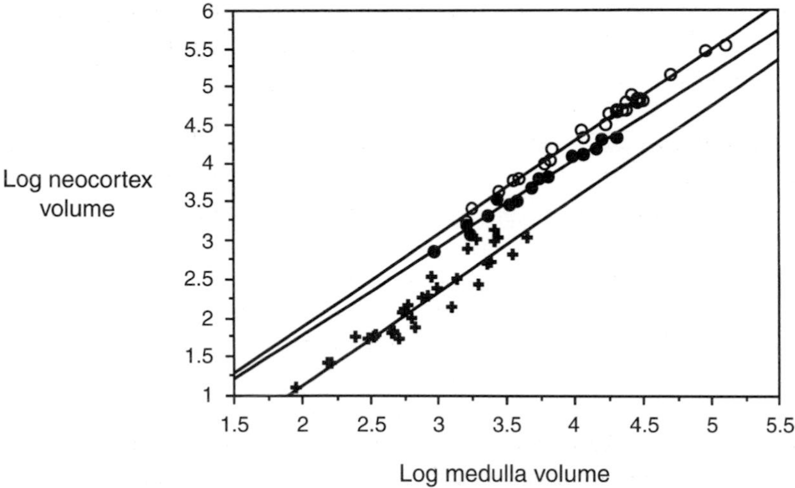

Figure 14.5 Taxonomic differences in relative neocortical volume. Details are as for Figure 14.3.

regions have evolved with the amygdala? As explained above (Sction 14.2.2), the method of independent contrasts can be used to test for correlated evolution, in this case between individual brain structures. Significant correlations between the contrast values for pairs of structures indicate that evolutionary changes in one brain structure were accompanied consistently by change in the other structure.

Major brain structures

We carried out a partial correlation analysis on 16 major brain structures in 43 primate species. The results are summarized in Figure 14.6. In the figure, a line between two structures indicates that evolutionary change in their size is significantly correlated when the effects of change in all other structures have been partialled out. The pattern is in many respects consonant with major functional and anatomical conections.

For the amygdala as a whole, the only significant partial correlation was with the 'palaeocortex', which consists almost entirely of olfactory cortex (see Table 14.1). The correlation is consistent with the long established role of the amygdala in olfactory-guided behaviour (Lehman *et al.*, 1980; Cousens and Otto, 1998; Zald and Pardo, 1997), and also with connectional data from primate brains (Turner *et al.*, 1978; Price, 1990; Carmichael *et al.*, 1994). Indeed, the periamygdaloid cortex typically is recognized as an integral part of the amygdala itself (Amaral *et al.*, 1992). Furthermore, studies of cerebral metabolism in rat amygdala kindling show that during focal seizures, the area which exhibits the most consistent increase in glucose utilization is the ipsilateral palaeocortex, and activation of microglia is seen in the piriform cortex after amygdala kindling (Loscher and Ebert, 1996).

When the CM and CBL nuclear groups are included as separate variables, their strongest correlations are with each other (r = 0.47, P <0.01). A near-significant partial correlation

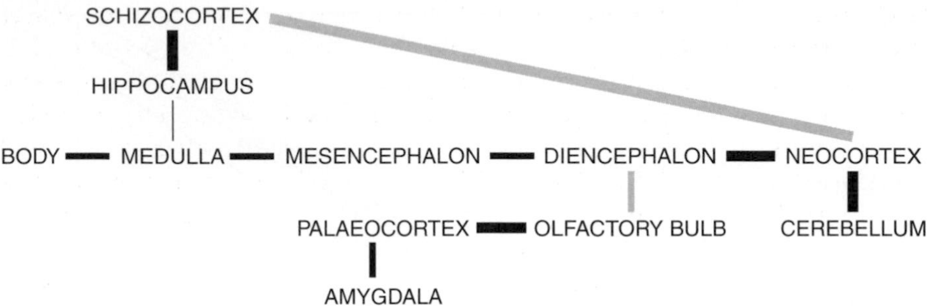

Figure 14.6 Correlated evolution among primate brain parts and body size. Structures connected by lines show significant partial correlations, in terms of evolutionary change in their volumes, after controlling for change in the other structures (based on 40 independent contrasts in structure volume and body size). Dashed lines are negative correlations. Five brain structures showed no significant partial correlations and are omitted from the figure. The patterns of correlated evolution reflect important anatomical and functional connections. For example, the neocortex receives most of its input from the thalamus, within the diencephalon. In turn, the neocortex has extensive connections with the cerebellum, and corticocerbellar circuits, such as those mediating hand–eye coordination, are particularly important in primates. The schizocortex (=entorhinal cortex and subiculum) is intimately connected with the hippocampus. The role of the palaeocortex in olfaction is reflected in its correlation with olfactory bulb size. See text for discussion of the connection between palaeocortex and amygdala.

also remains between the CM and palaeocortex ($r = 0.37$, $P < 0.07$), but none of the other correlations for these two groups approach significance. Hence, despite the differing pattern of grade shifts between orders and sub-orders, during the evolutionary radiation of primates, amygdaloid components have tended to evolve together, rather than separately with different inputs and projection targets. This conjoint development accords with the discovery of dense intrinsic connections within the amygdala (Aggleton, 1985; Amaral *et al.*, 1992; McDonald, 1992; Pitkänen, Chapter 2). This association also provides evidence of functional integrity within the amygdala, in spite of the evident differences between the connections of the component amygdaloid nuclei (Swanson and Petrovich, 1998).

Despite the known amygdala–palaeocortex connections, the partial correlation results are in some respects surprising. Given the connectional data for primates (Young *et al.*, 1994; Emery, 1997) and the pattern of grade shifts reported above, a correlation between neocortical and amygdaloid evolution might be expected. Specifically, we might expect basolateral and lateral nuclei to correlate strongly with the neocortex, as those nuclei have major connections with sensory, temporal, and prefrontal neocortex (Aggleton *et al.*, 1980; Turner *et al.*, 1980; Amaral *et al.*, 1992; Emery, 1997). The CM nuclei, in contrast, are more closely linked with palaeocortical, hypothalamic, and brainstem structures (Turner *et al.*, 1978; Price, 1990; Amaral *et al.*, 1992; Pitkänen, Chapter 2). One potential problem with the cortical correlations concerns the anatomical groupings used in the measurements by Stephan *et al.* (1987)

on which these analyses are based. The CBL is heterogenous, most notably because the connections of the cortical nucleus differ qualitatively from those of the basolateral group, and include olfactory inputs. Nevertheless, the cortical nucleus is small and it is possible that evolutionary changes in the larger basal and lateral nuclei are mainly responsible for overall differences in the size of this group. Another possible problem is that the large number of variables (16), all with fairly high bivariate correlations, and the relatively small number of cases (n = 40) make the analysis insensitive to real but comparatively weak relationships. A more selective analysis might reveal correlated evolution among neocortex and relevant amygdala components. Multiple regressions treating each amygdala component as a separate dependent variable and with just palaeocortex, neocortex, and body weight as independent variables support this prediction (Table 14.2). The CM correlates with body weight and palaeocortex, but not additionally with neocortex. The link between body weight and CM size might reflect the preponderance of connections with hypothalamic and brainstem sites, connections associated with autonomic and vegetative functions. Conversely, the CBL correlates with both neocortex and palaeocortex, and not with body weight. Of the two subcomponents of the CBL, LAB correlates more strongly with the neocortex than does MB.

Table 14.2 Mutiple regression analyses of the evolutionary relationships between size of amygdala components and body weight, neocortex size, and palaeocortex size in primates

	Standardized coefficient	*t-value*	*P-value*
(i) CM			
Adjusted r^2 = 0.88			
Body weight	0.394	2.47	0.018*
Neocortex	0.111	0.63	0.532
Palaeocortex	0.458	2.86	0.007**
(ii) CBL—total			
Adjusted r^2 = 0.94			
Body weight	0.116	0.94	0.354
Neocortex	0.487	3.55	0.001**
Palaeocortex	0.399	3.30	0.002**
(iii) MB			
Adjusted r^2 = 0.84			
Body weight	–0.001	–0.01	0.990
Neocortex	0.454	2.19	0.035*
Palaeocortex	0.428	2.35	0.024*
(iv) LAB			
Adjusted r^2 = 0.93			
Body weight	0.134	1.12	0.271
Neocortex	0.477	3.45	0.001**
Palaeocortex	0.428	2.35	0.024*

Each regression was based on 40 independent contrast values for each variable, computed from 43 species values. Regressions were set through the origin (Purvis and Rambaut 1995). Two-tailed tests: *P <0.05; **P <0.01.

Hence, whilst the two groups have a fairly close evolutionary relationship within primates, they also show a difference in the degree of co-evolution with the neocortex, reflecting the differences in the connections of their major component nuclei.

Connectional data are not available for insectivores, and the much smaller sample size (n = 22 independent contrasts) precludes a partial correlation analysis of the type summarized in Figure 14.6, since the number of variables would be too large relative to the number of cases for this to be meaningful. Multiple regressions similar to those reported in Table 14.2 show that both nuclear groups correlate with palaeocortex and with neocortex, and this is also true of the LAB component of the CBL (Table 14.3). The results are non-significant for the MB, unless body size is excluded from the analysis, in which case both palaeocortex and neocortex become significant.

Correlated evolution of vision and amygdala

The expansion of temporal cortex in primate evolution (see Preuss, 1993), together with the proliferation of its connections with the amygdala (Aggleton, 1993; Young *et al.*, 1994), may be indicative of the type of stimuli that the primate amygdala is specialized for handling.

Table 14.3 Multiple regression analyses of the evolutionary relationships between size of amygdala components and body weight, neocortex size, and palaeocortex size in insectivores

	Standardized coefficient	*t-value*	*P-value*
(i) CM			
Adjusted r^2 = 0.95			
Body weight	0.136	0.702	0.491
Neocortex	0.321	2.25	0.037*
Palaeocortex	0.632	3.63	0.002**
(ii) CBL			
Adjusted r^2 = 0.94			
Body weight	–0.158	–0.76	0.456
Neocortex	0.436	2.86	0.010*
Palaeocortex	0.749	4.02	<0.001***
(iii) MB			
Adjusted r^2 = 0.84			
Body weight	0.296	0.95	0.353
Neocortex	0.321	1.40	0.178
Palaeocortex	0.295	1.05	0.305
(iv) LAB			
Adjusted r^2 = 0.92			
Body weight	–0.314	–1.22	0.236
Neocortex	0.474	2.52	0.021*
Palaeocortex	0.731	4.19	<0.001***

Each regression was based on 22 independent contrast values for each variable. Regressions were set through the origin (Purvis and Rambaut 1995). Two-tailed tests: $*P < 0.05$; $**P < 0.01$; $***P < 0.001$.

Amygdala efferents terminate in almost every region of the ventral visual stream in the temporal lobe of primates (Amaral *et al.*, 1992). The ventral stream is known to be specialized for the visual analysis of fine detail and object identification (Ungerleider and Mishkin, 1982; Livingstone and Hubel, 1988), in contrast to the spatial vision and movement detection carried out in parietal regions of the dorsal stream, with which amygdala connections are lacking. It is assumed that a major function of the amygdala–temporal connections is the emotional modulation of social stimuli, such as facial expressions (Kling and Steklis, 1976; Young *et al.*, 1995; Adolphs and Tranel, Chapter 18). We showed above that the CBL and neocortex exhibit similar taxonomic grade shifts and consistently correlated evolution. Elsewhere it has been shown that the size of the lateral geniculate nucleus (LGN) also shows similar grade shifts (Barton, 2000), and that variation amongst primates in total neocortex size is largely a function of differential expansion of the visual system (Barton, 1998). Together, these findings provide circumstantial evidence that the co-evolution of amygdala and neocortex in primates is associated with specialization for processing fine-grained visual stimuli. If this is so, the neocortical areas that have expanded most with the amygdala would be those in the ventral stream, such as V4, inferotemporal cortex, and prefrontal areas with ventral stream inputs.

Unfortunately, quantitative comparative data on the size of visual areas in dorsal and ventral streams do not exist. There is, however, another level at which the link between visual specialization and amygdala evolution can be tested. Shulz (1967) measured the volume of and number of neurons in parvocellular and magnocellular layers of the LGN in 14 species. Parietal visual areas receive predominantly magnocellular input, whilst temporal cortex receives predominantly parvocellular input (Livingstone and Hubel, 1987; Shipp, 1995). If expansion of the CBL reflects its connections with temporal cortex, then its size should be correlated with the size of parvocellular rather than magnocellular layers of the LGN. To test this, we carried out multiple regressions on phylogenetic contrast data, with the volume of magnocellular and parvocellular layers as independent variables. Given the correlations with palaeocortex size (above), we also included this as an independent variable in each analysis. The results (Table 14.4) support the hypothesized association between amygdaloid and visual specialization. First, the size of both the total CBL and each of its separate components correlates with the size of the parvocellular—but not magnocellular—LGN, after taking the correlations with palaeocortex into account. Secondly, the correlation with parvocellular LGN is non-significant for the CM, reflecting its paucity of direct temporal cortex connections. In summary, CBL elements of the primate amygdala have evolved in concert with parvocellular LGN, consistent with the hypothesized role in amygdala evolution of ventral stream visual connections.

14.4 Lifestyle correlates of amygdala evolution

Previous comparative work has revealed a number of correlates of brain evolution (for reviews, see Harvey and Krebs, 1990; Allman, 1999; Barton, 1999). As mentioned above, the neocortex appears to have been a major focus of specialization in primate brain evolution, and neocortex size has been shown to correlate with activity period (nocturnal versus diurnal

Table 14.4 Results of multiple regression of amygdala components on visual components and palaeocortex in primates

	Standardized coefficient	*t-value*	*P-value*
(i) CM			
Adjusted r^2 = 0.95			
Palaeocortex	0.753	6.80	<0.0001***
Parvocellular	0.188	1.71	0.12
Magnocellular	–0.070	-0.40	0.70
(ii) CBL			
Adjusted r^2 = 0.98			
Palaeocortex	0.826	10.20	<0.0001***
Parvocellular	0.175	2.29	0.04*
Magnocellular	–0.025	–0.21	0.84
(iii) MB			
Adjusted r^2 = 0.94			
Palaeocortex	0.832	4.82	<0.001***
Parvocellular	0.428	2.82	0.02*
Magnocellular	–0.215	–0.90	0.39
(iv) LAB			
Adjusted r^2 = 0.92			
Palaeocortex	0.844	6.38	<0.001***
Parvocellular	0.289	2.21	0.05*
Magnocellular	0.031	0.16	0.88

Each regression was based on 13 independent contrast values for each variable. Two-tailed tests: *P <0.05; **P <0.01; ***P <0.001.

habits), diet (the extent of frugivory, i.e. fruit eating), and social group size (Sawguchi and Kudo, 1990; Dunbar, 1992; Barton, 1996). It is the latter correlation with social group size that has attracted most discussion (e.g. Dunbar, 1993; Whiten and Byrne, 1997). This is partly because the correlation appears to be particularly strong and consistent across taxonomic groups (Barton and Dunbar, 1997; Dunbar, 1998), but also because it substantiates a widely and long-held view that the complexity of social life has been a critical factor in cognitive evolution (e.g. Humphrey, 1976; Byrne and Whiten, 1988). Although opinions differ (see Dunbar, 1998), Barton (1996, 1998; Barton and Dunbar, 1997) has argued that the neocortical mechanisms involved include temporal lobe systems for monitoring and reacting to sociovisual stimuli, such as facial expressions, particularly in the context of complex multi-individual interactions. Clearly this is relevant to the interpretation of amygdala evolution (e.g. Brothers, 1990; Aggleton, 1993; LeDoux, 1998).

Joffe and Dunbar (1997) analysed comparative data on amygdala size in primates, finding no correlation with social group size. Re-analysis is warranted because these authors used data on only eight species. To test for evolutionary relationships between amygdala size and social group size, we once again carried out multiple regressions for each amygdala component, including group size, along with relevant allometric factors as independent variables. We assume that any such relationships reflect the joint expansion of neocortex and amygdala as discussed above. Since each amygdala component correlates with palaeocortex as well as neocortex, and since this correlation probably reflects the operation of rather different selection pressures, which we discuss below, palaeocortex size may be a confounding factor in seeking evolutionary relationships with group size. We therefore took account of the effects of palaeocortex size by entering it as an independent variable in the multiple regressions.

Table 14.5 indicates that, like neocortical and parvocellular LGN size, CBL size correlates with social group size once other factors are taken into account. The same is true for the MB and LAB components of the CBL, but, as expected, not for the CM. There is, however, a difficulty here in separating the effects of activity period from social group size, since diurnal species tend to live in larger groups. When activity period was entered as an

Table 14.5 Multiple regression analysis of amygdala size in relation to social group size and control variables

	Standardized coefficient	*t-value*	*P-value*
(i) CM			
Adjusted r^2 = 0.88			
Group size	–0.040	–0.38	0.70
Body weight	0.502	1.96	0.06†
Palaeocortex	0.571	2.89	0.007**
Medulla	–0.019	–0.06	0.95
(ii) CBL			
Adjusted r^2 = 0.92			
Group size	0.199	2.45	0.02*
Body weight	0.423	2.15	0.04*
Palaeocortex	0.762	5.03	<0.001***
Medulla	–0.143	–0.58	0.56
(iii) MB			
Adjusted r^2 = 0.84			
Group size	0.236	2.14	0.04*
Body weight	0.276	1.03	0.31
Palaeocortex	0.756	3.66	<0.001***
Medulla	–0.134	–0.40	0.69
(iv) LAB			
Adjusted r^2 = 0.84			
Group size	0.195	2.31	0.03*
Body weight	0.456	2.25	0.03*
Palaeocortex	0.744	4.84	<0.001***
Medulla	–0.152	–0.61	0.55

Each regression was based on 40 contrast values for each variable. The results show a significant positive relationship between social group size and the volume of the CBL with the effects of allometric variables taken into account. Two-tailed tests: $^{\dagger}P$ <0.1; *P <0.05; **P <0.01; ***P <0.001.

additional independent variable, its effect was significant in all four regressions, indicating increased amygdala size in diurnal compared with nocturnal primate lineages (CM, $t = 2.2$, $P = 0.03$; CBL, $t = 3.17$, $P = 0.003$; MB, $t = 2.43$, $P = 0.02$; LAB, $t = 2.07$, $P = 0.05$). Entry of activity period into the equations for group size and amygdala volume makes the previously significant correlations between CBL elements and social group size non-significant (CBL, $t = 1.73$, $P = 0.09$; MB, $t = 1.37$, $P = 0.18$; LAB, $t = 1.63$, $P = 0.11$). However, in the latter analysis, evolutionary transitions between discrete character states—nocturnal versus diurnal—were treated as a continuous variable. This is problematic, and probably overestimates the significance of such variables in independent contrasts analyses (Purvis, personal communication). When activity period was treated, more properly, as a dichotomous variable, using the BRUNCH option in CAIC and following appropriate allometric transformation (Purvis and Rambaut, 1995), three out of four contrasts between nocturnal and diurnal lineages showed larger amygdala components in the latter, but the overall differences were non-significant (one-sample *t*-tests on nocturnal–diurnal contrasts with expected value = 0, df = 3: CM, $t = 2.04$, $P = 0.13$; CBL, $t = 1.25$, $P = 0.3$; MB, $t = 1.9$, $P = 0.16$; LAB, $t = 1.18$, $P = 0.32$). On the other hand, when the effects of activity period were removed by restricting the multiple regression analysis to contrasts between taxa that show no difference in activity period, despite the fact that this reduces the sample size and amount of variance in group size, the effect of group size is still significant for the CBL ($t = 2.14$, $P = 0.04$) and its LAB component ($t = 2.15$, $P = 0.04$). Non-significant results are obtained for the MB($t = 1.23$, $P = 0.23$) and CM ($t = -0.29$, $P = 0.78$). In summary, there is evidence for a connection between sociality and the evolution of CBL size—specifically the LAB component—in primates. The effects of activity period and group size may not be entirely separable, since there is a strong correlation between the two, and the visual signals that are important in social groups can only be exploited fully under photic conditions.

Because neocortical evolution in primates has been linked to diet (specifically, the degree of frugivory), as well as to activity timing and group size (Barton, 1996), the possibility of a similar dietary correlation for the amygdala was investigated. A series of multiple regressions was run for each amygdaloid component, with and without other behavioural variables (group size and activity period), and testing for any effects of the procedure used for including variables by comparing stepwise and simultaneous multiple regressions. In none of these analyses did diet (expressed as the average percentage of feeding time devoted to fruit) come close to significance, despite evidence that the amygdala has a role in feeding (see below).

14.5 Synopsis

14.5.1 Palaeocortex, neocortex, and the amygdala

The results suggest that the connections of the amygdala with both palaeocortical and neocortical areas have been subject to natural selection during primate evolution. The selection pressures are likely to have been different in each case. Amygdalopalaeocortical expansion is likely to reflect increased importance of olfactory stimuli, whilst amygdaloneocortical expansion is likely to reflect increased emphasis on visual stimuli. Both types of expansion may be related to social information, but in different modalities. Olfactory communication is important in most mammalian taxa, including primates (Epple and Moulton, 1978; Eisenberg, 1981). There is, however, clearly variation in the relative importance of olfactory and visual stimuli. Amongst lemurs, for example, even diurnal species have poor visual acuity and immobile faces, limiting the utility of facial expression as a channel for communicating socioemotional signals. On the other hand, they have an elaborate system of olfactory signals which are used in the contexts of social dominance, sexual competition, and mating (Epple and Moulton, 1978; Kappeler, 1998). Although the importance of olfactory signals relative to visual signals tends to be greater in nocturnal species, the association with activity period is loose. New World monkeys, though diurnal (with one exception—the owl monkey), are like the nocturnal lemurs and lorises in possessing a well-developed vomeronasal organ with associated accessory olfactory bulb, and in engaging extensively in scent-marking as part of their communicative repertoire (Epple and Moutlon, 1978; Bhatnager and Meisami, 1998). These features are absent from Old World monkeys and apes. The role of the vomeronasal organ in communication in dominance interactions (Epple and Moulton, 1978) together with its projections to the medial nucleus of the amygdala (Bhatnager and Meisami, 1998) suggests that the correlated evolutionary expansions of amygdala and palaeocortex are olfactory analogues of the correlated expansions of amygdala and temporal neocortex. The first case would have involved enhancements of the sensitivity to, and powers of discrimination between, olfactory cues to social attributes such as individual identity, dominance, and aggressive motivation. The second case would have involved exactly the same kind of enhancements, but in the visual rather than the olfactory modality. The function and evolution of these systems in sexual as well as agonistic behaviour should also be considered. The accessory olfactory system is known to function in mate attraction (Epple and Moulton, 1978). Interestingly, the phylogenetic distribution of prominent visual sexual signals (marked perineal swelling and colour change) is a mirror-image of the distribution of the vomeronasal/accessory olfactory system. The first has evolved at least three times among catarrhine primates (Old World monkeys and apes), but is absent in New World monkeys and strepsirhines, which instead have the vomeronasal/accessory olfactory system. Therefore, there seems to be an evolutionary trade-off between visual and olfactory sexual signals, and the role of the primate amygdala in processing such signals perhaps deserves greater attention.

The present analyses have not considered the relevance of auditory signals in amygdala evolution. The reason for this omission is simply that comparative volumetric data on auditory inputs are lacking. Auditory signals are relayed to the basolateral nuclei, and could be part of the cause of enlargement in diurnal group-living monkeys and apes. For example, there may have been increased demands on the ability to recognize individuals by voice, and to link vocal signals with appropriate emotional responses. Many social signals in diurnal primates combine visual and auditory components. In humans, amygdala damage can cause a failure to identify not only visual (facial) but also auditory stimuli associated with fear (Scott *et al.*, 1997), a finding that is consistent with a functional magnetic resonance imaging (fMRI) study showing amygdala activation during vocal expressions of fear (Phillips *et al.*, 1998).

The amygdala also receives both olfactory and gustatory information. These senses are linked intimately with dietary function, yet the present analyses failed to find any correlations between amygdala volume and dietary specialization. While there is clear evidence that the amygdala has a role in food selection in monkeys, that role may be more specialized than previously suspected. Thus early studies of the Klüver–Bucy syndrome suggested that amygdala removal led to animals showing indiscriminate eating of food/non-food items, yet later research using more selective lesion techniques showed that while amygdalectomised monkeys are more willing to explore non-food items orally, they still show clear preferences between different foods (Aggleton and Passingham, 1981; Murray *et al.*, 1996). Dietary intake is not normal, however, as amygdala damage results in an increased willingness to eat novel foods, including meat (Baxter and Murray, Chapter 16). A much more subtle role is suggested by evidence that the amygdala enables monkeys to link a specific visual item with a specific food reinforcer. Thus it has been found that cytotoxic lesions of the amygdala disrupt discriminations in which the two objects to be discriminated have been associated with different food reinforcers, and the hedonic value of *one* of those reinforcers has been reduced by satiation (Malkova *et al.*, 1997; Baxter and Murray, Chapter 16). While normal monkeys prefer the object associated with the unsatiated food, amygdalectomy impairs this discrimination. Thus the amygdala may have an important, but specialized role in supporting the optimal selection of varied diets. However, this role may be of equal value to frugivores and folivores, explaining the lack of correlations with the degree of frugivory. Both folivores and frugivores learn to avoid unpalatable food types (Whitehead, 1985; Barton and Whiten, 1994). Even insectivores encounter potential prey items that are poisonous or unpalatable. It may be that the number and subtlety of the discriminations required for optimal foraging vary from species to species, but it is not yet clear what measure of diet would be the most appropriate for assaying this variation. Until we know that, the relationship between amygdala evolution and dietary specialization cannot be explored further.

14.5.2 Social evolution and the amygdala

A persistent theme in the preceding analyses has been the issue of whether the amygdala has an important role in visual aspects of social communication. The evidence of an association between the size of the CBL complex, visual structures in the 'ventral stream', and of social group size is supportive not only of the view that at least some amygdaloid regions are involved in the visual processing of social stimuli, but also that this may represent one of this structure's key functions. These findings can be integrated with other evidence from the analysis of amygdala damage in monkeys and humans, and from measures of amygdala activity (Aggleton and Young, 2000).

It has long been known that amygdala lesions can have catastrophic effects on social behaviour in monkeys, typically resulting in a loss of social status and a withdrawal from social interactions (Kling, 1972; Kling and Steklis, 1976). While the extent of this social disruption needs to be re-assessed in the light of evidence that conventional lesions of the amygdala disrupt fibres of passage that contribute to at least some 'amygdala' lesion effects (Aggleton and Young, 2000; Baxter and Murray, Chapter 16), recent lesion evidence still supports a role in affective processing. Thus, neurotoxic lesions of the rhesus monkey amygdala that spare fibres of passage alter emotional reactivity to visual stimuli, including reactions to socially relevant stimuli such as a monkey's head (Meunier *et al.*, 1999). Other evidence comes from recording studies which have revealed that there are neurons in the amygdala that respond selectively to faces (Leonard *et al.*, 1985; Brothers *et al.*, 1990; Rolls, Chapter 13). Some of these neurons respond to specific faces regardless of expression, while others respond best to particular facial expressions regardless of identity (Leonard *et al.*, 1985; Makamura *et al.*, 1992). These face-responsive cells were most prevalent in the accessory basal and lateral nuclei (Leonard *et al.*, 1985). This distribution is noteworthy as the basolateral nuclei (and most especially the accessory basal and lateral nuclei) receive dense inputs both from the inferior temporal cortex where facial identity may be processed (Hasselmo *et al.*, 1989), and from the superior temporal sulcus where units often respond to facial expressions (Hasselmo *et al.*, 1989). Cells that can respond selectively to more dynamic social stimuli, such as approach behaviour, have also been found in the medial amygdala (Brothers *et al.*, 1990), a region that includes the accessory basal nucleus. Similar units have been found in the adjacent perirhinal and entorhinal cortices (Brothers and Ring, 1993), cortical regions that are densely interconnected with the basolateral nuclei (Stefanacci *et al.*, 1996).

This electrophysiological evidence suggests that the basolateral nuclei of the amygdala, along with other closely related cortical regions in the medial temporal lobe, are particularly well placed to determine the nature of a visual (and auditory) social signal and the identity of the animal making the signal. This interpretation is fully consistent with the analyses made of the volume of the CBL group of nuclei, and can be contrasted with the results for the CM group of nuclei. Data from tests conducted on people with bilateral amygdala damage seem to indicate that while the amygdala is important for identifying facial expression, it is not crucial for facial identity (Adolphs *et al.*, 1994; Young *et al.*, 1995; 1996; Adolphs and Tranel, Chapter 18). Furthermore, the human amygdala appears to be of particular importance for the identification of fearful or angry faces (Adolphs and Tranel, Chapter 18), a conclusion that has been supported by fMRI studies (Morris *et al.*, 1996; Dolan, Chapter 19). Although recent studies have found a wider range of emotion recognition deficits in some patients with amygdala damage (Adolphs, 1999), consistent with electrophysiological and lesion data on monkeys, selective impairment of the recognition of fear and anger, both visually and auditorily, remains a consistent and striking pattern (Calder *et al.*, 1996; Scott *et al.*, 1997; Phillips *et al.*, 1998). A possible explanation for the associated deficits in fear and anger recognition is impairment of an evolved system for monitoring the reactions of conspecifics to danger. An alternative possibility is that a system mediating dominance interactions has been affected. In this view, fear and anger are conceived more accurately as submission and threat signals, respectively. Dominance interactions are, of course, a pervasive part of everyday life in the social groups of primates and other mammals, and success in managing these interactions is pivotal to reproductive success (Dunbar, 1988). Since submission and dominance form a continuum, and are evaluated by conspecifics within the context of a single type of interaction (agonistic), this idea can explain the associations reported in the neuropsychological literature. In contrast, it is not so clear why anger should be a common response to an external danger such as a predator. Nor is it clear that monitoring facial expressions of other group members would be an efficient way of noticing danger; non-human primates seem to rely primarily on specialized warning vocalizations which are quite different from expressions of anger or fear in a social context (Seyfarth *et al.*, 1980).

A view of the anthropoid brain as specialized for handling certain types of social information is emerging from the synthesis of connectional, neurophysiological, and comparative data (see also Brothers, 1990; Barton and Dunbar, 1997). First, a number of neocortical and amygdaloid areas show selective responsiveness to specific social stimuli, including visual stimuli that are probably more complex and dynamic than those processed in the brains of other mammals (Perrett *et al.*, 1989; Brothers *et al.*, 1990). The ability of the anthropoid brain to process such information depends in part on a high degree of visual acuity and the dedication of large areas of the neocortex to visual processing. Nocturnal species may show parallel specializations for processing social information in the olfactory domain. Secondly, the neocortex and amygdala are unusually profusely connected in monkeys compared with at least some other mammals (Young *et al.*, 1994), and the areas associated with the processing of sociovisual stimuli (temporal cortex and basolateral amygdala) show especially strong connectivity (Emery, 1997). Thirdly, as we have shown here, the neocortex and corticobasolateral complex of the amygdala have expanded conjointly during primate evolution, and this expansion is particularly marked in the haplorhines, which include the gregarious monkeys and apes. Finally, the size of the neocortex and corticobasolateral amygdala correlate with social group size. These adaptations allow group-living individuals to monitor and respond appropriately to the dynamically shifting dispositions, intentions, and actions of conspecifics (see Brothers, 1990), on which there is a particular premium during the rapid multi-individual interactions characteristic of the social groups of anthropoids, including humans (Barton and Dunbar, 1997). Reproductive success in such groups depends critically on social success (Humphrey, 1976; Strum, 1987; Whiten and Byrne, 1997), so the selection pressure for brains adept at handling social information is likely to have been intense.

Acknowledgements

We are grateful to Leslie Brothers and Andy Young for their very helpful comments on an earlier draft.

References

Adolphs, R. (1999) The human amygdala and emotion. *Neuroscientist*, 5, 125–137.

Adolphs, R., Tranel, D., Damasio, H., and Damasio, A. (1994) Impaired recognition of emotion in facial expressions following bilateral damage to the human amygdala. *Nature*, 372, 669–672.

Aggleton, J.P. (1985) A description of intra-amygdaloid connections in old world monkeys, *Experimental Brain Research*, 57, 390–399.

Aggleton, J.P. (1993) The contribution of the amygdala to normal and abnormal emotional states. *Trends in Neuroscience*, 16, 328–333.

Aggleton, J.P., Burton, M.J., and Passingham, R.E. (1980) Cortical and subcortical afferents to the amygdala of the rhesus monkey. *Brain Research*, 190, 347–368.

Aggleton, J.P. and Passingham, R.E. (1981) Syndrome produced by lesions of the amygdala in monkeys (*Macaca mulatta*). *Journal of Comparative and Physiological Psychology*, 95, 961–977.

Aggleton, J.P. and Young, A.W. (2000) The enigma of the amygdala: concerning its contribution to human emotion. In *Cognitive Neuroscience of Emotion* (eds R.D. Lane and L. Nadel), pp. 106–128, Oxford University Press, Oxford.

Allman, J.M. (1982) Reconstructing the evolution of the brain in primates through the use of comparative neurophysiological and neuroanatomical data. In *Primate Brain Evolution* (eds E. Armstrong and D. Falk), pp. 13–28. Plenum Press, New York.

Allman, J.M. (1987) Evolution of the brain in primates. In *The Oxford Companion to the Mind* (ed. R.L. Gregory), pp. 633–639. Oxford University Press, Oxford.

Allman, J.M. (1999) *Evolving Brains*. Scientific American Library, New York.

Amaral, D.G. and Price, J.L. (1984) Amygdala-cortical projections in the monkey (Macaca fascicularis) *Journal of Comparative Neurology*, **230**, 465–496.

Amaral, D.G., Price, J.L., Pitkänen, A., and Carmichael, S.T. (1992) Anatomical organization of the primate amygdaloid complex. In *The Amygdala: Neurobiological Aspects of Emotion, Memory, and Mental Dysfunction* (ed. J.P. Aggleton), pp. 1–66. Wiley-Liss, New York,

Barton, R.A. (1996) Neocortex size and behavioural ecology in primates. *Proceedings of the Royal Society of London, Series B*, 263, 173–177

Barton, R.A. (1998) Visual specialisation and brain evolution in primates. *Proceedings of the Royal Society of London, Series B*, 265, 1933–1937.

Barton, R.A. (1999) The evolutionary ecology of the primate brain. In *Comparative Primate Socioecology* (ed. P.C. Lee), pp. 167–203. Cambridge University Press, Cambridge.

Barton, R.A. (2000) Explaining large brains in primates: cognitive demands of foraging or of social life? In *On the Move: How and Why Animals Travel in Groups* (eds S. Boinski and P. Garber), pp. 204–237, Chicago University Press.

Barton, R.A. and Dunbar, R.I.M. (1997) Evolution of the social brain. In *Machiavellian Intelligence II* (eds A.Whiten, and R.W. Byrne), pp. 240–263. Cambridge University Press, Cambridge.

Barton, R.A., Purvis, A., and Harvey, P.H. (1995) Evolutionary radiation of visual and olfactory brain systems in primates, bats and insectivores. *Philosophical Transactions of the Royal Society of London, Series B*, 348, 381–392.

Barton, R.A. and Whiten, A. (1994) Reducing complex diets to simple rules: food selection in olive baboons. *Behavioural Ecology and Sociobiology*, 35, 283–293.

Baron, G., Stephan, H., and Frahm, H.D. (1996) *Comparative Neurobiology in Chiroptera. Vol. I: Macromorphology, Brain Structures, Tables and Atlases*. Birkhauser Verlag, Basel.

Bhatnagar, K.P. and Meisami, E. (1998) Vomeronasal organ in bats and primates: extremes of structural variability and its phylogenetic implications. *Microscopy Research and Technique*, 43, 465–475.

Brothers, L. (1990) The social brain: a project for integrating primate behavior and neurophysiology in a new domain. *Concepts in Neuroscience*, 1, 27–51.

Brothers, L. and Ring, B. (1993) Mesial temporal neurons in the macaque monkey with responses selective for aspects of social stimuli. *Behavioural Brian Research*, 57, 53–61.

Brothers, L., Ring, B., and Kling, A. (1990) Response of neurons in the macaque amygdala to complex social stimuli. *Behavioural Brain Research*, 41, 199–213.

Butler, A.B. and Hodos, W. (1996) *Comparative Vertebrate Neuroanatomy*. Wiley-Liss, New York.

Byrne, R.W. and Whiten, A. (1988) *Machiavellian intelligence*. Clarendon Press, Oxford.

Calder, A.J., Young, A.W., Rowland, D., Perrett, I., Hodges, J.R., and Etcoff, N.L. (1996) Facial emotion recognition after bilateral amygdala damage: differentially severe impairment of fear. *Cognitive Neuropsychology*, 13, 699–745.

Carmichael , S.T., Clugnet, M.-C., and Price, J.L. (1994) Central olfactory connections in the macaque monkey. *Journal of Comparative Neurology*, 346, 403–434.

Cheney, D.L. and Seyfarth, R.M. (1990) *How Monkeys See The World*. University of Chicago Press, Chicago.

Cousens, G. and Otto, T. (1998) Both pre- and post-training excitotoxic lesions of the basolateral amygdala abolish the expression of olfactory and contextual fear conditioning. *Behavioral Neuroscience*, 112, 1092–1103.

Crick, F. (1990) *The Astonishing Hypothesis: The Scientific Search for the Soul*. Simon and Schuster: London.

Damasio, A.R. (1995) *Descartes Error: Emotion, Reason and the Human Brain*. Picador: London.

de Olmos, J. (1990) Amygdaloid nuclear gray complex. In *The Human Nervous System* (ed. G. Paxinos), pp. 583–710. Academic Press, San Diego.

deVoogd, T.J., Krebs, J.R., Healy, S.D., and Purvis, A. (1993) Relations between song repertoire size and the volume of brain nuclei related to song: comparative evolutionary analyses amongst oscine birds. *Proceedings of the Royal Societyof London, Series B*, 254, 75–82.

deWaal, F.B.M. (1982) *Chimpanzee Politics*. Harper and Row, New York.

Dunbar, R.I.M. (1988) *Primate Social Systems*. Croom Helm, London.

Dunbar, R.I.M. (1992) Neocortex size as a constraint on group size in primates. *Journal of Human Evolution*, 20, 469–493.

Dunbar, R.I.M. (1993) Coevolution of neocortical size, group size and language in humans. *Behavioral and Brain Sciences*, 16, 681–735

Dunbar, R.I.M. (1998) The social brain hypthesis. *Evolutionary Anthropology*, 6, 178–190.

Eisenberg, J.F. (1981) *The Mammalian Radiations*. University of Chicago Press, Chicago.

Emery, N. (1997) Neuroethological studies of primate social perception. Unpublished PhD thesis. University of St Andrews.

Epple, G. and Moulton, D. (1978) Structural organization and communicatory functions of olfaction in nonhuman primates. In *Sensory Systems of Primates* (ed. C.R. Noback), pp. 1–22 Plenum Press, New York.

Felsenstein, J. (1985) Phylogenies and the comparative method. *American Naturalist*, 125, 1–15.

Finlay, B.L. and Darlington, R.B. (1995) Linked regularities in the development and evolution of mammalian brains. *Science*, 268, 1578–1584

Foldiak, P. and Young, M.P. (1995) Sparse coding in the primate cortex. In *The Handbook of Brain Theory and Neural Networks* (ed. M. Arbib), pp. 895–898. MIT Press, Cambridge, Massachusetts.

Hamann, S.B., Stefanacci, L., Squire, L.R., Adolphs, R., Tranel, D., Damasio, H., and Damasio, A. (1996) Recognizing facial emotion. *Nature*, 379, 497.

Hampton, R.R. and Shettleworth, S.J. (1996) Hippocampus and memory in a food-storing and in a nonstoring bird species. *Behavioral Neuroscience*, **110**, 946–964.

Harcourt. A.H. and DeWaal, F.B.M. (1992) *Coalitions and Alliances in Humans and Other Animals*. Oxford University Press, Oxford.

Harvey, P.H. and Krebs, J.R. (1990) Comparing brains. *Science*, 249, 140–146.

Harvey, P.H. and Pagel, M.D. (1991) *The Comparative Method in Evolutionary Biology*. Oxford University Press, Oxford..

Hasselmo, M.E., Rolls, E.T., and Baylis, G.C. (1989) The role of expression and identity in the face-selective responses of neurons in the temporal visual cortex of the monkey. *Behavioural Brain Research*, 32, 203–218.

Humphrey, T. (1936) The telencephalon of the bat I. The non-cortical nuclear masses and certain pertinent fiber connections. *Journal of Comparative Neurology*, 65, 603–711.

Humphrey, N.K. (1976) The social function of intellect. In *Growing Points in Ethology* (eds P.P.G. Bateson and R.A. Hinde), pp. 303–317. Cambridge University Press, Cambridge.

Jerison, H.J. (1973) *Evolution of the Brain and Intelligence*. Academic Press, New York.

Jerison, H.J. (1991) *Brain Size and The Evolution of Mind*. American Museum of Natural History, New York.

Joffe, T.H. and Dunbar, R.I.M. (1997) Visual and socio-cognitive information processing in primate brain evolution. *Proceedings of the Royal Society of London, Series B*, 264, 1303–1307.

Joffe, T.H. and Dunbar, R.I.M. (1998) Tarsier brain component composition and its implications for systematics. *Primates*, 39, 211–216.

Kaas, J.H. (1995) The evolution of isocortex. *Brain, Behavior and Evolution*, 46, 187–196.

Kaas, J.H. and Preuss, T.M. (1993) Archontan affinities as reflected in the visual system. In *Mammal Phylogeny* (eds F. Szalay, M. Novacek, and M. McKenna), pp. 115–128. Springer-Verlag, New York.

Kappeler, P.M. (1998) To whom it may concern: the transmission and function of chemical signals in *Lemur catta*. *Behavioral Ecology and Sociobiology*, 42, 411–421.

Kling, A. (1972) Effects of amygdalectomy on social-affective behaviour in non-human primates. In *The Neurobiology of the Amygdala* (ed. B.E. Eleftheriou), pp. 511–536. Plenum Press, New York.

Kling, A. and Steklis, H.D. (1976) A neural substrate for affiliative behavior in nonhuman primates. *Brain Behavior and Evolution*, 13, 216–238.

Krubitzer, L. (1998) What can monotremes tell us about brain evolution? *Philosophical Transactions of the Royal Society of London, Series B*, 353, 1127–1146.

Leonard, C.M., Rolls, E.T., Wilson, F.A.W., and Baylis, G.C. Neurons in the amygdala of the monkey with responses selective for faces. *Behavioural Brain Research*, 15, 159–176.

LeDoux, J.E. (1998) *The Emotional Brain*. Weidenfeld and Nicholson. London.

Lehman, M.N., Winans, S.S., and Powers, J.B. (1980) Medial nucleus of the amygdala mediates chemosensory control of male hamster sexual behavior. *Science*, 210, 557–560.

Livingstone, M.S. and Hubel, D.H. (1987) Psychophysical evidence for separate channels for the perception of form, colour, movement, and depth. *Journal of Neuroscience*, 7, 3416–3468.

Livingstone, M.S. and Hubel, D.H. (1988) Segregation of form, color, movement and depth: anatomy, physiology and perception. *Science*, 240, 740–749.

Loscher, W. and Ebert, U. (1996) The role of the piriform cortex in kindling. *Progress in Neurobiology*, 50, 427.

MacLean, P.D. (1970) The triune brain, emotion, and scientific bias. In *The Neurosciences, Second Study Program* (ed. F.O. Schmitt), pp. 336–349. Rockefeller University Press, New York.

Martin, R.D. (1990) *Primate Origins and Evolution: A Phylogenetic Reconstruction.* Chapman and Hall, London.

Martin, R.D. (1996) Scaling of the mammalian brain: the maternal energy hypothesis. *News in Physiological Sciences*, 11, 149–156.

Malkova, L., Gaffan, D., and Murray, E.A. (1997) Excitotoxic lesions of the amygdala fail to produce impairment in visual learning for auditory secondary reinforcement but interfere with reinforcer devaluation effects in rhesus monkeys. *Journal of Neuroscience*, 17, 6011–6020.

McDonald, A.J. (1992) Cell types and instrinsic connections of the amygdala. In *The Amygdala: Neurobiological Aspects of Emotion, Memory, and Mental Dysfunction* (ed. J.P. Aggleton), pp. 67–96. Wiley-Liss, New York.

Meunier, M., Bachevalier, J., Murray, E.A., Malkova, L., and Mishkin, M. (1999) Effects of aspiration versus neurotoxic lesions of the amygdala on emotional response in monkeys. *European Journal of Neuroscience*, in press.

Morris, J.S., Frith, C.D., Perrett, D.I., Rowland, D., Young, A.W., Calder, A.J., and Dolan, R.J. (1996) A differential neural response in the human amygdala to fearful and happy facial expressions. *Nature*, 383, 812–815.

Murray, E.A., Gaffan, E.A., and Flint, R.W. (1996) Anterior rhinal cortex and amygdala: dissociation of their contributions to memory and food preference in rhesus monkeys. *Behavioural Neuroscience*, 110, 30–42.

Pagel, M.D. (1992) A method for the analysis of comparative data. *Journal of Theoretical Biology*, 156, 434–442.

Passingham, R.E.P. (1982) *The Human Primate*. W.H. Freeman and Co., Oxford.

Perrett, D.I., Harries, M.H., Bevan, R., Thomas, S., Benson, P.J., Mistlin, A.J., Chitty, A.J., Hietanen, J., and Ortega, J.E. (1989) Frameworks of analysis for the neural representation of animate objects and actions. *Journal of Experimental Biology*, 146, 87–113.

Pinker, S. (1998) *How the Mind Works*. Penguin: London.

Phillips, M.L., Young, A.W., Scott, S.K., Calder, A.J., Andrew, C., Giampietro, V. *et al.* (1998) Neural reponses to facial and vocal expressions of fear and disgust. *Proceedings of the Royal Society of London, Series B*, 265, 1809–1817.

Price, J.L. (1990) Olfactory system. In *The Human Nervous System* (ed. G. Paxinos), pp. 979–998. Academic Press, San Diego.

Preuss, T.M. (1993) The role of the neurosciences in primate evolutionary biology. In *Primates and Their Relatives in Phylogenetic Perspective* (ed. R.S.D.E. Macphee), pp. 333–362. Plenum Press, New York.

Purvis, A. (1995) A composite estimate of primate phylogeny. *Philosophical Transactions of the Royal Society of London, Series B*, 348, 405–421.

Purvis, A. and Rambaut, A. (1995) Comparative analysis by independent contrasts (CAIC): an Apple Macintosh application for analysing comparative data. *Computer Applications in the Biosciences*, 11, 247–251.

Sawaguchi, T. and Kudo, H. (1990) Neocortical development and social structure in primates. *Primates*, 31, 283–290.

Scott, S., Young, A.W., Calder, A.J., Hellawell, D.J., Aggleton, J.P., and Johnson, M. (1997) Auditory recognition of emotion after amygdalotomy: impairment of fear and anger. *Nature*, 385, 254–257.

Seyfarth, R.M., Cheney, D.L., and Marler, P. (1980) Monkey responses to three different alarm calls: evidence for predator classification and semantic communication. *Science*, 210, 801–803.

Sherry, D.F., Vaccarino, A.L., Buckenham, K., and Herz, R.S. (1989) The hippocampal complex of food-storing birds. *Brain Behavior and Evolution*, 34, 308–317.

Shipp, S. (1995) The odd couple. *Current Biology*, 5, 116–119.

Shulz, H.-D. (1967) Metrische untersuchungen an den schichten des corpus geniculatum laterale tag- und nachtaktiver primaten. Doctoral dissertation, Johann Wolfgang Goethe-Universität Frankfurt.

Stefanacci, L., Suzuki, W.A., and Amaral, D.G. (1996) Organization of connections between the amygdaloid complex and perirhinal and parahippocampal cortices in macaque monkeys. *Journal of Comparative Neurology*, 375, 552–582.

Stephan, H., Frahm, H.D., and Baron, G. (1981) New and revised data on volumes of brain structures in insectivores and primates. *Folia Primatologica*, 35, 1–29.

Stephan, H., Frahm, H.D., and Baron, G. (1987) Comparison of brain structure volumes in insectivora and primates VII. Amygdaloid components. *Journal für Hirnforschung*, 28, 571–584.

Stephan, H., Baron, G., and Frahm, H.D. (1991) *Comparative Brain Research in Mammals. Vol. 1. Insectivores*. Springer, New York.

Strum, S. (1987) *Almost Human*. Random House, New York.

Swanson, L.W. and Petrovich, G.D. (1998) What is the amygdala? *Trends in Neuroscience*, 21, 323–331.

Turner, B.H., Gupta, K.C., and Mishkin, M. (1978) The locus and cytoarchitecture of the projection areas of the olfactory bulb in *Macaca mulatta*. *Journal of Comparative Neurology*, 177, 381–396.

Turner, B.H., Mishkin, M., and Knapp, M. (1980) Organization of the amygdalopetal projections from modality-specific cortical association areas in the monkey. *Journal of Comparative Neurology*, 191, 515–543.

Ungerleider, L.G. and Mishkin, M. (1982) Two cortical visual systems. In *Analysis of visual behaviour*, (eds D.J. Ingle, M.A. Goodale, and R.J.W. Mansfield), pp. 549–586. MIT Press, Cambridge, Mass.

Weiskrantz, L. (1956) Behavioral changes associated with ablations of the amygdaloid complex in monkeys. *Journal of Comparative Physiological Psychology*, 49, 381–391.

Whitehead, J.M. (1985) Development of feeding selectivity in mantled howling monkeys (*Alouatta palliata*). In *Primate Ontogeny, Cognition and Social Behaviour* (eds J. Else and P.C. Lee), pp. 105–117. Cambridge University Press, Cambridge.

Whiten, A. and Byrne, R.W. (1997) *Machiavellian Intelligence II: Extensions and Evaluations*. Cambridge University Press, Cambridge.

Young, A.W., Aggleton, J.P., Hellawell, D.J., Johnson, M., Broks, P., and Hanley, J.R. Face processing impairments after amygdalotomy. (1995) *Brain*, 118, 15–24.

Young, A.W., Hellawell, D. J., Van de Wal, C., and Johnson, M. (1996) Facial expression processing after amygdalotomy. *Neuropsychologia*, 34, 31–39.

Young, M.P., Scannell, J.W., Burns, G.A.P.C., and Blakemore, C. (1994) Analysis of connectivity: neural systems in the cerebral cortex. *Reviews in the Neurosciences*, 5, 227–249.

Zald, D.H., and Pardo, J.V. (1997) Emotion, olfaction, and the human amygdala: Amygdala activation during aversive olfactory stimulation. *Proceedings of National Academy of Sciences*, USA, **94**, 4119–4124.

15 The amygdala, social cognition, and autism

Jocelyne Bachevalier

University of Texas Health Science Center, Houston, TX 77030, USA

Summary

The regulation of social cognition is orchestrated by a multitude of interconnected structures of which the amygdala is one important constituent. This chapter reviews a significant amount of research in monkeys and humans, using different approaches, demonstrating that the amygdala decodes and integrates perceptual features from other individuals and allows the subject to act and adjust its behavioual responses according to the emotional and social context of a particular event. The role of the amygdala in social cognition in adult subjects implies that this brain structure must also be crucial for the emergence of affective states and the formation and maintenance of social bonds during the developmental period in primates. The data in this area are meagre but indicate that the amygdala has an early ontogenetic maturation, but its connections with other brain regions continue to be refined after birth, supporting the progressive development of affective responses in primates. Finally, the severe and persistent changes in emotional responses and social behaviour found after early damage to the amygdala together with recent evidence for the involvement of the amygdala and related structures in autism stress the urgent need to initiate many more developmental studies in primates to begin appreciating the role of the amygdala and other related brain regions early in life for the achievement of well-adapted social skills in adulthood. Such data may, in turn, provide progress in understanding the causes of developmental psychopathological disorders, such as autism.

15.1 Introduction

'I do not read subtle emotional cues. I have had to learn by trial and error what certain gestures and facial expressions mean . . . Since I don't have any social intuition, I rely on pure logic, like an expert computer program, to guide my behavior. I categorize rules according to their logical importance . . . It is a complex algorithmic decision-making tree . . . At age forty-seven, I have a vast databank, but

it has taken me years to build up my library of experiences and learn how to behave in an appropriate manner. I did not know until recently that most people rely heavily on emotional cues.'
(Grandin T., 1996).

This subjective experience of autism vividly describes the enormous handicap that a person with autism has to overcome when facing complex social environments. Autism, as well as schizophrenia and antisocial personality syndromes, is a mental illness associated with the disruption of a basic characteristic of the human species, i.e. its sophisticated and complex ability to generate displays of emotion and to respond to expressive behaviours of other individuals. The debilitating effects of such impaired or maladapted social skills recently have fostered a rising interest in the study of the neurobiology of social cognition in humans.

Reports of clinical cases with circumscribed lesions, as well as the results of neurostimulation, neurorecording, and neuroimaging of normal and diseased brain, have all provided evidence that there exists specific neural circuitry involved in the processing of social skills. Additional animal studies examining the neurobiology of social cognition continue to refine our knowledge of the brain systems that underlie such abilities and help us to understand how the functions of human social processes are realized. In this venture, non-human primates provide an excellent animal model to reach this goal.

Investigations of the social skills of non-human primates in the wild or in the laboratory have revealed that monkeys, like humans, live in social groups that are characterized by complex and dynamic social organization maintained through a variety of specific, long-term relationships between individual group members (deWaal, 1989; Cheney and Seyfarth, 1990). It is now clear that each member of a monkey troop establishes and maintains numerous long-term relationships with many other group members, and that the nature, intensity, and stability of each relationship varies according to the specific ages, sexes, and kinship relationship of that particular pair of monkeys. To maintain these relationships, monkeys, like humans, need to perceive and use sensory cues from other individuals in the troop and adapt their responses in order to function within the social environment. Indeed, the presence of a stable social hierarchy within a group indicates that the individuals comprising the social group recognize one another and respond differentially depending upon with whom they are interacting. Beginning at birth, the infant born into such a complex social group is faced with the developmental task of coming to respond differentially and appropriately to categories of social partners, as well as to individuals within those categories. Thus, during development, they progressively learn complex rules that ensure successful social relationships. Finally, although the ability to interpret mental states of others is still controversial in non-human primates, some studies have suggested that they too possess a rudimentary cognitive capacity for assessing intentions and motivations in others (Byrne and Whiten, 1988; Brothers, 1995). One cannot deny that the ability to communicate social intentions is likely to be far more complex in humans than in non-human primates. Nevertheless, it seems that the similarities between species in many phenotypic displays and basic behavioural processes outweigh the differences, suggesting that the neural mechanisms underlying social communications are likely to share common features across these species. In this respect, non-human primates are undoubtedly excellent animal models to investigate brain processes underlying social cognition.

The present chapter provides a review of data from non-human primate research implicating the amygdala in the regulation of social cognition. In reviewing the relevant literature, the similarities and differences in the research findings obtained with non-human primates and humans will be discussed. Furthermore, given the importance of the amygdala in the regulation of affective states and sociality in adulthood, one would expect this structure to have likewise a paramount influence on the development of social cognition in young primates. It is therefore remarkable that research in this area has been astonishingly neglected. It is only recently that researchers have begun to appreciate the importance of studying the development of social cognition and its neural substrate (Trevarthen, 1989; Schore, 1994; Brothers, 1995; Baron-Cohen *et al.*, 1999). This growing interest stems from recent evidence suggesting that early dysfunction of structures within the neural network subserving social cognition may be at the origin of some psychopathologies in children, including autism (Bachevalier, 1994; Brothers, 1995; Baron-Cohen *et al.*, 1999). Therefore, this chapter will also review the few studies that have attempted to study the development of the amygdala and of its functions in primates. The last part will focus on the implication of early amygdala dysfunction in autism.

15.2 Anatomical considerations

As originally proposed by Papez (1937) and further elaborated by MacLean (1949), social cognition is realized through a complex neural network of interconnected structures, which includes areas in the ventromedial aspect of the temporal and frontal lobes, and their connections with the hypothalamus and brainstem. This neural network is centred around the amygdala and appears to be involved in the regulation of behaviours by knowledge of the emotional responses and intentions of others (Brothers, 1989, 1995; Barbas, 1995). Although the present chapter will focus on the amygdala, the reader has to bear in mind that the amygdala is only one component of a more complex neural circuit important for the regulation of emotions and sociality.

Recent advances in the neuroanatomical organization of the primate amygdala have made a fundamental contribution to understanding its role in the regulation of emotions and affiliative behaviours (for reviews, see Amaral, 1992; Gloor, 1997; Emery and Amaral, 1999). Before discussing modern concepts of amygdala functions, a brief summary of the primate amygdala anatomy will be given to illustrate that this complex structure is strategically situated in the brain to orchestrate different aspects of social cognition.

The amygdala is composed of a set of nuclei with different cytological, histological, and connectional features. Within the amygdala, the lateral nucleus receives an enormous array of convergent sensory information from unimodal as well as polysensory areas of the neocortex and sends this information to the basal nucleus, which in turn projects back upon the sensory cortical areas. This pathway provides the amygdala with a wide array of highly processed sensory information, including visual cues of faces and facial expressions, and of body postures and motions, as well as auditory cues of specific vocal sounds and intonations (see Rolls, Chapter 13). Reciprocally, this pathway provides a route by which affective states could modulate cortical sensory stimuli (McGaugh *et al.*, 1992). Interestingly, because the projections from the amygdala to the cortical sensory areas are widespread, reaching not only the higher order areas but also the primary areas, emotional states could influence sensory inputs at even very early stages in their processing.

The basal nucleus in turn serves as an interface between sensory-specific cortical inputs and the central nucleus, which offers a relay to the brainstem and hypothalamus. These two neural centres are concerned with different aspects of emotional responses, including their behavioural and autonomic manifestations. Via this pathway, sensory stimuli could influence and activate emotional reactions (Amaral, 1992; Kling and Brothers, 1992).

The basal and accessory basal nuclei project substantially to the ventral striatum, thereby offering a way by which affective states may gain access to subcortical elements of the motor system and so affect actions related to emotional responses, including the modulation of facial and vocal expressions, and body postures and motions (Everitt and Robbins, 1992). These two amygdala nuclei are also interconnected with the anterior cingulate cortex, a cortical area implicated in the production of vocalizations in the monkeys (Robinson, 1967; Jürgens and Ploog, 1970; Ploog, 1986) and in the initiation of speech in humans (Barris and Schuman, 1953; Jürgens and von Cramon, 1982). This connectional system may be crucial for the emotional modulation of vocalizations and speech. In addition, the basal nucleus of the amygdala has dense interconnections with the orbital region of the prefrontal cortex. Through this pathway, the orbitofrontal cortex receives information about the emotional and affective content of sensory stimuli, and sends to the amygdala information about the social content of a situation. This route may permit the modulation of emotional responses according to rapid changes in a social situation (Barbas, 1995; Emery and Amaral, 1999).

Finally, the amygdala significantly interacts with the hippocampal formation, predominantly via the entorhinal cortex, though direct connections also exist (Saunders and Rosene, 1988; Saunders *et al.*, 1988; Amaral, 1992). This anatomical link between the amygdala and the hippocampus may allow affective states to act upon and modulate stored perceptions in cortical areas.

This general anatomical organization of the primate amygdala can also be found in humans, with the most prominent change being the allometric size of the lateral nucleus, which increases from non-human primates to humans (Braak and Braak, 1983; Stephan *et al.*, 1987; Sims and Williams, 1990; Gloor, 1997). Presumably, this expansion results from the increasing expansion and specialization of the cerebral cortex in the primate evolution, reaching its greatest complexity in humans. This enhanced specialization is likely to provide the amygdala with increasingly discrete and more highly processed sensory information (see Barton and Aggleton, Chapter 14). Although much less is known of the extent of interconnections of the human amygdala with the remainder of the brain, there are no reasons to believe that the connectional pattern of the human amygdala will be drastically different from that of other non-human primates; though the connections with certain cortical regions could be more extensive in humans than in non-human primates. Thus, using refined dissection techniques, Klinger and Gloor (1960) demonstrated in humans the existence of two important pathways connecting the amygdala to the cerebral cortex. One exits the lateral aspect of the amygdala and reaches the temporopolar cortex, while the other leaves the dorsal aspect of the amygdala and enters the insular gyrus. These two efferent pathways in humans correspond to the densest amygdalocortical pathways that have been described in non-human primates. Finally, as in non-human primates, the human amygdala projects to subcortical regions via two main pathways, the stria terminalis and the ventral amygdaloid system (Klinger and Gloor, 1960; Gloor, 1997). These pathways connect the amygdala to the basal forebrain, hypothalamus, thalamus, and brainstem. Thus, in humans and non-human primates, the amygdala stands in a strategic position to integrate exteroceptive and interoceptive signals, modulate sensory and autonomic processing, and act upon stored representations of emotional aspects of sensory information.

15.3 The amygdala and social cognition in primates

15.3.1 Non-human primates

Studies on the involvement of the amygdala in the regulation of emotional states and in social cognition began with the report of the dramatic effects of temporal lobectomy in monkeys (Brown and Schafer, 1888). Since then, results from studies using an array of techniques converged to suggest that the amygdala plays a crucial role in many aspects of social cognition. These encompass the regulation of emotional responses, the establishment and maintenance of social bonds, the decoding of sensory social signals from other individuals, and the development of appropriate sexual behaviours and proper maternal responses to infants. It is important to stress here that all behavioural lesion studies reporting striking emotional and social abnormalities following amygdalectomy (see below) were based upon aspiration lesions. As detailed by Baxter and Murray (Chapter 16), aspiration lesions necessarily include a portion of the entorhinal cortex as well as fibres of passage coursing through and around the amygdala and originating from medial temporal cortical areas (i.e. entorhinal and perirhinal cortex as well as some of inferior temporal cortical areas). Re-investigations of the memory loss following amygdala damage using cytotoxic lesions revealed that many of the memory deficits found after aspiration of the amygdala result instead from damage to the adjacent cortex. It is thus possible that the same conclusion could apply to the changes in emotions and social interactions found after aspiration lesions of the amygdala. However, a few recent studies (Emery *et al.*, 1998; Meunier *et al.*, 1999) have indicated that neurotoxic amygdala lesions in monkeys yield the same pattern of emotional and social changes as aspiration lesions, although some of the symptoms are less pronounced after neurotoxic than after aspiration lesions.

Emotional and behavioural responses.

Damage to the medial temporal lobe (Klüver and Bucy, 1938, 1939) and, more specifically, to the amygdala (for a review, see Aggleton, 1992) has long been associated with alterations in emotional and behavioural responses in monkeys. These changes include a tendency to become unnaturally fearless and tame, an excessive examination of objects, often with the mouth, and purposeless hyperactivity. Comparable changes in emotional reactivity have been described recently following selective, bilateral, neurotoxin lesions of the amygdala, which spare fibres coursing in and around the amygdaloid nuclei (Meunier *et al.*, 1999). With these more selective lesions, the severity of some of the symptoms (aggressivity, submission, and hyperorality) is consistently milder than after aspiration lesions. In addition, partial radiofrequency (Aggleton and Passingham, 1981) or neurotoxin (Meunier *et al.*, 1999) lesions have a lesser effect on fear reactions and manual exploration than aspiration lesions. Thus, although damage to the amygdaloid nuclei alone seems responsible for the changes in affect, additional damage to fibres to and from temporal cortical areas coursing in and around the amygdala and/or to the temporal cortical areas themselves may be required to produce the more severe symptoms observed by Klüver and Bucy (1939). In addition, the emotional changes following bilateral amygdala lesions do not reflect a complete lack of emotional responsivity but rather are more related to an increase in the threshold of a sensory signal necessary to trigger the emotional responses (Aggleton, 1992), and to a combination of inadequate and inappropriate use of emotional responses in response to external stimuli (Meunier *et al.*, 19990 Thus, given these profound alterations in emotional and behavioural responses, it is not surprising to find that bilateral amygdalectomy will also affect almost all aspects of social cognition (for reviews, see Kling and Brothers, 1992; Emery and Amaral, 1999).

Affiliation and social rank

The first demonstration that the amygdala is fundamental for the formation and maintenance of social bonds in non-human primates emerged from experiments using ablation techniques. Studies by Rosvold and colleagues (1954) and by Mirsky (1960) indicated that amygdalectomized monkeys when tested in their individual cage were less fearful towards the experimenter offering food, but fell from top to bottom in the hierarchy when socially grouped in a large enclosure. Since these original reports, several other studies have substantiated the marked changes in social interactions that follow amygdalectomy in monkeys. Thus, aspiration lesions of the anterior temporal cortex, which included the amygdala, yield marked decrements in aggression and dominance in squirrel monkeys placed in small laboratory cage groups (Plotnik, 1968). In rhesus monkeys observed in free-ranging social groups, these changes resulted in complete social isolation of the lesioned animals from the social groups (Kling and Brothers, 1992). While similar changes in social interactions were reported after damage to the anterior temporal cortex that spared the amygdala (Myers and Swett, 1970; Franzen and Myers, 1973), it is not yet known whether restricted (cytotoxic) damage to the amygdala, sparing the adjacent cortical areas as well as fibres of passage, will be sufficient to produce the changes in affiliative behaviour. Such studies currently are in progress in several laboratories. Thus, Emery and colleagues (1998) recently investigated the effects of neurotoxic amygdala lesions on dyadic interactions and showed that the lesioned animals appeared less aggressive and less fearful towards the other unlesioned controls, suggesting that the amygdaloid nuclei play a role in the development and maintenance of social bonds. Nevertheless, additional investigations of the effects of these selective amygdala lesions in more complex social group interactions are clearly needed.

The role of the amygdala in social interactions has also been demonstrated by electrophysiological recording studies in monkeys. Radiotelemetry recordings of the activity of neurons in the amygdala during social interactions showed the highest responses to ambiguous or threatening situations, such as threat face display, and the lowest to tension-lowering behaviours, such as grooming and huddling (Kling *et al.*, 1979).

It is clear from these earlier studies that the amygdala contributes significantly to affiliative behaviours. Several factors appear to influence the effects of amygdala lesions on social and emotional responses. Apart from the extent of the lesions discussed above, these factors include species-specific behaviours, sex of the subjects, age at the time of surgery, and amount of preoperative social experience with conspecifics in a social group. Thus, bilateral amygdalectomy appears to have less disruptive effects in species that display intense positive social behaviours of grooming and embracing, such as in *Macaca speciosa*, than in *Macaca mulatta* and *Macaca ira* (Kling and Cornell, 1971). Furthermore, male amygdalectomized monkeys showed less aggressive behaviours than female monkeys and, more often than females, fell in social rank (Rosvold *et al.*, 1954; Kling, 1974). In adult monkeys, the deleterious effects of amygdala lesions are present when the animals are placed in small laboratory groups and in free-ranging social groups, whereas in juvenile lesioned monkeys these effects emerged only when the social groups increased in complexity (Dicks *et al.*, 1969; Kling, 1972). Lastly, changes in social interactions following amygdalectomy depend on the length of time the social relationships had existed preoperatively, with greater and more rapid changes in lesioned animals being associated with less preoperative experience in a social group (Rosvold *et al.*, 1954).

Processing of sensory social signals

Primate visual and vocal communications are an essential component of successful social behaviour in all primates, though information from tactile and odour cues from other conspecifics is also likely to be involved. Earlier studies showed that electrical stimulation of the amygdala of monkeys living in social groups yields significant changes in vocalization in both rhesus (Robinson, 1967) and squirrel (Jürgens and Ploog, 1970; Jurgens, 1982) monkeys, suggesting that the amygdala appears to regulate vocal communications.

As yet, no lesion studies in monkeys have investigated the role of the amygdala in the discrimination of face identity, facial expressions, and body movements. Nevertheless, electrophysiological recording studies in awake monkeys strongly point to a role for the amygdala in the neural processes subserving these functions (for a review, see Rolls, 1986, 1994). Thus, amygdala neurons code not only for several aspects of a face, such as dimension (Yamane *et al.*, 1988), hairline, eyes, and mouth (Perrett *et al.*, 1982; Desimone *et al.*, 1984; Leonard *et al.*, 1985), but also for identity of a face (Perrett *et al.*, 1984; Baylis *et al.*, 1985) and for facial expressions (Perrett *et al.*, 1984; Hasselmo *et al.*, 1989a,b). Some of the amygdala neurons respond specifically to body movements, such as direction of rotation of head or direction of gaze, but not to movements of inanimate objects (Perrett *et al.*, 1985; Perret and Mistlin, 1990). Finally, amygdala recordings in monkeys viewing short video-clips of social interactions in a natural setting (Brothers *et al.*, 1990, 1995) showed neurons firing specifically to the identity of the individual or to active movements of a specific area of the face, such as the eyebrow region. It is clear from these studies that the amygdala appears to code and process facial movements, body postures, and gestures that are potent signals for the production and modulation of appropriate social and emotional responses towards other individuals.

Sexual behaviour

Another aspect of amygdalectomy is its effect on sexual behaviour. As originally described by Klüver and Bucy (1939), complete amygdalectomy is associated with hypersexuality. As for emotionality and affiliative behaviours, the changes in sexual behaviours also vary greatly according to the environment into which the lesioned animal is placed, the species studied, and, within a species, to the sex of the lesioned animals (Kling and Brothers, 1992). Thus, hypersexuality appears to be more apparent in lesioned monkeys placed in pairs than in those kept in small laboratory social groups or larger corral conditions (Kling and Dunne, 1976). In addition, in *Macaca arctoides*, hypersexuality is observed only towards conspecifics, while in *M.mulatta* it is also observed towards inanimate objects. Lastly, hypersexuality appears to be more frequent in lesioned female monkeys (Kling, 1974) than in lesioned male monkeys (Klüver and Bucy, 1939).

Maternal behaviour

A few observations have indicated that damage to the amygdala has extremely profound effects on maternal behaviours (for a review, see Kling, 1972). In general, even the most rudimentary elements of maternal behaviour are disrupted by the lesions. The lesioned females appear to consider their offspring as inanimate objects, which in some instances results in severe biting and death of the infant monkeys if not removed from the mother.

In summary, many factors appear to affect significantly the presence or severity of emotional and social abnormalities observed after amygdalectomy. Further, neurotoxic lesions of the amygdala indicate that this structure participates in the regulation of emotions and social interactions, though the adjacent cortical areas are likely to mediate these functions as well. Given the body of data in non-human primates demonstrating that the amygdala is fundamentally involved in detecting, processing, and responding to emotional and social signals, does it also play such a crucial role in humans?

15.3.2 Human studies

Emotional responses

The position of the amygdala in human social cognition is less clear, because selective damage to the amygdala is unusual and, in most cases, not selective. As reviewed by Halgren (1992) and Aggleton (1992), changes in emotional responses similar to those described in non-human primates have been found in humans with amygdala dysfunction, such as in patients suffering from viral encephalitis, in those who received bilateral temporal resections as a treatment either for psychosis or for otherwise untreatable epileptic seizures, such as case H.M, and in patients receiving chemotherapy for cancer treatment (Hayman *et al.*, 1998). The severity of the behavioural and emotional changes, however, varies greatly between cases. A small minority of these patients exhibited the fully fledged Klüver–Bucy syndrome, while the greater proportion developed only milder emotional changes. Thus, in general, amygdala damage in humans rarely produces the severe changes in emotional and behavioural responses observed in amygdalectomized monkeys. Hypersexuality is one of the symptoms reported least frequently in humans, although inappropriate sexual remarks and gestures are frequent (Lilly *et al.*, 1983; Hayman *et al.*, 1998). Changes in sexual preferences have also been reported (Rossitch and Oakes, 1989). In a detailed review of human cases with amygdala damage, Aggleton (1992) indicated that the differences between non-human primates and humans reside more in the magnitude of the effects than in the types of behavioural responses affected by the lesions. Overall, the data suggested that damage to temporal cortical areas together with that of the amygdala is necessary to produce more severe effects on emotional responses in humans as it does in monkeys.

Evidence for the involvement of the amygdala in the regulation of emotions in humans has also come from studies involving patients' reports of their subjective experiences upon stimulation of temporal lobe structures, including the amygdala (Gloor, 1997). They frequently touch on some aspects of the patients' relationship with other people and tend to involve actions, attitudes, or intentions of others, perceived by subjects to be directed at themselves. In addition, recording studies indicate that the human amygdala receives highly processed cognitive and visceral inputs and it affects the quality of awareness as well as the automatic states (for a review, see Halgren, 1992).

Affiliative behaviours

There are surprisingly few descriptions of changes in affiliative interactions after damage to the amygdala in humans. Almost all epileptic and schizophrenic cases that had received anterior temporal lobectomy display fewer social interactions (Scoville *et al.*, 1953; Terzian and Ore, 1955) or more antisocial behaviours (Hitchcock and Cairns, 1973). Again, as in the case of emotional responses, damage to the amygdala that does not encroach onto adjacent temporal cortical areas is not associated with drastic changes in sociality. Nevertheless, Tranel and Hyman (1990) described a patient with congenital bilateral calcification of the amygdala who displayed inappropriate and irrational social behaviour (see Adolphs and Tranel, Chapter 18). The patient is unusually forward with experimenters and has a tendency for coquettish, disinhibited behaviour, including inappropriate sexual remarks. In addition, when placed in difficult situations, this patient shows depressive symptoms. Nahm and collaborators (1993) also commented on the inappropriate social behaviour of a patient with bilateral damage to the amygdala. Furthermore, Broks and collaborators (1998) reported that two of four patients with amygdala damage due to herpes encephalitis displayed either difficulty in social interactions or social disinhibition. In a more recent investigation of the abilities to make social judgement, Adolphs and colleagues (1998) demonstrated that, as compared with normal subjects, three patients with bilateral amygdala damage showed deficits in making social judgement of approachability and trustworthiness from faces of unfamiliar people. Interestingly, the deficit appeared to be even greater with the most negative ratings of unapproachable and untrustworthy looking faces. Thus, the human amygdala appears critical for the retrieval of socially relevant knowledge on the basis of facial information. This view is supported by growing evidence indicating that the amygdala is implicated in the decoding and processing of visual cues from faces (for a review, see Dolan, Chapter 19).

Processing of social signals

Restricted bilateral damage to the amygdala in humans yields deficits in recognition of facial expressions (Adolphs *et al.*, 1994), as well as in the identification of facial expressions of emotions (Young *et al.*, 1996). This impairment was not found after unilateral damage to either the left or the right amygdala (Adolphs *et al.*, 1995). In addition, this deficit appears more severe for the recognition of negative emotional signals, such as fear and sadness (Calder *et al.*, 1996; Scott *et al.*, 1997; Broks *et al.*, 1998; but see Haman *et al.*, 1996). The role of the amygdala in the cognitive evaluation of facial expressions is supported further by other investigations in humans. First, electrophysiological recordings of amygdala neurons in epileptic patients have shown that neural activity in the amygdala can be evoked by neutral faces (Halgren *et al.*, 1994) and faces of family members and friends (Seeck *et al.*, 1993; Fried *et al.*, 1997). Within the processing of facial expressions, the amygdala appears to be activated preferentially by negative emotions, such as fearful rather than happy faces (Morris *et al.*, 1996) and by sad rather than angry faces (Blair *et al.*, 1999). Secondly, several recent neuroimaging studies have provided stronger support for the view that the amygdala is a key structure for extracting the affective significance of external stimuli, such as facial expressions (George *et al.*, 1995; Rauch *et al.*, 1995; Breiter *et al.*, 1996; Cahill *et al.*, 1996; Irwin *et al.*, 1996; Ketter *et al.*, 1996; see also Dolan, Chapter 19). Lastly, a recent magnetoencephalography study using healthy volunteers (Streit *et al.*, 1999) showed that recognition of facial emotions activates the amygdala. More importantly, the results of the neuroimaging and magnetoencephalography studies reported above show that neural activation during recognition of facial expressions is not limited to the amygdala, but extends to the inferior frontal cortex, different parts of the temporal cortex, and the parietal cortex. This supports the notion that the amygdala is one important component of a multifaceted neural network for social cognition.

In summary, the results from both non-human primates and humans indicate that there are many similarities in the role played by the amygdala in many aspects of social cognition. However, there are also differences. For example, it seems that the effects of amygdala damage on emotional responses and social relationships are less dramatic in humans than in non-human primates, although in both species the greatest effects are always seen when the pathology extends to temporal cortical areas. These differences could result from a number of factors that include not only the extent of the damage, but also the preoperative or psychopathological states existing in human cases, the effects of the operation in chronically psychotic individuals, the variability of environmental and cultural determinants of human behaviour, as well as the age at which amygdala damage was incurred. As suggested by Halgren (1992), the differences in the magnitude of the effects between the two species may also be consistent with the presence in humans of a more diffuse neural network, so that destruction of one component could be compensated significantly by other components in the system.

Despite these species differences, non-human primate and human studies have made parallel progress in our understanding of the role of the amygdala in social cognition. Indeed, one aspect of the research in which data from both species have not only reached a consensus but have also made complementary advances is the perception and processing of visual cues provided by a face. For example, while the results in non-human primates convey knowledge on the specific neural processes occurring within the amygdala which allow coding of information about faces, facial expressions, postures, and gestures, the findings in humans give support to the idea that the amygdala is involved more specifically in the processing of negative emotions than positive emotions. Together, the data emphasize the scientific merit of pursuing parallel studies in the two species.

15.4 Amygdala and social cognition during development

In the preceding pages, a comprehensive review of the role of the amygdala in social cognition in primates has been presented, indicating that the amygdala decodes and integrates perceptual features from other individuals and allows the animal to act and adjust its behavioural response according to the emotional and social context of a particular event. One area of research for which data are totally lacking concerns the role of the amygdala in the emergence of affective states and in the formation and maintenance of social bonds during the developmental period in primates. It would seem that, given the crucial role of the amygdala for social cognition in adult subjects, this structure should likewise play a critical role early in life in the development of social cognition. There exist at least three approaches to begin looking into this question. The first is to correlate the timing of developmental changes in affective expressions and social responses with the chronological maturation of the amygdala and its connections. The second is to assess the effects of neonatal amygdala lesions on the emergence and maturation of social cognitive skills. The third is to investigate the neural substrate of psychopathological diseases of human development, such as autism, in which the lack of appropriate social skills might be associated with an early dysfunction of one or more of the neural nodes in the network supporting emotional and social skills (Brothers, 1995). We recognize that these approaches will only link the amygdala indirectly to the emergence of emotional and social skills during development. Nevertheless, while awaiting more direct investigations, such as functional neuroimaging techniques in newborns actively engaging in emotional and social activities, the findings are helping to reveal the key role of the amygdala, as well as other associated neural structures, in the development of well-adapted emotional and social skills in young primates. The remainder of this chapter will thus summarize the few studies in non-human primates that link the amygdala to the early development of social cognition. This review will also reveal mounting evidence suggesting that an early dysfunction of the amygdala could be at the origin of autism.

15.4.1 Emergence of affective and social abilities

A large body of literature has given detailed behavioural descriptions of the timing of developmental changes in affective capabilities and social relationships in monkeys. All aspects of social cognition investigated thus far stressed the remarkable similarities between infant macaques and human infants in this domain of cognition (for reviews, see Hinde and Spencer-Booth, 1967; Suomi, 1977).

Newborn rhesus monkeys (*M.mulatta*) are born with all of their sensory systems largely functional. At the same time, while their motor capabilities are not as well developed, they exhibit a rather impressive repertoire of neonatal motor activities. Rhesus monkey neonates also display every human neonatal reflex sampled by contemporary neurological examination protocols, although the appearance of these reflexes is markedly accelerated in the monkey as compared with humans.

From birth to 2 months of age, the newborn rhesus monkeys interact mostly with the mother, and their specific affective states are not really differentiated to the human observer. They generally are described as relaxed, alert, or upset. It is only when they reached the second month postnatally that infant monkeys begin to expand their behavioural repertoires and exhibit more distinctive and diverse affective displays. Nevertheless, during the first 2 months, infant rhesus monkeys develop responsiveness to visual social cues from faces (Mendelson *et al.*, 1981). They appear to perceive a facial configuration and discriminate the direction of a conspecific's gaze by the first week postnatally, although they appreciate the social content of changes in gaze direction only by the third week postnatally. Concurrently, vocal recognition emerges as well (Mazataka, 1984). Vocal recognition was studied in 12- to 35-day-old infant Japanese macaques (*Macaca fuscata*) by presenting natural calls of mothers and non-mother cagemates to them in a habituation–dishabituation paradigm. Discriminability of the calls was measured by an increase in conditioned sucking response rate to a second stimulus call after habituation to the first stimulus call. By 3–4 weeks of age, the infants showed categorization of acoustic variants of vocalizations given by their cage mates, i.e. they reacted differently to calls from their mother and calls from other members. This early development of facial and vocal recognition in infant macaques is in line with that observed in human infants (for reviews, see Nelson, 1985, 1993; Fernald, 1993).

In the early weeks, infant rhesus monkeys explore their environment with eyes, hand, and mouth, but by the second month postnatally, they begin to leave their mothers for brief exploratory excursions in their close surrounding. Hence, the emerging affective state at this early age is one of inquisitiveness. During this increased exploration phase, infant rhesus monkeys, like human infants, still use their mothers as secure bases for their own exploration, and, when the infants become agitated by a sudden changes in the environment, the mothers will quickly retrieve their upset infants. Another affective trait that emerges during the second postnatal month is frustration. Frustration is caused generally by the mother, which restrains the infants from exploring the environment. The prevention of the exploratory activities results in a state of agitation.

Fear of strangers emerges at 3 months and is expressed by a well-defined behavioural expression, i.e. the fear grimace. This affective display has been studied extensively in infant rhesus (*M.mulatta*) and pigtailed (*Macaca nemestrina*) monkeys and characterizes a state of fear or wariness of social stimuli, which earlier in life elicited curious interest and sometimes exploration (Sackett, 1966). By this age, the infant rhesus monkeys can modulate their defensive activity adaptatively to meet changing environmental demands (Kalin and Shelton, 1989; Kalin *et al.*, 1991).

It is only by the age of 4 months of age that social play usually flourishes. This affiliative activity will grow rapidly in both scope and frequency of appearance until adolescence, and constitutes the most prominent behaviour pattern in a young monkey's interactions with its peers, siblings, and even some adults in its social group. Over this period of development, play behaviour becomes more complex and results in the development of a greater degree of affective or emotional differentiation.

As play behaviours develop, the infant–mother relationships change, with the mother beginning to reject more and more the nursing attempts from her infant. To cope with this new situation, the infant may seek comfort from other individuals in the social colony or begin to show some signs of aggressive responses towards peers or inanimate objects in their surroundings. Therefore, by 6–7 months, aggression becomes a clear-cut affective response in the rhesus monkey's behavioural repertoire and provides a way to a better control of behavioural activity.

Given the relatively precocious development of some aspects of affective states (recognition of social content of stimuli), one would expect the amygdala to be clearly functional by the end of the first month in rhesus monkeys. At the same time, other aspects of affective responses (i.e. fear responses) do not emerge before 3 months of age and others not before 6–7 months of age (aggressive responses). This progressive development of affective responses suggests that the maturation of the neural circuit supporting social cognition progresses in stages, as different components of the circuit reach full maturity. As summarized below, the experimental data to support this proposal are meagre, but certainly offer a point of departure to initiate further investigations of the development of the neural network supporting social cognition.

15.4.2 Maturation of the amygdala

Earlier reports indicate that the cytological constituents of the amygdaloid nuclei are in place at birth in monkeys (Kling, 1966). In a more recent study, Kordower and colleagues (1992) found that, in rhesus monkeys, neurons of the amygdala are generated during a 3 week period very early in gestation (e.g. embryonic days 30–50 of the rhesus monkey 165 day gestational period) and the neurogenesis seems to occur simultaneously within all amygdaloid nuclei. A similar early neurogenesis has been described for neurons of the amygdaloid complex in humans (Humphrey 1968; Nikolic and Kostovic, 1986). In addition, although the neurochemical development of the amygdala in monkeys is unknown, our own studies have indicated that the distribution of opiate receptors is almost identical in the amygdala of a 1-week-old monkey and in adult monkeys (Bachevalier *et al.*, 1986). Despite its early ontogenetic maturation, the connectional system of the amygdala with other brain areas appears to continue maturing postnatally in monkeys (Webster *et al.*, 1991).

As part of a long-term study designed to examine the ontogeny of visual memory in monkeys and its underlying neural circuitry, we have examined the connections between the inferior temporal cortex and the medial temporal lobe structures in infant monkeys and have compared them with those described in adult monkeys (Webster *et al.*, 1991). Inferior temporal areas TEO and TE were injected with wheat germ agglutinin conjugated to horseradish peroxidase and tritiated amino acids, respectively, or vice versa, in six 1-week-old and six 3- to 4-year-old rhesus macaques (*M.mulatta*), and the distribution of labelled cells and terminals was examined in medial temporal lobe structures. The results demonstrated that all projections from areas TEO and TE to the medial temporal lobe structures are secure in their adult locations in the infant monkey, including those from areas TEO and TE to the lateral nucleus of the amygdala. In addition, all medial temporal lobe inputs to areas TEO and TE that exist in adult monkeys are also present in infant monkeys. However, in addition to these adult-like projections, there exist projections in the infant from area TEO to the lateral basal nucleus of the amygdala that are not found in adult brains. Because the more anterior temporal cortical areas are not fully functional during the first 3 months postnatally (Bachevalier *et al.*, 1991; Rodman, 1994), the existence of transient corticoamygdala projections from cortical areas posterior to area TE suggests that, in the neonatal period, the amygdala receives less highly processed visual information. Through these routes, an infant monkey could begin to discriminate affective cues from faces of their mother and other conspecifics, and possibly recognize intonations of vocal communications as well. However, with the refinement of these corticoamygdala projections during the first 3 months of life, the infants may gain increasingly detailed information about the perceptual characteristics of social signals. This neuroanatomical refinement could well be at the origin of the switch of visual scanning of a face during the first few months after birth (Nelson, 1985, 1993).

The emergence of fear and defensive responses around the third month postnatally corresponds to the age at which rhesus mothers generally allow their infants to venture off with their peers and is in close association with the emergence of fear of strangers. This affective development indicates that, by this age, infant monkeys respond with different emotional displays to specific facial expressions from other conspecifics, suggesting that the innate wiring and learned skills needed to discriminate threatening cues are in place. It also suggests that some important changes in the neural organization of the network ensuring defensive responses have occurred. It is likely that these changes encompass a refinement of connectivity not only within the amygdala but also between the amygdala and other areas of the brain. Given the participation of the prefrontal cortex in the interpretation of sensory stimuli and in the inhibition of maladaptive responses in favour of appropriate ones, one would assume that important changes could occur between amygdala–prefrontal cortex interactions around this postnatal age. Very little is known in this respect, except that it is at around this age that the ability to perform an object reversal task emerges in monkeys (Goldman, 1971). Since this learning skill is known to depend on the integrity of the orbital prefrontal cortex in adult monkeys, one could assume that the maturation of the orbital prefrontal cortex and its connections with the amygdala would permit the animals to modulate their affective responses according to constant changes in social cues provided by others and to contend successfully with danger.

The paucity of data on the development of the amygdala and its connections with other brain structures important for social cognition emphasizes the need to design and carry out detailed analysis of the anatomical and chemical organization, as well as electrophysiological characteristics, of the amygdaloid nuclei during development. Findings from these studies will further our understanding of how the amygdala is connected to the remainder of the brain in early infancy, and how these maturational events progress and account for the emergence and maturation of affective responses and social skills in primates.

15.4.3 Amygdala lesions in infancy

The first observations of the effects of early amygdalectomy were made by Kling and collaborators (1967, 1972). They followed the development of four monkeys amygdalectomized during infancy over a period of 2 years and noted that, when returned to their mothers, the amygdalectomized infant monkeys could successfully be raised maternally. They displayed normal nipple orientation, sucking, and grasping, with a somatic and affective development grossly in the normal range. In addition, following repeated presentations of inedible objects, these lesioned animals did not display the typical compulsive oral behaviour seen in amygdalectomized adult monkeys. This apparent lack of effects of neonatal amygdalectomy in monkeys is in line with a number of studies showing that the behavioural effects of brain damage are minimized when the injury occurs early in life and can be accounted by an incomplete maturation of the brain at the time of the insult (Goldman, 1971). Nevertheless, the normal behavioural responses after early amygdala lesions could have resulted from the lack of specific quantification of behavioural responses and from the few aspects of amygdala functions investigated.

More systematic and detailed investigation of the effects of neonatal amygdala lesions in rhesus monkeys (Thompson *et al.*, 1969, 1977; Thompson and Towfighi, 1976; Thompson, 1981) clearly showed that bilateral amygdalectomy does not leave the subject unharmed, even when the surgery is performed during infancy. Thus, upon observation of six females that had sustained bilateral aspiration lesions of the amygdaloid complex during the third month postnatally, significant alterations in social affiliation were found and these changes became increasingly more evident with age. In the first few months post-surgery, the lesioned infant monkeys displayed more fear responses during social encounters than did control monkeys with whom they were paired, and the fear responses made by the lesioned monkeys towards controls increased whenever the control animals became more active, even though this activity was not overly aggressive. These enhanced fear reactions first appeared 3–5 months following surgery and intensified dramatically thereafter. Responses to novel stimuli in the absence of other monkeys revealed an opposite picture, however, with lesioned monkeys making fewer fear responses than controls and showing signs of hyperactivity. These findings indicate that the early amygdala lesions did not influence the emergence of fear responses around the appropriate age at which they normally appeared. Nevertheless, the early lesions did affect the magnitude of the fear responses displayed in the presence of a peer, suggesting that the lesioned animals may have difficulty in evaluating the social cues expressed by their unlesioned peers.

When re-tested at 3 and 6 years of age (Thompson *et al.*, 1977; Thompson, 1981), the monkeys operated on in infancy showed transient hyperactivity. They were also subordinate to normal controls but expressed less fear than did the controls when placed briefly with an unfamiliar aggressive animal. This increase in subordinate responses in the lesioned animals suggests that the amygdala lesions may have affected the normal development of aggressive responses, resulting in subordination and low social status in the lesioned animals. Lastly, the behavioural abnormalities in monkeys with early amygdala lesions did not differ from those of monkeys that had sustained the same lesions in adulthood. Thus, overall, these data suggest that the amygdala may be operating early in life to regulate affective responses and to establish and maintain social status.

These changes in emotionality and sociality seen after early damage to the amygdala were substantiated and extended by our own studies on the development of social interactions in infant monkeys that were amygdalectomized even earlier in life, i.e. in the first month postnatally (Bachevalier, 1994). Six newborn rhesus monkeys received bilateral aspiration lesions of the amygdaloid complex and six others served as age-matched unlesioned controls. The amygdaloid damage included all amygdaloid nuclei, the piriform cortex, and the rostral portion of the entorhinal cortex. Additional damage was found in the white matter coursing around the lateral edge of the amygdala and in inferior temporal cortical area TE (see Figures 5 and 6 in Bachevalier *et al.*, 1999).

All newborn monkeys were laboratory raised and, upon arrival in the primate nursery (NIMH, Bethesda, Maryland), they were assigned to social groups (dyads or triads) consisting of one normal and one or two lesioned animals. Infant monkeys were reared in individual wire cages that allowed visual, auditory, and some somatosensory contacts between animals from adjacent cages. They were handled several times per day by the experimenters. In addition, the animals forming each dyad or triad were placed for up to 4–6 h daily in a playpen, containing toys and towels, and located in the nursery. With these rearing procedures, the control animals developed relatively normal social skills and few stereotypies (Rosenblum, 1961; Sackett, 1982; Ruppenthal *et al.*, 1991; Schneider and Suomi, 1992; Suomi, 1997).

At the age of 2 months, 6 months, and 5–8 years, lesioned monkeys and their age-matched controls were placed in a play cage containing toys and towels. The behaviour of each pair was videorecorded for two periods of 5 min each, separated by a 5 min interval, for six consecutive days. At all ages, frequency and duration of behaviours for each animal on the videotapes were recorded independently by two observers, who assigned the behaviours to one of nine different behavioural categories. These behavioural categories included measures of general activity (passive behaviour, locomotion, and manipulations of toys or parts of the cage with the limbs or mouth), social behaviour (initiation of social contacts by the observed monkey and acceptance of social contacts initiated by the other monkey at 2 and 6 months of age, and proximity and contact as adults), social rank (aggressive gestures or withdrawal from social contacts), as well as emergence of abnormal behaviours (locomotor stereotypies and self-directed activities).

At 2 months of age, as compared with their unlesioned controls and the normal animals, amygdalectomized infant monkeys were more inactive and manipulated their environment less, although they displayed normal amounts of locomotor behaviours and no stereotypies. Amygdalectomized monkeys and their unlesioned controls also had normal amounts of total social contacts. However, the social interactions were initiated almost exclusively by the unlesioned monkeys. Interestingly, at this early age, it was the unlesioned controls that appeared to show increased amount of stereotypies, presumably in response to the abnormal social environment provided by the lesioned animals (e.g. inactivity and lack of social approaches and play).

At 6 months of age, the changes in general activity disappeared. In contrast, social interactions were reduced dramatically and this reduction of social bonds was accompanied by a significant increase of dominant approaches from the unlesioned controls and a mild increase in active withdrawals from social contacts by the lesioned animals. Presumably, as a result of a marked reduction in affiliative behaviours, both lesioned and control animals displayed increased amount of stereotyped behaviours, more so in the lesioned animals than in their unlesioned controls.

On reaching adulthood, the most striking changes between the two animals (one lesioned, one unlesioned) in the dyads were the almost complete lack of social interactions. Presumably, by this age, the normal animals had learned to cope with the abnormal affective and social responses of the lesioned animals, and did not interact any more with them. This, in turn, would reduce the tension in the animals in the group. Thus, as shown earlier by Thompson and collaborators (1981), early damage to the amygdala results in increasingly profound changes in affective responses and social behaviour, and these changes persisted until adulthood.

Not only did the early amygdala complex damage alter affiliative behaviour, but it also drastically altered vocal responses to social separations (Newman and Bachevalier, 1997). When separated from their mother or peers, infant monkeys emit frequent 'coo' calls (also called separation calls) to regain contact with their peers. A sonograph analysis of the 'coo' calls in early amygdalectomized monkeys and their unlesioned controls indicated that the slope of the 'coo' calls in animals with early amygdalectomy was significantly lower than those produced by normal monkeys or monkeys with early damage to inferior temporal cortex. This defect translated into a coo with little inflection, suggesting that animals with early amygdalectomy have a reduced ability to modulate their vocalizations as a means of conveying varying levels of affect. Because the ability to modulate the behavioural expression of affect is of obvious importance in a species with a rich and complex social structure such as the rhesus macaque, the poorly modulated calls found in early amygdalectomized subjects would thus be consistent with a more general deficiency in social affiliation found in these lesioned animals (Bachevalier, 1994).

As described for the adult monkeys (see above), when neonatal lesions were extended to include the ventromedial temporal cortical areas and hippocampus, the behavioural, emotional, and social changes were even more severe, including a lack of social skills, flat affect, and a significant increase in locomotor stereotypies and self-directed activities (Bachevalier, 1991, 1994). Nevertheless, these early lesions did not yield the lack of fear responses and hyperorality commonly seen after late medial temporal lobe lesions in monkeys (Nalwa and Bachevalier, 1991). Finally, when the animals with neonatal medial temporal lobe lesions were re-tested in social situations as they reached adulthood, the loss of social interactions was substantially more severe in magnitude in adults with early lesions than in adults with similar lesions acquired in adulthood, and the stereotypies were evident after early lesions but not after late lesions (Málková *et al.*, 1997). These later findings demonstrate that compensatory mechanisms do not always operate to ensure recovery of functions after early brain damage; indeed, in the case of the medial temporal lobe, the early lesions yielded more profound behavioural effects than late damage to the same neural system. The pattern of results thus suggest that, due to the immaturity of the brain at the time of the early medial temporal lobe lesions, the damage has affected other neural systems remote from the site of the lesions. Two of our most recent neurobiological investigations give credence to this proposal (Bertolino *et al.*, 1997; Saunders *et al.*, 1998).

In summary, early amygdalectomy in primates yields disorders of both social and non-social behaviours that appeared within a few months following surgery and became increasingly apparent with age. While the early appearance of behavioural abnormalities after neonatal amygdala damage substantiates the view that the amygdala is functional early after birth, these early symptoms might have been enhanced by the fact that the infants in both the study of Thompson *et al.* (1981) and our own investigations (Bachevalier, 1994) were peer-reared and were not provided with optimal social conditions at birth. It is therefore important to bear in mind that the effects of the neonatal amygdaloid lesions on emotional responses and social skills could have differed from those reported here had the monkeys been raised under more natural conditions. In this respect, the lack of effects of early amygdalectomy in infants that were returned to their mothers and social group (Kling and Green, 1967) is provocative and could indicate that environmental conditions could interact with the effects of amygdala lesions. However, before definitive conclusions can be made, replication of Kling's findings is needed.

Interestingly, there are also anecdotal reports indicating that early dysfunction of the medial temporal lobe, including the amygdala, yields significant changes in socioaffective states in children. Thus, neuropathology in medial temporal lobe structures has been identified in several children with Klüver–Bucy symptoms, such as placidity, blunted affect, hyperorality, and aberrant sexual behaviour (Chutorian and Antunes, 1981; Tonsgard *et al.*, 1987; Rossitch and Oakes, 1989; Lanska and Lanska, 1993; Caparros-Lefebvre *et al.*, 1996). These findings again suggest that early insult to the amygdala in human children may yield profound changes in emotionality and sociality. In fact, given the similarity in the behavioural changes found in monkeys with early medial temporal lobe damage (e.g. loss of social interactions and emergence of stereotypies) and the behavioural disturbances seen in autistic people, we as well as others (see below) propose that early insult to the amygdala contributes to the origin of autism.

15.5 The amygdala and autism

Autism is a lifelong developmental disorder that disrupts many essential cognitive functions that can be grouped into three main categories: impairment in social interactions with others; impairment in verbal and non-verbal communication; and impairment in play and imaginative activities. Associated features may include gross motor problems, unusual fears and anxiety, hyperorality, pica (peculiar preference for some food), and inability to modulate sensory inputs adequately. Impairments in social interactions and social understanding have been recognized since the description of the syndrome by Kanner (1943) and Asperger (1944) and cut across widely varying levels of cognitive and linguistic functioning (Fein *et al.*, 1987). The social–emotional abnormalities usually begin in the first years of life and persist into adulthood, even in patients with verbal skills and relatively high intelligence quotients. These abnormalities are characterized by an impairment of the social use of gaze, a failure of joint attention interactions, unresponsiveness to social stimulation, a preference for solitary play, lack of interest in peers, difficulty interpreting facial expressions, unusual affective behaviour, and difficulty initiating communication (Loveland and Landry, 1986; Sigman *et al.*, 1986; Buitelaar *et al.*, 1991; Tantam, 1992). In addition, many reports have now shown that persons with autism are impaired in face recognition, identification of facial expression of emotions, discrimination of faces, and memory of faces (Hobson *et al.*, 1988; Macdonald *et al.*, 1989; Yirmiya *et al.*, 1989; Adrien *et al.*, 1991; Green *et al.*, 1995; Celani *et al.*, 1999) as well as in recognizing how different expressions of particular emotions are associated with each other (Hobson, 1986). Thus, the nature of the core symptoms of autism and their early appearance suggest that a neurobiological theory of autism needs to focus on brain systems or circuits that are implicated in the regulation of social and emotional behaviour and are maturing early in development. In this respect, dysfunction of the amygdala as well as other components of the neural network supporting social cognition is an appealing proposal that has the potential to illuminate some of the most persisent issues in the field of autism research (Bachevalier, 1994; Brothers, 1995; Baron-Cohen *et al.*, 1999).

Following an analysis of the patterns of abnormal behaviour seen in autism and adults with certain forms of brain damage, Damasio and Maurer (1978) proposed that autism is consequent to dysfunction in a complex of bilateral central nervous system (CNS) structures that includes mesial frontal lobes, mesial temporal lobes, basal ganglia (in particular, the neostriatum), and thalami (dorsomedial and anterior nuclear groups). Aspects of this proposal have now been substantiated by several groups of researchers. For example, Hetzler and Griffin (1981) and deLong (1992) have hypothesized dysfunction in bilateral medial temporal lobe structures (hippocampus and amygdala) and drawn parallels between the amnesic and Klüver–Bucy syndromes, and autism. Fein and colleagues (1987) viewed the social and communication deficits in autism as resting on an amygdala-based failure to assign appropriate motivational significance to social objects. Brothers (1989) postulated that the amygdala is the source of empathy and suggested that lack of empathic concern for others is a central feature of autism. Fotheringham (1991) proposed that the core disorder in autism is a failure to appreciate the emotional significance of incoming stimuli and a failure to assign normal motivational value to the stimuli, and posited that these failures indicate dysfunction in the amygdala and its connections. A dysfunction of the amygdala and prefrontal cortex has also been emphasized by Bishop (1993), by Dawson and colleagues (1998), and more recently demonstrated by Baron-Cohen and collaborators (1999). Despite indirect evidence coupling autism and frontolimbic dysfunction, very few investigations have explored this possibility to date.

15.5.1 Association with temporal lobe dysfunction

Investigators have reported that some autistic children have subtle electroencephalogram (EEG) abnormalities in the temporal lobes (Hauser *et al.*, 1975; deLong, 1978), enlargement of the temporal horn of the lateral ventricles (Hauser *et al.*, 1975; Damasio *et al.*, 1980; Campbell *et al.*, 1982; Jacobson *et al.*, 1988), mild abnormalities of the ventricular system, including hydrocephalus (Hier *et al.*, 1979; Fernell *et al.*, 1991), increased incidence of herpes simplex types 1 and 2, which have a specific affinity for the medial temporal region (deLong *et al.*, 1981; Ghaziuddin *et al.*, 1992), and increased incidence of anoxia at birth, which is also often associated with medial temporal dysfunction (Coleman, 1978). Temporal lobe seizures constitute the most frequent variety in the autistic population and tend to be under-diagnosed (DeyKin and MacMahon, 1979). With careful monitoring, Payton and Minshew (1987) were able to identify limbic epilepsy in 57% (17 of 30) of prepubertal autistic children. More recently, Deonna and collaborators (1993) reported two children with autistic regression as the presenting syndrome. Both were found to have tuberous sclerosis, a developmental brain abnormality associated with early epilepsy. Their cerebral pathology was localized in the medial temporal lobe. Hoon and Reiss (1992) described a young male child with a left temporal oligodendroglioma, who demonstrated a constellation of autistic behaviours meeting the DSM-III-R criteria for pervasive developmental disorder. Finally, White and Rosenbloom (1992) described a child with infantile autism who was found to have a partial absence of the left temporal lobe upon computerized tomography (CT) scanning. These clinical findings, although intriguing, are only suggestive of the involvement of temporal lobe dysfunction in producing autistic symptoms.

15.5.2 Neuropathological studies

While initial neuropathological studies of seven cases (Darby, 1976; Williams *et al.*, 1980) were negative, more recent studies have identified microscopic abnormalities. Hof and collaborators (1991) reported neurofibrillary tangles in the ento- and perirhinal cortex as well as in the amygdala in a case of autism presenting with self-mutilating behaviour. Bauman and Kemper (1993) have investigated the brains of eight autistic subjects after autopsy, using the technique of gapless whole-brain serial sections, which involved posterior–anterior sections of the entire brain. The brains studied were normal in weight, gyral configuration, and myelination. In all eight subjects, microscopic cytoarchitectonic abnormalities (increased cell densities, small cell sizes) were found in limbic structures such as the hippocampus, amygdala, entorhinal cortex, septal nuclei, and mammillary bodies, along with a loss of Purkinje cells in the cerebellum. The overall size of the hippocampus was reduced and, in the amygdala, there was an indication that the more severe cases of autism had larger portions of the amygdala affected by abnormal cell-packing densities. Interestingly, in one such case of a higher functioning person as compared with the seven others, cytoarchitectonic abnormalities were confined more to the amygdaloid nuclei (Bauman and Kemper, 1993). Although the cytoarchitectonic findings on their higher functioning subjects await replication, the anatomical investigation of this series of autistic cases suggests that the extent of cognitive deficit seen in autism may well be related to the extent of hippocampal and adjacent medial temporal cortical damage that accompanies the amygdaloid damage. At the microscopic level, no changes have been reported in the architectonic organization of the orbitofrontal cortex or the dorsolateral prefrontal cortex. In addition, the neuropathological findings in the septum, the diagonal band of Broca, the deep cerebellar nuclei, and the inferior olive depended on the age of the subject. In younger brains, these areas show enlarged neurons, whereas in older brains, the neurons are reduced in size and/or number, or are absent. This suggests that the manifestations from a neurodevelopmental lesion are dynamic, changing during normal postnatal brain maturation. In conclusion, the neuropathological findings in autism are provocative, even though they need verification in many more autistic cases and with more refined neuroanatomical techniques.

15.5.3 Structural imaging studies

To our knowledge, there are only a few magnetic resonance imaging (MRI) studies of the medial temporal lobe region in autism. Filipek and colleagues (1992) found larger hemispheric and white matter volumes that were localized disproportionately to the temporal and posterior parietal region. In the second study (Reiss *et al.*, 1994), subjects with fragile X syndrome who met the diagnostic criteria for Autistic Disorder or Pervasive Developmental Disorder were found to have significantly increased amygdala–hippocampal boundary tissue. This increased volume could well reflect the neuropathological changes observed by Bauman and Kemper (1993). Up to now, we are aware of only one published report examining the volume of mesial temporal lobe structures in autism. Saitoh and colleagues (1995) measured the volume of the hippocampus proper, including the subiculum and dentate gyrus, in participants with autism and age-matched normal volunteers. No statistically significant volumetric differences were found. However, this study suffered from two methodological confounds. First, the volumetric measurements were made on 5 mm thick MRI slices. For a structure the size of the hippocampus and given the subtle nature of the hypothesized morphologic changes, 5 mm slices are inadequate to appreciate small but significant volumetric changes. Additionally, the volume of cerebral structures can be related substantially to a participant's IQ (Piven *et al.*, 1997), a variable that was not investigated by Saitoh's study (1995). Nevertheless, using thinner MRI slides, Piven and collaborators (1998) recently reported no differences in hippocampus volume in 35 autistic subjects, even when the volume measures were corelated with IQ. Amazingly, no studies so far have focused on the amygdala, the mesial temporal lobe structure most likely to be involved in social–emotional disorders, or the orbitofrontal cortex, another brain area crucial for the regulation of social behaviour. This obvious shortcoming highlights how much remains to be explored.

15.5.4 Functional and spectroscopic imaging studies

To date, results from functional neuroimaging in autism are inconsistent. This may be due to technical limitations, difficulty conceptualizing the illness, or heterogeneity of the disorder itself. Using fluoro-deoxyglucose positron emission tomography (FDG PET), the resting cerebral metabolism of autistic men was higher than that of controls (Rumsey *et al.*, 1985; Horwitz *et al.*, 1988). In contrast, 99mTc-HMPAO single-photon emission computerized tomography (SPECT) of four autistic adult men showed decreased perfusion throughout the brain, and focal decreases in the right temporal and bilateral frontal lobes (George *et al.*, 1992). However, the control volunteers were not matched for IQ or gender to the autistic patients. In addition, using 133Xe SPECT, children and adolescents with autism showed higher cerebral blood flow in the right than in the left hemisphere in sensorimotor cortex,

Broca's area, and parietotemporal cortex (Chiron *et al.*, 1995). A more recent study (Mountz *et al.*, 1995) found low regional cerebral blood flow in the temporal and parietal lobes. Again, this study was performed in only six patients with a wide variation in age and IQ; controls were not matched to patients on IQ. Furthermore, in resting PET and SPECT studies, no abnormalities in cerebral blood flow or metabolism were found in autistic children (De Volder *et al.*, 1987; Zilbovicius *et al.*, 1992) or adults (Herold *et al.*, 1988).

Such conflicting findings may arise from a number of variables. For example, in one intriguing 133Xe SPECT study, autistic children were studied longitudinally at age 3–4 years and again at age 6–7 years. Compared with age-matched controls, the younger autistic children showed frontal hypoperfusion; at the older age, frontal blood flow had normalized (Zilbovicius *et al.*, 1995). Participants' age may influence whether abnormalities are found, as may their intelligence level. Also, all the above studies were done at rest, which provides no control for the participants' affective or cognitive state. It is possible that brain differences would emerge if imaging were performed during a task that differentiates autistic and non-autistic individuals, or during a technique investigating brain systems thought to be involved in autism.

One study provides a step in this direction. Fifteen adults with autism were compared with schizophrenic patients and normal controls using PET during a continuous performance task. During this behavioural task, single digits were presented on a screen and the subjects were instructed to press a button every time a zero was detected (zeros were presented with a probability of occurrence of 0.25). Individuals with autism did not differ statistically from normal controls in their performance results. Likewise, there were no differences in cortical metabolism between individuals with autism and normal controls. Interestingly, when performance was correlated with metabolism, individuals with autism differed from controls in the direction of the correlation in the mesial frontal region (Siegel *et al.*, 1995). While this study represents an important research direction, it too is marred by not matching for IQ, which makes it impossible to determine whether group differences are associated with the illness under study, or are due to differences in cognitive ability. Moreover, individuals with autism were not significantly impaired in their performance on the continuous performance test. This suggests that, at least for this subgroup of participants, the task chosen did not tap a neural substrate associated with autism. For example, one specific brain region, the dorsolateral prefrontal cortex, has been studied using phosphorus-31 magnetic resonance spectroscopy in high-functioning autistic adolescent and adult men compared with age-, IQ-, and gender-matched controls (Minshew *et al.*, 1993). Although there were no abnormalities of phosphomonoesters or phosphodiesters (the building blocks and breakdown products of cell membranes), there were differences in high-energy phosphate compounds. These results await replication, and the meaning of the abnormality is unclear.

More recently, the brains of normal subjects, of high-functioning autistic persons, or of people with Asperger's syndrome were investigated through functional neuroimaging techniques while judging from the expressions of another person's eyes what that person was feeling or thinking about (Baron-Cohen *et al.*, 1999). During the behavioural task in normal subjects, there was activation of the cortex in the superior temporal gyrus, the amygdala, and orbital prefrontal regions, suggesting that these areas play a major role in the regulation of affective states and social cognition in humans. In contrast, in people with autism, the task activated the frontotemporal cortical region but not the amygdala, thus providing credibility to the notion that a dysfunction of the amygdala is associated with autism and Asperger's syndrome.

In summary, evidence for the involvement of the amygdala and related structures in autism is receiving growing support from numerous investigations. Nevertheless, much remains to be done to confirm this view and also to indicate what are the factors that initiate this devastating illness of the developing brain. Conversely, further detailed characterization of the social deficits in autistic people could provide insights into the cognitive processes mediated by the amygdala and associated brain structures.

15.6 Conclusions

Research in non-human primates has indicated that the amygdala plays a critical role in social cognition, although many more studies are still needed to understand the specific processes by which the amygdala achieves its functions. In addition, while the review presented here focuses on the amygdala, it is clear that the regulation of social cognition is orchestrated by a multitude of interconnected structures of which the amygdala is only one constituent. This complexity shows how studies of non-human primates will be needed to further our understanding of the neural processes subserving social cognition. This review has also highlighted that, because of the many similarities in the perception and modulation of social signals across primates, research in monkeys and humans should proceed in parallel, each informing and complementing the other with theoretical and empirical contributions. Finally, the chapter stresses the urgent need to initiate many more developmental studies in monkeys and humans to begin appreciating the role of the amygdala and other related brain regions early in life for the achievement of well-adapted social skills in adulthood. The joint effort of this research exploration will probably result in new and exciting results on the neurobiology of social cognition that in turn will provide significant progress in understanding the causes of developmental psychopathological disorders, such as autism.

Acknowledgements

Preparation of this chapter was supported by NIH grant PO1-HD35471.

References

Adolphs, R., Tranel, D., Damasio, H., and Damasio, A.R. (1994) Impaired recognition of emotion in facial expressions following bilateral damage to the human amygdala. *Nature*, 372, 669–672.

Adolphs, R., Tranel, D., Damasio, H., and Damasio, A.R. (1995) Fear and the human amygdala. *Journal of Neuroscience*, 15, 5880–5891.

Adolphs, R., Tranel, D., and Damasio, A.R. (1998) The human amygdala in social judgement. *Nature*, 393, 470–474.

Adrien, J.L., Faure, M., Perrot, A., Hameury, L., Garreau, B., Barthelemy, C., and Sauvage, D. (1991) Autism and family home movies: preliminary findings. *Journal of Autism Developmental Disorders*, 21, 43–48.

Aggleton, J.P. (1992) The functional effects of amygdala lesions in humans: a comparison with findings from monkeys. In *The Amygdala: Neurobiological Aspects of Emotion, Memory, and Dysfunction* (ed. J.P. Aggleton), pp. 485–503. Wiley-Liss, New York.

Aggleton, J.P. and Passingham, R.E. (1981) Syndrome produced by lesions of the amygdala in monkeys (*Macaca mulatta*). *Journal of Comparative and Physiological Psycholology*, 95, 961–977.

Amaral, D.G. (1992) Anatomical organization of the primate amygdaloid complex. In *The Amygdala: Neurobiological Aspects of Emotion, Memory, and Dysfunction* (ed. J.P. Aggleton), pp. 1–66. Wiley-Liss, New York.

Asperger, H. (1944) Die 'Autistischen Psychopathen' im kindesalter. *Archiv für Psychiatrie und Nervenkrankheiten*, 117, 76–136.

Bachevalier, J. (1991) An animal model for childhood autism: memory loss and socioemotional disturbances following neonatal damage to the limbic system in monkeys. In *Advances in Neuropsychiatry and Psychoparmacology, Volume 1: Schizophrenia Research* (eds C.A. Tamminga and S.C. Schulz), pp. 129–140. Raven Press, New York.

Bachevalier, J. (1994) Medial temporal lobe structures and autism: a review of clinical and experimental findings. *Neuropsychologia*, 32,627–648.

Bachevalier, J., Ungerleider, L.G., O'Neill, B.J., and Friedman, D.P. (1986) Regional distribution of [^{3}H]-naloxone binding in the brain of a newborn rhesus monkey. *Developmental Brain Research*, 25, 302–308.

Bachevalier, J., Hagger, C., and Mishkin, M. (1991) Functional maturation of the occipitotemporal pathway in infant rhesus monkeys. In *Alfred Benzon Symposium No. 31: Brain Work and Mental Activity—Quantitative Studies with Radioactive Tracers* (eds N.A. Lassen, D.H. Ingvar, M.E. Raichle, and L. Friberg), pp. 231–240. Munksgaard, Copenhagen.

Bachevalier, J., Beauregard, M., and Alvarado M.C. (1999) Long-term effects of neonatal damage to the hippocampal formation and amygdaloid complex on object discrimination and object recognition in rhesus monkeys. *Behavioral Neuroscience*, **113**, 1127–1151.

Barbas, H. (1995) Anatomic basis of cognitive–emotional interactions in the primate prefrontal cortex. *Neuroscience and Biobehavioral Reviews*, 19, 499–510.

Baron-Cohen, S., Ring, H.A., Wheelwright, S., Bullmore, E.T., Brammer, M.J., Simmons, A., and Williams, S.C.R. (1999) Social intelligence in the normal and autistic brain: an fMRI study. *European Journal of Neuroscience*, 11, 1891–1898.

Barris, R.W. and Schuman, H.R. (1953) Bilateral anterior cingulate gyrus lesions: syndrome of the anterior cingulate gyri. *Neurology*, 3, 44–52.

Bauman, M.L. and Kemper, T.L. (1993) Cytoarchitectonic changes in the brain of people with autism. In *The Neurobiology of Autism* (eds M.L. Bauman and T.L. Kemper), pp. 119–145. Johns Hopkins Press, Baltimore.

Baylis, L.L., Rolls, E.T., and Leonard, C.M. (1985) Selectivity between faces in the responses of a population of neurons in the cortex in the superior temporal sulcus of the monkey. *Brain Research*, 342, 91–102.

Bertolino, A., Saunders, R.C., Mattay, V.S., Bachevalier, J., Frank, J.A., and Weinberger, D.R. (1997) Altered development of prefrontal neurons in rhesus monkeys with neonatal mesial temporo-limbic lesions: a proton magnetic resonance spectroscopic imaging study. *Cerebral Cortex*, 7, 740–748.

Bishop, D.V.M. (1993) Annotation: autism, executive functions, and theory of mind: a neuropsychological perspective. *Journal of Child Psycholology and Psychiatiatry*, 54, 279–293.

Blair, R.J.R., Morris. J.S., Frith, C.D., Perrett, D.I., and Dolan, R.J. (1999) Dissociable neural responses to facial expressions of sadness and anger. *Brain*, 122, 883–893.

Braak, H. and Braak, E. (1983) Neuronal types in the basolateral amygdaloid nuclei of man. *Brain Research Bulletin*, 11, 349–365.

Breiter, H.C., Etcoff, N.L., Whalen, P.J., Kennedy, W.A., Rauch, S.L., Buckner, R., Strauss, M.M., Hyman, S.E., and Rosen, B.R. (1996) Response and habituation of the human amygdala during visual processing of facial expression. *Neuron*, 17, 875–887.

Broks, P., Young, A.W., Maratos, E.J., Coffey, P.J., Calder, A.J., Isaac, C.L., Mayes, A.R., Hodges, J.R., Montaldi, D., Cezayirli, E. Roberts, N., and Hadley, D. (1998) Face processing impairments after encephalitis: amygdala damage and recognition of fear. *Neuropsychologia*, 36, 59–70.

Brothers, L. (1989) A biological perspective on empathy. *American Journal of Psychiatry*, 146, 10–19.

Brothers, L. (1995) Neurophysiology of the perception of intention by primates. In *The Cognitive Neurosciences* (ed. M.S. Gazzaniga), pp. 1107–1117. MIT Press, Cambridge, Massachusetts.

Brothers, L., Ring, B., and Kling, A. (1990) Response of neurons in the macaque amygdala to complex social stimuli. *Behavioural Brain Research*, 41, 199–213.

Brown, S. and Schafer, A. (1888) An investigation into the functions of the occipital and temporal lobes of the monkey's brain. *Philosophical Transactions of the Royal Society of London, Series B*, 179, 303–327.

Buitelaar, J.K., van Engeland, H., de Kogel, K., de Vries, H., and van Hoof, C. (1991) Differences in the structure of social behaviour of autistic children and non-autistic retarded controls. *Journal of Child Psychology and Psychiatry*, 32, 995–1015.

Byrne, R. and Whiten, A. (1988) *Machavellian Intelligence: Social Expertise and the Evolution of Intellect in Monkeys, Apes, and Humans*. Clarendon Press, Oxford.

Cahill, L., Haier, R.J., Fallon, J., Alkire, M.T., Tang, C., Keator, D., Wu, J., and McGaugh, J.L. (1996) Amygdala activity at encoding correlated with long-term, free recall of emotional information. *Proceedings of the National Academy of Sciences of the United States of America*, 93, 8016–8021.

Calder, A.J., Young, A.W., Rowland, D., and Perrett, D.I. (1996) Facial emotion recognition after bilateral amygdala damage: differentially severe impairment of fear. *Cognitive Neuroscience*, 13, 699–745.

Campbell, M., Rosenbloom, S., Perry, R., George, A.E., Kricheff, I.I., Anderson, L., Small, A.M., and Jennings, S.J. (1982) Computerized axial tomography in young autistic children. *American Journal of Psychiatry*, 139, 510–512.

Caparros-Lefebvre, D., Girard-Buttaz, I., Reboul, S., Lebert, F., Cabaret, M., Verier, A., Steinling, M., Pruvo, J.P., and Petit, H. (1996) Cognitive and psychiatric impairment in herpes simplex virus encephalitis suggest involvement of the amygdalo-frontal pathways. *Journal of Neurology*, 243, 248–256.

Celani, G., Battachi, M.W., and Arcidiacono, L. (1999) The understanding of the emotional meaning of facial expressions in people with autism. *Journal of Autism and Developmental Disorders*, 29, 57–66.

Cheney, D.L. and Seyfarth, R.M. (1990) *How Monkeys See the World.* University of Chicago Press, Chicago, Illinois.

Chiron, C., Leboyer, M., Leon, F., Jambaque, I., Nuttin, C., and Syrota, A. (1995) SPECT of the brain in childhood autism: evidence for a lack of normal hemispheric asymmetry. *Developmental Medicine and Child Neurology*, 37, 849–860.

Chutorian A.B. and Antunes J.L. (1981) Klüver–Bucy syndrome and herpes encephalitis: case report. *Neurosurgery*, 8, 388–390.

Coleman, M. (1978) A report on the autistic syndrome. In *Autism: A Reappraisal of Concepts and Treatment* (eds M. Rutter and E. Schopler), pp. 185–199. Plenum Press, New York.

Damasio, A.R. and Maurer, R.G. (1978) A neurological model for childhood autism. *Archives of Neurology*, 35, 777–786.

Damasio, A.R., Maurer, R.G., Damasio, A.R., and Chui, H. (1980) Computerized tomographic scan findings in patients with autistic behavior. *Archives of Neurology*, 37, 504–510.

Darby, J.K. (1976) Neuropathological aspects of psychosis in children. *Journal of Autism and Childhood Schizophrenia*, 6, 339–352.

Dawson, G., Meltzoff, A.N., Osterling, J., and Rinaldi, J. (1998) Neuropsychological correlates of early symptoms of autism. *Child Development*, 69, 1276–1285.

Deonna, T., Ziegler, A-L., Moura-Serra, J., and Innocenti, G. (1993) Autistic regression in relation to limbic pathology and epilepsy: report of two cases. *Developmental Medicine and Child Neurology*, 35, 166–176.

deLong, G.R. (1978) A neuropsychological interpretation of infantile autism. In *Autism* (eds E. Schopler and G.B. Mesibov), pp. 207–218. Plenum Press, New York.

deLong, G.R. (1992) Autism, amnesia, hippocampus, and learning. *Neuroscience and Biobehavioral Review*, 16, 63–70.

deLong, G.R., Bean, S.C., and Brown F.R. (1981) Acquired reversible autistic syndrome in acute encephalopathic illness children. *Archives of Neurology*, 38, 191–194.

Desimone,R., Albright, T.D., Gross, C.G., and Bruce, C. (1984) Stimulus-selective properties of inferior temporal neurons in the macaque. *Journal of Neuroscience*, 4, 2051–2062.

De Volder, A., Bol, A., Michel, C., Congneau, M., and Goffinet, A.M. (1987) Brain glucose metabolism in children with the autistic syndrome: positron tomography analysis. *Brain Development*, 9, 581–587.

deWaal, F. (1989) *Peacemaking Among Primates*. Harvard University Press, Cambridge, Massachusetts.

Deykin, E.Y. and MacMahon, B. (1979) The incidence of seizures among children with autistic symptoms. *American Journal of Psychiatry*, 136, 860–864.

Dicks, D., Myers, R.E., and Kling, A. (1969) Uncus and amygdala lesions: effects on social behavior in the free-ranging rhesus monkey. *Science*, 165, 69–71.

Emery, N.J. and Amaral, D.G. (1999) The role of the amygdala in primate social cognition. In *Cognitive Neuroscience of Emotion* (eds R.D. Lane and L. Nadel), pp. 156–191. Oxford University Press, Oxford.

Emery, N.J., Machado, C.J., Mendoza, S.P., Capitanio, J.P., Mason, W.A., and Amaral, D.G. (1998) Role of the amygdala in dyadic social interactions and the stress response in monkeys. *Society for Neuroscience Abstracts*, 24, 780.

Everitt, B.J. and Robbins T.W. (1992) Amygdala–ventral striatal interactions and reward-related processes. In *The Amygdala: Neurobiological Aspects of Emotion, Memory, and Dysfunction* (ed. J.P. Aggleton), pp. 401–429. Wiley-Liss, New York.

Fein, D., Pennington, B., and Waterhouse, L. (1987) Implications of social deficits in autism for neurological dysfunction. In *Neurobiological Issues in Autism* (eds E. Schopler and G.B. Mesibov), pp. 127–144. Plenum Press, New York.

Fernald, A. (1993) Approval and disapproval: infant responsiveness to vocal affect in familiar and unfamiliar languages. *Child Development*, 64, 657–674.

Fernell, E., Gillberg, C., and Von Wendt, L. (1991) Autistic symptoms in children with infantile hydrocephalus. *Acta Paediatrica Scandinavica*, 80, 451–457.

Filipek, P.A., Richelme, C., Kennedy, D.N., Rademacher, J., Pitcher, D.A., Zidel, S.Y., and Caviness, V.S. (1992) Morphometric analysis of the brain in developmental language disorders and autism. *Annals of Neurology*, 32, 475.

Fotheringham, J.B. (1991) Autism and its primary psychosocial and neurological deficit. *Canadian Journal of Psychiatry*, 36, 686–692.

Franzen, E.A. and Myers, R.E. (1973) Neural control of social behavior: prefrontal and anterior temporal cortex. *Neuropsychologia*, 11, 141–157.

Fried, I., MacDonald, K.A., and Wilson C.L. (1997) Single neuron activity in human hippocamus and amygdala during recognition of faces and objects. *Neuron*, 18, 753–765.

George, M.S., Costa, D.C., Kouris, K., Ring, H.A., and Ell, P.J. (1992) Cerebral blood flow abnormalities in adults with infantile autism. *Journal of Nervous and Mental Diseases*, 180, 413–417.

George, M.S., Ketter, T.A., Parekh, P.I., Horowitz, B., Herscovitch, P., and Post, R.M. (1995) Brain activity during transient sadness and happiness in healthy women. *American Journal of Psychiatry*, 152, 341–351.

Ghaziuddin, M., Tsai, L.Y., Eilers, L., and Ghaziuddin, N. (1992) Brief report: autism and herpes simplex encephalitis. *Journal of Autism and Developmental Disorders*, 22, 107–113.

Gloor, P. (1997) *The Temporal Lobe and Limbic System*. Oxford University Press, Oxford.

Goldman, P.S. (1971) Functional development of the prefrontal cortex in early life and the problem of neuronal plasticity. *Experimental Neurology*, 32, 640–650.

Grandin, T. (1996) *Thinking in Pictures and Other Reports of My Life With Autism*. Vintage Books, New York.

Green, L., Fein, D., Joy, S., and Waterhouse, L. (1995) Cognitive functioning in autism: an overview. In *Learning and Cognition in Autism* (eds E. Schopler and G. Mesibov), pp. 13–31. Plenum Press, New York.

Halgren, E. (1992) Emotional neurophysiology of the amygdala within the context of human cognition. In *The Amygdala: Neurobiological Aspects of Emotion, Memory, and Dysfunction* (ed. J.P. Aggleton), pp. 191–228. Wiley-Liss, New York.

Halgren, E., Baudena, P., Heit, G., Clarke, J.M., and Marinkovic, K. (1994) Spatio-temporal stages in face and word processing. II. Depth-recorded potentials in the human frontal and Rolandic cortices. *Journal of Physiology*, 88, 1–50.

Hamann, S.B., Stefanacci, L., Squire, L.R., Adolps, R., Tranel, D., Damasio, H., and Damasio, A. (1996) Recognizing facial emotion. *Nature*, 379, 417.

Hasselmo, M.E., Rolls, E.T., and Baylis, G.C. (1989a) The role of expression and identity in the face-selective responses of neurons in the temporal visual cortex of the monkey. *Behavioural Brain Research*, 32, 203–218.

Hasselmo, M.E., Rolls, E.T., Baylis, G.C., and Nalwa, V. (1989b) Object-centered encoding by face-receptive neurons in the cortex in the superior temporal sulcus of the monkey. *Experimental Brain Research*, 75, 417–429.

Hauser, S.L., DeLong, G.R., and Rosman, N.P. (1975) Pneumoencephalographic finding in the infantile autism syndrome: a correlation with temporal lobe disease. *Brain*, 98, 667–668.

Hayman, L.A., Rexer, J.L., Pavol, M.A., Strite, D., and Meyers, C.A. (1998) Klüver–Bucy syndrome after bilateral selective damage of amygdala and its cortical connections. *Journal of Neuropsychiatry and Clinical Neuroscience*, 10, 354–358.

Herold, S., Frackowiak, R.S.J., LeCouteur, A., Rutter, M., and Howlin, P. (1988) Cerebral blood flow and metabolism of oxygen and glucose in young autistic adults. *Psychological Medicine*, 18, 823–831.

Hetzler, B.E. and Griffin, J.L. (1981) Infantile autism and the temporal lobe of the brain. *Journal of Autism and Developmental Disorders*, 9 153–157.

Hier, D.B., Lemay, M., and Rosenbergher, P.B. (1979) Autism and unfavorable left–right asymmetries of the brain. *Journal of Autism and Developmental Disorders*, 9, 153–159.

Hinde, R.A. and Spencer-Booth, Y. (1967) The behaviour of socially living rhesus monkeys in their first two and a half years. *Animal Behaviour*, 15, 169–196.

Hitchcock, E. and Cairns, V. (1973) Amygdalotomy. *Postgraduate Medical Journal*, 49, 894–904

Hobson, R.P. (1986) The autistic child appraisal of expressions of emotion. *Journal of Child Psychology and Psychiatry*, 27, 321–342.

Hobson, R.P., Ouston, J., and Lee A. (1988) Emotion recognition in autism: coordinating faces and voices. *Psychological Medicine*, 18, 911–923.

Hof, P.R., Knabe, R., Bovier, P., and Bouras, C. (1991) Neuropathological observations in a case of autism presenting with self-injury behavior. *Acta Neuropathologica*, 82, 321–326.

Hoon, A.H. and Reiss, A.L. (1992) The mesial-temporal lobe and autism: case report and review. *Developmental Medicine and Child Neurology*, 34, 252–265.

Horwitz, B., Rumsey, J.M., Grady, C.L., and Rapoport, S.I. (1988) The cerebral metabolic landscape in autism. Intercorrelations of regional glucose utilization. *Archives of Neurology*, 45, 749–755.

Humphrey, T. (1968) The development of the human amygdala during early embryonic life. *Journal of Comparative Neurology*, 132, 135–165.

Irwin, W., Davidson, R.J., Lowe, M.J., Mock, B.J., Sorenson, J.A., and Turski, P.A. (1996) Human amygdala activation detected with echo-planar functional magnetic resonance imaging. *NeuroReport*, 7, 1765–1769.

Jacobson, R., Le Couteur, A., Howlin, P., and Rutter, M. (1988) Selective subcortical abnormalities in autism. *Psychological Medicine*, 18, 39–48.

Jürgens, U. (1982) Amygdalar vocalization pathways in the squirrel monkey. *Brain Research*, 241, 189–196.

Jürgens, U. and Ploog, D. (1970) Cerebral representation of vocalization in the squirrel monkey. *Experimental Brain Research*, 10, 532–554.

Jürgens, U. and von Cramon, D. (1982) On the role of the anterior cingulate cortex in phonation: a case report. *Brain Language*, 15, 234–248

Kalin, N.H. and Shelton, S.E. (1989) Defensive behaviors in infant rhesus monkeys: environmental cues and neurochemical regulation. *Science*, 243, 1718–1721.

Kalin, N.H., Shelton, S.E., and Takahashi, L.K. (1991) Defensive behaviors in rhesus monkeys: their ontogeny and context-dependent selective expression. *Child Development*, 62, 1175–1183.

Kanner, L. (1943) Autistic disturbances of affective contact. *Nervous Child*, 2, 217–250.

Ketter, T.A., Andreason, P.J., George, M.S., Lee, C., Gill, D.S., Parekh, P.I., Willis, M.W., Herscovitch, P., and Post, R.M. (1996) Anterior paralimbic mediation of procaine-induced emotional and psychosensory experiences. *Archives of General Psychiatry*, 53, 59–69.

Kling, A.S. (1966) Ontogenetic and phylogenetic studies on the amygdaloid nuclei. *Psychosomatic Medicine*, 28, 155–161.

Kling, A.S. (1972) Effects of amygdalectomy on social-affective behavior in non-human primates. In *The Neurobiology of the Amygdala* (ed. B.E. Eleftheriou), pp. 511–536. Plenum Press, New York.

Kling, A.S. (1974) Differential effects of amygdalectomy in male and female nonhuman primates. *Archives of Sexual Behavior*, 3, 129–134.

Kling, A.S. and Brothers, L. (1992) The amygdala and social behavior. In *The Amygdala: Neurobiological Aspects of Emotion, Memory, and Dysfunction* (ed. J.P. Aggleton), pp. 353–377. Wiley-Liss, New York.

Kling, A. and Cornell, R. (1971) Amygdalectomy and social behavior in the caged stump-tailed (*M.speciosa*). *Folia Primatology*, 14, 91–103.

Kling, A. and Dunne, K. (1976) Social–environmental factors affecting behavior and plasma testosterone in normal and amygdala lesioned *M.speciosa*. *Primates*, 17, 23–42.

Kling, A. and Green, P.C. (1967) Effects of neonatal amygdalectomy in the maternally reared and maternally deprived macaque. *Nature*, 213, 742–743.

Kling, A.S., Steklis, H.D., and Deutsch, S. (1979) Radiotelemetered activity from the amygdala during social interactions in the monkeys. *Experimental Neurology*, 66, 88–96.

Klinger, J. and Gloor, P. (1960) The connections of the amygdala and the anterior temporal cortex in the human brain. *Journal of Comparative Neurology*, 115, 333–369.

Kordower, J.H., Piecinski, P., and Rakic. P. (1992) Neurogenesis of the amygdaloid nuclear complex in the rhesus monkey. *Developmental Brain Research*, 68, 9–15.

Klüver, H. and Bucy, P. (1938) An analysis of certain effects of bilateral temporal lobectomy in rhesus monkeys. *American Journal of Physiology*, 5, 33–54.

Klüver, H. and Bucy, P. (1939) Preliminary analysis of functioning of the temporal lobes in monkeys. *Archives of Neurology and Psychiatry*, 42, 979–1000.

Lanska, D.J. and Lanska, M.J. (1993) Klüver–Bucy syndrome in juvenile neuronal ceroid lipofuscinosis. *Journal of Child Neurology*, 9, 67–69.

Leonard, C.M., Rolls, E.T., Wilson, F.A.W., and Baylis, G.C. (1985) Neurons in the amygdala of the monkey with responses selective for faces. *Behavioural Brain Research*, 15, 159–176.

Lilly, R., Cummings, J.L., Benson, F., and Frankel, M. (1983) The human Klüver–Bucy syndrome. *Neurology*, 33, 1141–1145.

Loveland, K.A. and Landry, S. (1986) Joint attention and communication in autism and language-delay children. *Journal of Autism and Developmental Disorders*, 16, 335–349.

Macdonald, H., Rutter, M., Howlin, P., Rios, P., Le Conteur, A., Evered, C., and Folstein, S. (1989) Recognition and expression of emotional faces by autistic and normal adults. *Journal of Child Psychology and Psychiatry*, 30, 865–877.

MacLean, P.D. (1949) Psychosomatic disease and the 'visceral brain': recent developments bearing on the Papez theory of emotion. *Psychosomatic Medicine*, 11, 338–353.

Málková, L., Mishkin, M., Suomi, S.J., and Bachevalier, J. (1997) Socioemotional behavior in adult rhesus monkeys after early versus late lesions of the medial temporal lobe. *Annals of the New York Academy of Sciences*, 807, 538–540.

Mazataka, N. (1984) Development of vocal recognition of mothers in infant Japanese macaques. *Developmental Psychobiology*, 18, 107–114.

McGaugh, J.L., Introini-Collison, E.B., Cahill, L., Kim, M., and Liang, K.C. (1992) Involvement of the amygdala in neuromodulatory influences on memory storage. In *The Amygdala: Neurobiological Aspects of Emotion, Memory, and Dysfunction* (ed. J.P. Aggleton), pp. 401–430. Wiley-Liss, New York.

Mendelson, M.J. (1982) Clinical examination of visual and social responses in infant rhesus monkeys. *Developmental Psychology*, 18, 658–662.

Meunier, M., Bachevalier, J., Murray E.A., Málková, L., and Mishkin, M. (1999) Effects of aspiration vs neurotoxic lesions of the amygdala on emotional responses in monkeys. *European Journal of Neuroscience*, 11, 4403–4418.

Minshew, N.J., Goldstein, G., Dombrowski, S.M., Panchalingam, K., and Pettegrew, J.W. (1993) A preliminary ^{31}P MRS study of autism: evidence for undersynthesis and increased degradation of brain membranes. *Biological Psychiatry*, 33, 762–773.

Mirsky, A.F. (1960) Studies of the effects of brain lesions on social behaviors in *Macaca mulatta*: methodological and theoretical considerations. *Annals of the New York Academy of Sciences*, 85, 785–94.

Morris, J.S., Frith, C.D., Perrett, D.I., Rowland, D., Young, A.W., Calder, A.J., and Dolan R.J. (1996) A differential neural response in the human amygdala to fearful and happy facial expression. *Nature*, 383, 812–815.

Morris, J.S., Friston, K.J., Büchel, C., Frith, C.D., Young, A.W., Calder, A.J., and Dolan, R.J. (1998) A neuromodulatory role for the human amygdala in processing emotional facial expressions. *Brain*, 121, 47–57.

Mountz, J.M., Tolbert, L.C., Lill, D.W., Katholi, C.R., and Liu, H.-G. (1995) Functional deficits in autistic disorder: characterization by technetium-99m-HMPAO and SPECT. *Journal of Nuclear Medicine*, 36, 1156–1162.

Myers, R.E. and Swett, C. (1970) Social behavior deficits of free-ranging monkeys after anterior temporal cortex removal: a preliminary report. *Brain Research*, 18, 551–556.

Nahm, F.K.D., Tranel, D., Damasio, H., and Damasio, A.R. (1993) Cross-modal associations and the human amygdala. *Neuropsychologia*, 31, 727–744.

Nalwa, V. and Bachevalier, J. (1991) Absence of Klüver–Bucy symptoms after neonatal limbic lesions in infant rhesus monkeys. *Society for Neuroscience Abstracts*, 17, 664.

Nelson, C.A. (1985) The perception and recognition of facial expresions in infancy. In *Social Perception in Infants* (eds T.M. Field and N.A. Fox), pp. 101–125. Ablex Press, Norwod, New Jersey.

Nelson, C.A. (1993) The recognition of facial expressions in infancy: behavioral and electrophysiological correlates. In *Developmental Neurocognition: Speech and Face Processing in the First Year of Life* (B. de Boysson-Bardies, S. de Schonen, P. Jusczyk, P. MacNeilage, and J. Morton), pp. 187–193. Kluwer Academic Press, The Netherlands.

Newman, J.D. and Bachevalier, J. (1997) Neonatal ablations of the amygdala and inferior temporal cortex alter the vocal response to social separation in rhesus macaques. *Brain Research*, 758, 180–186.

Nikolic, I. and Kostovic, I. (1986) Development of the lateral amygdaloid nucleus of the human fetus: transient presence of discrete cytoarchitectonic units. *Anatomical Embryology*, 174, 355-360.

Papez, J.W. (1937) A proposed mechanism of emotion. *Archives of Neurology and Psychiatry*, 38, 725–744.

Payton, J.B. and Minshew, N.J. (1987) Early appearance of partial complex seizures in children with infantile autism. *Annals of Neurology*, 22, 408.

Perrett, D.L. and Mistlin, A.J. (1990) Perception of facial characteristics by monkeys. In *Comparative Perception* (eds M. Berkeley and W. Stebbins), pp. 53–71. John Wiley and Sons, New York.

Perrett, D.L., Rolls, E.T., and Caan, W. (1982) Visual neurons responsive to faces in the monkey temporal cortex. *Experimental Brain Research*, 47, 329–342.

Perrett, D.L., Smith, P.A.J., Potter, D.D., Mistlin, A.J., Head, A.S., Milner, A.D., and Jeeves, M.A. (1984) Neurones responsive to faces in the temporal cortex: studies of functional organization, sensitivity to identity and relation to perception. *Human Neurobiology*, 3, 197–208.

Perrett, D.L., Smith, P.A.J., Potter, D.D., Mistlin, A.J., Head, A.S., Milner, A.D., and Jeeves, M.A. (1985) Visual cells in the temporal cortex sensitive to faces view and gaze direction. *Proceedings of the Royal Society of London, Series B*, 223, 293–317.

Piven, J., Saliba, K., Bailey, J., and Arndt, S. (1997) An MRI study of autism: the cerebellum revisited. *Neurology*, 49, 546–551.

Piven, J., Bailey, J., Ranson, B.J., and Arndt, S. (1998) No difference in hippocampus volume detected on magnetic resonance imaging in autistic individuals. *Journal of Autism and Developmental Disorders*, 28, 105–110.

Ploog, D. (1986) Biological foundations of the vocal expressions of emotions. In *Emotion: Theory, Research, and Experience* (eds R. Plutchik and H. Kellerman), Vol. 3, pp. 173–197. Academic Press, New York.

Plotnik, R. (1968) Changes in social behavior of squirrel monkeys after anterior temporal lobectomy. *Journal of Comparative and Physiological Psychiatry*, 66, 369–372.

Rauch, S.L., Savage, C.R., Alpert, N.M., Miguel, E.C., Baer, L., Breiter, H.C., Fischman, A.J., Manzo, P.A., Moretti, C., and Jenike, M.A. (1995) A positron emission tomographic study of simple phobic symptom provocation. *Archives of General Psychiatry*, 52, 20–28.

Reiss, A.L., Lee, J., and Freund, L. (1994) Neuroanatomy of fragile X syndrome: the temporal lobe. *Neurology*, 44, 1317–1324.

Robinson, B.W. (1967) Vocalization evoked from forebrain *in Macaca mulatta. Physiology and Behavior*, 2, 345–354.

Rodman, H.R. (1994) Development of inferior temporal cortex in the monkey. *Cerebral Cortex*, 5, 484–498.

Rolls, E.T. (1986) A theory of emotion, and its application to understanding the neural basis of emotion. In *Emotions* (ed. Y. Oomura), pp. 325–344. Japan Scientific Society, Tokyo.

Rolls, E.T. (1994) A theory of emotion and consciousness, and its application to understanding the neural basis of emotion. In *The Cognitive Neurosciences* (ed. M.S. Gazzaniga), pp. 1091–1106. MIT Press, Cambridge, Massachusetts.

Rosenblum, L.A. (1961) The development of social behavior in the rhesus monkey. Unpublished doctoral dissertation, University of Wisconsin.

Rossitch, E., and Oakes, W.J. (1989) Klüver–Bucy syndrome in a child with bilateral arachnoid cysts: report of a case. *Neurosurgery*, 24, 110–112.

Rosvold, H.E., Mirsky A.F., and Pribram K.H. (1954) Influence of amygdalectomy on social behavior in monkeys. *Journal of Comparative and Physiological Psychology*, 47, 173–178.

Rumsey, J.M., Duara, R., Grady, C., Rapoport, J.L., Margolin R.A., Rapoport, S.I. and Cutler, N.R. (1985) Brain metabolism in autism. Resting cerebral glucose utilization rates as measured with positron emission tomography. *Archives of General Psychiatry*, 42, 448–455.

Ruppenthal, G.C., Walker, C.G., and Sackett, G.P. (1991) Rearing infant monkeys (*Macaca nemestrina*) in pairs produces deficient social development compared with rearing in single cages. *American Journal of Primatology*, 25, 103–113.

Sackett G.P. (1966) Monkeys reared in isolation with pictures as visual inputs: evidence for an innate releasing mechanism. *Science*, 154, 1468–1472.

Sackett, G.P. (1982) Can single processes explain effects of postnatal influences on primate development? In *The Development of Attachment and Affiliative Systems* (eds R.N. Emde and R.J. Harmon), pp. 3–12. Plenum Press, New York.

Saitoh, O., Courchesne, E., Egaas, B., Lincoln, A.J., and Schreibman, L. (1995) Cross-sectional area of the posterior hippocampus in autistic patients with cerebellar and corpus callosum abnormalities. *Neurology*, 45, 317–324.

Saunders, R.C. and Rosene D.L. (1988) A comparison of the efferents of the amygdala and the hippocampal formation in the rhesus monkey: I. Convergence in the entorhinal, prorhinal, and perirhinal cortices. *Journal of Comparative Neurology*, 271, 153–184.

Saunders, R.C., Rosene, D.C., and Van Hoesen, G.W. (1988) Comparison of the efferents of the amygdala and the hippocampal formation in the rhesus monkey: II. Reciprocal and non-reciprocal connections. *Journal of Comparative Neurology*, 271, 185–207.

Saunders, R.C., Kolachana, B.S., Bachevalier, J., and Weinberger, D.R. (1998) Neonatal lesions of the medial temporal lobe disrupt prefrontal cortical regulation of striatal dopamine. *Nature*, 393, 169–171.

Schneider, M.L. and Suomi, S.J. (1992) Neurobehavioral assessment in rhesus monkeys neonates (*Macaca mulatta*): developmental changes, behavioral stability, and early experience. *Infant Behavior and Development*, 15, 155–177.

Schore, A.N. (1994) *Affect Regulation and the Origin of the Self: The Neurobiology of Emotional Development*. Lawrence Erlbaum, Hillsdale, New Jersey.

Scott, S.K., Young, A.W., Calder, A.J., Hellawell, D.J., Aggleton, J.P., and Johnson, M. (1997) Impaired auditory recognition of fear and anger following bilateral amygdala lesions. *Nature*, 385, 254–257.

Scoville, W.B., Dunsmore, R.H., Liberson, W.T., Henry, C.E., and Pepe, A. (1953) Observations on medial temporal lobotomy and uncotomy in the treatment of psychotic states. *Research Publications, Association of Research on Nervous and Mental Diseases*, 31, 347–369.

Seeck, M., Mainwaring, N., Ives, J., Blume, H., Dubuisson, D., Cosgrove, R., Mesulam, M.M., and Schomer, D.L. (1993) Differential neural activity in the human temporal lobe evoked by faces of family members and friends. *Annals of Neurology*, 34, 369–372.

Siegel, B.V., Nuechterlein, K.H., Abel, L., Wu, J.C., and Buchsbaum, M.S. (1995) Glucose metabolic correlates of continuous performance test performance in adults with a history of infantile autism, schizophrenics, and controls. *Schizophrenia Research*, 17, 85–94.

Sigman, M., Mundy, P., Sherman, R., and Ungerer, J. (1996) Social interactions of autistic, mentally retarded, and normal children and their caregivers. *Journal of Child Psychology and Psychiatry*, 27, 647–656.

Sims, K.S. and Williams, R.S. (1990) The human amygdaloid complex: a cytologic and histochemical atlas using Nissl, myelin, acetylcholinesterase and nicotinamide adenine dinucleotide phosphate diaphorase staining. *Neuroscience*, 36, 449–472.

Stephan, H., Frahm, H.D., and Baron, G. (1987) Comparison of brain structure volumes in insectivores and primates. VII. Amygdaloid components. *Journal für Hirnforsch*, 28, 571–584.

Streit, M., Ioannides, A.A., Liu, L., Wölwer, W., Dammers, J., Gross, J., Gaebel, W., and Müller-Gärtner, H.W. (1999) Neurophysiological correlates of the recognition of facial expressions of emotion as revealed by magnetoencephalography. *Cognitive Brain Research*, 7, 481–491.

Suomi S.J. (1977) The development of attachment and other social behaviors in rhesus monkeys. In *Attachment Behavior* (eds L. Krames, T. Alloway, and Liner, P.), pp. 119–159. Plenum Press, New York.

Suomi, S.J. (1997) Long-term effects of different early rearing experiences on social, emotional, and physiological development in nonhuman primates. In *Neurodevelopment and Adult Psychopathology* (eds M.S. Keshavan and R.M. Murray), pp. 104–116. Cambridge University Press, Cambridge.

Tantam, D. (1992) Characterizing the fundamental social handicap in autism. *Acta Paedopsychologia*, 55, 83–91.

Terzian, H. and Delle-Ore, G. (1955) Syndrome of Klüver–Bucy reproduced in man by bilateral removal of temporal lobes. *Neurology*, 3, 373–380.

Thompson, C.I. (1981) Long-term behavioral development of rhesus monkeys after amygdalectomy in infancy. In *The Amygdaloid Complex* (ed. Y. Ben-Ari), pp. 259–270. Elsevier, Amsterdam.

Thompson, C.I. and Towfighi J.T. (1976) Social behavior of juvenile rhesus monkeys after amygdalectomy in infancy. *Physiology and Behavior*, 17, 831–836.

Thompson, C.I., Schwartzbaum, J.S., and Harlow, H.F. (1969) Development of social fear after amygdalectomy in infant rhesus monkeys. *Physiology and Behavior*, 4, 249–254.

Thompson, C.I., Bergland R.M., and Towfighi, J.T. (1977) Social and nonsocial behaviors of adult rhesus monkeys after amygdalectomy in infancy or adulthood. *Journal of Comparative and Physiological Psychology*, 91, 533–548.

Tonsgard, J.H., Harwicke, N., and Levine, S.C. (1987) Klüver–Bucy syndrome in children. *Pediatric Neurology*, 3, 162–165.

Tranel, D. and Hyman, B.T. (1990) Neuropsychological correlates of bilateral amygdala damage. *Archives of Neurology*, 47, 349–355.

Trevarthen, C. (1989) The relation of autism to normal socio-cultural development: the case for a primary disorder in regulation of cognitive growth by emotions. In *Autisme et Troubles du Developpement Global de L'Enfant* (eds G. Lelord, J.P. Muh, M. Petit, and D. Sauvage), pp. 1–26 Expansion Scientifique, Paris.

Webster, M.J., Ungerleider, L.G., and Bachevalier, J. (1991) Connections of inferior temporal areas TE and TEO with medial temporal-lobe structures in infant and adult monkeys. *Journal of Neuroscience*, 11, 1095–1116.

White, C.P. and Rosenbloom, L. (1992) Temporal-lobe structures and autism. *Developmental Medicine and Child Neurology*, 34, 558–559.

Williams, R.S., Hauser, S.L., Purpura, P.D., DeLong, R., and Swisher, C.N. (1980) Autism and mental retardation: neuropathologic studies in four retarded persons with autistic behavior. *Archives of Neurology*, 37, 749–753.

Yamane, S., Kaji, S., and Kawao, K. (1988) What facial features activate face neurons in the inferotemporal cortex of the monkey? *Experimental Brain Research*, 73, 209–214.

Yirmiya, N., Kasari, C., Sigman, M., and Mundy P. (1989) Facial expressions of affect in autistic, mentally retarded, and normal children. *Journal of Child Psychology and Psychiatry*, 30, 725–736.

Young, A.W, Hellawell, D.J., Van de Wakl, C., and Johnson, M. (1996) Facial expression processing after amygdalectomy. *Neuropsychologia*, 34, 31–39.

Zilbovicius, M., Garreau, B., Tzourio, N., Mazoyer, B., Bruck, B., Martinot, J.-L., Raynaud, C., Samson, Y., Syrota, A., and Lelord, G. (1992) Regional cerebral blood flow in childhood autism: a SPECT study. *Amerian Journal of Psychiatry*, 149, 924–930.

Zilbovicius, M., Garreau, B., Samson, Y., Remy, P., Barthelemy, C., Syrota, A., and Lelord, G. (1995) Delayed maturation of the frontal cortex in childhood autism. *American Journal of Psychiatry*, 152, 248–252.

16 Reinterpreting the behavioural effects of amygdala lesions in non-human primates

Mark G. Baxter[1] and Elisabeth A. Murray[2]

[1]Department of Psychology, Harvard University, Cambridge, MA 02138 and [2]Laboratory of Neuropsychology, National Institute of Mental Health, Bethesda, MD 20892, USA

Summary

Advances in neurosurgical methods that permit selective damage to the cell bodies of the amygdala, sparing the adjacent temporal cortex and white matter, have improved our understanding of the cognitive functions controlled by this structure. In this chapter, we attempt to summarize and integrate recent work with previous findings based on less selective removals of the amygdala. Recent anatomical and behavioural studies suggest that many behavioural impairments associated with removal of the amygdala by surgical aspiration can be accounted for by disconnection of inferior temporal cortex from its medial thalamic and prefrontal cortical targets rather than by damage to the cell bodies of the amygdala. Based on the currently available evidence, the amygdala appears to play little role in stimulus memory, a relatively restricted role in stimulus–reward associations, and a significant role in emotionality and stimulus–affect association.

16.1 Introduction

The amygdala in non-human primates classically has been thought to be involved in at least three broad domains of cognitive function, namely stimulus memory, stimulus–reward association, and stimulus–affect association (or emotionality). Given this diversity of amygdala contributions to behaviour, an integrated theoretical framework regarding amygdala function has been an elusive goal for neuropsychologists (e.g. Douglas and Pribram, 1966; Mishkin and Aggleton, 1981; Murray, 1990). Recent anatomical investigations, together with neuropsychological studies of the functions of the various ventromedial temporal cortical areas, have helped to clarify the contributions of amygdala versus temporal cortex to several cognitive functions, most notably to stimulus memory. In addition, new surgical methods have allowed investigators to make more selective lesions of the amygdala in non-human primates than heretofore possible, and this, too, has advanced our understanding of amygdala function. In this chapter, we summarize the current state of knowledge regarding the role of the non-human primate amygdala in the three behavioural domains noted above, with the aim of advancing towards the goal of a unified theoretical framework for amygdala function. We neglect the literature on social behaviour in non-human primates, which recently has been reviewed elsewhere (Emery and Amaral, 2000).

16.2 Disconnection of temporal cortex produced by amygdala aspiration

Neuropsychological investigations in non-humann primates, until recently, have relied almost exclusively on results obtained from aspiration lesions of the amygdala. The surgical approach typically used to remove the amygdala damages cortical areas of the temporal lobe subjacent to the amygdala, generally including temporal polar cortex and the anterior part of the entorhinal cortex. This extra-amygdalar damage, which is necessary to gain access to the amygdala, has been well documented. What is just now becoming appreciated, however, is that these lesions also result in damage to projections to and from more lateral portions of the temporal cortex, producing a disconnection of inferior temporal cortical areas from their inputs and targets. Therefore, the effects of aspiration of the amygdala on behaviour may not be accounted for fully by damage to the cell bodies of the amygdala, or direct damage to the cortex immediately subjacent to the amygdala, or the combination thereof, but may represent a more widespread disconnection syndrome.

Gower (1989) and Murray (1992) were among the first to make explicit proposals regarding the potential disconnection that could be produced by aspiration lesions of the amygdala. Although it had been well known that direct physical methods of producing lesions (e.g. radiofrequency or aspiration) could damage fibres of passage as well as cells in the structure of interest, the particular projection systems that could have been damaged by amygdala aspiration had not been identified. Murray suggested that efferents from the rhinal (i.e. entorhinal and perirhinal) cortex that travel just lateral to the amygdala would be transected by the amygdala aspiration lesion (see Figure 4 in Murray, 1992), resulting in a disconnection of the rhinal cortex from some of its targets. As we will discuss in the following sections, this would explain the similarity between certain behavioural effects of amygdala aspiration lesions and effects of lesions of the rhinal cortex.

To investigate this question directly, Goulet *et al.* (1998) placed bilaterally symmetrical injections of a fluorescent retrograde tracer into the medial, magnocellular part of the mediodorsal nucleus of the thalamus (MDmc) in rhesus monkeys that had received an amygdala aspiration lesion in one hemisphere. (This region of this thalamic nucleus is a target of efferents from the rhinal cortex, and was investigated because of the relative ease in achieving bilaterally symmetrical injections in this region, as opposed to other sites.)

Goulet *et al.* then determined the number of retrogradely labelled cells in the temporal cortex of each hemisphere of those monkeys. There were substantially fewer labelled neurons in the entorhinal cortex, perirhinal cortex, and area TE of the hemispheres with amygdala lesions, relative to the same cortical fields in intact hemispheres, indicating that the lesion damaged axons arising from neurons residing in these cortical fields that were projecting to the mediodorsal thalamus. Control regions showed no such hemispheric asymmetry in numbers of retrogradely labelled cells; thus, the result was unlikely to be due to hemispheric differences in the size or locus of the injection sites.

Preliminary data suggest that amygdala aspiration lesions also produce a similar disconnection of inferior temporal cortex from prefrontal cortical regions. Baxter *et al.* (1998) placed bilaterally symmetrical injections of fluorescent retrograde tracers into the ventral and orbital prefrontal cortex of rhesus monkeys who had received an amygdala aspiration lesion in one hemisphere combined with forebrain commissurotomy. Just as had been found by Goulet *et al.* (1998), substantially fewer retrogradely labelled cells were observed in the entorhinal cortex, perirhinal cortex, and area TE of hemispheres with the amygdala aspiration lesion relative to those same regions in intact hemispheres (Figure 16.1).

These findings indicate that amygdala aspiration lesions produce at least a partial disconnection of inferior temporal cortical areas from both thalamic and prefrontal targets. Disruption of inferior temporal cortical–thalamic–prefrontal networks caused by amygdala aspiration lesions could have wider ranging effects on behaviour than either damage to the cell bodies of the amygdala or direct damage to temporal cortex produced by the amygdala aspiration lesion. The implications of these findings for the interpretation of behavioural effects of amygdala aspiration lesions are taken up in the following sections.

It is worth noting that amygdala aspiration lesions also appear to disconnect the temporal cortex from inputs from the basal forebrain, hypothalamus, and substantia nigra, and potentially other subcortical inputs as well (D. Gaffan, personal communication). The results of crossed lesion experiments demonstrate that disconnection of temporal cortex from these structures, by combining a large lesion of inferior temporal cortex in one hemisphere with a small radiofrequency lesion in the hypothalamus of the other hemisphere, results in behavioural impairments like those associated with aspiration lesions of the amygdala (Easton and Gaffan, 1997), though, in accord with the more extensive inferior temporal cortex damage, the deficits appear to be more severe than after amygdalectomy (at least with regard to the particular behavioural domains examined in their study). Hence, at least some behavioural impairments that follow aspiration lesions of the amygdala appear to result from either partial disconnection of inferior temporal cortex from basal forebrain/hypothalamic/substantia nigra inputs, or from compromised outputs of inferior temporal cortex to prefrontal and thalamic targets, or the combination. If the latter, then whether the effects of these two different types of disconnection might represent disruption of different, perhaps serial, computational processes, or, alternatively, different parallel processes remains to be determined.

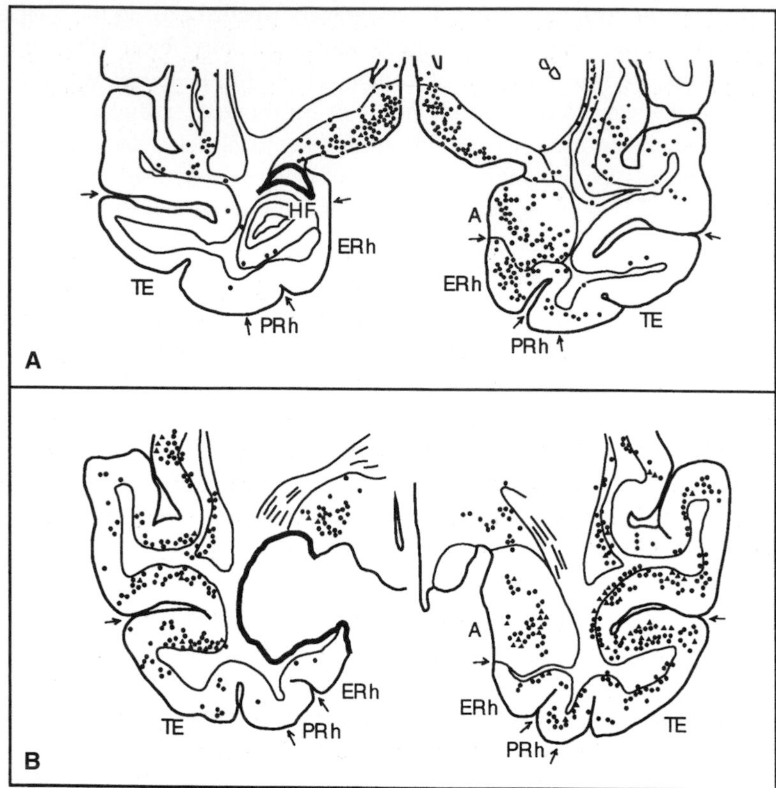

Figure 16.1 Comparison of intact (right) hemispheres and hemispheres with amygdala removals (left) from rhesus monkey brains with symmetrically placed bilateral injections of fluorescent retrograde tracers into the medial part of the mediodorsal thalamus (**A**) or ventral and orbital prefrontal cortex (**B**). The number of retrogradely labelled neurons is reduced dramatically in the entorhinal cortex, perirhinal cortex, and area TE of hemispheres with the amygdala aspiration lesion. Abbreviations: ERh, entorhinal cortex; PRh, perirhinal cortex; TE, area TE of von Bonin and Bailey (1947). Arrows indicate approximate boundaries between cytoarchitectonic fields. In both (A) and (B), a filled triangle represents five retrogradely labelled cells, whereas a filled circle represents one retrogradely labelled cell. Data are from Goulet *et al.* (1998) (A) and Baxter *et al.* (1998) (B).

16.3 Reinterpreting behavioural effects of 'amygdala' lesions

New methods that use magnetic resonance imaging (MRI) combined with stereotaxically guided injections of neurotoxins can yield selective damage to cell bodies in the amygdala, sparing the subjacent cortex and fibres of passage (Figure 16.2). Thus, it is now possible to examine the role of selective damage to the cells of the amygdala on behaviour in non-human primates. In the following sections, we compare the findings from these new studies with those from older experiments using less selective lesion methods.

16.4 Stimulus memory

Stimulus recognition memory refers to the process by which a novel stimulus becomes familiar. For over 30 years, the delayed matching- and non-matching-to-sample (DMS and DNMS) tasks have been used to investigate the neural basis of stimulus recognition memory in non-human primates. In the first phase of each DNMS trial, the monkey is allowed to view a sample object that covers the central well of a three-well test tray. The monkey displaces the object, obtains a food reward hidden underneath the object, and an opaque screen is lowered that occludes the monkey's view of the test tray. In the second phase of each trial, which takes place after a delay ranging from seconds to minutes, the opaque screen is raised and the monkey is allowed to choose between the sample object and a novel object, one covering each of the lateral wells of the test tray. The monkey can obtain another food reward by displacing the novel object.

The amygdala has been suggested to participate in several aspects of stimulus recognition memory. The amygdala and hippocampus were once thought to be equally important in mediating stimulus recognition. This conclusion arose from an influential study by Mishkin (1978), who found that combined, but not separate, damage to the amygdala and hippocampus produced a severe deficit in visual recognition memory. These two structures appeared to play equivalent roles in stimulus recognition memory (Saunders *et al.*, 1984). The deficit produced by combined amygdala plus hippocampal lesions was not restricted to the visual modality, as it extended to recognition of tactile stimuli as well (Murray and Mishkin, 1983, 1984). A subsequent investigation found that impairments in stimulus recognition memory could be produced by combined removal of the amygdala and portions of the rhinal cortex, sparing the hippocampus, but that combined removal of the hippocampus and portions of the rhinal cortex had relatively little effect on stimulus recognition memory, suggesting that the amygdala, but not the hippocampus, was critical for stimulus recognition memory (Murray and Mishkin, 1986). Hence, the data available at the time were consistent with the idea that damage to the amygdala was required to produce a global and severe deficit in stimulus memory.

Zola-Morgan *et al.* (1989) examined the effects of electrolytic lesions of the amygdala, and reported that amygdala lesions did not exacerbate the recognition memory impairment associated with damage to temporal cortex (perirhinal and parahippocampal cortex). Murray and Mishkin (1998) studied the effects of selective lesions of the amygdala and hippocampus using the neurotoxin ibotenic acid, and showed definitively that neither of these structures was required for recognition memory, even at delays extending as long as 40 min. Damage to the subjacent rhinal cortex, however, produced an impairment in DNMS nearly as severe as that caused by combined aspiration lesions of the amygdala and hippocampus (Meunier *et al.*, 1993). It now seems likely that the originally reported recognition memory impairment was caused by a combination of direct and indirect damage to the rostral and caudal portions

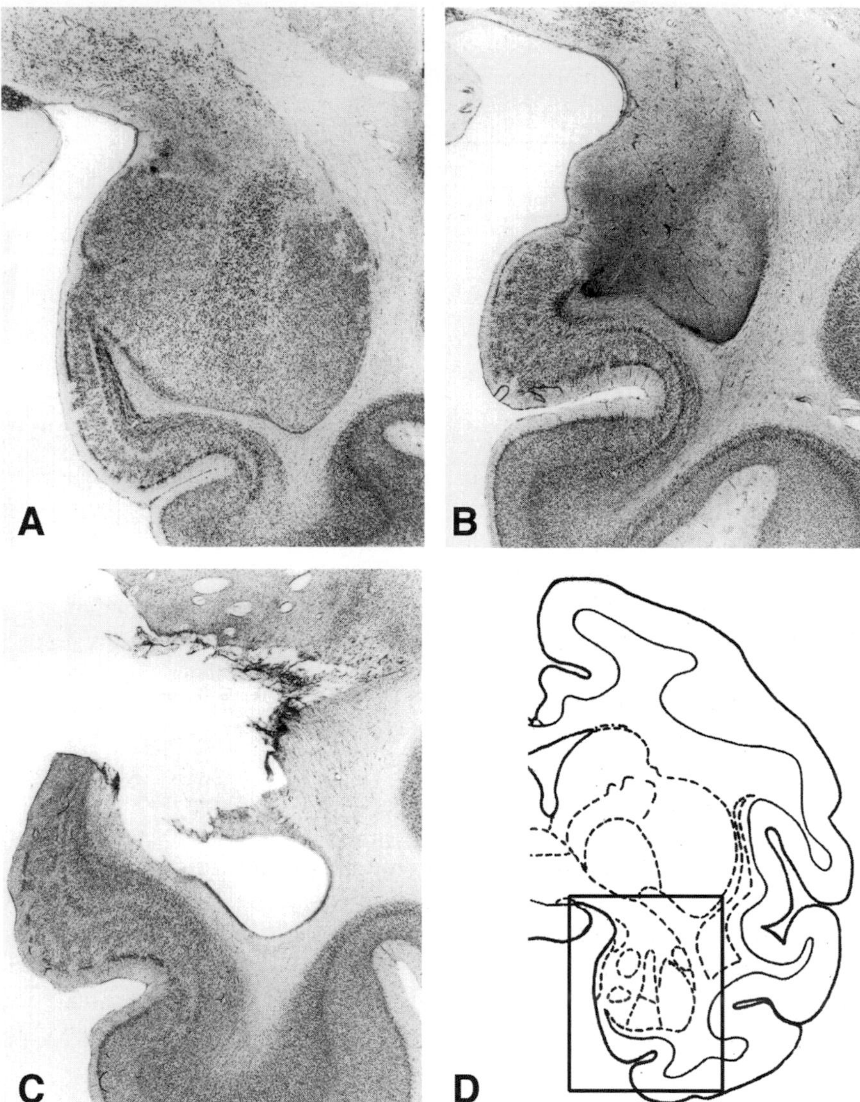

Figure 16.2 (A–C) Photomicrographs of Nissl-stained coronal sections through the mid-amygdala of rhesus monkeys (*Macaca mulatta*) comparing intact versus aspiration and excitotoxic amygdala lesions. (**A**) Bright-field photomicrograph of the temporal lobe in an intact monkey showing nuclei of the amygdala together with subjacent entorhinal and perirhinal cortex. (**B**) Photomicrograph of the same region shown in (A) following stereotaxically guided injections of ibotenic acid. Note the massive cell loss, gliosis, and atrophy in regions of amygdala, together with relative sparing of adjacent white matter and underlying cortex. (**C**) Photomicrograph of the same region as shown in (A) following an aspiration lesion of the amygdala. Note that the aspiration lesion invades the white matter of the

of the ventromedial temporal cortex, mainly the perirhinal cortex, rather than to combined damage to the amygdala and hippocampus. The reader is referred to Murray (1992), Goulet *et al.* (1998), and Murray and Mishkin (1998) for a more detailed discussion of this topic.

Although the most recent studies reviewed above indicated that the amygdala, either alone or together with the hippocampus, was not critical for the recognition of trial-unique objects, it was thought that the amygdala was essential for recognition of *familiar* stimuli. On a version of the DNMS task in which the same two objects are used throughout testing, the monkey cannot rely on familiarity with the stimulus to make a correct choice, but must recall which of the two familiar stimuli served as a sample more recently. This version of the task is more difficult as it requires identification of which stimulus was presented more recently, rather than merely which stimulus has been presented previously at all. Damage to the amygdala (but not the hippocampus) produced a severe impairment in relearning of DMS with a single pair of objects (Correll and Scoville, 1965; Mishkin and Oubre, 1976). A subsequent experiment (Murray *et al.*, 1996), however, demonstrated that neurotoxic lesions of the amygdala do not produce a consistent effect on relearning of DNMS with a single pair of objects, but removal of the anterior portion of the rhinal cortex (subjacent to the amygdala) does. Therefore, learning to discriminate which of two familiar stimuli appeared most recently, a function that was once attributed to the amygdala, appears to be a property of the rhinal cortex. We hasten to add that the effect of rhinal cortex lesions seems to be limited to learning/relearning (as opposed to performance over delays) of the single-pair DNMS task, or is perhaps a transient deficit; Eacott *et al.* (1994) found no effect of rhinal cortex lesions on DMS with a single pair of objects, but those monkeys had received extensive postoperative training on DMS and had experienced a gradual reduction in the set size used in testing.

The previous discussion shows that stimulus recognition memory can proceed in the absence of the amygdala. However, the foregoing discussion is concerned only with *intramodal* stimulus recognition, i.e. recognizing a visual stimulus when it is presented again in the visual modality, or a tactile stimulus when it is presented again in the tactile modality. The amygdala has also been implicated strongly in *crossmodal* recognition, i.e. recognizing (identifying) a stimulus in a modality different from that in which it was first encountered. For example, in tactual-to-visual crossmodal DNMS, a monkey encounters the sample stimulus tactually (i.e. sample displacement in the dark), then must make a recognition judgement (choosing the novel stimulus) based on visual properties of the objects (i.e. choice test in the light; the monkey is not permitted to compare the objects tactually before choosing). Like DNMS with familiar stimuli, the amygdala was accorded a central role in crossmodal recognition: aspiration lesions of the amygdala alone produced an inability to perform the crossmodal DNMS task postoperatively (Murray and Mishkin, 1985), even if it had been acquired preoperatively (Málková and Murray, 1996). This crossmodal impairment was

---

temporal stem just lateral to the amygdala. Also, although the entorhinal cortex is largely intact in this example, aspiration lesions often include much of this region. Compare and contrast with Figure 16.1. (**D**) Drawing of a standard coronal brain section from a rhesus monkey (right hemisphere only) at the same level as shown in (A–C). The approximate region shown in the photomicrographs (A–C) is outlined.

striking and fairly selective, as the same monkeys were able to perform well on the intramodal versions of DNMS using the same objects, test apparatus, and short intratrial delays (Murray and Mishkin, 1985). In contrast, lesions of the hippocampus had no such detrimental effect on crossmodal DNMS (Murray and Mishkin, 1985).

To evaluate the contribution of the amygdala to this task more directly, Goulet and Murray (1995) tested monkeys with either neurotoxic lesions of the amygdala, or aspiration lesions of the anterior portion of the rhinal cortex (i.e. that part of the rhinal cortex that ordinarily would be most disrupted by aspiration amygdala lesions), on crossmodal DNMS. After postoperative retraining on visual and tactual versions of DNMS, the monkeys were retested on crossmodal non-matching. After extensive retraining, it appears that monkeys with neurotoxic lesions of the amygdala performed equivalently to controls, whereas monkeys with removal of the anterior portion of the rhinal cortex were severely impaired (Figure 16.3). Hence, once again, properties of object recognition (or identification) once attributed to the amygdala appear instead to reside in the rhinal cortex. Indeed, the rhinal cortex has been implicated strongly in certain aspects of object identification (for reviews, see Murray and Bussey, 1999, Murray, 2000).

Both of the versions of DNMS that originally appeared to rely on the amygdala, based on studies using aspiration lesions, employed sets of objects that were used repeatedly throughout testing, i.e. only two objects were used for single-pair DMS (Correll and Scoville, 1965; Mishkin and Oubre, 1976) and typically the same 40 objects were used throughout

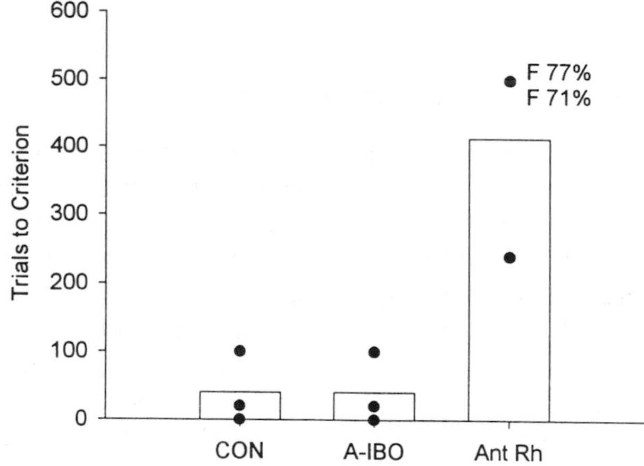

Figure 16.3 Performance on crossmodal DNMS by unoperated control monkeys (CON) and monkeys with either neurotoxic lesions of the amygdala (A-IBO) or aspiration lesions of the anterior rhinal cortex (Ant Rh), following postoperative retraining on both crossmodal and subsequently the intramodal versions of DNMS. CON and A-IBO monkeys show normal reacquisition of crossmodal DNMS on this second postoperative administration of the test, but monkeys with rhinal cortex damage are severely impaired, with two of them failing to re-acquire the task within the training limit of 500 trials (F; final levels of performance are given as percentage correct). Data are from Goulet and Murray (1995).

crossmodal DNMS testing (Murray and Mishkin, 1985). Both of these variants of DNMS were severely impaired by amygdala aspiration lesions, whereas the trial-unique version of DNMS was much less affected. As indicated earlier, these tasks are not testing 'recognition memory' in the usual sense, i.e. the ability to judge whether a given stimulus has been experienced before, but rather other aspects of sensory processing. Despite the common feature of small stimulus sets used in the two tasks, which suggests that a single mechanism may be disrupted, there may be two separate reasons for the behavioural impairments. For single-pair DNMS (or DMS), demands on stimulus identification are relatively low but demands on recency judgements are high. Consequently, it is possible that there is a specialization of this region (i.e. the anterior rhinal cortex) for dealing with recency judgements of familiar stimuli, a possibility that remains to be tested directly experimentally. Brown and colleagues (Fahy *et al.*, 1993), who recorded the activity of single neurons in awake, behaving monkeys performing a visual recognition memory task, found some neurons in the temporal polar cortex (area TG) that were concerned exclusively with encoding recency information for familiar objects, although the significance of this conclusion is limited by the relatively small number of cells recorded. Alternatively, the deficit on single-pair DNMS (DMS) may be a transient one due to partial disruption of object identification abilities. In contrast, the disruption on tactual-to-visual (crossmodal) DNMS after rhinal cortex damage is severe and persistent, and is thought to be due to a failure to link already stored stimulus representations located in different modality-specific neocortical fields (Murray and Bussey, 1999, Murray, 2000).

16.5 Stimulus–reward association

The amygdala has also been implicated in stimulus–reward learning, the capacity to associate previously neutral stimuli with an affective valence. Although simple discrimination learning was unaffected by amygdala lesions (Douglas *et al.*, 1969; Overman *et al.*, 1990; Schwartzbaum, 1965; cf. Gaffan, 1994b), more complex tasks involving interproblem transfer of training were impaired, for instance discrimination learning set and discrimination reversals (Schwartzbaum and Poulos, 1965; Barrett, 1969). Such an inability to associate stimuli with reward was thought perhaps to underlie some of the symptoms associated with temporal lobe removal and amygdalectomy, operations that appear to disrupt knowledge of the emotional significance of stimuli (Brown and Schäfer, 1888; Klüver and Bucy, 1938, 1939; Weiskrantz, 1956; Horel *et al.*, 1975).

Aspiration lesions of the amygdala produce a marked impairment in discrimination learning set, in which normal monkeys become very efficient at solving novel visual discrimination problems after they have been presented with a large number of such problems. Gaffan and Murray (1990) replicated the original finding of Schwartzbaum and Poulos (1965), who reported that monkeys with bilateral aspiration lesions of the amygdala were impaired on discrimination learning set. Thus, after the operation, amygdalectomized monkeys did not solve new problems as rapidly as they had preoperatively (Gaffan and Murray, 1990). In addition, bilateral lesions of the ventromedial prefrontal cortex or mediodorsal thalamus also produced a deficit equivalent in magnitude to that produced by bilateral amygdala lesions (Gaffan and Murray, 1990). However, surprisingly, crossed lesions of the amygdala and either the ventromedial prefrontal cortex or mediodorsal thalamus produced only a mild deficit, suggesting that these three structures each contribute in different ways to discrimination learning set performance. Gaffan *et al.* (1993) later reported that crossed lesions of the amygdala in one hemisphere, and *both* the ventromedial prefrontal cortex and mediodorsal thalamus in the opposite hemisphere, produced as severe an impairment in discrimination learning set as bilateral amygdala lesions alone. This suggested the critical interaction was between the amygdala and frontal–thalamic structures, and implicated an amygdala–thalamic–prefrontal network in stimulus–reward learning. The effects of neurotoxic lesions of the amygdala, or cortical lesions restricted to rhinal cortex, on discrimination learning set remain undetermined. Given the pattern of results, especially in relation to the foregoing discussion of recognition memory and the known disconnection effects of amygdala lesions, there is a distinct possibility that this kind of learning, too, is dependent on the rhinal cortex rather than the amygdala. We will return to this topic in a later section.

Another commonly used measure of stimulus–reward association is the win–stay, lose–shift task, in which objects are first presented one at a time, either rewarded (i.e. baited with a food reward) or non-rewarded (i.e. unbaited). One version of this task employs a 'constant alternative', in this case a grey plaque. Thus, in a choice test, the monkey is allowed to choose between one of the previously presented objects and a flat grey plaque. If the object was baited when encountered previously, it again covers a food reward on this choice test, and the grey plaque is unbaited. Conversely, if the object was not baited when encountered previously, it is also not baited on the choice test, and the grey plaque covers a food reward. Spiegler and Mishkin (1981) reported that monkeys with amygdala aspiration lesions were significantly impaired on this task. This was thought to reflect an impairment in stimulus–reward association, rather than stimulus memory, because, as previously mentioned, monkeys with amygdala aspiration lesions were unimpaired on visual DNMS with trial-unique objects, a test of stimulus recognition memory (Mishkin, 1978). A similar pattern of results was observed in a version of this task in which choices were given between a pair of objects, one of which had been rewarded when previously encountered alone, and the other of which had not (Phillips *et al.*, 1983).

Once again, the effects of neurotoxic amygdala lesions, or selective removal of the rhinal cortex, on these tasks have not yet been examined. It would be interesting to investigate the effects of neurotoxic amygdala lesions on win–stay, lose–shift performance; based on our anatomical findings, and on the pattern of impairment observed in other studies, it would be predicted that no impairment would be observed. Instead, it seems likely that the rhinal cortex again is critically involved. Support for this hypothesis comes from the finding that although aspiration of the hippocampus has little effect on win–stay, lose–shift performance (Spiegler and Mishkin, 1981), combined aspiration lesions of the two structures produce a devastating impairment larger than that produced by either lesion alone (Spiegler and Mishkin, 1979; Phillips and Mishkin, 1984). Thus, just as was the case for DNMS, it may be that damage to the anterior and posterior portions of the rhinal cortex, rather than damage to the amygdala and hippocampus, led to impairment on this task. This possibility is consistent with the idea that win–stay, lose–shift represents a type of stimulus–stimulus association learning (between the object and the visual properties of the food reward), a capacity that is also severely disrupted by combined amygdala plus hippocampal aspiration lesions or rhinal cortex lesions (Murray *et al.*, 1993; Buckley and Gaffan, 1998).

Object reversals are thought to be a particularly sensitive measure of stimulus–reward association learning because of the requirement continually to form and break stimulus–reward bonds. In this task, the monkey learns a single object discrimination problem to a set criterion, and then the discrimination is reversed (i.e. the previously rewarded object is now unrewarded, and vice versa) and relearned to criterion. This cycle repeats a number of times. Monkeys whose amygdala has been removed by aspiration (Schwartzbaum and Poulos, 1965) or with stereotaxic radiofrequency lesions (Aggleton and Passingham, 1981), or with lesions of the temporal polar cortex plus amygdala (Jones and Mishkin, 1972), were severely impaired on object reversals. It was reported recently that lesions restricted to the rhinal cortex produce a substantial impairment in object reversal learning (Murray *et al.*, 1998), but one not so severe in magnitude as had been observed in previous studies. The effects of neurotoxic amygdala lesions on object reversal learning have not yet been examined.

Discrimination learning tasks with secondary reinforcers have been used in an attempt to dissociate psychological processes linking neutral stimuli with 'reinforcement' from those linking neutral stimuli with food. In these tasks, a monkey learns that some originally neutral sensory event (a visual or auditory cue) is associated with a reinforcing event (food delivery). The sensory cue itself then acquires reinforcing properties, or becomes associated with the event of food delivery, and becomes a 'secondary reinforcer'. The monkey is then required to solve visual discrimination problems, and the only feedback provided is from the secondary reinforcers. Only after solving the discrimination, as evinced by performing several consecutive correct responses, is the monkey given food reward.

Gaffan and Harrison (1987) trained monkeys to solve visual discrimination problems for auditory secondary reinforcement. This task is particularly useful, because the sensory modalities of the discriminanda, secondary reinforcers, and reward are all different, preventing the monkey from solving the task by making any simple intramodal associations. In addition, this design permits independent manipulation of the sensory processing of the discriminanda and reinforcers using lesions. The monkeys were confronted with two novel visual stimuli on each trial, one arbitrarily designated correct. Touching the correct stimulus led to the presentation of an auditory reward signal (i.e. one that had been associated with food reward); touching the incorrect stimulus led to the presentation of an auditory non-reward signal (i.e. one that had not been associated with food). The monkey was required to choose the correct stimulus four times in a row in order to receive food reward. Aspiration lesions of the amygdala produced a devastating impairment in this task.

More recently, Málková *et al.* (1997) examined the performance on this task of monkeys with selective neurotoxic lesions of the amygdala. Surprisingly, these monkeys were unimpaired in learning visual discrimination problems for auditory secondary reinforcement. Baxter *et al.* (1999) subsequently tested monkeys with rhinal cortex lesions on this same task, and found a small, but statistically significant impairment. Extension of the temporal cortex lesion laterally to include area TE did produce a severe impairment in performance on this task

(Figure 16.4). Thus, it appears that neither damage to the amygdala alone, nor damage to the rhinal cortex alone, is sufficient to produce a severe impairment in visual discrimination learning for an auditory secondary reinforcer.

The currently available evidence suggests that neither damage to the amygdala nor damage to the rhinal cortex is sufficient to account for all the effects of amygdala aspiration lesions on various tasks measuring stimulus–reward association. Because aspiration lesions of the amygdala indirectly damage TE cortex, and produce a combination of direct and indirect damage to entorhinal and perirhinal cortex, the removal probably yields a disconnection of widespread regions of inferior temporal cortex from mediodorsal thalamus and ventromedial prefrontal cortex. Thus, an inferior temporal cortical–thalamic–prefrontal network may be the critical substrate for these functions. This notion finds support in the study by Gaffan *et al.* (1993), in which lesions of both the mediodorsal thalamus and ventromedial prefrontal cortex, crossed with amygdala aspiration, were required to produce severe impairments in

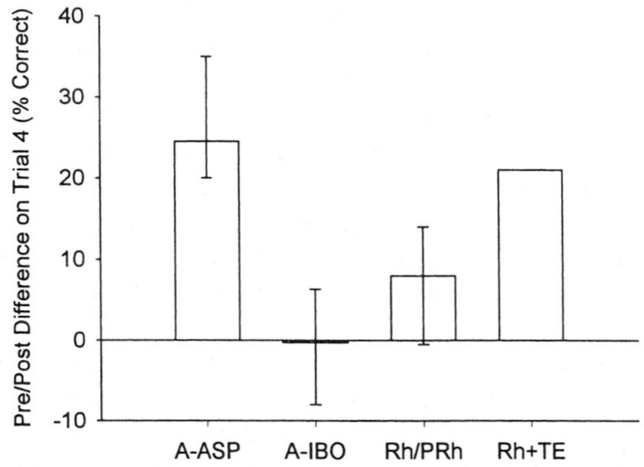

Figure 16.4 Comparison of performance of cynomolgus monkeys with aspiration lesions of the amygdala (A-ASP, n = 3, Gaffan and Harrison, 1987), rhesus monkeys with ibotenic acid lesions of the amygdala (A-IBO, n = 4, Málková *et al.*, 1997), and rhesus monkeys with lesions of rhinal or perirhinal cortex (Rh/PRh, n = 6, Baxter *et al.*, 1999) on visual discrimination learning for auditory secondary reinforcement. The height of each bar represents the group mean difference in trial 4 performance of problems given pre- and postoperatively. The vertical bars show the range of scores within each group. A severe impairment is evident in the monkeys with aspiration lesions of the amygdala, but there is no impairment in monkeys with ibotenic acid lesions of the amygdala and only a mild (but statistically significant) impairment in monkeys with lesions of rhinal or perirhinal cortex. Additional data are included for one rhesus monkey (Rh + TE) tested in this task, who received a rhinal cortex lesion that deliberately was extended more laterally to include cortical area TE (Baxter and Murray, unpublished observations). This monkey showed an impairment comparable with that observed in the monkeys with aspiration lesions of the amygdala in the original study by Gaffan and Harrison (1987).

discrimination learning set performance. Based on the evidence we have reviewed so far, it now seems likely that this effect is due to an *inferior temporal cortex* disconnection from the mediodorsal thalamus and ventromedial prefrontal cortex, rather than an amygdala disconnection from these regions. Furthermore, disruption by amygdala aspiration lesions of subcortical inputs to the temporal cortex that presumably carry information about primary reinforcement, mentioned previously, cannot account for these impairments, because the hemisphere with lesions of the thalamus and frontal cortex still has an intact amygdala and inferior temporal cortex. In any event, the essential notion is that the rhinal cortex participates in stimulus–reward learning (probably to the extent that it is required to identify the stimuli to be associated with reward; see discussion in Baxter *et al.*, 1999; Murray and Bussey, 1999), but it is not a critical substrate of stimulus–reward learning in the temporal lobe. Instead, visual stimulus–reward learning functions, at least those indexed by tasks such as visual discrimination learning, reversal learning, win–stay/lose–shift, etc., occur throughout inferior temporal cortex, via interactions with thalamus and prefrontal cortex, or with basal forebrain and hypothalamus, or with both sets of structures, but do not require the amygdala. This hypothesis would also explain the mild effect of rhinal cortex lesions on discrimination learning for auditory secondary reinforcement (Baxter *et al.*, 1999). The strong prediction is that rhinal cortex lesions would also produce a mild impairment on discrimination learning set for primary reinforcement, and that disconnection of inferior temporal cortex from mediodorsal thalamus and ventromedial prefrontal cortex would also produce a severe impairment in discrimination learning for auditory secondary reinforcement. In other words, both types of discrimination learning seem to operate via one and the same mechanism, requiring inferior temporal cortex, but not the amygdala, and interaction with other structures.

All of this having been said, it is worth noting that there is evidence for the participation of the amygdala in association of objects with the specific *value* of reinforcing events. Hatfield *et al.* (1996) tested rats in a food devaluation procedure, in which a light conditioned stimulus (CS) was paired with food reward. After developing conditioned responding to the light (evidenced by food cup entries during presentation of the light), the food reward was devalued by allowing the rats to consume the food in their home cages, and then giving them an injection of lithium chloride (LiCl) to produce malaise. In a subsequent test session, control rats demonstrated substantially fewer conditioned responses to the light CS if the food consumption in their home cages was followed immediately by an LiCl injection. Rats with neurotoxic lesions of the basolateral amygdala failed to show this effect. This suggested that the basolateral nucleus of the amygdala was important for adjusting behaviour in response to the current value of the reward (see Gallagher, Chapter 8).

Málková *et al.* (1997) tested a similar behaviour in their monkeys with neurotoxic amygdala lesions. In their task, monkeys learned a set of 60 object discrimination problems. Each positive object was consistently baited with one of two distinct food rewards (food-1 or food-2). After the object discrimination problems were learned to criterion, a number of critical test sessions were presented. In the critical test sessions, the monkey was offered a choice between pairs of positive (i.e. previously baited) objects, consisting of an object that had been rewarded consistently with food-1, and an object that had been rewarded consistently with food-2. Some of the critical test sessions were preceded by a selective satiation procedure, which was intended to devalue one of the two food rewards. Others, serving as baseline sessions, were not preceded by selective satiation. In practice, selective satiation was achieved by allowing monkeys to eat their fill of either food-1 or food-2 before being taken to the test apparatus. On test days in which the monkeys were sated with one of the foods before a critical test session, intact monkeys chose more of the objects baited with the other (non-sated) food than they did during baseline test sessions without satiation. Monkeys with neurotoxic amygdala lesions did not show this effect; their choices after satiation did not differ reliably from those made without satiation. Thus, although the amygdala does not seem to be necessary for associating objects with reinforcement, it does seem to be important for providing updated information about the current value of a particular reinforcer, or for allowing the current value of the reinforcer to gain access to the stimulus representation. (It is not the case that the amygdala is required simply for discriminating between the different food reinforcers, because monkeys with neurotoxic amygdala lesions also exhibited stable preferences for objects rewarded with a particular food during baseline sessions.)

Remarkably, monkeys with lesions of the rhinal cortex show intact reinforcer devaluation effects in this same task (Thornton *et al.*, 1998). This represents a double dissociation of the effects of amygdala removal and rhinal cortex ablations: amygdala removal disrupts the effects of reinforcer devaluation, but not visual discrimination learning for auditory secondary reinforcement; conversely, rhinal cortex lesions disrupt visual discrimination learning for auditory secondary reinforcement, but not the effects of reinforcer devaluation (Figure 16.5). Taken together, the currently available evidence suggests that the amygdala plays a much more restricted role in stimulus–reward association than previously thought, probably serving to modify behaviour based on the current reinforcing value of particular stimuli rather than acting to form stimulus–reward bonds in the first place. This may take place via a prefrontal–amygdala–temporal neocortical circuit; neurons in the orbital frontal cortex discriminate between different reinforcers in a behavioural task (Schultz *et al.*, 1998; Tremblay and Schultz, 1999) and there are substantial reciprocal connections among the amygdala, the orbital frontal cortex, and the temporal neocortex (especially the perirhinal cortex), where object representations are stored (Aggleton *et al.*, 1980; Carmichael and Price, 1995; Stefanacci *et al.*, 1996). Indeed, there is now evidence that interactions between orbital frontal cortex and amygdala are required to mediate the reinforcer devaluation effects in monkeys (Baxter *et al.*, 2000).

16.6 Stimulus–affect association

The behavioural changes perhaps most commonly associated with damage to the amygdala involve alterations in emotional behaviour. The Klüver–Bucy syndrome associated with temporal lobectomy (Klüver and Bucy, 1938, 1939) comprises a variety of behavioural changes, including reduced fearfulness, hypersexuality, oral tendencies, 'psychic blindness' (i.e. the apparent inability to determine the significance of an object from its visual

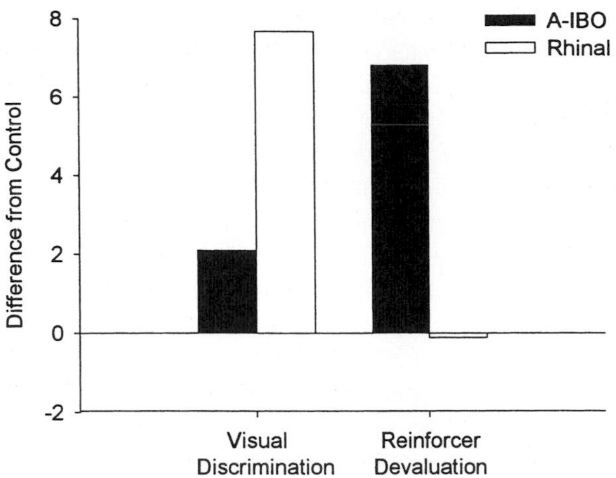

Figure 16.5 An illustration of the double dissociation between amygdala and rhinal cortex on two tasks: visual discrimination learning for auditory secondary reinforcement and reinforcer devaluation. The ordinate represents a difference score between performance of lesioned and intact monkeys, which is the difference between preoperative and postoperative performance on trial 4 of each problem for the visual discrimination task, and the difference between mean devaluation scores between lesioned monkeys and unlesioned controls for the reinforcer devaluation task. Lesions of the rhinal cortex impair visual discrimination learning but are without effect on reinforcer devaluation, whereas the opposite pattern of results is seen following ibotenic acid lesions of the amygdala. Data are adapted from Málková *et al.* (1997), Thornton *et al.* (1998), and Baxter *et al.* (1999).

characteristics), and 'hypermetamorphosis' (i.e. an abnormal tendency to attend to and react to all visual stimuli). Subsequent experiments attempted to fractionate the aspects of this syndrome with respect to the temporal cortex and amygdala: behavioural alterations were found after more selective ablations of the amygdala, as well as after removal of temporal polar cortex (Weiskrantz, 1956; Horel and Keating, 1972; Horel *et al.*, 1975; Iwai *et al.*, 1986).

Aggleton and Passingham (1981) employed a stereotaxic surgical method based on X-ray photographs to place radiofrequency lesions in different subnuclei of the amygdala. They found that subtotal lesions of the amygdala restricted to the basolateral, lateral, or dorsal amygdala, or the white matter of the temporal stem, had little effect on emotional behaviour. In contrast, more extensive lesions of the entire amygdala produced emotional changes. Deficits in object reversal learning were only observed in monkeys that showed changes in emotional behaviour, suggesting that these two effects of temporal lobe damage shared the same anatomical substrate. These findings were replicated in a later study by Zola-Morgan and colleagues (1991), who reported emotional changes following radiofrequency lesions intended to destroy the entire amygdala.

As already indicated, the interpretation of these experiments is limited by the probable damage to fibres of passage caused by the radiofrequency lesion method. Recent investigations have begun to examine the effects of neurotoxic amygdala lesions on emotional behaviour. Meunier *et al.* (1999) systematically examined the effects of neurotoxic amygdala lesions on emotional responses of monkeys to a variety of stimuli. Emotional responses were videotaped and later scored in several categories. Monkeys with neurotoxic amygdala lesions showed similar changes in emotional behaviour to monkeys with aspiration lesions of the amygdala, namely reduced fear and aggressiveness, increased submission, and excessive manual and oral exploration. However, the magnitude of some of these effects in monkeys with complete neurotoxic lesions of the amygdala was somewhat less than in monkeys with aspiration lesions of the amygdala, suggesting a role for the temporal cortex in emotional behaviour as well. Interestingly, lesions restricted to the rhinal cortex produced a different pattern of results, which appeared to be an enhancement of fearful reactions (Meunier *et al.*, 1991).

Amygdala lesions also produce an alteration in so-called 'food preference' behaviour, which typically examines monkeys' choices between different foods, or between food versus non-food items. Monkeys with aspiration lesions of the amygdala are abnormally willing to eat meat, which intact monkeys usually reject (Aggleton and Passingham, 1981; Baylis and Gaffan, 1991). Murray *et al.* (1996) examined food preference behaviour in monkeys with either neurotoxic lesions of the amygdala or lesions of the anterior rhinal cortex. Monkeys with neurotoxic amygdala lesions were more likely to eat meat and were also more likely to take non-food objects during food preference testing. Monkeys with anterior rhinal cortex lesions showed food preferences that were indistinguishable from those of controls. Interestingly, Parker and Gaffan (1998) report that monkeys with complete removals of rhinal cortex are more likely to make 'strange' choices during food preference testing, i.e. choices of foods that are inconsistent with their overall preferences. This behaviour is exhibited by monkeys with aspiration lesions of the amygdala but not by monkeys with lesions restricted to perirhinal cortex (Gaffan, 1994a). These findings might suggest that these aspects of food preference are dissociable from one another: making consistent food choices might be more reliant on the rhinal cortex, whereas the selection of preferred foods versus non-foods and meat might rely more on the cells of the amygdala. In fact, monkeys with neurotoxic lesions of the amygdala do not make more 'strange' choices when tested in the Gaffan protocol than intact control monkeys (L. Málková, D. Gaffan, and E.A. Murray, unpublished observations), and monkeys with complete lesions of the rhinal cortex (including anterior and posterior portions) are not more likely to take meat than controls (J. Bachevalier, personal communication).

16.7 Additional considerations

It is important to note that the three behavioural domains under discussion, stimulus memory, stimulus–reward association, and stimulus–affect association, do not comprise the limit of the functions of the amygdala in primates, but simply those domains which have been most accessible to experimental study in non-human primates. For instance, lesion studies in rats and neuroimaging studies in humans have accorded the amygdala a role in fear conditioning

(Davis *et al.*, 1993; LeDoux, 1995; LaBar *et al.*, 1998); studies in monkeys have not examined the acquisition of fearful responses, or emotional *learning* more generally, following selective amygdala damage. Furthermore, studies in rats point to the involvement of the amygdala in certain aspects of attentional processing, specifically, the ability to increase attention to a stimulus whose predictive relationship with other events has been made unpredictable (Gallagher and Holland, 1994; Holland and Gallagher, 1999; Gallagher, Chapter 8). Moreover, the amygdala has been implicated in olfactory and pheromonal sensory processing, which are probably linked to amygdala contributions to reproductive behaviour (see Kling and Brothers, 1992), and plays a central role in the modulation of memory, by serving to enhance storage of significant events (McGaugh, 1990; Cahill and McGaugh, 1998; McGaugh *et al.*, Chapter 11; Cahill, Chapter 12). The involvement of the amygdala in these latter functions has not yet been examined systematically in non-human primates. Finally, based on evidence implicating the amygdala in social behaviour (as noted at the outset), investigation of the effects of neurotoxic lesions of the amygdala on social behaviour will represent an important direction for future research.

16.8 Summary and future directions

A summary of the behavioural data discussed in the preceding three sections is presented in Table 16.1. It can be seen that aspiration lesions of the amygdala produce behavioural impairments in a wide variety of domains, but the impairments produced by selective damage to the cell bodies of the amygdala are relatively restricted. Damage to or dysfunction of the inferior temporal cortex, including the rhinal cortex, can account for many of the impairments associated with amygdala aspiration lesions. Taken together, these data indicate that the role of the amygdala in primate behaviour is much more restricted than has been appreciated previously. With regard to the three behavioural domains traditionally associated with the amygdala in non-human primates, it would be fair to summarize the recent findings by stating that the amygdala plays little or no role in stimulus memory (including stimulus recognition and stimulus–stimulus association, and excluding a possible modulatory role that has not yet been investigated in non-human primates; see McGaugh *et al.*, Chapter 11; Cahill, Chapter 12), plays some role in stimulus–reward association, but in a different way from that which was conceived originally, and is critically involved in stimulus–affect association, or in eliciting the appropriate emotional response to environmental stimuli.

The recent work has some implications for the neurobiology of stimulus–reward processing. Traditionally, the function of stimulus–reward association has been viewed as psychologically and neuroanatomically discrete. The findings discussed in this chapter suggest important dissociations between different aspects of stimulus–reward learning. The association of a previously neutral visual stimulus with reward seems to take place in a more distributed fashion within inferior temporal cortex, through interaction with prefrontal/thalamic or subcortical networks (or both). Interestingly, although earlier physiological studies failed to uncover any evidence for stimulus–reward association mechanisms within the inferior temporal cortex (Jarvis and Mishkin, 1977; Rolls, 1981), more recent studies have identified

Table 16.1 Comparison of the effects of neurotoxic and aspiration lesions of the amygdala, and of rhinal cortex lesions, on a variety of behavioural tasks administered to monkeys

	A(ASP)	*Rh*	*A(IBO)*
DNMS single pair (relearning)[a,b]	++	+	–
Cross-modal DNMS[c,d,e]	+++	++	–
Visual discrimination learning set[f,g]	++	?	?
Win–stay, lose–shift[h,i]	++	?	?
Object reversals[g,j,k]	+++	++	?
Visual discrimination for auditory secondary reinforcement[l,m,n]	+++	+	–
Reinforcer devaluation[n,o]	? (++)	–	++
Food choices[b,p,q]	++	+/–	+
Emotional changes[r,s]	+++	+*	++

– Indicates no effect; + indicates a deficit, with the number of symbols indicating the relative magnitude of the deficit within a row; ? indicates not known. (++) indicates expected effect based on A-IBO lesions.
Abbreviations: A(ASP), aspiration lesions of the amygdala; Rh, aspiration removals of the entorhinal and perirhinal (i.e. rhinal) cortex; A(IBO), selective excitotoxic lesions of the amygdala.
*The available data for Rh lesions indicate that the direction of the effect is opposite that of A lesions: Rh lesions produce an enhancement of fear responses, whereas A lesions attenuate them.
[a]Mishkin and Oubre (1976), [b]Murray *et al.* (1996), [c]Murray and Mishkin (1985), [d]Goulet and Murray (1995), [e]Málková and Murray (1996), [f]Gaffan and Murray (1990), [g]Schwartzbaum and Poulos (1965), [h]Spiegler and Mishkin (1981), [i]Phillips *et al.* (1983), [j]Jones and Mishkin (1972), [k]Murray *et al.* (1998), [l]Gaffan and Harrison (1987), [m]Baxter *et al.* (1999), [n]Málková *et al.* (1997), [o]Thornton *et al.* (1998), [p]Parker and Gaffan (1998), [q]Baylis and Gaffan (1991), [r]Meunier *et al.* (1999), [s]Meunier *et al.* (1991).

such a potential mechanism. Erickson *et al.* (2000), who recorded from neurons in perirhinal cortex of monkeys performing a discrimination learning task, found cells that reflect stimulus–reward history by virtue of a 'target effect'. When a monkey is viewing a visual display containing two items, perirhinal neuronal activity is greater when the preferred stimulus is the target (i.e. the S+) relative to when the non-preferred stimulus is the target, even though the sensory conditions for the two different trial types are the same. This effect is due, at least in part, to suppression of the neuronal response to the non-target (i.e. the S–) that develops with learning. Thus, some perirhinal cortex neurons reflect the behavioural status of a visual stimulus, as well as its identity. The amygdala apparently is not required for this association function. However, the amygdala does seem to be engaged when an adjustment of behaviour is required, based on the current value of a particular reinforcer, as evinced by impairments in the reinforcer devaluation task. Hence, the neural systems that mediate the simple association of a neutral stimulus with a reinforcer appear incapable of altering that representation in response to a rapid change in the value of the reinforcer.

With regard to the goal set forth at the beginning of the chapter, namely to achieve a unified neuropsychological framework for amygdala function, we are perhaps closer than before, by being better able to understand the neural substrates of deficits produced by aspiration lesions of the amygdala which have been particularly difficult to account for, i.e. all of the visual stimulus memory and some of the visual stimulus–reward functions earlier attributed to the amygdala can now be seen as belonging instead to the nearby inferior temporal neocortex. In addition, to the extent that the representations of hedonic aspects of reward resemble the representations of emotional states, the (remaining) stimulus–reward functions of the amygdala can be grouped with the stimulus–affect functions. Furthermore, the altered food choices seen after amygdala damage might likewise be interpreted as a failure of the visual and tactual properties of certain foods (e.g. meat) to elicit the appropriate emotional response(s). In this view, the primary function of the amygdala is to act as an interface between emotion (including the hedonic aspects of reward) and objects, both animate and inanimate. Nevertheless, integrating even just those findings based on selective damage to the amygdala remains a daunting task. One simple possibility, an alternative to that just proposed, is that the anatomical diversity of inputs and outputs to different subnuclei of the amygdala will preclude a simple attribution of function to the structure as a whole (Swanson and Petrovich, 1998), a view supported by studies in rats that find very different (and doubly dissociable) behavioural effects of lesions of the basolateral and central nuclei of the amygdala (Killcross *et al.*, 1997; Holland and Gallagher, 1999; Gallagher, Chapter 8). Indeed, even the central role accorded to the amygdala as critical to the perception and expression of fear-related behaviour has been called into question recently, by the finding of representations of fear that exist outside the amygdala (Vazdarjanova and McGaugh, 1998). Taking these considerations into account in future studies of amygdala function, and achieving better ways to identify and measure emotion and affective valence (e.g. Davidson and Sutton, 1995), may refine further our understanding of the neuropsychological function(s) of this structure.

Acknowledgements

We thank J.P. Aggleton, D. Gaffan, and M. Mishkin for helpful comments on an earlier version of this chapter.

References

Aggleton, J.P. and Passingham, R.E. (1981) Syndrome produced by lesions of the amygdala in monkeys (*Macaca mulatta*). *Journal of Comparative and Physiological Psychology*, 95, 961–977.

Aggleton, J.P., Burton, M.J., and Passingham, R.E. (1980) Cortical and subcortical afferents to the amygdala of the rhesus monkey (*Macaca mulatta*). *Brain Research*, 190, 347–368.

Barrett, T.W. (1969) Studies of the function of the amygdaloid complex in *Macaca mulatta. Neuropsychologia*, 7, 1–12.

Baxter, M.G., Saunders, R.C., and Murray, E.A. (1998) Aspiration lesions of the amygdala interrupt connections between prefrontal cortex and temporal cortex in rhesus monkeys. *Society for Neuroscience Abstracts*, 24, 1905.

Baxter, M.G., Hadfield, W.S., and Murray, E.A. (1999) Rhinal cortex lesions produce mild deficits in visual discrimination learning for an auditory secondary reinforcer in rhesus monkeys. *Behavioral Neuroscience*, 113, 243–252.

Baxter, M.G., Parker, A., Lindner, C.C.C., Izquierdo, A., and Murray, E.A. (2000) Control of response selection by reinforcer value requires interaction of amygdala and orbital prefrontal cortex. *Journal of Neuroscience*, **20**, 4311–4319.

Baylis, L.L. and Gaffan, D. (1991) Amygdalectomy and ventromedial prefrontal ablation produce similar deficits in food choice and in simple object discrimination learning for an unseen reward. *Experimental Brain Research*, 86, 617–622.

Brown, S. and Schäfer, E.A. (1888) An investigation into the functions of the occipital and temporal lobes of the monkey's brain. *Philosophical Transactions of the Royal Society of London, Series B*, 179, 303–327.

Buckley, M.J. and Gaffan, D. (1998) Perirhinal cortex ablation impairs configural learning and paired-associate learning equally. *Neuropsychologia*, 36, 535–546.

Cahill, L. and McGaugh, J.L. (1998) Mechanisms of emotional arousal and lasting declarative memory. *Trends in Neurosciences*, 21, 294–299.

Carmichael, S.T. and Price, J.L. (1995) Limbic connections of the orbital and medial prefrontal cortex in macaque monkeys. *Journal of Comparative Neurology*, 363, 615–641.

Correll, R.E. and Scoville, W.B. (1965) Performance on delayed match following lesions of medial temporal lobe structures. *Journal of Comparative and Physiological Psychology*, 60, 360–367.

Davidson, R.J. and Sutton, S.K. (1995) Affective neuroscience: the emergence of a discipline. *Current Opinion in Neurobiology*, 5, 217–224.

Davis, M., Falls, W.A., Campeau, S., and Kim, M. (1993) Fear-potentiated startle: a neural and pharmacological analysis. *Behavioural Brain Research*, 58, 175–198.

Douglas, R.J. and Pribram, K.H. (1966) Learning and limbic lesions. *Neuropsychologia*, 4, 197–220.

Douglas, R.J., Barrett, T.W., Pribram, K.H., and Cerny, M.C. (1969) Limbic lesions and error reduction. *Journal of Comparative and Physiological Psychology*, 68, 437–441.

Eacott, M.J., Gaffan, D., and Murray, E.A. (1994) Preserved recognition memory for small sets, and impaired stimulus identification for large sets, following rhinal cortex ablations in monkeys. *European Journal of Neuroscience*, 6, 1466–1478.

Easton, A. and Gaffan, D. (1997) Hypothalamic–cortical disconnection impairs visual reward-association learning in rhesus monkeys. *Society for Neuroscience Abstracts*, 23, 11.

Emery, N.J. and Amaral, D.G. (2000) The role of the amygdala in primate social cognition. In *Cognitive Neuroscience of Emotion* (eds R.D. Lane and L. Nadel), pp. 156–191 Oxford University Press, Oxford.

Erickson, C.A., Jagadeesh, B., and Desimone, R. (2000) Learning and memory in the inferior temporal cortex of the macaque. In *The Cognitive Neurosciences*, 2nd edn (ed. M. Gazzaniga), pp. 743–752. MIT Press, Cambridge, Massachusetts.

Fahy, F.L., Riches, I.P., and Brown, M.W. (1993) Neuronal activity related to visual recognition memory: long-term memory and the encoding of recency and familiarity information in the primate anterior and medial inferior temporal and rhinal cortex. *Experimental Brain Research*, 96, 457–472.

Gaffan, D. (1994a) Dissociated effects of perirhinal cortex ablation, fornix transection and amygdalectomy: evidence for multiple memory systems in the primate temporal lobe. *Experimental Brain Research*, 99, 411–422.

Gaffan, D. (1994b) Role of the amygdala in picture discrimination learning with 24-h intertrial intervals. *Experimental Brain Research*, 99, 423–430.

Gaffan, D. and Harrison, S. (1987) Amygdalectomy and disconnection in visual learning for auditory secondary reinforcement by monkeys. *Journal of Neuroscience*, 7, 2285–2292.

Gaffan, D. and Murray, E.A. (1990) Amygdalar interaction with the mediodorsal nucleus of the thalamus and the ventromedial prefrontal cortex in stimulus–reward associative learning in the monkey. *Journal of Neuroscience*, 10, 3479–3493.

Gaffan, D., Murray, E.A., and Fabre-Thorpe, M. (1993) Interaction of the amygdala with the frontal lobe in reward memory. *European Journal of Neuroscience*, 5, 968–975.

Gallagher, M. and Holland, P.C. (1994) The amygdala complex: multiple roles in associative learning and attention. *Proceedings of the National Academy of Sciences of the United States of America*, 91, 11771–11776.

Goulet, S. and Murray, E.A. (1995) Effects of lesions of either the amygdala or anterior rhinal cortex on crossmodal DNMS in rhesus macaques. *Society for Neuroscience Abstracts*, 21, 1446.

Goulet, S., Doré, F.Y., and Murray, E.A. (1998) Aspiration lesions of the amygdala disrupt the rhinal corticothalamic projection system in rhesus monkeys. *Experimental Brain Research*, 119, 131–140.

Gower, E.C. (1989) Efferent projections from limbic cortex of the temporal pole to the magnocellular medial dorsal nucleus in the rhesus monkey. *Journal of Comparative Neurology*, 280, 343–358.

Hatfield, T., Han, J.-S., Conley, M., Gallagher, M., and Holland, P. (1996) Neurotoxic lesions of basolateral, but not central, amygdala interfere with Pavlovian second-order conditioning and reinforcer devaluation effects. *Journal of Neuroscience*, 16, 5256–5265.

Holland, P.C. and Gallagher, M. (1999) Amygdala circuitry in attentional and representational processes. *Trends in Cognitive Sciences*, 3, 65–73.

Horel, J.A. and Keating, E.G. (1972) Recovery from a partial Klüver–Bucy syndrome in the monkey produced by disconnection. *Journal of Comparative and Physiological Psychology*, 79, 105–114.

Horel, J.A., Keating, E.G., and Misantone, L.J. (1975) Partial Klüver–Bucy syndrome produced by destroying temporal neocortex or amygdala. *Brain Research*, 94, 347–359.

Iwai, E., Nishio, T., and Yamaguchi, K. (1986) Neuropsychological basis of a K–B sign in Klüver–Bucy syndrome produced following total removal of inferotemporal cortex of macaque monkeys. In *Emotion—Neural and Chemical Control* (ed. Y. Oomura), pp. 299–311. Japan Scientific Society Press, Tokyo.

Jarvis, C.D. and Mishkin, M. (1977) Responses of cells in the inferior temporal cortex of monkeys during visual discrimination reversal. *Society for Neuroscience Abstracts*, 3, 564.

Jones, B. and Mishkin, M. (1972) Limbic lesions and the problem of stimulus–reinforcement associations. *Experimental Neurology*, 36, 362–377.

Killcross, S., Robbins, T.W., and Everitt, B.J. (1997) Different types of fear-conditioned behaviour mediated by separate nuclei within amygdala. *Nature*, 388, 377–380.

Kling, A.S. and Brothers, L.A. (1992) The amygdala and social behavior. In *The Amygdala: Neurobiological Aspects of Emotion, Memory, and Mental Dysfunction* (ed. J.P. Aggleton), pp. 353–377. Wiley-Liss, New York.

Klüver, H. and Bucy, P.C. (1938) An analysis of certain effects of bilateral temporal lobectomy in the rhesus monkey, with special reference to 'psychic blindness'. *Journal of Psychology*, 5, 33–54.

Klüver, H. and Bucy, P.C. (1939) Preliminary analysis of functions of the temporal lobes in monkeys. *Archives of Neurology and Psychiatry*, 42, 979–1000.

LaBar, K.S., Gatenby, J.C., Gore, J.C., LeDoux, J.E., and Phelps, E.A. (1998) Human amygdala activation during conditioned fear acquisition and extinction: a mixed-trial fMRI study. *Neuron*, 20, 937–945.

LeDoux, J.E. (1995) Emotion: clues from the brain. *Annual Review of Psychology*, 46, 209–235.

Málková, L. and Murray, E.A. (1996) Effects of partial versus complete lesions of the amygdala on cross-modal associations in cynomolgus monkeys. *Psychobiology*, 24, 255–264.

Málková, L., Gaffan, D., and Murray, E.A. (1997) Excitotoxic lesions of the amygdala fail to produce impairments in visual learning for auditory secondary reinforcement but interfere with reinforcer devaluation effects in rhesus monkeys. *Journal of Neuroscience*, 17, 6011–6020.

McGaugh, J.L. (1990) Significance and remembrance: the role of neuromodulatory systems. *Psychological Science*, 1, 15–25.

Meunier, M., Bachevalier, J., Murray, E.A., Merjanian, P.M., and Richardson, R. (1991) Effects of rhinal cortical or limbic lesions on fear reactions in rhesus monkeys. *Society for Neuroscience Abstracts*, 17, 337.

Meunier, M., Bachevalier, J., Mishkin, M., and Murray, E.A. (1993) Effects on visual recognition of combined and separate ablations of the entorhinal and perirhinal cortex in rhesus monkeys. *Journal of Neuroscience*, 13, 5418–5432.

Meunier, M., Bachevalier, J., Murray, E.A., Málková, L., and Mishkin, M. (1999) Effects of aspiration versus neurotoxic lesions of the amygdala on emotional responses in rhesus monkeys. *European Journal of Neuroscience*, **11**, 4403–4418.

Mishkin, M. (1978) Memory in monkeys severely impaired by combined but not by separate removal of amygdala and hippocampus. *Nature*, 273, 297–298.

Mishkin, M. and Aggleton, J. (1981) Multiple functional contributions of the amygdala in the monkey. In *The Amygdaloid Complex* (ed. Y. Ben-Ari), pp. 409–420. Elsevier/North-Holland Biomedical Press, Amsterdam.

Mishkin, M. and Oubre, J.L. (1976) Dissociation of deficits on visual memory tasks after inferior temporal and amygdala lesions in monkeys. *Society for Neuroscience Abstracts*, 2, 1127.

Murray, E.A. (1990) Representational memory in nonhuman primates. In *Neurobiology of Comparative Cognition* (eds R.P. Kesner and D.S. Olton), pp 127–155. Lawrence Erlbaum, Hillsdale, New Jersey.

Murray, E.A. (1992) Medial temporal lobe structures contributing to recognition memory: the amygdaloid complex versus the rhinal cortex. In *The Amygdala: Neurobiological Aspects of Emotion, Memory, and Mental Dysfunction* (ed. J.P. Aggleton), pp. 453–470. Wiley-Liss, New York.

Murray, E.A. (2000) Memory for objects in nonhuman primates. In *The Cognitive Neurosciences*, 2nd edn. (ed. M. Gazzaniga), pp. 753–763. MIT Press, Cambridge, Massachusetts.
Murray, E.A. and Bussey, T.J. (1999) Perceptual–mnemonic functions of the perirhinal cortex. *Trends in Cognitive Sciences*, 3, 142–151.
Murray, E.A. and Mishkin, M. (1983) Severe tactual memory deficits in monkeys after combined removal of the amygdala and hippocampus. *Brain Research*, 270, 340–344.
Murray, E.A. and Mishkin, M. (1984) Severe tactual as well as visual memory deficits follow combined removal of the amygdala and hippocampus in monkeys. *Journal of Neuroscience*, 4, 2565–2580.
Murray, E.A. and Mishkin, M. (1985) Amygdalectomy impairs crossmodal association in monkeys. *Science*, 228, 604–606.
Murray, E.A. and Mishkin, M. (1986) Visual recognition in monkeys following rhinal cortical ablations combined with either amygdalectomy or hippocampectomy. *Journal of Neuroscience*, 6, 1991–2003.
Murray, E.A. and Mishkin, M. (1998) Object recognition and location memory in monkeys with excitotoxic lesions of the amygdala and hippocampus. *Journal of Neuroscience*, 18, 6568–6582.
Murray, E.A., Gaffan, D., and Mishkin, M. (1993) Neural substrates of visual stimulus–stimulus association in rhesus monkeys. *Journal of Neuroscience*, 13, 4549–4561.
Murray, E.A., Gaffan, E.A., and Flint, R.W., Jr (1996) Anterior rhinal cortex and amygdala: dissociation of their contributions to memory and food preference in rhesus monkeys. *Behavioral Neuroscience*, 110, 30–42.
Murray, E.A., Baxter, M.G., and Gaffan, D. (1998) Monkeys with rhinal cortex damage or neurotoxic hippocampal lesions are impaired on spatial scene learning and object reversals. *Behavioral Neuroscience*, 112, 1291–1303.
Overman, W.H., Ormsby, G., and Mishkin, M. (1990) Picture recognition vs. picture discrimination learning in monkeys with medial temporal removals. *Experimental Brain Research*, 79, 18–24.
Parker, A. and Gaffan, D. (1998) Lesions of the primate rhinal cortex cause deficits in flavour–visual associative memory. *Behavioural Brain Research*, 93, 99–105.
Phillips, R.R. and Mishkin, M. (1984) Further evidence of a severe impairment in associative memory following combined amygdalo-hippocampal lesions in monkeys. *Society for Neuroscience Abstracts*, 10, 136.
Phillips, R.R., Malamut, B.L., and Mishkin, M. (1983) Memory for stimulus–reward associations in the monkey is more severely affected by amygdalectomy than by hippocampectomy. *Society for Neuroscience Abstracts*, 9, 189.
Rolls, E.T. (1981) Processing beyond the inferior temporal visual cortex related to feeding, memory, and striatal function. In *Brain Mechanisms of Sensation* (eds Y. Katsuki, R. Norgren and M. Sato), pp. 241–269. Wiley, New York.
Saunders, R.C., Murray, E.., and Mishkin, M. (1984) Further evidence that amygdala and hippocampus contribute equally to recognition memory. *Neuropsychologia,* 22, 785–796.
Schultz, W., Tremblay, L., and Hollerman, J. R. (1998) Reward prediction in primate basal ganglia and frontal cortex. *Neuropharmacology*, 37, 421–429.

Schwartzbaum, J.S. (1965) Discrimination behavior after amygdalectomy in monkeys: visual and somesthetic learning and perceptual capacity. *Journal of Comparative Physiological Psychology*, 60, 314–319.

Schwartzbaum, J.S. and Poulos, D.A. (1965) Discrimination behavior after amygdalectomy in monkeys: learning set and discrimination reversals. *Journal of Comparative and Physiological Psychology*, 60, 320–328.

Spiegler, B.J. and Mishkin, M. (1979) Associative memory severely impaired by combined amygdalo-hippocampal removals. *Society for Neuroscience Abstracts*, 5, 323.

Spiegler, B.J. and Mishkin, M. (1981) Evidence for the sequential participation of inferior temporal cortex and amygdala in the acquisition of stimulus–reward associations. *Behavioural Brain Research*, 3, 303–317.

Stefanacci, L., Suzuki, W.A., and Amaral, D.G. (1996) Organization of connections between the amygdaloid complex and the perirhinal and parahippocampal cortices in macaque monkeys. *Journal of Comparative Neurology*, 375, 552–582.

Swanson, L.W. and Petrovich, G.D. (1998) What is the amygdala? *Trends in Neuroscience*, 21, 323–331.

Thornton, J. Málková, L., and Murray, E.A. (1998) Rhinal cortex ablations fail to disrupt reinforcer devaluation effects in rhesus monkeys (*Macaca mulatta*). *Behavioral Neuroscience*, 112, 1020–1025.

Tremblay, L. and Schultz, W. (1999) Relative reward preference in primate orbitofrontal cortex. *Nature*, 398, 704–708.

Vazdarjanova, A. and McGaugh, J.L. (1998) Basolateral amygdala is not critical for cognitive memory of contextual fear conditioning. *Proceedings of the National Academy of Sciences of the United States of America*, 95, 15003–15007.

von Bonin, G. and Bailey, P. (1947) *The Neocortex of Macaca mulatta*. University of Illinois Press, Urbana, Illinois.

Weiskrantz, L. (1956) Behavioral changes associated with ablation of the amygdaloid complex in monkeys. *Journal of Comparative and Physiological Psychology*, 49, 381–391.

Zola-Morgan, S., Squire, L.R., and Amaral, D.G. (1989) Lesions of the amygdala that spare adjacent cortical regions do not impair memory or exacerbate the impairment following lesions of the hippocampal formation. *Journal of Neuroscience*, 9, 1922–1936.

Zola-Morgan, S., Squire, L.R., Alvarez-Royo, P., and Clower, R.P. (1991) Independence of memory functions and emotional behavior: separate contributions of the hippocampal formation and the amygdala. *Hippocampus*, 1, 207–220.

17 Amygdala and the memory of reward: the importance of fibres of passage from the basal forebrain

Alexander Easton and David Gaffan

Department of Experimental Psychology, University of Oxford, Oxford, UK

Summary

The understanding of the role played by the amygdala in the memory of reward has changed substantially in the years since the review of Gaffan (1992) in the previous edition of this book. It appeared from the data available at that time that the amygdala played a crucial part in the association of stimuli with the value of reward. As discussed here, this view has been changed by the use of excitotoxins in lesioning the amygdala, which have shown that the effects discussed previously are dependent mainly on fibres of passage through the amygdala. In particular, we will argue that fibres of passage from the basal forebrain through the amygdala are crucial for the reinforcement of visual learning.

17.1 The learning of object–reward associations

One way to approach this issue of how we learn object–reward associations is to start with the cortical areas involved in object representations. The inferior temporal cortex (which includes both visual area TE and the perirhinal cortex) has been seen to serve both perceptual object representations and mnemonic processes (Buckley and Gaffan, 1998; Murray and Bussey, 1999). The way in which objects are represented within the inferior temporal cortex is now well understood (for a review, see Tanaka, 1996), but the question of how these objects are associated with reward remains less clear. In monkeys, bilateral lesions of the inferior temporal cortex impair the learning of object–reward associations (Gaffan *et al.*, 1986), and large bilateral lesions of the entire frontal cortex (sparing primary motor cortex) prevent the learning of even single object–reward association problems (Parker and Gaffan, 1998b). The interaction between these temporal and frontal cortical areas is thus likely to be of great importance in the learning of these associations, but by which routes do they communicate with one another?

The major direct, monosynaptic, route of corticocortical communication between inferior temporal cortex and frontal cortex is via the uncinate fascicle (Ungerleider *et al.*, 1989). Section of this pathway bilaterally in the monkey, however, does not affect object–reward association learning but does impair performance on certain visually cued conditional tasks (Eacott and Gaffan, 1992; Gutnikov *et al.*, 1997). Therefore, the communication between these cortical areas in object–reward association learning is not by means of a monosynaptic cortical pathway. Indeed, communication does not even rely on communication between frontal cortex and inferior temporal cortex within the same hemisphere. Crossed unilateral ablations of frontal cortex in one hemisphere and inferior temporal cortex in the opposite hemisphere, combined with section of the forebrain commissures, prevent any interaction between these cortical areas within the same hemisphere. Nonetheless, monkeys with this exact cortical disconnection can learn object–reward associations at a normal rate (Parker and Gaffan, 1998b). The communication between frontal cortex and inferior temporal cortex in object–reward learning therefore relies on subcortical structures, and the information can be transferred interhemispherically via these structures.

Recent excitotoxic lesion studies have demonstrated that in the monkey the association of objects with rewards is not critically dependent on the cells of the amygdala. Rather, as outlined by Baxter and Murray (Chapter 16), the amygdala itself seems to be important to reward association memory only when alteration in the current value of the reinforcer can alter behaviour. In contrast, object–reward association learning relies more generally on interactions with inferior temporal cortex and prefrontal, thalamic, or basal forebrain circuits. We will emphasize the importance of the projections into temporal cortex from the basal forebrain through the amygdala, and of frontal projections into basal forebrain, in object–reward association learning.

17.2 The amygdala and learning about the intrinsic reward value of objects

The extensive emotional changes in monkeys after bilateral temporal lobe ablations (Klüver and Bucy, 1939) have been shown to result also from bilateral aspiration lesions limited to the amygdala and overlying cortical areas (Weiskrantz, 1956). Animals with such lesions show increased tameness, abnormal food choices, and apparent indifference to desirable food rewards. One might expect, therefore, that reinforcement learning would be severely affected by such lesions.

The effects of bilateral aspiration lesions of amygdala on object–reward association learning has in fact proved variable, ranging from a significant impairment (Schwartzbaum and Poulos, 1965; Barrett, 1969) to almost no impairment (Douglas *et al.*, 1969; Horel *et al.*, 1975). Tests in an automated apparatus where responses are to objects on a computer touchscreen and a food reward is delivered to a central hopper, independently of where the touched object is, show a significant, though mild, effect of amygdala lesions (Gaffan and Murray, 1990). The same holds true when crossed lesions are made of amygdala in one hemisphere and inferior temporal cortex in the opposite hemisphere (Gaffan *et al.*, 1988). Here the interaction between amygdala and inferior temporal cortex is disrupted bilaterally and the effect on reward-association learning can be measured without any additional motivational problems which may result from bilateral amygdala lesions.

A study by Gaffan and Harrison (1987) showed a very severe impairment in learning a visual object–reward association by means of an auditory secondary reinforcer. Correct responses to an object were followed by a reinforcing auditory stimulus, and incorrect choices by a non-reinforcing auditory stimulus. A food reward was delivered only after a predetermined number of consecutive responses to the correct object, and so within-trial learning was dependent only on secondary reinforcement and not the primary reinforcement of food reward. It was proposed that this severe impairment indicated a role for the amygdala in associating objects with the intrinsic reward value of that object (Gaffan and Harrison, 1987; Gaffan, 1992).

17.3 Functions of fibres of passage

Recent lesion techniques have allowed the exploration of these ideas with excitotoxic lesions of the amygdala, which spare both fibres passing through the region and cortical tissue damaged on the approach of an aspiration lesion. Malkova *et al.* (1997) studied the auditory secondary reinforcement task of Gaffan and Harrison (1987) which had proved to be very sensitive to the effects of aspiration amygdalectomy. Importantly, it was seen that the excitotoxic lesions of amygdala had no effect at all on the performance of animals on this task. The impairments after amygdala lesions in this task (Gaffan and Harrison, 1987) must, therefore, have been a reliance on structures which send their projections through the amygdala. A similar effect had been seen previously in rats with excitotoxic lesions of the amygdala which were not impaired at learning a conditioned taste aversion while rats with electrolytic lesions of the amygdala were (Dunn and Everitt, 1988).

What fibres that course through the amygdala might be important in the learning of reward described above? The study of Dunn and Everitt (1988) showed that projections to insula cortex from basal forebrain (hypothalamus and substantia innominata) were interrupted by electrolytic lesions of the amygdala, but not by excitotoxic lesions. These basal forebrain structures also project to inferior temporal cortex (including perirhinal cortex) in the monkey via the amygdala (Kitt *et al.*, 1987), and their axons are interrupted by surgical section of the amygdala and the temporal stem white matter dorsolaterally adjacent to the amygdala (Easton and Gaffan, unpublished observations). In the monkey, it has also been shown that projections from inferior temporal cortex (including rhinal cortex) to both the medial part of the magnocellular division of nucleus medialis dorsalis (MD) of the thalamus (Goulet *et al.*, 1998) and ventral and orbital prefrontal cortex (Baxter *et al.*, 1998) are disrupted by conventional aspiration lesions of the amygdala. Can any of these fibres of passage through the amygdala be responsible for the impairments seen after aspiration amygdalectomy on reward learning?

As described above, the frontal cortex is necessary for object–reward association learning (Parker and Gaffan, 1998b). Section of the uncinate fascicle, which is the major route of direct corticocortical projections between frontal cortex and inferior temporal cortex

(Ungerleider *et al.*, 1989), does not impair object–reward association learning (Eacott and Gaffan, 1992), nor the auditory secondary reinforcer task described above (Gaffan and Eacott, 1995). The disruption of direct projections from inferior temporal cortex to frontal cortex is thus unlikely to be the explanation of the reward learning impairments seen after aspiration amygdalectomy.

What of the inferior temporal projections to MD of the thalamus? The projection of inferior temporal cortical regions to MD are localized only to the medial part of the magnocellular division (Russchen *et al.*, 1987). Bilateral lesions of MD confined only to this medial part of the magnocellular division have little effect on object–reward association learning (Parker *et al.*, 1997), which limits the relevance of the inputs to MD from amygdala and rhinal cortex. However, the entire extent of the magnocellular division of MD both receives projections from and sends projections to the frontal cortex (Goldman-Rakic and Porrino, 1985; Russchen *et al.*, 1987), and Parker and Gaffan (1998a) have proposed that lesions of magnocellular MD have their effect through disruption of normal frontal cortex function. Recognition memory (as assessed by delayed match-to-sample in our automated apparatus) is only affected very mildly by lesions of magnocellular MD restricted to the medial region, which receives inferior temporal cortical input (Parker *et al.*, 1997). In contrast, larger lesions extending into the entire magnocellular division of MD have a far greater effect on recognition memory (Parker and Gaffan, 1998a). Parker and Gaffan (1998a) propose that as the large effect is only seen after lesions of MD that extend beyond the medial portion of the magnocellular division (the only portion to receive inputs from amygdala and rhinal cortex), then the effect is due to the afferent and efferent connections of MD and frontal cortex. The slightly smaller effect of large MD lesions on recognition memory than disconnection of frontal cortex directly from perirhinal cortex (Parker and Gaffan, 1998a) is the result of the cortical lesions removing all the cortical tissue which needs to interact in this task. In contrast, the magnocellular MD lesions only disrupt frontal activity and so may allow some preservation, however small, of frontal function. This preservation of frontal function can explain the smaller effect on recognition memory. The effect of aspiration amygdala lesions on object–reward association learning, therefore, is unlikely to be due to disruption of a projection from inferior temporal cortex to only the medial part of the magnocellular division of MD.

The proposal outlined by Baxter and Murray (Chapter 16) that one effect of aspiration amygdala lesions on reward-association learning is to interrupt inferior temporal cortex communication with both frontal lobe and the medial portion of the magnocellular division of MD can now be considered fully. Gaffan *et al.* (1993) showed that aspiration lesions of the amygdala in one hemisphere when crossed with ablation of either ventromedial prefrontal cortex or the medial part of the magnocellular division of MD in the opposite hemisphere produced only a mild impairment in object–reward association learning. In contrast, a disconnection of amygdala in one hemisphere from both ventromedial prefrontal cortex and the medial part of the magnocellular division of MD in the opposite hemisphere produced a more severe impairment. This result may suggest that the combined disruption of projections from inferior temporal cortex to the frontal cortex and the magnocellular portion of MD by aspiration amygdalectomy is the cause of the object–reward association learning impairments after amygdalectomy. However, we have already seen that the effects of MD ablations in learning are likely to be due to their effect on frontal cortex function (Parker and Gaffan, 1998a). It would then hold true that a small disruption of frontal cortex function by the medial magnocellular MD lesion of Gaffan *et al.* (1993), when combined with a small lesion of frontal cortex tissue, actually results in a larger disruption of frontal cortex function than is produced by any one of these lesions on their own. As such, the effect of this combined disconnection in the experiment of Gaffan *et al.* (1993) may be the result of effectively disconnecting an aspiration amygdalectomy in one hemisphere from a relatively large frontal cortex disruption in the opposite hemisphere. However, disconnections of frontal cortex from inferior temporal cortex by crossed unilateral lesions do not impair object–reward association learning (Parker and Gaffan, 1998b), so why do Gaffan *et al.* (1993) see an impairment after their disconnection pattern?

17.4 Perceptual demand increases reliance on perirhinal cortex

A possible explanation for this difference can come from examining the different perceptual demands of the object–reward association learning task in the experiments of Gaffan *et al.* (1993) and Parker and Gaffan (1998b). Perirhinal cortex lesions in monkeys do not impair learning of new two-choice discriminations postoperatively when there has been limited preoperative training and there are few discrimination problems being learnt concurrently (Buckley and Gaffan, 1997). The performance of these animals is outlined in Figure 17.1 where the second column (PRh) represents the average errors per problem in learning 20 concurrent discrimination problems. Learning of discriminations by perirhinal lesioned animals can be impaired, however, by increasing the perceptual demands of the task. Increasing the number of objects for each trial (e.g. a 15-choice object–reward association with only one rewarded object and 14 non-rewarded distracters), or increasing the number of problems being learnt concurrently within a session leads to an impairment in learning after perirhinal cortex removals (Buckley and Gaffan, 1997). This increase in the perceptual demands of the task taxes the perirhinal cortex more due to its own involvement in some forms of object perception (Buckley and Gaffan, 1998; Murray and Bussey, 1999). An alternative way to increase the perceptual demands of an object–reward association task is to increase the number of problems the animal is exposed to, which requires a high degree of object identity processing in order to discriminate new objects from those previously experienced.

Experiments which previously have shown no effect of perirhinal cortex lesions in new object–reward association learning (Gaffan and Murray, 1992; Buckley and Gaffan, 1997; Thornton *et al.*, 1997) have all had limited preoperative training of the animals on the task. Easton and Gaffan (2000) tested the new concurrent learning of 10 two-choice discrimination problems after extensive preoperative training. Preoperatively the animals were trained in both concurrent object–reward association learning (with many sets of 10 concurrent problems and a minimum of 100 trials per session) and a scene-based object-in-place task (with many sets of 20 pairs of objects each repeated eight times per session) which used

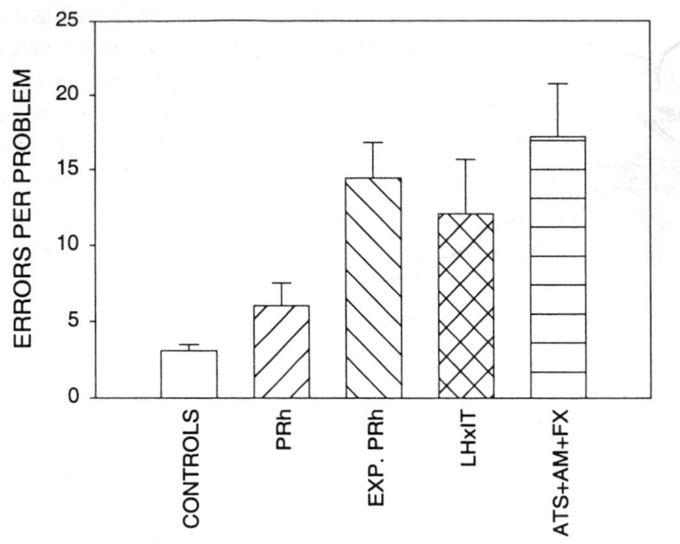

Figure 17.1 Comparison of performances on object–reward association learning with different lesions. Performance is shown as the average errors per problem in learning several concurrent problems, with error bars representing the standard error of the mean. CONTROLS = performance of normal, experienced, animals. PRh = postoperative performance of animals with perirhinal lesions and limited preoperative experience (Buckley and Gaffan, 1997). EXP. PRh = postoperative performance of animals with perirhinal lesions and extensive preoperative experience (Easton and Gaffan, 2000). LHxIT = postoperative performance of animals with crossed unilateral lesions of lateral hypothalamus (basal forebrain) and inferior temporal cortex (Easton and Gaffan, in press). ATS+AM+FX = postoperative performance of animals with bilateral combined lesions of the anterior temporal stem, amygdala, and fornix to isolate the inferior temporal cortex from its basal forebrain afferents (Gaffan *et al.*, in press). It can be seen both that experience alters the reliance of object–reward association learning on the perirhinal cortex, and that disconnecting the inferior temporal cortex from its basal forebrain afferents severely impairs object–reward association learning.

similar visual objects to the object–reward association task. Thus, the animals were exposed preoperatively to many thousands of trials with many hundreds of similar visual objects. The discrimination of newly presented objects then would be expected to tax the perceptual mechanisms of the perirhinal cortex more than in the previous studies. Indeed, this is the result we obtained. The third column of Figure 17.1 (EXP. PRh) shows the average errors per problem in the learning of 10 concurrent discrimination problems. The animals with perirhinal lesions were now very severely impaired, making on average more than five times as many errors postoperatively as preoperatively. This impairment, not seen in previous studies with perirhinal lesions (compare groups PRh and EXP. PRh in Figure 17.1), supports the reliance on perirhinal cortex for perceptually demanding object–reward learning.

This may help us to explain the apparent difference between the effect of the disconnections of Gaffan *et al.* (1993) and Parker and Gaffan (1998b) on reward-association learning. The animals of Parker and Gaffan (1998b) had been exposed preoperatively to a relatively limited number of visual problems (the pre-training of 20 concurrent two-choice discrimination problems and two sets of reward–visual conditional problems with two visual objects per problem; a total of 44 objects). The animals of Gaffan *et al.* (1993) had been exposed preoperatively to many more problems (the learning of 45 sets of five concurrent problems; 450 objects). This larger number of experienced objects in Gaffan *et al.* (1993) may have increased the reliance of the task on the perirhinal cortex and so altered the effects of disconnection in object–reward association.

17.5 The basal forebrain and reward learning

What then about the projections from basal forebrain to inferior temporal cortex that pass through both the amygdala and the white matter surrounding the amygdala (Kitt *et al.*, 1987; Seldon *et al.*, 1998)? Aspiration lesions of the amygdala are going to damage both those fibres passing through the amygdala and those adjacent to the amygdala in the white matter of the temporal stem which is likely to be damaged or disrupted either mechanically by the lesion or as a result of interrupted blood flow. If, as we have proposed above, the learning of object–reward associations is by interaction between the frontal cortex and inferior temporal cortex with subcortical and interhemispheric communication, then the primate basal forebrain is anatomically suited to this function. The frontal cortex projects both to the cholinergic cells of the basal forebrain and to the lateral hypothalamus (Mesulam and Mufson, 1984; Ongur *et al.*, 1998; Rempel-Clower and Barbas, 1998), and these regions in turn project to inferior temporal cortex (Mesulam *et al.*, 1983; Webster *et al.*, 1993). There are also projections from lateral hypothalamic cells to contralateral cells of the substantia innominata (Cullinan and Zaborszky, 1991). These crossed projections, along with the strong interconnection of basal forebrain with midbrain areas (Russchen *et al.*, 1985) which are themselves bilaterally integrated, allow the basal forebrain to be a route of communication between frontal cortex and inferior temporal cortex both within the same hemisphere and between hemispheres. Indeed, both the cholinergic cells of the basal forebrain (Mesulam *et al.*, 1983) and the acetylcholinesterase staining cells of the lateral hypothalamus (Saper, 1990) have a widespread projection to many cortical areas. In contrast, they receive projections from a far more limited set of cortical areas (Mesulam and Mufson, 1984). Mesulam and Mufson (1984) propose that this pattern of afferents and efferents allows a few specific regions of cortex to influence widespread cortical activity. If this route of interaction is important in learning of object–reward associations, then disrupting it should impair the learning of object–reward associations at least as badly as aspiration amygdalectomy.

Easton and Gaffan (in press b) disconnected the basal forebrain of monkeys from the inferior temporal cortex, by crossed unilateral lesions, in a task of object–reward association. The basal forebrain lesion consisted of a small heat lesion of the lateral hypothalamus, which also had the effect of sectioning the medial forebrain bundle. The medial forebrain bundle is the route by which hypothalamic cells interact with cells of the cholinergic basal forebrain (Cullinan and Zaborszky, 1991) and by which basal forebrain areas interact with structures of the midbrain and brainstem (Russchen *et al.*, 1985). This heat lesion, therefore, both damages cells of the lateral hypothalamus which receive frontal cortex projections and project in turn to the inferior temporal cortex (Webster *et al.*, 1993; Ongur *et al.*, 1998; Rempel-Clower and Barbas, 1998), and also disrupts basal forebrain activity in general on the side of the lesion by damaging the medial forebrain bundle. After this hypothalamic–cortical disconnection, we found an impairment in object–reward association learning as severe, if not more so, as that seen after aspiration amygdalectomy (Gaffan and Murray, 1990). This is outlined in Figure 17.1 where the fourth column (LHxIT) shows the substantial impairment in learning 10 concurrent visual discriminations. The explanation for this more severe impairment after hypothalamic–cortical disconnection is, presumably, that there is a disruption of the projections of hypothalamus and basal forebrain beyond only those fibres that pass through or near the amygdala.

Basal forebrain projects to structures of the medial temporal lobe and inferior temporal cortex by three main routes: the fornix, amygdala, and anterior temporal stem (Kitt *et al.*, 1987; Seldon *et al.*, 1998). Aspiration amygdala lesions will disrupt those fibres of passage through the amygdala, and may also disrupt some fibres in the temporal stem, but fibres through the fornix, and some in the temporal stem, will remain unaffected by aspiration amygdalectomy. Gaffan *et al.* (in press) showed that combined sections of the amygdala and temporal stem had a severe but temporary effect on object–reward association. Note that in these animals the amygdala was only sectioned and not removed, and so fibres of passage will have been cut, but there would be some sparing of amygdala function. Addition of fornix section to this amygdala and temporal stem section both stabilized and increased the severity of the learning impairment (Gaffan *et al.*, in press), presumably by sectioning the remaining fibres from basal forebrain to medial temporal lobe structures. This combined lesion of fornix, amygdala, and temporal stem produced an impairment in object–reward association learning which was not significantly different from that after hypothalamic–cortical disconnection (Easton and Gaffan, in press b). The performance of these animals is shown in the fifth column of Figure 17.1 (ATS+AM+FX). The impairment is seen to be very similar to that after basal forebrain disconnection from inferior temporal cortex (compare groups LHxIT and ATS+AM+FX in Figure 17.1). Therefore, we propose that the reward learning impairments seen after aspiration but not excitotoxic lesions of the amygdala are the result of interrupting fibres of passage from basal forebrain to inferior temporal cortex.

17.6 The subcortical communication of frontal and inferior temporal cortex via the basal forebrain

We propose that these basal forebrain fibres are part of a subcortical communication route between frontal cortex and inferior temporal cortex which are important for many aspects of learning. Indeed, Easton and Gaffan (in press b) have shown that the hypothalamic lesion when disconnected from frontal cortex produces the same size of impairment in object–reward association learning as does disconnection from inferior temporal cortex. This supports the proposal that the basal forebrain is a route of communication between these two cortical areas. Also, isolation of inferior temporal cortex from its basal forebrain inputs, either by combined section of the fornix, amygdala, and temporal stem (Gaffan *et al.*, in press; see Figures 17.1 and 17.2), or hypothalamic–cortical disconnection (Easton and Gaffan, 2000; in press a; see Figures 17.1 and 17.2), or even a disconnection from an immunotoxic lesion of only the cholinergic cells of the basal forebrain (Easton *et al.*, 2000; see Figure 17.2), results in a dense amnesia. This amnesia covers the learning of all the visual tasks we have tested; object–reward associations (Easton and Gaffan, in press b; Gaffan *et al.*, in press; see Figure 17.1), a scene-based object-in-place task which is in some ways analogous to human episodic memory (Gaffan *et al.*, in press; Easton and Gaffan, 2000; see Figure 17.2),

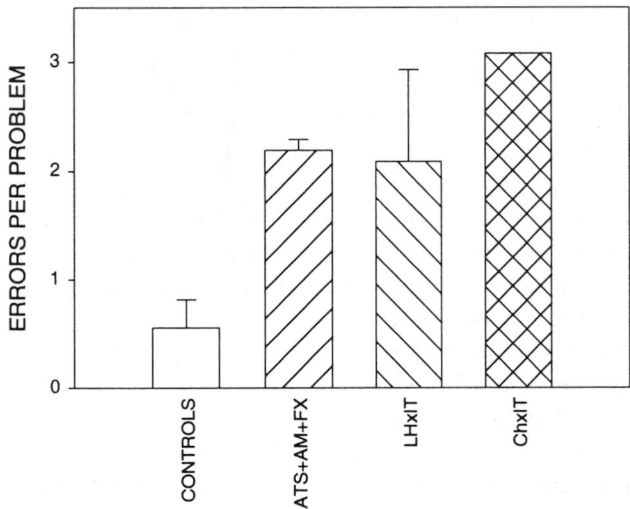

Figure 17.2 Comparison of performances on a scene-based object-in-place task. Performance is shown as average errors per problem in learning several concurrent problems, with error bars representing the standard error of the mean. The task limits the presentation of each problem to only eight trials, so chance performance is 3.5 errors per problem (as performance on the initial trial is not controlled by memory). CONTROLS = performance of normal animals. ATS+AM+FX = performance of animals with bilateral combined lesions of the anterior temporal stem, amygdala, and fornix to isolate the inferior temporal cortex from its basal forebrain afferents (Gaffan *et al.*, in press). LHxIT = performance of animals with crossed unilateral lesions of lateral hypothalamus and inferior temporal cortex (Easton and Gaffan, 2000). ChxIT = performance of an animal with crossed unilateral lesions of the cholinergic basal forebrain and inferior temporal cortex (Easton *et al.*, 2000). All groups disconnecting the basal forebrain from inferior temporal cortex are very severely impaired at this task, with group ChxIT approaching chance performance.

and recognition memory (Gaffan *et al.*, in press; Parker, Easton and Gaffan, 2000). In contrast, the retention of preoperatively taught object–reward associations is relatively preserved (Gaffan *et al.*, in press; Easton and Gaffan, 2000).

The scene-based object-in-place task (Figure 17.2) is a task whereby each trial consists of a unique complex background scene, with two unique visual objects in unique positions on that scene. Only one of these objects is rewarded, and the rewarded object always appears in the same position on the same background scene. Because of the spatial and object components of each problem and the ease with which normal animals learn this task, it has been proposed as being in some ways analogous to episodic memory in monkeys (Gaffan, 1994, 1998). As one object per scene is always rewarded, however, this can in some ways be considered as an object–reward association task. The severe impairment in this task after lesions which disrupt the basal forebrain projection to inferior temporal cortex thus further supports the proposal that the basal forebrain is crucial to the interaction between frontal and inferior temporal cortex in object–reward association learning.

One obvious objection to the hypothalamic lesion studies outlined above is that a heat lesion of the lateral hypothalamus will disrupt the fibres of the medial forebrain bundle which include dopaminergic cells with reward-signalling properties (Hollerman and Schultz, 1998). Indeed, it is also possible that the hypothalamic lesions of Easton and Gaffan (2000; in press a,b) and the temporal stem lesions of Gaffan *et al.* (in press) have the effect of disrupting communication of inferior temporal cortex, thalamus, and frontal cortex. We have addressed the role of nucleus MD of the thalamus above, and the effects of lesions of one of the main terminals of the dopaminergic projections (the ventral striatum) have no effect on object–reward association learning in the monkey when disconnected from aspiration amygdalectomy (Gaffan *et al.*, 1993). We have, however, investigated this question further using crossed unilateral lesions of the frontal and inferior temporal cortex in the scene task described above (Easton and Gaffan, 1999). This disconnection will disrupt all intrahemispheric communication between frontal and inferior temporal cortex. As such, only communication between hemispheres, such as the route we propose through basal forebrain, will be available for the intact frontal cortex to communicate with the intact inferior temporal cortex. The effect of this crossed cortical disconnection was to produce a significant impairment in the task, though milder than the impairment seen after any of the basal forebrain disruptions. As such, the role of thalamic and dopaminergic fibres cannot be ignored, but the stable and substantial impairments seen after basal forebrain lesions, including section of the medial forebrain bundle by a heat lesion of the lateral hypothalamus, are most likely to be due to the interhemispheric communication of reinforcement by basal forebrain, as outlined below.

Figure 17.3A summarizes our proposal for basal forebrain influence on frontal and inferior temporal interactions. The objective properties of a specific reward event, which could be a primary reward such as a 190 mg food pellet or a secondary reward that is associated with food, are shown as an afferent input to the basal forebrain ('reward' in the figure). In addition, frontal cortex input to the basal forebrain modulates the response of the basal forebrain to this specific reward event according to the current goals of the animal ('goal'). If the reward event is relevant to current goals, it produces the arousal signal ('reinforcement') which is sent to temporal cortex and facilitates associative memory. Similarly, the absence of a food reward can be a memorable event when an animal is seeking food, and memory of non-reward is modulated by cortical interaction with the basal forebrain in the same way, but not shown in the figure. Figure 17.3B outlines the situation in the case of crossed unilateral lesions of frontal cortex and inferior temporal cortex (Parker and Gaffan, 1998b). The frontal cortex still signals the current goals to the basal forebrain which, due to its interconnections with structures in the contralateral hemisphere, can signal the reward-related information interhemispherically. As a result, the goal information from the intact frontal cortex is still able to signal reinforcement to the intact inferior temporal cortex. Figure 17.3C outlines the situation in the case of crossed unilateral lesions of lateral hypothalamus (basal forebrain) and inferior temporal cortex (Easton and Gaffan, in press a,b). The frontal cortex on the side of the intact basal forebrain remains able to signal the current goal to that basal forebrain. However, on the side of the intact lateral hypothalamus, interhemispheric communication is disrupted by the contralateral basal forebrain lesion, and intrahemispheric communication is made impossible by the inferior temporal cortex lesion in this hemisphere. The goal signal from frontal cortex is thus unable to send reinforcement signals to the intact inferior temporal cortex in this case. Figure 17.3D outlines the situation in the case of crossed unilateral lesions of lateral hypothalamus (basal forebrain) and frontal cortex (Easton and Gaffan, in press b). Now the inferior temporal cortex can receive reinforcement signals from the intact basal forebrain, but this is not under the control of frontal cortex. The intact frontal cortex cannot signal the current goal to the lesioned basal forebrain, and the lesioned frontal cortex cannot signal the current goal at all. As a result, the only reinforcement signal that reaches inferior temporal cortex is not set by the current goals of the task. This model of basal foıebrain function in object–reward association learning therefore supports the experimental evidence that crossed unilateral lesions of frontal cortex and inferior temporal cortex have no effect on object–reward association learning (Parker and Gaffan, 1998b), while crossed unilateral lesions of inferior temporal or frontal cortex and lateral hypothalamus impair object–reward association learning (Easton and Gaffan, in press b).

17.7 Reinforcement of visual memories in inferior temporal cortex

The ablation experiments and the anatomical data we have reviewed make a strong case for the idea that memory of reward, both in the scenes task and with simple objects, relies on the basal forebrain input into medial and inferior temporal cortex. Electrophysiological data, however, make it clear that if this idea is true, the synaptic interaction between basal forebrain and temporal cortex in memory cannot be a Hebbian associative mechanism. The Hebb model of synaptic plasticity (Hebb, 1949) requires that the events to be recalled, in this case reward or non-reward, are encoded in the depolarization and therefore in the action potentials of the postsynaptic cell, while, in contrast, the retrieval cue, here an object either alone or as part of a scene, is encoded in the depolarization of the presynaptic cell. The earlier proposal which we now reject, to the effect that object–reward associations are stored in the synapses of the inferior temporal cortical projection into the amygdala (Gaffan, 1992; Gaffan

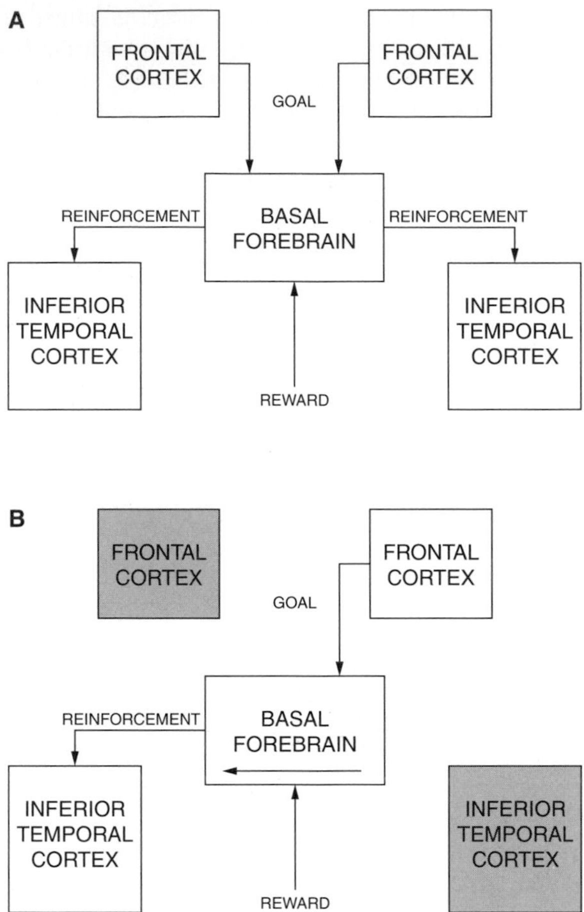

Figure 17.3 Proposed role of the basal forebrain in the subcortical communication of frontal lobe and inferior temporal cortex. Lesions in the model are indicated by shading. (**A**) The intact brain, where frontal lobe signals the current goals to basal forebrain which also receives peripheral reward signals. In turn, reinforcement is signalled from basal forebrain to the inferior temporal cortex to set the visual memory. (**B**) The case of crossed unilateral disconnections of frontal lobe and inferior temporal cortex. The interhemispheric communication of reinforcement by the basal forebrain allows the intact frontal lobe to communicate with the intact inferior temporal cortex. Object–reward association learning is unimpaired by this combination of lesions (Parker and Gaffan, 1998b). (**C**) The case of crossed unilateral disconnections of basal forebrain and inferior temporal cortex. There is now no route possible by which either frontal lobe can influence the intact inferior temporal cortex via the basal forebrain. Object–reward association learning is impaired by this combination of lesions (Easton and Gaffan, in press b). (**D**) The case of crossed unilateral disconnections of basal forebrain and frontal cortex. Now reinforcement signals can reach inferior temporal cortex from the intact

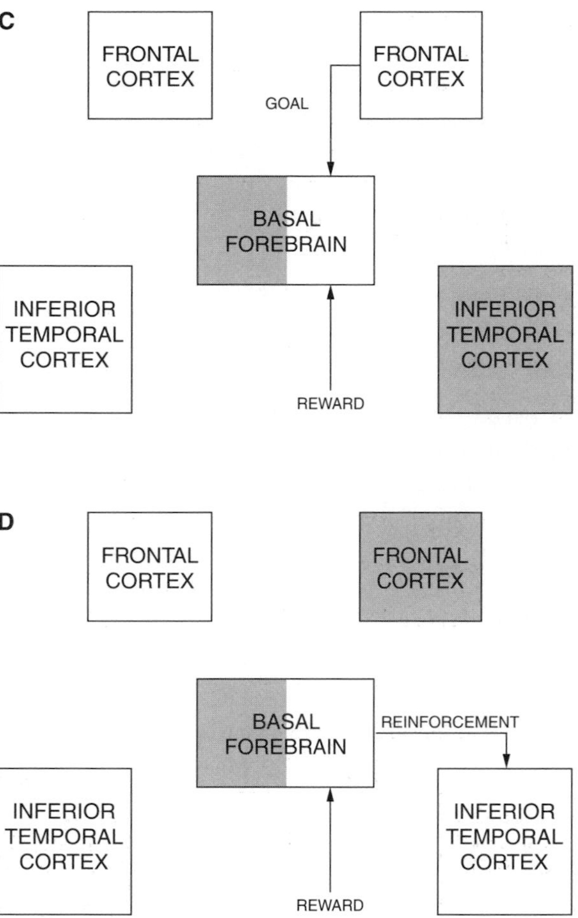

basal forebrain, but this reinforcement signal is not guided by signals of the current goal from frontal cortex. Object–reward association learning is impaired by this combination of lesions (Easton and Gaffan, in press b).

et al., 1988) was a Hebbian hypothesis. However, in our present model, the temporal cortical cells which encode object identity are postsynaptic to the basal forebrain cells which encode reward and non-reward. This is the wrong way round for the Hebb model. That model could still be applied perhaps if the basal forebrain input into temporal cortex elicited powerful activity reflecting reward or non-reward in the temporal cortex cells themselves, but there is no evidence that reward and non-reward are powerfully encoded in inferior temporal cortical action potentials (Rolls *et al.*, 1977).

Instead, we propose that the basal forebrain input to inferior temporal cortex acts to facilitate the synaptic plasticity of corticocortical synapses. The inferior temporal cortical cells which encode object identity will then provide, through corticocortical projections, the retrieval cue for representations of reward and non-reward events that are encoded elsewhere in the cortex, for example in the prestriate or parietal cortex (Brown *et al.*, 1995; Gaffan and Hornak, 1997). According to this model, the inferior temporal cortex cells are presynaptic in the corticocortical synaptic changes which encode the memory of an object's association with reward. The synapses between basal forebrain cells and inferior temporal cortex cells do not need to be plastic themselves in this model. Furthermore, according to this idea, the basal forebrain input to the cortex acts like a reinforcement signal in the literal sense (Hull, 1943), in that it facilitates the storage of an association but does not itself enter into that association, neither as a retrieval cue nor as a recall target. Therefore, the basal forebrain cells do not need to encode the difference between a reward and a non-reward in order to perform their facilitative function. They could simply encode the necessity to remember the current event, without specifying what that event is. This is consistent with electrophysiological data indicating that many basal forebrain cells encode arousal rather than specific kinds of reward or punishment (Semba, 1991). However, specific encoding of reward events enters into the associative process elsewhere. We have already suggested that reward is represented cortically in associative memory. Reward must also be one of the inputs to the basal forebrain that can produce arousal. This proposal fits with the role of goals, reward, and reinforcement described above and outlined in Figure 17.3.

17.8 What is the role of the amygdala?

It seems likely from the experiments outlined above that the effects of aspiration amygdalectomy on reward learning were due to the partial interruption of basal forebrain efferents to inferior temporal cortex. We do not propose, however, that the basal forebrain is itself a reward structure in the brain. It is true that cells of both the hypothalamus and the cholinergic basal forebrain respond to reward (Fukuda *et al.*, 1986, 1993; Wilson and Rolls, 1990; Masuda *et al.*, 1997). We propose, however, that as the effect of isolating medial temporal lobe and inferior temporal cortex from the basal forebrain is to produce a dense amnesia (Gaffan *et al.*, in press), the role of the basal forebrain is to modulate cortical activity based on current reward criterion and goals, as directed by frontal cortex control (see Figure 17.3). Object–reward association learning, therefore, will be disrupted by basal forebrain lesions, but so are non-object–reward association tasks such as delayed match-to-sample (Gaffan *et al.*, in press; Parker, Easton, and Gaffan, 2000).

In contrast to the basal forebrain, the effects of excitotoxic amygdala lesions still appear to centre on reward and emotional behaviour. Malkova *et al.* (1997) showed that although their excitotoxic lesions of the amygdala did not impair object–reward learning, they did impair reinforcer devaluations. Discrimination problems were taught preoperatively, with each object presented being rewarded, but by different foodstuffs. Animals tended to choose that object of a pair which was associated with its preferred reward. After devaluation of that preferred reward (through satiation to that food), normal monkeys tended to choose the object associated with the non-devalued food reward. In contrast, monkeys with excitotoxic amygdala lesions chose inconsistently. Malkova *et al.* (1997) interpret this result as supporting the amygdala's role in associating stimuli with the value of a reward as proposed by Gaffan and Harrison (1987). Similarly, the effects of excitotoxic amygdala lesions on the emotional behaviour of monkeys reflect those effects of aspiration amygdala lesions, i.e. an increased tameness and abnormal social interactions with other monkeys (Amaral *et al.*, 1997; Meunier *et al.*, 1999).

It appears, then, that when a question is asked about the learning of reward in the monkey, one should be careful about the exact nature of that question. If the question posed can be solved simply by the reinforcement of behaviour, then the basal forebrain appears to be of importance. In contrast, when the question relies on more hedonistic values of reward (i.e. 'Is this food still pleasant rather than simply reinforcing?', or 'What are the rewarding consequences of social interaction?'), then the amygdala appears to be of importance.

References

Amaral, D.G., Capitanio, J.P., Machado, C.J., Mason, W.A., and Mendoza, S.P. (1997) The role of the amygdaloid complex in rhesus monkey social behavior. *Society for Neuroscience Abstracts*, 23, 570.

Barrett, T.W. (1969) Studies of the function of the amygdaloid complex in *Macaca mulatta*. *Neuropsychologia*, 7, 1–12.

Baxter, M.G., Saunders, R.C., and Murray, E.A. (1998) Aspiration lesions of the amygdala interrupt connections between prefrontal cortex and temporal cortex in rhesus monkeys. *Society for Neuroscience Abstracts*, 24, 1905.

Brown, V.J., Desimone, R., and Mishkin, M. (1995) Responses of cells in the tail of the caudate nucleus during visual discrimination learning. *Journal of Neurophysiology*, **74**, 1083–1094.

Buckley, M.J. and Gaffan, D. (1997) Impairment of visual object-discrimination learning after perirhinal cortex ablation. *Behavioral Neuroscience*, 111, 467–475.

Buckley, M.J. and Gaffan, D. (1998) Perirhinal cortex ablation impairs configural learning and paired-associate learning equally. *Neuropsychologia*, 36, 535–546.

Cullinan, W.E. and Zaborszky, L. (1991) Organization of ascending hypothalamic projections to the rostral forebrain with spatial reference to the innervation of cholinergic projection neurons. *Journal of Comparative Neurology*, 306, 631–667.

Douglas, R.J., Barrett, T.W., Pribram, K.H., and Cerny, M.C. (1969) Limbic lesions and error reduction. *Journal of Comparative and Physiological Psychology*, 68, 437–441.

Dunn, L.T. and Everitt, B.J. (1988) Double dissociations of the effects of amygdala and insular cortex lesions on conditioned taste aversion, passive avoidance, and neophobia in the rat using the excitotoxin ibotenic acid. *Behavioral Neuroscience*, 102, 3–23.

Eacott, M.J. and Gaffan, D. (1992) Inferotemporal–frontal disconnection: the uncinate fascicle and visual associative learning in monkeys. *European Journal of Neuroscience*, 4, 1320–1332.

Easton, A. and Gaffan, D. (1999) Interaction of frontal lobe and inferior temporal cortex in object-in-place memory. *Society for Neuroscience Abstracts*.

Easton, A., and Gaffan, D. (in press-a). Comparison of perirhinal cortex ablation and crossed unilateral lesions of medial forebrain bundle from inferior temporal cortex in the Rhesus monkey: effects on learning and retrieval, *Behavioral Neuroscience*.

Easton, A., and Gaffan, D. (in press-b). Crossed unilateral lesions of the medial forebrain bundle and either inferior temporal or frontal cortex impair object–reward association learning in Rhesus monkeys. *Neuropsychologia*.

Easton, A., Ridley, R.M., Baker, H.F., and Gaffan, D. (2000). Crossed unilateral lesions of the cholinergic basal forebrain (by ME20.41gG-saporin) and fornix from inferior temporal cortex produce severe learning impairments in Rhesus monkeys. *Society for Neuroscience Abstracts*, **26**.

Fukuda, M., Ono, T., Nishino, H., and Nakamura, K. (1986) Neuronal responses in monkey lateral hypothalamus during operant feeding behaviour. *Brain Research Bulletin*, 17, 879–884.

Fukuda, M., Masuda, R., Ono, T., and Tabuchi, E. (1993) Responses of monkey basal forebrain neurons during a visual discrimination task. *Progress in Brain Research*, 95, 359–369.

Gaffan, D. (1992) Amygdala and the memory of reward. In *The Amygdala: Neurobiological Aspects of Emotion, Memory, and Mental Dysfunction* (ed. J.P. Aggleton), pp. 471–483. Wiley-Liss, New York.

Gaffan, D. (1994) Scene-specific memory for objects: a model of episodic memory impairment in monkeys with fornix transection. *Journal of Cognitive Neuroscience*, 6, 305–320.

Gaffan, D. (1998) Idiothetic input into object–place configuration as the contribution to memory of the monkey and human hippocampus: a review. *Experimental Brain Research*, 123, 201–209.

Gaffan, D. and Eacott, M.J. (1995) Visual learning for an auditory secondary reinforcer is intact after uncinate fascicle section: indirect evidence for the involvement of the corpus striatum. *European Journal of Neuroscience*, 7, 1866–1871.

Gaffan, D. and Harrison, S. (1987) Amygdalectomy and disconnection in visual learning for auditory secondary reinforcement by monkeys. *Journal of Neuroscience*, 7, 2285–2292.

Gaffan, D. and Hornak, J. (1997) Visual neglect in the monkey: representation and disconnection. *Brain*, 120, 1647–1657.

Gaffan, D. and Murray, E.A. (1990) Amygdalar interaction with the mediodorsal nucleus of the thalamus and the ventromedial prefrontal cortex in stimulus–reward associative learning in the monkey. *Journal of Neuroscience*, 10, 3479–3493.

Gaffan, D. and Murray, E.A. (1992) Monkeys (*Macaca fascicularis*) with rhinal cortex ablations succeed in object discrimination learning despite 24-hr intertrial intervals and fail at matching to sample despite double sample presentations. *Behavioral Neuroscience*, 106, 30–38.

Gaffan, D., Murray, E.A., and Fabre-Thorpe, M. (1993) Interaction of the amygdala with the frontal lobe in reward memory. *European Journal of Neuroscience*, 5, 968–975.

Gaffan, D., Parker, A., and Easton, A. (in press). Dense amnesia in the monkey after transection of fornix, amygdala and anterior temporal stem. *Neuropsychologia*.

Gaffan, E.A., Harrison, S., and Gaffan, D. (1986) Single and concurrent discrimination learning by monkeys after lesions of inferotemporal cortex. *Quarterly Journal of Experimental Psychology*, 38B, 31–51.

Gaffan, E.A., Gaffan, D., and Harrison, S. (1988) Disconnection of the amygdala from visual association cortex impairs visual reward-association learning in monkeys. *Journal of Neuroscience*, 8, 3144–3150.

Goldman-Rakic, P.S. and Porrino, L.J. (1985) The primate mediodorsal (MD) nucleus and its projections to the frontal lobe. *Journal of Comparative Neurology*, 242, 535–560.

Goulet, S., Dore, F.Y., and Murray, E.A. (1998) Aspiration lesions of the amygdala disrupt the rhinal corticothalamic projection system in rhesus monkeys. *Experimental Brain Research*, 119, 131–140.

Gutnikov, S.A., Ma, Y., and Gaffan, D. (1997) Temporo-frontal disconnection impairs visual–visual paired association learning but not configural learning in *Macaca* monkeys. *European Journal of Neuroscience*, 9, 1524–1529.

Hebb, D.O. (1949) *Organization of Behavior*. Wiley, New York.

Hollerman, J.R. and Schultz, W. (1998) Dopamine neurons report an error in the temporal prediction of reward during learning. *Nature Neuroscience*, 1, 304–309.

Horel, J.A., Keating, E.G., and Misantone, L.G. (1975) Partial Klüver–Bucy syndrome produced by destroying temporal neocortex or amygdala. *Brain Research*, 94, 347–359.

Hull, C.L. (1943) *Principles of Behavior*. Appleton Century Crofts, New York.

Kitt, C.A., Mitchell, S.J., DeLong, M. R., Wainer, B.H., and Price, D.L. (1987) Fiber pathways of basal forebrain cholinergic neurons in monkeys. *Brain Research*, 406, 192–206.

Klüver, H. and Bucy, P. (1939) Preliminary analysis of functions of the temporal lobes in monkeys. *Archives of Neurology and Psychiatry*, 42, 979–1000.

Malkova, L., Gaffan, D., and Murray, E.A. (1997) Excitotoxic lesions of the amygdala fail to produce impairment in visual learning for auditory secondary reinforcement but interfere with reinforcer devaluation effects in rhesus monkeys. *Journal of Neuroscience*, 17, 6011–6020.

Masuda, R., Fukuda, M., Ono, T., and Endo, S. (1997) Neuronal responses at the sight of objects in monkey basal forebrain subregions during operant visual tasks. *Neurobiology of Learning and Memory*, 67, 181–196.

Mesulam, M.-M. and Mufson, E.J. (1984) Neural inputs into the nucleus basalis of the substantia innominata (Ch4) in the rhesus monkey. *Brain*, 107, 253–274.

Mesulam, M.-M., Mufson, E.J., Levey, A.I., and Wainer, B.H. (1983) Cholinergic innervation of cortex by the basal forebrain: cytochemistry and cortical connections of the septal area, diagonal band nuclei, nucleus basalis (substantia innominata), and hypothalamus in the rhesus monkey. *Journal of Comparative Neurology*, 214, 170–197.

Meunier, M., Bachevalier, J., Murray, E.A., Malkova, L., and Mishkin, M. (1999) Effects of aspiration versus neurotoxic lesions of the amygdala on emotional responses in monkeys. *European Journal of Neuroscience*, **11**, 4403–18.

Murray, E.A. and Bussey, T.J. (1999) Perceptual–mnemonic function of the perirhinal cortex. *Trends in Cognitive Sciences*, 3, 142–151.

Ongur, D., An, X., and Price, J.L. (1998) Prefrontal cortical projections to the hypothalamus in macaque monkeys. *Journal of Comparative Neurology*, 401, 480–505.

Parker, A., Easton, A., and Gaffan, D. (2000). Disconnection of the medial forebrain bundle from either inferior temporal or frontal cortex severely impairs object recognition memory in Rhesus monkeys. *Society for Neuroscience Abstracts*.

Parker, A. and Gaffan, D. (1998a) Interaction of frontal and perirhinal cortices in visual object recognition memory in monkeys. *European Journal of Neuroscience*, 10, 3044–3057.

Parker, A. and Gaffan, D. (1998b) Memory after frontal–temporal disconnection in monkeys: conditional and nonconditional tasks, unilateral and bilateral frontal lesions. *Neuropsychologia*, 36, 259–271.

Parker, A., Eacott, M.J., and Gaffan, D. (1997) The recognition memory deficit caused by mediodorsal thalamic lesion in non-human primates: a comparison with rhinal cortex lesion. *European Journal of Neuroscience*, 9, 2423–2431.

Rempel-Clower, N.L. and Barbas, H. (1998) Topographic organization of connections between the hypothalamus and prefrontal cortex in the rhesus monkey. *Journal of Comparative Neurology*, 398, 393–419.

Rolls, E.T., Judge, S.J., and Sanghera, M.K. (1977) Activity of neurones in the inferior temporal cortex of the alert monkey. *Brain Research*, 130, 2229–2238.

Russchen, F.T., Amaral, D.G., and Price, J.L. (1985) The afferent connections of the substantia innominata in the monkey, *Macaca fascicularis*. *Journal of Comparative Neurology*, 242, 1–27.

Russchen, F.T., Amaral, D.G., and Price, J.L. (1987) The afferent input to the magnocellular division of the mediodorsal thalamic nucleus in the monkey, *Macaca fascicularis*. *Journal of Comparative Neurology*, 256, 175–210.

Saper, C.B. (1990) Hypothalamus. In *The Human Nervous System* (ed. G. Paxinos), pp. 389–411. Academic Press, London.

Schwartzbaum, J.S. and Poulos, D.A. (1965) Discrimination behavior after amygdalectomy in monkeys: learning set and discrimination reversals. *Journal of Comparative and Physiological Psychology*, 60, 320–328.

Seldon, N.R., Gitelman, D.R., Salamon-Murayama, N., Parrish, T.B., and Mesulam, M.-M. (1998) Trajectories of cholinergic pathways within the cerebral hemispheres of the human brain. *Brain*, 121, 2249–2257.

Semba, K. (1991) The cholinergic basal forebrain: a critical role in cortical arousal. In *The Basal Forebrain. Anatomy to Function* (eds T.C. Napier, P.W. Kalivas, and I. Hanin), pp. 197–217. Plenum, New York.

Tanaka, K. (1996) Inferotemporal cortex and object vision. *Annual Review of Neuroscience*, 19, 109–139.

Thornton, J.A., Rothblat, L.A., and Murray, E.A. (1997) Rhinal cortex removal produces amnesia for preoperatively learned discrimination problems but fails to disrupt postoperative acquisition and retention in rhesus monkey. *Journal of Neuroscience*, 17, 8536–8549.

Ungerleider, L.G., Gaffan, D., and Pelak, V.S. (1989) Projections from inferior temporal cortex to prefrontal cortex via the uncinate fascicle in Rhesus monkeys. *Experimental Brain Research*, 76, 473–484.

Webster, M.J., Bachevalier, J., and Ungerleider, L.G. (1993) Subcortical connections of inferior temporal areas TE and TEO in macaque monkeys. *Journal of Comparative Neurology*, 335, 73–91.

Weiskrantz, L. (1956) Behavioral changes associated with ablation of the amygdaloid complex in monkeys. *Journal of Comparative and Physiological Psychology*, 49, 381–391.

Wilson, F.A. and Rolls, E.T. (1990) Learning and memory is reflected in the reponses of reinforcement-related neurons in the primate basal forebrain. *Journal of Neuroscience*, 10, 1254–1267.

18 Emotion recognition and the human amygdala

Ralph Adolphs and Daniel Tranel

Department of Neurology, Division of Cognitive Neuroscience, University of Iowa College of Medicine, Iowa City, Iowa, USA

Summary

We have conducted a systematic series of investigations aimed at understanding the role of the human amygdala in processing emotion, by studying a rare individual (subject S.M.) with selective bilateral damage to the amygdala. We assessed S.M.'s ability to recognize emotions in facial expressions, lexical stimuli, and auditory stimuli on a variety of tasks that investigated naming, recognition, and categorization. Many of these findings have now been replicated in additional subjects with bilateral amygdala lesions, from both our laboratory and those of others. Also, functional imaging studies in normal subjects have begun to provide convergent results. This chapter provides a comprehensive review of recent findings regarding the role of the human amygdala in recognition of emotion, focusing in particular on the experiments we have conducted with S.M.

18.1. Introduction

What is an emotion? One could take the question as asking what people normally think constitutes an emotion, i.e. what is the folk-psychological concept of an emotion? This question is not as irrelevant to our aims as it might seem. In fact, in several of the experiments reviewed below, we asked normal subjects to tell us what they know about emotions, and compared their knowledge with that of subjects with amygdala damage.

The folk-psychological concept of emotion derives both from observations of people's behaviour and from perception of a feeling associated with being in a given emotional state. These relate, respectively, to classification on the basis of social behaviour and on the basis of perception of body states. Both views have a respectable history: Charles Darwin discussed emotions in terms of social behaviour (Darwin, 1872/1965), and William James emphasized the relationship between emotions and perceptions of body states (James, 1884). It should also be clear that the acquisition of a mature concept of an emotion by these mechanisms would require consolidation of a vast amount of knowledge over the course of many years; precisely how we learn any concept is a challenging issue in developmental psychology (see Saarni *et al.*, 1997).

18.1.1 Recognizing emotions

In this chapter, we will concentrate on the amygdala's role in the retrieval of knowledge about emotions using a variety of tasks that assess subjects' ability to access conceptual knowledge and to classify emotions into categories. It is clear from a number of studies, in both animals and in humans, that the amygdala subserves a much more diverse set of roles than emotion recognition, many of which are discussed in detail in this volume. However, it is the amygdala's role in the recognition of emotions that has been studied most intensively in humans, and for which the findings are especially well established from both lesion and functional imaging studies.

What types of knowledge normally constitute the concept of a given emotion? How is such knowledge instantiated in the brain? When we speak of 'happiness' or 'fear', we are using a single word as shorthand for a cluster of phenomena (experiences, behaviours, reactions, body states, etc.) that, all together, are pieces of knowledge which comprise a normal concept of happiness or of fear. When we attempt to assess knowledge of emotions in subjects, the particular tasks we use aim to engage the subject in retrieving such knowledge components.

The retrieval of conceptual knowledge is perhaps most easily understood with regard to lexical stimuli, such as words. In such an experiment, a subject would read or hear a word denoting an emotion, e.g. the word 'anger', and would then be asked to retrieve knowledge regarding the emotion concept denoted by that word. One could ask, for instance, if anger is a pleasant or an unpleasant emotion, if anger is more similar to disgust than it is to happiness, if anger is arousing or relaxing, and so on. All of these items of knowledge are components of the concept of the emotion 'anger'. One could do the same experiment without using the word, and instead show subjects a facial expression of anger, asking the same questions of it as one might ask about the word. Below we report findings from several such experiments, in which subjects were asked what they knew about a variety of stimuli that convey information about emotions.

18.1.2 The amygdala and emotion

Processing of emotion draws upon a diverse set of widely distributed neural structures, whose specific involvement depends on the precise aspect of processing, and on the nature of the emotion under consideration. However, the amygdala is the single structure whose role in emotional processing has been investigated most intensively, in both humans and animals. Early lesion studies of the animal amygdala pointed towards its role in recognizing the emotional and social relevance of sensory stimuli (Klüver and Bucy, 1939; Weiskrantz, 1956), and more recent studies have demonstrated a clear role for the amygdala in the acquisition, consolidation, and retrieval of emotional information (Davis, 1992a; McGaugh *et al.*, 1996; Le Doux, 1996; Adolphs, 1999).

Systematic studies of the amygdala in humans are much more recent, and have been more difficult methodologically, for a number of reasons. As far as lesion studies are concerned, a primary concern is that nearly all subjects with substantial lesions to the amygdala (typically a consequence of either surgical treatment for epilepsy or aggression, or a result of acute encephalitis) also have considerable damage to other structures surrounding the amygdala. Thus, all subjects with amygdala damage due to encephalitis also have damage to hippocampus and adjacent cortices; consequently, such subjects often exhibit an amnesic syndrome that makes it difficult to attribute task impairments solely to the amygdala damage. Similarly, the largest sample of subjects with unilateral amygdala damage, namely those with neurosurgical temporal lobectomy, have extensive damage to temporal neocortex and white matter surrounding the amygdala.

The only subject, to our knowledge, with amygdala damage that is both complete and that does not include substantial damage to other structures, is subject S.M. As we describe below, S.M. offers a unique opportunity to investigate the role of the human amygdala in emotional processing, in the absence of confounding damage to other structures. Given the detailed experimental results we report with this subject, it then becomes useful to compare the data from other subjects with non-selective amygdala damage with those from S.M., to investigate possible similarities that could be attributed to amygdala damage in both cases. Similarly, data from functional imaging studies, which can tell us what structures are sufficient to carry out a given task, but not which are necessary, can be compared and contrasted with data from S.M. We thus believe that our findings from subject S.M. will offer a valuable point of comparison and interpretation for other data from humans, and will motivate specific hypotheses that could be corroborated by additional lesion studies, or by hypothesis-driven functional imaging studies in normal subjects.

18.2 Neuroanatomy and neuropsychological background of S.M.

Subject S.M. is a 32-year-old woman with a very rare, heritable illness that affects primarily epithelial tissue, Urbach–Wiethe disease. The disease, also known as lipoid proteinosis, typically exhibits a variable phenotype of thickened skin, thickened vocal cords, beaded appearance of the eyelids, and a diagnostic staining of epithelial tissue with lipophilic dyes (Hofer, 1973). In roughly half the cases, patients develop avascular and atrophic mineralizations of medial temporal neural tissue. This involves variable calcification of hippocampal, amygdaloid, and adjacent parahippocampal, periamygdaloid, entorhinal, and perirhinal cortices. The phenotype becomes evident in early childhood, although it is not known at what age central nervous system abnormalities may develop.

In the case of S.M., we have reason to believe that she sustained her amygdala damage in early childhood, and perhaps earlier. Her neuroanatomical and neuropsychological profile has remained entirely stable during the time we have studied her (15 years). In particular, magnetic resonance imaging (MRI) scans taken at various times show selective and complete bilateral damage of the amygdala, as well as some minor damage to anterior entorhinal cortices. There is no damage to other structures anywhere in her brain, and there is no damage to the hippocampus, as also confirmed by her normal performance on standard tasks of declarative memory.

We averaged the signal from three co-registered volumetric MRI sets (three sets of serial MRI scans that cover the entire brain) to obtain a three-dimensional reconstruction of S.M.'s brain with superior spatial resolution. This reconstruction, and selected sections through it, are shown in Figure 18.1. The amygdala shows a structural lesion in its entirety, and we confirmed that this structural lesion was in fact a functional lesion with 14-deoxyglucose positron emission tomography (PET) (co-registered onto MRI data). The PET showed severe hypometabolism bilaterally in the entire amygdala (at rest), but normal glucose uptake elsewhere in the brain. The brain of S.M. provides the only known case of selective and complete bilateral amygdala damage in a human. It is important to note here that all the findings we summarize below pertain to a subject with complete damage to all nuclei within the amygdala; however, the amygdala is not a homogeneous structure, either functionally or hodologically (Swanson and Petrovich, 1998), and the details of functional contributions made by different nuclei in humans will be important issues for future research.

S.M.'s neuropsychological background has been described in detail (Tranel and Hyman, 1990), and is updated and summarized in Table 18.1. She has a high school education and lives independently. We briefly summarize her neuropsychological profile below; Table 18.1 provides quantitative information.

18.2.1 Behavioural observations

In all testing sessions in our laboratory, S.M. has been alert, fully oriented, and entirely cooperative. Her attention and cognitive 'stamina' are intact. We noted previously that her interpersonal behaviour was remarkable for a somewhat coquettish, disinhibited style, and this has remained constant across the years. She tends to be quite friendly with experimenters and administrative personnel with whom she comes into contact in our laboratory, and she has a very comfortable, 'hands on' style of interaction that goes somewhat beyond the norm for conventional midwestern culture. She is not, however, blatantly inappropriate, and she is capable of restraining herself in order to meet specific task and situational demands. It is especially important to point out that, while S.M. may exhibit some slightly inappropriate social behaviour, she does not exhibit any of the features of the classic Klüver–Bucy syndrome (Klüver and Bucy, 1939). We discuss her social cognition in more detail in Section 18.6 below.

18.2.2 Intellect and academic achievement

Part A of Table 1 presents data from the Wechsler Adult Intelligence Scale-Revised and from the Wide Range Achievement Test-Revised. S.M.'s IQ scores have remained essentially stable across time. There is a slight trend for higher scores in more recent assessments, attributable to mild practice effects; the data clearly show no hint of decline over more than a decade. Overall, her intellectual abilities range from the lower end of the average range to the upper end of the low average range, well within expectations given her educational

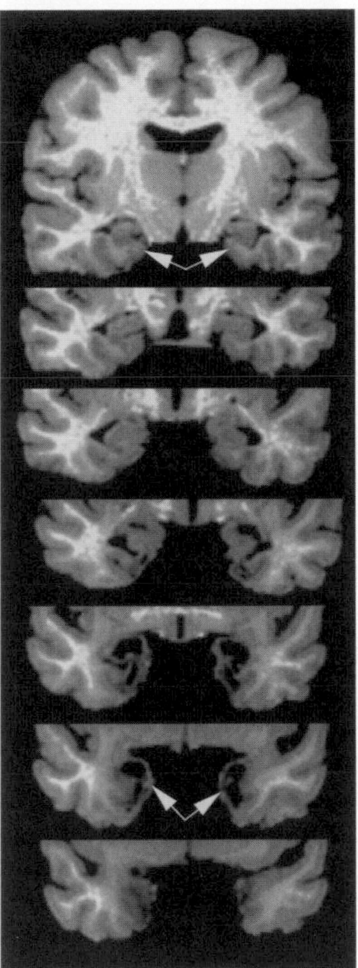

Figure 18.1 The brain of S.M. Neuroanatomical data from three co-registered MRIs. Low signals (black regions) indicate the calcified tissue of the amygdala. MR images were acquired in three separate volumetric data sets that were averaged linearly in order to yield a single, mean volumetric data set with improved spatial resolution. Data from Human Neuroanatomy and Neuroimaging Laboratory, Department of Neurology, University of Iowa.

and occupational background. Academic achievement skills range from average (spelling) to borderline (reading, arithmetic), commensurate with her educational background.

18.2.3 Memory (Table 18.1, Part B)

S.M.'s performances on all major components of the Wechsler Memory Scale-Revised are squarely within expectations, given her intellectual abilities. Her ability to acquire and retain

Table 18.1 Neuropsychological profile for subject S.M.

Test/Function	*Score/Result*	
Part A. Intellect and academic achievement		
Wechsler Adult Intelligence Scale-Revised (age-corrected scaled scores)		
Verbal IQ	86	(82)
Information	8	(7)
Digit Span	9	(9)
Vocabulary	7	
Arithmetic	6	(6)
Comprehension	7	
Similiarities	10	(8)
Performance IQ	95	(90)
Picture Completion	10	
Picture Arrangement	14	(13)
Block Design	9	(9)
Object Assembly	7	
Digit–Symbol Substitution	7	(6)
Full Scale IQ	88	
Wide Range Achievement Test-Revised (standard scores)		
Reading	79	
Spelling	91	
Arithmetic	72	
Part B. Memory		
Wechsler Memory Scale-Revised		
Verbal Memory Index	90	
Visual Memory Index	93	
General Memory Index	89	(89)
Attention/Concentration Index	87	
Delayed Recall Index	88	
Rey Auditory–Verbal Learning Test (#/15)		
Trial 1	5	(5)
Trial 2	6	(9)
Trial 3	8	(11)
Trial 4	10	(14)
Trial 5	13	(13)
30-min delayed recall	10	(10)
30-min delayed recognition (#/30)	29	(29)
Benton Visual Retention Test		
Number correct	5	(5)
Number errors	7	(10)
Complex Figure Test, 30-min recall	14/36	(9.5/36)

Table 18.1 continued

Test/Function	*Score/Result*	
Part C. Speech and linguistic functions		
Speech		Hoarse
Linguistic functions		
Boston Naming Test	46/60	
Sentence repetition	15th	
Reading comprehension	9/10	
Writing	Normal	
Controlled Oral Word Association	3rd	(6th)
Token Test	95th	
Part D. Visuoperceptual/visuospatial/visuoconstructional functions		
Facial Recognition Test (%ile)	85th	(90th)
Judgment of Line Orientation (%ile)	22nd	(11th)
Hooper Visual Organization Test		(25.5/30)
Complex Figure Test, copy	32/36	(31/36)
Drawing to dictation		
Clock	Normal	
House	Normal	
Person	Normal	
3-Dimensional Block Construction	29/29	
Grooved Pegboard (%ile)		
Right hand	5th	
Left hand	9th	
Part E. Executive control and related functions		
Wisconsin Card Sorting Test		
Number correct	68	
Errors	27th %ile	
Perseverative responses	53rd %ile	
Non-perseverative errors	18th %ile	
Perseverative errors	84th %ile	
Categories	>16th %ile	
Trail-making Test (%ile)		
Part A	16th	(47th)
Part B	37th	(13th)
Tower of Hanoi (no.of moves; means for age-matched controls in brackets)		
Trial 1	120	[87.1]
Trial 2	97	[70.2]
Trial 3	57	[66.8]
Trial 4	88	[68.9]
Tower of London		
Minimum moves	86	
Excess moves	20	
% above optimal strategy	23	

Table 18.1 continued

Test/Function	*Score/Result*
Part F. Standardized personality assessment	
MMPI-2 (T-scores)	
Scale	
L	66
F	48
K	59
1	72
2	51
3	68
4	75
5	66
6	56
7	67
8	68
9	53
0	49

S.M. was evaluated initially in the Benton Neuropsychology Laboratory on several occasions between November 1986 and June 1988, and data from those testing sessions were published in 1990 (Tranel and Hyman, 1990). Since then, S.M. has been re-evaluated a number of times with standard neuropsychological testing, in order to establish the stability of her neuropsychological profile. Here we report an updated, comprehensive overview of her current neuropsychological status (data collected between 1997 and 1999). For purposes of comparison, previously published results (collected between 1986 and 1988) are presented in parentheses for those instruments for which such data are available (for tests for which more than one score was published previously, the best score is presented here). The table presents the complete summary of current neuropsychological data for S.M.

verbal information, for example as reflected in the Rey Auditory–Verbal Learning Test performance, is intact. As noted previously (Tranel and Hyman, 1990), she displays a mild weakness in the domain of non-verbal, visual memory (Benton Visual Retention Test, Complex Figure Test recall); however, the magnitude of this impairment is smaller, and its meaning more equivocal, than documented previously. Specifically, she is not impaired on all similar tasks that assess visual memory (e.g. her performance on the Warrington Faces Recognition Memory Task is well within the normal range; see Tranel and Hyman, 1990; and her performance on the complex figure recall, although impaired, is variable; see Table 18.1). Overall, it can be concluded that her ability to acquire and retain declarative knowledge, particularly of the verbal type, is intact.

18.2.4 Speech and linguistic function (Table 18.1, Part C)

S.M.'s speech is markedly hoarse, as is characteristic of subjects with Urbach–Wiethe disease; with this exception, her speech is normal in every respect. Naming, repetition, comprehension, reading, and writing are all intact. She performs defectively on the Controlled Oral Word Association Test, which we interpret as a mild weakness in 'executive function' (see below).

18.2.5 Visuoperceptual, visuospatial, and visuoconstructional functions

As shown in Part D of Table 18.1, all aspects of S.M.'s visuoperceptual, visuospatial, and visuoconstructional abilities are fully intact. We have emphasized this feature in many of the previous publications relevant to S.M. (e.g. Adolphs *et al.*, 1994, 1998), and it is important to reiterate that there is no indication that she suffers from any type of basic visual information processing disturbance that might contribute to her many defective performances on tests of facial emotion recognition and cognate experiments reviewed in this chapter. In fact, she appears to have normal ability to discriminate stimuli in all sensory modalities, with the one exception of a borderline anosmia.

18.2.6 Executive control and related functions

We noted previously that S.M. had some difficulties on tasks of 'executive function,' which tap abilities such as judgement, planning, and decision making. The current data continue to support this impression, albeit somewhat more equivocally than before. For example, S.M. performed entirely normally on the Wisconsin Card Sorting Test, considered by many to be the 'gold standard' of executive functioning. Also, her current performance on the Trail-making Test (especially the critical Part B) is well within the normal range. In contrast, she evidenced some difficulty with the two 'tower' tasks (Tower of Hanoi; Tower of London), and she produced a relatively poor performance on the Controlled Oral Word Association Test.

18.2.7 Personality assessment

Part F of Table 18.1 summarizes the T-scores from the MMPI-2, a standard measure of personality and psychopathology. The most important conclusion to be drawn from these data is that S.M. does not evidence any form of significant psychopathology; her profile is not suggestive, nor is there any evidence from her everyday life of a formal psychiatric diagnosis. It is interesting, however, that she has some mild indication of antisocial behaviour (Scale 4), comprising features such as rebelliousness, disregard of social convention, and lack of respect for authority figures.

18.3 Recognition of emotion in facial expressions

18.3.1 Recognition of prototypical facial expressions of emotion

Recently, the human amygdala has been studied fairly extensively with regard to its involvement in recognition of certain emotions in facial expressions, notably fear. Several lesion studies have now demonstrated that bilateral amygdala damage impairs recognition of emotions in facial expressions (Adolphs *et al.*, 1994, 1995, 1999b; Calder *et al.*, 1996b; Young *et al.*, 1995, 1996; Broks *et al.*, 1998). While recognition of several emotions of negative valence can be variably impaired, the most consistent impairment is an inability to recognize fear. These findings have been corroborated recently by a number of functional imaging studies, using both PET and fMRI, which we briefly review first (see also Dolan, Chapter 19).

Functional imaging studies in normal individuals have shown that visual (Breiter *et al.*, 1996; Morris *et al.*, 1996, 1998a; Phillips *et al.*, 1997), auditory (Phillips *et al.*, 1998), olfactory (Zald and Pardo, 1997), and gustatory (Zald *et al.*, 1998) stimuli all appear to engage the amygdala when signalling unpleasant and arousing emotions. These studies have examined the encoding and recognition of emotional stimuli, as well as emotional experience and emotional response (for a review,see Davidson and Irwin, 1999), but it has been exceedingly difficult to disentangle all these different components. While there is now clear evidence of amygdala activation during encoding of emotional material (e.g. Cahill *et al.*, 1996; Canli *et al.*, 1998; Hamann *et al.*, 1999), it is less clear whether the amygdala is also activated during retrieval. It is also quite unclear whether or not the amygdala plays a critical role in emotional experience (e.g. Adolphs, 1999), since many functional imaging studies of emotional experience reporting amygdala activation have been conducted in psychiatric populations without an activation task, again making it difficult to interpret some of the data (for a discussion and an example of a study that considered this issue, see Beauregard *et al.*, 1998).

Several studies (Breiter *et al.*, 1996; Morris *et al.*, 1996, 1998a; Phillips *et al.*, 1997) have now found increased amygdala activation when subjects were shown facial expressions of fear, either passively (Breiter *et al.*, 1996) or while performing an unrelated task (gender discrimination) (Morris *et al.*, 1996). While neither study asked subjects to *retrieve* knowledge, during the scan session they would have been *acquiring* knowledge about the stimuli (for instance, they would be able to recognize many of the stimuli later, or they would be able to recall what emotions they saw during the scan session), and it remains unclear which of these different components of emotion might have contributed to the amygdala activation reported.

A further insight has come from studies which used stimuli that could not be perceived consciously. Whalen and colleagues reported amygdala activation when subjects viewed facial expressions of fear that were presented so briefly that they could not be recognized consciously (Whalen *et al.*, 1998), showing that the amygdala plays a role in non-conscious processing of emotional stimuli. There is some evidence that the left amygdala may be more involved in processing supraliminal stimuli, while the right amygdala may be more involved in processing subliminal stimuli (Morris *et al.*, 1998b) (but see Davidson and Irwin, 1999, for some caveats). Specifically, there is a correlation between activation of visual structures involved in non-conscious processing (superior colliculus and pulvinar nucleus) and activation of right amygdala, when processing emotional faces that are presented subliminally. No such correlation was observed for the left amygdala, or if supraliminal stimuli were used (Morris *et al.*, 1999). An important function of the amygdala may be to trigger responses and to allocate processing resources to stimuli that may be of special importance to the organism, and ecological considerations as well as the data adduced above all appear to argue for such a role especially with regard to rapid responses that need not involve conscious awareness. Normally, such fast, pre-conscious processing would contribute essentially to the ongoing behaviour and knowledge retrieval triggered by an emotionally salient stimulus, and would be expected to operate in parallel with, and feed back upon, other processing loops. We elaborate on this picture in the final section of this chapter.

While functional imaging studies typically have not used tasks in which subjects were asked explicitly to recognize emotion, lesion studies have investigated such explicit recognition tasks. The two primary tasks that have been used across studies are (i) choosing a label from a list of six emotion words to describe a facial expression (a six-alternative, forced-choice label–face matching task) and (ii) rating the intensity of all six basic emotions shown by a facial expression (the subjects were supplied with labels of the six emotions in this task). Comparisons between different studies have been difficult, because different sets of stimuli, and different methods, have been used. For example, several studies by Young and colleagues (Young *et al.*, 1995, 1996; Calder *et al.*, 1996b; Broks *et al.*, 1998) have used certain sets of face stimuli, and task (i) above, whereas other studies (Adolphs *et al.*, 1994, 1995; Hamann *et al.*, 1996) have used a different set of stimuli and task (ii) above.

A recent collaborative study (Adolphs *et al.*, 1999b) using task (ii) with nine subjects who had bilateral amygdala damage has confirmed that, as a group, patients with bilateral amygdala damage are impaired in recognizing some negative emotions in this task, including, but not limited to, fear (Figure 18.2). Despite this group finding, there is considerable variability in the data obtained from different subjects.

All studies have used stimuli chosen from a standardized set of facial expressions developed by Paul Ekman (Ekman and Friesen, 1976), a set of stimuli that has also been the most commonly used in psychological studies of facial affect in normal individuals. With respect to the two tasks described above, task (ii) is a very detailed assessment of a subject's ability to retrieve knowledge about the emotion signalled by a face; it is both much longer and more difficult than task (i). In five replications of task (ii) with S.M., she was specifically and severely impaired with regard to faces of fear every time. When shown emotional facial expressions, S.M. consistently failed to rate the emotions surprise, fear, and anger as very intense. She was particularly impaired in rating the intensity of fear, on several occasions failing to recognize any fear whatsoever in prototypical facial expressions of fear. We examined S.M.'s ability to recognize all the different basic emotions in facial expressions, and found a severe and specific impairment in recognizing emotions signalled by fearful facial expressions (Adolphs *et al.*, 1994, 1995). Not only did S.M. fail to attribute fear to fearful faces, but she also did not judge them to express surprise or anger, two closely related emotions normally judged also to be expressed by fearful faces (Adolphs *et al.*, 1995) (Figure 18.3A). A further analysis of these data, and findings from a separate task involving direct similarity judgements, showed that S.M. also could not recognize some emotions as similar to one another (Adolphs *et al.*, 1994) (Figure 18.3B). The most robust derived measure from task (ii) is the correlation of a subject's ratings of a face with the mean ratings given to that face by normal subjects. When such correlations are averaged over all the faces that express a particular emotion, S.M. stands out as specifically impaired in her ability to assign normal ratings to faces of fear, but normal in her ability to recognize emotions other than fear (Figure 18.3C).

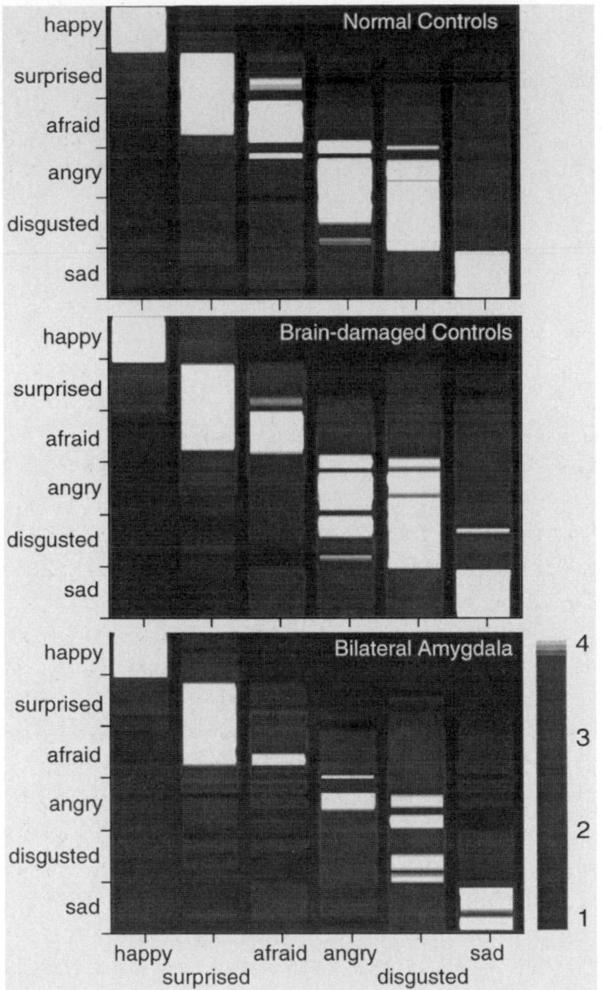

Figure 18.2 Impaired recognition of emotions from facial expressions in subjects with bilateral amygdala damage. Raw rating scores of facial expressions of emotion are shown from eight subjects with bilateral amygdala damage (from Adolphs *et al.*, 1999b). The emotional stimuli (36 faces; six each of each of the six basic emotions indicated) are ordered on the *y*-axis according to their perceived similarity (stimuli perceived to be similar, e.g. happy and surprised faces, are adjacent; stimuli perceived to be dissimilar, e.g. happy and sad faces, are distant; see Adolphs *et al.*, 1995). The six emotion labels on which subjects rated the faces are displayed on the *x*-axis. Greyscale brightness encodes the mean rating given to each face by a group of subjects, as indicated in the scale. Thus, a darker line would indicate a lower mean rating than a brighter line for a given face; and a thin bright line for a given emotion category would indicate that few stimuli of that emotion received a high rating, whereas a thick bright line would indicate that many or all stimuli within that emotion

We followed up on these findings with several additional tasks. First, we confronted her with explicit questions about the degree of fear shown by the stimuli. We showed S.M. the same stimuli, and asked the single question, 'Does this person look as though they might be feeling any fear at all, even the smallest amount?' The findings with this question confirmed S.M.'s impaired ability to recognize fear: for 5/6 of the stimuli depicting prototypical fear, she responded that, while she was not sure what the emotion was, there was no trace of fear whatsoever.

We have also examined S.M.'s spontaneous naming of the emotions shown in faces (here, she was asked to come up with the single word that she thought best described the emotion displayed by the face; this experiment was done prior to all the others so as not to 'prime' the labels). This labelling experiment used stimuli identical to those we have used for experiment (ii). The results are shown in Figure 18.4: S.M.'s spontaneous naming was impaired, compared with normal controls, in that she virtually never used the label 'fear', typically mislabelling such faces as surprised, angry, or disgusted.

While the data from S.M. clearly point to a specific and disproportionate impairment in recognizing fear, data from other subjects with bilateral amygdala damage argue for a more general impairment in recognizing negative emotions. It is thus somewhat unclear how specific the amygdala's role may be in recognition of certain emotions. A group analysis of the data from nine subjects with bilateral amygdala damage showed that subjects with bilateral amygdala damage were impaired in rating facial emotion, compared with brain-damaged controls (Adolphs *et al.*, 1999b). Furthermore, across all normal and amygdala-damaged subjects, happy expressions and fearful expressions stood out as being rated differently from the other emotions: happy faces were recognized the most consistently (no subject was impaired in recognizing happiness), whereas fearful faces exhibited a large variance (several subjects with bilateral amygdala damage were severely impaired in recognizing fear). One interpretation of these results could be that fear is simply the most difficult emotion to recognize, and happiness the easiest. In fact, it may well be that happiness is the easiest basic emotion to recognize, because (i) it contains a stereotypical feature (the smile) that permits unambiguous classification, and (ii) there are fewer positive than negative emotions, meaning that happiness requires a level of categorization that may be superordinate to the level of categorization required to recognize fear or anger. A second interpretation of the above findings is that impaired recognition of fear is due to damage to a more general neural system for recognizing emotions that signal potential harm to the organism, which would include fear and anger. A third possibility is that the amygdala is critical specifically for recognition of fear.

While distinguishing among these possibilities will require further investigation, we believe that the available data are most consonant with the second alternative. An examination of

---

category received high ratings. Because very few mean ratings were <1 or >4, we truncated the graphs outside these values. Data from subjects with bilateral amygdala damage indicate abnormally low ratings of negative emotions (thinner bright bands across any horizontal position corresponding to an expression of a negative emotion). (From Adolphs *et al.*, 1999b; copyright Elsevier Science Publishers, 1999.) See also colour plate section.

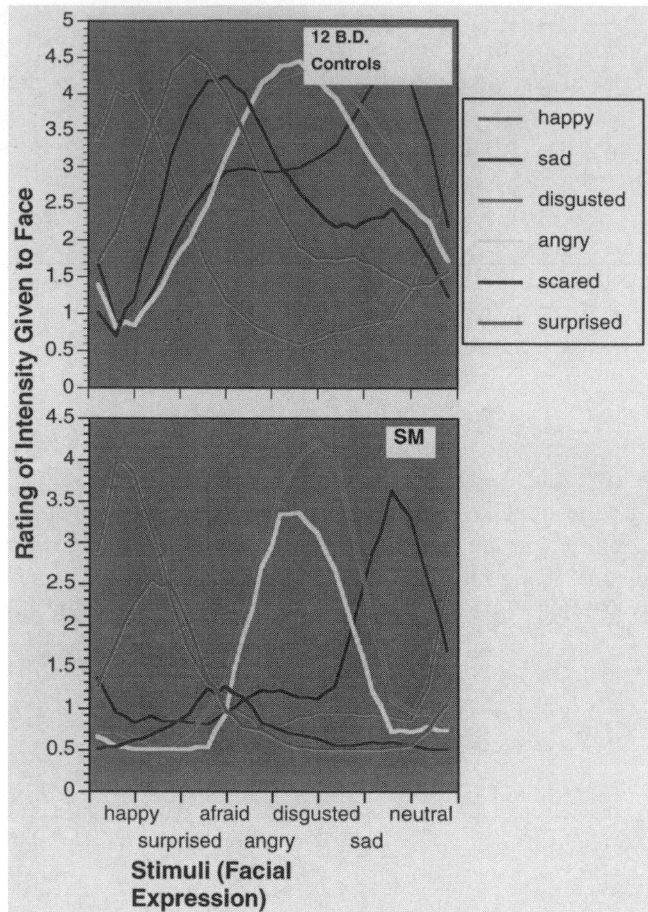

Figure 18.3 Impaired recognition of emotional facial expressions in subject S.M. See also colour plate section.(**A**) Impaired recognition of fear in facial expressions in S.M. Twelve brain-damaged control subjects (without damage to amygdala) and subject S.M. were shown 39 facial expressions of emotion from Ekman and Friesen (1976), and asked to rate the 39 faces with respect to the intensity of one of the six basic emotions displayed (happiness, surprise, fear, anger, disgust, and sadness) on a scale of 0 (=not at all showing this emotion) to 5 (=most intense rating possible for this emotion). These data are shown for S.M. (bottom*)* and 12 brain-damaged controls (top*)*, with the ratings that subjects gave to the 39 faces depicted by the coloured lines. Each differently coloured line corresponds to subjects' ratings on one of the six different emotions. The stimuli (39 facial expressions) are ordered along the *x*-axis by their judged similarity (more similar emotional expressions are adjacent on the *x*-axis, while dissimilar ones are further apart; the order of the stimuli on the *x*-axis corresponds to the order obtained by proceeding clockwise around a circumplex model of emotion (Russell, 1980; Adolphs *et al.*, 1995). (Modified from Adolphs *et al.*, 1995; copyright Society

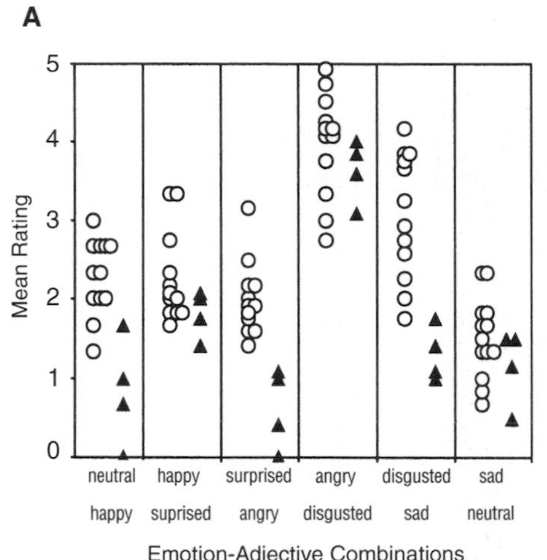

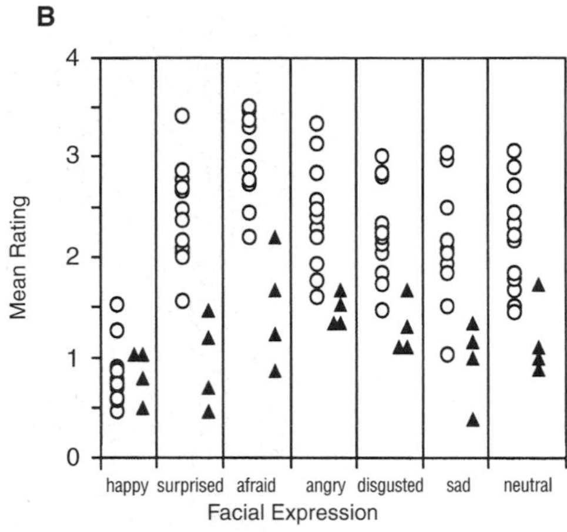

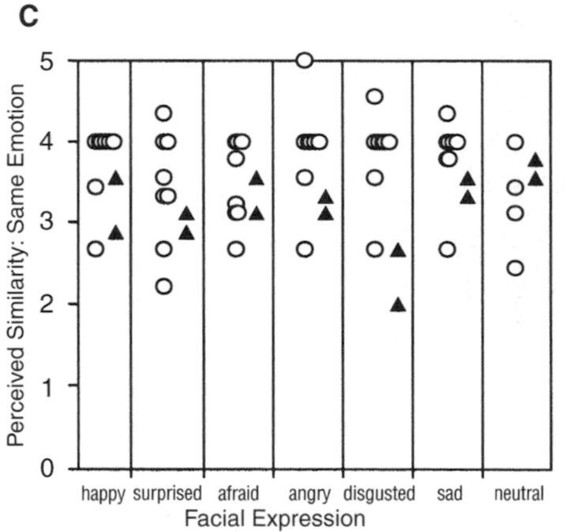

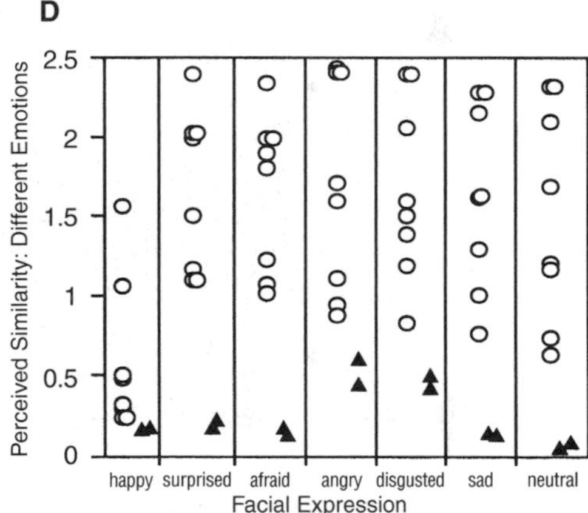

for Neuroscience, 1995.) (**B**) Impaired recognition of multiple emotions in facial expressions. (a) Mean ratings of facial expressions on adjectives denoting adjacent emotions. The emotion–adjective combinations are shown on the *x*-axis; data were averaged over six faces within each emotion category except neutral (three faces), and over the two cases where emotional expression and adjective are interchanged. S.M.'s (▲, four experiments) low ratings compared with the controls' ratings (○, n = 12) correspond to the gaps in her MDS plots. (b) Mean ratings of all the emotions other than the prototypical emotion recognized in an expression. S.M. tends not to recognize any emotions other than the prototypical ones. (c) Direct similarity ratings of faces expressing the same emotion. (d) Direct similarity ratings between faces expressing different emotions. Each category shows average similarity ratings of all 54 possible pairings of expressions (3 expressions of the given emotion×6 other emotions×3 expressions). S.M. fails to recognize similarity between expressions of different

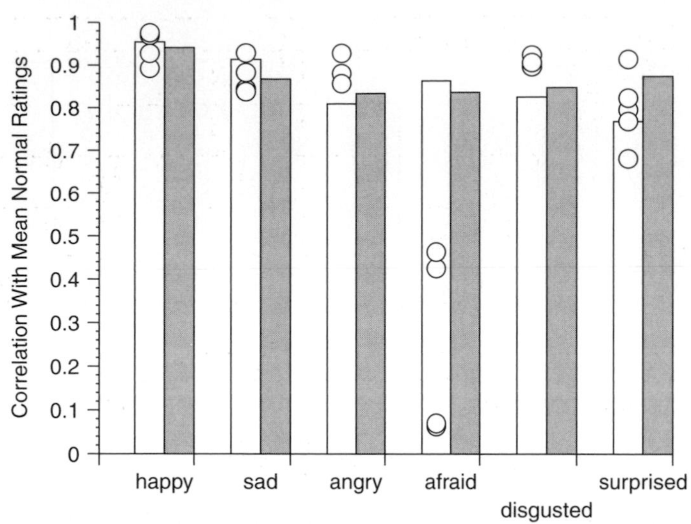

emotions (number of SD difference from control mean: happy = 0.8, surprised = 2.8, afraid = 3, angry = 1.6, disgusted = 2.1, neutral = 2.5). For (c) and (d), subjects directly judged similarity of emotion expressed by 21 of the faces used in all other experiments (three of each of the seven emotion categories) on a five-point scale. All possible pairwise combinations (231) of facial expressions were presented as adjacent photographs, a pair at a time. (From Adolphs *et al.*, 1994; copyright MacMillan Magazines, 1994.) (**C**) Recognition of emotional facial expressions in a control subject with Urbach–Wiethe disease but no amygdala damage. Correlations with mean ratings are shown for 18 normal controls (grey bars), subject E.S. (white bars), and from four experiments with S.M. (circles). Both E.S. and S.M. have Urbach–Wiethe disease, but the disease resulted in bilateral amygdala damage only in S.M.; E.S. has no detectable brain lesions. S.M. was severely impaired in recognizing fear in facial expressions, whereas E.S. was normal.

the data from many subjects with bilateral amygdala damage argues against the third of the above possibilities (see Figure 18.2). A strong argument against the first possibility comes from findings of double-dissociations in humans: recognition of expressions of disgust can be selectively impaired (e.g. Gray *et al.*, 1997), as can recognition of fear (Adolphs *et al.*, 1994). These data make it unlikely that impaired recognition of specific emotions can be explained by task difficulty alone, although, as we mentioned above, we do find it plausible that happiness may be disproportionately easy to recognize. This leaves the second of the possibilities outlined above as the most plausible option to explain the impairments seen, an interpretation which is also most consistent with the large body of work from animal studies that implicate the amygdala in the detection of potentially harmful or threatening stimuli (e.g. Weiskrantz, 1956; Aggleton, 1992; Le Doux, 1996). Taken together, the data argue that the human amygdala is a component of a neural system specialized for rapidly triggering physiological states related to stimuli that signal threat or danger (Adolphs *et al.*, 1999b).

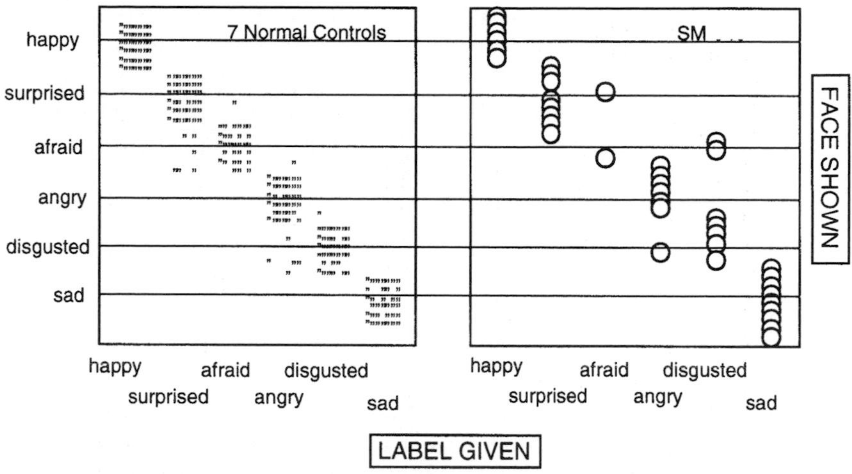

Figure 18.4 Impaired labelling of facial expressions of fear following amygdala damage. Seven normal control subjects and S.M. were shown 39 facial expressions of emotion from Ekman and Friesen (1976) (six of each of the basic emotions, and three neutral faces) and asked to provide spontaneously a label of the emotion. S.M. was impaired in labelling faces expressing fear (she only labelled a single face of fear correctly in the figure). Subjects' labels are shown as data points when synonymous with the words in the figure (e.g. when calling angry faces 'mad'); labels that are not clear synonyms (e.g. calling a sad face 'guilty') were omitted from the figure (accounting for the absent data points for some of the control subjects).

Such physiological states involve both specific sets of behavioural responses, as well as the modulation of cognitive processes, including those involved in knowledge retrieval necessary for normal performance on the above tasks.

18.3.2 Control tasks and control subjects

The above finding—that S.M. is impaired in recognizing fear in emotional facial expressions—is one of the most robust and specific findings in the literature concerning the consequences of amygdala damage in humans. Her impairment was specific to processing knowledge of emotion, since her ability to discriminate faces perceptually was entirely normal, and since she had no difficulty in recognizing a person's identity or gender from the face. These latter abilities were assessed with standardized, sensitive tasks in which subjects were asked to discriminate morphs of faces on the basis of emotion, gender, or identity. S.M.'s performance on all these discrimination tasks was normal, including normal discrimination of all basic emotions. The impairment reported above thus conforms to the strict definition of agnosia: an impairment in retrieving conceptual knowledge about a stimulus, in the setting of normal perception. Moreover, the agnosia is specific to certain types of knowledge and not to others: S.M. is unable to recognize certain emotions signalled by the expressions shown in faces, despite normal ability to recognize other information from faces.

Might it simply be the case that S.M. does not know the meaning of the word 'fear', or that she has no knowledge concerning the concept of fear at all? We can rule out this possibility, since S.M. is able to use the word 'fear' appropriately in conversation, and since she is in fact able to retrieve considerable knowledge regarding the concept of fear. Thus, when asked what sorts of events would make people feel afraid, or what people do when they are afraid, she is able to retrieve a large store of appropriate knowledge. She knows, as a matter of declarative fact, that afraid people will tend to scream and run away, that being in a dark alley alone at night will tend to make one feel afraid, and so on. Like most of us, she has acquired all this knowledge from a variety of sources, including reading books, talking to other people, and watching movies. So why can she not recognize facial expressions of fear? We propose that this particular knowledge, what facial expressions of fear look like, is knowledge that cannot be encoded easily into language, and that it is not a component of the declarative facts one has ready for retrieval. Roughly, we propose that what distinguishes S.M.'s impairment is an inability to trigger processes that permit a reconstruction or a simulation of some components of the physiological state normally associated with the facial expression of fear, while she is nonetheless able to retrieve most knowledge pertaining to fear that has been encoded lexically. We take up this issue in more detail in the final section of this chapter.

Given S.M.'s rare disease, we felt it important also to control for the possibility that there could be some unknown effects of the disease on task performance that were not related directly to her focal brain lesions. Urbach–Wiethe disease typically results in a phenotype that includes multiple disorders of epithelial tissue, in addition to the focal neurological abnormalities that are present in about 50% of cases. The ideal control in this respect would be a subject who also has Urbach–Wiethe disease, but who is one of the 50% of subjects with this disease that do not develop medial temporal calcification as part of the phenotype.

We have studied one such rare subject, E.S., a 70-year-old male who exhibits all the symptoms of Urbach–Wiethe disease, but whose MRI scans are negative for any macroscopic brain lesions. Like S.M., E.S. has thickening of the skin, a very hoarse voice, and increased susceptibility to infection from skin wounds. Moreover, like S.M., E.S. knows that he has Urbach–Wiethe disease, and he has some difficulty with vocal communication in real life, due to his hoarse voice. He thus provides a similar psychosocial background associated with the disease, and also a similar constellation of pathologies separate from the amygdala lesions.

Figure 18.3C shows E.S.'s entirely normal performance on the identical emotion recognition task previously described with S.M. Unlike S.M., who performed abnormally on multiple administrations of this task, E.S. performed entirely normally. The fact that he has had Urbach–Wiethe disease for a much longer duration than has S.M. further strengthens the interpretation that S.M.'s impaired recognition of fearful facial expressions is a specific consequence of her amygdala lesions, and is not attributable to social or extraneural physiological abnormalities associated with the disease.

18.3.3 Emotion recognition in computer-generated morphs of facial expressions

While the above findings demonstrate S.M.'s impaired recognition of fear in prototypical facial expressions, they leave open the question of precisely how specific the impairment is to the particular stimuli depicting fear that we used. Is the impairment evident only for prototypical expressions of fear? Where precisely does S.M.'s category of fear begin and end? We have begun to address this issue with the use of computer-generated images that are interpolations between basic emotion prototypes, using a technique called 'morphing'. Such stimuli have been used extensively with normal subjects to investigate the structure of emotion categories (Etcoff and Magee, 1992; Calder *et al.*, 1996a; Young *et al.*, 1997), and recently also in studies of the amygdala (Calder *et al.*, 1996b; Morris *et al.*, 1996).

We created our stimuli from one individual's face (P.E.) from the Ekman and Friesen (1976) set. We generated linear morphs between two different expressions. Morphs were generated by specifying corresponding features between the two faces. Each image was then subjected to a morphing algorithm consisting of two components. (i) All pixels in the images were partitioned by a Delauney tesselation, and subsequently warped in a manner analogous to stretching a rubber sheet that continuously deforms one image into the other. This component is a spatial transformation. (ii) All pixel greyscale values (their brightness) were set to a weighted average of their values in the two images. This component is a luminance transformation, essentially a continuous fade between corresponding pixels.

We conducted two experiments with S.M. in order to probe in detail her emotion recognition of morphed facial expressions. We generated a continuum of morphs around a circumplex order of the basic emotions (neutral–happy–surprised–afraid–angry–disgust–sadness–neutral). In the first experiment, subjects were shown these morphs, in randomized order, and asked to rate them with respect to the intensity of each of the six basic emotions, exactly as before [the 'task (ii)' described above]. S.M.'s data were correlated with those obtained from 12 normal controls, and the results confirmed her impaired recognition of fear (Figure 18.5A). These data rule out the possibility that it might have been some idiosyncratic feature of specific faces in the Ekman stimulus set that made them especially difficult for her to recognize, since here the same individual's face was used in all the morphed stimuli. The only dimension on which the stimuli varied was emotional expression, and S.M. showed a disproportionate impairment in recognition of those morphs close to the prototype of fear, consistent with previous findings.

In the second experiment (carried out on a separate visit), we used the same emotion morphs as above, but S.M. controlled the images dynamically by scrolling through morph space on a computer. All the morphed images had been joined into a scrollable movie (in the order given above), through which S.M. could move both forwards or backwards (or stop on a given image). There was no time limit. We asked her to scroll ahead until the image looked like it had changed to another emotion, and to indicate where she thought the emotion prototypes were located. This method in essence permitted S.M. to show us where her emotion category boundaries and prototypes were located, with respect to a circumplex model of affect (Russell, 1980). She accurately picked out happiness, surprise, and sadness.

However, she omitted the category 'fear' entirely, lumped fear and some angry faces together as 'anger', and lumped some anger and all disgust faces together as 'frustrated'. The detailed structure of her data is represented in Figure 18.5B.

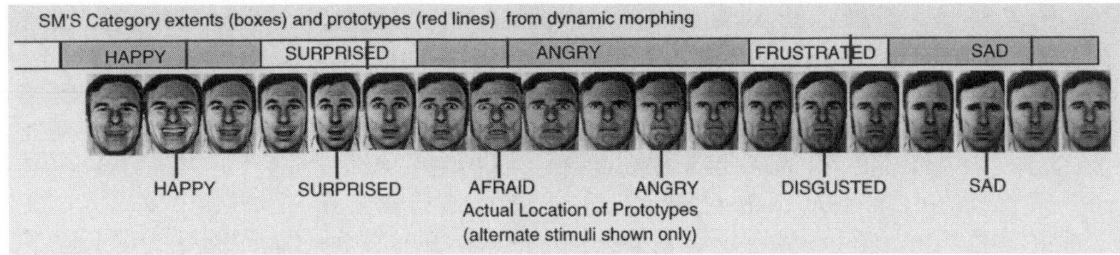

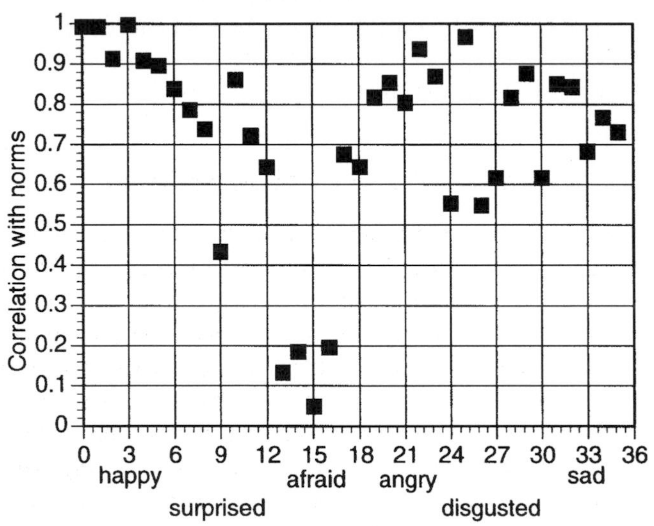

Figure 18.5 Recognition of emotion categories from continuously morphed facial expressions. Subjects were shown six morphs between each of neutral–happy–surprised–afraid–angry–disgusted–sad–neutral for a total of 42 stimuli. (**A**) Correlations of ratings given by S.M. to the 42 morphs with the mean ratings given by 12 normal controls. Ratings were obtained as before. S.M. was most impaired in rating those morphs close to the prototype of fear. (**B**) S.M.'s emotion categories revealed by interactive scrolling through morph space. S.M. controlled a slider which allowed her to move forwards and backwards along the 42 morphed facial expressions. We asked her to pick out the boundaries (labelled boxes) and most typical instances (thick grey lines) of all the different emotions she perceived. S.M. entirely omitted the category 'fear'. The *x*-axes in (A) and (B) both plot the morphed stimuli (neutral stimuli are omitted); every other stimulus is shown at the bottom, together with the actual emotion prototype as indicated by the labels.

18.3.4 Recognition without naming

Many of the above tasks depend, at least in part, on knowing the names for the emotions. In order to assess S.M.'s recognition of emotional facial expressions without requiring her to attach any names to them, we asked her to sort photographs of facial expressions into piles on the basis of the similarity of the emotion displayed. We used a subset of 18 of the faces used in the previous tasks (three of each emotion). S.M. was asked to sort the photographs into three, four, seven, and 10 different piles, with a short break and re-randomization of the stimuli between each sorting. The photographs were sorted such that faces of people who looked like they felt similar should be together in the same pile, and faces of people who looked like they felt different should be put into different piles. Naming the emotion was not asked for in this task.

We calculated a derived similarity score between all pairwise combinations of the faces as the weighted sum of their co-occurences in a pile (Figure 18.6). S.M.'s derived similarity measure differed the most from normal controls for afraid faces, differing up to nearly two standard deviations (SDs) in terms of sorting the three fear faces together (within-category similarity), and differing by more than 4 SDs in how she sorted some fear faces together with faces other than fear (between-category similarity) (Table 18.2).

18.4 Recognition of emotion in auditory stimuli

It is of interest to determine the functional role of the human amygdala with respect to stimuli in different sensory modalities. While functional imaging studies have now examined the amygdala's role in processing visual, auditory, olfactory, and gustatory stimuli, lesion studies have thus far focused mainly on visual stimuli (facial expressions). Two recent case studies examined the amygdala's role with respect to the auditory modality. One study reported impaired recognition of emotional prosody following partial and non-selective bilateral damage to the amygdala for the treatment of epilepsy (Scott *et al.*, 1997), whereas another case study with bilateral damage more restricted to the amygdala found no such impairment (Anderson and Phelps, 1998). One functional imaging study to date has reported amygdala activation in response to emotional auditory stimuli (Phillips *et al.*, 1998). A possible explanation for the discrepant findings may be that the impairments that have been reported (Scott *et al.*, 1997) are due not to amygdala damage, but instead resulted from damage to the right basal ganglia (for a discussion, see Anderson and Phelps, 1998; Adolphs and Tranel, 1999a). On the other hand, neither of the cases reported in these studies (Scott *et al.*, 1997; Anderson and Phelps, 1998) had complete damage to the amygdala, and it is conceivable that the impaired subject had lesions to some portions of the amygdala that may have been spared in the other subject.

We investigated recognition of emotional prosody in two subjects with complete bilateral amygdala damage, R.H. and S.M. (Adolphs and Tranel, 1999a). R.H. had complete bilateral amygdala damage, in addition to some damage to surrounding temporal lobe structures, following herpes simplex encephalitis. To facilitate comparison, we used an auditory recognition task identical in protocol to the task we have used previously to demonstrate impaired

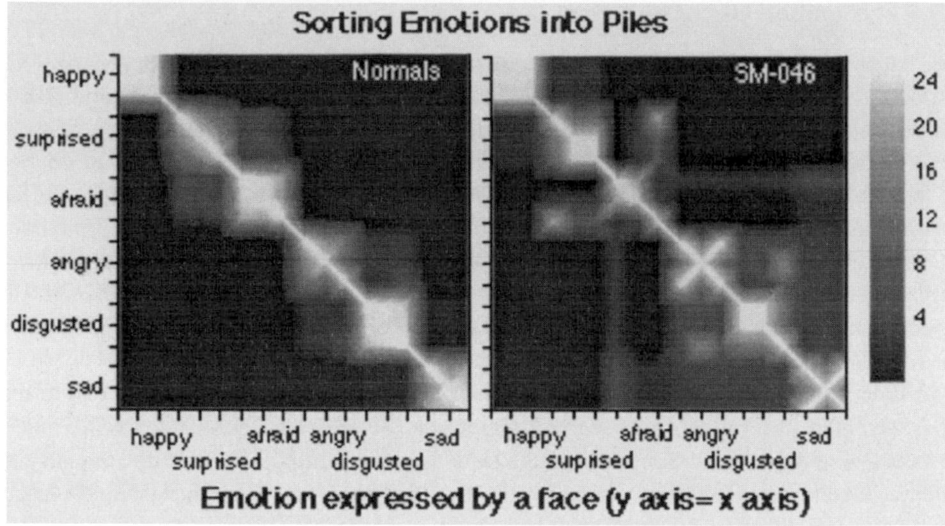

Figure 18.6 Emotion categories derived from sorting photographs of faces into piles. Normal subjects (left, $n = 7$) distinguished the six basic emotions, as well as superordinate categories that revealed the similarity between surprise and fear, and between anger and disgust. S.M. (right) showed an unusual structure in which she did not distinguish negative emotions normally. All subjects were asked to sort photographs of 18 facial expressions (three of each emotion) into three, four, seven, and 10 piles (in random order) on the basis of the similarity of the emotion expressed. A measure of similarity between each pair of faces was calculated from this task by summing the occurrences of that pair of faces in a pile, weighted by the number of possible piles, to yield a number between 1 and 24 (a face sharing no pile with any other face yielded the number 1 because it would have shared a single pile that included all the faces) (Ward, 1977; Russell, 1980). Faces are ordered identically on the *x*- and *y*-axes. Pixel brightness represents the similarity between face x and face y. Bright regions correspond to faces judged to be more similar to one another. The diagonal shows each face's similarity to itself (maximal similarity); plots are symmetric about the diagonal. See also colour plate section.

recognition of emotion in facial expressions [task (ii) described above]. Subjects were asked to judge the intensity of emotion displayed in human voices reading semantically neutral sentences. Fifteen brain-damaged subjects without damage to amygdala and 14 normal subjects served as controls.

Subjects with bilateral amygdala damage rated the intensity of each prototypical emotion expressed in prosody within 2 SDs of the mean ratings given by normal controls, similar to or better than the performance of brain-damaged controls. While there was a considerable range in the ratings given, and a fair degree of variance in normal ratings, there was no evidence that subjects with bilateral amygdala damage were impaired on this measure. Particularly striking were the data from three experiments with S.M., who performed within

Table 18.2 Recognition of similarity within and between emotion categories

Emotion	*Within*	*Between*
Happy	0.65	0.42
Sad	0.98	4.06
Angry	0.95	1.02
Afraid	1.86	4.15
Disgusted	0.99	1.08
Surprised	0.73	4.15

S.M.'s performance on a task of sorting facial expressions of emotion into piles on the basis of similarity. For each of the six basic emotion categories, we give the mean deviance of S.M.'s derived similarity measure (in SD) from that of normal controls, for all those faces within the same emotion category ('within') and the similarity between faces showing the given emotion and all those faces showing other emotions ('between'). Higher numbers thus indicate more abnormal performance. Subjects were asked to sort photographs of 18 facial expressions (three of each emotion) into three, four, seven, and 10 piles (in random order) on the basis of the similarity of the emotion expressed. A measure of similarity between each pair of faces was calculated from this task by summing the occurrences of that pair of faces in a pile, weighted by the number of possible piles, to yield a number between 0 and 24.

1 SD of normal control ratings on all emotions, including fear, an emotion which she cannot recognize in facial expressions. A subsequent correlation analysis confirmed these findings: S.M. was entirely normal in recognizing all emotions from prosody in three replications of the experiment (Figure 18.7).

One possible explanation for these findings could be that it is simply easier to recognize emotion in prosody than in facial expressions. Clear evidence against this account comes from normal subjects' performances: we did not have ceiling effects for the stimuli, especially with regard to negative emotions, which were not trivial to recognize even for normal subjects. It is thus all the more striking that subjects with bilateral amygdala damage performed normally on the task. Another strong argument against the possibility that difficulty alone could account for impaired recognition of emotion in either facial expressions or in prosody is the presence of double dissociations. S.M. was clearly impaired in recognizing emotion in facial expressions, but not in prosody. Conversely, we have found several subjects with damage to right neocortex who were severely impaired in recognizing emotion in prosody, but entirely normal when judging facial expressions. The presence of double dissociations clearly indicates that level of difficulty alone cannot account for the current findings.

In a follow-up experiment, we presented S.M. with bimodal stimuli: visual stimuli showing facial expressions (the same ones as before) accompanied by prosodic stimuli that corresponded to the same emotion as the face expressed. S.M.'s recognition of fear signalled by such bimodal stimuli was essentially normal ($r = 0.75$ correlation with normal ratings of the faces), showing that she can use her intact recognition of emotion in prosody in order to compensate for her impaired recognition of fear in facial expressions. Taken together, these findings provide strong support for the idea that the human amygdala is not essential to recognize basic emotions, including fear, in auditory prosodic stimuli of natural human voices. It remains an open question whether recognition of auditory stimuli other than prosody might rely more on the amygdala.

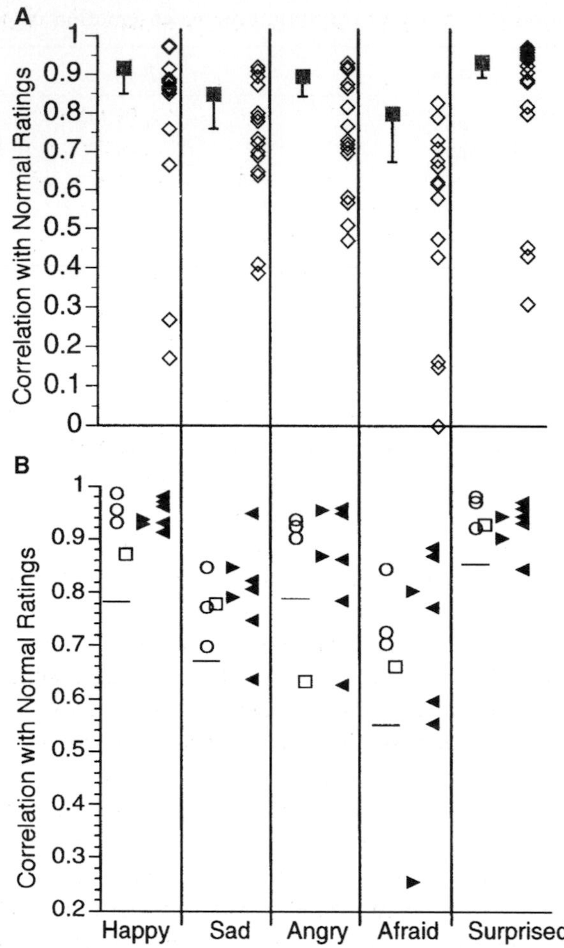

Figure 18.7 Normal recognition of emotional prosody following amygdala damage. Correlation of subjects' ratings of prosodic stimuli with the mean ratings given by normal controls. Data are from two subjects with complete bilateral amygdala damage (S.M. and R.H.), two with unilateral right amygdala damage, five with unilateral left amygdala damage, and 15 brain-damaged controls without damage to amygdala. Subjects heard 28 semantically neutral sentences that had been read by the same person in different prosodic tones of voice: happy, sad, anger, fear, or sleepiness, eight times, and rated them on a scale of 0 (= 'not at all') to 5 (= 'very much') with respect to the labels, 'awake', 'happy', 'sleepy', 'sad', 'angry', 'afraid', 'disgusted', and 'surprised'. This procedure was identical to the one we have used previously with visual stimuli of emotional facial expressions. (**A**) Correlation of ratings given by brain-damaged controls (open diamonds). Several brain-damaged controls were impaired. Grey squares indicate means and SD given by 14 normal controls (each normal control's ratings were correlated with the mean ratings of the remaining 13). (**B**) Correlation

18.5 The amygdala's role in processing stimuli with high emotional arousal

Subject S.M.'s impairment in recognizing emotional facial expressions is disproportionately severe with respect to fear. However, she also has lesser impairments in recognition of highly arousing emotions that are similar to fear, such as anger (see Figure 3A), consistent with findings from other subjects with bilateral amygdala damage, whose impairments include a variety of negative emotions (see Figure 18.2). The data so far are thus compatible both with neural systems that process a specific basic emotion, fear, and with neural systems specialized to process highly arousing, unpleasant emotions, of which fear and anger may be two instances. A direct dissociation on the basis of arousal has been demonstrated in rats: amygdala lesions interfere with avoidance of water that has been paired with electric shock (a highly arousing, unpleasant stimulus), but do not interfere with avoidance of water that has been made to taste bitter (an unpleasant, but not highly arousing stimulus) (Cahill and McGaugh, 1990). In both humans and rats, the amygdala plays a key role in conditioned fear (LeDoux *et al.*, 1990; Davis, 1992a; Bechara *et al.*, 1995), as well as in fearful and aggressive behaviours (Blanchard and Blanchard, 1972; Kling, 1986; Lee *et al.*, 1988; Davis, 1992b), further suggesting that the amygdala may be critical for processing a class of emotions that are highly arousing and related to threat and danger (Kesner, 1992; Goldstein *et al.*, 1996).

To investigate the amygdala's role in processing emotional arousal and valence directly, we asked subjects to rate facial expressions of emotion (the same stimuli as those for which data were shown in Figures 18.2–18.4) with respect to these two factors. In addition, we asked subjects to rate the arousal and the valence of the emotion depicted by single words and by sentences describing emotional events. We asked subjects to rate all these stimuli with respect to their valence (pleasantness/unpleasantness) and arousal on a nine-point scale. Our rating instrument consisted of a one-dimensional grid onto which the subject placed an 'x'; this was a simpler modification of a previously developed rating instrument called the 'Affect Grid', which has demonstrated reliability and construct validity (Russell *et al.*, 1989). Subjects were told that, for the valence scale, ratings greater than five corresponded to feelings that were more pleasant than neutral, and that ratings less than five corresponded to feelings that were less pleasant than neutral. Similarly, for the arousal scale, subjects were told that ratings greater than five corresponded to a higher energy/arousal/wakefulness than one's average arousal state, and that ratings lower than five corresponded to a lower energy/arousal or greater sleepiness/relaxation than one's average arousal state. Subjects were told that any given level of arousal could be either a pleasant or an unpleasant emotion. In addition to subject S.M., 24 (for rating faces) or 18 (for rating stories) normal control subjects were studied in order to provide normative data on all tasks.

---

of ratings given by two subjects with complete bilateral amygdala damage [S.M., ○, and R.H., □, and by two subjects with unilateral right (filled triangles pointing right) and five with unilateral left (filled triangles pointing left) amygdala damage]. (From Adolphs and Tranel, 1999b; copyright Elsevier Science Publishers, 1999.)

S.M.'s ratings of the valence of emotional facial expressions were within 2 SDs of the control mean for all six basic emotions, indicating a largely normal performance. In contrast, she was clearly severely impaired in her ratings of arousal, differing from the control mean by more than 4 SDs for certain emotional facial expressions. We calculated the difference between S.M.'s arousal rating and the mean rating given to that face by the 24 normal control subjects (Figure 18.8A). This analysis showed clearly that she assigned abnormally low arousal ratings to negative emotions. The two negative emotions normally judged to be the most arousing, fear and anger, received the most abnormal ratings. The specificity of the impairment is especially striking when comparing pleasant and unpleasant emotions that are both highly arousing: for example, S.M.'s ratings of the arousal of surprise were normal, whereas her ratings of fear were severely impaired. Additionally, this specificity for only certain emotions argues that S.M.'s performance cannot be due simply to a failure to understand the rating attribute.

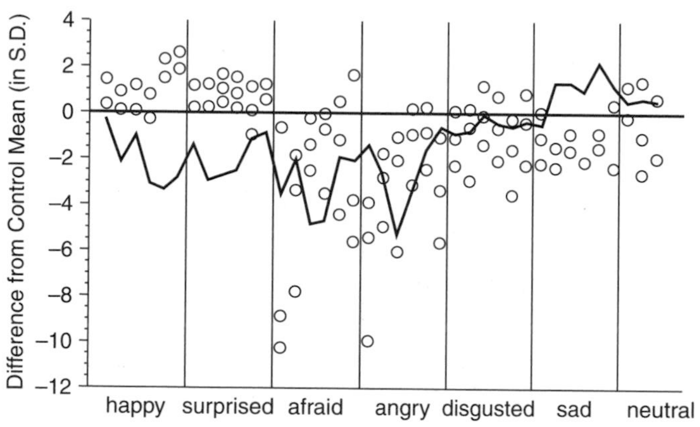

Figure 18.8 Impaired recognition of the arousal of stimuli with negative valence in subject S.M. (**A**) Comparisons between 24 normal controls and S.M. in rating the magnitude of arousal signalled by 39 facial expressions. Each circle plots the difference between S.M.'s arousal rating and control subjects' mean arousal rating for a given face in SD units. The stimuli are rank-ordered on the *x*-axis according to their perceived similarity (Adolphs *et al.*, 1994, 1995); expressions of emotions judged to be more similar are adjacent on the axis. The solid grey curve on the plot indicates the measure expected for completely random ratings, i.e. it represents the expected (average) difference of random ratings from the mean control ratings. S.M. gave abnormally low ratings of arousal to faces expressing negative emotions (○), and this finding could not be accounted for solely by larger variance in her ratings. (**B**) S.M.'s (●; three experiments) and normal controls' (bars; $n = 18$; mean ±SD) ratings of emotional stories and words depicting basic emotions. The words were the labels, 'happy, surprised, afraid, angry, disgusted, and sad'. The stories depicted either a situation typical of an emotion (e.g. 'The alley was very dark, and the footsteps behind Linda were getting louder') or a behaviour typically associated with an emotion (e.g. 'Jody giggled and laughed'), but there was no mention of the label of the emotion. Ratings >5 denote more

We carried out an additional experiment with S.M. and 18 normal control subjects, in which we asked subjects to rate the arousal and valence of lexical stimuli that denote emotions. S.M. showed a severe impairment in her ability to recognize the arousal signalled by stories and by words denoting negative emotions. She rated stories depicting anger or fear as 'relaxing,' ratings that were typically more than 5 SDs below the mean for the normal controls (Figure 18.8B). For two of the stories depicting fear (marked with asterisks in Figure 18.8B), every normal subject gave arousal ratings of 9 (the highest possible rating), whereas S.M. gave ratings of 6 (to the sentence, 'As the car was speeding down the mountain, Mike stepped down to find that he had no brakes') and 3 (to the sentence, 'Sally waved her hands in the air and called for help, as the boat was sinking'). However, she gave normal ratings of valence to all emotions.

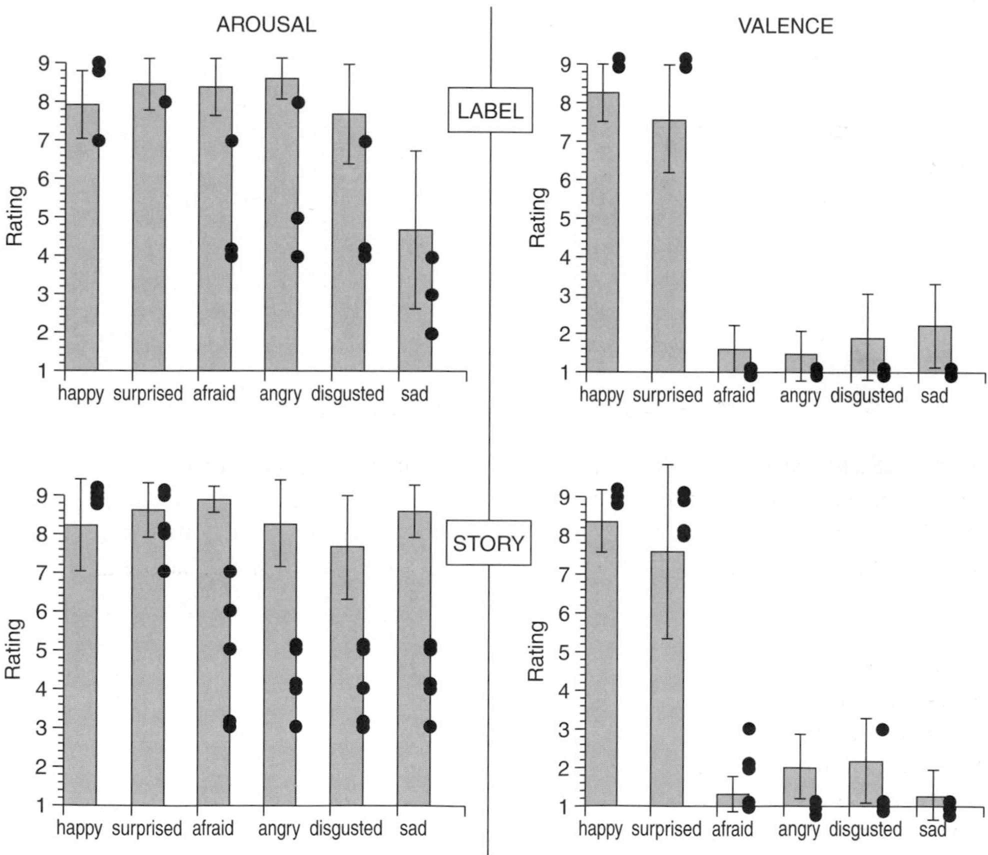

pleasant, or more arousing, emotions than neutral; those <5 denote more unpleasant or more relaxing emotions than neutral. (From Adolphs *et al.*, 1999a; copyright Blackwell Scientific Publishers, 1999.)

In a third experiment, S.M. was shown short clips from movies designed to elicit specific, basic emotions. We used stimuli from Gross and Levenson, which previously had been shown to elicit the most specific, negative emotional experiences in subjects (Gross and Levenson, 1995). In this experiment, S.M. was asked to indicate how the stimuli made her feel, a different question from the one asked with all other stimuli, and one which provides pilot data on the complex question of S.M.'s emotional experience. When shown clips that normally elicit anger, disgust, or sadness, S.M. gave them normal ratings of negative valence (they all received the most negative rating possible), but endorsed average emotional arousal (ratings of 5 for all), just as we had found with respect to her recognition in the experiments above. When shown clips that normally elicit fear ('The Shining' and 'The Silence of The Lambs'), S.M. gave neutral ratings (5) on both the valence scale and the arousal scale. When we asked her what emotion she felt while watching these two clips, she replied 'neutral', but added that, in general, most people watching these clips would feel afraid. That is, it appears that S.M. is able to recognize the emotion that is intended by these complex stimuli, but that she is not able to trigger a normal emotional response personally. It is possible that the latter impairment may account for some of her recognition impairment, and specifically for her impaired ability to attribute arousal to negatively valenced stimuli.

We should also point out that S.M. does appear to experience strong negative emotions in response to some stimuli, notably those depicting injury or harm to other people. These generally corresponded to scenes of anger, but not to scenes of fear. Thus, when she was shown some of the anger movie clips above (e.g. an episode from the film 'Cry Freedom', which showed ethnic violence in South Africa), she became visibly upset and requested we discontinue the film. On the other hand, she has never made similar comments to stimuli depicting fear, but all of these have been devoid of actual physical harm to people. Instead, such stimuli rely on the tension caused by the possibility or prediction of harmful events. The amygdala may be of special importance in linking stimuli to such predictive harmful outcomes (Schoenbaum *et al.*, 1998), a role in which it is likely to participate together with other structures, notably the ventromedial prefrontal cortices (Bechara *et al.*, 1994, 1996, Damasio, 1994; Schoenbaum *et al.*, 1999).

The data provide further detail to previously reported impairments in recognizing facial expressions of fear in subjects with bilateral amygdala damage. It is not the case that bilateral amygdala damage impairs all knowledge regarding fear; rather, it impairs the knowledge that fear is highly arousing, which may be an important correlate of the ability to predict potential harm or danger. S.M.'s inability to recognize emotional arousal in negatively valenced stimuli, and her inability to recognize fear (Adolphs *et al.*, 1994, 1995) may be consequences of a common underlying impairment in processing a class of stimuli that signal potential danger. The amygdala may be of special importance in triggering, rapidly and automatically, a concerted physiological change in response to an emotionally salient stimulus. A key component of such an emotional response may be physiological arousal, including the well-documented increases in autonomic arousal that can be triggered by the amygdala. A key issue for further research will be an elucidation of how emotional arousal, as a component of an emotional response triggered by the amygdala, can also come to depend on the amygdala as a component of conceptual knowledge regarding the emotion. One possibility deserving further investigation is that, in S.M.'s case, amygdala damage early in life impaired her experience of emotional arousal in conjunction with certain classes of sensory stimuli, and that she consequently failed to develop normal knowledge of which stimuli are emotionally arousing (see Phelps and Anderson, 1997; Adolphs, 1999; Adolphs *et al.*, 1999a). Data from our laboratory which compared performances on the above task (rating the arousal of facial expressions) obtained from subjects who acquired amygdala damage early in life, and from subjects that acquired such damage in adulthood, provide preliminary support for this interpretation (Adolphs *et al.*, 1997b). Further experiments, also in non-human primates (Bachevalier, 1991, Chapter 15), will be necessary to specify the amygdala's role during development, a topic of considerable complexity.

18.6 Recognition of social information

Humans are the most social of primates, with brains adapted for the rapid retrieval of knowledge, formation of judgements, and generation of behaviours necessary for survival in a complex social environment. Like other primates, humans possess a vast store of knowledge, including both facts and emotional reactions, which is called upon during social encounters. Along with language, the human face is a key channel by which such knowledge can be triggered. To examine the role of the amygdala in this process, we asked subjects to rate photographs of the faces of unfamiliar people, solely on the basis of their appearance, with respect to two attributes important in real-life social encounters: approachability and trustworthiness.

We studied three subjects with complete bilateral amygdala damage (subjects S.M., J.M., and R.H.), four subjects with unilateral right amygdala damage, and three subjects with unilateral left amygdala damage on this task. J.M., like R.H., had complete bilateral amygdala and damage to surrounding structures in temporal lobe following encephalitis. Both J.M. and R.H. had sustained their damage as adults. Data from subjects with amygdala damage were compared with those from 46 normal control subjects and from 10 brain-damaged control subjects whose lesions did not involve the amygdala. All subjects with bilateral amygdala damage had normal ability to discriminate faces on the basis of identity, gender, and pattern of expression, and were able to discriminate direction of gaze normally, to ensure that there were no visuoperceptual impairments that might account for the results we report below.

Ratings of approachability and of trustworthiness were analysed separately for the 50 faces to which normal controls assigned the most negative ratings, and for the 50 most positive faces. Subjects with bilateral amygdala damage rated the 50 most negative faces more positively than did either normal ($P < 0.01$) or brain-damaged controls ($P < 0.05$; Mann–Whitney U-tests on subjects' mean ratings, Bonferroni corrected for multiple comparisons) (Figure 18.9). Groups with unilateral amygdala lesions did not differ from controls on either rating. All subject groups gave similar ratings to the 50 most positive faces ($P > 0.1$ for both approachability and trustworthiness when comparing bilateral amygdala subjects with the control groups). There was no effect of subject gender on rating the faces ($P > 0.7$, ANOVA

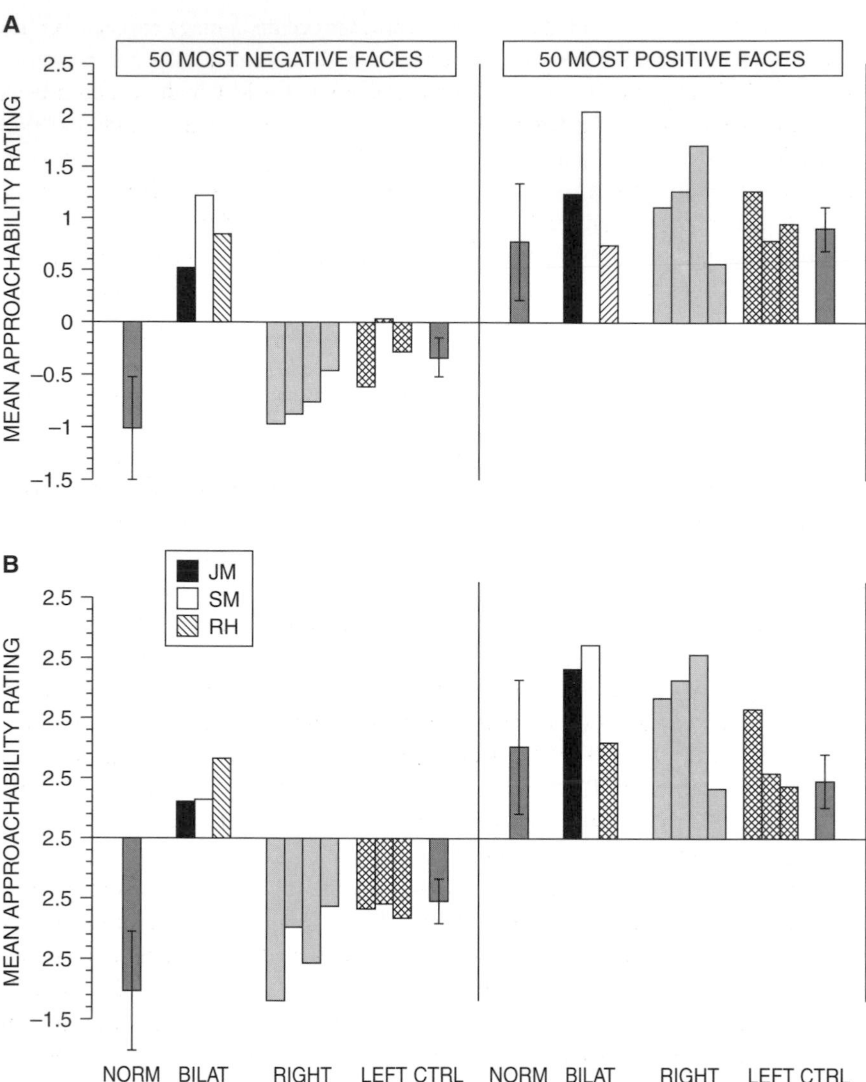

Figure 18.9 Impaired social judgment following bilateral amygdala damage. Mean judgements of approachability (top) and trustworthiness (bottom) of the faces of 100 unfamiliar people. Data are broken down into those obtained from the 50 faces which received the most negative (left) and most positive (right) mean ratings from normal controls on each of these attributes. Each face was judged on a scale of –3 (very unapproachable) to +3 (very approachable). Means and SD are shown for data from 46 normal controls ('NORM'). Individual means are shown for each of three subjects with bilateral amygdala damage ('BILAT'), four subjects with unilateral right ('RIGHT') and three with unilateral left ('LEFT') amygdala damage. Means and SEM are shown for 10 brain-damaged controls with no damage to amygdala ('CTRL'). (From Adolphs *et al*., 1998; copyright MacMillan Magazines, 1998.)

on normal data). Subject S.M. spontaneously commented during the experiment that, in real life, she would not know how to judge if a person were trustworthy. The findings are consonant also with S.M.'s tendency to approach and engage in physical contact with other people rather indiscriminately, as we mentioned in Section 18.2 above (Tranel and Hyman, 1990; Adolphs *et al.*, 1994).

An examination of the ratings given by subject with bilateral amygdala damage showed two effects: they tended to rate all faces more positively than did controls, and they also showed the largest deviation from control ratings, and the largest variance, specifically when rating the most negative faces. This analysis suggests an overall positive bias, as well as a specific impairment in rating the most negative faces. To determine whether these two effects were independent, and to control for a possible ceiling effect that might result from using a bounded rating scale, we gave S.M. a two-alternative forced-choice task, using the same face stimuli, in which these possible confounds were eliminated. We asked S.M. to choose the more approachable face in pairwise comparisons between each of five of the faces paired with each of the remaining 99 faces (a total of 5x99 = 495 pairwise comparisons). We compared S.M.'s choices on this task with the choices that would be expected on the basis of the mean approachability rating given to the faces in each pair by normal controls. S.M. made the largest number of abnormal choices in comparisons involving those of the five faces that normally receive the most negative ratings (Figure 18.10A), findings which cannot be accounted for solely on the basis of a general positive bias. We further analysed S.M.'s choices regarding the 50 least, and the 49 most, approachable of the other 99 faces. In this analysis, S.M.'s choices consistently correlated better with mean normal ratings for the 49 most approachable than for the 50 least approachable faces (logistic regression of S.M.'s binary data with the mean normal control data; Figure 18.10B). These analyses confirm that S.M.'s judgements are disproportionately impaired relative to individuals that are normally classified as unapproachable and untrustworthy.

We addressed three further questions. (i) Does the impairment extend to stimuli other than faces? One might expect impairments in judging other stimuli, given the amygdala's importance in emotional response to a large variety of stimuli in nearly all modalities (Weiskrantz, 1956; Sawa and Delgado, 1963; Blanchard and Blanchard, 1972; Nishijo *et al.*, 1988; Brothers *et al.*, 1990; Grant *et al.*, 1996; Scott *et al.*, 1997; Zald and Pardo, 1997). While such impairments following amygdala damage are most apparent in the social domain (i.e. with regard to stimuli depicting, or behaviours directed at, other animals), there is evidence that the amygdala also plays a role in preferences for non-social stimuli. For instance, amygdalectomized monkeys will approach unfamiliar objects more readily, and appear less cautious in novel environments than do normal monkeys (Amaral *et al.*, 1997). Consonant with these findings, neurophysiological activity of neurons within the primate amygdala is also modulated by the affective significance of a variety of non-social sensory stimuli (Nishijo *et al.*, 1988; Muramoto *et al.*, 1993). All these data provide support for the view that the amygdala plays a critical role both in social behaviour and in emotional response to non-social stimuli. However, nearly all available evidence has come from studies in non-human animals.

To address this question, we asked two of the subjects with bilateral amygdala damage, S.M. and R.H., to rate how much they liked visual stimuli other than faces (Adolphs and

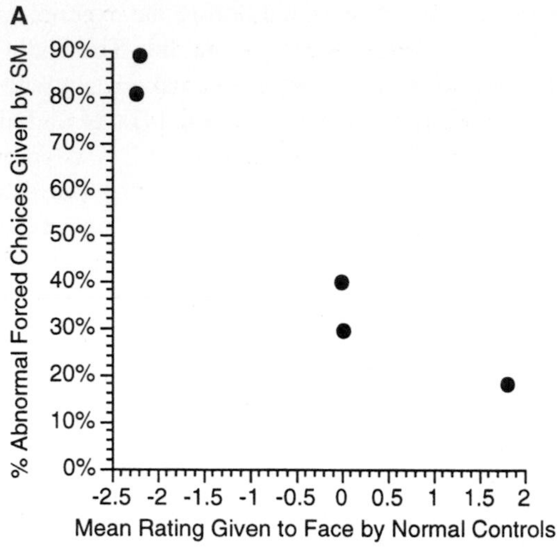

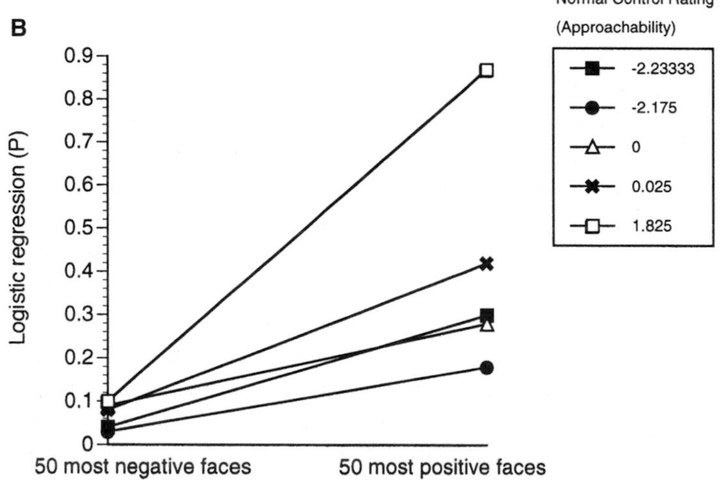

Figure 18.10 S.M.'s judgments of approachability in a two-alternative forced-choice task. (**A**) Proportion of S.M.'s choices that differed from the choices predicted from normal control ratings, for each of five faces (•) that were compared with the remaining 99 faces. The mean rating of approachability given to each of the five faces by normal controls is shown on the *x*-axis, and the proportion of incorrect choices made by S.M. for all 99 pairings with each of the five faces is given on the *y*-axis. S.M. made the largest proportion of incorrect choices in comparisons involving those of the five faces normally considered most unapproachable (data points on left side of graph). (**B**) Logistic regression of S.M.'s data for the pairwise comparisons of each of the five faces (five lines) with the remaining 50 most negative (left), and 49 most positive faces (right). Values on the *y*-axis are *P*-values computed from a maximum-likelihood estimated logistic regression of S.M.'s binary data on the mean normal

Tranel, 1999b). We used three types of stimuli: landscapes, complex coloured patterns (pictures of coloured spheres), and simple black and white patterns (lines on a white background). Both subjects endorsed more positive ratings for each of these classes of stimuli than did normal controls (Figure 18.11), showing that the impairment is not limited to faces. A statistical evaluation of these findings showed that amygdala subjects were significantly impaired in rating that half of the unrecognizable figures and of the spheres that normally receive the most negative ratings ($t = -15.3$, $P < 0.001$ for figures; $t = -10.0$, $P < 0.05$ for spheres) but not those that normally receive the most positive ratings ($P > 0.4$; one-tailed *t*-tests on subjects' mean ratings for the given classes of stimuli, with *P*-values Bonferroni-corrected for multiple comparisons). Due to the small number of stimuli and the large variance in ratings given by subjects (including controls), no statistical significance could be attached to the data from Mondrians or from landscapes (all $P > 0.1$).

Regressions of the deviations of ratings given by amygdala subjects on the rank order of the ratings given to stimuli by normal controls revealed statistical significance in several cases, as indicated in Figure 18.11. Moreover, all regressions were in the same direction for the four different classes of stimuli: subjects with amygdala damage gave abnormally positive ratings to stimuli that normal controls gave the most negative ratings, just as they did with regard to judging social attributes from faces. The human amygdala thus appears to play a general role in guiding preferences for visual stimuli that normally are judged to be aversive, or to predict aversive consequences. This function may be especially critical, or may be most perspicuous, with regard to judgement of social stimuli such as faces.

(ii) Does the impairment extend to judging biographical verbal descriptions of people? Milder, or absent, impairments might be expected when judging lexical stimuli, as these may provide explicit pointers to the relevant knowledge, and might thus compensate for a knowledge retrieval impairment, as we have conjectured previously (Adolphs *et al.*, 1995). We investigated this issue by asking subject S.M. to rate the likeability of people as described by written adjectives. S.M. was entirely normal in judging both these classes of stimuli (within 1.5 SD of norms on all stimuli; Figure 18.12). These data show that the above impairments are unlikely to be due to a simple failure to understand the task, or to a general agnosia for socially relevant knowledge. Instead, the findings argue that the amygdala helps link percepts of external sensory stimuli with the retrieval of pertinent knowledge, the formation of advantageous decisions, and the choice of adaptive behavioural responses that are appropriate to the emotional or social relevance of the stimulus (Damasio, 1994, 1995).

(iii) A final question concerns the nature of the cues in faces on the basis of which the above judgements are made, no doubt a topic of daunting complexity. We undertook a preliminary and entirely empirical investigation of this issue, in which we chose the 10 faces which S.M. had rated most abnormally on the above tasks, and systematically manipulated individual features in each face. We showed subjects 109 pairs of faces in which each pair

---

control data. The inset indicates the mean normal rating of each of the five faces (same as their *x*-axis value in A). S.M.'s choices could be well predicted from mean normal data for the 49 most positive, but not for the 50 most negative faces, consistent with the findings from (A).

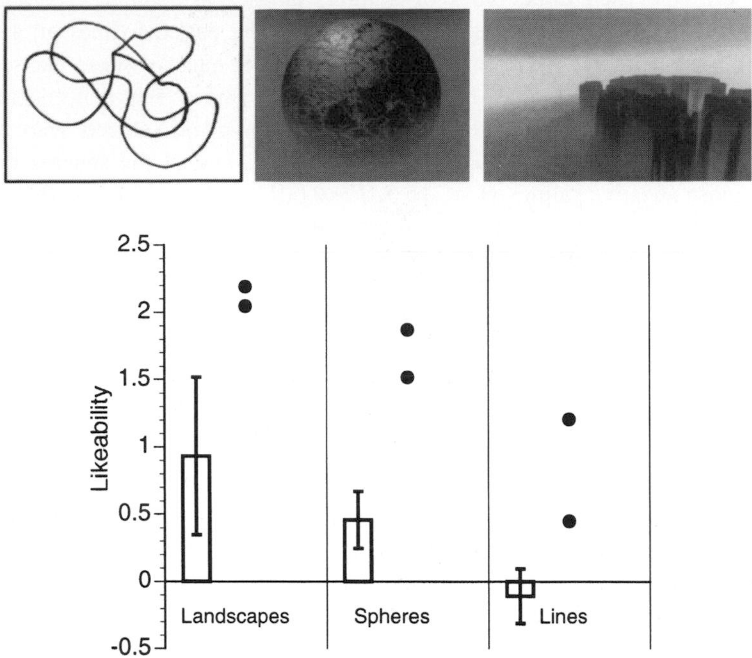

Figure 18.11 Preferences for unfamiliar visual stimuli following amygdala damage. **(A)** Examples of stimuli used. From left to right: nonsense line figure, sphere, landscape. **(B)** Mean ratings of likeability from normal controls (bars, mean ± SD) and S.M. (•). S.M. gave abnormally positive ratings to all classes of stimuli. (From Adolphs and Tranel, 1999b; copyright MIT Press, 1999.) See also colour plate section.

showed the same individual with a difference in only a single feature. We manipulated either direction of gaze, expression of the eyes, expression of the mouth, or visibility of the eyes, all features that could conceivably contribute to subjects' judgements on the previous tasks. In a two-alternative forced-choice task, S.M. and 16 normal controls were asked to choose the face they liked most in the pair. S.M. performed entirely normally on this task. Logistic linear analysis, with subjects' binary choices as the dependent variable and the manipulated features as factors, showed that S.M. did not differ from controls in her choices with respect to any of the above features that we had manipulated. These findings indicate that insensitivity to particular features, in isolation, is unlikely to account for the findings.

The above findings suggest a role for the human amygdala in triggering socially relevant knowledge in response to visual stimuli. With regard to faces, the amygdala's role appears to be relatively specific for those faces that normally are classified to be unapproachable and untrustworthy, findings consistent with the amygdala's demonstrated role in processing threatening and aversive stimuli. The result that unilateral amygdala damage causes no comparable impairment is parallel to previous reports that bilateral, but not unilateral, amygdala damage

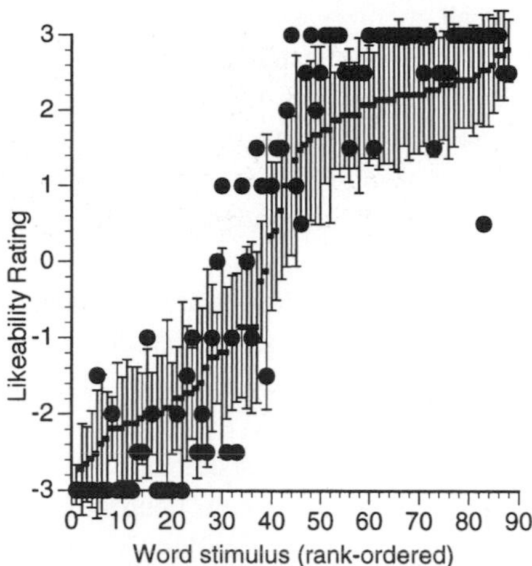

Figure 18.12 Preferences for people described by lexical stimuli. Ratings given by S.M. (two experiments; •) and 20 normal controls (small black squares and SDs) to 88 adjectives describing personality, selected from a standardized set (Anderson, 1968). Stimuli are rank-ordered on the x-axis according to the mean ratings of likeability given by normal controls. (From Adolphs *et al.*, 1998; copyright MacMillan Magazines, 1998.)

impairs recognition of emotional facial expressions (Adolphs *et al.*, 1995). While the detailed mechanism by which the amygdala enacts these functions remains unclear, the above experiment with individual features of faces suggests that the amygdala may trigger knowledge retrieval on the basis of global face configurations. As such, the role of the amygdala in human social behaviour may be most important not in innate feature detection, but in the evaluation of complex stimuli that have acquired relevance through prior experience with similar exemplars.

18.7 Influences of emotional processing on other aspects of cognition

We cannot here review in detail additional abnormalities in the emotional modulation of other aspects of cognition. However, we would like to mention briefly two additional domains: memory and decision making.

Several recent functional imaging studies have reported that encoding and consolidation of declarative knowledge into long-term memory activated the amygdala, when the material that is being encoded is emotionally arousing (Cahill *et al.*, 1996; Canli *et al.*, 1998; Hamann *et al.*, 1999), lending support to the idea that the amygdala plays an important modulatory role during the encoding of emotionally arousing material into declarative long-term memory (Cahill and McGaugh, 1996, 1998; Cahill, Chapter 12). There is a good correlation between increased activity within the amygdala during encoding, and the subsequent performance of subjects on recognition or recall memory tasks: emotionally arousing stimuli activate the amygdala during encoding, and are remembered better. In contrast, encoding of material that is emotionally neutral correlates with activation of the hippocampus, but not the amygdala (Alkire *et al.*, 1998). Furthermore, the amygdala activation observed correlated with activation of the hippocampus (Hamann *et al.*, 1999), consistent with findings from animal studies that emotional arousal engages amygdala-dependent modulation of the hippocampal memory system (Packard *et al.*, 1994).

These findings from functional imaging studies are consonant with a role for the amygdala in modulation of motivated learning in animal studies (McGaugh *et al.*, 1996; Cahill and McGaugh, 1998; see also McGaugh *et al.*, Chapter 11), and have also been corroborated by lesion studies in humans. Subject S.M., as well as another subject with the same disease and similar brain lesions, is impaired specifically in remembering stimuli that are emotionally arousing, but shows normal memory for neutral material (Adolphs *et al.*, 1997a). The mechanisms for the emotional facilitation of declarative memory consolidation in humans are not well understood; one possibility may be that the amygdala modulates consolidation that occurs during sleep, perhaps especially rapid eye movement (REM) sleep. In support of this idea, the amygdala is highly activated during REM sleep (Maquet *et al.*, 1996), and sleep is known to consolidate a variety of forms of memory (Stickgold, 1999), perhaps especially emotionally salient memories (Smith and Lapp, 1991).

We have examined in detail the sleep stages that subject S.M. experiences during a typical night's sleep. S.M. appears to have normal frequency and duration of the different stages of sleep (time spent in each stage: 7% stage I, 54% stage II, 17% stage III/IV, and 22% REM). She reports frequent dreams, and appears to have a normal diurnal sleep–wake cycle. While the amygdala may thus be involved in memory reprocessing during some of the stages of sleep, it does not appear to play a necessary role in controlling sleep stage durations or transitions themselves. These issues remain important avenues for future research.

A second important line of research concerns the amygdala's role in guiding decision making. It is known that emotional processing contributes importantly to decision making under conditions of uncertainty, a function that has been best studied with regard to the ventromedial prefrontal cortices (Damasio, 1994). Recent studies suggest that the amygdala does contribute importantly to making decisions on the basis of prior emotional associations with similar situations. Thus, like subjects with ventromedial prefrontal damage, S.M. is also impaired in a gambling task on which choices must be made on the basis of hunches under conditions of uncertainty (Bechara *et al.*, 2000). Amygdala and ventromedial prefrontal cortices may play complementary roles in guiding choices by feelings (Bechara *et al.*, 2000), an architecture that also receives considerable support from studies in animals (Gaffan *et al.*, 1993; Schoenbaum *et al.*, 1998).

18.8 Conclusions

The established role of the human amygdala in recognizing facial expressions of fear, its role in recognizing untrustworthiness and unapproachability from faces, and the evidence for a role in preferences for non-social stimuli, all make plausible the following hypothesis. Stimuli that have been associated with negative (aversive) consequences in the past (possibly either in individual experience or through phylogeny) activate the amygdala to trigger responses such that the organism can avoid the aversive consequence that is predicted by the stimulus. In animals, the amygdala may trigger predominantly behavioural reactions; in humans, it may trigger both behaviour and conscious knowledge that the stimulus predicts something 'bad'. In our tasks, the latter may appear primarily as the triggering of a feeling that one does not like, or wishes to avoid, the stimulus or the situation with which the stimulus is associated.

With regard to the best established finding from subjects with bilateral amygdala damage—their impaired recognition of fear in certain stimuli—it is important to be clear on what such subjects do and do not know with regard to fear. Does S.M. not know what fear is? Does she not have a concept of fear, or not know what the label 'fear' refers to? As we mentioned above (see Section 18.3.2), we think that neither is the case. S.M. can use the word 'fear' appropriately in conversation, and she is able to retrieve some knowledge pertaining to the concept of fear. In our view, she has two primary impairments: (i) an inability to trigger certain responses, including those normally involved in reconstructing conceptual knowledge regarding the emotion, when shown non-lexical stimuli, such as facial expressions, and (ii) a lack of knowledge, which may be a result both of an impaired acquisition of conceptual knowledge during development concerning some aspects of emotion concepts, as well as a consequence of (i).

This brings us to an important question that applies to S.M.'s amygdala damage, but not to the amygdala damage of other subjects who have been reported in the literature: are her recognition impairments due primarily to impaired acquisition or to impaired retrieval of knowledge? As we pointed out, we cannot be sure of the onset of S.M.'s lesion, but it is plausible that she sustained her amygdala damage early in life, and plausibly early enough that such developmental damage might have interfered with her acquisition and consolidation of knowledge regarding emotions. We (Adolphs *et al.*, 1996) and others (Phelps and Anderson, 1997) have previously conjectured that the human amygdala may be more crucial for the acquisition of knowledge regarding emotions, rather than for subsequent retrieval (see also McGaugh *et al.*, Chapter 11; Cahill, Chapter 12; Bachevalier, Chapter 15). Some comparisons of case studies have hinted that amygdala damage can impair recognition of fear in facial expressions if sustained early in life, but not if sustained in adulthood (Adolphs *et al.*, 1994; Anderson *et al.*, 1996; Hamann *et al.*, 1996; but see Calder *et al.*, 1996b), and both functional imaging (Cahill *et al.*, 1996) and lesion studies (Cahill *et al.*, 1995; Adolphs *et al.*, 1997a) have demonstrated the human amygdala's involvement in encoding declarative knowledge regarding emotionally arousing material. One explanation of the findings with S.M. is thus that she never acquired normal conceptual knowledge of emotion to begin with, such as, for instance, knowledge concerning the arousal of unpleasant emotions, and hence that she is unable to retrieve such knowledge subsequently on the experimental tasks. This possible role of the amygdala in declarative knowledge may bear some analogy to the established role of the hippocampus (Zola-Morgan and Squire, 1990): both structures may be most important with regard to the acquisition, but not the retrieval, of declarative knowledge; and both structures may participate in the consolidation of long-term memory over the course of many years (Rempel-Clower *et al.*, 1996), e.g. during development. In the case of the amygdala, this role may be both more specific (pertaining to stimuli that signal threat or danger) and less direct (pertaining to modulation of declarative memory systems rather than direct encoding; McGaugh *et al.*, 1996, Chapter 11; Cahill, Chapter 12).

However, S.M.'s impaired knowledge as evidenced on the tasks we have reviewed above need not be interpreted as due to impaired acquisition, or as directly impaired retrieval of declarative knowledge. There is another possibility, which views knowledge as information that is created on-the-fly, and which acknowledges a more indirect and modulatory role for the amygdala in knowledge reconstruction. We find it plausible that S.M.'s emotion recognition impairments may be due, at least in part, to an impaired ability to reconstruct or simulate an emotional state normally associated with the emotion depicted by the stimulus. Consider how we normally recognize another individual's feeling from looking at their face, or how we decide whether someone would be friendly or trustworthy from their face. Clearly, these are difficult tasks requiring, at a minimum, that perceptual representations of the stimulus trigger considerable emotional and social knowledge. What form might such emotional and social knowledge take? One possibility is that visual representations of an individual's face trigger components of an emotional response within ourselves that in essence attempt to simulate the other individual's mental state, i.e. we obtain information about another individual's mental state by simulating components of what it would be like to be the other person. This idea, the 'simulation theory', has received some support among philosophers and cognitive scientists who study how we represent and interpret the mental states of other people (see, for example, Gallese and Goldman, 1999), and we believe that such reconstruction of knowledge by simulation may play a very general role in how we access conceptual knowledge. Within this framework, one attractive hypothesis views the human amygdala as one component of the neural systems whereby we can trigger a physiological response, or the internal representation (i.e. the somatic image) of a physiological response in sensory neocortices, whose structure attempts to simulate the internal state of another person, i.e. the amygdala (together with other neural structures, such as cortical regions located in right hemisphere) allows us to engage a certain dispositional (emotional or social) state, and this state can then be used to guide behaviour or to reconstruct conceptual knowledge, depending on the precise demands made by the experimental task in question. The work reviewed in this chapter is consistent with such a role for the amygdala, specifically with regard to states associated with threat and danger towards an individual. Future studies, using functional imaging as well as the lesion method, could begin to address these ideas explicitly, by jointly investigating the amygdala in emotional recognition, expression, and experience, and assessing the extent to which its role in all three domains is correlated.

Acknowledgements

The research reported in this chapter was supported by NIH grant PO1-NS19632 to Antonio R. Damasio; and by NIH grant R29-MH57905, a Sloan Foundation Research Fellowship, and an EJLB Foundation Research Scholars Award to R.A. We would like to thank Antonio R. Damasio, Hanna Damasio, Antoine Bechara, Denise Krutzfeldt, Kris Kinsey, and Jeremy Nath, for advice and assistance with various aspects of the reported studies.

References

Adolphs, R. (1999) The human amygdala and emotion. *The Neuroscientist*, 5, 125–137.

Adolphs, R. and Tranel, D. (1999a) Intact recognition of emotional prosody following amygdala damage. *Neuropsychologia*, 37, 1285–1292.

Adolphs, R. and Tranel, D. (1999b) Preferences for visual stimuli following amygdala damage. *Journal of Cognitive Neuroscience*, 11, 610–616.

Adolphs, R., Tranel, D., Damasio, H., and Damasio, A. (1994) Impaired recognition of emotion in facial expressions following bilateral damage to the human amygdala. *Nature*, 372, 669–672.

Adolphs, R., Tranel, D., Damasio, H., and Damasio, A.R. (1995) Fear and the human amygdala. *Journal of Neuroscience*, 15, 5879–5892.

Adolphs, R., Damasio, H., Tranel, D., and Damasio, A.R. (1996) Cortical systems for the recognition of emotion in facial expressions. *Journal of Neuroscience*, 16, 7678–7687.

Adolphs, R., Cahill, L., Schul R., and Babinsky, R. (1997a) Impaired declarative memory for emotional material following bilateral amygdala damage in humans. *Learning and Memory*, 4, 291–300.

Adolphs, R., Lee, G.P., Tranel, D., and Damasio, A.R. (1997b) Bilateral damage to the human amygdala early in life impairs knowledge of emotional arousal. *Society for Neuroscience Abstracts*, 23, 1582.

Adolphs, R., Tranel, D., and Damasio, A.R. (1998) The human amygdala in social judgment. *Nature*, 393, 470–474.

Adolphs, R., Russell, J.A., and Tranel, D. (1999a) A role for the human amygdala in recognizing emotional arousal. *Psychological Science*, 10, 167–171.

Adolphs, R., Tranel, D., Hamann, S., Young, A., Calder, A., Anderson, A., Phelps, E., and Damasio, A.R. (1999b) Recognition of facial emotion in nine subjects with bilateral amygdala damage. *Neuropsychologia*, 37, 1111–1117.

Aggleton, J.P (1992) *The Amygdala: Neurobiological Aspects of Emotion, Memory, and Mental Dysfunction*. Wiley-Liss, New York.

Alkire, M.T., Haier, R.J., Fallon, J.H. , and Cahill, L. (1998) Hippocampal, but not amygdala, activity at encoding correlates with long-term, free recall of nonemotional information. *Proceedings of the National Academy of Sciences of the United States of America*, 95, 14506–14510.

Amaral, D.G., Capitanio, J.P., Machado, C.J., Mason, W.A., and Mendoza, S.P. (1997) The role of the amygdaloid complex in rhesus monkey social behavior. *Society for Neuroscience Abstracts*, 23, 570.

Anderson, A., LaBar, K.S., and Phelps, E.A. (1996) Facial affect processing abilities following unilateral temporal lobectomy. *Society for Neuroscience Abstracts*, 22, 1866.

Anderson, A.K. and Phelps, E.A. (1998) Intact recognition of vocal expressions of fear following bilateral lesions of the human amygdala. *NeuroReport*, 9, 3607–3613.

Anderson, N.H. (1968) Likableness ratings of 555 personality-trait words. *Journal of Personality and Social Psychology*, 9, 272–279.

Bachevalier, J. (1991) An animal model for childhood autism: memory loss and socioemotional disturbances following neonatal damage to the limbic system in monkeys. In *Advances in Neuropsychiatry and Psychopharmacology, Volume 1: Schizophrenia Research* (eds C.A. Tamminga and S.C. Schultz), pp. 129–140. Raven Press, New York.

Beauregard, M., Leroux, J.-M., Bergman, S., Arzoumanian, Y., Beaudoin, G., Bourgouin, P., and Stip, E. (1998) The functional neuroanatomy of major depression: an fMRI study using an emotional activation paradigm. *NeuroReport*, 9, 3253–3258.

Bechara, A., Damasio, A.R., Damasio, H., and Anderson, S.W. (1994) Insensitivity to future consequences following damage to human prefrontal cortex. *Cognition*, 50, 7–15.

Bechara, A., Tranel, D., Damasio, H., Adolphs, R., Rockland, C., and Damasio, A.R. (1995) Double dissociation of conditioning and declarative knowledge relative to the amygdala and hippocampus in humans. *Science*, 269, 1115–1118.

Bechara, A., Lee, G.P., Adolphs, R., Tranel, D., and Damasio, A.R. (1996) Insensitivity to future consequences following bilateral damage to the human amygdala: contrasts with ventromedial frontal lobe lesions. *Society for Neuroscience Abstracts*, 22, 1109.

Bechara, A., Damasio, H., Damasio, A.R., and Lee, G.P. (2000) Different contributions of the human amygdala and ventromedial prefrontal cortex to decision-making. *Journal of Neuroscience*, in press.

Blanchard, D.C. and Blanchard, R.J. (1972) Innate and conditioned reactions to threat in rats with amygdaloid lesions. *Journal of Comparative and Physiological Psychology*, 81, 281–290.

Breiter, H.C., Etcoff, N.L., Whalen, P.J., Kennedy, W.A., Rauch, S.L., Buckner, R.L., Strauss, M.M., Hyman, S.E. , and Rosen, B.R. (1996) Response and habituation of the human amygdala during visual processing of facial expression. *Neuron*, 17, 875–887.

Broks, P., Young, A.W., Maratos, E.J., Coffey, P.J., Calder, A.J., Isaac, C., Mayes, A.R., Hodges, J.R., Montaldi, D., Cezayirli, E., Roberts, N., and Hadley, D. (1998) Face processing impairments after encephalitis: amygdala damage and recognition of fear. *Neuropsychologia*, 36, 59–70.

Brothers, L., Ring, B., and Kling, A. (1990) Response of neurons in the macaque amygdala to complex social stimuli. *Behavioral Brain Research*, 41, 199–213.

Cahill, L. and McGaugh, J.L. (1990) Amygdaloid complex lesions differentially affect retention of tasks using appetitive and aversive reinforcement. *Behavioral Neuroscience*, 104, 532–543.

Cahill, L. and McGaugh, J.L. (1996) Modulation of memory storage. *Current Opinion in Neurobiology*, 6, 237–242.

Cahill, L. and McGaugh, J.L. (1998) Mechanisms of emotional arousal and lasting declarative memory. *Trends in Neurosciences*, 21, 294–299.

Cahill, L., Babinsky, R., Markowitsch, H.J., and McGaugh, J.L. (1995) The amygdala and emotional memory. *Nature*, 377, 295–296.

Cahill, L., Haier, R.J., Fallon, J., Alkire, M.T., Tang, C., Keator, D., Wu, J., and McGaugh, J.L. (1996) Amygdala activity at encoding correlated with long-term, free recall of emotional information. *Proceedings of the National Academy of Sciences of the United States of America*, 93, 8016–8021.

Calder, A.J., Young, A.W., Perrett, D.I., Etcoff, N.L., and Rowland, D. (1996a) Categorical perception of morphed facial expressions. *Visual Cognition*, 3, 81–117.

Calder, A.J., Young, A.W., Rowland, D., Perrett, D.I., Hodges, J.R., and Etcoff, N.L. (1996b) Facial emotion recognition after bilateral amygdala damage: differentially severe impairment of fear. *Cognitive Neuropsychology*, 13, 699–745.

Canli, T., Zhao, Z., Desmond, J., Glover, G., and Gabrieli, J.D.E. (1998) Amygdala activation at encoding correlates with long-term recognition memory for emotional pictures: an fMRI study. *Society for Neuroscience Abstracts*, 24, 935.

Damasio, A.R. (1994) *Descartes' Error: Emotion, Reason, and the Human Brain*. Grosset/Putnam, New York.

Damasio, A.R. (1995) Toward a neurobiology of emotion and feeling: operational concepts and hypotheses. *The Neuroscientist*, 1, 19–25.

Darwin, C. (1872/1965) *The Expression of the Emotions in Man and Animals*. University of Chicago Press, Chicago.

Davidson, R.J. and Irwin, W. (1999) The functional neuroanatomy of emotion and affective style. *Trends in Cognitive Sciences*, 3, 11–22.

Davis, M. (1992a) The role of the amygdala in conditioned fear. In *The Amygdala: Neurobiological Aspects of Emotion, Memory, and Mental Dysfunction* (ed. J.P. Aggleton), pp. 255–306. Wiley-Liss, New York.

Davis, M. (1992b) The role of the amygdala in fear and anxiety. *Annual Review of Neuroscience*, 15, 353–375.

Ekman, P. and Friesen, W. (1976) *Pictures of Facial Affect*. Consulting Psychologists Press, Palo Alto, California.

Etcoff, N.L. and Magee, J.J. (1992) Categorical perception of facial expressions. *Cognition*, 44, 227–240.

Gaffan, D., Murray, E.A., and Fabre-Thorpe, M. (1993) Interaction of the amygdala with the frontal lobe in reward memory. *European Journal of Neuroscience*, 5, 968–975.

Gallese, V. and Goldman, A. (1999) Mirror neurons and the simulation theory of mind-reading. *Trends in Cognitive Sciences*, 2, 493–500.

Goldstein, L.E., Rasmusson, A.M., Bunney, B.S., and Roth, R.H. (1996) Role of the amygdala in the coordination of behavioral, neuroendocrine, and prefrontal cortical monoamine responses to psychological stress in the rat. *Journal of Neuroscience*, 16, 4787–4798.

Grant, S., London, E.D., Newlin, D.B., Vellemagne, V.L., Liu, X., Contoreggi, C., Phillips, R.L., Kimes, A.S., and Margolin, A. (1996) Activation of memory circuits during cue-elicited cocaine craving. *Proceedings of the National Academy of Sciences of the United States of America*, 93, 12040–12045.

Gray, J.M., Young, A.W., Barker, W.A., Curtis, A., and Gibson, D. (1997) Impaired recognition of disgust in Huntington's disease gene carriers. *Brain*, 120, 2029–2038.

Gross, J.J. and Levenson, R.W. (1995) Emotion elicitation using films. *Cognition and Emotion*, 9, 87–107.

Hamann, S.B., Stefanacci, L., Squire, L.R., Adolphs, R., Tranel, D., Damasio, H., and Damasio, A. (1996) Recognizing facial emotion. *Nature*, 379, 497.

Hamann, S.B., Ely, T.D., Grafton, S.T., and Kilts, C.D. (1999) Amygdala activity related to enhanced memory for pleasant and aversive stimuli. *Nature Neuroscience*, 2, 289–293.

Hofer, P.-A. (1973) Urbach–Wiethe disease: a review. *Acta Dermatologia Venerologia*, 53, 5–52.

James, W. (1884) What is an emotion? *Mind*, 9, 188–205.

Kesner, R.P. (1992) Learning and memory in rats with an emphasis on the role of the amygdala. In *The Amygdala: Neurobiological Aspects of Emotion, Memory, and Mental Dysfunction* (ed. J.P. Aggleton), pp. 379–400. Wiley-Liss, New York.

Kling, A.S. (1986) The anatomy of aggression and affiliation. In *Emotion: Theory, Research, and Experience* (eds R. Plutchik and H. Kellerman), pp. 237–264. Academic Press, New York.

Klüver, H. and Bucy, P.C. (1939) Preliminary analysis of functions of the temporal lobes in monkeys. *Archives of Neurological Psychiatry*, 42, 979–997.

Le Doux, J. (1996) *The Emotional Brain*. Simon and Schuster, New York.

LeDoux, J.E., Cicchetti, P., Xagoraris, A., and Romanski, L.M. (1990) The lateral amygdaloid nucleus: sensory interface of the amygdala in fear conditioning. *Journal of Neuroscience*, 10, 1062–1069.

Lee, G.P., Arena, J.G., Meador, K.J., Smith, J.R., Loring, D.W., and Flanigin, H.F. (1988) Changes in autonomic responsiveness following bilateral amygdalotomy in humans. *Neuropsychiatry, Neuropsychology, and Behavioral Neurology*, 1, 119–129.

Maquet, P., Peters, J.-M., Aerts, J., Delfiore, G., Degueldre, C., Luxen, A., and Franck, G. (1996) Functional neuroanatomy of human rapid-eye-movement sleep and dreaming. *Nature*, 383, 163–166.

McGaugh, J.L., Cahill, L., and Roozendaal, B. (1996) Involvement of the amygdala in memory storage: interaction with other brain systems. *Proceedings of the National Academy of Sciences of the United States of America*, 93, 13508–13514.

Morris, J.S., Frith, C.D., Perrett, D.I., Rowland, D., Young, A.W., Calder, A.J., and Dolan, R.J. (1996) A differential neural response in the human amygdala to fearful and happy facial expressions. *Nature*, 383, 812–815.

Morris, J.S., Friston, K.J., Buchel, C., Frith, C.D., Young, A.W., Calder, A.J., and Dolan, R.J. (1998a) A neuromodulatory role for the human amygdala in processing emotional facial expressions. *Brain*, 121, 47–57.

Morris, J.S., Oehman, A., and Dolan, R.J. (1998b) Conscious and unconscious emotional learning in the human amygdala. *Nature*, 393, 467–470.

Morris, J.S., Ohman, A., and Dolan, R.J. (1999) A subcortical pathway to the right amygdala mediating 'unseen' fear. *Proceedings of the National Academy of Sciences of the United States of America*, 96, 1680–1685.

Muramoto, K., Ono, T., Nishijo, H., and Fukuda, M. (1993) Rat amygdaloid neuron responses during auditory discrimination. *Neuroscience*, 52, 621–636.

Nishijo, H., Ono, T., and Nishino, H. (1988) Single neuron responses in amygdala of alert monkey during complex sensory stimulation with affective significance. *Journal of Neuroscience*, 8, 3570–3583.

Packard, M.G., Cahill, L., and McGaugh, J.L. (1994) Amygdala modulation of hippocampal-dependent and caudate nucleus-dependent memory processes. *Proceedings of the National Academy of Sciences of the United States of America*, 91, 8477–8481.

Phelps, E.A. and Anderson, A.K. (1997) What does the amygdala do? *Current Biology*, 7, R311–R314.

Phillips, M.L., Young, A.W., Senior, C., Brammer, M., Andrew, C., Calder, A.J., Bullmore, E.T., Perrett, D.I., Rowland, D., Williams, S.C.R., Gray, J.A., and David, A.S. (1997) A specific neural substrate for perceiving facial expressions of disgust. *Nature*, 389, 495–498.

Phillips, M.L., Young, A.W., Scott, S.K., Calder, A.J., Andrew, C., Giampietro, V., Williams, S.C.R., Bullmore, E.T., Brammer, M., and Gray, J.A. (1998) Neural responses to facial and vocal expressions of fear and disgust. *Proceedings of the Royal Society of London, Series B*, 265, 1809–1817.

Rempel-Clower, N.L., Zola, S.M., Squire, L.R., and Amaral, D.G. (1996) Three cases of enduring memory impairment after bilateral damage limited to the hippocampal formation. *Journal of Neuroscience*, 16, 5233–5255.

Russell, J.A. (1980) A circumplex model of affect. *Journal of Personality and Social Psychology*, 39, 1161–1178.

Russell, J.A., Weiss, A., and Mendelsohn, G.A. (1989) Affect grid: a single-item scale of pleasure and arousal. *Journal of Personality and Social Psychology*, 57, 493–502.

Saarni, C., Mumme, D.L., and Campos, J.J. (1997) Emotional development: action, communication, and understanding. In *Handbook of Child Psychology, Volume 3: Social Emotional, and Personality Development* (ed. W. Damon), pp. 237–309. John Wiley, New York.

Sawa, M. and Delgado, J.M.R. (1963) Amygdala unitary activity in the unrestrained cat. *Journal of Electroencephalography and Clinical Neurophysiology*, 15, 637–650.

Schoenbaum, G., Chiba, A.A., and Gallagher, M. (1998) Orbitofrontal cortex and basolateral amygdala encode expected outcomes during learning. *Nature Neuroscience*, 1, 155–159.

Schoenbaum, G., Chiba, A.A., and Gallagher, M. (1999) Neural encoding in orbitofrontal cortex and basolateral amygdala during olfactory discrimination learning. *Journal of Neuroscience*, 19, 1876–1884.

Scott, S.K., Young, A.W., Calder, A.J., Hellawell, D.J., Aggleton, J.P., and Johnson, M. (1997) Impaired auditory recognition of fear and anger following bilateral amygdala lesions. *Nature*, 385, 254–257.

Smith, C. and Lapp, L. (1991) Increases in number of REMs and REM density in humans following an intensive learning period. *Sleep*, 14, 325–330.

Stickgold, R. (1999) Sleep: off-line memory reprocessing. *Trends in Cognitive Sciences*, 2, 484–492.

Swanson, L.W. and Petrovich, G.D. (1998) What is the amygdala? *Trends in Neurosciences*, 21, 323–331.

Tranel, D. and Hyman, B.T. (1990) Neuropsychological correlates of bilateral amygdala damage. *Archives of Neurology*, 47, 349–355.

Ward, L.M. (1977) Multidimensional scaling of the molar physical environment. *Multivariate Behavioral Research*, 12, 23–42.

Weiskrantz, L. (1956) Behavioral changes associated with ablation of the amygdaloid complex in monkeys. *Journal of Comparative Physiology and Psychology*, 49, 381–391.

Whalen, P.J., Rauch, S.L., Etcoff, N.L., McInerney, S.C., Lee, M.B., and Jenike, M.A. (1998) Masked presentations of emotional facial expressions modulate amygdala activity without explicit knowledge. *Journal of Neuroscience*, 18, 411–418.

Young, A.W., Aggleton, J.P., Hellawell, D.J., Johnson, M., Broks, P., and Hanley, J.R. (1995) Face processing impairments after amygdalotomy. *Brain*, 118, 15–24.

Young, A.W., Hellawell, D.J., Van de Wal, C., and Johnson, M. (1996) Facial expression processing after amygdalotomy. *Neuropsychologia*, 34, 31–39.

Young, A.W., Rowland, D., Calder, A.J., Etcoff, N.L., Seth, A., and Perrett, D.I. (1997) Facial expression magamix: tests of dimensional and category accounts of emotion recognition. *Cognition*, 63, 271–313.

Zald, D.H. and Pardo, J.V. (1997) Emotion, olfaction, and the human amygdala: amygdala activation during aversive olfactory stimulation. *Proceedings of the National Academy of Sciences of the United States of America*, 94, 4119–4124.

Zald, D.H., Lee, J.T., Fluegel, K.W., and Pardo, J.V. (1998) Aversive gustatory stimulation activates limbic circuits in humans. *Brain*, 121, 1143–1154.

Zola-Morgan, S.M. and Squire, L.R. (1990) The primate hippocampal formation: evidence for a time-limited role in memory storage. *Science*, 250, 288–289.

19 Functional neuroimaging of the human amygdala during emotional processing and learning

Raymond J. Dolan

Wellcome Department of Cognitive Neurology, Queen Square, London WC1N 3BG, UK

Summary

The functions of the amygdala traditionally have been studied using animal models or reports on patients with focal lesions. Functional neuroimaging techniques, such as positron emission tomography (PET) and functional magnetic resonance imaging (fMRI), now provide non-invasive tools to study human amygdala function *in vivo*. This chapter provides an account of recent studies on human amygdala function using neuroimaging techniques where the prime focus will be fear processing. These studies highlight a key role for the amygdala during the perception of fear and in fear-related learning. Two striking observations emerge from these studies. First, activation of amygdala does not depend on conscious awareness of a fear-eliciting stimulus. Secondly, during fear learning, using classical Pavlovian conditioning, the amygdala's role would seem to be time limited.

19.1 Introduction

The role of the amygdala in human psychological function has been inferred principally from animal studies and neuropsychological descriptions in humans of the effects of amygdala lesions. With advances in neuroimaging, it is now possible to study human amygdala function in the intact human brain under controlled psychological conditions. Data from neuroimaging-based studies, using positron emission tomography (PET) and functional magnetic resonance imaging (fMRI), indicate involvement of the amygdala in a wide range of psychological tasks. The most compelling of these data relate to its role in perceptual processing of fear-related stimuli, particularly faces (Breiter *et al.*, 1996; Morris *et al.*, 1996). The present chapter, however, will consider the amygdala's involvement in emotional learning and memory as revealed by neuroimaging studies in my own, and others', laboratories. These data also serve to illustrate how functional neuroimaging has become a powerful investigative tool in unravelling the functional architecture of the human brain.

From a psychological perspective, learning and memory reflect the influence of prior experience. Memory is expressed through enhanced motor skill, perceptual fluency, or increased knowledge about the world available to conscious awareness. However, the type of memory that forms the basis of much of this chapter is that implemented by changes in expectations about whether sensory or cognitive events predict future reward or punishment. The type of learning associated with this predictive function is generally referred to as associative memory, and the best characterized, both psychologically and neurobiologically, is classical conditioning.

The majority of experiments under consideration in this chapter involve the use of standard classical conditioning paradigms. The experimental questions addressed involve characterizing changes in brain function as a consequence of associative learning. In standard classical conditioning paradigms, a sensory cue (referred to as the CS+) comes to predict reward or punishment (referred to as the unconditioned stimulus; US). For this type of learning to occur, the cue (conditioned stimulus; CS) consistently must precede the reward or punishment. An often mistaken assumption is that conditioning is primarily passive and reflex-like in operation. More complex cognitive models show this to be a mistaken view, and the critical component in conditioning is now assumed to be the predictive power of a CS (Holland, 1993).

The essential cognitive nature of conditioning is reinforced by observations that the ability of a CS to elicit a conditioned response (CR) depends upon establishing an association between the CS and a representation of the US. Key experiments that speak to this point include those demonstrating that altering the value of a US is reflected in spontaneous changes in conditioned responses to a previously paired CS+ when it is presented subsequently alone (Holland, 1990; Stanhope, 1992). Consequently, altering the value of a US representation outside the learning context, for example by repeated presentation of a shock but now at lower intensity than during conditioning, is reflected in spontaneous changes in elicited responses to the presentations of the CS+. The fact that responses to a CS are sensitive to the current value of the reinforcer that established learning can only be explained on the basis that the CS activates a central representation of the reinforcer.

The type of associative learning under consideration can occur without explicit awareness of the relationship between the CS and US. For example, patients with amnesia, with intact amygdala and damaged hippocampi, acquire reliable discriminatory skin conductance responses (SCRs) to a CS but cannot report which stimuli have been paired with the US (Fried *et al.*, 1997). Conversely, patients with amygdala damage fail to acquire conditioned SCRs to stimuli paired with an aversive US, despite intact declarative knowledge concerning the CS contingencies (Bechara *et al.*, 1995; LaBar, 1995). Psychophysical experiments in neurologically intact subjects show that discriminatory SCRs to aversively conditioned stimuli can occur when the eliciting stimulus (CS+) has been masked backwardly to prevent conscious awareness of its occurrence (Esteves *et al.*, 1994; Parra *et al.*, 1997).

19.2 The amygdala is sensitive to sensory stimuli that represent fear

Faces represent one of the most important sources of social information. Facial expressions of emotion provide one of the most critical signals through which internal emotional states and intentions of conspecifics become available as external signals. One of the most potent forms of facial expression is that of fear. Neuropsychological evidence has suggested that the amygdala is crucial to its recognition in faces (Adolphs *et al.*, 1995; Calder *et al.*, 1996). To address how facial emotional expressions of fear are processed in the intact brain, we carried out a functional neuroimaging experiment that compared neutral with either happy or fearful facial expressions. In our experimental design, we also introduced a parametric variation in the degree to which each class of emotion was expressed by a computer graphical manipulation (or morphing) of the faces (Perrett *et al.*, 1994). Comparing the neural response associated with processing fearful and happy expressions revealed activation of left amygdala and left periamygdaloid cortex specific to the fear condition (Morris *et al.*, 1996). Using a similar design, but without an intensity variation, this finding has been replicated by others (Breiter *et al.*, 1996). The introduction of an intensity variation, with respect to the intensity of expressed emotion, allowed us to determine brain regions conjointly responsive to emotion category (fearful versus happy) and expression intensity (low versus high). Strikingly, the neural responses in the left amygdala increased monotonically with increasing intensity of expression (Morris *et al.*, 1996). Thus, this experiment indicated that the amygdala was exquisitely sensitive to expressions of fear in human faces consistent with a role in modulating social interactions. In the light of this preliminary finding, and given an extensive literature on face processing *per se*, our subsequent studies have used this class of stimulus extensively.

19.3 The role of the amygdala in classical conditioning

An extensive animal literature has emphasized the role of the amygdala in the acquisition of fear conditioning behavioural responses (Le Doux, 1993). We were interested in the question of whether the amygdala was involved similarly in human associative learning. An immediate question in implementing a functional neuroimaging conditioning paradigm that addresses this issue is how to unconfound neural responses associated with a CS+ from neural responses evoked by a reward or punishment. Recall that in standard delay conditioning, the CS and US are presented, by necessity, in close temporal contiguity. Consequently, we used an event-related fMRI paradigm that enabled us to measure, on a trial-by-trial basis, responses to discrete stimulus events, in this case presentation of faces. Using a discriminative conditioning paradigm, where one set of stimuli predict the occurrence (CS+) and the other the absence (CS–) of an aversive (US) event (white noise 10% above threshold), our approach was to use a partial reinforcement strategy. Consequently, only half the face (CS+) presentations were paired with noise (Büchel *et al.*, 1998). This approach means that it is possible to separate neural responses elicited by distinct event types and directly compare evoked haemodynamic responses (an index of neural activity) elicited by a CS+ in the absence of noise with responses evoked by a CS– (faces never paired with noises and which serves as the control condition). In effect, there were three visual events, (i) CS–, (ii) CS+ paired, and (iii) CS+ unpaired, to be modelled in the data analysis. On-line SCRs were obtained simultaneously and provided independent evidence that learning took place.

The critical comparison of interest in the study was differential responses evoked by the CS+ compared with those evoked by the CS– acquired over the same time course. This comparison revealed greater activation in anterior cingulate gyrus and bilateral anterior insula specific to the CS+ condition. Note that this analysis involved a categorical comparison of the two event types (CS+ versus CS–) which assumes that learning-related neural responses do not vary as a function of time. Consequently, this analysis best characterizes time-invariant neural responses which are more likely to reflect neural events associated with the consequences of learning. Consequences of learning in this instance would include increased autonomic responses and preparatory motor activity. In this context, it is of interest that animal data strongly implicate the anterior cingulate in the expression of amygdala-dependent conditioned responses (Porembra and Gabriel, 1997).

As already indicated, the region where animal studies predict a primary involvement in associative learning is the amygdala. We failed to detect differential amygdala effects in a categorical comparison of evoked responses to CS+ and CS– stimuli. Animal studies and reports of direct intracranial recordings in human subjects have reported rapid adaptation in amygdala responses (Fried *et al.*, 1997; Quirk *et al.*, 1997). Consequently, we carried out an analysis that accounted for this type of time-dependent response profile. Specifically, we employed a statistical model that allows for adaptation over time, in effect modelling for a time by condition interaction. Testing for such effects revealed a highly robust differential response in bilateral amygdala, reproducible across all subjects, involving an early increase and subsequent decrease in response specific to processing the CS+ (see Figure 19.1).

The significant time by condition interaction suggests a time-limited role for the amygdala in associative learning. This finding speaks to a number of issues. Neurophysiological studies in animals have suggested a time-limited role for the amygdala during learning in so far as one of its main functional roles is neuromodulatory with respect to other brain systems (McGaugh *et al.*, 1996). Our data would accord entirely with such a model in so far as they suggest that neuromodulatory effects are manifest early and expressed in more stable patterns of activity in other brain regions. For example, the time-invariant response in the cingulate would accord with the notion that more stable associative learning effects are expressed in this brain region which might be critical in emotional expression (Porembra and Gabriel, 1997).

From a theoretical perspective, Pearce and Hall (1980) have proposed a distinction between two kinds of attentional processing of CSs during associative learning: automatic processing mediating conditioned responses and controlled 'attentional' processing which determines the extent of new learning (Pearce and Hall, 1980). Specifically, this model suggests that controlled attentional processing of a CS is reduced whenever that CS predicts its consequences. In early stages of learning, a CS can elicit considerable controlled processing because it is a relatively poor predictor of the US. As a consequence, early CS–US pairings result

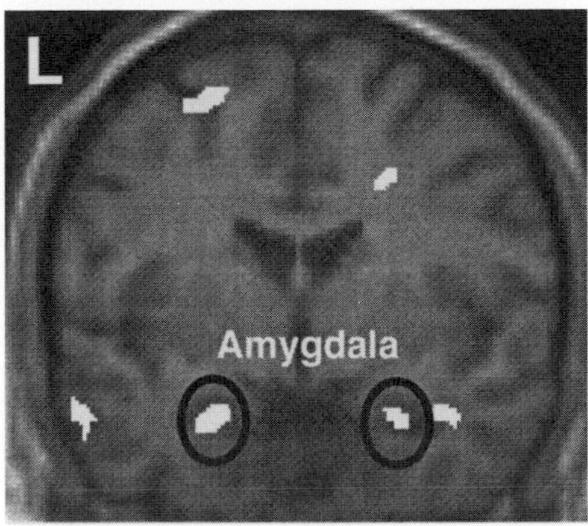

Figure 19.1 The effects of delay fear conditioning. (**A**) Left amygdala neural response to a CS+, as a function of time, during conditioning for an individual subject. Note that an early enhanced response attenuates with time and repeated presentation of CS+. (**B**) Bilateral amygdala responses in the same subject are depicted as regions of activation superimposed on the same individual's structural MRI scan. See also colour plate section.

in substantial learning. However, as learning is acquired, the CS is a better predictor of the US and, according to this model, it becomes less able to engender new learning. Extending this theoretical model to our physiological data, it is difficult to ignore a parallel with the time-limited role of the amygdala and the proposed temporally modulated 'attentional' processing of the CS associated with enhanced learning (see also Gallagher, Chapter 8). This theoretical proposal speaks to a consideration, outlined earlier, that during associative learning the amygdala initiates neurobiological changes that mediate learning, but these changes are expressed and consolidated elsewhere in the brain. More specifically, enhanced activation in cingulate to a CS+ may reflect rapid formation and maintenance of learnt stimulus–response associations.

19.4 Amygdala–hippocampal interactions during trace conditioning

In standard classical conditioning paradigms, there is temporal contiguity between presentation of the CS and US. A variant of classical conditioning is what is termed trace conditioning in which a temporal gap is introduced between the CS and US presentations. While the amygdala alone is sufficient for delay conditioning, there is evidence that in trace conditioning the hippocampus is crucial. Its putative role in this context involves bridging the temporal gap between the CS offset and onset of a US. For example, in trace eyeblink conditioning, animal and human studies indicate that the integrity of the hippocampus is crucial (McGlinchey-Berroth *et al.*, 1997; Clark and Squire, 1998).

We used an aversive trace-conditioning paradigm in conjunction with event-related fMRI to compare neural responses to a CS+ and CS–. The layout of the experiment was identical in all respects to the experiment described in the previous section. The CS stimuli again involved faces, and conditioning was implemented using a partial reinforcement schedule that allowed sampling of evoked responses to a CS+ that was not paired with the aversive noise US. Significant learning was again evident as indexed by differential SCRs to CS+ compared with CS– trials.

In this trace-conditioning paradigm, comparison of the CS+ and CS– conditions revealed significant differential augmented responses specific to the CS+ in bilateral anterior cingulate and anterior insulae. In view of our previous finding of time-dependent responses in the amygdala, we again tested explicitly for regions showing this type of response profile. In this analysis, the amygdala and anterior hippocampal regions both showed significant time by condition interactions for the CS+ relative to the CS– condition. The interaction for both regions reflected an adaptation in the neural response in the amygdala and anterior hippocampus to presentation of the CS+, relative to the CS–, as a function of time (see Figure 19.2).

The findings of this trace-conditioning study were identical to those of our previous classical conditioning study, using fMRI, except with respect to the involvement of the hippocampus. Note that a time-limited response to repeated stimulus presentation would not be detected when using blocked experimental designs as is always the case with PET. Thus, the striking finding in the present study is the identical temporal response profiles in the hippocampus and amygdala. This suggests that their functional roles may be similar. A time-limited role for the hippocampus has been shown previously during episodic learning (Strange *et al.*, 1999). Its functional role in the present context is likely to involve providing a mnemonic bridge in the temporal discontinuity between the CS+ and the US that is a prerequisite for associative learning (Eichenbaum and Otto, 1992).

19.5 The expression of conditioned responses

The previous section describes an experiment where learning took place in a context where subjects can clearly report the contingencies between the CS and US. Therefore, even though this type of associative learning frequently is assumed to be a manifestation of implicit memory, it is clear that in standard experimental paradigms process purity is unlikely. In other words, it is impossible to determine contributions to neural responses that represent implicit compared with explicit forms of memory. Associative learning can take place even when a subject's awareness of the contingencies between a CS and a US are non-existent, implying that implicit forms of memory are sufficient. In other words, associative learning, using delay conditioning paradigms, does not require awareness of stimulus contingencies. This provides a distinction from a closely associated form of learning, trace conditioning, where, in certain instances, such as eyeblink conditioning, explicit awareness of stimulus contingencies may be necessary (Clark and Squire, 1998). Two sorts of empirical data speak to the issue of associative learning without awareness in delay conditioning. First, patients with intact amygdala and damaged hippocampi, who are amnesic, acquire reliable

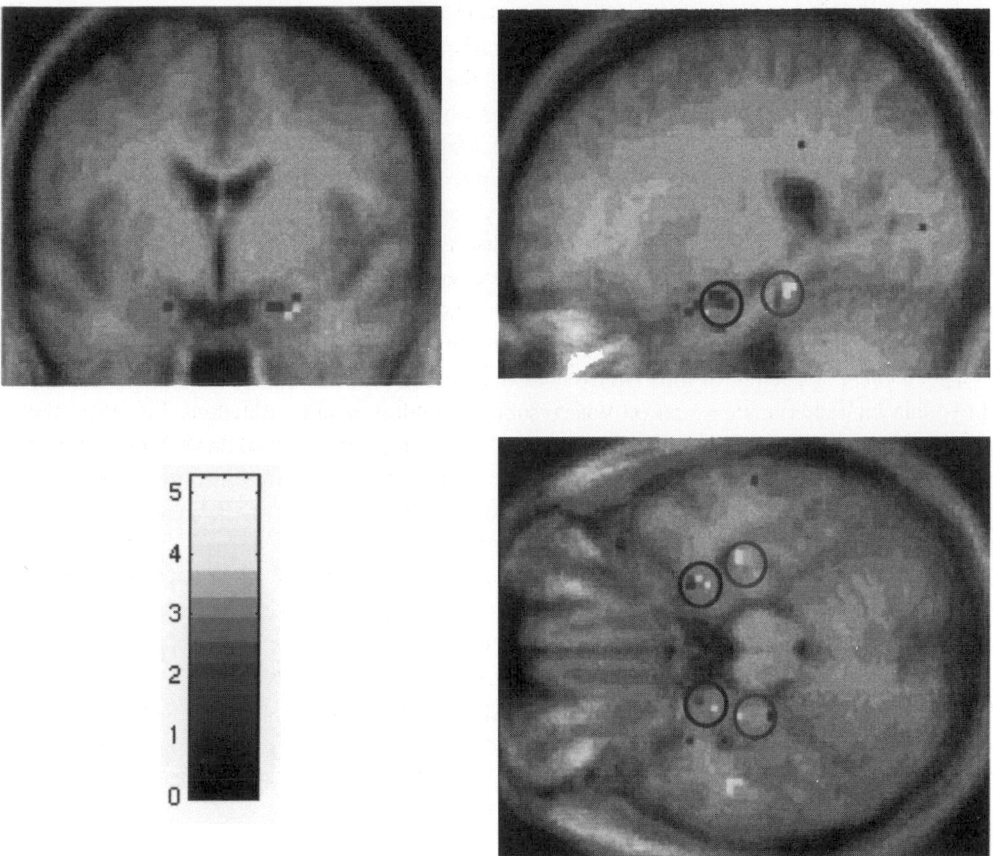

Figure 19.2 Amygdala–hippocampal neural responses during trace conditioning. The data are from an individual subject and illustrate regions where there is a significant time by condition interaction specific to CS+ presentation during conditioning. The coronal section shows a bilateral amygdala response as seen in delay conditioning. The transverse and sagittal sections show amygdala (blue circles) and hippocampus (red circles) in the same contrast. See also colour plate section.

discriminatory SCRs in delay conditioning paradigms (Bechara *et al.*, 1995; Fried *et al.*, 1997). Secondly, subjects make discriminatory SCRs to aversively conditioned stimuli that have been masked backwardly to prevent conscious awareness of their occurrence (Esteves *et al.*, 1994; Parra *et al.*, 1997).

To study mechanisms involved in the expression of associative learning, in the absence of awareness of stimulus contingencies, we used a backward masking paradigm. In brief, at study, we presented to volunteer subjects pictures of two angry faces (unmasked) one of which was paired (CS+), and the other unpaired (CS–), with a US consisting of a 100 dB white noise burst. The faces were then presented sequentially (for 30 ms) during scanning, without the US, while neural activity was measured by PET. Importantly, in half the presentations, subjects' awareness of occurrence of target faces (CS+ and CS–) was prevented by backward masking with neutral faces (presented for 45 ms; see Figure 19.3). In the remaining conditions, the CS+ and CS– effectively became the masks for presentation of neutral faces. The task requirement in all conditions was for subjects to report the occurrence of an angry face, however fleeting. The responses of the subjects in the explicit task indicated that they were unable to detect the target-masked angry faces. In the masked condition, 0% of the angry faces were reported, whereas the detection rate for unmasked angry faces was 100%. Mean SCRs were significantly greater for CS+ than CS– faces ($P < 0.001$), both for masked (mean CS+ SCR = 0.605 μS; mean CS– SCR = 0.473 μS) and unmasked (mean CS+ SCR = 0.748 μS; mean CS– SCR = 0.426 μS) presentations.

The critical question in this study was whether a differential neural response in the amygdala characterizes a situation where subjects cannot report awareness of target stimuli that previously had acquired behavioural value through associative learning. Contrasting neural responses associated with the masked CS+ and CS– conditions revealed a highly significant response in the right amygdala specific to presentation of the masked CS+ faces

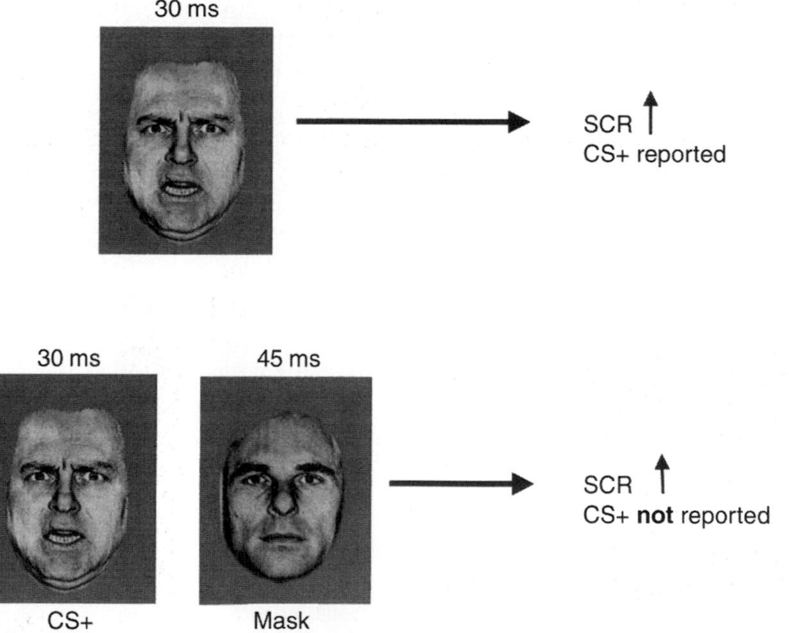

Figure 19.3 The masking paradigm used in the imaging analysis. A conditioned angry face presented alone for 30 ms is reportable by subjects and elicits an enhanced skin conductance response (SCR). When presented for the same duration but now immediatley followed by a neutral face (i.e. backwardly masked) presented for 45 ms only, the latter face is reportable. However, an enhanced SCR can still be elicited by the masked target face.

(see Figure 19.4). It is important to recall that the only difference between the CS+ and CS– conditions was the subjects' prior experience of an association between the CS+ faces and an aversive noise. Consequently, the neural response in the right amygdala must reflect engagement of a system that is critical in discriminating between stimuli on the basis of their associative behavioural significance. Interestingly, when we compared unmasked presentation of the CS+ and CS–, a significant differential enhanced neural response was observed in the left amygdala to the CS+.

These findings suggest that neural processing in the human amygdala is involved in the behavioural expression of previously learnt stimulus-relevant associations. This differential amygdala response during masked presentations, when subjects were unable to report the occurrence of the target stimuli, indicates that the amygdala can mediate consequences of associative learning in the absence of conscious (reportable) awareness of stimulus contingencies. These data extend functional neuroimaging findings that the amygdala can discriminate between salient, but categorically distinct, facial emotions (Whalen and Kapp, 1991). The data also provide a mechanistic account of behavioural observations that indicate unconscious processing of previously learnt aversive stimuli (Esteves *et al.*, 1994; Öhman and Soares, 1994; Parra *et al.*, 1997).

A common theme in both studies is the idea that the amygdala assigns emotional value or behavioural significance to sensory events. Cognitively, a stimulus that predicts future adversity can be construed as a danger signal. Activation of the amygdala in response to such a stimulus is likely to provide a mechanism by which autonomic and associative, including mnemonic, processes are triggered rapidly in order to ensure appropriate and rapid responses to danger. The survival value of this basic mechanism is self-evident. Thus, the role of the amygdala may be to act as a link between stimuli that predict future reward or punishment and stored representations of the relevant contingency (Adolphs *et al.*, 1995).

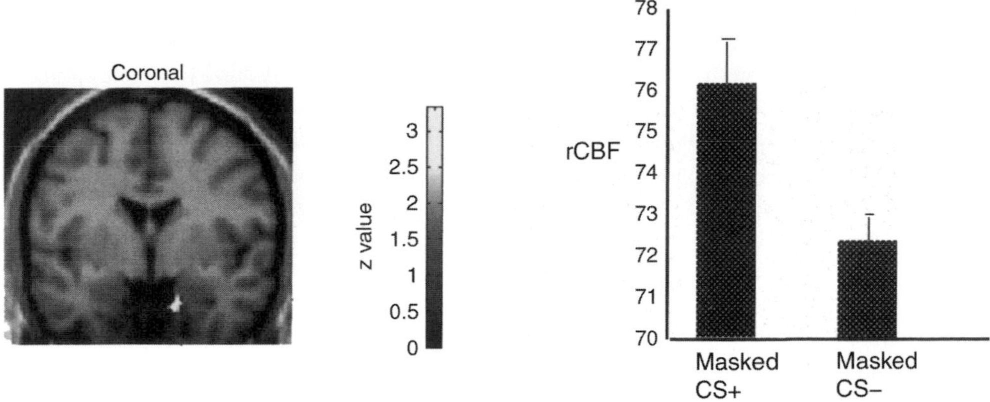

Figure 19.4 The left hand panel shows activation of the right amygdala superimposed on a coronal MRI image in a comparison of masked CS+ and masked CS– conditions. The right hand panel shows the adjusted regional cerebral blood flow (rCBF) responses in right amygdala for the same comparisons. See also colour plate section.

19.6 Cortical and subcortical interactions of the amygdala during the expression of learning

Animal data highlight the importance of the amygdala in fear processing and thalamoamygdala interactions in fear learning (LeDoux *et al.*, 1988, 1990; Campeau and Davis, 1995; LeDoux, 1995; LeBar and LeDoux, 1996). The amygdala receives a major visual input from the anterior temporal lobe and this is the most likely pathway through which visual CSs access the amygdala (Amaral *et al.*, 1992). This raises the question of what pathway mediates processing of masked or 'unseen' behaviourally relevant stimuli, as described in the previous section.

Single unit recording in monkeys has shown that transient responses in V1, normally occurring immediately after the offset of a target stimulus, are inhibited by masks that render the target invisible to human subjects (Macknik and Livingstone, 1988). These transient V1 afterdischarges appear to be a critical component of neural processes associated with conscious perception. The disruption of these responses by visual backward masking may provide, therefore, a temporary functional equivalent of the permanent loss of visual awareness seen with striate cortex lesions. Indeed, psychophysical experiments have demonstrated blindsight-like effects in healthy subjects using visual backward masking techniques (Meeres and Graves, 1990).

Studies of patients with lesions to striate cortex provide evidence for a parallel visual system in the brain associated with different levels of conscious visual awareness. Despite having no conscious perception of stimuli in their blind fields, patients with striate cortex lesions nevertheless can exhibit residual visual abilities or 'blindsight' by accurately 'guessing' the location of visual targets (Weiskrantz *et al.*, 1974). This has led to the suggestion that preserved abilities of these patients are mediated by a parallel 'secondary' visual pathway comprising the superior colliculus and pulvinar nucleus of the posterior thalamus (Zihl and von Crammon, 1979; Gross, 1991). We conjectured that, given the evidence of a pulvinar–amygdala projection in primates (Jones and Burton, 1976), the anatomical pathways that have been proposed as providing a second visual pathway in blindsight (i.e. superior colliculus and pulvinar) might also be implicated in processing masked conditioned ('unseen') stimuli. Animal models of auditory fear conditioning have proposed that a subcortical anatomical pathway involving the medial geniculate nucleus (MGN) and its projections to the lateral nucleus of the amygdala provide a rapid processing system for auditory CSs (LeDoux, 1996). In auditory fear conditioning paradigms, post-training lesions of the auditory cortex result in loss of an animal's ability for discriminatory conditioned responding though crude non-discriminatory responding is preserved (Jarrell *et al.*, 1987). This suggests that an intact subcortical input to the amygdala can provide a sufficient input for mediating components of associative learning. One caveat to this proposal is the lack of strong evidence for an MGN amygdala anatomical projection in primates.

To address the nature of the amygdala's functional interactions with cortical and subcortical regions, we extended the analysis of the neuroimaging data described in the previous section (Morris *et al.*, 1998b). The key question in this analysis related to whether the right amygdala showed a distinct pattern of interaction, with cortical or subcortical regions, under the context of processing masked conditioned stimuli compared with all other experimental conditions. This analysis is predicated on an assumption that brain regions constituting a functionally cooperative network should manifest context-specific patterns of covariance (Friston *et al.*, 1997). In agreement with our *a priori* prediction, regions in bilateral pulvinar and superior colliculus demonstrated positive co-variation with activity in the right amygdala during masked ('unseen') presentations of the CS+ faces (Morris *et al.*, 1998b) (see Figure 19.5).

These results provide support for a hypothesis that behaviourally relevant features of the visual environment may be detected and processed, without conscious awareness, by a subcortical colliculopulvinar–amygdala pathway that also controls reflexive and autonomic responses. Explicit detection of face stimuli involves specialized cortical processing areas, for example fusiform gyrus and temporal pole, regions associated with detailed analysis of the visual scene leading to object categorization (Dolan *et al.*, 1997). The backward masking employed in this study disrupts processing in these cortical pathways while leaving the subcortical pathway unaffected. Unlike the retinogeniculostriate pathway, which comprises relatively slowly conducting wavelength-sensitive neurons, the retinocollicular–pulvinar pathway is characterized by a rapidly conducting non-wavelength-sensitive transient response profile (Schiller and Malpeli, 1977). This response profile is in keeping with an idea that this pathway is suited to processing briefly presented visual stimuli and is less vulnerable to the influence of a backward mask. However, it needs to be born in mind that the context-dependent interactions that we noted may be a downstream effect from the amygdala itself reflecting the fact that the behaviourally relevant visual input through the cortical route is severely degraded due to masking.

19.7 The amygdala's contribution to experience-dependent sensory plasticity

One model of associative learning is auditory receptive field plasticity (Edeline and Weinberger, 1993). In this model, which describes the best characterized forms of physiological memory, there is a rapid and enduring learning-induced modification of receptive fields in primary auditory cortex. An outstanding question is whether similar plasticity is evident in the human brain and the degree to which it is dependent on functional interactions with the amygdala as suggested by animal models (Weinberger, 1995). We addressed both these questions in a discriminative conditioning paradigm where we presented subjects with auditory stimuli consisting of high- (8000 Hz) and low-frequency (200 Hz) pure tones.

Three different types of sequence presentation were employed: *non-conditioning*, during which only the pure tones were played; *unpaired* in which four 100 dB white noise bursts (1 s duration) were played midway between tones (equal frequency between low–high, high–low, high, and low consecutive tone pairs to ensure no differential conditioning to one frequency); and *conditioning*, in which four 100 dB white noise bursts were played immediately after the offset of tones of one frequency to produce discriminatory classical conditioning to either high (half the subjects) or low tones (the remaining subjects) in a 4:10 partial reinforcement schedule. The tone frequency paired with noise represented the conditioned stimulus (CS+); the tone frequency unpaired with noise was the CS–.

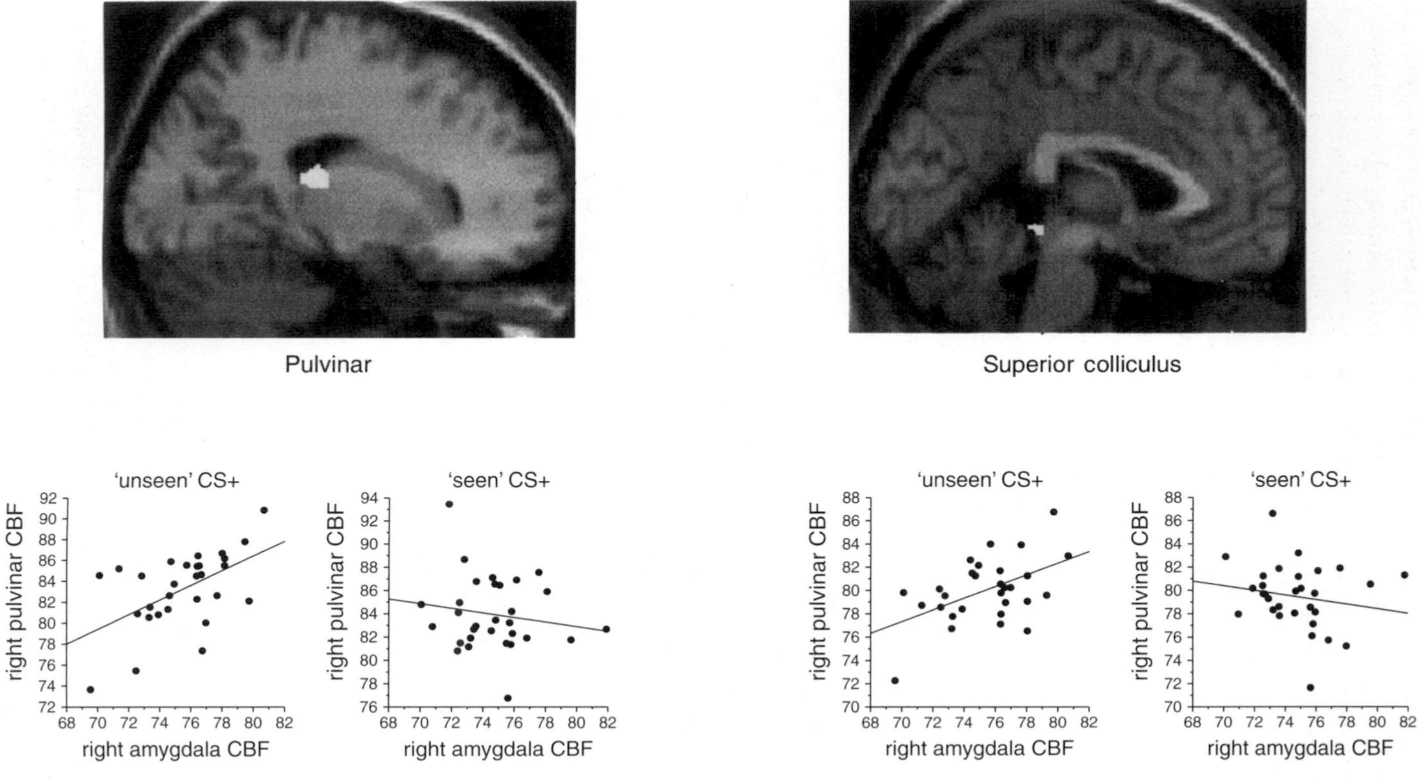

Figure 19.5 Regions which show significant covariance in response to activity in the right amygdala during masked CS+ compared with masked CS– presentations. The sagittal MRI sections illustrate activations in pulvinar and superior colliculus, respectively. The plots are regressions of right amygdala activity on pulvinar and superior colliculus activity for the same contrasts. See also colour plate section.

The primary interest of the experiment was whether there were adaptive changes in primary auditory cortex as a function of a tone predicting an aversive event. Consequently, we first identified auditory cortex regions that showed a tonotopic response to each of the two frequencies independently of conditioning (i.e. responses to 200 and 8000 Hz). Having identified tonotopic responsiveness in auditory cortex, the critical question remained whether these same regions showed frequency-specific modulation solely as a function of conditioning. As predicted by the animal model, both high and low response regions showed significant modulation involving decreases in the neural response to conditioned tones (CS+) (Weinberger, 1995). In other words, an association of low tones with the aversive noise attenuated the neural response of low-frequency-selective regions of auditory cortex. Responses to high-frequency tones were unaffected in this region (see Figure 19.6). Similarly, in the high-frequency-selective regions, conditioning-related decreases were seen in response to high tones with no change in response to low tones within these same regions (Morris *et al.*, 1998a).

The reversal of frequency selectivity in auditory cortex seen in this study is entirely consistent with experience-dependent receptive field plasticity in auditory cortex seen in a wide

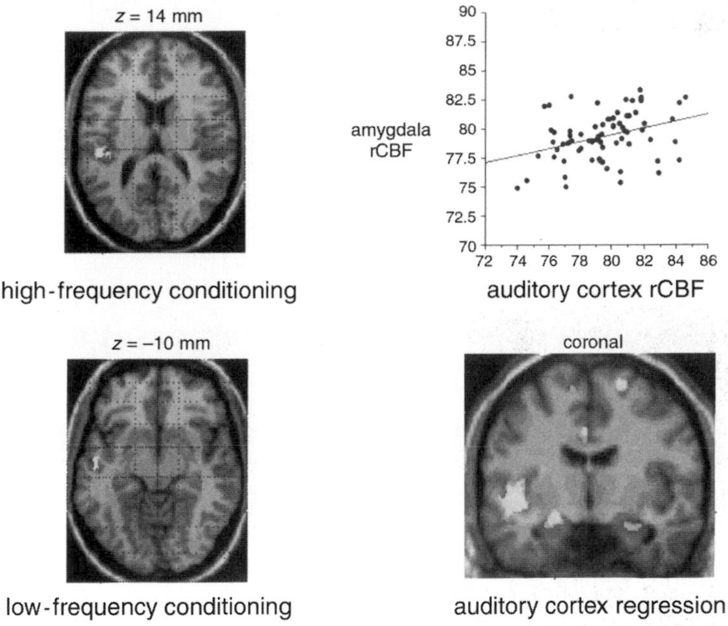

Figure 19.6 The left transverse slices through the brain illustrate auditory cortical regions which show learning-related modulation of responses as a function of conditioning to high- (left upper panel) and low- (left lower panel) frequency tones, respectively. The right lower panel shows bilateral amygdala regions which co-vary significantly in response with conditioning-related responses in auditory cortex. The plot (right upper panel) illustrates this significant co-variation in a positive regression of auditory cortex activity on activity in left amygdala. See also colour plate section.

range of animal species (Weinberger and Diamond, 1987; Edeline and Weinberger, 1992; Recanzone *et al.*, 1993; Scheich *et al.*, 1993). In two-tone discrimination learning, a small and narrowly tuned increase in the response of auditory cortex is seen for the CS+ frequency together with decreased responses to a broad range of surrounding frequencies (Edeline and Weinberger, 1992). The surprising frequency-specific attenuation of response to the CS+ tones that we observed may reflect activity of these intrinsic inhibitory processes. Frequency-specific augmented responses are likely to be spatially restricted and their effects will be masked by the greater extent of surround inhibition leading to a net decrease in activity within the limited spatial resolution of PET.

The outstanding question in these data is the degree to which experience-dependent plasticity is dependent on influences from the amygdala. Strong functional interactions with the amygdala can be predicted on the basis of an influential model of experience-dependent receptive field plasticity (Weinberger *et al.*, 1990). To test for functional interactions between auditory cortex and amygdala, we identified brain regions which positively co-varied in activity with conditioning-related activity in left auditory cortex. Strikingly, bilateral amygdala showed significant co-variation with auditory cortex in this analysis. This functional coupling is consistent with the idea that direct or indirect neuromodulatory influences from the amygdala are important in the expression of experience-dependent sensory plasticity. The amygdala sends direct projections to auditory cortex (Amaral and Price, 1984), though a critical pathway in mediating these plastic effects may be projections from the amygdala to the nucleus basalis of Meynert (NBM) (Roberts *et al.*, 1992). The NBM in turn projects to widespread cortical regions including auditory cortex (Bigl *et al.*, 1982). Stimulation of NBM, that coincides in time with presentation of a sensory stimulus, is itself sufficient to induce learning-related cortical plasticity (Kilgard and Merzenich, 1998).

19.8 Intra-amygdala differential neural responses during conditioning and representation of a US

As outlined, the type of learning expressed during classical conditioning is driven primarily by information concerning the reinforcer. Consequently, an important determinant of the associated behavioural response during first-order conditioning is the nature of the representation of the reinforcer. Little is known concerning how the US representation is instantiated in brain responses. Konorski has put forward a view that the representation encodes specific sensory features of processing the US (Konorski, 1967). In the experiments described up to this point, the US involved presentation of a loud aversive noise. Therefore, if accessing an auditory US representation involves reactivation of its sensory processing, then it follows that a visual CS+ should elicit a differential response, relative to a CS–, in auditory-related cortices.

To address whether accessing an auditory US representation, by a visual CS+, involves differential responses in auditory cortex, we presented volunteer subjects with a pseudo-random sequence of two angry target faces (CS+ and CS–). The explicit instruction to subjects was to index an occurrence, via a button press, of either of these two target faces. Half the presentations of the angry faces were masked backwardly using non-repeated neutral faces that prevented explicit awareness of these angry face targets or their association with the US noise. The masked CS+ face was always followed by an aversive 100 dB noise. The unmasked CS+, as well as both masked and unmasked CS– faces were never paired with noise. Subjects' SCRs were measured throughout the experiment. The unmasked CS+ and CS– conditions were identical, therefore, except for the association, albeit a masked association, between the CS+ and noise. Subjects' button press responses revealed that they failed to detect the masked target faces. However, significant differences in SCRs and reaction times were present between the CS+ and CS– conditions, revealing that visual–auditory associative learning occurred despite the lack of awareness of the CS+ and noise pairing. Thus, the learning that is taking place is primarily implicit in so far as subjects are unaware of the contingencies between the CS and the US.

Increased neural activity during unmasked CS+ presentations (relative to CS–) was observed in left basomedial amygdala, right pulvinar, superior colliculus, and right extrastriate cortex. Decreased responses to unmasked CS+ (relative to CS–) faces were seen in left anterosuperior amygdala. The segregated amygdala responses we observed are in keeping with considerable evidence that distinct subnuclei of the amygdala play specific roles during conditioning (Killcross *et al.*, 1997). Visual, auditory, and somatosensory information is conveyed to the lateral nucleus of the amygdala through segregated, modality-specific cortical cascades (McDonald and Jackson, 1987; McDonald, 1998). Polysensory and mnemonic inputs from parahippocampal, temporal polar, and prefrontal cortices terminate in basal, accessory basal, and superficial amygdala nuclei. However, extensive intra-amygdala connections are thought to be crucial in the establishment of stimulus–reinforcement associations (Collins and Pare, 1999). The profile of intra-amygdala differential responses we observed may reflect these latter processes.

The most surprising finding was a differential responses to presentation of a visual CS+, relative to the visual CS–, in left auditory cortex and left medial geniculate. In simple terms, there was a significant deactivation to a visual CS+, relative to CS–, in regions involved in early auditory processing. Note that the only auditory stimulus in this experiment was the noise US, and presentation of the CS+ was unpaired. Theoretically, this response is of considerable importance in two respects. First, the fact that we observed an auditory response to a visual stimulus can be interpreted as evidence that the unmasked CS+ reactivates perceptual processing of aspects of the US. Secondly, the data also indicate that CS+-elicited differential auditory cortex responses might also represent information in the temporal domain. Specifically, it may encode the time of occurrence of the US. In other words, the modulation of the auditory cortex may occur at a time when the US might be anticipated, as has been seen in single unit recording studies (Armony *et al.*, 1998).

19.9 Is the amygdala involved in episodic memory function?

An extensive functional neuroimaging literature has provided detailed descriptions of brain regions involved in encoding and retrieving emotionally neutral episodic memories (Cabeza and Nyberg, 1997). It is generally accepted that there is enhanced learning for events with strong emotional valence (Bower, 1992) and preferential recall for emotionally laden autobiographical events (Holmes, 1970; Brewer, 1988).These observations raise the issue of whether distinct memory-related brain systems are engaged when the content of memory is emotional (see also McGaugh *et al.*, Chapter 11; Cahill, Chapter 12; Adolphs and Tranel, Chapter 18).

The probable involvement of the amygdala in mediating emotional memory is suggested by a number of lines of evidence. For example, there is an extensive animal literature that associates the amygdala with consolidation of emotional long-term memories (McGaugh *et al.*, 1992; Cahill and McGaugh, 1998). Neuropsychological studies of patients with bilateral amygdala damage, indicating impaired recall for emotional material, as well as data showing preservation of the enhanced recall for emotional material in amnesics, have likewise been interpreted as supporting an encoding deficit (Babinsky *et al.*, 1993; Markowitsch *et al.*, 1994; Hamann *et al.*, 1997).

Functional neuroimaging studies have provided evidence for an amygdala contribution to episodic memory encoding. Enhanced free recall for emotional, relative to neutral, film clips is significantly correlated with an index of increased right amygdala activity at encoding (Cahill *et al.*, 1996). It has also been demonstrated that amygdala activity at encoding is correlated with enhanced episodic recognition memory for emotional material, pleasant or unpleasant, but not for recognition of emotionally neutral material (Hamann *et al.*, 1999). Thus, while there is compelling evidence for an amygdala role during encoding of emotional material, we were interested in whether the amygdala might also be involved during retrieval.

To address this question, we chose to study items comprising visual images of objects or scenes drawn from the International Affective Pictorial System (IAPS) (Lang *et al.*, 1995). This consists of an extensive library of images standardized with respect to emotional valence and arousal (Lang *et al.*, 1995). We chose items from two discrete valence categories, reflecting either neutral or emotional content. The emotional content pictures consisted of either positively or negatively valenced (i.e. pleasant or unpleasant) items. Twelve study sets were constructed containing lists of 20 items, and for each of these study lists a corresponding test list was constructed. These test lists varied with respect to the number of study items they contained (high target density = 80% targets; low target density = 0% targets).

Five minutes prior to each scanning, subjects were shown a study set of pictures consisting of either emotional or neutral items. The task requirement was to make a valence rating, on a nine-point scale, for each of the pictures. The psychological task at test involved either a visual recognition or judgement task. During scanning, subjects were presented with test lists, some of which they had seen previously at study. As already outlined, the proportion of study list items contained in these test lists varied from either 85 or 0%, constituting high and low target conditions, respectively. This manipulation of target density was crossed with valence (emotional or neutral conditions) and with task (recognition or judgement condition). In the memory recognition task, subjects responded with a yes/no response to indicate whether they had seen each individual item at study. In the judgement task, subjects made an outdoor/indoor judgement.

Our experimental approach involved comparing conditions where the valence of pictorial material (emotional versus neutral), task requirement (recognition memory or judgement task), and density of target items (high versus low) were manipulated experimentally. In essence, our design involved three factors (task, valence, and target density) each with two levels. As this design involved presentation of old and new items at test (corresponding to high and low target density conditions), it is important to control for mere effects, such as increased arousal, elicited by on-line processing of targets and foils particularly during emotional recognition. This issue is addressed by the judgement condition, where valence and target density were varied in a manner identical to the memory conditions.

We assessed the influence of emotional item target density on retrieval-related activations from the three-way interaction in the factorial design. Specifically, we examined the influence of target density on the differences between emotional and neutral conditions in a comparison of memory and judgement conditions. The only significant effect was an activation in left amygdala extending into the left uncus. The specificity of this amygdala response was also established by a contrast restricted to the memory conditions alone involving a comparison of target density (high versus low) for emotional compared with neutral memory conditions. Again, the only significant effect was in the left amygdala. Furthermore, this effect was independent of the valence of the retrieved material (i.e. there was no interaction in left amygdala as a function of whether the retrieved material was pleasant or unpleasant). Finally, testing the simple main effect of high versus low target density for emotional items alone showed that the amygdala response remained significant. Thus, the response profile in the amygdala indexed actual retrieval of emotional items.

A well-established view links the amygdala to effects on emotional memory encoding. For example, an extensive animal literature associates the amygdala with consolidation of emotional long-term memories (McGaugh *et al.*, 1992; Cahill and McGaugh, 1998). Neuropsychological studies of patients with bilateral amygdala damage, indicating impaired recall for emotional material, as well as data showing preservation of the enhanced recall for emotional material in amnesics, have likewise been interpreted as supporting an encoding deficit (Babinsky *et al.*, 1993; Markowitsch *et al.*, 1994; Hamann *et al.*, 1997). While these latter data are compatible with an amygdala influence at encoding, it is important to bear in mind that encoding or retrieval deficits are difficult to distinguish on the basis of neuropsychological data alone. In this regard, our neuroimaging data are not compatible with an exclusive role for the amygdala at encoding.

The critical question arising out of these findings is what functional role does the amygdala fulfil in emotional memory retrieval? First, the relationship between target density and amygdala activation at retrieval does not easily accord with a time-limited modulatory role that characterizes the amygdala response during emotional learning. Secondly, recent neuropsychological data on patients with amygdala damage highlight deficits in social judgements in response to faces, indicating that the amygdala is required for retrieval of components of social knowledge in response to visual stimuli (Adolphs *et al.*, 1998). This social knowledge may well be evaluative in nature and we note that this idea is implicit in an early conceptualization of amygdala function as attaching emotional significance to sensory stimuli (Weiskrantz, 1956). Our memory data are broadly compatible with this formulation, with the added caveat that eliciting stimuli include not only sensory events but also memories. In this light, we suggest that a model for the functional role of the amygdala during memory retrieval is automatically to index retrieved memories with representations of their past behavioural significance.

19.10 Conclusions

This chapter has focused on the contribution of functional neuroimaging in furthering our understanding of the human amygdala. Rather than provide an exhaustive listing of studies which have described amygdala activation, the emphasis has been on its role in mediating components of fear-related behavioural responses. The data emphasize a role for the amygdala in (i) the acquisition and expression of conditioned fear responses, (ii) the expression of experience-dependent receptive field plasticity, and (iii) both encoding and retrieval of episodic emotional memories. Future directions for neuroimaging approaches to the study of the functions of the human amygdala are likely to capitalize on enhanced spatial resolution enabling the attribution of condition-specific activations to distinct amygdala nuclei. In parallel, the exploitation of techniques that can characterize functional interactions in the human brain will allow better characterization of dynamic intra-amygdala and amygdala cortical and subcortical interactions associated with learning.

References

Adolphs, R., Tranel, D., Damasio, H., and Damasio, A.R. (1995) Fear and the human amygdala. *Journal of Neuroscience*, 15, 5879–5891.

Adolphs, R., Tranel, D., and Damasio, A.R. (1998) The human amygdala in social judgment. *Nature*, 1998, 393, 470–474.

Amaral, D.G. and Price, J.L. (1984) Amygdalo-cortical projections in the monkey (*Macaca fascicularis*). *Journal of Comparative Neurology*, 230, 465–496.

Amaral, D., Price, J.L., Pitkanen, A., and Carmichael, S.T. (1992) Anatomical organization of the primate amygdaloid complex. In *The Amygdala: Neurobiological Aspects of Emotion, Memory, and Mental Dysfunction* (ed. J.P. Aggleton), pp. 1–66. Wiley-Liss, New York.

Armony, J.L., Quirk, G.J., and LeDoux, J.E. (1998) Differential effects of amygdala lesions on early and late plastic components of auditory cortex spike trains during fear conditioning. *Journal of Neuroscience*, 18, 2592–2601.

Babinsky, R., Calabrese, P., Durwen, H.F., Markowitsch, H.J., Brechtelsbauer, D., Heuser, L., and Gehlen, W. (1993) The possible contribution of the amygdala to memory. *Behavioural Neurology*, 6, 167–170.

Bechara, A., Tranel, D., Damasio, H., Adolphs, R., Rockland, C., and Damasio, A.R. (1995) Double dissociation of conditioning and declarative knowledge relative to the amygdala and hippocampus in humans. *Science*, 269, 1115–1118.

Bigl, V., Woolf, N.J., and Butcher, L.L. (1982) Cholinergic projections from the basal forebrain to frontal, parietal, temporal, occipital, and cingulate cortices: a combined fluorescent tracer and acetylcholinesterase analysis. *Brain Research Bulletin*, 8, 727–749.

Bower, G.H. (1992) How might emotions affect learning. In *The Handbook of Emotion and Memory: Research and Theory* (ed. S.A. Christianson), pp. 3–31 Lawrence Erlbaum Associates, Hilsdale, New Jersey.

Breiter, H.C., Ectoff, N.L., Whalen, P.J., Kennedy, D.N., Rauch, S.L., Buckner, R.L., Strauss, M.M., Hyman, S.E., and Rosen, B.R. (1996) Response and habituation of the human amygdala during visual processing of facial expression. *Neuron,* 2, 875–887.

Brewer, G.H. (1988) Memory for randomly sampled autobiographical events. In *Remembering Reconsidered: Ecological and Traditional Approaches to the Study of Memory* (eds U. Neisser and E. Winograd), pp. 21–90 Cambridge University Press, New York.

Büchel, C., Morris, J., Dolan, R.J., and Friston, K.J. (1998) Brain systems mediating aversive conditioning: an event related fMRI study. *Neuron*, 20, 947–957.

Cabeza, R. and Nyberg, L. (1997) Imaging cognition: an empirical review of PET studies with normal subjects. *Journal of Cognitive Neuroscience*, 9, 1–26.

Cahill, L. and McGaugh, J.L. (1998) Mechanisms of emotional arousal and lasting declarative memory. *Trends in Neuroscience*, 21, 294–299.

Cahill, L., Haier, R.J., Fallon, J., Alkire, M.T., Tang, C., Keator, D., Wu, J., and McGaugh, J.L. (1996) Amygdala activity at encoding correlated with long-term, free recall of emotional information. *Proceedings of the National Academy of Sciences of the United States of America*, 93, 8016–8021.

Calder, A.J., Young, A.W., Rowland, D., Perrett, D.I., Hodges, J.R., and Etcoff, N.L. (1996) Facial emotion recognition after bilateral amygdala damage: differentially severe impairment of fear. *Cognitive Neuropsychology*, 13, 699–745.

Campeau, S. and Davis, M. (1995) Involvement of subcortical and cortical afferents to the lateral nucleus of the amygdala in fear conditioning measured with fear potentiated startle in rats trained concurrently with auditory and visual conditioned stimuli. *Journal of Neuroscience*, 15, 2301–2311.

Clark, R.E. and Squire, L.R. (1998) Classical conditioning and brain systems: the role of awareness. *Science*, 280, 77–81.

Collins, D.R. and Pare, D. (1999) Reciprocal changes in firing probability of lateral and central medial amygdala neurons. *Journal of Neuroscience*, 19, 836–844.

Dolan, R.J., Fink, G.R., Rolls, E., Booth, M., Holmes, A., Frackowiak, R.S.J., and Friston, K.J. (1997) How the brain learns to see objects and faces in an impoverished context. *Nature*, 389, 596–599.

Edeline, J.-M. and Weinberger, N.M. (1992) Associative retuning in the thalamic source of input to the amygdala and auditory cortex: receptive field plasticity in the medial division of the medial geniculate body. *Behavioral Neuroscience*, 106, 81–105.

Edeline, J.-M. and Weinberger, N.M. (1993) Receptive field plasticity in the auditory cortex during frequency discrimination training: selective retuning independent of task difficulty. *Behavioral Neuroscience*, 107, 82–103.

Eichenbaum, H. and Otto, T. (1992) The hippocampus—what does it do? *Behavioral and Neural Biology*, 57, 2–36.

Esteves, F., Dimberg, U., and Öhman, A. (1994) Automatically elicited fear: conditioned skin conductance responses to masked facial expressions. *Cognition and Emotion*, 9, 99–108.

Fried, I., Macdonald, K.A., and Wilson, C.L. (1997) Single neuron activity in hippocampus and amygdala during recognition of faces and objects. *Neuron*, 18, 875–887.

Friston, K.J., Büchel, C., Fink, G., Morris, J.S., Rolls, E.T., and Dolan, R.J. (1997) Psychophysiological and modulatory interactions in neuroimaging. *Neuroimage*, 6, 218–229.

Gross, C.G. (1991) Contribution of striate cortex and the superior colliculus to visual function in area MT, the superior temporal polysensory area and the inferior temporal cortex. *Neuropsychologia*, 29, 497–515.

Hamann, S.B., Cahill, L., and Squire, L.R. (1997) Emotional perception and memory in amnesia. *Neuropsychology*, 11, 104–113.

Hamann, S.B., Ely, T.D., Grafton, S.T., and Kilts, C.D. (1999) Amygdala activity related to enhanced memory for pleasant and aversive stimuli. *Nature Neuroscience*, 2, 289–293.

Holland, P.C. (1990) Event representation in pavlovian conditioning: image and action. *Cognition*, 37, 105–131.

Holland, P.C. (1993) Cognitive aspects of classical conditioning. *Current Biology*, 3, 230–236.

Holmes, D. (1970) Differential change in affective intensity and the forgetting of unpleasant experiences. *Journal of Personality and Social Psychology*, 15, 234–239.

Jarrell, T.W., Gentile, C.G., Romanski, L.M., McCabe, P.M., and Schneiderman, N. (1987) Involvement of cortical and thalamic auditory regions in retention of differential conditioning to acoustic conditioned stimuli in rabbits. *Brain Research*, 412, 285–294.

Jones, E.G. and Burton, H. (1976) A projection from the medial pulvinar to the amygdala in primates. *Brain Research*, 104, 142–147.

Kilgard, M.P. and Merzenich, M.M. (1998) Cortical map reorganisation enabled by nucleus basalis activity. *Science*, 279, 1714–1718.

Killcross, S., Robbins, T.W., and Everitt, B.J. (1997) Different types of fear-conditioned behaviour mediated by separate nuclei within amygdala. *Nature*, 388, 377–380.

Konorski, J. (1967) *Integrative Activity of the Brain. An Interdisciplinary Approach.* University of Chicago Press, Chicago.

LaBar, K.S. and LeDoux, J.E. (1996) Partial disruption of fear conditioning in rats with unilateral amygdala damage—correspondence with unilateral temporal lobe damage in humans. *Behavioral Neuroscience*, 110, 991–997.

LaBar, K.S., LeDoux, J.E., Spencer, D.D., and Phelps, E.A. (1995) Impaired fear conditioning following unilateral temporal lobectomy. *Journal of Neuroscience*, 15, 6846–6855.

Lang, P.J., Bradley, M.M., and Cuthbert, B.N. (1995) *The International Affective Picture System (IAPS): Photographic Slides*. University of Florida, Gainesville.

LeDoux, J.E. (1993) Emotional memory systems in the brain. *Behaviour and Brain Research*, 58, 69–79.

LeDoux, J.E. (1995) In search of an emotional system in the brain: leaping from fear to emotion and consciousness. In *The Cognitive Neurosciences* (ed. M. Gazzaniga), pp. 1049–1061. MIT Press, Cambridge, Massachusetts.

LeDoux, J. (1996) *The Emotional Brain*. Simon and Schuster, New York.

LeDoux, J.E, Cicchetti, P., Xagoraris, A., and Romanski, L.M. (1990) The lateral amygdaloid nucleus: sensory interface of the amygdala in fear conditioning. *Journal of Neuroscience*, 10, 1062–1069.

LeDoux, J.E., Iwata, J., Cicchetti, P., and Reis, D. (1988) Differential projections of the central amygdaloid nucleus mediate autonomic and behavioural correlates of conditioned fear. *Journal of Neuroscience*, 8, 2517–2529.

Macknik, S.L. and Livingstone, M.S. (1998) Neuronal correlates of visibility and invisibility in the primate visual system. *Nature Neuroscience*, 1, 144–149.

Markowitsch, H.J., Calabrese, P., Wurker, M., Durwen, H.F., Kessler, J., Babinsky, R., Brechtelsbauer, D., Heuser, L., and Gehlen, W. (1994) The amygdala's contribution to memory—a study on two patients with Urbach–Wiethe disease. *NeuroReport*, 5, 1349–1352.

McDonald, A.J. (1998) Cortical pathways to the mammalian amygdala. *Progress in Neurobiology*, 55, 257–332.

McDonald, A.J. and Jackson, T.R. (1987) Amygdaloid connections with posterior and temporal cortical areas in the rat. *Journal of Comparative Neurology*, 262, 59–77.

McGaugh, J.L., Introini-Collison, I.B., Cahill, L., Kim, M., and Liang, K.C. (1992) Involvement of the amygdala in neuromodulatory influences on memory storage. In *The Amygdala: Neurobiological Aspects of Emotion, Memory, and Mental Dysfunction* (ed. J.P. Aggleton), pp. 143–167. Wiley-Liss, New York.

McGaugh, J.L., Cahill, L., and Roozendaal, B. (1996) Involvement of the amygdala in memory stroage: interaction with other brain systems. *Proceedings of the National Academy of Sciences of the United States of America*, 93, 13508–13514.

McGlinchey-Berroth, R., Carrillo, M.C., Gabrieli, J.D., Brawn, C.M., and Disterhoft, J.F. (1997) Impaired trace eyeblink conditioning in bilateral, medial-temporal lobe amnesia. *Behavioral Neuroscience*, 111, 873–882.

Meeres, S.L. and Graves, R.E. (1990) Localization of unseen visual stimuli by humans with normal vision. *Neuropsychologia*, 28, 1231–1237.

Morris, J., Frith, C.D., Perrett, D., Rowland, D., Young, A.W., Calder, A.J., and Dolan, R.J. (1996) A differential neural response in the human amygdala to fearful and happy facial expressions. *Nature*, 383, 812–815.

Morris, J.S., Friston, K.J., and Dolan, R.J. (1998a) Experience-dependent modulation of tonotopic neural responses in human auditory cortex. *Proceedings of the Royal Society of London, Series B*, 265, 649–657.

Morris, J.S., Ohman, A., and Dolan, R.J. (1998b) Conscious and unconscious emotional learning in the human amygdala. *Nature*, 393, 467–470.

Morris, J., Ohman, A. and Dolan, R.J. (1999) A subcortical pathway to the right amygdala mediating 'unseen' fear. *Proceedings of the National Academy of Sciences of the United States of America*, 96, 1680–1685.

Öhman, A. and Soares, J.F. (1994) 'Unconscious anxiety': phobic responses to masked stimuli. *Journal of Abnormal Psychology*, 103, 231–240.

Parra, C., Esteves, F., Flykt, A., and Öhman, A. (1997) Pavlovian conditioning to social stimuli: backward masking and dissociation of implicit and explicit cognitive processes. *European Psychology*, 2, 106–117.

Pearce, J.M. and Hall, G. (1980) A model for Pavlovian learning: variations in the effectiveness of conditioned but not of unconditioned stimuli. *Psychological Review*, 82, 532–552.

Perrett, D., May, K.A., and Yoshikawa, S. (1994) Female shape and judgements of female attractiveness. *Nature*, 368, 239–242.

Poremba, A. and Gabriel, M. (1997) Amygdalar lesions block discriminative avoidance and cingulothalamic training-induced neuronal plasticity in rabbits. *Journal of Neuroscience*, 17, 5237–5244.

Quirk, G.J., Armony, J.L., and LeDoux, J.E. (1997) Fear conditioning enhances different temporal components of tone-evoked spike trains in auditory cortex and lateral amygdala. *Neuron*, 19, 613–624.

Recanzone, G.H., Schreiner, C.E., and Merzenich, M.M. (1993) Plasticity in the frequency representation of primary auditory cortex following discrimination training in adult owl monkeys. *Journal of Neuroscience*, 13, 87–103.

Roberts, A.C., Robbins, T.W., Everitt, B.J., and Muir, J.L. (1992) A specific form of cognitive rigidity following excitotoxic lesions of the basal forebrain in marmosets. *Neuroscience*, 47, 251–264.

Scheich, H., Simonis, C., Ohl, F., Tillein, J., and Thomas, H. (1993) Functional organization and learning-related plasticity in auditory cortex of the Mongolian gerbil. *Progress in Brain Research*, 97, 135–143.

Schiller, P.H. and Malpeli, J.G. (1977) Properties and tectal projections of monkey retinal ganglion cells. *Journal of Neurophysiology*, 40, 428–445.

Stanhope, K.J. (1992) The representation of the reinforcer and force of the pigeon's keypeck in first- and second-order conditioning. *Quarterly Journal of Experimental Psychology*, 44B, 137–158.

Strange, B.A., Fletcher, P.C., Henson, R.N., Friston, K.J., and Dolan, R.J. (1999) Segregating the functions of human hippocampus *Proceedings of the National Academy of Sciences of the United States of America*, 96, 4034–4039.

Weinberger, N.M. (1995) Retuning the brain by fear conditioning. In *The Cognitive Neurosciences* (ed. M. Gazzaniga), pp. 1071–1090. MIT Press, Cambridge, Massachusetts.

Weinberger, N.M. and Diamond, D.M. (1987) Physiological plasticity of single neurones in auditory cortex: rapid induction by learning. *Progress in Neurobiology*, 29, 1–55.

Weinberger, N.M., Ashe, J.H., Metherate, R., McKenna, T.M., Diamond, D.M., and Bakin, J.S. (1990) Retuning auditory cortex by learning: a preliminary model of receptive field plasticity. *Concepts in Neuroscience*, 1, 91–132.

Weiskrantz, L. (1956) Behavioural changes associated with ablation of the amygdaloid complex in monkeys. *Journal of Comparative Physiology and Psychology*, 49, 381–391.

Weiskrantz, L., Warrington, E.K., Sanders, M.D., and Marshall, J. (1974) Visual capacity in the hemianopic field following a restricted occipital ablation. *Brain*, 97, 709–728.

Whalen, P.J. and Kapp, B.S. (1991) Contributions of the amygdaloid central nucleus to the modulation of the nictitating membrane reflex in the rabbit. *Behavioral Neuroscience*, 104, 141–153.

Zihl, J. and von Crammon, D. (1979) The contribution of the 'second' visual system to directed visual attention in man. *Brain*, 102, 835–856.

20 The amygdala and Alzheimer's disease

Tiffany W. Chow and Jeffrey L. Cummings

UCLA School of Medicine, 710 Westwood Plaza, Los Angeles, CA 90095-1769, USA

Summary

The amygdala is affected whenever neurodegenerative disorders involve the temporal lobes. Alzheimer's disease is the most common dementia involving the amygdala. Symptoms of amygdalar dysfunction usually manifest as components of the Klüver–Bucy syndrome: visual agnosia, hyperorality, hypermetamorphosis, blunting of fear or rage, and hypersexuality. Despite the pathological changes seen in the amygdala due to Alzheimer's disease, patients rarely present with a Klüver–Bucy syndrome. Similar pathology in frontal and temporal cortices may prohibit these abnormal behaviors from emerging.

20.1 Introduction

Alzheimer's disease (AD) is the most common cause of dementia in the elderly, rendering patients dysfunctional due to multifaceted cognitive impairments. The typical clinical presentation of AD begins with insidious onset of a gradually progressive memory loss. Patients remain indifferent to their cognitive impairment, which eventually includes difficulty with language, visuospatial orientation, calculations, planning and organization, and reasoning. Many patients with AD manifest neuropsychiatric symptoms such as apathy, delusions, anxiety, changes in eating habits, purposeless repetitive behaviours, and autonomic changes. Neurological symptoms of AD may include anosmia, Parkinsonism, and myoclonus late in the course of the illness. The symptoms of AD reflect diffuse involvement of cortical regions and the limbic system.

Pathological hallmarks of AD include neurofibrillary tangles (NFTs) and extracellular plaques. Formerly referred to as senile plaques, these collections of amyloid protein and degenerated neurites currently are classified as neuritic plaques. Braak and Braak (1991) described the longitudinal appearance of these neuropathological hallmarks in entorhinal cortex, followed by hippocampus, then amygdala. Thus, the paralimbic areas, including the amygdalar complex, are among the first to manifest the pathological changes of AD.

The involvement of the amygdala in degenerative dementia was recorded as early as 1938 by Brockhaus and has been noted consistently since, yet the hippocampus has garnered more attention in AD research than the amygdala. The specific role of the amygdala in AD is often clouded because of its frequent grouping with the hippocampus as 'medial temporal structures' (Brun and Englund, 1981; Mielke *et al.*, 1996; Heun *et al.*, 1997; O'Brien *et al.*, 1997b; Pantel *et al.*, 1997). The review by Corsellis (1970) of the literature on limbic degeneration in AD highlighted the role of the hippocampus in memory loss and reported a striking degree of damage in the neighbouring amygdala. The severity of amygdalar involvement prompted him to propose the amygdala as the region of the brain most susceptible to plaques and NFTs. Despite the neuropathology seen in the amygdala, its role in AD has not been as clear-cut as the correlation between hippocampal changes and memory loss. Conceptions regarding which symptoms of AD correlate with amygdalar damage currently are evolving.

As a collection of nuclei involved in several functional systems, the function of the amygdala has been summarized as assignment of emotional valence to environmental stimuli, which facilitates memory and other cognitive processes (Clark, 1995). A variety of lesional and stimulation studies provide the evidence for this function. For example, the conditioned fear pathway relies upon the amygdala (LeDoux, Chapter 7). Normal rats learned to associate an auditory tone (conditioned stimulus) with an electric shock from the floor of the cage. Subsequently, subjecting the same rats to the conditioned stimulus elicited autonomic changes and restless behaviour, even in the absence of the shock (Davis, Chapter 6). Amygdalectomized rats did not learn the association between the tone and the shock, and therefore did not react to the tone. Rats who learned the association prior to amygdalectomy lost expression of fear when exposed to the tone after the procedure (Clark, 1995). The lateral and central amygdalar nuclei may play the largest part in mediating fear conditioning (see Pitkänen *et al.*, 1997; LeDoux, Chapter 7). When the amygdala is lesioned or resected bilaterally in non-human primates, Klüver–Bucy syndrome (KBS) may result (Weiskrantz, 1956; Akert *et al.*, 1961). The syndrome is characterized by visual agnosia, hyperorality, hypermetamorphosis, blunting of fear or rage, and hypersexuality (Clark, 1995; Fudge *et al.*, 1998).

In humans, lesions of the amygdala lead to a less dramatic syndrome than the complete KBS, but stimulation experiments have elicited marked behavioural changes. Unilateral amygdalectomy during the course of neurosurgery to control epilepsy abolished autonomic responses to emotionally provocative stimuli, although memory remained intact (Tranel and Hyman, 1990; LaBar *et al.*, 1994). Other patients with amygdalar degeneration have demonstrated impaired ability to recognize fearful or angry facial expressions in others (Adolphs *et al.*, 1994; Aldophs and Tranel, Chapter 18). Patients with Urbach–Weithe syndrome develop mineralization of the amygdala bilaterally and, as a result, lose the ability to augment learning of emotionally laden stimuli (Cahill *et al.*, 1995). Bilateral amygdalectomy results in abnormal perception and expression of emotion, and not the complete manifestation of KBS (Terzian and Dalle Ore, 1955; Aggleton, 1992; Hayman *et al.*, 1998). Bilateral amygdalectomy of five patients with schizophrenia led to hyperorality and placidity (Sawa *et al.*, 1954). More extensive bilateral temporal lobectomy has resulted in partial or complete KBS. Infectious disease, trauma, and neurodegenerative diseases that involve bilateral temporal lobes have also led to KBS (Gascon and Giles, 1973; Marlow *et al.*, 1975; Hierons *et al.*, 1978; Cummings and Duchen, 1981; Lilly *et al.*, 1983). Changes in human behaviour are also seen when the amygdala is stimulated. Stimulation of amygdala results in fear, anxiety, complex hallucinations, and deja vu (Fudge *et al.*, 1998).

In summary, the amygdalar complex merges the individual's emotional and cognitive systems, and so impacts both on learning processes and behavioural expression. This chapter describes the neuroanatomy of the amygdala relevant to AD, the neurochemistry of amygdalar connectivity, neuropathological and neuroimaging changes in AD, and the role of the amygdala in the symptomatology of AD and other dementias.

20.2 Neuroanatomy of the amygdalar complex

Brain regions that constitute the limbic system share expression of a limbic system-associated membrane protein from an early stage in development (Levitt, 1984). Besides the limbic lobe structures, there are many paralimbic structures that contribute to the functionally designated 'limbic system' (see Table 20.1). Paralimbic components in the temporal lobe include the entorhinal cortex, hippocampus, and amygdala. The amygdala rests anterior to the temporal horn of the lateral ventricle, on the dorsomedial aspect of the medial temporal lobe. Rather than acting as one nucleus, it represents a complex of nuclei nestled together as an almond-shaped grey matter structure. The amygdala is often discussed as a functional unit of the central nervous system (CNS), but its nuclei have dense intrinsic and extrinsic connections. Figure 20.1 illustrates the positions of the nuclei relative to one another in the amygdala. Although nomenclature varies, in most descriptions, the nuclei are categorized as the basolateral nuclear group, the corticomedial nuclear group, and the central nucleus. The central nucleus is sometimes included in the corticomedial nuclear group, but its connectivity differs from that of the corticomedial nuclear group. The basolateral nuclear group is the largest part of the amygdala and sends mainly unreciprocated efferents to the corticomedial nuclear group, which is situated closer to the putamen and tail of the caudate.

Table 20.2 lists the principal afferent and efferent projections for the major nuclear groups (Amaral, 1992; Parent, 1996; Swanson and Petrovich, 1998). In general, the afferents maintain the amygdala's connections to the phylogenetic origin of each nucleus. The nuclei of the amygdala arose from (i) neocortex, (ii) claustrum, and (iii) striatum. Several areas maintain reciprocal afferent and efferent connections with the amygdala. The most significant of these in AD may be the nucleus basalis of Meynert, which will be discussed below. Other reciprocal loop connections exist between the amygdala and nucleus accumbens, ventral striatum, olfactory bulb, hypothalamus, thalamus and the ventral tegmental area. In some cases, the reciprocal connections are weighted more heavily to efferent than afferent processes. For example, amygdalar efferents to the hippocampus are more prominent than the reciprocal afferents (Parent, 1996).

The amygdalar efferents in Table 20.2 are categorized as intrinsic or extrinsic. Most of the intrinsic efferents between nuclei are reciprocal, but the lateral nucleus receives relatively few intrinsic afferents, emphasizing the overall direction of information flow from the basolateral nuclear group to the corticomedial nuclear group (Aggleton, 1985; Amaral *et al.*, 1992).

Table 20.1 The limbic system

- Limbic lobe
  - Cingulate gyrus
  - Fornix
  - Parahippocampal gyrus (includes entorhinal cortex)
  - Orbitofrontal cortex
  - Temporal pole
- Paralimbic structures
  - Septal nuclei
  - Hypothalamus
  - Epithalamus
  - Anterior nuclei of the thalamus
  - Hippocampus
  - Amygdalar complex
    - Basolateral nuclear group (BLA)
      - Basal nucleus, i.e. basolateral nucleus
        - Magnocellular division (BNmc)
        - Intermediate division
        - Parvicellular division (BNpc)
      - Paralaminar nucleus ('BNpl' in Figure 20.1)
      - Accessory basal nucleus
        - Magnocellular division (ABNmc)
        - Ventromedial division
        - Parvicellular division (ABNpc)
      - Lateral nucleus (LN)
        - Dorsomedial division
        - Ventrolateral division
    - Corticomedial nuclear group
      - Anterior amygdaloid area (AAA)
      - Central nucleus (CeA)
      - Cortical nuclei, i.e. periamydaloid cortex (CoN or PAC)
        - PAC2
        - PAC3
        - PACs
      - Medial nucleus (MN)
    - Nucleus of the lateral olfactory tract

The extrinsic efferents leave the amygdalar complex via the stria terminalis and the ventral amygdalofugal pathway. Processes extend from each of the amygdalar nuclei into either of these tracts, sometimes switching tracts, until they arrive at neocortical or subcortical destinations. The largest extrinsic connection joins the basolateral nuclear group with the acetylcholinesterase-poor striosomes of the striatum (Amaral *et al.*, 1992).

It is helpful to group the efferents by their contributions to other functional systems. These systems are referred to as autonomic, frontotemporal, main olfactory, and accessory

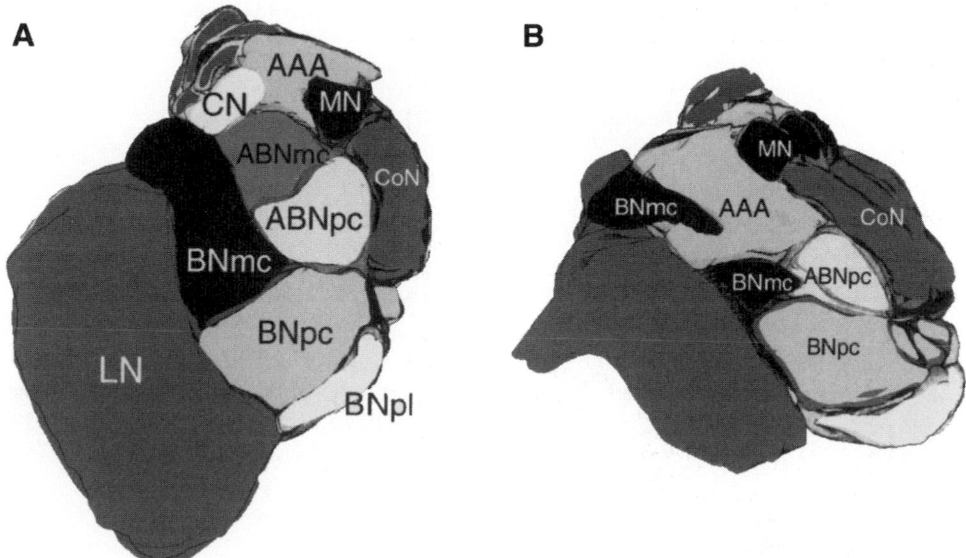

Figure 20.1 Three-dimensional reconstructions of the amygdala showing the rostral aspect from a normal control patient (**A**) and from a patient with Alzheimer's disease (**B**) (Scott *et al.*, 1991). AAA = anterior amygdaloid area, ABNmc = accessory basal nucleus—magnocellular portion, ABNpc = accessory basal nucleus—parvocellular portion, BNmc = basal nucleus—magnocellular portion, BNpc = basal nucleus—parvocellular portion, BNpl = basal nucleus—paralaminar portion, CN = central nucleus, CoN = cortical nucleus, LN = lateral nucleus, and MN = medial nucleus. (Reprinted from Smith *et al.*, 1991, with permission of the author and publisher.)

olfactory (Swanson and Petrovich, 1998). The amygdala drives physiological responses associated with emotion through the autonomic system. The central nucleus has been identified as a striatal derivative that differentiated and became integrated with the autonomic system. Both the central and medial nuclei send efferent projections to hypothalamus and brainstem regions as part of this system. Stress responses such as heightened arousal, increased vigilance, tachycardia, ulcer formation, analgesia and corticosteroid-releasing hormone levels are the result of amygdalar input to the autonomic nervous system (Clark, 1995).

The frontotemporal system places the claustrum-derived basolateral nuclear group between frontal and temporal cortical input and the striatum. In contrast to the other three systems, efferent flow from the amygdalar component of the frontotemporal system goes to striatum and not hypothalamus. It is of interest in the case of AD that it is the basolateral nuclear group that has reciprocal connections with nucleus basalis of Meynert.

The cortical nucleus contributes to the main olfactory system (named for its major projection from the main olfactory bulb).

The cortical and medial amygdalar nuclei are the only major projection fields of the accessory olfactory bulb. Other primary sensory regions (medial prefrontal and agranular insular

Table 20.2 Non-neocortical afferents and efferents of the amygdalar complex.

Afferent connections	*Amygdalar nuclei*	*Efferent connections*
Anterolateral portion of nucleus basalis of Meynert* Hippocampus* Piriform cortex (indirect olfactory pathway) Posterior thalamic nuclei Ventromedial hypothalamic nucleus and lateral hypothalamic area	Basolateral nuclear group	INTRINSIC Corticomedial nuclear group EXTRINSIC Amygdalostriatal projection: Nucleus accumbens Tail of caudate Ventral striatum Entorhinal cortex Hippocampus* Hypothalamus Mediodorsal thalamus (→prefrontal cortex) Nucleus basalis of Meynert*
Olfactory bulb* Lateral olfactory tract Ventromedial hypothalamic nucleus and lateral hypothalamic area* Vomeronasal region	Corticomedial nuclear group	INTRINSIC Basal and accessory basal nuclei EXTRINSIC Olfactory bulb* Substantia innominata→ stria terminalis→ anterior hypothalamus→ medial forebrain bundle Ventromedial hypothalamus
Midline thalamic nuclei* Ventral tegmental area* Ventromedial hypothalamic nucleus and lateral hypothalamic area*	Central nucleus	EXTRINSIC Brainstem (periaqueductal grey, peripeduncular nucleus, reticular formation, substantia nigra, nucleus solitarius, vagal nerve nucleus, ventral tegmental area). Lateral and ventromedial hypothalamus Midline thalamic nuclei Nucleus basalis of Meynert Tuberomammillary and supramamillary nuclei→ midbrain tegmentum

*Reciprocal afferents and efferents from amygdala.

cortical), the hippocampus, and the hypothalamus also contribute to the accessory olfactory system. The accessory olfactory system conveys pheromonal information along further projections from the amygdala to the striatum, nucleus accumbens, claustrum, and thalamus.

20.3 Neurochemistry of the amygdala

Amygdalar neurochemistry features catecholaminergic, hormonal, and peptide neurotransmitters (see Table 20.3). The primary transmitter deficit in AD is cholinergic. The most significant cholinergic projection in the forebrain is from the anterolateral portion of the

Table 20.3 Neurochemistry of the amygdala

	Source of afferent projections	*Amygdalar nuclei*
Acetylcholine (ACh)	Nucleus basalis of Meynert	Basolateral nuclear group, lateral part of central nucleus, lateral olfactory tract nucleus and periamygdalar cortex
Corticotropin-releasing factor (CRF)		Basolateral nuclear group
Dopamine (DA)	Ventral tegmental area Substantia nigra	Lateral, central, and basal nuclei
Oestrogen (in the monkey)		Corticomedial nuclear group
γ-Aminobutyric acid (GABA)	Nucleus basalis of Meynert	Basolateral nuclear group; central and medial nuclei
Glutamate	Layers III and V of frontal, cingulate, insular, and temporal cortex CA1 hippocampal neurons Deep layers of entorhinal cortex Claustrum Midbrain peripeduncular nuclei	Basolateral nuclear group
Neurotensin		Central, medial>other nuclei>>accessory basal and lateral nuclei.
NADPH diaphorase		Basolateral nuclear groups>corticomedial groups>>central nucleus.
Noradrenaline (NA)	Locus coeruleus	Central and corticomedial nuclear groups
Serotonin (5-HT)	Dorsal raphe	Lateral, basal (magnocellular), and central nuclei. Lateral, basal and cortical nuclei feature 5-HT_1 receptors.

From Amaral *et al.* (1992), Fallon and Ciofi (1992), and Parent (1996).

nucleus basalis of Meynert to the basal nucleus magnocellular region of the amygdala (Parent, 1996). Enzymes related to acetylcholine (ACh) processing [acetylcholinesterase (AChE) and choline acetyl transferase (ChAT)] are present in the lateral part of the central nucleus, the lateral olfactory tract nucleus, and the periamygdalar cortex, which constitutes part of the transition zone between amygdala and hippocampus. The presence of ChAT signifies that ACh synthesis occurs in the amygdala.

Tyrosine hydroxylase, a marker for dopaminergic neurons, is exchanged reciprocally between amygdala and midbrain areas. The dopaminergic ventral tegmental area and substantia nigra are in communication with the lateral, central, and basal amygdalar nuclei (Fallon and Ciofi, 1992). In the rat, extracellular dopamine release in the basolateral nucleus of the amygdala increases in response to stress and may augment dopaminergic prefrontal cortical stress responses. (Inglis and Moghaddam, 1999). Noradrenaline (NA) from the locus coeruleus reaches central and corticomedial nuclear groups. Amygdalar levels of serotonin (5-HT) are more abundant than those of NA (Parent, 1996). Serotonin has been found in lateral, basal (magnocellular portion), and central nuclei. 5-HT_1 receptors are featured in the lateral, basal, and cortical nuclei (Fallon and Ciofi, 1992, Parent, 1996).

Glutamatergic afferents extend mainly to the basolateral nuclear group from frontal, cingulate, insular, and temporal cortex, hippocampus, entorhinal cortex, claustrum, and midbrain peripeduncular nuclei (Parent, 1996). Glutamatergic intrinsic efferents run from the basolateral nuclear group to the central nucleus. These efferents may play a role in learning, since *N*-methyl-D-aspartate antagonists block the registration of the conditioned fear response in rats (Miserendino *et al.*, 1990). Glutamic acid decarboxylase converts glutamate to γ-aminobutyric acid (GABA) in central and medial nuclei (Swanson and Petrovich, 1998). Benzodiazepine–$GABA_A$ receptors appear in clusters of neurons within all nuclei of the amygdala. They are most prominent in the basolateral nuclear group (see File, Chapter 5).

Several hormones have been described in the amygdala: corticotrophin-releasing factor (CRF) is found in the basolateral nuclear group; oestradiol and aromatase (the enzyme that converts androgens to oestrogens) are present in the corticomedial nuclear group. Oestradiol-containing neurons send efferent processes to other areas of the limbic system and the thalamus (Pfaff and Keiner, 1973). Neurotensin is a neuropeptide most abundant in the central and medial amygdalar nuclei (Parent, 1996).

20.4 Changes in the amygdala in Alzheimer's disease

Post-mortem examination of the amygdala in AD reveals neuronal loss, NFTs, neuritic plaques, diffuse plaques, and Lewy bodies (Figures 20.2–20.6). Brun's series of seven AD brain autopsies showed that the most extensive atrophic changes were found consistently in amygdala (grouped with uncus), hippocampus, and subicular and entorhinal cortex (Brun and Gustafson, 1976). Figure 20.5 shows senile plaques in the entorhinal cortex, as seen in the amygdala in Figures 20.3 and 20.4; in addition, the meningeal vessel walls appear thickened with amyloid. Amyloid angiopathy and plaques with amyloid cores represent the aggregation of abnormal β-amyloid fragments and appear commonly in AD in all cerebral regions.

The amygdala loses 2% of its volume during the course of normal ageing and 25.8% in patients with AD (see Figure 20.1) (Herzog and Kemper, 1980). Others have confirmed this degree of amygdalar atrophy (Hooper and Vogel, 1976; Brady and Mufson, 1990; Scott *et al.*, 1991, 1992). Scott *et al.* (1991) were able to demonstrate the most severe amygdalar volumetric loss (71%) in the magnocellular regions of the basal and accessory basal nuclei. Significant loss occurs in the lateral nucleus as well. This volumetric loss may be due to neuronal shrinkage, measured as 'packing density', in addition to neuronal loss. The neuronal

Figure 20.2 Coronal sections of brain. Amygdala (indicated by arrows) in a patient with AD (**A**), in comparison with a control patient (**B**). The specimen from the AD patient shows atrophy. Figures 20.3–20.6 are from the amygdala shown in (A). Photographs courtesy of Dr. Harry Vinters, UCLA Neuropathology.

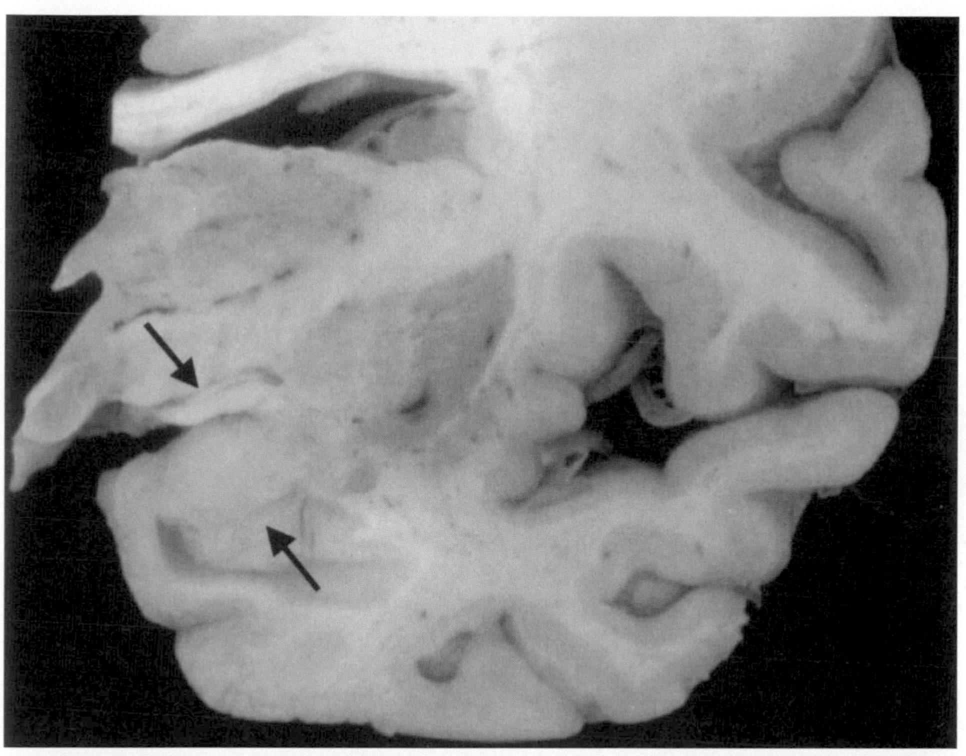

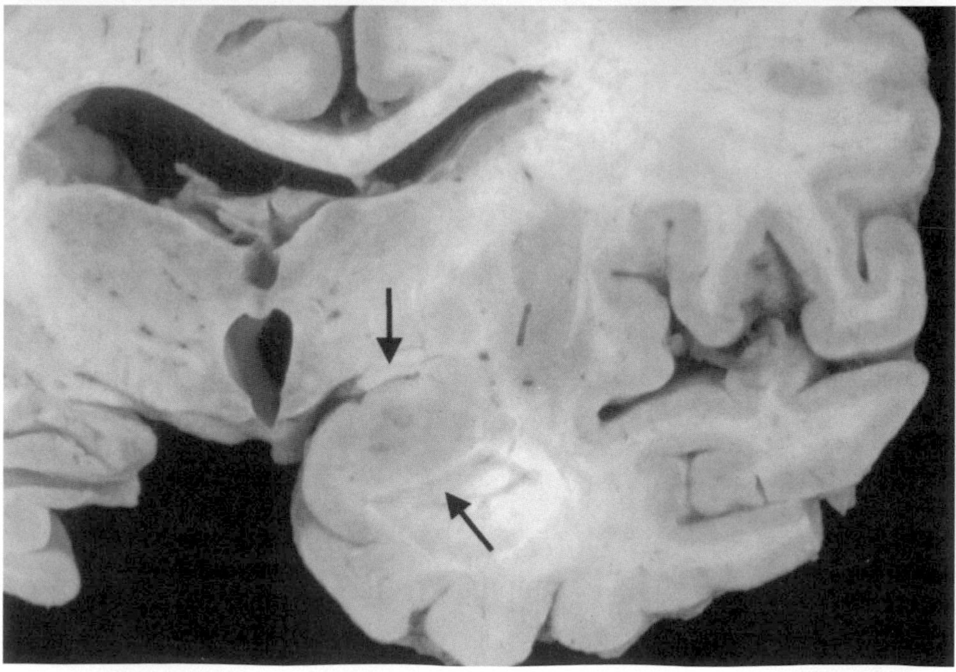

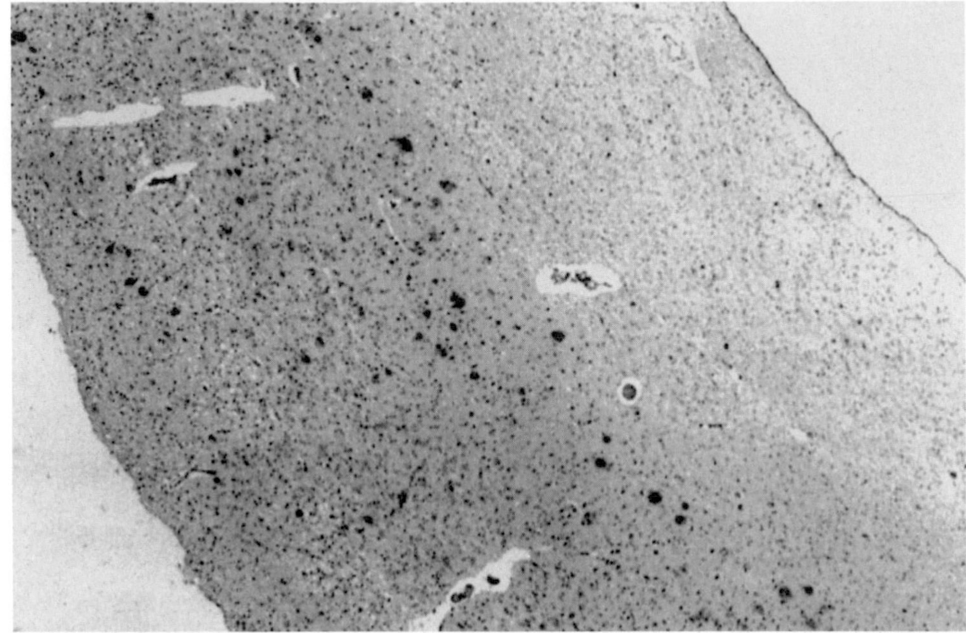

Figure 20.3 Section of a basolateral nuclear group located in the medial inferior amygdala, immunostained with an antibody to A-β1–42. The ependymal lining with the adjacent ventricular cavity is on the upper right of the micrograph. Note numerous A-β-immunoreactive senile plaques (magnification ×50). Photograph courtesy of Dr Harry Vinters, UCLA Neuropathology.

loss is more selective in some amygdalar nuclei. Whereas the magnocellular portion of the basal nucleus loses neuronal and glial cells, the deep portion of the cortical nucleus loses neurons specifically (Scott *et al.*, 1992).

In addition to atrophy, one would expect to find more NFTs and plaques in the amygdala, since it is affected early and progressively during the course of AD (Braak and Braak, 1991). Jamada and Mehraein (1968) observed higher densities of NFTs and plaques in amygdala than in other neocortical areas of AD brains, raising the question of whether this might be a target region for degenerative changes (Jamada and Mehraein, 1968).

NFTs in the amygdala have been qualitatively and quantitatively reported (Brady and Mufson, 1990; Esiri *et al.*, 1990; Bancher and Jellinger, 1994; Bierer *et al.*, 1995; Jellinger and Bancher, 1998). Braak and Braak (1991) described the longitudinal development of NFTs in AD cases. They divided the course into stages in which different regions developed isolated, small, moderate, or large numbers of NFTs. Their staging shows that the amygdala is among the first regions to develop isolated NFTs, preceded only by entorhinal cortex (Braak and Braak, 1991). In one study, NFTs were up to 10 times more numerous than plaques in the amygdala from AD brains and were most abundant in medial temporal areas,

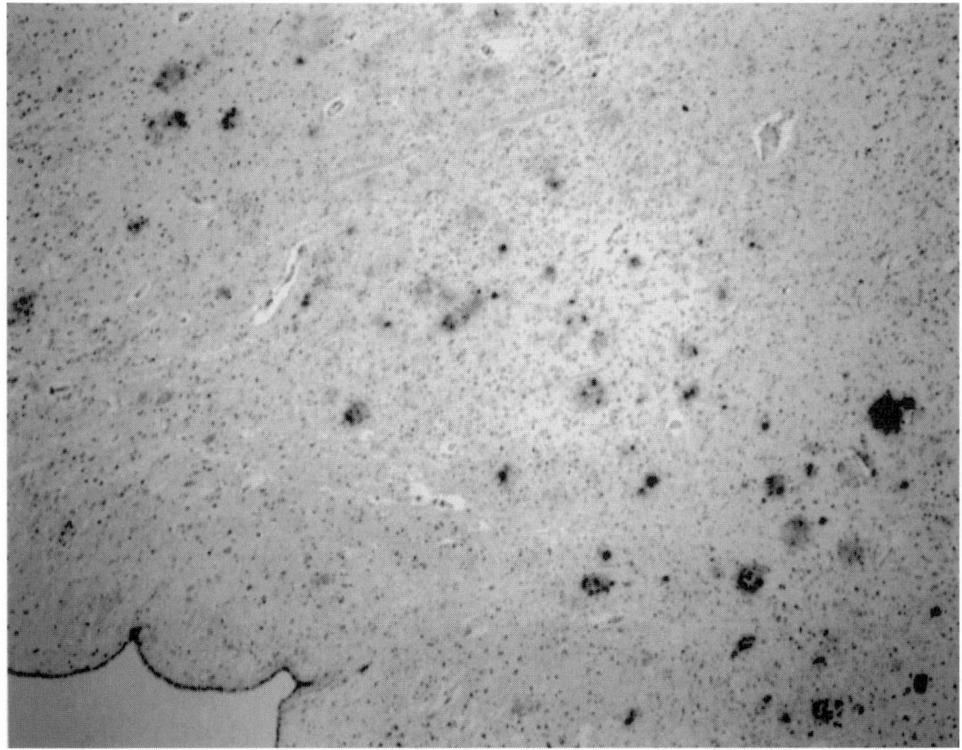

Figure 20.4 Inferior amygdala (basal nuclear group), adjacent to the ependymal/ventricular lining, shows prominent A-β1–40-immunoreactive neuritic plaques. Photograph courtesy of Dr Harry Vinters, UCLA Neuropathology.

which included the amygdala (Esiri *et al.*, 1990). Tangle-predominant-type AD patients autopsied by Bancher (1994) and Jellinger (1998) developed numerous to abundant amygdalar NFTs. The NFTs in these brains were concentrated almost exclusively in limbic areas, resembling Braak and Braak AD Stages III and IV. An abundance of NFTs accompanies the degree of atrophy seen in the amygdala in AD and tangle-predominant dementia.

There is some controversy as to whether NFTs and neuritic plaques arrange themselves separately in amygdalar subregions. Braak and Braak (1991) reported that in Stage IV of AD pathology, NFTs dominated in the basolateral nuclear group, with neuritic plaques predominant in the corticomedial nuclear group. Brady and Mufson (1990) reported co-existence of intraneuronal NFTs and neuritic plaques in the corticomedial nuclear group, while extraneuronal NFTs or ghost tangles were situated in the basolateral nuclear group. Corsellis (1970) and Hooper (1976) reported significantly more neuronal loss, neuritic plaques, and NFTs in the corticomedial than the basolateral nuclear group. Since the medial and central nuclei appear earlier phylogenetically than the basolateral nuclei, it is hypothesized that the more primitive cortical region is more vulnerable to the degenerative changes of AD (Corsellis, 1970).

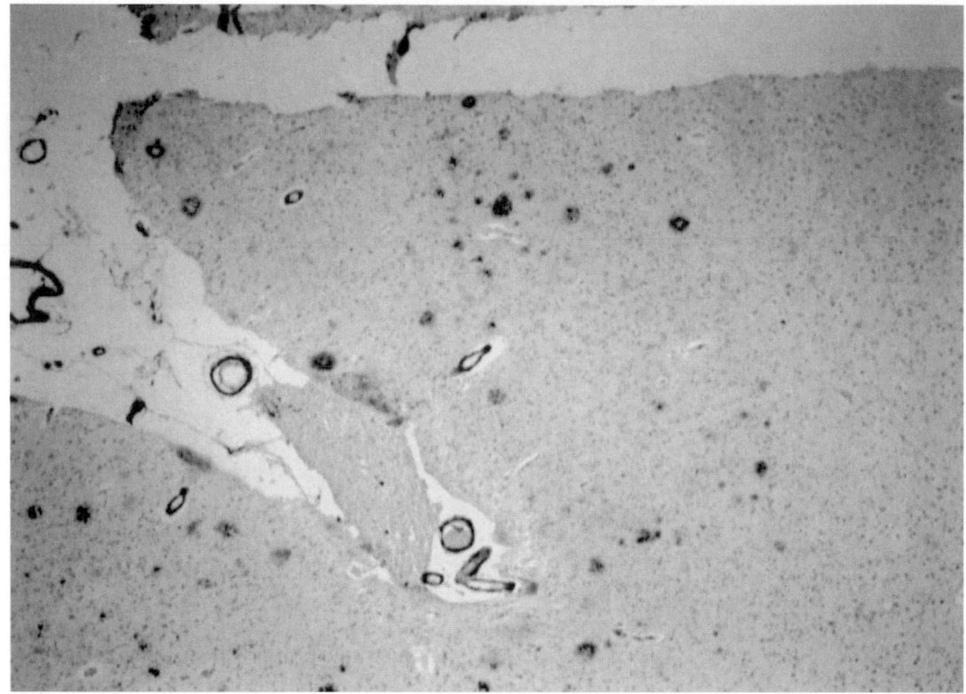

Figure 20.5 Temporal cortex adjacent to amygdala shows A-β1–40-immunoreactive senile plaques and meningocortical amyloid angiopathy (magnification ×50). Photograph courtesy of Dr Harry Vinters, UCLA Neuropathology.

Neuritic plaques consistently are more prominent in the corticomedial nuclear group of the amygdala (Corsellis, 1970; Hooper and Vogel, 1976; Brashear *et al.*, 1988; Brady and Mufson, 1990; Braak and Braak, 1991). Neuritic plaques have been seen in the amygdala of aged, non-demented individuals and, when seen in this context, they occur in the cortical, accessory basal, medial, and central nuclei. Lateral nuclei were involved only in those cases with more numerous plaques (Mann *et al.*, 1987), and those plaques tend to be diffuse, rather than neuritic plaques (Brady and Mufson, 1990). The magnocellular basal nucleus features smaller plaques than the more mature ones seen in the cortical and central nuclei, implying that plaques form first in corticomedial and central nuclear groups; then the process spreads to the basolateral areas. The topographic distribution of neuritic plaques supports the notion that derivations from more primitive cortex are more susceptible to degeneration.

In addition to the hallmark pathology of AD, other degenerative changes are found in the amygdala. Mild to moderate granulovacuolar degeneration (Hooper and Vogel, 1976), ubiquitin-positive granular structures, Lewy bodies, and argyrophilic grains are reported. Ubiquitin-positive granular structures appear in normal ageing in transentorhinal cortex and amygdala (Iseki *et al.*, 1998). When present, they are highest in density in the accessory basal and basal nuclei. In patients at later stages of AD, however, they decrease in number,

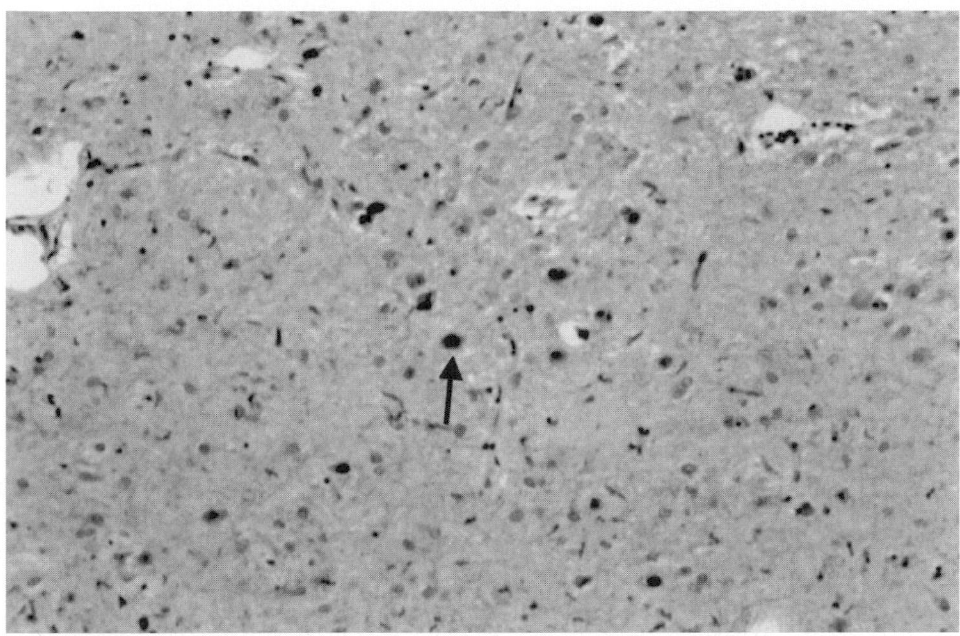

Figure 20.6 Section of amygdala immunostained with antibody to α-synuclein. The arrow indicates one of many immunoreactive neurofibrillary tangles (magnification ×255). Photograph courtesy of Dr Harry Vinters, UCLA Neuropathology.

possibly due to the degeneration of ubiquitin-positive granular structure-containing cells after NFT densities increase (Iseki *et al.*, 1998). Ubiquitin-positive granular structures differ from Lewy bodies in that they consist of neurofilaments, mitochondria, lamellar components, and vesicles with synaptic structures; Lewy bodies are also ubiquitin immunoreactive but consist only of neurofilamentous structures, and they increase in number and distribution over the course of illness.

α-Synuclein antibody staining detected numerous amygdalar Lewy bodies in 22% of 74 late-onset familial AD brains. Not only was the finding unexpected, but the highest numbers of Lewy bodies were found in the amygdala, supporting the significance of this location as a primary site for neuropathological changes of AD (Lippa *et al.*, 1998). Argyrophilic tau-immunoreactive grains are a non-specific finding in the aged brain. They have been found at post-mortem in the amygdalas of elderly patients with and without dementia. Demented patients with argyrophilic grains have had diagnoses of AD, progressive supranuclear palsy, corticobasal degeneration, or frontotemporal dementia (Jellinger, 1998). The amygdala reflects degeneration seen throughout the dementing CNS and is often one of the first regions to show changes.

The amygdala may be affected due to its connectivity to other structures that degenerate in AD, i.e. through an 'innocent bystander' or remote effect. Connections link the basal and accessory basal nuclei with entorhinal cortex; magnocellular basal and accessory basal nuclei send efferents to temporal and frontal neocortex; and the amygdala receives afferents from the nucleus basalis of Meynert (Scott *et al.*, 1991). Each of these extrinsic areas also shows early neuropathological changes in AD. Indeed, the numbers of NFTs in neocortical regions correspond to the density of each region's afferent and efferent connections with the amygdala (Esiri *et al.*, 1990). It has not been determined whether the amygdala's extrinsic connectivity provides an incoming or outgoing conduit for AD pathology.

20.5 Neurochemistry of the amygdala in AD

The cholinergic hypothesis of AD dictates that a deficiency of ACh from the nucleus basalis of Meynert would deactivate the amygdala. Assays of ChAT activity showed percentage decreases in the medial temporal area that correlate with the NFT burden in this region as a whole (Esiri *et al.*, 1990). At the level of the amygdaloid complex, neuritic plaque counts were lowest in the basolateral nuclear group, the region with highest AChE reactivity. This finding implies that loss of AChE reactivity might precede the initiation of plaque formation, but, as discussed above, the basolateral nuclear group may be less vulnerable to AD changes (Brashear *et al.*, 1988).

NA release within the amygdala mediates influences on memory storage, possibly through modulation of cholinergic activation, so that loss of neurochemical or structural connectivity to the locus coeruleus may add indirectly to the hindrance of cholinergic activation from the nucleus basalis of Meynert (McGaugh *et al.*, 1996) In addition, the locus coeruleus itself suffers neuronal loss in AD to compound the decrease in cholinergic activation (Zweig *et al.*, 1988; Chan-Palay and Asan, 1989; Forstl *et al.*, 1992).

Derangements in other neurotransmitters have not been reported in AD, but neuronal loss in the amygdala is likely to lead to decreases in other neurotransmitters. Based on what is known about the neurochemistry of the amygdala, the degree of atrophy and concentration of neuropathologic markers in centromedial nuclear groups could be speculated to decrease amygdalar dopaminergic, GABA, NA, and 5-HT release (see Table 20.3).

Similar deficiencies would be expected at the hormonal level. CRF receptors are expressed by the amygdala, and deficits in brain CRF have been reported in AD (De Souza, 1995). It remains to be determined if this contributes to symptomatology in AD but, normally, CRF levels increase in response to stress. Nerve growth factor (NGF) receptors are present in the amygdala; their distribution does not correlate with that of ChAT- and AChE- containing nuclei (Amaral *et al.*, 1992).

Neurotensin immunoreactivity is decreased in all nuclei of the amygdala in AD (Benzing *et al.*, 1992). If neurotensin is the peptide messenger for connections between the amygdala and the autonomic, endocrine, and memory systems (Parent, 1996), the decrease may account for some manifestations of AD.

Catalase is a detoxifying enzyme expressed in response to free radical damage. Catalase activity in the amygdala of AD brains (in addition to other regions) is significantly reduced compared with elderly normal controls. Whether this difference indicates a pathogenic, causative, or resultant effect in degeneration of the amygdala is not clear (Gsell *et al.*, 1995).

Nicotinamide adenine dinucleotide phosphate diaphorase (NADPH-d) is a nitric oxide synthase present in selected neurons within each of the amygdalar nuclei. Interestingly, the specific neurons throughout the amygdala which express this enzyme tend to be immune to changes of AD (Unger and Lange, 1992).

20.6 Neuroimaging evidence of amygdalar involvement in AD

Diffuse cerebral atrophy in advanced AD patients is appreciated on structural and functional neuroimaging studies. Mesial temporal atrophy has been described as an early finding. Since the amygdala has shown clear changes in AD on pathology, it has been hoped that amygdalar volumes as measured by neuroimaging studies can be used to differentiate between normally ageing patients and those in the earliest stage of AD. Available therapies for AD maintain but generally do not restore function, emphasizing the importance of the early detection and initiation of treatment for AD. Early diagnosis through non-invasive procedures such as magnetic resonance imaging (MRI) would be ideal, and if the amygdala is one of the first areas of the brain to atrophy, it makes a reasonable region of interest for detection of AD.

The region measured as amygdala differs among various MRI studies. Most use the following criteria: the amygdaloid complex includes the basolateral and corticomedial nuclear groups, as well as the central nucleus, the gyrus semilunaris, and the gyrus ambiens. The anterior boundary is defined as the plane including the most anterior portion of the temporal stem, where the amygdala appears as a thickening of the anterior grey matter (Cuenod *et al.*, 1993). The amygdala may be differentiated from the hippocampus at the level of the alveus hippocampi, the semiannular sulcus, or the uncal recess of the inferior horn of the lateral ventricle (Mori *et al.*, 1997). The inferior border is delineated by a line drawn between the uncal notch to the uncal recess of the lateral ventricle. The entorhinal sulcus runs superior to the amygdala (Hashimoto *et al.*, 1998).

Most attempts to diagnose early AD through structural MRI have been unsuccessful. One study showed that the amygdalar atrophy seen on MRI brain scans from AD patients was significantly more severe than that of patients with vascular dementia, Parkinson's disease, Korsakoff's syndrome, and progressive supranuclear palsy (Maunoury *et al.*, 1996), and mild to moderate AD patients had more amygdalar atrophy than normal controls (Mauri *et al.*, 1998), but other studies have not reproduced this finding. MRI has shown amygdalar reductions in volume of up to 32% (Deweer *et al.*, 1995; Heun *et al.*, 1997; Jack *et al.*, 1997; O'Brien *et al.*, 1997a; Pantel *et al.*, 1997; Hashimoto *et al.*, 1998; Mori *et al.*, 1999), but this finding alone was not reliable enough to distinguish AD patients from others. Laakso and colleagues (1995) found that amygdalar volumes as seen on MRI did not differ significantly between AD patients at an early stage and normal elderly controls. Volumetric changes on MRI do not seem to correspond to the early development of the histopathological changes of AD. This may be due to the fact that the amygdala is losing volume in both non-demented and AD patients, thereby decreasing the apparent volumetric difference in comparative studies.

Investigations attempting to prove the usefulness of MRI volumetric studies in distinguishing AD patients from normal controls *in vivo* have found the hippocampus and entorhinal cortex to be more reliable regions for comparison than the amygdala (Laakso *et al.*, 1995; Jack *et al.*, 1997; O'Brien *et al.*, 1997a).

Mori and colleagues (1999) made the observation that Japanese AD patients had less difficulty with emotional memories of the catastrophic Kobe earthquake than with declarative episodic memories of the event. Differences in amygdalar volume for this sample of AD patients correlated more significantly with the emotional memory deficit than did hippocampal volumes, supporting the role of the amygdala in the emotional aspect of memory function.

Functional neuroimaging with positron emission tomography (PET) might be useful to correlate cognitive or behaviour changes in AD patients with amygdalar activity. In a fluorodeoxyglucose PET study, verbal learning task activation revealed hypometabolism in the left amygdala for AD patients relative to normal controls. Compared with abnormalities in other cortical regions of interest, the left amygdalar abnormality was a highly sensitive indicator of disease states, but patients with other illnesses were not included in the study, and specificity could not be determined (Valladares-Neto *et al.*, 1995). Use of PET activation studies to explore amygdalar function in AD is fraught with uncertainty. Any metabolic derangement detected in this region may be due to non-compliance with the task by a cognitively impaired patient, primary dysfunction of the amygdala itself, or dysfunction secondary to amygdalar afferent connectivity from damaged neocortical or limbic areas (diaschisis).

20.7 Clinical correlates of amygdalar involvement in AD

The clinical presentation of AD includes cognitive, behavioural, and neurological deficits. The role of the amygdala in effecting these changes has been the subject of enthusiastic speculation. Memory loss, a cardinal feature of AD, may be worsened by loss of facilitation by the damaged amygdala. In many cases, emotional or behavioural changes in AD do not parallel the degree of memory loss observed. This may provide evidence for an amygdalar role outside of hippocampal memory and learning processes (Parent, 1996).

The damage to both amygdalae due to AD should cause KBS. Diffuse atrophy and functional disconnection of multiple regions of the brain may prevent patients from being able to manifest KBS fully. AD patients remain indifferent to their cognitive impairment and are apathetic, which may signify decreased emotional expression due to amygdalar dysfunction. This would be consistent with the amygdalectomy patients who manifested inability to recognize and express emotional content. As demonstrated by Inglis and Moghaddam (1999), the normal CNS stress response is mediated by dopamine release in the amygdala; impaired ability of the amygdala to respond to dopamine release within the basolateral amygdalar nuclear group may hinder responses to stressful stimuli and contribute to the apathy evident in AD patients. Apathy may be the most common representation of KBS caused by AD. In Cummings and Duchen's series (1981) of five patients with KBS due to frontotemporal dementia, all patients had apathy, whereas other elements of the syndrome were not as consistently present. Hyperorality was seen frequently in this small sample. Humans with dementia as the underlying aetiology of KBS may lose limbic and cognitive systems necessary for a more consistent expression of hypersexuality, hypermetamorphosis, hyperorality, and agnosias.

Burns and colleagues (1990) were able to detect partial KBS in 81% of their population of possible and probable AD patients. The most common features reported were apathy, hypermetamorphosis, and rages. Hyperorality and sexual disinhibition occurred less frequently in the AD patients. The high proportion of KBS was biased by the authors' interpretation of Capgras syndrome as a manifestation of the visual agnosia initially described by Klüver and Bucy, and they also included urinary incontinence as a feature of KBS. Capgras syndrome is a misidentification syndrome in which the patient believes that others are claiming false identities, and will challenge them, no matter how familiar the visitor might have been in the past. Capgras syndrome has been observed in the context of delirium and AD.

In addition to overall systems dysfunction due to AD, normal changes of ageing may provide another explanation for the partial manifestation of KBS in AD patients. Hypersexuality in amygdalectomized patients may rely upon an intact testosterone axis. Elderly males who have low levels of testosterone may not develop hypersexuality, even after bilateral amygdalar changes of AD.

Alternatively, paranoid delusions, anxiety, hallucinosis, reduplicative paramnesias, purposeless repetitive behaviours, and autonomic instability in patients with AD may be the manifestations of disinhibited amygdalar input to the autonomic system. Without normal regulation of this system, increased levels of arousal and sympathetic tone may dictate the patient's behaviour. A similar experimental stimulation of the amygdala in untrained animals results in physiological and behavioural fear responses (Clark, 1995).

Neurological symptoms of AD may be related to amygdalar changes. As discussed above, the main olfactory and accessory olfactory bulbs project directly to both the basolateral and corticomedial nuclear groups. In addition to the degeneration of primary olfactory sensation, disruption of the amygdalar component of the main olfactory and accessory olfactory systems may contribute to the variable anosmia experienced by AD patients (reviewed by Thompson *et al.*, 1998). The amygdala has many connections with the striatum and with the substantia nigra, and this may relate to the Parkinsonism seen at later stages of AD.

Some studies have attempted to confirm the role of the amygdala in the clinical decline of AD. As in the attempt to use amygdalar atrophy as a neuroimaging diagnostic tool, MRI studies are not as helpful as post-mortem studies in proving clinical correlations between the amygdala and cognitive or behavioural deficits. MRI volumetric studies have not shown a correlation between reductions in amygdalar volume and scores on the Mattis dementia rating scale (Mattis, 1976) or the Raven coloured progressive matrices (Raven, 1962), but the density of NFTs and neuritic plaques in amygdalar regions showed correlation with patients' Clinical Dementia Rating scores (Hughes *et al.*, 1982; Bierer *et al.*, 1995; Haroutunian *et al.*, 1998). The amygdala harbours obvious changes in AD but retains an enigmatic role in clinical symptomatology.

20.8 Amygdalar involvement in other dementias

The amygdala is also involved in numerous other neurodegenerative disorders, including vascular dementia (VaD), dementia with Lewy bodies (DLB), Parkinson's disease (PD) with dementia, and frontotemporal dementia (Corsellis, 1970). VaD patients have atrophy of hippocampal–amygdalar complexes similar to the atrophy seen in AD (Pantel *et al.*, 1998). Hashimoto and colleagues (1998) compared MRI amygdalar volumes among 27 AD patients, 27 DLB patients, and 27 normal elderly controls. Normalized volumes were significantly smaller (21%) in the demented patients than in controls but did not differ by diagnosis. Ubiquitin-positive granular structures are found in AD and DLB and decrease as both dementias progress. Iseki and colleagues (1996) reported a series of brain autopsies from patients with courses of dementia ranging from 1 to 18 years. Although ubiquitin-positive granular structures were found in normally ageing brains, their numbers were lower at advanced stages of AD and DLB; as neurons degenerated, the intraneuronal ubiquitin-positive granular structures became undetectable (Iseki *et al.*, 1996).

High densities of Lewy bodies and Lewy neurites appear in amygdala from PD patients with and without dementia, but there is no significant difference from controls in the degree of atrophy, implying that dementia in this disease is not related to amygdalar changes (Churchyard and Lees, 1997).

Frontotemporal dementia patients frequently manifest features included in KBS, such as hypersexuality, aggressivity, hyperorality, emotional blunting, loss of social awareness, and hypermetamorphosis (Balajthy, 1964; Miller *et al.*, 1991, 1993, 1995a,b, 1997; Mendez *et al.*, 1993; Brun *et al.*, 1994; Lynch *et al.*, 1994; Levy *et al.*, 1996; Edwards-Lee *et al.*, 1997). Neuronal loss and gliosis of the amygdala have been reported in all nuclear subdivisions on multiple post-mortem examinations of frontotemporal dementia patients (Cummings and Duchen, 1981; Brun, 1987, 1993, 1994; Neary *et al.*, 1993; Kertesz *et al.*, 1994; Hooten and Lyketsos, 1996; Jackson and Lowe, 1996; Yamaoka *et al.*, 1996), but these findings appear in the context of extensive frontal and temporal cortex pathology. Pick bodies have been reported in the amygdalas of patients with Pick's disease (Cummings and Duchen, 1981). Derangement of the temporolimbic system leads to the Klüver–Bucy signs observed in frontotemporal dementia, and involvement of the amygdala may contribute to this symptom complex.

Patients with amyotrophic lateral sclerosis (ALS) may develop dementia with pathological changes in the amygdala. These patients often manifest a frontal dysexecutive syndrome, which may evolve into dementia. While Anderson and colleagues (1995) demonstrated ubiquitin-immunoreactive inclusions in the amygdalas of ALS cases with and without dementia (Anderson *et al.*, 1995), demented ALS patients differed by showing neuronal loss in the basolateral nuclei of the amygdala, subiculum, nucleus accumbens, and other frontal and temporal cortical regions (Kato *et al.*, 1994). Dickson and colleagues (1986) reported atrophy of the corticomedial nuclear group of the amygdala in one demented ALS patient with symptoms of KBS.

One case of KBS has been reported due to Huntington's disease (Janati, 1985), although the amygdala does atrophy in this, as well as in the other neurodegenerative dementias. It is possible that both patients with AD and those with Huntington's disease, a neurodegenerative disease of the basal ganglia, and frontal and temporal lobes, lose the ability to manifest KBS due to the degree of cortical deterioration.

20.9 Conclusions

The nuclear groups of the amygdala share connectivity with multiple regions affected heavily in AD. There is evidence that neuritic plaques are concentrated topographically in the corticomedial nuclear group of the amygdala; NFTs have not shown a predilection for a particular group of nuclei. The dominance of neuritic plaques in the corticomedial group may stem from these neurons' more primitive phylogenetic origins.

Deterioration of amygdalar contributions to cognitive, emotional, behavioural, and autonomic systems may be related to the progression of deficits in AD patients. AD symptomatology includes elements of KBS that may be due to the virtual amygdalectomy brought about over the course of the illness. It has, however, been difficult to correlate amygdalar changes with functional deficits using structural MRI or PET. Functional MRI studies with the amygdala as a region of interest may enhance understanding of the clinical consequences of amygdalar involvement in AD. New radioisotope markers for AD pathology and high-resolution imaging techniques may give neuroimaging researchers another means of associating amygdalar changes with clinical changes during life.

Acknowledgements

The authors are grateful to Harry Vinters, MD, for providing the photomicrographs used in Figures 20.2–20.6. This work has been funded by an Alzheimer's Disease Center (AG10123) grant from the National Institute on Aging, the Sidell-Kagan Research Fund, and the Department of Veteran Affairs Geriatric Neurology Fellowship.

References

Adolphs, R., Tranel, D., Damasio, H., and Damasio, A. (1994). Impaired recognition of emotion in facial expressions following bilateral damage to the human amygdala. *Nature*, 372, 669–672.

Aggleton, J.P. (1992) The functional effects of amygdala lesions in humans: a comparison with findings from monkeys. In *The Amygdala: Neurobiological Aspects of Emotion, Memory, and Dysfunction* (ed. J.P. Aggleton), pp. 485–503. Wiley-Liss, New York.

Aggleton, J.P. (1985) A description of intra-amygdaloid connections in old world monkeys. *Experimental Brain Research*, **57**, 390–399.

Akert, K., Gruesen, R.A., Woolsey, C.N., and Meyer, D.R. (1961) Klüver–Bucy syndrome in monkeys with neocortical ablations of temporal lobe. *Brain*, 84, 480–498.

Amaral, D.G., Price, J.L., Pitkanen, A., and Carmichael, S.T. (1992) Anatomical organization of the primate amygdaloid complex. In *The Amygdala: Neurobiological Aspects of Emotion, Memory, and Mental Dysfunction* (ed. J.P. Aggleton), pp. 1–66. Wiley-Liss, New York.

Anderson, V.E.R., Cairns, N.J., and Leigh, P.N. (1995) Involvement of the amygdala, dentate, and hippocampus in motor neuron disease. *Journal of the Neurological Sciences*, 129, 75–78.

Balajthy, B. (1964) Symptomatology of the temporal lobe in Pick's convolutional atrophy. *Acta Medical Academy of Sciences of Hungary*, 20, 301–316.

Bancher, C. and Jellinger, K.A. (1994) Neurofibrillary tangle predominant form of senile dementia of Alzheimer type: a rare subtype in very old subjects. *Acta Neuropathologica*, 88, 565–570.

Benzing, W.C., Mufson, E.J., Jennes, L., Stopa, E.G., and Armstrong, D.M. (1992) Distribution of neurotensin immunoreactivity within the human amygdaloid complex: a comparison with acetylcholinesterase- and Nissl-stained tissue sections. *Journal of Comparative Neurology*, 317, 283–297.

Bierer, L.M., Hof, P.R., Purohit, D.P., Carlin, L., Schmeidler, J., Davis, K.L., and Perl, D.P. (1995) Neocortical neurofibrillary tangles correlate with dementia severity in Alzheimer's disease. *Archives of Neurology*, 52, 81–88.

Braak, H. and Braak, E. (1991) Neuropathological stageing of Alzheimer-related changes. *Acta Neuropathologica*, 82, 239–259.

Brady, D.R. and Mufson, E.J. (1990) Amygdaloid pathology in Alzheimer's disease: qualitative and quantitative analysis. *Dementia*, 1, 5–17.

Brashear, H.R., Godec, M.S., and Carlsen, J. (1988) The distribution of neuritic plaques and acetylcholinesterase staining in the amygdala in Alzheimer's disease. *Neurology*, 38, 1694–1699.

Brockhaus, H. (1938) Zuranatomie des mandelkerngebietes. *Journal of Psychological Neurology*, 49, 1–136.

Brun, A. (1987) Frontal lobe degeneration of non-Alzheimer type. I. Neuropathology. *Archives of Gerontology and Geriatrics*, 6, 193–208.

Brun, A. (1993) Frontal lobe degeneration of non-Alzheimer type revisited. *Dementia*, 4, 126–131.

Brun, A. and Englund, E. (1981) Regional pattern of degeneration in Alzheimer's disease: neuronal loss and histopathological grading. *Histopathology*, 5, 549–564.

Brun, A. and Gustafson, L. (1976) Distribution of cerebral degeneration in Alzheimer's disease. A clinco-pathological study. *Archiv für Psychiatrie und Nervenkrankheiten*, **223**.

Brun, A., Englund, B., Gustafson, L., Passant, U., Mann, D.M.A., Neary, D., and Snowden, J.S. (1994) Clinical and neuropathological criteria for frontotemporal dementia. The Lund and Manchester Groups. *Journal of Neurology, Neurosurgery and Psychiatry*, 57, 416–418.

Burns, A., Jacoby, R., and Levy, R. (1990) Psychiatric phenomena in Alzheimer's disease. IV. Disorders of behavior. *British Journal of Psychiatry*, 157, 86–94.

Cahill, L., Babinsky, R., Markowitsch, H.J., and McGaugh, J.L. (1995) The amygdala and emotional memory. *Nature*, 377, 295–296.

Chan-Palay, V. and Asan, E. (1989) Alterations in catecholamine neurons of the locus ceruleus in senile dementia of the Alzheimer type and in Parkinson's disease with and without dementia and depression. *Journal of Comparative Neurology*, 287, 373–392.

Churchyard, A. and Lees, A.J. (1997) The relationship between dementia and direct involvement of the hippocampus and amygdala in Parkinson's disease. *Neurology*, 49, 1570–1576.

Clark, G.A. (1995) Fear and loathing in the amygdala. *Current Biology*, 5, 246–248.

Corsellis, J.A.N. (1970) The limbic areas in Alzheimer's disease and in other conditions associated with dementia. In *Alzheimer's Disease: A Ciba Foundation Symposium* (eds G.E.W. Wolstenholme and M.O'Connor), pp. 37–50. J. and A. Churchill, London.

Cuenod, C.-A., Denys, A., Michot, J.-L., Jehenson, P., Forette, F., Kaplan, D., Syrota, A., and Boller, F. (1993) Amygdala atrophy in Alzheimer's disease: an *in vivo* magnetic resonance imaging study. *Archives of Neurology*, 50, 941–945.

Cummings, J.L. and Duchen, L.W. (1981) Klüver–Bucy syndrome in Pick disease: clinical and pathologic correlations. *Neurology*, 31, 1415–1422.

De Souza, E.B. (1995) Corticotropin-releasing factor receptors: physiology, pharmacology, biochemistry and role in central nervous system and immune disorders. *Psychoneuroendocrinology*, 20, 789–819.

Deweer, B., Lehericy, S., Pillon, B., Baulac, M., Chiras, J., Marsault, C., Agid, Y., and Dubois, B. (1995) Memory disorders in probable Alzheimer's disease: the role of hippocampal atrophy as shown with MRI. *Journal of Neurology, Neurosurgery and Psychiatry*, 58, 590–597.

Edwards-Lee, T., Miller, B.L., Benson, D. F., Cummings, J.L., Russell, G. L., Boone, K., and Mena, I. (1997) The temporal variant of frontotemporal dementia. *Brain*, 120, 1027–1040.

Esiri, M.M., Pearson, R.C.A., Steele, J.E., Bowen, D.M., and Powell. (1990) A quantitative study of the neurofibrillary tangles and the choline acetyltransferase activity in the cerebral cortex and the amygdala in Alzheimer's disease. *Journal of Neurology, Neurosurgery, and Psychiatry*, 53, 161–165.

Fallon, J.H. and Ciofi, P. (1992) Distribution of monoamines within the amygdala. In *The Amygdala: Neurobiological Aspects of Emotion, Memory, and Mental Dysfunction* (ed. J.P. Aggleton), pp. 97–114. Wiley-Liss, New York.

Forstl, H., Burns, A., Luthert, P., Cairns, N., Lantos, P., and Levy, R. (1992) Clinical and neuropathological correlates of depression in Alzheimer's disease. *Psychological Medicine*, 22, 877–884.

Fudge, J.L., Powers, J.M., Haber, S.N., and Caine, E.D. (1998) Considering the role of the amygdala in psychotic illness: a clinicopathological correlation. *Journal of Neuropsychiatry and Clinical Neurosciences*, 10, 383–394.

Gascon, G.G. and Giles, F. (1973) Limbic dementia. *Journal of Neurology, Neurosurgery, and Psychiatry*, 36, 421–430.

Gsell, W., Conrad, R., Hickethier, M., Sofic, E., Frolich, L., Wichart, I., Jellinger, K., Moll, G., Ransmayr, G., Beckmann, H., and Riederer, P. (1995) Decreased catalase activity but unchanged superoxide dismutase activity in brains of patients with dementia of Alzheimer type. *Journal of Neurochemistry*, 64, 1216–1223.

Haroutunian, V., Perl, D.P., Purohit, D.P., Marin, D., Khan, K., Lantz, M., Davis, K.L., and Mohs, R.C. (1998) Regional distribution of neuritic plaques in the nondemented elderly and subjects with very mild Alzheimer disease. *Archives of Neurology*, 55, 1185–1191.

Hashimoto, M., Kitagaki, H., Imamura, T., Hirono, N., Shimomura, T., Kazui, H., Tanimukai, S., Hanihara, T., and Mori, E. (1998) Medial temporal and whole-brain atrophy in dementia with Lewy bodies: a volumetric MRI study. *Neurology*, 51, 357–362.

Hayman, L.A., Rexer, J.L., Pavol, M.A., Strite, D., and Meyers, C.A. (1998) Klüver–Bucy syndrome after bilateral selective damage of amygdala and its cortical connections. *Journal of Neuropsychiatry and Clinical Neurosciences*, 10, 354–358.

Herzog, A.G. and Kemper, T.L. (1980) Amydaloid changes in aging and dementia. *Archives of Neurology*, 37, 625–629.

Heun, R., Mazanek, M., Atzor, K.R., Tintera, J., Gawehn, J., Burkart, M., Gansicke, M., Falkai, P., and Stoeter, P. (1997) Amygdala–hippocampal atrophy and memory performance in dementia of Alzheimer type. *Dementia and Geriatric Cognitive Disorders*, 8, 329–336.

Hierons, R., Janota, I., and Corsellis, J.A.N. (1978) The late effects of necrotizing encephalitis of the temporal lobes and limbic areas: a clinico-pathological study of 10 cases. *Psychology and Medicine*, 8, 21–42.

Hooper, M.W. and Vogel, S.F. (1976) The limbic system in Alzheimer's disease. *American Journal of Pathology*, 85, 1–13.

Hooten, W.M. and Lyketsos, C.G. (1996) Frontotemporal dementia: a clinicopathological review of four postmortem studies. *Journal of Neuropsychiatry and Clinical Neurosciences*, 8, 10–19.

Hughes, C.P., Berg, L., Danziger, W.L., Coben, L.A., and Martin, R.L. (1982) A new clinical scale for the staging of dementia. *British Journal of Psychiatry*, 140, 566–572.

Inglis, F.M. and Moghaddam, B. (1999) Dopaminergic innervation of the amygdala is highly responsive to stress. *Journal of Neurochemistry*, 72, 1088–1094.

Iseki, E., Odawara, T., Li, F., Kosaka, K., Nishimura, T., Akiyama, H., and Ikeda, K. (1996) Age-related ubiquitin-positive granular structures in non-demented subjects and neurodegenerative disorders. *Journal of the Neurological Sciences*, 142, 25–29.

Iseki, E., Li, F., Odawara, T., Hino, H., Suzuki, K., Kosaka, K., Akiyama, H., Ikeda, K., and Kato, M. (1998) Ubiquitin-immunohistochemical investigation of atypical Pick's disease without Pick bodies. *Journal of the Neurological Sciences*, 159, 194–201.

Jack, C.R., Jr, Petersen, R.C., Xu, Y.C., Waring, S.C., O'Brien, P.C., Tangalos, E.G., Smith, G.E., Ivnik, R.J., and Kokmen, E. (1997) Medial temporal atrophy on MRI in normal aging and very mild Alzheimer's disease. *Neurology*, 49, 786–794.

Jackson, M. and Lowe, J. (1996) The new neuropathology of degenerative frontotemporal dementias. *Acta Neuropathologica*, 91, 127–134.

Jamada, M. and Mehraein, P. (1968) Verteilungmuster der senilen veranderungen im gehirn. *Archive für Psychiatrische und Nervenkrankheiten*, 211, 308–324.

Janati, A. (1985) Klüver–Bucy syndrome in Huntington's chorea. *Journal of Nervous and Mental Disease*, 173, 632–635.

Jellinger, K.A. (1998) Dementia with grains (argyrophilic grain disease). *Brain Pathology*, 8, 377–386.

Jellinger, K.A. and Bancher, C. (1998) Senile dementia with tangles (tangle predominant form of senile dementia). *Brain Pathology*, 8, 367–376.

Kato, S., Oda, M., Hayashi, H., Kawata, A., and Shimizu, T. (1994) Participation of the limbic system and its associated areas in the dementia of amyotrophic lateral sclerosis. *Journal of the Neurological Sciences*, 126, 62–69.

Kertesz, A., Hudson, L., Mackenzie, I.R., and Munoz, D.G. (1994) The pathology and nosology of primary progressive aphasia. *Neurology*, 44, 2065–2072.

Laakso, M.P., Soininen, H., Partanen, K., Helkala, E.L., Hartikainen, P., Vainio, P., Hallikainen, M., Hanninen, T., and Riekkinen, P.J., Sr (1995) Volumes of hippocampus, amygdala and frontal lobes in the MRI-based diagnosis of early Alzheimer's disease: correlation with memory functions. *Journal of Neural Transmission. Parkinsons Disease and Dementia Section*, 9, 73–86.

LaBar, K.S., Phelps, E.A., and LeDoux, J.E. (1994) Fear conditioning following unilateral temporal lobectomy in humans: impaired conditional discrimination. *Society for Neurosciences Abstracts*, 20, 360.

Levitt, P. (1984) A monoclonal antibody to limbic system neurons. *Science*, 223, 299–301.

Levy, M., Miller, B.L., Cummings, J.L., Fairbanks, L.A., and Craig, A. (1996) Alzheimer's disease and frontotemporal dementias: behavioral distinctions. *Archives of Neurology*, 53, 687–690.

Lilly, R., Cummings, J L., Benson, D.F., and Frankel, M. (1983) The human Klüver–Bucy syndrome. *Neurology*, 33, 1141–1145.

Lippa, C.F., Fujiwara, H., Mann, D.M., Giasson, B., Baba, M., Schmidt, M.L., Nee, L.E., O'Connell, B., Pollen, D.A., St. George-Hyslop, P., Ghetti, B., Nochlin, D., Bird, T.D., Cairns, N.J., Lee, V.M., Iwatsubo, T., and Trojanowski, J.Q. (1998) Lewy bodies contain altered alpha-synuclein in brains of many familial Alzheimer's disease patients with mutations in presenilin and amyloid precursor protein genes. *American Journal of Pathology*, 153, 1365–1370.

Lynch, T., Sano, M., Marder, K.S., Bell, K.L., Foster, N.L., Defendini, R.F., Sima, A.A., Keohane, C., Nygaard, T.G., Fahn, S., Mayeux, R., Rowland, L.P., and Wilhelmsen, K.C. (1994) Clinical characteristics of a family with chromosome 17-linked disinhibition–dementia–Parkinsonism–amyotrophy complex [see comments]. *Neurology*, 44, 1878–1884.

Mann, D.M.A. (1992) The neuropathology of the amygdala in ageing and in dementia. In *The Amygdala: Neurobiological Aspects of Emotion, Memory, and Mental Dysfunction* (ed. J.P. Aggleton), pp. 575–593. Wiley-Liss, New York.

Mann, D.M.A., Tucker, C.M., and Yates, P.O. (1987) The topographic distribution of senile plaques and neurofibrillary tangles in the brains of non-demented persons of different ages. *Neuropathology and Applied Neurobiology*, 13, 123–139.

Marlow, W.B., Mancall, E.L., and Thomas, J.J. (1975) Complete Klüver–Bucy syndrome in man. *Cortex*, 11, 53–59.

Mattis, S. (1976) Dementia rating scale. In *Geriatric Psychiatry* (eds R. Bellack and B. Keraso), pp. 77–121. Grune and Stratton, New York.

Maunoury, C., Michot, J.L., Caillet, H., Parlato, V., Leroy-Willig, A., Jehenson, P., Syrota, A., and Boller, F. (1996) Specificity of temporal amygdala atrophy in Alzheimer's disease: quantitative assessment with magnetic resonance imaging. *Dementia*, 7, 10–14.

Mauri, M., Sibilla, L., Bono, G., Carlesimo, G.A., Sinforiani, E., and Martelli, A. (1998) The role of morpho-volumetric and memory correlations in the diagnosis of early Alzheimer dementia. *Journal of Neurology*, 245, 525–530.

McGaugh, J. L., Cahill, L., and Roozendaal, B. (1996) Involvement of the amygdala in memory storage: interaction with other brain systems. *Proceedings of the National Academy of Sciences of the United States of America*, 93, 13508–13514.

Mendez, M.F., Selwood, A., Mastri, A.R., and Frey, W.H. (1993) Pick's disease versus Alzheimer's disease: comparison of clinical characteristics. *Neurology*, 43, 289–292.

Mielke, R., Schroder, R., Fink, G.R., Kessler, J., Herholz, K., and Heiss, W.-D. (1996) Regional cerebral glucose metabolism and postmortem pathology in Alzheimer's disease. *Acta Neuropathologica*, 91, 174–179.

Miller, B.L., Cummings, J.L., Villanueva-Meyer, J., Boone, K., Mehringer, C.M., Lesser, I.M., and Mena, I. (1991) Frontal lobe degeneration: clinical, neuropsychological and SPECT characteristics. *Neurology*, 41, 1374–1382.

Miller, B.L., Chang, L., Mena, I., Boone, K., and Lesser, I.M. (1993) Progressive right frontotemporal degeneration: clinical, neuropsychological, and SPECT characteristics. *Dementia*, 4, 204–213.

Miller, B.L., Cummings, J.L., Boone, K., Chang, L., Schuman, S., Pahana, N., and Darby, A. (1995a) Clinical and neurobehavioral characteristics of fronto-temporal dementia and Alzheimer disease. *Neurology*, 45, A318.

Miller, B.L., Darby, A.L., Swartz, J.R., Yener, G.G., and Mena, I. (1995b) Dietary changes, compulsions and sexual behavior in frontotemporal degeneration. *Dementia*, 6, 195–199.

Miller, B.L., Ikonte, C., Ponton, M.P., Levy, M., Boone, K., Darby, A., Berman, N., Mena, I., and Cummings, J.L. (1997) A study of the Lund–Manchester research criteria for frontotemporal dementia: clinical and single-photon emission CT correlations. *Neurology*, 48, 937–942.

Miserendino, M.J.D., Sananes, C. B., Melia, K.R., and Davis, M. (1990) Blocking acquisition but not expression of conditioned fear-potentiated startle by NMDA antagonists in the amygdala. *Nature*, 345, 716–718.

Mori, E., Yoneda, Y., Yamashita, H., Hirono, N., Ikeda, M., and Yamadori, A. (1997) Medial temporal structures related to memory impairment in Alzheimer's disease: an MRI volumetric study. *Journal of Neurology, Neurosurgery, and Psychiatry*, 63, 214–221.

Mori, E., Ikeda, M., Hirono, N., Kitagaki, H., Imamura, T., and Shimomura, T. (1999) Amygdalar volume and emotional memory in Alzheimer's disease. *American Journal of Psychiatry*, 156, 216–222.

Neary, D., Snowden, J.S., and Mann, D.M.A. (1993) The clinical pathological correlates of lobar atrophy. *Dementia*, 4, 154–159.

O'Brien, J.T., Desmond, P., Ames, D., Schweitzer, I., Chiu, E., and Tress, B. (1997a) Temporal lobe magnetic resonance imaging can differentiate Alzheimer's disease from normal ageing, depression, vascular dementia and other causes of cognitive impairment. *Psychological Medicine*, 27, 1267–1275.

O'Brien, J.T., Desmond, P., Ames, D., Schweitzer, I., and Tress, B. (1997b) Magnetic resonance imaging correlates of memory impairment in the healthy elderly: association with medial temporal lobe atrophy but not white matter lesions. *International Journal of Geriatric Psychiatry*, 12, 369–374.

Pantel, J., Schroder, J., Essig, M., Popp, D., Dech, H., Knopp, M.V., Schad, L.R., Eysenbach, K., Backenstrass, M., and Friedlinger, M. (1997) Quantitative magnetic resonance imaging in geriatric depression and primary degenerative dementia. *Journal of Affective Disorders*, 42, 69–83.

Pantel, J., Schroder, J., Essig, M., Jauss, M., Schneider, G., Eysenbach, K., von Kummer, R., Baudendistel, K., Schad, L.R., and Knopp, M.V. (1998) *In vivo* quantification of brain volumes in subcortical vascular dementia and Alzheimer's disease. An MRI-based study. *Dementia and Geriatric Cognitive Disorders*, 9, 309–316.

Parent, A. (1996) Limbic system. In *Carpenter's Human Neuroanatomy*, 9th edn. pp. 744–794. Williams and Wilkins, Media.

Pfaff, D.W. and Keiner, M. (1973) Atlas of estradiol concentrating cells in the central nervous system of the female rat. *Journal of Comparative Neurology*, 151, 121–159.

Pitkänen, A., Savander, V., and LeDoux, J.E. (1997) Organization of intra-amygdaloid circuitries in the rat: an emerging framework for understanding functions of the amygdala. *Trends in Neuroscience*, 20, 517–523.

Raven, J., Raven, J.C., and Court, J.H. (1998) *Manual for Raven's Progressive Matrices and Vocabulary Scales. Section 2. The Coloured Progressive Matrices*. Oxford Psychologists Press, Oxford.

Sawa, M., Ieki, Y., Arita, M., and Harada, T. (1954) Preliminary report on the amygdalectomy on the psychotic patients, with interpretation of oral–emotional manifestations of schizophrenia. *Folia Psychiatrica et Neurologica Japonica*, 7, 309–329.

Scott, S.A., DeKosky, S.T., and Scheff, S.W. (1991) Volumetric atrophy of the amygdala in Alzheimer's disease: quantitative serial reconstruction. *Neurology*, 41, 351–356.

Scott, S.A., DeKosky, S.T., Sparks, D.L., Knox, C.A., and Scheff, S.W. (1992) Amygdala cell loss and atrophy in Alzheimer's disease. *Annals of Neurology*, 32, 555–563.

Swanson, L.W. and Petrovich, G.D. (1998) What is the amygdala? *Trends in Neuroscience*, 21, 323–331.

Terzian, H. and Dalle Ore, G. (1955) Syndrome of Kluver and Bucy: reproduced in man by bilateral removal of the temporal lobes. *Neurology*, 5, 373–380.

Thompson, D., Knee, K., and Golden, C.J. (1998) Olfaction in persons with Alzheimer's disease. *Neuropsychology Review*, 8, 11–23.

Tranel, D. and Hyman, B.T. (1990) Neuropsychological correlates of bilateral amygdala damage. *Archives of Neurology*, 47, 349–355.

Unger, J.W. and Lange, W. (1992) NADPH-diaphorase-positive cell population in the human amygdala and temporal cortex: neuroanatomy, peptidergic characteristics and aspects of aging and Alzheimer's disease. *Acta Neuropathologica*, 83, 636–646.

Valladares-Neto, D.C., Buchsbaum, M.S., Evans, W.J., Nguyen, D., Nguyen, P., Siegel, B.V., Stanley, J., Starr, A., Guich, S., and Rice, D. (1995) EEG delta, positron emission tomography, and memory deficit in Alzheimer's disease. *Neuropsychobiology*, 31, 173–181.

Weiskrantz, L. (1956) Behavioral changes associated with ablation of the amygdaloid complex in monkeys. *Journal of Comparative and Physiological Psychology*, 49, 381–391.

Yamaoka, L.H., Welsh-Bohmer, K.A., Hulette, C.M., Gaskell, P.C., Jr, Murray, M., Rimmler, J.L., Helms, B.R., Guerra, M., Roses, A.D., Schmechel, D.E., and Pericak-Vance, M.A. (1996) Linkage of frontotemporal dementia to chromosome 17: clinical and neuropathological characterization of phenotype. *American Journal of Human Genetics*, 59, 1306–1312.

Zweig, R.M., Ross, C.A., Hedreen, J.C., Steele, C., Cardillo, J.E., Whitehouse, P.J., Folstein, M.F., and Price, D.L. (1988) The neuropathology of aminergic nuclei in Alzheimer's disease. *Annals of Neurology*, 24, 233–242.

Index